Paul word

Ex Libris
Medicus
1957

Edward
Shapiro
MD

DISEASES OF THE HEART
AND CIRCULATION

DISEASES OF
THE HEART AND
CIRCULATION

by

PAUL WOOD, O.B.E.
M.D. (Melbourne), F.R.C.P. (London)

Director, Institute of Cardiology, London
Physician, National Heart Hospital
Physician in charge of the Cardiac Department, Brompton Hospital

SECOND, REVISED AND ENLARGED EDITION

J. B. LIPPINCOTT COMPANY
East Washington Square   *Philadelphia*

First published 1950
2nd (revised) impression 1952
2nd (revised and enlarged) edition 1956

Published and distributed in the United
States of America for Eyre & Spottiswoode
by J. B. Lippincott Company. 1956

PRINTED IN GREAT BRITAIN

To

SIR JOHN PARKINSON

PREFACE TO SECOND EDITION

DURING the last five years cardiology has continued to advance rapidly in the direction outlined in the first edition, i.e. in respect of investigatory techniques, physiological concepts, and treatment (both surgical and medical).

Classical electrocardiography has perhaps halted, and vectorcardiography, introduced long ago by Mann in 1920, has not added a great deal to our knowledge. Angiocardiography and tomography have continued to enlighten radiology, and cardiac catheterisation has become a routine diagnostic method, and a proved tool for physiological investigation. The technique of phonocardiography has improved sufficiently to make visual sound records superior to auscultation. Electrokymography has been disappointing, and ballistocardiography is still impeded by technical difficulties.

The chief advances in cardiological physiology have been in connexion with congenital heart disease and acquired valve disease.

Direct cardiac surgery, led in this country by Sir Russell Brock, has developed fast: both pulmonary and mitral valvotomy have proved brilliantly successful; infundibular resection has achieved far better results than many predicted; and aortic valvotomy is promising. Hypothermia is slightly ahead of artificial circulations as an aid to cardiac surgery under direct vision, and atrial septal defects are now being successfully repaired.

Medical treatment has advanced chiefly in relation to hypertension.

In presenting this second edition I am aware that these recent advances are over-emphasised, but that is a fault that can hardly be avoided, for they provide the chief reasons for re-writing much of the book.

April 1956

PAUL WOOD

PREFACE TO FIRST EDITION

THE rapid advance in cardiology during the first half of the twentieth century may be fairly ascribed to the introduction of new techniques. Riva-Rocci's mercurial sphygmomanometer (1896), Mackenzie's polygraph (1902), Einthoven's string galvanometer (1903), and Röntgen's beam (1895) opened the new era, and in the hands of men such as Sir Clifford Allbutt, Sir James Mackenzie, Sir Thomas Lewis and Sir John Parkinson respectively, soon solved or clarified innumerable problems. Further impetus resulted from the elaboration and perfection of these methods, particularly from unipolar lead electrocardiography and angio-cardiography, for which we have to thank Frank Wilson (1932 *et seq.*), Castellanus (1937), and Robb and Steinberg (1938). More recently still Forsmann's courageous use of the cardiac catheter on himself (1929) led to its clinical application on a wide scale, particularly owing to the efforts of Cournand (1941) in the U.S.A. and of McMichael and Sharpey-Schafer (1944) in England. Thus electrocardiography, cardiac radiology, and the physiology of the heart and circulation have advanced side by side. At the same time the surgeons have invaded what was once forbidden territory and are rapidly turning miraculous operations on the heart into the commonplace. Amongst the many pioneers who have helped to develop safe routine cardiac surgery must be included Claud S. Beck, E. D. Churchill, Lawrence O'Shaughnessy, R. E. Gross, Alfred Blalock, C. Crafoord, and R. C. Brock, although so many distinguished surgeons have played their part that it may seem invidious to mention names. It is, perhaps, not really a coincidence that more precise methods of diagnosis became available just when surgery demanded them.

The more conservative physicians may have witnessed these and many other less important technical developments with some misgiving, but relatively few have expressed reactionary views. Yet there is already plenty of evidence to show that we are in danger of losing our clinical heritage and of pinning too much faith in figures thrown up by machines. Medicine must suffer if this tendency is not checked.

In presenting this book I have attempted to maintain a proper balance between man and his instruments, between experienced opinion and statistics, between traditional views and the heterodox, between bedside medicine and special tests, between the practical and the academic; and so to link the past with the present.

January 1950   PAUL WOOD

ACKNOWLEDGMENTS

I wish to thank my colleagues at the Postgraduate Medical School of London, at the Institute of Cardiology, at Brompton Hospital and at the Rheumatic Fever Centre at Taplow, for playing an important, though unwitting part in the preparation of this book; for one is constantly absorbing ideas, knowingly and unknowingly, from one's associates. In particular, I would like to mention the names of Sir Francis Fraser, Professor John McMichael and Professor E. P. Sharpey-Schafer, who influenced me considerably at Hammersmith; and Sir John Parkinson, Dr. Maurice Campbell, Dr. D. Evan Bedford, and Dr. William Evans, who have helped me so much at the National Heart Hospital.

I must thank many kind friends for supplying the originals of some of the figures: Sir John Parkinson, Dr. Maurice Campbell, Dr. William Evans, Dr. Jenner Hoskin, Dr. Graham Hayward, Dr. Charles Baker, Dr. Frances Gardner, Dr. Wallace Brigden, Dr. Philip Ellman, Dr. Aubrey Leatham, Dr. Raymond Daley, Dr. Derek Abrahams, Dr. Max Zoob, Dr. Arthur Hollman, Dr. J. S. McCann, and Dr. E. D. H. Cowen.

In any work of my own that is included, I received valuable help from a series of teams which included registrars, house physicians and medical technicians, and I must thank all of them; unfortunately, they are too numerous to mention by name.

Then, I would like to pay a special tribute to my private secretary, Miss Elizabeth Turner, on whose able shoulders a great deal of the work necessarily fell. Her efficiency, enthusiasm, and unflagging industry merit the highest praise.

Finally, and most important, I want to express my gratitude to my wife, not only for her unfailing moral support, but for undertaking far more than her fair share of domestic responsibility, so that I was able to write the book in my "spare" time.

AUTHOR'S NOTE

THE method of numbering the figures was adopted so that desirable changes could be made from time to time without upsetting the order of the illustrations in subsequent chapters. The number before the decimal point represents the chapter in which the illustration occurs, whilst the number after the decimal point is serial for that chapter. Thus, figure 3.15 refers to the fifteenth illustration in chapter 3. From the author's point of view the system proved highly convenient; it is hoped that the reader will not find it irksome.

The method of mounting the electrocardiograms has been adopted because it is the only way in which a simple and harmonious design can be made to indicate the approximate position of the leads. The apices of the triangle represent the relative positions of the three conventional limb electrodes: unipolar limb leads (Goldberger's augmented leads are used throughout) and standard leads are placed accordingly. Chest leads (V_1–V_6) are shown horizontally across the centre. In adopting such a convention no theoretical assumptions are necessary; nor have they been made.

In the title of the book the word circulation refers to the general circulation, not to peripheral vascular disease. A chapter on the latter was originally included, but was finally abandoned as separate monographs on the subject appeared in greater profusion.

Anatomy and pathology have been discussed only when clinically relevant.

The arrangements of the contents has been determined chiefly by physiological and etiological considerations, rather than by morbid anatomy. Thus there is no chapter devoted to valve disease as a whole. It is believed that the advantages of such an arrangement outweigh the disadvantages.

Special attention has been paid to the index, so that it serves a dual role. It may be used both conventionally and as a guide to differential diagnosis.

The book has been written primarily for graduates interested in clinical cardiology; but the needs of students, general practitioners, and specialist physicians in other fields of medicine have been constantly borne in mind. To expect that consulting cardiologists themselves might also find it of value would be presumptuous, and it is certainly not intended for the advanced academic research worker.

CONTENTS

CHAPTER IX. RHEUMATIC FEVER AND ACTIVE RHEUMATIC CARDITIS

CHAPTER X.   CHRONIC RHEUMATIC HEART DISEASE

CHAPTER XI.   NON-RHEUMATIC MYOCARDITIS AND MISCELLANEOUS CARDIOPATHIES

Chapter XVI. HYPERTENSIVE HEART DISEASE

Chapter XVII. PULMONARY EMBOLISM

Chapter XVIII. PULMONARY HYPERTENSION

THE ILLUSTRATIONS

CHAPTER II

CHAPTER VIII.—*continued*

INTRODUCTION

HEART disease is by far the most common cause of natural death in civilised communities in the more temperate zones of the world. It is responsible for at least two-fifths of all such deaths and for an annual mortality rate in the general population of about 0.45 per cent. Both incidence and mortality curves have been rising steadily for many years, a fact which is not fully explained by ageing populations and by the control of infectious fevers, pulmonary tuberculosis, and pyogenic infections. The incidence and mortality of cancer, for example, show no comparable increase. Ischæmic heart disease, particularly, is becoming more frequent.

It is by no means easy to estimate the prevalence of each kind of heart disease, for selection plays havoc with most personal and hospital statistics, whilst random samples usually suffer from inaccurate diagnosis. For example, amongst a consecutive series of 10,000 cases of cardiovascular disease that I have seen personally during the last few years, 900 or 9 per cent had congenital heart disease, which is about six times the number that would be expected in a random sample of cardiovascular cases. The other side of the picture is illustrated by the Registrar-General's statistical review for 1953, in which the chief cause of all deaths is myocardial degeneration, a diagnosis which is not recognised in cardiovascular clinics, whilst cor pulmonale is not mentioned at all. Nevertheless, an attempt has been made to assess the prevalence of the more important forms of heart disease, based on the literature, my own data and the Registrar-General's statistical reviews. A few general observations may be made first.

The population of England and Wales in 1953 was approximately 44,000,000. There were 503,529 deaths during this year. Of these, 183,917 were due to heart disease, 68,069 to a cerebral vascular accident, and 30,392 to bronchitis and emphysema. At least half of all the deaths were therefore cardiovascular, and over half if cor pulmonale had been included. For comparison, there were 89,680 deaths from neoplasm (of which 15,132 were due to carcinoma of the lung), 20,759 from pneumonia, and 8,902 from tuberculosis.

The ensuing table is no more than an approximate estimate of the incidence of the more important kinds of heart disease, and the many blanks represent lack of reliable information.

INCIDENCE OF CHIEF FORMS OF HEART DISEASE

	PERCENTAGE OF CLINICAL CASES OF HEART DISEASE	PERCENTAGE OF POPULATION	PERCENTAGE OF CARDIAC DEATHS	PERCENTAGE OF ALL DEATHS
Bacterial endocarditis .	1.0	—	0.17	0.07
Congenital heart disease (surviving infancy) .	1.5	0.1	0.9	0.36
Cor pulmonale . .	5.0	—	5–15	2–6
Dissecting aneurysm .	0.2	—	0.45	0.18
Hyperkinetic circulatory states . . .	0.3	—	—	—
Hypertension . .	25.0	3.0	10.0	4.0
— cerebral vascular accidents . .	—	—	—	13.5
Ischæmic heart disease .	30.0	2.0	31.2	12.5
Miscellaneous and uncertain . .	6.5	—	—	—
— "degenerative" .	—	—	35.0	14.0
Myocarditis and other rare or obscure cardiopathies . .	0.3	—	—	—
Pericarditis (primary) .	1.0	—	—	—
Pulmonary embolism .	—	—	6.5	2.6
Pulmonary hypertension (primary or thrombo-embolic). . .	0.2	—	—	—
Rheumatic carditis .	5.0	0.5	0.15	0.06
Rheumatic heart disease (chronic) . .	15.0	1.5	4.5	1.8
Rhythm changes— primary . . .	5.0	—	—	—
Syphilitic aortitis . .	1.0	—	0.5	0.2
Thyrotoxic heart disease	2.0	—	0.2	0.08

DISEASES OF THE HEART AND CIRCULATION

CHAPTER I

THE CHIEF SYMPTOMS OF HEART DISEASE

HISTORY-TAKING

TO take an accurate and relevant history is one of the most difficult and important arts in medicine. Sometimes, a complete diagnosis can be made from the history alone, and not infrequently the possibilities can be whittled down to two or three. A good history should at least indicate the system involved, or it should point unerringly to some group or groups of diseases. A common mistake is the failure to analyse any given symptom sufficiently; in cardiovascular work this applies especially to pain, breathlessness, palpitations, and syncope. The student is usually taught to encourage the patient to tell his story in his own words, and to record them more or less verbatim. Yet such an account may be verbose, irrelevant, inaccurate, and misleading. It is an axiom that the leading question must be avoided at all cost; yet again, an experienced physician must know that the ability to put the appropriate leading question at the right moment, and the intelligent interpretation of its reply, are invaluable. It is not pretended that leading questions may not lead to false information, if the power of their suggestion is not appreciated by the questioner; and it is agreed that much may be lost by failure to allow the patient freedom and time to express his complaints in his own way; but the average patient will not mention half the available information until he is pressed, and the data freely given must be checked as at the bar. For example, in the differential diagnosis between a neural and non-neural somatic lesion, an accurate description of the quality of the pain may determine the issue immediately; yet the majority of patients will volunteer no information concerning the quality of pain, and if asked to describe it will do so inadequately. They may say it is aching or sharp, but fail to enlarge on this, even when urged to do so. In answer to the leading question, "Does it tingle?", however, they may reply at once in the affirmative. It is essential to realise that the matter does not end there: that such a positive reply to a leading question demands the most penetrating cross-examination, until the questioner is satisfied that the pain really does tingle, and that the patient is not merely saying so because it seems the easier answer. It is scarcely too much to say that the best history-taker is he who can best interpret the answer to a leading question. Appropriate leading questions can only be asked, however, when the proffered history has provided sufficient data upon which to work, and if the physician has sufficient knowledge of the possibilities then entailed. It is this latter factor which makes it easier for the expert than for the student.

SYMPTOMS

The symptoms of heart disease vary considerably according to the nature of the cardiopathy and the kind of physiological disturbance in the circulation that results: each will be discussed in particular relation to the form of heart disease in which it occurs in subsequent chapters, but it may help here to survey the subject in general.

To begin with, it should be thoroughly understood that cardiovascular disease may be severe without any symptoms whatever: good examples of this axiom are coarctation of the aorta, pulmonary stenosis, atrial septal defect, aortic stenosis, malignant hypertension, primary pulmonary hypertension, and aortic aneurysm; even cardiac infarction may be silent.

A second point of general interest is that patients rarely appreciate what is a heart symptom and what is not. The most classical example of this is the well-known paradox that patients with angina pectoris (including doctors) often complain of indigestion, whereas those with dyspepsia or left inframammary pain may be convinced that their hearts are at fault. Headaches and dizziness are frequently attributed to high blood pressure when there is no hypertension; palpitations, which are usually innocent, are a common source of anxiety; fatigue and lack of energy resulting from psychological conflict are often ascribed to failing circulation. On the other hand, breathlessness due to mitral stenosis or left ventricular failure may be attributed to bronchitis, an attack of paroxysmal cardiac dyspnœa to bronchial asthma, and coughing from pulmonary venous congestion to over-smoking. A man with gross congestive heart failure has even been known to present himself first at a skin clinic on account of pruritis (due to jaundice).

Finally, after recording the symptoms faithfully in chronological order, the absence of any important symptom that might reasonably have been expected under the clinical circumstances should also be noted. In a case presenting with mitral stenosis, for example, with effort breathlessness of moderate grade as the only positive symptom, an experienced physician would record the absence of hæmoptysis, winter bronchitis, orthopnœa, paroxysmal cardiac dyspnœa, angina pectoris, recurrent palpitations, peripheral embolism and œdema, because all these are important symptoms of mitral stenosis, each having its own particular meaning. On the other hand, he would not record the absence of syncope, squatting, transient cyanosis, headache, heat intolerance, Raynaud's phenomenon, and a host of other negatives which under the clinical circumstances are irrelevant. The recording of a negative implies that the appropriate leading question has been asked.

PAIN

Cardiac pain is ischæmic, being due to stimulation of afferent nerve endings in the myocardium by metabolites resulting from oxygen deficiency in working muscle.

The commonest cause is occlusive coronary atherosclerosis. In *simple angina pectoris* the coronary flow is adequate at rest, but becomes inadequate when the demands of the myocardium are increased by exercise. In *acute coronary insufficiency* the flow suddenly becomes inadequate at rest, usually as a result of thrombosis, but is still sufficient to prevent necrosis. In *acute cardiac infarction* failure of the coronary flow to part of the heart muscle leads to ischæmic necrosis (gangrene).

Pain in angina pectoris is characteristically central in position, pressing in quality, brief in duration, and closely related to effort. It is felt more across the chest than in the mid-line, and may radiate to the shoulders, down both arms, into the neck or jaws, and through to the back. It is usually described as heavy or squeezing, but may be bursting, burning, or like indigestion. It occurs especially on walking, particularly after meals, on a cold day, against the wind, or uphill. It forces the patient to stop or slow down, and disappears in two or three minutes when he stands still. In acute coronary insufficiency the pain also occurs at rest, lasts longer, and is often more severe; and in cardiac infarction it continues for hours, even for a day or two.

The chief cause of a sudden increase in the frequency or duration of cardiac pain is coronary thrombosis, whether it leads to cardiac infarction or not. Coronary occlusion due to subintimal hæmorrhage is rare. Diabetes mellitus, myxœdema, xanthomatosis and familial or idiopathic hypercholesterolæmia are often complicated by angina because they encourage atherogenesis. Thromboangiitis obliternans, polycythæmia vera, shock and trauma may be complicated by cardiac infarction because they encourage coronary thrombosis. Infarction secondary to subintimal hæmorrhage may be caused by injury to the chest or too vigorous anticoagulant therapy.

Angina may also be caused by any condition which adversely disturbs the balance between cardiac work and coronary blood flow. There are four classical examples: (1) severe hypertension may cause angina when the coronary arteries are normal because the work of the heart is increased by the high peripheral resistance; (2) any of the hyperkinetic circulatory states, such as thyrotoxicosis, may encourage angina by increasing cardiac work in respect of the volume pumped; (3) angina in syphilitic aortitis is due to reduction of coronary flow owing to obstruction at the mouths of the coronary arteries; (4) angina during a paroxysmal rhythm change with rapid ventricular rate is due to the poor coronary flow that results from the shortened periods of diastole.

In the presence of healthy coronary arteries, physiological work and normal coronary flow, angina may yet occur if the oxygen supply is deficient. This is the chief cause of cardiac pain in severe anæmia, although extra work due to a raised cardiac output is contributory. Angina similarly provoked might be expected in anoxic cor pulmonale, but it is uncommon and when present may well be due to coincidental coronary disease. Angina rarely occurs from anoxia in cyanotic congenital heart disease. Finally, mechanical obstruction to the circulation may cause angina by strictly limiting the cardiac output and hence the coronary flow, while increasing the work of the heart. Examples include aortic stenosis, mitral valve disease, pulmonary hypertension, massive pulmonary embolism, and pulmonary stenosis.

Pericardial pain is usually sharper, more left-sided than central, and may be referred to the neck or flank. It is relatively long-lasting and independent of effort.

Pain from *aneurysm of the aorta* is usually due to pressure erosion and from *dissecting aneurysm* to a variety of causes including stripping of the adventitia, involvement of the segmental arteries, coronary occlusion, and hæmopericardium.

Despite the characteristic nature and behaviour of cardiac pain, the vast majority of lay persons believe it is situated in the region of the left breast. *Innocent left inframammary pain* is therefore one of the commonest symptoms that brings a patient to seek medical advice. This pain is a long-lasting dull ache, momentarily accentuated from time to time by sudden sharp jabs; it is situated well to the left, bears no direct relationship to effort, may prevent the patient lying on the left side, and is often associated with superficial tenderness. Thus it differs radically from angina pectoris in site, quality, duration and behaviour, i.e. in all four major characteristics.

Other varieties of chest pain which may have to be distinguished from angina pectoris include pain referred from the spine, œsophagus, stomach, duodenum, gall bladder, and mediastinum; and local pain arising from structures in the chest wall such as muscles and ligaments.

DYSPNŒA

Breathlessness is the most common and perhaps the most important of all symptoms relating to heart disease, and also the most complex. The physiology of cardiac dyspnœa is discussed more fully in the chapters on special techniques (respiratory function), heart failure, and mitral stenosis.

Shortness of breath, like all other symptoms, is subjective, and the intensity of the sensation depends in no small measure on the patient's acuteness of perception. Individual variation is great and explains why under exactly similar physiological circumstances one patient appears to be incapacitated, while another carries on his normal occupation with relative tranquillity.

Hysterical dyspnœa or hyperventilation is rather different, for here the added stimulus to breathe is purely cortical and the activity may continue in the presence of true alkalæmia and oxygen supersaturation. A similar situation may occur in encephalitis. Hyperventilation may also be caused by various proprioceptive impulses, such as pain, and especially from activity of voluntary muscle, as on exercise (Comroe and Schmidt, 1943).

The simplest form of dyspnœa is suffocation. The intense desire for breath is due to direct stimulation of the respiratory centre by a *rising*

Œdema with a high protein content (3 to 4 G. per cent) results. Such œdema may be associated with *burns, trench feet, insect bites* and *allergy* (e.g. Quincke's disease). *Lymphatic œdema* has a similar high protein content, but is also rich in cholesterol (White and Sachs, 1950).

Œdema due to *sodium and water retention* is associated with hydræmia. This raises the hydrostatic filtering pressure of the capillaries and lowers the osmotic pressure. Physiologically, the amount of water retained or excreted is controlled by the hypothalmus via the neurohypophysis: osmoreceptors in the hypothalmus react to dilution of the plasma by inhibiting the liberation of anti-diuretic hormone by the neurohypophysis so that diuresis results; on the other hand, if the plasma becomes more concentrated an increased quantity of anti-diuretic hormone is liberated, and the flow of urine is suppressed (Verney, 1946). Physiological hydræmia, sometimes accompanied by slight œdema, occurs during the *premenstrual phase* in women (Frank, 1931), and has been attributed to elevation of the œstradiol progesterone ratio (Greene and Dalton, 1953). This also may act by stimulating the liberation of anti-diuretic hormone.

Famine œdema is complex. It may be associated with thiamine deficiency (wet beri-beri) or with serious reduction of plasma proteins (Denz, 1947), but in other cases neither of these factors can be held responsible; this last group is characterised by diuresis in the horizontal position and with enlargement of the adrenal glands (Sinclair, 1948).

Renal œdema is discussed in Chapter VI.

In practice the causes of œdema most often confused with cardiac œdema are Milroy's lymphatic deficiency, premenstrual hydræmia, bilateral phlebothrombosis, and chronic nephritis.

FATIGUE

Since fatigue cannot be seen like laboured breathing or œdema, it is apt to be underestimated as a symptom of heart failure; yet it is as closely related to a low cardiac output as dyspnœa is to pulmonary venous congestion. Thus patients with tight mitral stenosis and a low pulmonary vascular resistance complain of dyspnœa, for the chief physiological result of the situation is pulmonary venous congestion; but if the pulmonary vascular resistance is extreme, congestion of the lungs is relieved at the expense of right ventricular failure and a low cardiac output, and dyspnœa is replaced by fatigue.

Patients complain of heaviness of the limbs on exertion, weakness or lack of vigour, or general tiredness and exhaustion. The physiology of such fatigue is too complex and ill understood to discuss here with profit. The practical problem is to distinguish cardiac fatigue from that due to anxiety or other mental conflict. This is rarely difficult, for cardiac fatigue is related to effort, and is always associated with genuine signs of congestive heart failure.

CYANOSIS

Cyanosis is a physical sign rather than a symptom, but since it often looms large in a patient's history it may be best considered here.

It is well known that a blue colour is imparted to the skin when the capillary blood contains 5 G. or more of reduced hæmoglobin per cent (Lundsgaard, 1919). Thus with a normal quota of hæmoglobin (15 G. per cent), at least one-third of it must be in the reduced form in the capillaries for cyanosis to appear. Normal arterial blood is 95 per cent saturated with oxygen, i.e. 14.25 of the 15 G. per cent of hæmoglobin in the arterial blood is oxyhæmoglobin and only 0.75 G. reduced hæmoglobin. The normal mixed venous blood is about 70 per cent saturated with oxygen, i.e. 10.5 G. per cent of the hæmoglobin in venous blood is oxyhæmoglobin and 4.5 G. reduced hæmoglobin. The amount of reduced hæmoglobin in capillary blood is assumed to be the mean between arterial and venous contents: thus in a normal individual at rest capillary blood would be assumed to contain $\dfrac{0.75\ G.+4.5\ G.}{2}$ of reduced hæmoglobin per cent, or 2.6 G. per cent. The colour of the normal skin and mucous membranes is therefore pink, not blue.

A corollary of Lundsgaard's thesis is that cyanosis cannot appear in anæmic subjects if the hæmoglobin is less than 33 per cent, for even if all the hæmoglobin was then in the reduced form in the capillaries the total amount would still be less than the critical level of 5 G. per cent. In polycythæmia, on the other hand, a total of 5 G. per cent of reduced hæmoglobin in the capillaries is readily achieved.

While the colour of the skin and mucous membranes depends on the amount of reduced hæmoglobin in the capillaries, the intensity of the hue is determined by the physical state of the capillaries: if they are dilated the colour is rich, if they are constricted the colour is pale.

Cyanosis may be central or peripheral. Central cyanosis means that the arterial oxygen saturation is low. It can usually be detected clinically when the arterial oxygen saturation falls below 85 per cent. With a normal hæmoglobin arterial blood contains 3 G. per cent of reduced hæmoglobin when 80 per cent saturated with oxygen. If the cardiac output is normal the mixed venous blood is then about 60 per cent saturated and contains 6 G. of reduced hæmoglobin per cent. The capillary mean thus works out at $\dfrac{3+6}{2}$ G. per cent or 4.5 G. per cent.

With 85 per cent arterial oxygen saturation, a normal cardiac output and 100 per cent hæmoglobin, mean capillary blood contains about $\dfrac{2.25+5.25}{2}$ or 3.75 G. of reduced hæmoglobin per cent. Yet in Fallot's tetralogy under just these conditions cyanosis can be detected clinically.

In a group of fifteen "acyanotic" cases of Fallot's tetralogy studied by the author the arterial oxygen saturation ranged between 87 and 97 per cent, at rest; anything less than this gave rise to clinical cyanosis, except in one case with anæmia.

Cyanosis in cor pulmonale due to emphysema may also be clinically detected when the arterial oxygen saturation falls below 85 per cent, even when the cardiac output is raised and the arterio-venous oxygen difference reduced. In six such cases studied by the writer and in which the arterial oxygen saturation ranged between 78 and 87 per cent, the mean capillary blood contained an average of 3.9 G. of reduced hæmoglobin per cent.

These observations do not tally with Lundsgaard's figure of 5 G. per cent quoted earlier, but the calculations are based on mixed venous samples obtained from the right atrium, not from blood obtained directly from the skin veins. We have no data on how such samples would effect the calculations. It is observed, however, that ordinary venous blood containing 4.5 G. per cent of reduced hæmoglobin is obviously blue.

Central cyanosis occurs in congenital heart disease with right to left shunt, as in Fallot's tetralogy, in arterio-venous fistula of the lung, and in certain pulmonary diseases, such as severe emphysema, which interfere with alveolar function, so that blood passing through the lung is incompletely oxygenated. Central cyanosis is usually associated with polycythæmia, although this may be masked by a high blood volume as in many cases of cor pulmonale. If sufficiently severe and long-lasting it is also associated with clubbing of the fingers and toes.

Peripheral cyanosis may be a manifestation of a low cardiac output, the tissues extracting more oxygen from each 100 ml. of blood because of the limited supply; but heart failure must be extreme before the mean capillary blood contains sufficient reduced hæmoglobin to cause cyanosis in warm territories such as the conjunctivæ. Thus of 20 cases with an extreme pulmonary vascular resistance (averaging 15 units or 1,200 dynes.sec./cm.5) due to primary pulmonary hypertension (6 cases) or secondary to mitral stenosis (14 cases), chosen at random provided the cardiac output was below 4 litres per minute (in fact it averaged 3 l./min.), the mean capillary blood contained an average of 4.17 G. of reduced hæmoglobin per cent. None of these cases had cyanosis of the conjunctivæ or other mucous membranes, yet the amount of reduced hæmoglobin in the capillaries calculated in the customary fashion was often as high or even higher than that found in cases of Fallot's tetralogy with arterial oxygen saturations around 80 per cent and obvious though mild central cyanosis. Mixed venous samples had a higher content and arterial samples a lower content of reduced hæmoglobin in these low output cases than in the examples of Fallot's tetralogy mentioned. It follows that cyanosis in warm areas depends much more on the content of reduced hæmoglobin in the arterial blood than in the venous blood. It is extremely rare for the arterial oxygen saturation to fall below 85 per cent in these uncomplicated low output states.

In view of these findings the term peripheral cyanosis has come to have a narrower meaning than that originally intended: it may be defined as cyanosis of cold surfaces due to reduction of peripheral blood flow. Thus it is seen chiefly in the skin of the fingers, ears, nose, cheeks, and outer side of the lips; it is not seen in the conjunctivæ, palate, or inner side of the lips or cheeks. In heart failure with a low cardiac output considerable vasoconstriction occurs in certain territories in order to maintain the blood pressure; the skin, being relatively unimportant, is one of these territories, and the vasoconstriction is most intense in exposed surfaces, which are necessarily cooler. The diminished blood flow leads to increased oxygen extraction by the tissues and the subpapillary venous plexuses of the skin must contain a high proportion of reduced hæmoglobin.

At the bedside considerable difficulty may be experienced in attempting to distinguish between central and peripheral cyanosis. Cyanosis of the conjunctivæ, palate, tongue, and inner side of the lips and cheeks is always central. In congenital heart disease cyanosis is certainly central if it is associated with clubbing and polycythæmia, and probably central if it deepens on effort. In suspected cor pulmonale cyanosis is surely central if associated with warm hands, capillary pulsation, digital throbbing, distended forearm veins, and a water-hammer type of pulse, all manifestations of peripheral vasodilatation. Peripheral cyanosis is limited to the ears, nose, cheeks, outer side of the lips, hands, feet and digits, and these parts are cold. Clubbing is not associated, but polycythæmia may be present if the cardiac output has been low for a sufficient time. If doubt still exists despite close attention to these details, direct measurement of the arterial oxygen saturation is advised, the critical distinguishing level being 85 per cent with normal hæmoglobin.

SYNCOPE

There are many causes of transient loss of consciousness, and a complete list would include the causes of epilepsy, coma, concussion, and asphyxia; but syncope has come to mean transient loss of consciousness of sudden onset due to inadequacy of the cerebral blood flow. As so defined, syncope may be divided into cardiac, vasomotor or vaso-vagal, cerebral and anoxic forms.

Cardiac syncope

Cardiac syncope occurs when the heart, through some fault in itself or in its great vessels, fails to maintain an adequate cerebral circulation. These faults are listed for convenience as follows:

1. Cardiac standstill—vagal inhibition.
2. Ventricular asystole—Stokes-Adams fit.
3. Ventricular fibrillation.
4. Ball-valve thrombus or pedunculated myxoma.

5. Aortic stenosis.
6. Paroxysmal rhythm changes with extremely rapid ventricular rates.
7. Massive pulmonary embolism.
8. Cardiac compression from hæmopericardium.
9. Low cardiac output states under certain conditions.

The practical mechanism whereby the heart fails to fulfil its task varies according to the lesion.

In *cardiac standstill, ventricular asystole, ventricular fibrillation, ball-valve thrombus,* and *pedunculated myxoma,* loss of consciousness is abrupt and without warning. The attack may occur at any time while the patient is walking, standing, sitting, or lying. At first, the patient is grey or white, flaccid, pulseless, and motionless. The heart sounds are inaudible, but respirations may continue. In about 10 to 15 seconds anoxic twitchings begin and may develop into convulsions if the attack lasts long enough. If recovery does not occur within two minutes, death usually results. Cardiac and ventricular asystole usually recover well within that time, commonly within 5 to 20 seconds, but ventricular fibrillation is usually, though not necessarily, fatal. Ball-valve thrombus and pedunculated myxoma are rare. Return to consciousness is abrupt and complete and is followed by a vivid flush, hyper-oxygenated blood being flung into a dilated vascular system (reactive hyperæmia).

Similar attacks of uncertain mechanism may occur in *aortic stenosis.* As a rule, however, syncope in aortic stenosis is vasomotor, the valve lesion acting merely as a predisposing factor, or it is due to a low fixed cardiac output (*vide infra*).

Heart rates up to 200 per minute in *paroxysmal tachycardia* are usually well tolerated, but syncope may result if the rate is much faster. Speeds of over 300 per minute have been recorded. The heart has no time to fill or empty properly at these high rates, and both cardiac output and blood pressure fall precipitously.

Massive pulmonary embolism may cause syncope when more than two-thirds of the circulation is blocked. The onset is sudden, but rarely so abrupt as in the group just mentioned. Moreover, it may be preceded by pain or tightness in the chest. The duration of unconsciousness is longer, being usually measured in minutes or even hours. Recovery is at first only partial, extreme faintness persisting. During the attack the patient is limp, grey, sweating and breathless. The pulse is thready or imperceptible, the heart sounds faint or inaudible, the blood pressure low or unobtainable.

Smaller pulmonary emboli, insufficient seriously to embarrass the circulation, occasionally cause reflex syncope. Such reactions may be prevented by means of atropine. Similar attacks may be encountered in cases of acute myocardial infarction. These should not be regarded as examples of cardiac syncope, for the mechanism is vasomotor.

Cardiac compression must be gross to reduce the cardiac output sufficiently to cause loss of consciousness. This condition may be fulfilled by hæmopericardium due to rupture of an aneurysm, dissecting or saccular, or to perforation of the heart from bullet or stab wounds, or spontaneously through a myocardial infarct or ventricular aneurysm.

Since the cardiac output varies with the blood pressure and inversely with the total peripheral resistance $\left(\text{C.O.} = \dfrac{\text{B.P.}}{\text{R}}\right)$, syncope on effort, or as a result of any other agent that lowers "R", may occur in any condition characterised by a *low fixed cardiac output*; e.g. severe aortic, mitral, pulmonary, or tricuspid stenosis, and severe pulmonary hypertension; for if the cardiac output cannot rise the blood pressure must fall.

Syncope on effort in certain obstructive lesions of the circulation, such as primary pulmonary hypertension and severe pulmonary stenosis with closed septa, may also be due to acute right ventricular failure (Howarth and Lowe, 1953).

Yet another type of "cardiac syncope" is encountered in congenital heart disease with right to left shunt, but this is really anoxic.

All these forms of cardiac syncope and their treatment are considered individually elsewhere (see Index).

Vasomotor syncope

Under this heading may be grouped all varieties of syncope in which the cerebral blood flow fails as a result of a sudden fall in blood pressure due to collapse of the peripheral resistance. This includes the common faint.

ETIOLOGY. Vasomotor syncope may be initiated by a critical fall in central venous pressure, by chemical agents that cause sudden profound vasodilatation, or by stimulation of an assortment of receptors which excite a vaso-vagal reaction (Lewis, 1932). Particular causes are listed below:

Causing critical fall in central venous pressure
1. Hæmorrhage
2. Loss of plasma into wounds, burns, crush injuries or gassed lungs
3. Loss of plasma into the skin or tissues as a result of allergy, e.g. generalised urticaria and Quincke's œdema
4. Venous tourniquets on the thighs
5. Orthostatic hypotension
6. Other forms of postural hypotension

Chemical agents causing sudden profound vasodilatation
1. Acetylcholine and other cholinergic substances
2. Histamine
3. Tetraethylammonium, hexamethonium, and ansolysen.
4. Nitrites
5. Diodone and similar radio-opaque substances.
6. Quinidine and procaine amide.

Stimulation of other receptors that excite a vaso-vagal reaction

1. Psychogenic disturbances
2. Carotid sinus compression
3. Extreme pain
4. Cardiac infarction and other sudden visceral catastrophies.

This list is by no means complete, but it includes most of the common causes of vasomotor syncope.

MECHANISM. Syncope from hæmorrhage has been thoroughly investigated in blood-donors. As the blood volume diminishes, the venous pressure falls and the cardiac output is reduced. Compensatory vasoconstriction may temporarily maintain the blood pressure. The faint, which is associated with a sudden fall in blood pressure and pronounced bradycardia, appears to be due to sudden vasodilatation in muscle (Barcroft *et al.*, 1944). This vasodilatation is mediated by vasomotor nerves (Barcroft and Edholm, 1944). Whether this reflex is excited by the fall in venous pressure or otherwise is unknown; but it is clear that diminution in the blood volume is not directly responsible for the faint, for the cardiac output may not alter at the critical moment – the peripheral resistance simply collapses.

This sequence of events has also been demonstrated when syncope results from the prolonged application of venous tourniquets to the thighs, and probably occurs in all cases of syncope initiated by a critical fall in central venous pressure (Sharpey-Schafer, 1944). Venous tourniquets on the thighs act as a "bloodless venesection" by trapping blood in the legs. Fainting in soldiers on parade, who may have to stand at attention for long periods, is believed to depend on similar factors. The fall in central venous pressure initiating orthostatic syncope following lumbo-dorsal sympathectomy is due to abolition of veno-motor tone in the lower half of the body. Veno-motor paralysis may also be partly responsible for fainting following the injection of ganglionic blocking agents. Spontaneous, toxic, and convalescent orthostatic syncope may also be due to loss of veno-motor tone.

Other forms of postural syncope include fainting in pregnant women when they lie on their backs too long, and fainting in certain subjects on adopting the lordotic position. The fall in central venous pressure is then attributed to compression of the inferior vena cava by a pregnant uterus, or by the liver which is forced against the spine (Bull, 1948).

Syncope from chemical agents which cause sudden profound vasodilatation is directly due to collapse of the peripheral resistance. The blood pressure falls steeply, but the cardiac output may be raised, and there may be tachycardia instead of bradycardia. Heat, gross aortic incompetence, and other vasodilatation-states predispose to syncope by lowering the peripheral resistance.

Loss of consciousness produced by the intravenous injection of acetylcholine, *mecholin* (acetyl-beta-methylcholine) and *doryl* (carbo-aminoacetylcholine) is preceded by flushing and a feeling of warmth due to vasodilatation, and by sweating. There is commonly abdominal colic, nausea or vomiting, and desire to micturate or defæcate. The blood pressure is low, but the pulse rate accelerates. Patients may complain bitterly after regaining consciousness, saying they feel "dreadfully weak", as if they had been ill for months. Ordinary therapeutic doses of mecholin and doryl rarely cause syncope; the dose must be large and given intravenously. Symptoms are relieved at once by 1 to 2 mg. of atropine.

Syncope from histamine, nitrites and diodone is also preceded by flushing, headache and tachycardia. Flush syncope may occur spontaneously in women at the menopause or in men at the climacteric. Both hot flushes and syncope disappear following treatment with stilbœstrol, 0.5 to 1 mg. daily.

Syncope is not uncommon in hypertensive subjects being treated with hexamethonium or ansolysen. It is usually postural and may be severe. There is not only collapse of the peripheral resistance, but the central venous pressure falls, blood being pooled in the periphery. The patient should be laid on a couch and tilted head-down by means of blocks under the foot-end; mephentermine 5 mg. may be given intravenously and repeated when necessary, or noradrenalin may be given by intravenous drip in a strength of 4 or 5 mg. per litre, the rate being governed by the blood pressure response.

The severe collapse that sometimes follows the intravenous injection of too large a dose of quinidine is usually due to its vasodilating action, but cardiac standstill or ventricular asystole is occasionally responsible. Too large a dose of procaine amide may have a similar effect on the peripheral resistance.

The simple psychogenic faint is initiated by emotional disturbance, or by stimulation of the afferent component of a conditioned reflex; both result in a powerful autonomic discharge. The type of emotion usually responsible is a mixture of fear, amazement, and curiosity, as may arise when a nurse sees a thoracic paracentesis for the first time, or when a hypersensitive subject witnesses a street accident. The vasomotor centre appears to be suddenly depressed, and there are associated cholinergic manifestations: the chief result is gross vasodilatation. This is certainly not in the skin, which is pale and cold, but may be in muscle or in the splanchnic bed. The peripheral resistance collapses and the blood pressure sinks rapidly. As the cerebral blood flow depends chiefly upon the blood pressure, it becomes inadequate, and consciousness is lost. Spontaneous recovery is inevitable for three reasons: first, unconsciousness abolishes the trigger; secondly, liberated acetylcholine, upon which many of the features of the attack may depend, is rapidly destroyed by choline esterase; thirdly, the horizontal position naturally adopted by an unconscious subject increases the cardiac output and is favourable to the cerebral blood flow.

Carotid sinus syncope is said to be of four main types which may be reproduced by carotid sinus compression (Weiss and Baker, 1933; Ferris, Capps and Weiss, 1935). First, syncope may be due to cardiac standstill. Second, loss of consciousness may be associated with a gross fall of blood pressure and with marked slowing of the pulse rate. If the latter is restored to normal by atropine, consciousness is not regained; if the blood pressure is restored by any means, consciousness returns even though the pulse remains slow. It is the low blood pressure and not the slow pulse rate which is responsible for the syncope. This type corresponds to vaso-vagal syncope. Third, carotid sinus pressure may induce syncope associated with a profound fall in blood pressure without slowing of the pulse rate. It is doubtful if there is any fundamental difference between these two forms of attack, for not infrequently the first type merges into the second; indeed it has been suggested that initial slowing of the heart occurs in all cases, but that subsequent quickening resulting reflexly from the low blood pressure may occur so rapidly as to mislead the observer.

Weiss and Baker describe a fourth type of syncope resulting from carotid sinus pressure, in which the blood pressure and pulse rate are unchanged, and refer to it as cerebral syncope. This appears to be allied to epilepsy; for no reduction of cerebral blood flow can be demonstrated.

Spontaneous carotid sinus syncope may occur in rare instances. The organ is hypersensitive and may be excited by sudden pressure of the neck against a tight collar. The condition may be cured by carotid sinus denervation.

Reflex syncope from pain, myocardial infarction, pulmonary embolism, etc., is similar in mechanism to the simple psychogenic faint.

CLINICAL FEATURES. Spontaneous vasomotor syncope is ushered in with numerous signs and symptoms of autonomic disturbance, e.g. yawning, pallor, sweating, coldness of the skin, a sinking feeling in the pit of the stomach, general muscular weakness, subjective changes of temperature, a feeling as if the blood was all rushing downwards, epigastric discomfort and nausea, desire to micturate or defæcate, a feeling of light-headedness, and so forth.

Patients are aware of imminent loss of consciousness, and although the onset of the faint may be described as quick or sudden, it is never abrupt.

Susceptible individuals faint when standing up, rarely when sitting, and practically never when lying; they faint in company or when in reach of company, rarely when alone. They are especially liable to attacks in closed spaces, in church, in the cinema, and in circumstances that provoke emotional disturbance.

The muscles are flaccid in vasomotor syncope, so that the patient collapses like a house of cards, his final position being determined by gravity: he lies limp and inert, in a sprawled or crumpled position, and may well be on his back. He is deathly white, and often cold and clammy. The eyes may be open or closed, the position of the upper lid being governed by gravity. The pupils are dilated, and may be insensitive to light, the reflexes and tendon jerks absent or depressed. The tongue is never bitten, but urine may be voided. The essential feature is the low blood pressure which may be in the region of 50 or 60 mm. Hg; more often it cannot be determined. The pulse rate is slow, normal or quick. In severe attacks slight twitching may be seen but is uncommon.

The duration of vasomotor syncope is variable, and though usually measured in minutes it may last much longer, even up to an hour. Consciousness is regained gradually, and the patient then feels weak and ill; he may complain of headache, nausea, or vomiting, of a continued feeling of faintness or light-headedness, of trembling and shaking, or of cold sweats. He rarely recovers completely for half an hour or so, and usually likes to lie down until he is better.

Historically the chief difficulty is to distinguish vasomotor syncope from cardiac or cerebral syncope and from epilepsy.

Ménière's syndrome or aural vertigo is usually recognised by its spinning quality, but occasionally there is no spinning, but merely unsteadiness, imbalance, or sudden attacks in which the subject is thrown violently forwards or backwards. Consciousness is rarely lost, however, and either tinnitus or deafness is usually associated.

Cerebral syncope

Cerebral syncope may result from cerebral vascular spasm or transient occlusion. The fault is local.

Hyperventilation syncope is the best example. Forced breathing results in carbon dioxide washout with secondary alkalæmia. Carbon dioxide ordinarily helps to maintain an adequate degree of cerebral vasodilatation (Norcross, 1938); its lack causes cerebral vasoconstriction. This induces dizziness within a minute in most normal individuals undergoing forced breathing. If hyperventilation is maintained long enough syncope may occur. Spontaneous attacks are seen in hysteria and sometimes in encephalitis lethargica. There is usually associated vasoconstriction in the extremities, with pallor, cyanosis, and tingling of the fingers and toes, and there may be tetany. The blood pressure is maintained or raised owing to vasoconstriction, the latter tending to prevent reduction of cerebral blood flow.

Forced breathing may be used as a test in cases of syncope, to discover whether an attack can be reproduced. It should be remembered, however, that epilepsy is sometimes excited by hyperventilation, so that the diagnosis depends upon the nature of the induced attack, not upon the simple fact that consciousness is lost. The effects of spontaneous hyperventilation may be quickly abolished by the inhalation of carbon dioxide. This may be accomplished by breathing in and out of a paper bag or long rubber tube.

Loss of consciousness due to hypertensive encephalopathy or to cerebral vascular lesions with or without associated spasm of cerebral vessels is usually called coma, unless convulsive epilepsy occurs. Embolism, however, especially when due to air or fat, may provoke an attack which fulfills the definition of syncope. The onset is abrupt, and recovery may be remarkably quick and complete if the embolism moves on, or if spasm passes off suddenly.

Loss of consciousness occasionally occurs in Ménière's syndrome, but is then probably a vaso-vagal reaction.

Bilateral carotid compression, an old ju-jitsu trick, is a most effective way of inducing unconsciousness in an adversary.

Anoxic syncope

Loss of consciousness resulting from most causes of anoxia is described as asphyxia or coma. Anoxic syncope, however, may occur in congenital heart disease with right to left shunt, especially in Fallot's tetralogy, and is attributed to diminished peripheral resistance, increased pulmonary resistance, or a fall in total cardiac output. A vaso-vagal turn may have a disastrous effect in Fallot's tetralogy, for the drop in blood pressure at once increases the amount of blood shunted from right to left, and the sudden fall in arterial oxygen saturation may further depress the vasomotor centre, so that a vicious circle is established; patients may die in this way. In four cases of anoxic syncope investigated by the writer, however, an increase of pulmonary resistance seemed to be responsible for the attacks. Loss of consciousness was associated with extreme cyanosis, disappearance of the characteristic pulmonary systolic thrill and murmur, and no fall in blood pressure. In one instance the arterial blood was almost completely unsaturated. Raising the blood pressure well above normal by means of methedrine had no effect on the arterial oxygen saturation and did not restore consciousness. These cases behaved as if there were transient functional pulmonary atresia: whether the obstruction was due to temporary closure of the infundibulum itself or to pulmonary vasoconstriction could not be determined. No structural block, by a clot for example, was found at necropsy in the case that died in the attack. The writer has also witnessed syncope in Fallot's tetralogy resulting from an ill-advised venesection: since the blood pressure fell sharply, however, the increased cyanosis that accompanied loss of consciousness could well have been due to a vaso-vagal mechanism and not to reduction of total cardiac output *per se*.

Tussive syncope (from a prolonged attack of coughing) may be anoxic or asphyxial in one sense, but is more properly ascribed to failure of cardiac filling due to an extremely high intrathoracic pressure which totally obstructs the venous return at the thoracic inlet.

PALPITATIONS

Palpitations may be rapid and regular, with abrupt onset and offset, as in paroxysmal tachycardia; rapid and chaotic, as in auricular fibrillation; or fleeting and repetitive, as with ectopic beats; in such cases the abnormal rhythm can usually be recognised from the description of the sensation. Palpitations may be heavy, rather than fast or irregular, however, and then an increased stroke volume may be responsible. Physiological or patho-logical hyperkinetic circulatory states, aortic or mitral incompetence, patent ductus, ventricular septal defect and atrial septal defect may cause heavy thudding of this kind. In both types the sensation seems to be caused by a radical change in the natural stroke action of the heart; it is the unusual movement of the heart within the thorax that is felt, not an increased force of cardiac contraction, nor more forcible valve closure. Thus palpitations are not a feature of aortic stenosis or pulmonary stenosis, nor of malignant hypertension or primary pulmonary hypertension. The point may be fur-ther elaborated in respect of palpitations due to ectopic beats. It is usually said that it is not the ectopic beat which is felt, but the strong beat following the compensatory pause. Anyone who has himself experienced ectopic palpitations is invited to question this. He may well beg to disagree: the quick beat, out of time, with the heart improperly filled, gives rise to the first sensation, and this alone may be felt; or it may be followed by a second sensation due to the beat of the over-filled heart after the pause. A run of ectopics makes it only too obvious that the quick beat is felt.

A third type of throbbing is vascular. This may be arterial, as in aortic incompetence, or venous, as in gross tricuspid incompetence. It is again the unusual movement within the tissues that is felt. Tactile perceptors in the skin may be stimulated by pressure from within, as can be demon-strated easily enough during the passage of a venous catheter, for this procedure causes no sensation at all unless the catheter tip comes into indirect contact with the skin in the arm, neck or thorax.

Patients may also complain of a beat in the head which is really a sound. It may be single, an internal phase III Korotkow sound, associated with vasodilatation, or it may be double, when both first and second heart sounds are heard. The symptom usually occurs in bed at night.

Palpitations of any kind naturally draw the patient's attention to his heart, and he may soon begin to question its integrity; this leads to anxiety, and since emotional turmoil is the commonest cause of the symptom, at once closes a vicious circle.

HÆMOPTYSIS

Although hæmoptysis may occur in a wide variety of cardiovascular diseases, it only does so under strictly defined circumstances:

(1) A necrotic arterial lesion may rupture, as in disseminated lupus. Pulmonary tuberculosis may accidentally complicate any form of heart disease: this accounted for hæmoptysis in two out of three cases of A.S.D. in the writer's series in which this symptom occurred (2 per cent). An arterio-venous aneurysm may rupture, or a syphilitic or mycotic aneurysm may rupture into the bronchus. Pulmonary lesions like bronchiectasis or bronchial carcinoma should not be overlooked when hæmoptysis occurs unexpectedly in association with heart disease. All these hæmorrhages are essentially necrotic.

(2) Hæmoptysis may occur suddenly as the first symptom of mitral stenosis, and may be precipitated by effort or pregnancy. This kind of pulmonary apoplexy has been attributed to rupture of small pulmonary or broncho-pulmonary anastomotic venules as a result of a sudden rise of left atrial pressure. Such hæmorrhages tend to cease as the pulmonary veins thicken in response to the rise of pressure within them, or when the pulmonary vascular resistance exceeds 10 units (800 dynes sec./cm.5) and so protects the pulmonary venous system from developing too high a pressure (Wood, 1954).

(3) Bloodstained sputum may accompany an attack of paroxysmal cardiac dyspnœa in mitral stenosis or left ventricular failure, and may be attributed to intense pulmonary venous congestion (congestive hæmoptysis). In these cases the dyspnœa is much more important than the hæmoptysis. Blood-spitting in an attack of bronchitis complicating mitral stenosis has a similar significance, and the pink frothy sputum of acute pulmonary œdema is closely related.

(4) Frank hæmoptysis may be caused by pulmonary infarction. This is usually a late manifestation of heart disease, for the phlebothrombosis in the legs from which the responsible embolus springs is apt to be a complication of congestive heart failure proper. Emboli from right-sided bacterial endocarditis may also cause hæmoptysis from small areas of infarction.

Hæmoptysis rarely, if ever, results from uncomplicated pulmonary plethora in patent ductus, V.S.D. and A.S.D.; nor is it a symptom of pulmonary hypertension, primary, secondary or hyperkinetic. It may occur with passive pulmonary hypertension, but here it is the high pulmonary venous pressure that matters, not the arterial.

"Hæmoptysis" in essential hypertension is sometimes due to posterior epistaxis; in other cases, however, this can be excluded, and the site of the hæmorrhage is then a matter for conjecture. It is not common.

RECURRENT BRONCHITIS

Trivial upper respiratory tract infections may rapidly develop into florid bronchitis in two main types of disturbed physiology in cardiovascular disease, pulmonary plethora and pulmonary venous congestion.

Pulmonary plethora, i.e. an increased pulmonary blood flow, occurs typically in patent ductus, and ventricular or atrial septal defect; pulmonary venous congestion in left ventricular failure and mitral valve disease. It is suggested that the violent reaction to trivial infection is due to the hyperæmic state of the pulmonary circulation. Most diseases require both an etiological agent and some tissue reaction; a pathogenic agent alone may be harmless. Thus spirochætal aortitis does not occur in congenital syphilis, although the aorta may contain numerous spirochætes, because there is no tissue reaction; again, amœbæ do not necessarily cause dysentery when they take up their abode in the human colon, but only when reactive ulcerative colitis develops. Hyperæmia is one of the fundamental reactions to infective agents and a major part of what is known as inflammation; if the lung is already hyperæmic an inflammatory reaction would be expected to be intense.

Recurrent bronchitis is not a feature of pulmonary ischæmia in congenital anomalies with right to left shunt, or in low output states; for example, it is uncommon in Fallot's tetralogy and primary pulmonary hypertension.

Recurrent bronchitis is of course an important feature of anoxic cor pulmonale, but here it has a causal rôle.

Both chronic cough and bronchitis may also result from compression of the right or left main bronchus from aneurysm of the aorta or pulmonary artery, or from aneurysmal dilatation of the left atrium.

INSOMNIA

Many patients with heart failure complain bitterly of insomnia. Since the physiology of sleep is still improperly understood, little would be gained by discussing the mechanism of the insomnia. But there are two obvious symptoms which may interrupt sleep in cases of heart failure—paroxysmal cardiac dyspnœa and Cheyne-Stokes breathing.

Nocturnal dyspnœa in left ventricular failure and mitral valve disease may be abolished by means of a low sodium diet and mercurial diuretics, and it has been well said that the best cure for insomnia in these cases is mersalyl (Evans).

Cheyne-Stokes breathing tends to wake the patient during the dyspnœic phase of each respiratory cycle. The symptom can be very troublesome because it is aggravated by morphine, barbiturates and indeed by sleep itself. Fortunately, however, it can usually be abolished by aminophylline, preferably given as a suppository in a dose of 0.4 G. at night. Aminophylline has the double advantage of preventing paroxysmal cardiac dyspnœa as well.

Thus although barbiturates may have to be used for the insomnia of heart failure, better results are usually achieved by the efficient treatment of the heart failure itself.

SYSTEMIC EMBOLISM

Under certain circumstances a clot may form in the left side of the heart, or in a pulmonary vein, and if liberated must find its way into some cerebral, visceral or peripheral artery. The chief causes of thrombosis in the cavity of the left ventricle are cardiac infarction and isolated myocarditis; in the left atrium, mitral valve disease and auricular fibrillation; and in the aortic or mitral valve, bacterial endocarditis. The commonest cause of embolism is undoubtedly mitral valve disease with auricular fibrillation.

There is increasing evidence that only a fresh clot is liable to be set free, and that in mitral valve disease this fresh clot is most likely to form within the first few days of the onset of uncontrolled auricular fibrillation, whether paroxysmal or permanent. The embolism may occur while the auricle is still fibrillating, or soon after normal rhythm is resumed spontaneously or in response to quinidine therapy.

Cerebral embolism

The clinical features of cerebral embolism differ from those of cerebral thrombosis in three ways: first, the attack is abrupt rather than sudden in onset, often with loss of consciousness; second, the symptoms are maximal at the start; and third, remarkable recovery may take place within a few minutes or hours. In addition, one of the known underlying causes of systemic embolism should be apparent.

Treatment consists of doing everything possible to promote an effective cerebral circulation, and to prevent secondary thrombosis. The patient should be nursed flat if the state of the heart allows it. Uncontrolled auricular fibrillation and congestive heart failure should be treated quickly and efficiently to encourage the maximum cardiac output. Oxygen with 5 per cent carbon dioxide may be inhaled with advantage, and the blood pressure must be maintained, if necessary by means of a noradrenaline intravenous infusion at a rate of approximately 10 μg. per minute, mephentermine (wyamine) 35 mg. intramuscularly, or some other pressor amine; for the cerebral blood flow depends chiefly upon the arterial carbon dioxide content and the blood pressure. Vasodilators (to relieve vascular spasm) are not recommended, for they are more likely to act peripherally than on the cerebral vessels, and by lowering the blood pressure may have an adverse effect on cerebral flow. Anticoagulants have often been withheld on the grounds that they might induce hæmorrhage in an area of cerebral softening; but there is little factual evidence to support this view, and in the writer's opinion they should be given, both to prevent secondary thrombosis and further embolism.

Visceral embolism

An embolus may lodge in a mesenteric, splenic, renal, coronary or other visceral artery.

Mesenteric embolism is characterised by sudden severe epigastric pain with or without shock. The patient presents with an acute abdomen, but on examination there is no guarding and but little tenderness. Within a few hours malena appears, the blood being dark red in colour. Symptoms and signs of sub-acute or complete intestinal paralysis follow, with vomiting and increasing distension. The outlook is bad in the more severe cases, death occurring in a few days. In less severe cases, however, despite evidence of ileus and even though malena may be extensive, recovery may occur within the week.

As with cerebral embolism the object of treatment is to encourage the circulation in the territory concerned. Auricular fibrillation and heart failure require urgent treatment. Operation is often advised but the results are not encouraging; success depends upon extensive gut resection and end-to-end anastomosis, procedures rarely tolerated by these sick patients. Conservative treatment has been rewarded by as good if not better results, provided other measures have been taken to promote the circulation and to combat ileus. A gastric suction tube should be inserted early and pain relieved by pethidine or morphine. Anticoagulants are probably better withheld in view of the hæmorrhage, although they have been given with success. As with all emboli an apparently grave situation in the early stages may suddenly become favourable, perhaps because the embolus moves on, because associated vascular spasm passes off, or because an adequate collateral circulation develops.

Renal embolism results in hæmaturia and renal colic. If the other kidney is healthy there are no serious sequelæ. Most renal infarcts are quite small, and even though the other kidney is diseased there is little danger of renal failure; occasionally, however, the whole kidney is thrown out of action by a large embolus and anuria results.

Infarction of the spleen from embolism may be silent; on the other hand it may give rise to perisplenitis with pain and friction in the left hypochondrium, or to sudden enlargement of the organ due to hæmorrhage. Treatment is conservative.

The clinical features of *coronary embolism* are indistinguishable from those of coronary thrombosis. The diagnosis should only be considered when there is an obvious underlying cause for embolism in a patient in whom coronary thrombosis is unlikely, e.g. in a young person with mitral stenosis or bacterial endocarditis.

Peripheral embolism

It is a common experience to encounter peripheral embolism in a hospital where large numbers of patients with mitral stenosis and auricular fibrillation are gathered together. The following remarks are based on such experience. It is not sufficiently understood that if an embolus occludes the radial, ulnar, posterior or anterior tibial arteries, or even if it lodges at the bifurcation of the brachial or popliteal vessels, there are as a rule no symptoms. The embolus is then only discovered by accident or if especially looked for. These cases prove conclusively that pain is not a feature of the mere lodgment of an embolus in an artery. If the clot comes to rest higher up, however, symptoms may follow according to its position and to the efficacy of the collateral circulation. In the arm symptoms are usually absent or trivial, whatever the site of the embolism. In the leg significant or serious symptoms are likely to follow occlusion of the femoral artery above the origin of its deep branch which is given off about an inch below Poupart's ligament. Below this point an adequate collateral circulation is usually established by the deep femoral artery. When collateral vessels are atherosclerotic or otherwise diseased, however, as is common in the aged, these principles do not apply, for then a relatively small embolism may precipitate gangrene. Each case must be considered carefully on its merits. Pain is due to ischæmia of working muscle in the affected territory. Thus an embolus may lodge quietly in a resting limb and cause no pain until the limb is actively moved. If there is sufficient ischæmia of nervous tissue, pain at rest, paræsthesia or peripheral anæsthesia may be present. On examination the affected limb is colder than its fellow and may be pale or cyanosed. The distal vessels are impalpable. Methodical palpation of the vessels in a proximal direction may reveal the site of the embolism, for above it pulsation is normal.

The problem in every case is whether to advise embolectomy or conservative treatment. Good judgment would take into account the site of the embolus, the age of the patient, the presence or absence of peripheral vascular disease such as atherosclerosis, the objective findings concerning the immediate state of the peripheral circulation, and the fact that if an operation is to be performed it should not be delayed more than six hours. There are three other points of peculiar importance which should also be considered. First, an embolus often moves on from a position of danger to one of safety. It is not wise to attempt to milk it down the limb because the embolus may then break up, and its fragments may block several distal vessels and so interfere seriously with collateral circulatory efficiency. Second, there may be considerable vascular spasm associated with an embolus, so that initial ischæmia may be disproportionate to the size of the vessel blocked. Third, in cases associated with heart failure and auricular fibrillation with rapid ventricular rate, an inadequate collateral circulation may be made sufficient by improving the cardiac output. Dramatic effects may be obtained in such cases by intravenous digoxin or strophanthin, when a critical situation may be turned within half an hour.

The fact is that most of these cases do better than is generally supposed. The wisest course is to start intensive medical treatment immediately the diagnosis is made. Morphine or pethidine, heating the body with an electric cradle or hot water bottles, and various vasodilators such as eupaverine or priscol are helpful. Hypertonic saline is rarely practical in cardiac cases. If after two hours of such treatment the peripheral circulation, as judged by the colour, temperature and function of the limb, remains in jeopardy, the surgeon should be invited to perform embolectomy. Once this decision has been made the physician should increase rather than decrease his efforts to make the operation unnecessary, and in close co-operation with the surgeon should be prepared to ask for a little more time if there is any sign of improvement. A good surgeon, however, will be anxious to avoid delay if in his own opinion conservative measures are proving ineffective.

Reluctance to advise embolectomy is based on three precepts: first, if an operation is to be performed heparin may have to be withheld, yet anticoagulants are highly desirable to prevent post-embolic thrombosis and further embolism; second, it is embarrassing to witness exposure of a vessel which is found to be pulsating freely by the time it is reached; third, arteriotomy is not devoid of the risk of post-operative thrombosis. Nevertheless, embolectomy is essential if the limb is really in danger.

OTHER SYMPTOMS

Pulmonary embolism, usually secondary to phlebothrombosis in the legs, is a common complication of heart failure with a low cardiac output, and is discussed fully in Chapter XVII.

Cardiac cachexia, sometimes obscured by œdema and swelling of the abdomen, is a common late manifestation of chronic heart failure. It occurs especially in lingering cases of aortic, mitral, or tricuspid stenosis.

Cerebral symptoms include varying grades of dementia in advanced hypertension, attacks of encephalopathy in malignant hypertension, and confusional or frankly psychotic states attributed to anoxia, diminished cerebral blood flow, or impaired hepatic function as, for example, in cor pulmonale, following operations on the heart in which the blood pressure has dropped to low levels for too long a period, and in severe low-output heart failure respectively.

Swelling of the abdomen due to gross enlargement of the liver, with or without ascites, may complicate chronic heart failure from any cause, but is seen especially in constrictive pericarditis, severe tricuspid stenosis, and advanced cases of functional tricuspid incompetence associated with chronic right ventricular failure. Cirrhosis of the liver in alcoholics with heart failure may provide independent grounds for ascites, and thrombosis of the hepatic vein may complicate heart failure.

Jaundice and vomiting complicating heart failure are discussed in Chapter VII.

Oligemia and nocturia are also discussed under "Heart Failure", and nocturia again in the chapter on "Hypertension".

REFERENCES

Barcroft, H., and Edholm, O. G. (1944): (Unpublished report to the Medical Research Council.)

——, ——, McMichael, J., and Sharpey-Schafer, E. P. (1944): "Posthæmorrhagic fainting. Study by cardiac output and forearm flow", *Lancet*, **1**, 489.

Bull, G. M. (1948): Personal communication.

Christie, R. V. (1934): "The elastic properties of the emphysematous lung and their clinical significance", *J. Clin. Invest.*, **13**, 295.

——, and Meakins, J. C. (1934): "The intrapleural pressure in congestive heart failure and its clinical significance", *J. Clin. Invest.*, **13**, 323.

Comroe, J. H., Jr., and Schmidt, C. F. (1943): "Reflexes from the limbs as a factor in the hyperpnœa of muscular exercise", *Amer. J. Physiol.*, **138**, 536.

Denz, F. A. (1947): "Hunger Oedema", *Quart. J. Med.*, **16**, 1.

Ferris, E. B., Capps, R. B., and Weiss, S. (1935): "Carotid sinus syncope and its bearing on the mechanism of the unconscious state and convulsions", *Medicine*, **14**, 377.

Frank, R. T. (1931): "Hormonal causes of premenstrual tension", *Arch. Neurol. Psychiat.*, **26**, 1053.

Gesell, R. (1925): "The chemical regulation of respiration", *Physiol. Rev.*, **5**, 551.

Greene, R., and Dalton, K. (1953): "The premenstrual syndrome", *Brit. med. J.*, **1**, 1007.

Haldane, J. S., and Priestley, J. G. (1905): "The regulation of the lung-ventilation", *J. Physiol.*, **32**, 225.

Hering, E., and Breuer, J. (1868): "Die Seibststeuerung der Athmung durch den Nervus vagus", *S. B. Akad. Wiss. Wien*, **57**, 672.

Heymans, C., and Bouckaert, J. J. (1939): "Les chémorécepteurs du sinus carotidien", *Ergebn. d. Physiol.*, **41**, 28.

Howarth, S., and Lowe, J. B. (1953): "The mechanism of effort syncope in primary pulmonary hypertension and cyanotic congenital heart disease", *Brit. Heart J.*, **15**, 47.

Krogh, A. (1929): "The anatomy and physiology of capillaries", Yale University Press, New Haven.

Landis, E. M. (1930): "Micro-injection studies of capillary blood pressure in human skin", *Heart*, **15**, 209.

Lewis, T. (1932): "Vaso-vagal syncope and the carotid sinus mechanism", *Brit. med. J.*, **i**, 873.

Lundsgaard, C. (1919): "Studies on Cyanosis", *J. exp. Med.*, **30**, 259 and 271.

Norcross, N. C. (1938): "Intra-cerebral blood flow: an experimental study", *Arch. Neurol. and Psychiat.*, **40**, 291.

Sharpey-Schafer, E. P. (1944): "Circulatory dynamics of hæmorrhage", *Brit. med. Bull.*, **2**, 171.

Sinclair, H. M. (1948): "Nutritional œdema", *Proc. R.. Soc. Med.*, **41**, 541.

Starling, E. H. (1895–6): "On the absorption of fluids from the connective tissue species", *J. Physiol.*, **19**, 312.

Verney, E. B. (1946): "Absorption and excretion of water. The antidiuretic hormone", *Lancet*, **2**, 781.

Weiss, S., and Baker, J. P. (1933): "The carotid sinus reflex in health and disease. Its rôle in the causation of fainting and convulsions", *Medicine*, **12**, 297.

White, A. G., and Sachs, B. A. (1950): "Studies in œdema: cholesterol and its relation to protein nitrogen in œdema fluid", *Science* **112**: 18.

Wood, Paul (1954): "An appreciation of mitral stenosis", *Brit. med. J.*, **1**, 1051, and 1113.

CHAPTER II

PHYSICAL SIGNS

THERE are two methods of examining a patient: the first begins at the top of the head and ends with the toes, a method often adopted for the sake of convenience; the second is to examine the various systems of the body, one by one, in logical sequence. The procedure recommended here is concerned only with the cardiovascular system, but it is essential, of course, that all other systems be examined.

GENERAL INSPECTION

While extracting the history the physician should be making a preliminary general inspection. He should pay particular attention to the head and neck, looking for goitre and for the eye signs of thyrotoxicosis, for Corrigan's sign, and especially for jugular pulsation. He will note the general build and appearance of the patient, his attitude and demeanour, and should form some idea of his character. He should observe plethora, pallor, or cyanosis. He may see that respiration is hurried, irregular, shallow, or wheezy; or he may detect the tell-tale sigh of emotional tension. He is sure to glance at the hands, noting their posture, shape, colour, and behaviour; he may discern clubbing of the fingers, spooning of the nails, tremor, or palmar sweating. All these things and many others he will learn to observe without effort, taking note of them without seeming to do so, and in such a limited survey may be put on the track of the correct diagnosis, and be forewarned where to look most diligently for further signs.

THE ARTERIAL PULSE

It is customary to examine the pulse first at the wrist, and to consider it in terms of speed, rhythm, tension, amplitude, and quality; at the same time it is convenient to note the state of the arterial wall. Whilst speed and rhythm may be checked by auscultation of the heart, and tension by sphygmomanometry, the quality and amplitude of the pulse wave can only be analysed in peripheral vessels, and are features of great diagnostic importance.

The most convenient and revealing pulse to examine is the right brachial; it is best felt with the thumb of the right hand, the physician being on the patient's right side. The quality of the brachial pulse can only be learned by experience. What is felt is a pressure wave, and to appreciate it fully it is necessary to vary the pressure which the thumb exerts upon the artery until maximum movement is detected. This implies exerting a force equal to the diastolic arterial pressure. The upstroke of the pulse or percussion wave is smooth and fairly sharp without being abrupt, and occupies about 0.08 sec. (range 0.06 to 1.0 sec.); the peak of the wave is momentarily sustained, so that arterial pressure curves have a rounded summit occupying 0.06 to 0.12 sec.; and the downstroke is initially fairly quick but not precipitous, the whole movement being smooth and uniform (fig. 2.01).

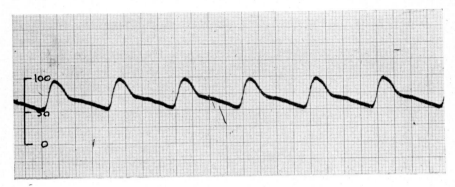

Fig. 2.01—Normal arterial pulse in a child.

Pulsus parvus

A pulse wave of small amplitude means that systolic and diastolic pressures are nearer one another than usual, i.e. they are approaching the mean arterial pressure. This is a sign of vasoconstriction and generally implies a low cardiac output. In normal subjects it may be due to cold or anxiety. It occurs locally in the arteries of the legs in coarctation of the

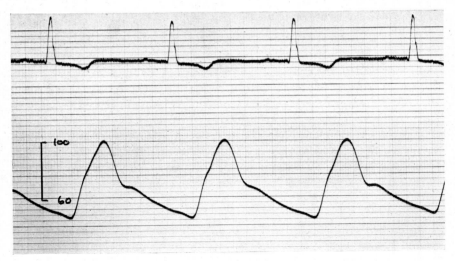

Fig. 2.02—The anacrotic pulse of aortic stenosis: the percussion wave is dwarfed and occupies 0.1 second; the large blunt peak builds up slowly, the maximum pressure not being reached until 0.24 second after the onset (major time intervals 0.1 sec.).

aorta, and in any artery distal to partial occlusion. In disease it is characteristic of severe hypertension, aortic stenosis, cardiac infarction, mitral
stenosis, extreme pulmonary hypertension, severe pulmonary stenosis,
tricuspid stenosis, Pick's disease, pericardial effusion, myocarditis and any
form of low-output failure.

Bounding pulse

A large pulse wave of good form means a high pulse pressure associated
with an increased blood
flow, and is seen characteristically in the hyper-
kinetic circulatory states.

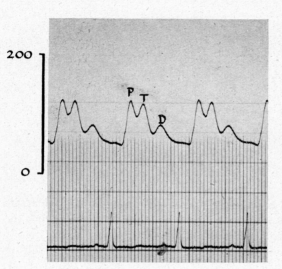

Anacrotic pulse

A slow upstroke asso-
ciated with a pulse wave
of low amplitude is typical
of aortic stenosis (fig. 2.02).
Sometimes a notch can be
felt on the upstroke: this
is the *anacrotic* pulse (or in
full, anadicrotic—*ava*, up;
δίς, twice; χροτος, beat).

Pulsus bisferiens

In combined aortic
stenosis and incompetence
a double beat during sys-
tole may be very pro-
nounced (fig. 2.03): it

Fig. 2.03—Pulsus bisferiens: external arteriogram showing two peaks in systole, P being the
percussion wave and T the tidal wave; they are
followed by the dicrotic wave.

shows up well in the ordinary external arteriogram when some pressure is
applied to the surface of the artery by means of the pick-up device, but
the trough between the two peaks usually disappears in intra-arterial pressure tracings, being replaced by a short plateau or shoulder (fig. 2.04).
The second component of the beat has been attributed to a tidal wave,
the onset of the percussion wave being reflected back from the periphery
before the tail of the percussion wave has passed, the meeting of the two
having a summation effect (Bramwell, 1947).

Dicrotic pulse

In the better-known form of twice-beating pulse the percussion wave is
followed by a palpable secondary wave after aortic valve closure (fig. 2.05).
In normal individuals the downstroke of the pulse wave is interrupted by
a notch (dicrotic notch) representing aortic valve closure, but the small
positive pressure wave (dicrotic wave) that follows the notch or distorts

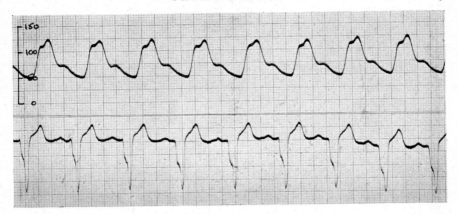

Fig. 2.04—Intra-arterial pressure tracing of the pulsus bisferiens. The dip between percussion and tidal waves is replaced by a plateau.

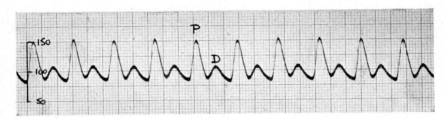

Fig. 2.05—Intra-arterial pressure tracing of a typical dicrotic pulse (D).

the contour of the descent cannot be felt clinically. The dicrotic pulse is encountered chiefly in patients sick with some fever such as typhoid; the peripheral resistance is low, the blood pressure low, the arteries lax, and the cardiac output probably normal.

Water-hammer pulse

This aptly describes the combination of an abrupt percussion wave, ill-sustained crest, and rapid collapse (fig. 2.06). A water-hammer is a hermetically sealed tube containing a vacuum partly filled with water; when the tube is inverted quickly the water drops abruptly and imparts a palpable shock to that end of the container. A pulse having this characteristic quality indicates a low filling resistance in the reservoir into which the left ventricle pumps its contents. In health a low resistance is always peripheral and means vasodilatation, usually due to heat, exercise, emotional disturbance, pregnancy, or alcohol. Peripheral vasodilatation is characteristic of the hyperkinetic circulatory states such as thyrotoxicosis, anæmia, beri-beri, hepatic failure, and anoxic cor pulmonale. Peripheral resistance is lowered by a leak in the arterial side of the circulation, e.g.

in arterio-venous fistula, patent ductus, aortic incompetence, mitral incompetence, and possibly ventricular septal defect. The physiological counterpart of an arterio-venous fistula may also occur in the thyroid gland in thyrotoxicosis (spontaneously or as a result of anti-thyroid drugs), in the uterus during pregnancy, and in bone in Paget's disease. Again, peripheral

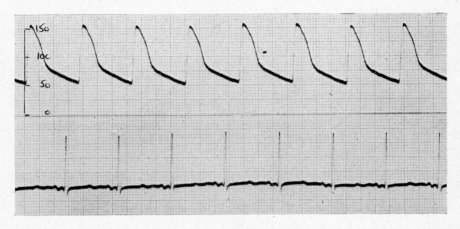

Fig. 2.06—Intra-arterial pressure tracing of a water-hammer pulse in a case of patent ductus arteriosus. Note the singularly abrupt wave front.

vasodilatation tends to accompany most of the conditions mentioned, with the teleological effect of encouraging forward flow in competition with the leak. Finally, a water-hammer pulse often accompanies complete heart block, in which an unusually large volume of blood is flung into a relatively empty arterial reservoir each beat.

The amplitude of the water-hammer pulse varies considerably in these different conditions, being highest in aortic incompetence, heart block, and the hyperkinetic circulatory states (physiological or pathological), and lowest in mitral incompetence. The collapse occurs in the latter part of systole, and the dicrotic notch is usually displaced towards the base-line. In the majority the systolic blood pressure is somewhat raised and the diastolic low.

Pulsus alternans

Alternate larger and smaller beats with normal rhythm are characteristic of severe systemic hypertension or left ventricular failure. The mechanism is discussed in Chapter VII. Similar alternation may occur in the pulmonary arterial pulse, right ventricle and right atrium in severe pulmonary hypertension or stenosis (fig. 2.07). There is no change in alternate electrocardiographic complexes, and as a rule the phenomenon cannot be recognised by means of auscultation. A bout of alternation is frequently precipitated by an ectopic beat in susceptible cases.

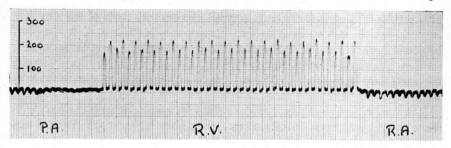

Fig. 2.07—Right ventricular alteration in a case of severe pulmonary stenosis. (Paper speed 2.5 mm. per sec.)

Pulsus paradoxus

The pulse normally quickens during inspiration and slows during expiration, but it does not alter appreciably in volume; in chronic constrictive pericarditis and in tense pericardial effusion, however, it may become very small or disappear altogether during inspiration. The mechanism is discussed in Chapter XIII.

Pulsus bigeminus

Alternate ventricular ectopic beats results in coupling, each pair of beats consisting of a normal or large pulse followed by a small one.

The pulse in other arteries

The pulse should be checked in all the palpable major arteries on both sides, i.e. in the radials, brachials, carotids, femorals, popliteals, posterior tibials, and dorsal arteries of the feet.

Difficulty in locating the radial artery may be due to its taking an aberrant dorso-lateral course. *Weakness on one or other side* usually denotes proximal compression, as from aneurysm of the aorta, but a weak left radial pulse may be due to an ectopic origin and aberrant course of the left subclavian artery.

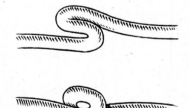

The carotids may present an unusual degree of pulsation associated with coarctation of the aorta, Corrigan's sign of aortic incompetence, kinking from atherosclerosis, or a thrill or shudder indicating aortic stenosis.

Fig. 2.08—Two types of kinked carotid.

CORRIGAN'S SIGN consists of abrupt distension and quick collapse of the carotids, the movement being of high amplitude. It is discovered by inspection (Corrigan, 1832), not by palpation, and should not strictly be confused with a palpable water-hammer pulse.

CAROTID KINKING superficially resembles a rounded pulsating aneurysm at the base of the right common carotid. A short segment of the vessel is looped back sharply on itself to give this impression (fig. 2.08). It is caused by elevation of the aortic arch as a result of hypertension or atherosclerosis, so that the carotids, particularly the right, come to be too long for the distance they occupy. The lesion is seen especially in obese women in whom the heart is also elevated.

Routine palpation of the arteries in the legs would insure the immediate recognition of coarctation of the aorta in nearly all cases, *diminished and delayed femoral pulsation* being characteristic and almost pathognomonic. The presence of pulsation in the vessels of the feet should always be recorded, if only for subsequent reference.

THE EXTREMITIES

Further information of the kind partly given by the arterial pulse may be obtained from examining the extremities, particularly the fingers, hands and forearms.

Signs of vasodilatation

DIGITAL THROBBING indicates vasodilatation, and may be detected by picking up all the fingers of the patient's right hand with all the fingers of the examiner's right hand, so that the two sets grip each other gently, finger to finger, in a flexed position.

CAPILLARY PULSATION has a similar significance, and is best demonstrated by transilluminating the tip of the middle finger or thumb by pressing a pocket torch into the pad underneath and shading the nail bed from daylight with the flexed fingers of the examiner's other hand.

WARM HANDS are associated with these signs of vasodilatation, and if the blood flow is increased *the forearm veins are usually distended.*

Vasodilatation occurs in all the physiological and pathological hyperkinetic circulatory states and in all conditions which may give rise to the water-hammer pulse.

Signs of vasoconstriction

COLD HANDS are associated with peripheral vasoconstriction, and when the blood flow is diminished the *forearm veins become spidery.* Peripheral vasoconstriction may be due to cold, when it helps to prevent loss of heat from exposed surfaces; to apprehension, as part of a general response; or to a low cardiac output, when it helps to maintain the blood pressure.

Other circulatory signs

THE COLOUR OF THE HANDS gives less information concerning blood flow and arterial tone. As a general rule the colour is pink when there is vasodilatation and pale or blue when there is vasoconstriction. But the palms of the hands may be bright red in certain cases of low output heart failure, when hepatic function is sufficiently disturbed; and the hands are pale in anæmia and blue in anoxic cor pulmonale although the cardiac output may be high and the arterioles dilated. Richly coloured, often cyanosed hands are seen in polycythæmia vera.

DIFFERENTIAL CYANOSIS between the hands and feet, the hands being pink and the feet blue, is pathognomonic of pulmonary hypertension with right to left shunt via a patent ductus arteriosus.

THE RAYNAUD PHENOMENON (Raynaud, 1862), defined by Hunt (1936) as "intermittent pallor or cyanosis of the extremities, precipitated by exposure to cold without blockage of the large peripheral vessels and with nutritional lesions, if present at all, limited to the skin", cannot be described here in detail. It must be stated, however, that at least one-third of patients with myxœdema suffer from this disorder, and that it is not infrequently the first symptom of the disease. Hypersensitivity to cold and a reduced peripheral blood flow are presumably responsible. Raynaud's phenomenon is not uncommon in other low output states, such as hypertensive heart failure and advanced mitral stenosis; on the other hand, it is rare in thyrotoxicosis and other hyperkinetic circulatory states.

THE SCLERODERMA OF THE FINGERS (acrosclerosis) that may be associated with Raynaud's disease is usually regarded as a vasomotor trophic change, but may be associated with more widespread lesions, particularly in the skin of the face and neck, and in the submucosal connective tissue of the mouth and œsophagus (Olsen, O'Leary, and Kirklin, 1945). Scleroderma, however, may also involve the heart (Weiss et al., 1943). In the majority of such cases the extremities have shown pigmentation, a rheumatoid type of arthritis and Raynaud's syndrome in addition to the smooth, glossy, drumtight skin of scleroderma (fig. 2.09).

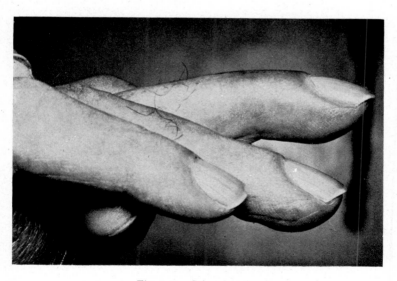

Fig. 2.09—Sclerodactyly.

Changes in the nails

CLUBBING OF THE FINGERS AND TOES may occur in cyanotic forms of congenital heart disease, bacterial endocarditis, and anoxic cor pulmonale; also, of course, in suppurative lesions of the lungs, such as pulmonary abscess and bronchiectasis, and bronchial carcinoma; clubbing may also be hereditary, and has been reported in association with sprue, cirrhosis of the liver, post-operative myxœdema, and syphilitic aneurysm (where it may be unilateral). Advanced clubbing is obvious, the tips of the digits beyond the root of the nail being swollen, rounded and congested, there being an overgrowth of the soft tissues of the nail bed and hyperæmia. The best sign of mild clubbing is probably obliteration of the normal angle between the base of the nail and the skin proximal to it (fig. 2.10). Clubbing is rare in infancy, even when cyanosis is intense, but is common enough in Fallot's tetralogy by the age of two or three. It may develop very quickly under appropriate circumstances, in two to three weeks for example in cases of pulmonary abscess, and may disappear equally quickly when its cause is radically removed, e.g. when the arterial oxygen saturation is restored to normal by means of pulmonary valvotomy or infundibular resection in cases of Fallot's tetralogy. The precise cause of clubbing is still unknown, but it appears to be related to an increase of blood flow in the terminal digits (Mendlowitz, 1938).

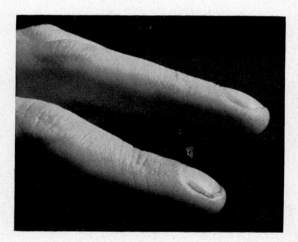

Fig. 2.10—Clubbed fingers showing disappearance of the normal angle between the skin and nail.

KOILONYCHIA (spooning of the nails) is a well-known sign of iron deficiency anæmia: the nails are flattened, even concave, fragile, and tend to split longitudinally (fig. 2.11). They are rapidly restored to normal as the anæmia improves with iron therapy. Koilonychia has also been reported

in thyrotoxicosis, without anæmia (Cooke and Luty, 1944), and is sometimes encountered in apparently normal individuals.

OPAQUE WHITE NAILS have been reported in hepatic cirrhosis (Terry,
1954), including cardiac cirrhosis.

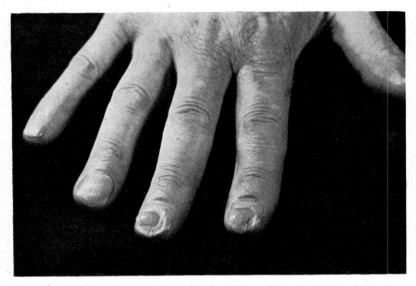

Fig. 2.11—Koilonychia. The spoon-shaped nails are holding a drop of water.

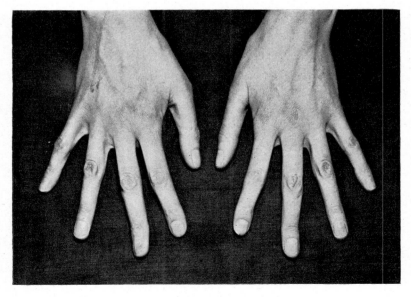

Fig. 2.12—Arachnodactyly.

Congenital deformities

ARACHNODACTYLY or spider fingers (fig. 2.12), first described by Marfan (1896), is an hereditary and familial disorder of mesoblastic growth, and in its complete form is characterised by elongated spidery fingers and toes, thin facies, tall lean build, muscular hypotonia (and its consequences, e.g. scoliosis and flat feet), dislocation of the lenses, high-arched palate, deformed teeth, and pigeon chest (Rados, 1942). Cardiac anomalies, especially hypoplasia of the aorta (with or without dilatation, aneurysm, dissection or rupture), and atrial septal defect are associated in 40 to 45 per cent of cases, and patients have an increased liability to rheumatism and rheumatic mitral or aortic valve disease (Reynolds, 1950; Goyette and Palmer, 1953).

SYNDACTYLY and POLYDACTYLY may also be hereditary or familial, and may be associated with congenital heart disease.

Arthritis of the hands and feet

RHEUMATIC FEVER in adults not infrequently attacks the small joints of the hands and may be mistaken for rheumatoid.

RHEUMATOID itself may cause pericarditis, with or without effusion.

Historical or objective evidence of previous *gout* should be noted, partly because in susceptible individuals an attack may be readily provoked by dehydration resulting from mercurial diuretics or a strict low sodium régime, unless special precautions are taken.

PULMONARY OSTEOARTHROPATHY associated with central cyanosis and an increased blood flow to the extremities is an uncommon complication of advanced anoxic cor pulmonale (see Chapter XVIII). The wrists, elbows, ankles and knees may all be involved, as well as the small joints of the hands and feet.

Heberden's nodes or other evidence of osteoarthritis are of no cardio-vascular significance.

Nodes

OSLER'S NODES are small, tender, erythematous, transient and often palpable skin lesions characteristic of bacterial endocarditis. They occur especially in the pads of the fingers or toes, the palms of the hands or soles of the feet, and are due to infected emboli (Osler, 1909).

RED TENDER MACULES, biopsies of which may also yield positive cultures, are equally if not more common in bacterial endocarditis.

LARGER INFLAMMATORY NODES, resembling a septic finger in the pre-suppurative stage, constitute a third type of peripheral lesion in this disease.

DISSEMINATED LUPUS may give rise to painful erythematous or hæmorrhagic necrotic nodes in the extremities (and elsewhere).

ERYTHEMA NODOSUM in the legs or forearms is too well known to warrant description (fig. 2.13). It seems to be a non-specific allergic type of tissue reaction to a variety of antigenic agents including tuberculosis, meningococcal septicæmia, streptococcal infection, and a host of drugs, particularly sulphathiazol. It is not uncommon in sarcoidosis and is sometimes associated with rheumatic fever. Not infrequently none of these agents or relationships can be demonstrated with certainty.

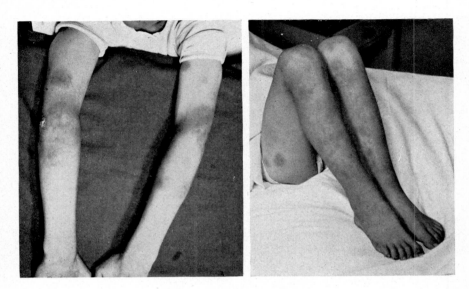

Fig. 2.13—Typical distribution of erythema nodosum.

RHEUMATIC NODULES are illustrated and discussed in Chapter IX. Similar and larger nodules may occur in rheumatoid arthritis.

Heberden's nodes and chalky deposits of gout have already been mentioned.

SPIDER NÆVI are not nodes, but may be mentioned here for convenience. They are characteristic of advanced disease of the liver, and are usually associated with bright red palms and other evidence of vasodilatation (see Chapter XX).

A GLOMUS TUMOUR is a minute subcutaneous erythematous or bluish point, usually under a nail, and often exquisitely painful. It is mentioned here because it may be mistaken for an Osler's node. It is essentially a small innocent tumour of one of the rounded arterio-venous shunt arrangements known as glomera (*glomus*, a ball), which are so numerous in the tips of the fingers and palms.

Nervous disorders

MOIST PALMS provide good evidence of an anxiety state.

TREMOR should be interpreted with care. Thyrotoxic tremor is fine, regular, and constant. The tremor of an anxiety state is fine or coarse, irregular and inconstant. Coarse tremor may be due to alcohol, paralysis agitans, disseminated sclerosis, fatigue or senility; occasionally it is congenital.

TETANY of the hands is commonly due to hysterical hyperventilation, which causes tissue alkalæmia; it is quickly relieved by the inhalation of carbon dioxide. The sign is valuable when it is clinically uncertain whether overbreathing is due to pulmonary or cardiac disease, or to hysteria. A venous tourniquet applied to the limb will augment carpal spasm (Trousseau's sign); or tapping the facial nerve with the finger may cause an obvious facial twitch (Chvostek's sign).

PERIPHERAL NEURITIS with motor weakness, impairment of sensation and loss of tendon jerks may give the clue to the nature of an obscure cardiopathy such as periarteritis, beri-beri, and diphtheria. The signs of neurosyphilis may disclose the cause of aortic incompetence or a mediastinal mass; signs of subacute combined degeneration of the cord may at once explain a hyperkinetic circulatory state; transient paraplegia immediately distinguishes dissecting aneurysm from coronary thrombosis; evidence of poliomyelitis, however slight, may reveal the true nature of a myocarditis.

Pigmentation

Brownish pigmentation of the skin may be due to Addison's disease, hæmochromatosis, or scleroderma.

Loss of hair

Loss of axillary hair is characteristic of hæmochromatosis.

A host of other signs may be found in the extremities, but most of those which have a bearing on the cardiovascular system have been mentioned, and underline the importance of examining the hands and feet very closely.

THE BLOOD PRESSURE

The blood pressure was first measured directly in a live mare by Stephen Hales (1733): a brass pipe, 1/6th of an inch in diameter, was inserted into the left crural artery and connected to a vertical glass tube; blood rose in the tube to a height of 8 feet 3 inches above the level of the left ventricle.

An excellent detailed account of the subsequent history of sphygmomanometry may be found in a monograph by Master, Garfield and Walters (1952).

Technique of measurement

CLINICAL ESTIMATION. Approximate estimation of the blood pressure by clinical means is not only possible, but should be practised regularly; with experience it is easy to tell whether it is low, normal, or high, and the procedure takes but a moment. The physician should stand in front and to the right of the patient, and should compress the right brachial artery with his right thumb, while feeling the right radial pulse with the fingers of his left hand; the force required to obliterate the pulse represents the systolic blood pressure. The alternative method of placing three fingers on the radial artery, the first to compress the vessel above, the second to feel the pulse, and the third to obliterate the ulnar collateral below, is both difficult and cumbersome.

SPHYGMOMANOMETRY. In cardiovascular work, however, the blood pressure should always be measured with a mercurial manometer or reliable aneroid instrument. The patient must be comfortable, whether lying or sitting, and must have had time to recover from any recent excitement or exertion. The arm should be bared to the shoulder to avoid constriction from clothing and to facilitate proper application of the cuff. The latter should be fitted closely and evenly round the arm, so that its lower edge is one inch above the bend of the elbow, and the middle of the rubber bag lies over the brachial artery. Preliminary readings should be taken by palpation: the cuff is inflated rapidly until the brachial pulse is obliterated, and is then deflated slowly; the point at which the brachial pulse first reappears represents the systolic pressure; as the cuff is further deflated, brachial pulsation gradually assumes a water-hammer quality, and then abruptly resumes its normal character; the reading corresponding to this sudden change represents the diastolic blood pressure. When approaching an end-point the pressure must be altered slowly in the cuff. The palpatory method avoids the pitfall of the auscultatory gap, and is uninfluenced by subjective auditory defects; nevertheless, it should be checked by auscultation. The stethoscope should be applied lightly and accurately over the brachial artery, just below but not in contact with the cuff. The latter is then inflated to a pressure of some 30 mm. Hg above the systolic pressure as found by palpation, and slowly deflated. The accepted systolic blood pressure is the highest level at which successive sounds (phase I of Korotkow) are heard. As the pressure is further lowered in the cuff, the dull thud of the upper limits is replaced first by a murmur (phase II of Korotkow), and then by louder and sharper sounds (phase III); the point at which these slapping sounds suddenly become muffled (phase IV) is usually taken as the diastolic pressure. When there is vasodilatation, especially when associated with aortic incompetence, sounds may still be heard when the cuff pressure is reduced to zero, but normally they disappear a few mm. Hg below the change-over.

The above recommendations are freely borrowed from the joint report of the committees appointed by the British Cardiac Society and the American Heart Association for the standardisation of methods of measuring the arterial blood pressure (1939).

SIZE OF THE CUFF. The cuff method of measuring the blood pressure is not entirely accurate. Riva-Rocci's cuff (1899) was only 4.5 cm. wide and gave falsely high readings, as shown by von Recklinghausen (1901) who introduced the standard 5 inch cuff (12.7 cm.). During the last twenty years it has been pointed out repeatedly that this cuff was designed for an adult with an average-sized arm; when applied to a large arm or thigh the reading obtained is too high, and when applied to a small arm the reading is too low (Ragan and Bordley, 1941). For infants the cuff should not exceed 2.5 cm. (Woodbury, Robinow and Hamilton, 1938), for young children it should be about 3 inches wide, and for the outsized adult 7 or 8 inches wide. Even with these precautions cuff readings only approximate those recorded directly by means of arterial puncture, the systolic level averaging 8 mm. Hg too low and the diastolic (taken at the point of muffling) 8 mm. Hg too high (Bordley et al., 1951). The point at which sounds cease altogether is actually nearer the true diastolic pressure, and is gradually gaining favour on that account, but it is technically a less satisfactory end-point.

AUSCULTATORY SILENT GAP. When there is hypertension, sounds occasionally disappear as the cuff is inflated but reappear at higher levels. In standing patients the gap is encouraged by allowing the arm to hang down, and discouraged by elevating the arm (Berry, 1940). Similarly, the gap is favoured by inflating the cuff slowly and may be abolished by inflating it rapidly (Ragan and Bordley, 1941). The phenomenon may be related to the development of a very high venous pressure distal to the cuff which causes the diastolic arterial pressure to rise well above its proper level, thus diminishing the pulse pressure.

IRREGULARITIES. When there are ectopic beats, the higher pressure of the beat that follows the ectopic should be ignored. In auricular fibrillation only approximate readings can be obtained; the systolic pressure should be taken at the point where the majority of beats come through, the diastolic where the majority of beats become muffled. As the blood pressure normally varies by a few mm. Hg with respiration, it may be suitably recorded to the nearest multiple of five.

Normal range

THE NORMAL SYSTOLIC BLOOD PRESSURE lies between 95 and 150 mm. Hg. Whilst it is true that apparently normal subjects between the ages of 40 and 65 tend to have higher systolic pressures than those between 20 and 40, insurance companies well recognise the value of low figures, and it is probable that the higher average pressures of the middle-aged and elderly are due to atherosclerosis (Lewis, 1938).

THE NORMAL DIASTOLIC BLOOD PRESSURE lies between 60 and 90 mm. Hg. The mean pressure approximates to the diastolic plus one-third of the pulse pressure.

Although these figures have been standard for a long time, a determined attempt to raise the upper limits of normal has recently been made by Master, Garfield and Walters (1952). In their well-reasoned monograph these authors have made a strong plea for accepting a figure of 100 plus the age of the patient in years plus 5 to 10 mm. Hg as the upper limit of normal systolic pressure for middle-aged men (aged 40 to 65), and a figure 5 mm. Hg higher for women between the ages of 50 and 65. They also provided good evidence for raising the upper limit of the normal diastolic pressure from 95 to 100 mm. Hg in men and women over 50 years of age.

IN CHILDREN the blood pressure averages 90/60 between the ages of 3 and 9, 95–100/60–65 between the ages of 10 and 12, and 105/65 between the ages of 13 and 15 (Judson and Nicholson, 1914).

A COMMON SOURCE OF ERROR in blood pressure estimation results from failure to obtain a reasonably basal reading; this may be due to impatience, or to lack of recognition of emotional or other physiological factors. Whenever the pressure is found to be raised, the cuff should be left in position so that a second reading may be taken at the end of the examination. Casual measurements in healthy young adults who are a little anxious often register 160/90 mm. Hg, but if the patient is put at ease, and allowed to rest quietly on a couch, this figure may fall steadily to normal levels. It must be thoroughly understood that the maximum normal blood pressure of 150/90 mm. Hg is meant to be at ease. The question of pre-hypertensive levels will be discussed later.

Slight *disparity between readings taken from each arm* is common, especially in atherosclerotic and hypertensive subjects, but the difference rarely exceeds 5 mm. Hg (Amsterdam and Amsterdam, 1943). The blood pressure is sometimes taken in the legs with the cuff above the knee and the stethoscope in the popliteal fossa. In the average normal individual in the horizontal position, *the blood pressure in the legs* reads 20 to 40 mm. Hg above that in the arms. The discrepancy is due to using the standard cuff as previously described, and is not found when records are obtained by means of direct arterial puncture (Loman *et al*, 1936). *In the standing position* the systolic pressure in the arms, measured at heart level, usually shows no appreciable change, but in 33 per cent of normal subjects it drops about 10 to 15 mm. Hg; the diastolic pressure rises about 5 mm. Hg in 48 per cent of normal subjects, drops about 5 mm. Hg in 12 per cent, and remains unchanged in 40 per cent (Currens, 1948). *At death* all intra-vascular pressures level out at 14 to 22 mm. Hg. This is known as the static pressure and may be reached during periods of prolonged asystole (Dowling *et al.*, 1952; Anderson, 1954).

THE OCULAR FUNDI

Before leaving the peripheral vascular system, the ocular fundi should be examined. The ophthalmoscope should be used with both eyes open, and with either hand, so that one may hold the instrument with the right hand when examining the patient's right eye, and with the left hand when examining his left eye. There are four features of particular interest to the cardiologist: the appearances of the disc, the state of the arteries, the presence of hæmorrhages, and the presence of exudates.

PAPILLŒDEMA may occur in acute or chronic renal hypertension, and necessarily in malignant hypertension (by definition). In these cases the swelling of the disc is usually attributed to the high cerebro-spinal fluid pressure that is commonly found, but it is by no means clear just why the C.S.F. pressure should be raised. Papillœdema may also occur in anoxic cor pulmonale (see frontispiece), and here again the C.S.F. pressure is high, possibly because of increased filtration through the choroid plexus resulting from cerebral vasodilatation due to carbon dioxide retention. Papillœdema is seen occasionally in bacterial endocarditis when it is usually associated with acute nephritis; also in temporal arteritis and rarely in periarteritis nodosa. When found in association with other kinds of cardio-vascular disease, cerebral tumour is more likely to be responsible. It does not occur in congestive heart failure or in chronic constrictive pericarditis; nor even in the majority of cases of superior vena cava obstruction, despite jugular venous pressures up to 30 mm. Hg, and correspondingly high C.S.F. pressures.

THE CALIBRE OF THE RETINAL ARTERIES should be compared with that of the veins and expressed as an A/V ratio, the normal being 4/5 or 5/5. It should be understood that only the blood stream flowing through the artery or vein is seen, the wall of the vessel itself being normally invisible. The lighter longitudinal band in the centre represents reflection of light from that part of the vessel which lies in a plane more or less at right-angles to the beam from the ophthalmoscope. The state of the arteries in hypertension is described in Chapter XVI. Here it may be added that both arteries and veins become very small in cases of optic atrophy, that a thrombosed artery is represented by a white streak, that remarkably large veins may be physiological, and that vasodilatation causes venous rather than arterial pulsation (this is well seen in cases of aortic incompetence).

HÆMORRHAGES. Retinal hæmorrhages are discussed in relation to hypertension in Chapter XVI. They may also occur in bacterial endocarditis, diabetes mellitus, acute nephritis, periarteritis nodosa, disseminated lupus, temporal arteritis, and any condition which may give rise to petechiæ. Extensive hæmorrhage may follow venous thrombosis. Sometimes its cause is not apparent.

EXUDATES. Retinal exudates associated with hypertension are described in Chapter XVI. Exudate may also occur in any of the conditions specified in the preceding paragraph.

JUGULAR VENOUS PRESSURE

General considerations

The jugular venous pulse should be analysed clinically in terms of pressure and wave form; it is hard to conceive of any physical sign that is more informative.

It should first be understood that the mean intravascular pressure generated by left ventricular systole and maintained by aortic valve closure gradually falls as energy is expended overcoming the peripheral resistance, so that from a level of about 90 mm. Hg in the aorta and major arteries it falls to around 70 mm. Hg in the smallest arteries, 30 mm. Hg in the smallest arterioles, about 10 mm. Hg in the venules and around zero in the great veins. When there is arteriolar vasodilatation the venous pressure tends to rise a little, and when there is arteriolar vasoconstriction it tends to fall. If the venous return from any part is totally obstructed, the pressure in the veins distal to the obstruction rises rapidly to arterial level, provided the arteries are not also obstructed. The central venous pressure is also influenced by right atrial contraction and relaxation, closure of the tricuspid value, right ventricular diastolic tone, and the intrathoracic pressure (normally negative).

As seen at the bedside the jugular venous pulse is the oscillating top of the distended proximal portion of the internal jugular veins, and represents volumetric changes which faithfully reflect the right atrial pressure at all stages of the cardiac cycle. Thus if the mean pressure in the right atrium is 10 cm. of water the jugular veins will be distended to an average point in the neck exactly 10 cm. vertically above the centre of the right atrium (disregarding the specific gravity of blood, which is 1.056). The veins above this level are collapsed, for the actual pressure within them is less than atmospheric. This introduces another facet of the subject, which it may be as well to clarify at once. The pressure at any given point in the circulation is always expressed in relation to a fixed geographical reference point, usually the heart itself. In the simple illustration just mentioned, the actual pressure at the top of the jugular venous pulse is zero, but if the base-line of the manometric system is set at heart level, the reading becomes 10 cm. of water, which represents the 10 cm. height of water in the tube connecting the manometric base-line to the needle in the vein. Similarly, the actual pressure in the inferior vena cava at a point 15 cm. below heart level in the same illustration is 25 cm. of water; but the reading is still 10 in relation to heart level, because the 15 cm. column of water in the connecting tube exerts a negative pressure of 15 cm. of water on the manometric system. In this way the influence of gravity is removed from all pressure measurements, a highly desirable condition, because in a closed circuit such as the circulation the effects of gravity in the arterial and venous pressures are necessarily opposed and tend to cancel each other out; in so much as the blood vessels do not behave like rigid tubes, this annulment of the effects of gravity is far from perfect, but natural adjustments normally compensate for the disparity.

Recognition of venous pulsation

Venous pulsation in the neck can be recognised and distinguished from arterial pulsation in the following ways:

1. The movement is soft, diffuse and undulant.
2. The pulse that is seen cannot usually be felt.
3. With normal rate and rhythm there are two crests and two troughs per cardiac cycle.

Veins collapse in systole

4. When timed against the carotid pulse only the first trough appears to coincide with systole. This is the *x* descent which follows the presystolic *a* wave. The second crest *v* appears to be late systolic or early diastolic, and the second trough, *y*, is obviously diastolic (fig. 2.14).

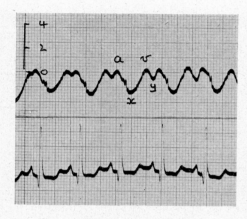

Fig. 2.14—Normal central venous pulse recorded simultaneously with the electro-cardiogram. The *x* descent is interrupted by a small *c* wave or by a first heart sound artefact. The rate of 116 beats per minute is too fast for the full development of *y*.

5. The top level of pulsation normally drops to a lower level on inspiration and rises to a higher level on expiration, passively following the changes in intrathoracic pressure.

6. The jugular venous pressure usually rises on abdominal compression. This may increase the intrathoracic pressure or raise the total intra-abdominal venous pressure, and it matters little to what part of the abdomen pressure is applied (fig. 2.15).

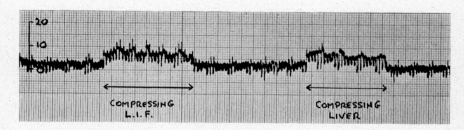

Fig. 2.15—Rise of venous pressure on abdominal compression: compressing the left iliac fossa is as effective as compressing the liver. (Time marking 1 mm. per sec.)

7. The jugular venous pressure varies with posture, being higher in the horizontal position and lower in the vertical, owing to the influence of gravity.

8. Cervical venous pulsation ceases if the jugular veins are compressed at the root of the neck.

9. Light pressure of the finger against the root of the external jugular vein distends the upper part of the vessel. On removing the finger the vein collapses to the level of the mean jugular venous pressure.

Clinical measurement of jugular venous pressure

The most satisfactory reference point from which to measure the jugular venous pressure is the sternal angle. Lewis chose this point because its relation to the right atrium is more or less stable, being about 5 cm. above the centre of the right atrium in both the horizontal and vertical positions. The patient should be propped up at 30, 60 or 90 degrees, whichever position reveals maximum venous pulsation. The vertical distance between the top of the oscillating venous column and the sternal angle represents the central venous pressure and is recorded in centimetres (of blood) above the sternal angle. The incline of the patient when the measurement was made should also be recorded, because the venous pressure varies with posture as previously stated (this has nothing to do with the relationship of the sternal angle to the right atrium).

The *normal jugular venous pressure* ranges between plus 3 cm. and about minus 7 cm. with reference to the sternal angle with the patient horizontal. The mean right atrial pressure averaged minus 1.5 mm. Hg with reference to the sternal angle in 50 normal controls studied by the author.

Causes of an elevated venous pressure

The venous pressure may rise under a variety of physiological and pathological conditions in addition to heart failure.

1. *Physical effort* raises the venous pressure owing partly to the squeezing action of skeletal muscular contraction on the veins, and partly to peripheral vasodilatation; the effect may be masked by reduction of the mean intrathoracic pressure resulting from hyperventilation. The venous pressure rises sharply during a rigor.

2. *Hyperkinetic circulatory states* due to heat, fever, pregnancy, anæmia, arterio-venous aneurysm, beri-beri, thyrotoxicosis, Paget's disease of bone, hypoxia, or advanced disease of the liver are all associated with a rise of venous pressure which may be partly attributed to vasodilatation. The cardiac output is raised and it may be difficult to be sure whether the heart is overloaded or not. Amyl nitrite, acetyl-beta-methylcholine, and other vasodilators in therapeutic doses may have a similar effect.

3. *An increased blood volume* is usually due to sodium retention and occurs physiologically in women during the pre-menstrual phase and in

pregnancy; it occurs pathologically in acute nephritis without denoting heart failure, and can be induced artificially by feeding with salt and desoxycorticosterone acetate, by pitressin, A.C.T.H. therapy, and of course by large intravenous infusions.

4. *A sufficiently slow heart rate*, whether due to heart block or not, is usually associated with a rise of venous pressure owing to right ventricular resistance to overfilling. To maintain an adequate cardiac output per minute the stroke output may have to be doubled. Thus a rise of venous pressure does not necessarily mean congestive failure in cases of complete heart block.

5. *An increased intrathoracic pressure* raises the jugular venous pressure but not the right ventricular filling pressure. The effect is produced momentarily during the act of coughing, and artificially by means of the Valsalva manœuvre. Pleural effusion may have a similar effect and may be wrongly attributed to heart failure in consequence.

6. *An increased intra-abdominal pressure* probably acts indirectly by raising the intrathoracic pressure. Tight corsets, abdominal binders, trousers too tight round the waist, obesity alone, ascites, pregnancy, or even gross flatulence may each have this effect. To witness alleged "heart failure" immediately relieved by undoing the top trouser buttons can be both embarrassing and instructive.

7. *A raised intrapericardial pressure* from effusion increases the filling resistance of the right ventricle and so raises the jugular venous pressure. Chronic constrictive pericarditis has the same effect.

8. *Partial obstruction of the superior vena cava* raises the jugular venous pressure without abolishing pulsation; only when the block is complete or very nearly so does venous pulsation cease. *Obstruction of the inferior vena cava* may raise the jugular venous pressure indirectly by interfering with renal function and sodium excretion.

9. *In tricuspid stenosis* the raised venous pressure is associated with a normal right ventricular diastolic pressure.

10. *Space-filling lesions affecting the right side of the heart* prevent proper filling of the right ventricle and include massive thrombosis of the right atrium, tumour, constrictive endocarditis, aneurysm of the interventricular septum, and Bernheim's syndrome.

11. *Giant* a *waves, cannon waves,* and *tricuspid incompetence* raise the jugular venous pressure during a particular phase of the cardiac cycle, and will be considered in relation to the venous pulse (*vide infra*).

12. *Congestive heart failure* itself, of course, is the most important cause of an elevated venous pressure and is discussed in detail in Chapter VII; hydræmia from sodium retention, resistance to right ventricular over-

filling, and sometimes functional tricuspid incompetence are all implicated.

In all the pathological conditions mentioned above (apart from coughing and the Valsalva manœuvre) venous pulsation is preserved, and with the exception of partial S.V.C. obstruction the jugular venous pressure represents the right atrial pressure. When the cervical veins are distended but do not pulsate, they are either obstructed at the root of the neck or there is total obstruction of the superior vena cava. Obstruction of one or more cervical veins at the root of the neck may be due to kinking or local compression from neighbouring structures and may disappear at once if the relationship between the head and neck and the shoulder girdle is altered.

Therapeutic methods of raising the central venous pressure include the horizontal posture (more effective if the legs are raised), leg binders exerting a subarterial pressure on as large a surface as possible from the toes to the hips, overalls that can be inflated to any desired pressure, intravenous infusions and salt with desoxycorticosterone. Selective chemical venoconstrictors have not yet been discovered. Arteriolar vasodilators are usually contra-indicated because the blood pressure is too low in these cases and there is already too much blood laked in the periphery; moreover, many such substances are also venodilators.

Venous pressure lowering agents include the erect or semi-erect posture (sitting or propped up with the legs hanging down), venous tourniquets applied to the thighs, venesection, dehydration by means of sodium depletion (low sodium diet, kation exchange resins, carbonic anhydrase inhibitors, and mercurial diuretics), and chemical venodilators such as theophylline, tetraethylammonium and hexamethonium.

THE JUGULAR VENOUS PULSE

Precise analysis of the cervical venous pulse and measurement of the height of each individual wave with reference to the sternal angle is not only possible at the bedside but highly desirable. In the previous section on the jugular venous pressure there was a noticeable lack of precision concerning the wave responsible for the pressure actually measured; this defect will now be remedied.

Definition of waves

The jugular venous pulse consists essentially of four waves, *a*, *x*, *v* and *y* (fig. 2.16). The first and third waves (*a* and *v*) are crests, the second and fourth (*x* and *y*) troughs. A fifth wave, known as *c*, another crest, may interrupt the *x* descent, and a final upward movement, often quite sharp, follows *y*. There is some advantage in allotting the letter *z* to the point reached by this last movement before the inscription of the *a* wave of the next cardiac cycle.

The a wave is due to right atrial systole and disappears in auricular fibrillation.

The x descent is due chiefly to atrial relaxation and also disappears in auricular fibrillation (fig. 2.17); for this reason it is difficult to believe that withdrawal of the atrioventricular septum towards the cavity of the right ventricle, a movement known as descent of the base, is mainly responsible for x.

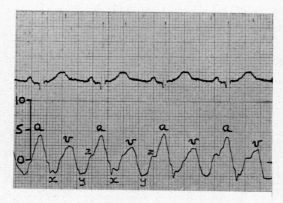

Fig. 2.16—Normal right atrial pressure tracing: c is represented by a small notch towards the end of the x descent; the rise of pressure from the trough y to the zero point z before atrial contraction is well shown.

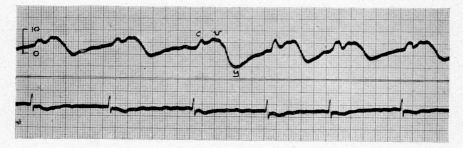

Fig. 2.17—Pressure pulse from the right atrium in a case of mitral stenosis with auricular fibrillation showing absence of the x descent.

The c *wave*, which may interrupt the x descent, was first attributed to tricuspid valve close (Potain, 1867), and later to a carotid artefact (Mac-kenzie, 1902). While admitting that a c wave due to mitral valve closure is usually prominent in direct left atrial pressure tracings in cases of mitral stenosis (fig. 2.18), the writer has found relatively few conspicuous c waves due to tricuspid valve closure in well over a thousand right atrial pressure tracings obtained from a wide variety of cases including 50 normal subjects. There is a great deal of difference between the forceful closure of the mitral valve in mitral stenosis and the gentle apposition of the tricuspid leaflets in normal hearts. Clinically c is unobstrusive in the majority of jugular venous pulses, the trough *x* usually accompanying the early part of systole in cases with normal rhythm (figs. 2.14 and 2.16). The *c* wave of external jugular phlebograms is always far more prominent (fig. 2.19), and as shown by Mackenzie represents the carotid pulse itself.

There is some evidence that well-defined "*c*" waves due to tricuspid valve closure may occur in atrial septal defect, and they might be expected in any condition in which the tricuspid valve is wide open at the moment the ventricle contracts.

The v *wave* represents a rising right atrial pressure due to temporary obstruction of the blood flow during ventricular systole. When there is

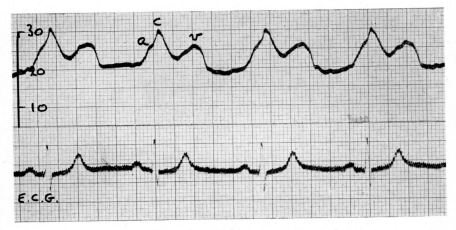

Fig. 2.18—Left atrial pressure tracing showing a powerful *c* wave closely following *a* in a case of mitral stenosis.

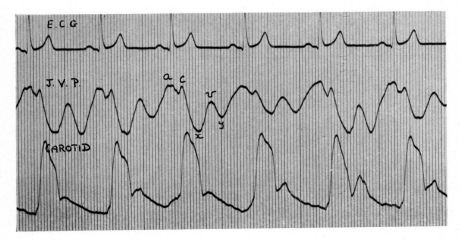

Fig. 2.19—Conspicuous *c* wave in an external jugular phlebogram recorded simultaneously with the carotid pulse (see text).

normal rhythm it appears in late systole, for it is at first overpowered by the *x* descent of atrial relaxation; when there is auricular fibrillation, however, it starts with the first heart sound and occupies the whole of systole (fig. 2.17).

The y *descent* begins as soon as the tricuspid valve opens, i.e. at the end of the period of isometric ventricular relaxation. This, of course, is the down-slope of *v*, just as the *x* descent is the down-slope of *a*. As the tricuspid valve opens there is a potential pressure gradient between the slightly raised right atrial pressure and the rapidly falling right ventricular pressure, but they equalise rapidly and appear to fall together to the trough *y*.

Return of pressure to the point z is gradual or rapid according to the ease with which the right ventricle dilates. In normal hearts the ascent is gradual for there is little resistance to right ventricular filling.

Normal venous pulse

The normal jugular venous pulse oscillates gently around a mean level a little below zero with reference to the sternal angle. Typical figures for *a*, *x*, *v*, *y* and *z* are 0, −4, 0, −3, −1 mm. Hg respectively, *a* and *v* being about equal in amplitude, and the greatest excursion being the *x* descent. Only with heart rates below 90 beats per minute is there time for full inscription of all five waves. With heart rates between 90 and 110 the zero point is not defined, *a* succeeding *y* immediately. With rates higher than 110 there is no time for the proper development of *y*, *a* succeeding *v* just as the *y* descent starts; and at a rate of around 150 *v* and *a* are wholly superimposed. These figures are only approximate for they vary considerably according to the length of the P-R interval and the duration of ventricular systole.

Clinically it is usually easy to measure the height of *a* and *v* in centimetres above the sternal angle, and *z* is not difficult with slow rates; but the troughs *x* and *y* may have to be estimated only approximately. In clinical notes the form of the venous pulse should be drawn and a figure representing the approximate pressure of each wave should be inscribed in the appropriate place.

Abnormalities of the jugular venous pulse

A giant *a* wave (fig. 2.20), measuring between 6 and 15 mm. Hg above *v*, is characteristic of severe pulmonary hypertension, severe pulmonary stenosis, tricuspid stenosis or tricuspid atresia (provided there is no free right to left shunt in any of them). It is presystolic, abrupt and collapsing in quality (venous Corrigan), palpable, transmitted to the liver, and usually associated with right atrial gallop and a conspicuous P pulmonale. It alters little, if at all, with change of posture, and increases in amplitude both with inspiration (fig. 2.21) and abdominal compression. The powerful right atrial contraction responsible for the giant *a* wave seems to be due to increased resistance to right ventricular filling over a long period of time.

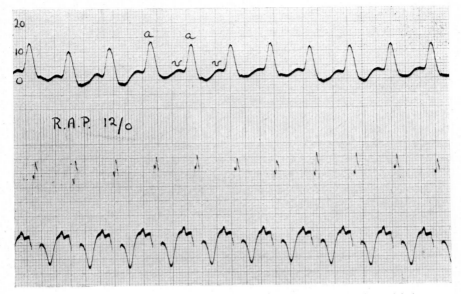

Fig. 2.20—Giant *a* wave in pulmonary valve stenosis with reversed interatrial shunt.

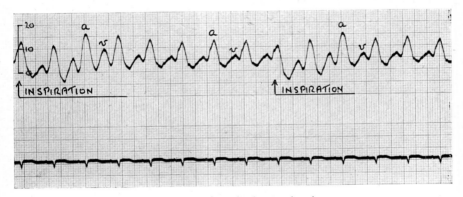

Fig. 2.21—The effect of respiration on the giant *a* wave.

It does not occur in ordinary cases of heart failure in which the right ventricular diastolic pressure is raised; and it is usually absent in both Eisenmenger's complex and Fallot's tetralogy. Teleologically in pulmonary hypertension and pulmonary stenosis it serves to increase the contractile force of the right ventricle in accordance with Starling's law, which states that within certain limits the force of cardiac contraction is a function of fibre length. When nodal rhythm has occurred fortuitously during cardiac catheterisation in several of these cases, the right ventricular systolic pressure has fallen abruptly by 20 to 30 mm. Hg (fig. 2.22).

A prolonged a-c *interval* occurs in partial heart block. Clinically the interval between *a* and the carotid pulse can be graded easily enough into

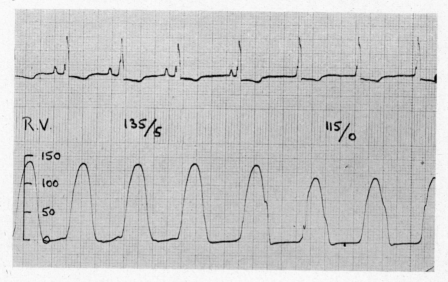

Fig. 2.22—Right ventricular pressure tracing from a case of severe pulmonary valve stenosis showing a sudden fall in pressure of at least 20 mm. Hg with the onset of nodal rhythm (see text).

short (P-R interval around 0.12 sec.), average (P-R 0.16 sec.), rather long (P-R 0.20 sec.) and obviously prolonged (P-R 0.24 sec.). When P-R is longer than 0.24 second *a* tends to fuse with *v*, as it does with sinus tachycardia and normal conduction.

Independent a *waves* occur in complete heart block. They are usually of small amplitude and likely to be overlooked unless the venous pulse is studied very carefully.

Cannon waves are more obvious and occur whenever the right atrium contracts against a closed tricuspid valve, i.e. when the P wave of the electrocardiogram falls between the end of QRS and the end of T. This occurs irregularly in complete heart block (fig. 2.23) and with multiple ectopic beats, and regularly with nodal rhythm, paroxysmal nodal tachycardia, and partial heart block with an extremely long P-R interval.

A cannon wave is *not* a summation effect, but a particular form of giant *a*. The whole of the energy released by right atrial contraction is translated into pressure because forward flow is impossible The word is used in the sense of rebound, apt enough since the tricuspid valve is shut in the face of the oncoming wave from the atrium.

In complete heart block cannon waves are *not* synchronous with "cannon sounds"; on the contrary, the first heart sound associated with a cannon wave is relatively quiet. The cannon sound in heart block refers to the explosive first sound that is heard when the atria contract about 0.10 second before the ventricles, so that the mitral cusps, flung wide open by atrial contraction, are slammed shut by the quickly succeeding ventricular systole —another kind of rebound altogether, if the word is still used in that sense.

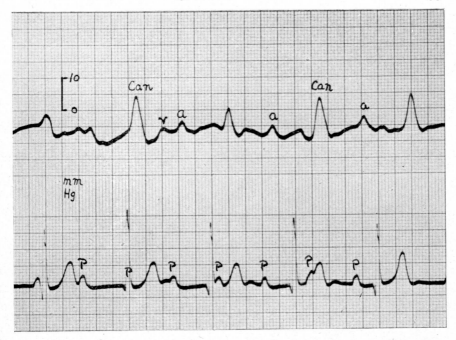

Fig. 2.23—Irregular cannon waves in the central venous pulse in a case of complete heart block: cannons are seen whenever P falls between Q and the peak of T in the electro-cardiogram.

In 2-1 heart block alternate *a* waves usually broaden *v*, and are inconspicuous, but if they fall a little earlier regular cannon waves may be observed.

Ectopic beats may cause cannon waves in several different ways. An atrial ectopic may coincide with the previous ventricular systole. Nodal ectopics usually cause the atria and ventricles to beat together as in nodal rhythm. Ventricular ectopics cause cannon waves when they are only slightly premature, so that they coincide with normal atrial contraction excited by discharge of the sinus node.

Paroxysmal tachycardia need not necessarily be nodal to cause cannon waves. Atrial tachycardia may do so when there is 2-1 fatigue block (if atrial contraction is forceful enough) or when P-R is prolonged so that P falls before the end of the preceding T wave; and ventricular tachycardia may cause irregular cannon waves when atrial contraction is independent.

Absence of a conspicuous x *descent* is invariable in auricular fibrillation; instead there is a broad positive systolic wave *v*, sometimes initiated by a small *c* wave (fig. 2.17). If the *x* descent were due chiefly to downward movement of the atrial floor during ventricular systole, it should be influenced but little by auricular fibrillation.

The *x* descent is diminished in tricuspid incompetence, but may still be recognised when the rhythm is normal (fig. 2.24). The *x* descent is similarly absent from direct and indirect left atrial pressure pulses in cases of auricular fibrillation, but may be present in mitral incompetence when the rhythm is normal.

Large v *waves* are especially characteristic of tricuspid incompetence with auricular fibrillation (fig. 2.25), and are transmitted to the liver. The

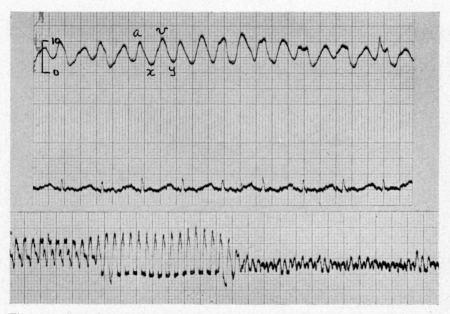

Fig. 2.24—Case of tricuspid valve disease (due to lupus) with stenosis and incompetence and with normal rhythm showing an *x* descent before the *v* wave. The bottom tracing is a continuous record of the pressures obtained as the catheter was withdrawn from the pulmonary artery (left) to the right atrium (right): note the pressure gradient across the tricuspid valve.

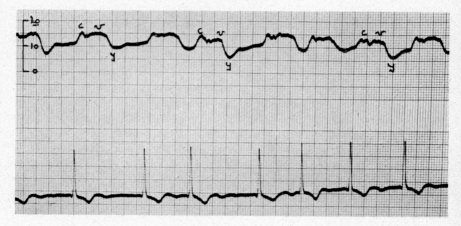

Fig. 2.25—Case of tricuspid incompetence with auricular fibrillation showing a large *v* wave.

high amplitude of the systolic wave is augmented by the deep *y* trough which follows.

A deep y *descent*, or diastolic collapse of the venous pulse, was first described in relation to chronic constrictive pericarditis (Friedreich, 1864). In these cases the venous pressure is high throughout the cardiac cycle except for a short period immediately following the opening of the tricuspid valve, when blood from the right atrium pours into the relaxing right ventricle. Right atrial and ventricular pressures equalise rapidly and the small cavity of the right ventricle is quickly filled; further filling is resisted by the rigid pericardium, so the pressure rises again sharply during the rest of diastole (fig. 2.26).

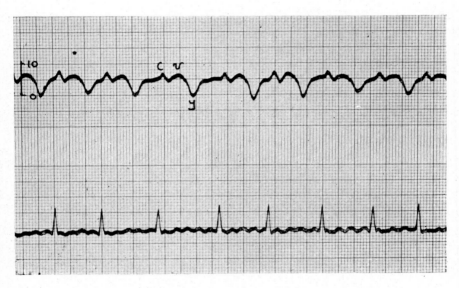

Fig. 2.26—The steep *y* descent in a case of Pick's disease.

It was at first thought that the rigid pericardium, tensed inwards during systole (either alone or in conjunction with the chest wall), recoiled like a spring in early diastole, and so created a powerful negative pressure which explained the diastolic venous collapse; but although such a mechanism may exist, it is superfluous to the thesis, for the same phenomenon occurs in any condition in which the venous pressure is very high, provided there is no obstruction at the tricuspid valve (fig. 2.27). In severe right ventricular failure, for example, the same high potential pressure gradient between atrium and ventricle must exist immediately the tricuspid valve opens, ventricular filling and equalisation of pressures are just as rapid, and further filling is resisted by the already overstretched fibres of the failing myocardium: the stroke output in these cases is just as small as in Pick's disease.

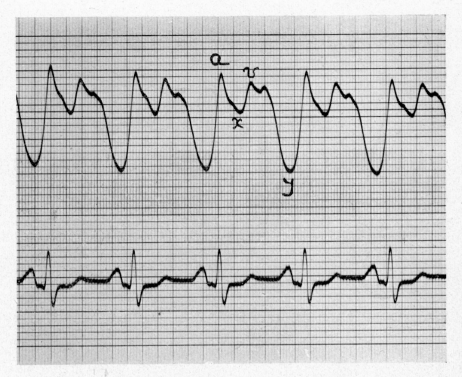

Fig. 2.27—Jugular phlebogram showing a steep *y* descent and deep *y* trough in a case of mitral stenosis with extreme pulmonary hypertension.

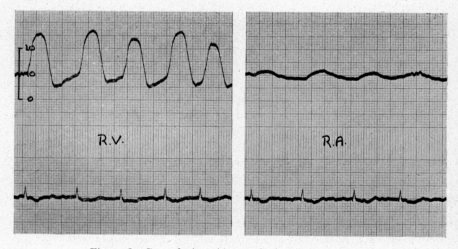

Fig. 2.28—Case of tricuspid stenosis showing a slow *y* descent.

A slow y *descent* following *v*, despite a high venous pressure, is characteristic of tricuspid stenosis (fig. 2.28), for rapid equalisation of jugular and right ventricular pressures is then impossible. The same sluggish *y* descent is seen in left atrial pressure tracings in cases of mitral stenosis (Owen and Wood, 1955). Again, in tricuspid stenosis there is no rapid rise of pressure following the *y* trough as there is in heart failure and Pick's disease, so that *z* is little if at all higher than *y*.

OTHER CLASSICAL SIGNS OF HEART FAILURE

If the jugular venous pressure is raised in a manner suggesting heart failure, a *distended and often tender liver* can usually be palpated. If the liver edge cannot be felt the epigastrium and right hypochondrium should be percussed; a good resonant note up to the right costal margin anteriorly excludes significant enlargement. A high venous pressure without hepatic enlargement suggests obstruction of the superior vena cava; enlargement of the liver without a rise of venous pressure should never be attributed to heart failure.

Œdema does not necessarily accompany a raised venous pressure due to heart failure, as explained in Chapter I; on the other hand, cardiac œdema does not occur without a raised venous pressure. The swelling is maximal round the ankles in ambulant patients, but may be chiefly sacral in those confined to bed. Its mechanism is discussed in Chapters I and VII.

Physical signs of "pulmonary venous congestion" due to left ventricular failure are usually wanting. Basal rales are notoriously unreliable, being absent in the majority of cases and often having another interpretation when present. In acute pulmonary œdema, however, fine crepitations can be heard over a wide area of both lungs. The explanation for these two statements is simple enough: a rise of pulmonary venous pressure up to 30 mg. Hg causes no exudation of serum into the alveoli, and therefore does not give rise to crepitations; only when the pulmonary venous pressure exceeds the osmotic pressure of the plasma does such exudation occur, i.e. in acute pulmonary œdema. When basal rales are heard in either left ventricular failure or mitral stenosis in the absence of pulmonary œdema, increased bronchial secretions are culpable; but although "pulmonary venous congestion" may be responsible for the increased bronchial activity, the sign is so common in simple bronchitis or bronchiolitis that it cannot be accepted as reliable evidence of heart failure.

EXAMINATION OF THE HEART

Having gleaned as much information as possible from general inspection, from examining the peripheral vascular system and the extremities, and from searching for signs of failure, one may turn with advantage to the heart itself, and duly inspect, palpate, percuss and auscultate.

Inspection

The position and character of the cardiac impulse, if visible, and of any other thoracic pulsation, should be noted. In this way, left or right ventricular hypertrophy, gallop rhythm, dilatation of the pulmonary artery, and aortic aneurysm may be detected. Præcordial deformity may be observed, and if due to the heart indicates its enlargement during the period of thoracic growth. Depression of the sternum, or other thoracic deformity, should be noted, for it may alter the shape or position of the heart. Systolic indrawing of the thoracic wall is not abnormal if it occurs over the right ventricle, and is exaggerated in this situation when the left ventricle is alone enlarged: and it may be seen in the anterior axillary line or beyond when there is gross enlargement of the right ventricle. As a sign of adherent pericardium it should be looked for posteriorly over the last two ribs, as described by Broadbent (1895).

Palpation

The apex beat, which is a geographical point, should be determined by locating the exact site of the left ventricular impulse. The physician's hand should be placed over the region of the fifth left intercostal space in the nipple line in order to ascertain its approximate position: the middle finger should then be directed vertically over it, and shifted about until the maximum thrust is located. This, rather than the lowest left point of such pulsation, is the apex beat. Its position should be recorded with reference to the intercostal spaces, to the mid-line, and to the mid-clavicular line. If it is located beyond these confines, the possibility of displacement from scoliosis, elevation of the diaphragm, or from pulmonary or pleural lesions should be considered before concluding that the heart is enlarged.

The character of the cardiac impulse is as important, if not more important, than its position (the apex beat); it should be sensed both with the palm of the hand and with the finger-tip. A steady heaving impulse means left ventricular hypertrophy, and is felt in aortic stenosis and systemic hypertension. A hyperdynamic impulse is also forceful, but has greater amplitude and is more abrupt and lively; it signifies an overfilled ventricle usually working against a low resistance, as in aortic incompetence, mitral incompetence, patent ductus, ventricular septal defect, and the hyperkinetic circulatory states. Both heaving and hyperdynamic left ventricular impulses are usually associated with increased retraction of the chest wall overlying the right ventricle, slight retraction in this region being normal. A steady heave over the right ventricle about the left parasternal line is felt in pulmonary hypertension and pulmonary stenosis. A hyperdynamic right ventricular lift is more tumultuous and is characteristic of the overfilled right ventricle of atrial septal defect. A strong impulse over the right ventricle is usually associated with conspicuous retraction further to the left where the apex beat (left ventricular impulse) might have been expected. This rocking movement is very easily seen, and is the reverse of the left ventricular rock described above. When the left ventricle is small or rotated posteriorly, and the right ventricle unimpressive, no cardiac impulse may be felt at all, only the tap of the first heart sound being appreciated; this is typical of uncomplicated mitral stenosis when the first heart sound is accentuated.

Palpation of the heart sounds in general can hardly be avoided: not only the first, but also systolic ejection clicks, both elements of the second sound, the opening snap of mitral stenosis, the third sound, and any kind of gallop are all frequently palpable when present.

Palpation may next be used to detect the presence of thrills, preferably in forced expiratory apnoea. This manoeuvre brings the heart and great vessels closer to the chest wall, encourages the lung to retract from its buffering position, and lessens the chance of confusing cardiac with respiratory phenomena. Tricuspid thrills alone are better appreciated during inspiration. The vibration sense of normal individuals varies considerably, but increased perception comes with experience and good technique.

Practically all important murmurs, including certain functional murmurs, may be accompanied by a thrill. Indeed, of the twenty-one different types of murmur described later in this chapter, only the Carey Coombs murmur of active rheumatic carditis and the cardio-respiratory murmur are never so accompanied.

Percussion

The value of percussing the heart has given rise to much dispute, many modern cardiologists maintaining that its place has been taken by the far more accurate and fertile method of radiography. The older school, however, modestly suggest that it is a useful bedside method, which gives reliable and helpful information if practised diligently, and if its limitations are appreciated. Certainly, if a fluoroscope is available, percussion is pointless; but a fluoroscope may not be available, or the patient may be so ill that only a portable X-ray machine can be used, and the distorted skiagram so obtained is liable to gross misinterpretation. In such cases percussion may be of value, and by constant practice the physician should learn what can, and what cannot, be expected from it.

The approximate position of the left border of the heart may be checked when the apex beat is difficult to locate, and dullness beyond the known or probable confines of the apex beat may sometimes be detected in cases of pericardial effusion.

It is impossible to determine the right border of the heart by percussion, unless there is aneurysmal dilatation of the right atrium. On the other hand, pericardial effusion, even of moderate degree, can often be demonstrated.

It was once customary to speak of relative and absolute cardiac dullness, the latter being the note heard over the area of heart not covered by lung, but it is doubtful whether this distinction can be maintained. Diminution or absence of cardiac dullness, however, is a useful sign of emphysema.

Percussion at the base may be rewarded in pericardial effusion, there being characteristic dullness in the second left interchondral space when the patient lies flat; also in substernal goitre, and in anterior aneurysm of the aorta, when a band of dullness extends laterally from the manubrium sterni.

AUSCULTATION

When a man buys a tool for some specific purpose, he usually takes care that it is the best available for the particular job in hand. It is therefore strange that a superstition has grown up within the medical world that the older and more disreputable a stethoscope, the better; that it is not the stethoscope which matters, but the man behind it. This, of course, is nonsense. When a student fails to hear a murmur which is heard easily by another, exchange of stethoscopes quickly leads to mutual understanding. There is another curious tradition, fostered by many who appreciate the value of a good stethoscope, that the chest-piece must be bell-shaped, and that any other type, especially the flat diaphragm (Bowles), is pernicious. This doctrine is as unreasonable as the first; for there is no doubt that certain high-pitched sounds, especially aortic diastolic murmurs and faint tubular breathing, which can be heard with ease through a Bowles, may be inaudible through a bell. The physical laws which govern auscultation have been studied by Rappaport and Sprague (1941 and 1951). The diameter of the Bowles chest-piece should be about $1\frac{1}{2}$ inches; the cup should be shallow and its edge sharp (fig. 2.29a). Good material for the diaphragm is photographic or X-ray film, washed clean in hot water, and cut to shape. The rubber tubing should be thick, about 10 inches long, and should fit snugly to the connections. The internal calibre of the whole system, including the metal binaurals and the hole in the centre of the chest-piece, should be one-eighth of an inch. A good bell stethoscope (fig. 2.29 b) is better for detecting low-pitched sounds, such as soft mitral diastolic murmurs; moreover, its range of sensitivity may be increased by varying the force with which it is applied to the chest wall. Light contact accentuates low-pitched sounds, firm pressure high-pitched sounds. The cup should not be too deep, and its diameter not less than one inch.

There are two other types of stethoscope which deserve comment: the monaural wooden instrument of by-gone days, and

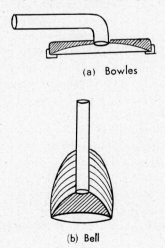

(a) Bowles

(b) Bell

Fig. 2.29—Binaural stethoscopes.

the differential stethoscope (symballophone). The rigid wooden stethoscope is rarely used nowadays, but by combining aural and tactile senses it facilitates the recognition of gallop rhythm. The differential stethoscope is constructed as shown in figure 2.30, and may be used to compare the timing of sounds originating at different sites, and to determine the direction in which a murmur is propagated (Kerr *et al.*, 1937).

Auscultation of the heart can only be learned at the bedside, but the following advice may be helpful to students. The præcordium should be examined all over, not just at areas where individual valve sounds are expected; gallop rhythm, pericardial friction, and certain important murmurs will not then escape notice. It is enough to listen to one thing at a time: thus, when an expert hears a soft elusive mitral diastolic murmur, hitherto overlooked, it is not necessarily because he has better ears or a better stethoscope, but because he has acquired a more selective power of concentration. Basal murmurs and pericardial friction are heard most easily in expiratory apnœa; tricuspid murmurs during inspiration; mitral murmurs in the left lateral position, especially when the heart slows down after exercise. Heart sounds should be timed against carotid pulsation; if difficulty is experienced due to tachycardia, the heart may be slowed by carotid sinus compression.

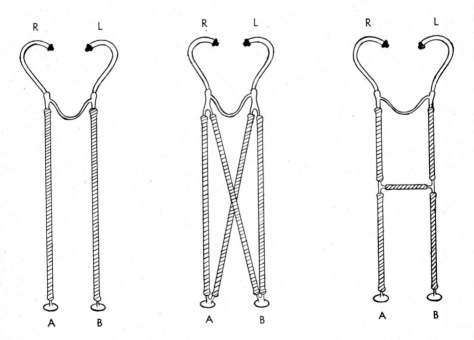

Fig. 2.30—The differential stethoscope (3 varieties). Sounds travelling from A to B reach the right ear before the left, giving the impression of movement in that direction.

Valve areas

Certain favourable areas have come to be recognised at which each valve may be auscultated selectively. Traditionally, these areas are the second right costal cartilage (aortic area), second left intercostal space (pulmonary area), apex beat or fifth left intercostal space in the mid-clavicular line (mitral area), and fourth left intercostal space near the sternal edge (tri-cuspid area). Blind faith in the integrity of these sites has led to much misunderstanding: for example, the pulmonary second sound should not mean the second heart sound in the pulmonary area, but the pulmonary element of the second heart sound, for aortic valve closure is also well heard in the second left space and normally just precedes pulmonary valve closure; again, aortic valve sounds and murmurs are well heard over the right carotid artery in the neck, in the third left space at the sternal edge, and over the left ventricle at the apex beat, as well as at the aortic area. Thus the aortic second sound should mean the sound made by aortic valve closure, wherever it is heard. Similarly, a mitral systolic murmur should mean a murmur created by turbulence at the mitral orifice during ventricular systole, not any systolic murmur (aortic, for example) which happens to be heard at the mitral area (apex beat). It follows that analysis of heart sounds and murmurs requires more than geographical data; their quality and timing are very important and will be discussed in some detail.

THE HEART SOUNDS

Atrial gallop. The first mechanical event in the cardiac cycle is atrial contraction, which may give rise to an audible *presystolic sound* (fig. 2.31a). Vibrations associated with atrial systole were recorded in 68 per cent of

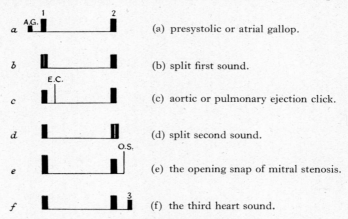

(a) presystolic or atrial gallop.

(b) split first sound.

(c) aortic or pulmonary ejection click.

(d) split second sound.

(e) the opening snap of mitral stenosis.

(f) the third heart sound.

Fig. 2.31—The heart sounds.

normal schoolboys by Bridgman (1914), and were found to be invariable in normal subjects when records were obtained from the surface of the left atrium by means of œsophageal phonocardiography (Taquini, 1936).

These low-frequency presystolic vibrations cannot be heard clinically in normal people, but may become audible when the atria contract more forcibly as a result of increased ventricular resistance to late diastolic filling, e.g. over the left ventricle in severe hypertension and over the right ventricle in severe pulmonary hypertension. The presystolic sound is sufficiently separated from the first heart sound to give rise to what is known as triple rhythm, or to be more precise to presystolic or atrial gallop. The extra sound is probably caused by sudden distension of the ventricle concerned, for it is not heard over the left ventricle in mitral stenosis, nor over the right ventricle in tricuspid stenosis, despite very forcible atrial contraction; moreover, low-frequency phonocardiographic vibrations accompanying atrial contraction itself just precede the sound in question, there being really two sets of vibrations connected with atrial systole, the first inaudible and normal, the second being responsible for presystolic gallop (Orías and Braun-Menendez, 1939).

The first heart sound proper is due almost entirely to mitral and tricuspid valve closure. Its intensity depends chiefly upon the position of the cusps at the beginning of ventricular systole, partly upon the volume of lung covering the heart or upon the thickness of the chest wall, and least, if at all, upon the strength of ventricular contraction.

The position of the valve leaflets at the beginning of ventricular systole depends partly upon the P-R interval: the loudest first sound is produced when atrial contraction forces the leaflets wide open immediately before the ventricles contract (P-R around 0.10 sec.); but when there is a relatively long delay between atrial and ventricular excitations (P-R=0.2 sec.), the cusps may float into apposition before the ventricles contract and hence shut quietly (Dock, 1933). The loud first sound of mitral stenosis and of the hyperkinetic circulatory states is similarly produced in that a high filling pressure keeps the cusps fully open until the last possible moment. Conversely, the soft first sound of shock is probably due to a low filling pressure.

Splitting of the first heart sound (fig. 2.31b) is common in health and is due to separation of mitral and tricuspid components, the mitral valve tending to close about 0.02–0.03 second before the tricuspid (Leatham, 1954); it is best heart in the tricuspid area, the mitral sound being louder and therefore more easily heard at a distance from its source.

Systolic ejection clicks (fig. 2.31c), loudest in expiration, may be aortic or pulmonary, occurring just after the opening of the aortic or pulmonary valve respectively (Lian *et al.*, 1941 and 1951). The first heart sound proper occurs at the beginning of the period of isometric contraction, an ejection click at the end of that period. Aortic ejection clicks are usually associated with dilatation of the ascending aorta from any cause; they are best heard in the third left space at the sternal edge or at the apex beat. Pulmonary ejection clicks are common in pulmonary hypertension, mild pulmonary stenosis, and idiopathic dilatation of the pulmonary artery

(Leatham and Vogelpoel, 1954); they are also best heard in the third left space at the sternal edge, but are not transmitted to the apex beat.

If the definition of the first heart sound is extended to include vascular vibrations occurring at the end of the isometric contraction phase (Braun-Menendez, 1938), then an ejection click may be regarded as the second component of a widely split first sound. There is an obvious advantage, however, in using the term aortic or pulmonary ejection click to describe this vascular sound, and restricting the term split first sound to mean separation of mitral and tricuspid components only.

The second heart sound is due to aortic and pulmonary valve closure. The aortic element is heard best in the aortic area, in the neck, and at the apex beat, and the pulmonary element in the pulmonary area. In normal individuals both elements can usually be heard in the second and third left interchondral spaces close to the sternal border. In children and adolescents the split is often obvious (grade II), particularly towards the end of inspiration. The first element is aortic, the second pulmonary. The lag of P2 during inspiration has been attributed to prolongation of right ventricular systole from increased filling (Leatham, 1954). In atrial septal defect the split fails to widen on inspiration.

Pathological splitting (grade III) is due to delay in pulmonary valve closure, and is usually due to right bundle branch block, delay in the emptying time of an overfilled right ventricle, or pulmonary stenosis. In these cases the split may approach 0.1 second in width (grade I=0.02–0.03 sec.; grade II=0.04–0.05 sec.). Slight delay in aortic valve closure may bring the two elements together and so cause a single second heart sound. In aortic stenosis and left bundle branch block the aortic element may lag behind the pulmonary element; a reversed split so caused tends to close on inspiration and widen on expiration, and can thus be recognised by its paradoxical behaviour (Leatham, 1954).

Recognition of a split second heart sound at once proves that both semilunar valves are functioning and thus excludes persistent truncus arteriosus, pulmonary atresia and severe pulmonary stenosis, although a very faint and delayed P2 can sometimes be heard in the last. When the split is wide the intensity of the pulmonary element helps to distinguish pulmonary stenosis (P_2 quiet) from right bundle branch block or atrial septal defect (P_2 normal or rather loud).

Accentuation of the second heart sound may result from systemic or pulmonary hypertension: the clinical circumstances and the site of maximal intensity may decide which, but sometimes it is only possible to be sure if there is sufficient splitting. If the ascending aorta or pulmonary artery is unusually close to the anterior surface of the chest, either because it is abnormal or because it is scantily covered by lung and chest wall, the second heart sound is also loud. Conversely, *a soft or absent second heart sound* is usual in emphysema.

About midway between the second and third heart sounds, or about

0.08–0.1 second after A_2, may be heard the *opening snap of mitral stenosis* (fig. 2.31e); the sharp extra sound is due to the abrupt flapping back of the mitral cusps at the end of the period of isometric relaxation, i.e. when the rapidly falling left ventricular pressure drops below the raised left atrial pressure. The opening snap is best heard in expiration at the lower left sternal edge over the root of the aorta, and over the left ventricle at the apex beat. It is discussed more fully in relation to mitral valve disease in Chapter X.

The physiological third heart sound (fig. 2.31f) was well described by Gibson (1907). It is soft, low pitched, and often accompanied by a palpable shock; it is more or less localised to the apex beat, varies in intensity with respiration, and is accentuated when the subject lies on the left side. It may be heard in the great majority of children, in about 50 per cent of young adults, occasionally in the middle-aged, and rarely in the elderly. Phonocardiography shows that the third sound coincides with the latter half of the descending limb of the v wave of the jugular phlebogram, i.e. with the end of the period of rapid ventricular filling (Ohm, 1913); it is attributed to sudden distension of the left ventricle at this time (about 0.15 sec. after the onset of A_2).

The third heart sound is accentuated by any condition which encourages rapid left ventricular filling, e.g. mitral incompetence, ventricular septal defect, patent ductus, Pick's disease, the hyperkinetic circulatory states, and left ventricular failure. In the last of these examples the triple rhythm produced by the development of the third heart sound is called diastolic gallop and will be discussed more fully in Chapter VII.

MURMURS

There are at least twenty different heart murmurs which can be recognised by means of simple auscultation:

1. *The apical presystolic murmur of mitral stenosis* (fig. 2.32a). This is a left atrial systolic murmur, left atrial contraction increasing the blood flow through the narrow mitral orifice towards the end of diastole. It sounds crescendo, especially when it suddenly augments a fading diastolic rumble and ends abruptly with an accentuated first heart sound, but is not necessarily so. The murmur is best heard with the bell stethoscope when the patient lies on the left side, and is often accompanied by a thrill.

2. *The presystolic murmur of Austin Flint* (1862, 1886) may be heard in any form of well-developed aortic incompetence and is generally believed to be due to vibrations of the anterior (aortic) cusp of the mitral valve which is agitated by the opposing forces of aortic reflux and left atrial contraction (Da Costa, 1908). It is indistinguishable in quality and timing from the presystolic murmur of mitral stenosis. Phonocardiograms have confirmed the reality of the murmur in cases which have been proved later to have normal mitral valves at necropsy (Currens *et al.*, 1953).

3. *The presystolic murmur of tricuspid stenosis* is similar in quality, timing and mechanism to its mitral counterpart, but is heard at the tricuspid area instead of at the apex beat, and is appreciably louder during inspiration.

4. *The apical pansystolic murmur of mitral incompetence* (fig. 2.32b). This begins early, immediately after the first heart sound, as soon as the pressure

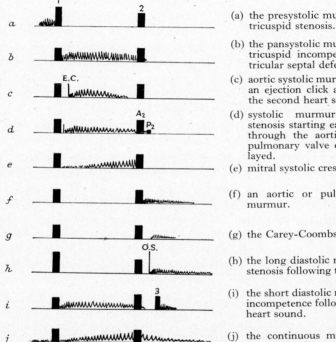

a	(a) the presystolic murmur of mitral or tricuspid stenosis.
b	(b) the pansystolic murmur of mitral or tricuspid incompetence or of ventricular septal defect.
c	(c) aortic systolic murmur opening with an ejection click and fading before the second heart sound.
d	(d) systolic murmur in pulmonary stenosis starting earlier and spilling through the aortic second sound, pulmonary valve closure being delayed.
e	(e) mitral systolic crescendo murmur.
f	(f) an aortic or pulmonary diastolic murmur.
g	(g) the Carey-Coombs murmur.
h	(h) the long diastolic murmur of mitral stenosis following the opening snap.
i	(i) the short diastolic murmur of mitral incompetence following a loud third heart sound.
j	(j) the continuous murmur of patent ductus arteriosus.

Fig. 2.32—The chief murmurs.

in the left ventricle rises above that in the left atrium. It also ends late, embracing the aortic element of the second sound, for the left ventricular pressure is still well above that in the left atrium when the aortic valve closes. A thrill is common in organic cases, but rare when the leak is functional.

5. *The pansystolic murmur of tricuspid incompetence* is similar to its mitral counterpart, except that it is heard best in the tricuspid area and is much louder during inspiration.

6. *The pansystolic murmur of ventricular septal defect* (Roger, 1879) is very like the murmur of mitral (or tricuspid) incompetence in quality and timing, for the ordinary relationship between left and right ventricular pressure is not very greatly different from the relationship between left ventricular and left atrial pressure. The murmur is heard best, however,

in the third and fourth intercostal spaces at the left sternal edge, and is not accentuated by inspiration. A thrill can be felt in 90 per cent of cases.

7. *The aortic systolic murmur* (fig. 2.32c). This is heard over the carotids, in the aortic area, in the third left intercostal space at the sternal edge, and at the apex beat. It does not begin with the first heart sound proper, but after a short interval, when the aortic valve opens, an interval which becomes obvious enough when an aortic ejection click signals the opening of the valve. The murmur is also relatively short, ending just before aortic valve closure. Turbulence may be due to increased flow as in the hyperkinetic circulatory states, to dilatation of the ascending aorta, or to aortic valve disease—especially stenosis. An aortic systolic thrill usually means stenosis, but may occur exceptionally with the other conditions mentioned.

8. *The pulmonary systolic murmur* (fig. 2.32d). This is more or less confined to the pulmonary area and third left intercostal space at the sternal edge, but may be much lower when the turbulence is infundibular. It also begins a little while after the first heart sound proper, its onset coinciding with the pulmonary ejection click when that is present, i.e. with the opening of the pulmonary valve at the end of the period of isometric contraction. It usually lasts longer than the aortic systolic murmur, for the pulmonary valve shuts later than the aortic. Turbulence may be due to increased flow, as in atrial septal defect, to dilatation of the pulmonary artery, or to pulmonary or infundibular stenosis. A thrill is nearly always present when there is stenosis, but is by no means rare in uncomplicated A.S.D.

9. *The crescendo mitral systolic murmur* (fig. 2.32e). To the human ear this seems to begin rather late in systole and waxes greatly to end abruptly with the second heart sound just when it has reached its maximum. It is usually due to trivial mitral incompetence, although some authorities have stated it is commonly "innocent" (Evans, 1948). Just how its curious crescendo quality is produced is unknown.

10. *The late basal or posterior systolic murmur of coarctation of the aorta* is attributed to turbulence set up at the stricture itself rather than in collateral vessels. The murmur sounds a little late and may spill through the second sound into early diastole. It is heard in the epigastrium or over the lumbar spine when the stricture is in the abdominal aorta.

11. *The diastolic murmur of aortic incompetence* (fig. 2.32f) is relatively high pitched and best heard with the diaphragm type of chest-piece. It is situated in the aortic area, down the left border of the sternum, and over the left ventricle at the apex beat. The murmur begins immediately after the aortic second sound and when loud persists throughout diastole, in diminuendo fashion. When the leak is very slight, however, the murmur may be faint and short, and then its greatest intensity is appreciably after the second heart sound; indeed, when only maximum vibrations can be

heard, the murmur appears to be separated from the second heart sound by a distinct gap. This is because the greatest backward flow does not occur until the left ventricular pressure has fallen to zero. A diastolic aortic thrill favours syphilis or a perforated cusp, but not exclusively. A whining diastolic murmur has a similar meaning.

12. *The diastolic murmur of pulmonary incompetence* is similar in quality and timing to the aortic diastolic murmur, but is usually confined to the second and third left intercostal spaces. It is nearly always functional, being due to pulmonary hypertension as described by Graham Steell (1888), or to dilatation of the pulmonary artery without hypertension; occasionally it is due to organic disease of the valve as in pulmonary stenosis after bacterial endocarditis or valvotomy. It may be accompanied by a thrill.

13. *The soft apical diastolic murmur of active mitral valvulitis* was well described by Carey Coombs (1924). It is low pitched, relatively short, diminuendo, and separated from the second heart sound by an appreciable gap representing the time interval between aortic valve closure and rapid ventricular filling (fig. 2.32g). The murmur is best heard with the bell stethoscope when the patient lies on the left side, and is attributed to turbulence set up by inflammatory thickening of the mitral cusps. It is one of the few murmurs practically never accompanied by a thrill.

14. *The functional apical diastolic murmur* due to a torrential mitral blood flow is similar to the Carey Coombs murmur in all respects. It may be heard in patent ductus, ventricular septal defect, complete heart block, thyrotoxicosis, and anæmia. The mitral diastolic murmur sometimes associated with coarctation of the aorta and congenital aortic stenosis is not yet fully understood, but is probably either rheumatic or due to some degree of fibroelastosis.

15. *The apical diastolic murmur of mitral stenosis* is louder and usually rougher than those just described, and is commonly preceded by the mitral opening snap (fig. 2.32h). The murmur is long and in well-developed uncomplicated cases continues to the next first heart sound. A thrill is frequently associated. In many cases of organic mitral incompetence a rough mitral diastolic murmur is also heard, but it is short and follows a loud third heart sound instead of a snap (fig. 2.32i).

16. *The diastolic murmur of atrial septal defect* gives rise to the same triple rhythm cadence as mitral diastolic murmurs, for it is almost certainly due to a torrential tricuspid blood flow. The murmur may be heard best at the apex beat, where it may encourage a false diagnosis of Lutembacher's syndrome, or near the left sternal edge, sometimes as high as the third space, but may be maximum anywhere over the dilated right ventricle. It is characteristically accentuated by inspiration, which increases the tricuspid blood flow but not that through the atrial septal defect.

17. *The continuous "machinery" murmur of patent ductus* (Gibson, 1900), often accompanied by a thrill, is more or less localised to the pulmonary area. It waxes during systole and early diastole, and wanes in late diastole (fig. 2.32j). A similar murmur is heard in aorto-pulmonary septal defect.

18. *Continuous murmurs*, waxing and waning in similar fashion, are also heard on either or both sides of the chest, usually high up anteriorly, in cases of pulmonary atresia, and are due to broncho-pulmonary anastomatic (arterial) communications, single or multiple.

19. *The jugular venous hum*, discussed at length by Potain in 1867, is also continuous and phasic in quality. Although best heard over the jugular veins themselves, it may be first detected when auscultating the aortic or pulmonary area. It is loudest in the sitting or standing position, is sharply accentuated during inspiration, and usually disappears when the subject lies flat. The murmur is also abolished immediately if the jugular blood flow is temporarily halted by digital compression on the vein (usually the right), or by the Valsalva manœuvre.

20. Other *continuous "machinery" murmurs* over the heart may be caused by perforation of an aortic sinus into the pulmonary artery, right ventricle or atrium, or by coronary arterio-venous fistula; and over any part of the chest by pulmonary arterio-venous fistula.

So-called functional murmurs have led to great confusion. In a sense all murmurs are an expression of function, and in a very strict sense some very important valve murmurs are functional, e.g. certain mitral diastolic murmurs and the Graham Steell murmur. If the term is used at all, it should mean either murmurs due to turbulence set up by increased blood flow alone, the anatomy of the heart at the site of origin of the murmur being normal, or murmurs due to functional changes in anatomy. In the first group, functional murmurs so defined include aortic and pulmonary systolic murmurs associated with hyperkinetic circulatory states, the pulmonary systolic murmur of atrial septal defect, the mitral diastolic murmur of patent ductus, ventricular septal defect, etc., and the jugular venous hum; and in the second group we have the Austin Flint murmur, the systolic murmurs of functional mitral or tricuspid incompetence, basal systolic murmurs associated with functional dilatation of the aorta or pulmonary artery, and the Graham Steell murmur of functional pulmonary incompetence.

To dismiss a murmur as functional is unpardonable. A functional murmur is not insignificant, and is certainly not meaningless; nor does it refer exclusively to extracardiac murmurs, although at least one of these is functional, e.g. the cardio-respiratory murmur. This is attributed to systolic decompression of some segment of lung which is compressed by the expanding heart during diastole; thus it is a vesicular murmur similar to the sound of inspiration. It varies with posture and respiration.

EXAMINATION OF OTHER SYSTEMS

Thorough examination of all the other systems of the body should never be neglected in a presumed cardiological case, not only as a matter of principle, but also because important clues to cardiovascular diagnosis may lie outside that system. Partly to emphasise this point a special section has already been devoted to examining the extremities. Space forbids dealing with these other systems in a comprehensive manner, and since to do so in a niggardly fashion would be valueless, no purpose would be served by pursuing the subject further.

REFERENCES

Amsterdam, B., and Amsterdam, A. L. (1943): "Disparity in blood pressures in both arms in normals and hypertensives and its clinical significance: a study of 1,000 normals and 272 hypertensives", *N.Y. State J. Med.*, **43**, 2294.
Anderson, R. M. (1954): "Intrinsic Blood Pressure", *Circulation*, **9**, 641.

Berry, M. R. (1940): "The mechanism and prevention of impairment of auscultatory sounds during determination of blood pressure in standing patients", *Proc. Staff Meet. Mayo Clinic*, **15**, 699.
Bordley, J., Connor, C. A. R., Hamilton, W. F., Kerr, W. J., and Wiggers, C. J. (1951): "Recommendations for human blood pressure determinations by sphygmomanometers", *Circulation*, **4**, 503.
Bramwell, C. (1937): "Arterial pulse in health and disease", *Lancet, ii*, 239, 301, 366.
Braun-Menendez, E. (1938): "The heart sounds in normal and pathological conditions", *Lancet, ii*, 761.
Bridgman, E. W. (1914): "Notes on a normal, presystolic sound", *Arch. Intern. Med.*, **14**, 475.
Broadbent, W. (1895): "An unpublished physical sign", *Lancet, ii*, 200.

Cooke, L., and Luty, S. M. (1944): "Koilonychia and its recovery in cases of thyrotoxicosis", *Brit. med. J., ii*, 207.
Coombs, C. F. (1924): "Rheumatic heart disease", Bristol.
Corrigan, D. J. (1832): "On permanent patency of the mouth of the aorta, or inadequacy of the aortic valves", *Edin. med. and surg. J.*, **37**, 225.
Currens, J. H. (1948): "A comparison of the blood pressures in the lying and standing positions; a study of 500 men and 500 women", *Amer. Heart J.*, **35**, 646.
——, Thompson, W. B., Rappaport, M. B., and Sprague, H. B., (1953): "Clinical and phonocardiographic observations on the Flint murmur", *New England J. Med.*, **248**, 583.

Da Costa, J. G. (1908): "Physical Diagnosis", p. 354, Saunders, Philadelphia.
Dock, W. (1933): "Mode of production of the first heart sound", *Arch. Int. Med.*, **51**, 737.
Dowling, C. V., *et al.* (1952): "The effect on blood pressure in the right heart, pulmonary artery and systemic artery of cardiac standstill produced by carotid sinus stimulation", *Circulation*, **5**, 742.

Evans, W. (1948): "Cardiography", Butterworth, London.

Flint, A. (1862): "On cardiac murmurs", *Am. J. med. Sc.*, **44**, 29.
——, (1886): "Mitral cardiac murmurs", *Am. J. med. Sc.*, **91**, 27.
Friedreich, N. (1864): *Virchows Arch. Path. Anat.*, **29**, 296.

Gibson, A. G. (1907): "The significance of a hitherto undescribed wave in the jugular pulse", *Lancet, ii*, 1380.

Gibson, G. A. (1900): "Clinical lectures on circulatory affections; Lecture 1, persistence of the arterial duct and its diagnosis", *Edin. med. J.*, **8**, 1.

Goyette, E. M., and Palmer, P. W. (1953): "Cardiovascular lesions in arachnodactyly", *Circulation*, **7**, 373.

Hales, S. (1733): "Statical essays: containing hæmastaticks; or, an account of some hydraulic and hydrostatical experiments made on the blood and blood vessels of animals", W. Innys and R. Manly, London.

Hunt, J. H. (1936): "Raynaud's Phenomena: critical review", *Quart. J. Med.*, **5**, 399.

Joint Report of the Committees Appointed by the Cardiac Society of Great Britain and Ireland, and the American Heart Association (1939): "Standardisation of methods of measuring the arterial blood pressure", *Brit. Heart J.*, **1**, 261.

Judson, C. F., and Nicholson, P. (1914): "Blood pressure in normal children", *Am. J. Dis. Child.*, **8**, 257.

Kerr, W. T., Althausen, T. L., Bassett, A. M., and Goldman, M. J. (1937): "The symballophone: a modified stethoscope for the lateralisation and comparison of sounds", *Amer. Heart J.*, **14**, 594.

Korotkow (1905): Berichte d. Kaiserl. Militararztl. Akad., St. Petersburg, **12**, 395.

Leatham, A. (1954): "Splitting of the first and second heart sounds", *Lancet*, ii, 607.

——, and Vogelpoel, L. (1954): "The early systolic sound in dilatation of the pulmonary artery", *Brit. Heart J.*, **16**, 21.

Lewis, W. H., Jr. (1938): "Changes in age in the blood pressure of adult men", *J. Physiol.*, **122**, 491.

Lian, C., and Danset, P. (1951): "Notions Cardiologiques Nouvelles", Masson et Cie, Paris.

——, Minot, G., and Welti, J. J. (1941): "Phonocardiographie", Masson et Cie, Paris.

Loman, J., Dameshek, W., Myerson, A., and Goldman, D. (1936): "Effect of alterations in posture on the intra-arterial blood pressure in man. I. Pressure in the carotid, brachial and femoral arteries in normal subjects", *Arch. Neurol. Psychiat.*, **35**, 1216.

Mackenzie, James (1902): "The study of the pulse arterial venous and hepatic and of the movements of the heart", Young J. Pentland, London.

Marfan, A. B. (1896): "Un cas de déformation congénitale des quatre membres, plus prononcée aux extrémités, caractérisée par l'allongement des os avec un certain degré d'amincissement", *Bull. et Mém. Soc. méd. d'hôp. de Paris*, **13**, 220.

Master, A. M., Garfield, C. I., and Walters, M. B. (1952): "Normal blood pressure and hypertension", Henry Kimpton, London.

Mendlowitz, M. (1938): "Some observations on clubbed fingers", *Clin. Sc.*, **3**, 387.

Ohm, R. (1913): "Venenpulz und Herztone", *Dtsch. Med. Wsch.*, **39**, 1493.

Olsen, A. M., O'Leary, P. A., and Kirklin, B. R. (1945): "Esophageal lesions associated with acrosclerosis and scleroderma", *Arch. Int. Med.*, **76**, 189.

Orias, O., and Braun-Menendez, E. (1939): "The heart sounds in normal and pathological conditions", Oxford University Press, London.

Osler, W. (1909): "Chronic infectious endocarditis", *Quart. J. Med.*, **2**, 219.

Owen, S. G., and Wood, P. H. (1955): "A new method of determining the degree or absence of mitral obstruction: an analysis of the diastolic part of indirect left atrial pressure tracings", *Brit. Heart J.*, **17**, 41.

Potain, P. C. E. (1867): "Des mouvements et des bruits qui se passent dans les veines jugulaires", *Bull. et Mém. Soc. méd. hôp. de Paris*, **4**, 3.

Rados, A. (1942): "Marfan's syndrome (arachnodactyly) coupled with dislocation of lens", *Arch. Ophthal.*, **27**, 477.

Ragan, C., and Bordley, J. (1941): "The accuracy of clinical measurements of
arterial blood pressure", *Bull. John S. Hopkins Hosp.*, **69**, 504.

Rappaport, M. B., and Sprague, H. B. (1941): "Physiologic and physical laws
that govern auscultation, and their clinical application", *Amer. Heart J.*, **21**, 257.

——, —— (1951): "The effects of tubing bore on stethoscope efficiency", *Amer.
Heart J.*, **42**, 605.

Raynaud, M. (1862): "Local asphyxia and symmetrical gangrene of the extremities", Rignaux, Paris.

Reynolds, G. (1950): "The Heart in Arachnodactyly", *Guy's Hosp. reports*, **99**,
178.

Riva-Rocci, S. (1899): "De la mésuration de la pression arterielle en clinique",
La Presse Medicale, **22**, 307.

Roger, H. (1879): "Recherches cliniques sur la communication congenital des
deux cœurs, par inocclusion du septum interventriculaire", *Bull. Acad. Med. d
Paris*, **8**, 1074.

Steel, G. (1888): "The murmur of high pressure in the pulmonary artery", *Med.
Chronicle, Manchester*, **9**, 182.

Taquini, A. C. (1936): "Exploración del corazón por via esofágica", Buenos
Aires.

Terry, R. (1954): "White nails in hepatic cirrhosis", *Lancet*, **1**, 757.

von Recklinghausen, H. (1901): "Ulber Blutdruckmessung beim Menschen",
Arch. f. Exper. Path., **46**, 88.

Weiss, S., Stead, E. A. Jr., Warren, J. V., and Bailey, O. T. (1943): "Scleroderma
Heart Disease", *Arch. Int. Med.*, **71**, 749.

Woodbury, R. A., Robinow, M., and Hamilton, W. F. (1938): "Blood pressure
studies on infants", *Am. J. Physiol.*, **122**, 472.

CHAPTER III

ELECTROCARDIOGRAPHY

ELECTROCARDIOGRAPHY was discovered in relation to the frog's heart by Kölliker and Müller (1856), and was proved applicable to the study of the heart in man by Waller (1887), who used a capillary electrometer and an antero-posterior chest lead. It was elaborated by Einthoven (1903), inventor of the string galvanometer and author of the famous triangle which bears his name, and used extensively by Lewis (1925) in his well-known researches on abnormalities of rhythm. In recent years many attempts have been made to place electrocardiography upon a more scientific and less empirical basis, and considerable success has been achieved in this respect, especially by Wilson and his colleagues (1930 *et seq.*). It is not easy (or necessary) for the ordinary physician, unless he also be a physicist and mathematician, to grasp the electrical details involved; but the following simplified account will be readily understood.

Certain molecules in the resting cardiac muscle cell dissociate into positive and negative ions. The positively charged ions (cations) are distributed on the outer surface, the negatively charged ions (anions) within (Curtis and Cole, 1941). Such a cell is in a state of electrical balance and is said to be polarised (fig. 3.01a). When the cell is excited its polarity is reversed, the negative charges coming to the surface, the positive charges passing within, and the cell is said to be depolarised (fig. 3.01b). It should be clear that when a number of cells are clustered together, all in the resting polarised state or all in the excited depolarised state, there can be no potential differences anywhere on their collective surface. If a group of cells were in the process of being excited, however, those already depolarised would possess negative surface charges, whereas those still polarised would have positive surface charges, and the collective surfaces of the two sets would yield a potential difference (fig. 3.01c). This constitutes a doublet (Craib, 1930), dipole (Ashman, 1948), or double layer (Bayley, 1943). Thus, when an excitatory wave flows through cardiac muscle, its head is electrically positive and its tail negative (fig. 3.01d). If electrodes are placed at A and B and connected to a galvanometer, an electrical current flows from B to A through the galvanometer, and from A to B through the tissue. The excitatory process, or accession wave as it is called, causes a very rapid or almost instantaneous reversal of cellular polarity, so that the duration of the galvanometric deflection is brief, and practically indicates the speed of the wave if the muscle thickness is known, or the muscle thickness if the speed of the wave is known. When the impulse reaches B (fig. 3.01e) the whole muscle-block AB has a negative collective

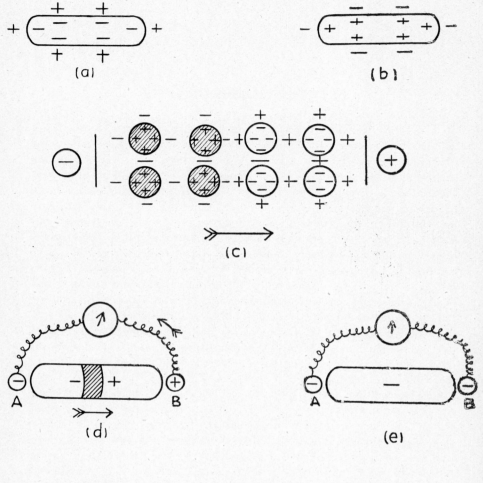

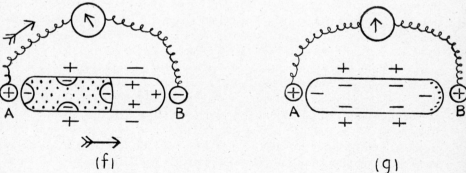

Fig. 3.01—Accession and regression waves (stages of excitation and recovery) in cardiac muscle (see text).

(a) Resting polarised cell.   (b) Excited depolarised cell.

(c) Excitation proceeding through a group of cells.

(d) Spread of the accession wave through a block of cardiac muscle.

(e) Muscle-block fully excited (depolarised).

(f) Spread of the regression wave or recovery process.

(g) Muscle-block fully recovered (re-polarised).

surface, if recovery has not yet commenced at A, and there is no potential difference between A and B. Within a short time, however, recovery begins at A (fig. 3.01f), and the cells become repolarised, their collective surfaces becoming positively charged again. While the recovery process, or regression wave as it is called, is spreading from A towards B, a current again flows through the galvanometer, but in the opposite direction. The regression wave travels at the same speed as the accession wave, but causes a slower change of polarity, so that the galvanometric deflection is not so brief. If the movements of the galvanometer are graphically recorded, the passage of an excitatory impulse from A to B results therefore in a diphasic curve such as that shown in figure 3.02, the first deflection being quick or sharp, the second slow or blunt. Moreover, if the neuro-muscular tissue is uniform in all relevant respects, the area occupied by the first deflection, which may be measured by means of a planimeter with suitable magnification, is exactly equal, though of opposite sign, to the area occupied by the second deflection. In modern electrocardiographic parlance the first deflection is represented by the P wave when it reflects atrial excitation, and by the QRS complex when it reflects ventricular excitation; while the second is represented by the Ta and T waves respectively. The QRS complex is written as the accession wave flows through the heart muscle from endocardial to epicardial surfaces; not as the excitatory impulse passes down the bundle of His, bundle branches and Purkinje network. As the heart is not a uniform muscle-block, but a bi-ventricular organ composed of numerous intertwining S-shaped muscle bundles (Robb and Robb, 1938), the initial ventricular deflection (QRS) is not monophasic, as in figure 3.02, but complex, and usually biphasic or triphasic; nor is the second ventricular deflection (T) of equal area and opposite sign. On account of this complexity, it is impossible, in the light of present knowledge, to determine by scientific theory precisely what an electrocardiogram should look like; it is only possible to find out by the practical method. For this reason, electrocardiography has largely remained an empirical study.

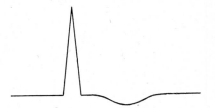

Fig. 3.02—The diphasic curve produced by the processes of excitation and recovery in heart muscle.

Einthoven's string galvanometer consists of an exceedingly fine fibre, such as silver-coated glass, suspended between the poles of an electro-magnet; when a current passes through the fibre, the latter is deflected towards one or other pole, according to the direction of the current. By suitable magnification and illumination the movements of the shadow of this string may be recorded on a moving photographic film. Valve-amplifying oscillographs of various forms, operated by potential differences, may be used instead of Einthoven's instrument. Time-marking is so arranged that fine vertical lines appear on the film at intervals of

0.04–0.05 second, preferably with thicker lines every 0.20 second. Horizontal lines for measuring voltage are spaced at intervals of 1 mm.

Practical points to bear in mind include satisfactory insulation of the machine and lead-wires to prevent 50-cycle A.C. interference, proper standardisation of the galvanometer so that a deflection of 1 cm. represents a potential difference of 1 mv., and the elimination of skin resistance by means of electrode jelly. The paste described by Jenks and Graybiel (1935) has proved effective: it consists of sodium chloride 2950 G. (6.5 lb.), powdered pumice 3600 G. (8 lb.), gum tragacanth 226 G. (8 oz.), potassium bitartrate 114 G. (4 oz.), glycerol 710 ml. (24 oz.), phenol 28.5 G. (1 oz.), and water to 7.5 litres (2 gallons). The electrolytes are dissolved in one gallon of water, while the gum and glycerol are heated for six hours in the other; the two are then mixed, stirred, and reheated for one hour. Phenol and pumice (and more water if necessary) are then added, and mixed until the preparation has the consistency of cream. Fresh soft green soap (B.P.) is very little inferior, especially after rubbing the skin with some abrasive (Bell, Knox and Small, 1939). A number of satisfactory pastes or gels are marketed.

CHEST LEADS

Analysis of electrocardiograms has become simplified since the introduction of Wilson's neutral electrode (Wilson, 1934). Previously all electrocardiograms were bipolar, and registered the potential differences between two electrodes placed at different sites on the surface of the body, each gathering different potential values. According to Einthoven's theory, however, the algebraic sum of the potentials at the left arm, right arm and left leg always equal zero, these points representing the apices of an equilateral triangle in the frontal plane of the body, the heart lying at its centre, and the limbs being regarded as extensions of the lead wires.[*] Thus it is only necessary to link up these three points to a common terminal (preferably through a resistance of 5,000 ohms in order to neutralise differences in skin resistance) to provide an electrode that remains at zero potential throughout the cardiac cycle. If this neutral or indifferent electrode is linked to one arm of the galvanometer, the instrument will record the potential variations of an "exploring" electrode linked to the other arm. This is the basis of all V leads, V standing for potential value or voltage at any particular point. It has been agreed that positivity of this exploring electrode should be represented by an upright electrocardiographic deflection.

It is now necessary to consider the variations in potential that may be recorded if the exploring electrode is placed over the surface of the left ventricle in man (Wilson et al., 1944). As the accession wave spreads from endocardial to epicardial surfaces, the left ventricular cavity (in contact with the tail of the wave) becomes electrically negative, and the surface of the heart (in contact with the head of the wave) becomes electrically positive. The galvanometer therefore records an upright or positive deflection, R (fig. 3.03b). When the accession wave reaches the surface, the exploring

---

[*] The mathematical proof of this equation is given by Wilson et al. (1946), Goldberger 1947), and by others.

electrode undergoes an abrupt reversal of polarity, and the galvanometer registers a sharp downward deflection (the intrinsic deflection). As both the cavity and surface of the left ventricle are then at the same negative potential, the electrical field is abolished, and the galvanometer comes to rest (fig. 3.03c). A complication arises, however, because the accession wave starts at some point (such as the left side of the interventricular septum) remote from the muscle underlying the electrode. The left ventricular cavity thus becomes negative before the muscle under the electrode

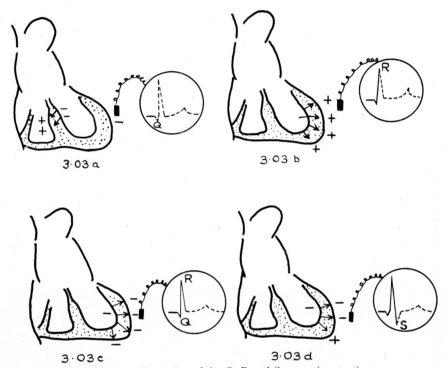

3·03 a   3·03 b

3·03 c   3·03 d

Fig. 3.03—Formation of the Q, R and S waves (see text).

begins to be activated, and this negative potential is passively transmitted to the surface to be recorded as an initial downward deflection, Q (fig. 3.03a). Since leads taken from the right ventricular cavity show an initial positive deflection in practically all instances, it is believed that the excitation wave starts on the left side of the septum. Again, if the accession wave is still spreading through muscle remote from the exploring electrode when the galvanometer has registered the local intrinsic deflection, the electrical field is maintained, and continued negativity of the cavity is passively transmitted to the surface under the electrode, to be recorded as a final downward deflection, S (fig. 3.03d).

When the exploring electrode is placed over the right ventricle, similar principles hold good; but the right ventricle is much thinner than the left, and therefore the local potential differences are smaller and are normally overpowered by left ventricular events. An initial R wave is almost invariable and represents the positive potential produced in the right ventricular cavity as the accession wave spreads through the septum from left to right; in other words it is the head of the left ventricular Q wave. Further development of R, as excitation passes through the anterior wall of the right ventricle, is more or less prevented by the stronger negative potential induced by the tail of the accession wave that is spreading through the left ventricle; this is represented by a large S wave. Q is never seen over a normal right ventricle. The second ventricular deflection, T, is upright over the left ventricle, but may be inverted over the right (in leads V_1 and V_2).

With the aid of unipolar intramural electrodes Prinzmetal and his colleagues (1953) have proved that the inner third of the myocardium is electrically silent, as if the Purkinje network penetrated to this depth. Subendocardial leads always yield monophasic QS waves and R only begins to develop when the electrode is nearly half-way between endocardial and epicardial surfaces. As the electrode approaches the surface R increases rapidly in amplitude while S diminishes.

In clinical electrocardiography multiple chest leads are designated leads V_{1-7}. The figures indicate the position of the proximal electrode with reference to the chest-wall, and represent respectively the right and

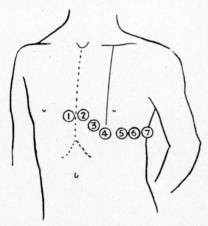

Fig. 3.04—Multiple chest leads V_1-V_7. Position of the exploring electrode.

left borders of the sternum, the left para-sternal and mid-clavicular lines, and the anterior, mid, and posterior axillary lines, at the level of a line passing from the fourth intercostal space at points 1 and 2, to the fifth intercostal space at point 4, and thence horizontally (fig.3.04). For routine purposes leads V_1, V_3 and V_5, or V_2, V_4 and V_6 are usually sufficient; but in particular instances other combinations or all seven leads are preferable. A typical record obtained with this technique is illustrated in fig. 3.05. Over the left ventricle (V_5 and V_6) there is a small Q wave, a large R wave, no S wave, an iso-potential R-T junction, and an upright T wave. In the transition zone (V_3-V_4) Q has disappeared, a conspicuous S wave has developed, and T is sharply upright. Over the right ventricle (V_1) there is again no Q wave, R is small, S large, and T is flattened. In normal subjects the P wave is upright or occasionally diphasic (3 per cent) in V_3, but often diphasic (20 per cent) or inverted (15 per cent) in V_1. Q is usually present

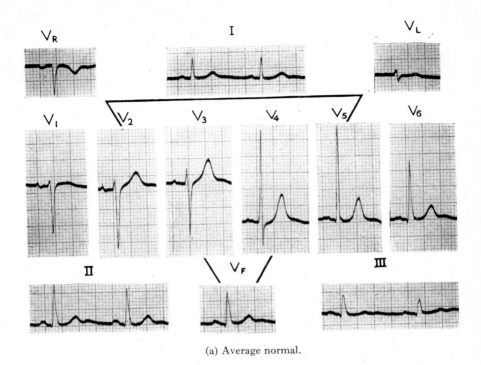

(a) Average normal.

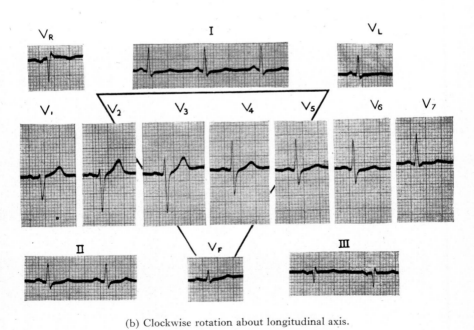

(b) Clockwise rotation about longitudinal axis.

Fig. 3.05—Normal chest lead electrocardiogram

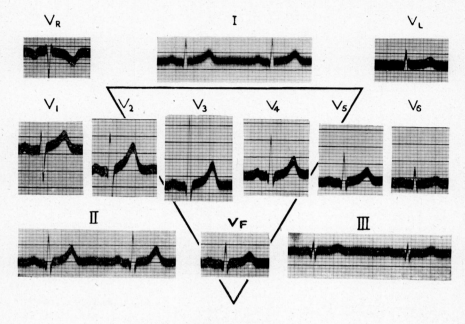

(c)—Anti-clockwise rotation.

Fig. 3.05—Normal chest lead electrocardiogram (V_1–V_6).

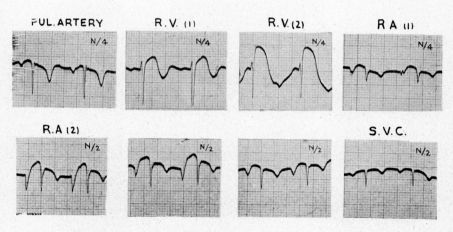

Fig. 3.06—Right ventricular and pulmonary artery cavity leads.

in V_6, occurs in V_5 in 45 per cent of cases, but is rarely seen farther to the right. S is usually absent in V_{6-7}, is absent in V_5 in 17 per cent of cases, but is invariably found in V_3 and V_1. T is always upright in V_4–V_6, may be occasionally diphasic in V_3, and is inverted in V_1 in 62 per cent of cases.

If there is clockwise rotation about the longitudinal axis (viewed from below), the anterior surface of the septum is shifted to the patient's left: this means that S is dominant in V_4, the transition zone being shifted to V_4 or V_5. In such cases Q may not appear until V_6 or V_7. Similar graphs are obtained when the heart is horizontal in position, the septum then being displaced to the patient's left (fig. 3.05b).

Anticlockwise rotation about the longitudinal axis brings the anterior surface of the septum to the patient's right. The QR pattern may then be seen from V_6 to V_3, and the transition zone is shifted to V_2 (fig. 3.05c).

In addition to leads V_1–V_7, other positions of the exploring electrode have been used with advantage under exceptional circumstances. An œsophageal lead may also be helpful in doubtful cases of posterior myocardial infarction, and an intracardiac lead may provide interesting information; but these are rarely necessary for clinical purposes.

The œsophageal lead takes its potential from the surface of the left atrium when high, and from the posterior surface of the left ventricle when low. Left atrial potentials are transmitted from the cavity of the left ventricle, and show monophasic Q waves and inverted T waves, the cavity of the left ventricle being negative throughout the inscription of the initial and second ventricular deflections. The posterior surface of the left ventricle gives rise to a QR complex similar to that obtained anteriorly or laterally. Œsophageal patterns therefore show monophasic Q waves or QR deflections, Q dominating when the electrode is relatively high up, R when the electrode is relatively low down. T is usually negative when the electrode is high, positive when low.

Intracardiac leads from the cavity of the right ventricle show a small initial R wave followed by a deep S wave as already described. If the catheter is passed through a patent foramen ovale into the left ventricle, a monophasic Q wave is obtained. When the catheter is passed into the pulmonary artery, the small R wave seen within the cavity of the right ventricle disappears in favour of a monophasic Q wave (fig. 3.06); this is because the pulmonary artery takes its potentials from the surface of the left auricle.

There are thus only a limited number of basic QRS patterns upon which all ventricular deflections encountered in clinical electrocardiography depend (fig. 3.07): the QR complex of a left ventricular surface lead (T normally upright); the RS complex of a right ventricular surface lead (T usually upright); the monophasic Q wave of a left ventricular cavity lead (T normally inverted); the RS complex of a right ventricular cavity lead (T normally inverted); and the balanced QR pattern of a combined left ventricular cavity and surface lead from the back of the heart (Goldberger, 1947).

The direction of the second ventricular deflection, T, is opposite to theoretical prediction in all the basic patterns, and suggests that the

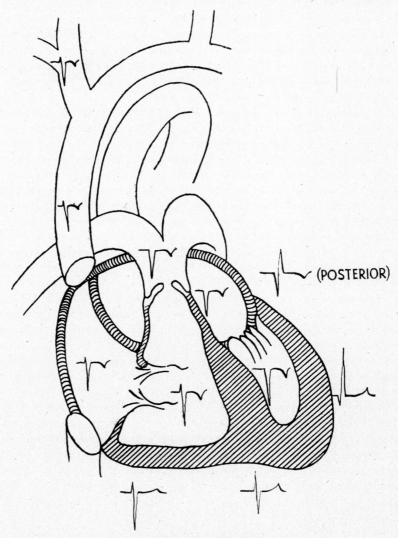

(POSTERIOR)

Fig. 3.07—The basic QRS-T patterns.

recovery wave starts at the surface of the ventricles and is directed towards the cavities.

Instead of V leads, many workers, including Wolferth and Wood (1932–33) who re-introduced chest leads to clinical electrocardiography, have coupled the exploring electrode with a relatively indifferent electrode placed on the right arm (CR) or on the left leg (CF). Agreement will never be reached as to which of these is the more informative and it is expected that they will both be abandoned in favour of V leads. They will be con- sidered in greater detail in subsequent paragraphs.

UNIPOLAR LIMB LEADS

The potential values in the right arm (V_R), left arm (V_L), and left leg (V_F), may be obtained by placing the exploring electrode on the desired limb and linking it with Wilson's neutral electrode. As unipolar limb leads are of low voltage, it is customary to alter the standardisation so that a potential difference of 1 millivolt causes a deflection of 15 mm. (instead of 10 mm.). Alternatively, Goldberger's augmented leads may be used. With this technique the V lead is attached to the limb, the potential values of which are being measured, whilst the wire connecting this limb with the central neutral terminal is detached and left hanging free. The potentials are thus increased by 50 per cent (Goldberger, 1942), thus:

$$\text{Since } V_R + V_L + V_F = O$$
$$\text{then } V_L + V_F = -V_R$$

Now when an electrode on the right arm is paired with a central terminal linked to the left arm and left leg, the galvanometer records $V_R - \dfrac{V_L + V_F}{2}$, the latter being the mean potentials of the left arm and left leg.

$$\text{Now} \quad V_R - \frac{V_L + V_F}{2}$$

$$= V_R - \frac{(-V_R)}{(\ 2\ )}$$

$$= V_R + \tfrac{1}{2}V_R = 1\tfrac{1}{2}V_R$$

There has been some confusion concerning the equation $V_L + V_R + V_F$ = zero. This statement is obvious in relation to the technique used for obtaining the unipolar limb lead potentials, for the "neutral" electrode (e) employed with this technique is the mean of the potential values in each of the three limbs, i.e. $e = \dfrac{L + R + F.}{3}$

$$\text{Now } V_L = L - e$$
$$V_R = R - e$$
$$V_F = F - e$$
$$\text{So that } V_L + V_R + V_F = L + R + F - 3e$$
$$= L + R + F - \frac{3(L + R + F)}{3}$$
$$= \text{zero.}$$

It should be readily appreciated that this self evident fact has no bearing on whether the common terminal is neutral or otherwise, but would be true for any value of e. Thus the statement does not imply the truth of

Einthoven's hypothesis nor the validity of the theory underlying Wilson's neutral electrode.

Unipolar limb leads are useful in determining the electrical position of the heart, in explaining the difference between CR, CF, and V chest leads, and in demonstrating the basis of the standard leads. V_R usually shows inversion of all complexes because it reflects the negative potential of the cardiac cavities transmitted through the great vessels (figs. 3.07 and 3.08).

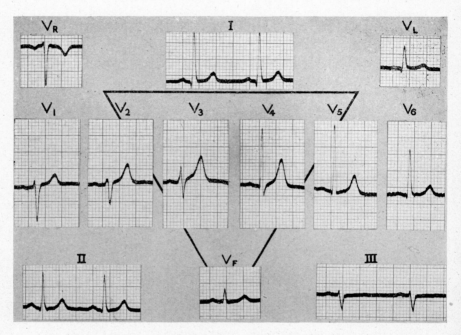

Fig. 3.08—Unipolar limb leads (V_L, V_R, V_F) and standard leads 1, 2, and 3.
(a) Normal (the heart is more horizontal than vertical).

When the heart is normal in size and position, V_L and V_F are mainly positive, dominant left ventricular surface potentials being transmitted more or less equally to both of them (fig. 3.08a). When the heart is electrically horizontal, however, left ventricular surface potentials are transmitted more strongly to the left arm, and right ventricular surface potentials to the left leg. There is then a small Q and tall R wave in lead V_L, and a small R and deep S wave in lead V_F (fig. 3.08b). When the heart is electrically vertical, the negative potentials of the cavities are transmitted more strongly to the left arm, and the left ventricular surface potentials more strongly to the left leg. There is then a small R and deep S wave in V_L, and a small Q and tall R wave in V_F (fig. 3.08c). In normal subjects the electrical position of the heart is more or less in line with its anatomical position.

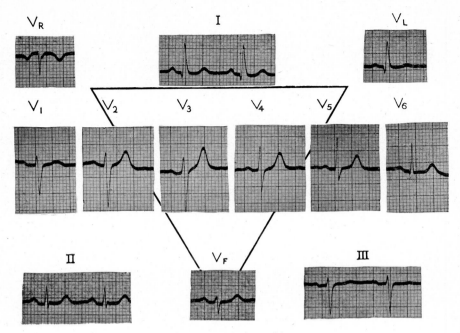

Fig. 3.08 (b)—Horizontal heart.

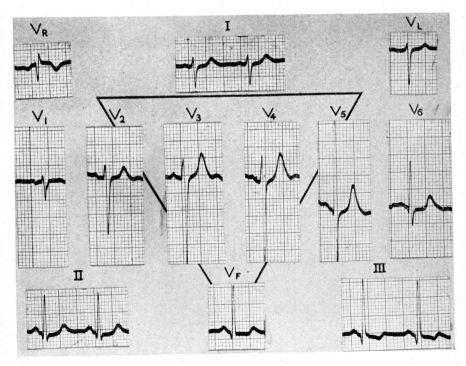

Fig. 3.08 (c)—Vertical heart.

The differences between CR, CF and V chest leads may now be appreciated: CR leads are V leads minus the potentials in V_R, whilst CF leads are V leads minus the potentials in V_F. As V_R potentials are negative, their subtraction from V in CR records makes all deflections more positive – not only is R taller in lead CR_1, but T is invariably upright in adults and in children over eight years of age. Again, since V_F potentials are normally positive, their subtraction from V in CF records makes all deflections more negative. As the voltage is usually higher in V_R than in V_F, however, CR leads show greater differences from V leads than do CF leads.

STANDARD LEADS

Einthoven's bipolar leads, introduced at the beginning of the century and adopted as the standard leads throughout the world, consist of the left and right arm (lead I), the left leg and the right arm (lead II), and the left leg and left arm (lead III). Electrocardiograms derived from these leads can be calculated, of course, from the deflections obtained with unipolar limb leads; for lead I equals $V_L–V_R$; lead II equals $V_F–V_R$; lead III equals $V_F–V_L$. The subtraction of the negative potentials in V_R from the positive potentials in V_L and V_F result in strongly positive QRS and T deflections in leads I and II. Again, as the voltage of R in V_F is usually higher than that in V_L, QRS is also normally positive in lead III.

By definition there is an obvious relationship between the three standard leads:

$$\text{lead II} = \text{lead I} + \text{lead III}$$

This merely states that

$$V_F–V_R \text{ (lead II)} = V_L–V_R \text{ (lead I)} + V_F–V_L \text{ (lead III)}$$
$$= V_F–V_R.$$

and has nothing to do with Einthoven's theory or triangle.

The relationship between the standard leads and the Wilson unipolar limb leads is as follows:

$$V_L = \frac{I - III}{3}$$

$$V_R = \text{minus} \; \frac{I + II}{3}$$

$$V_F = \frac{II + III}{3}$$

The augmented values obtained with Goldberger's technique may be derived from the standard leads by changing the denominator in the above equations from 3 to 2.

NORMAL APPEARANCES
(Fig. 3.08)

P wave

P represents the excitation process as it spreads from the sinoauricular node through both atria. It is usually blunt, and is upright in leads I and

II, but may be inverted in lead III. Its height should not exceed 2.0 mm., and its duration 0.1 second. Following P, slight depression of the base-line, sometimes hidden by the QRS complex, may be evident, and represents atrial recovery or repolarisation. It has been termed the atrial T wave or Ta wave.

P–R interval

No deflection is caused by the passage of the excitatory impulse down the bundle of His, its main branches, and Purkinje network, so that there is an iso-potential interval between atrial and ventricular events: this is the P–R interval, and is conveniently measured from the beginning of P to the beginning of QRS. It commonly ranges between 0.12 and 0.20 second, but occasionally, even in young subjects, it may measure 0.21 or 0.22 second, without evidence of heart disease or of general ill health.

The P–R interval is little affected by spontaneous variations in heart rate, but may be slightly reduced by atropine, and slightly lengthened by carotid sinus compression. Vagal tone has a much greater effect on the sinus node than on A–V conduction.

The QRS complex

Q, R, and S, when all are present, form a triphasic complex representing the spread of the accession wave through the ventricles, and are convenient symbols for describing the shape of the initial ventricular deflection. Each is applied to a wave so defined by its direction and by its time-relationship to the others. Thus any upward deflection is called R, or if there are two such, R and R'. A downward deflection is called Q if it precedes R, or if it is the only wave present, and S if it follows R.

Q rarely measures more than 1 or 2 mm. in leads I and II, and is often absent altogether; in lead III, however, it may be conspicuous, and may measure up to one-third of the amplitude of R. R should exceed 5 mm. in height in the most favourable lead, unless the spatial vector is unusually postero-anterior. Slight notching or slurring near its base is common and has no significance. Distortion of the apex of R is rare in normal subjects, but may be disregarded when unaccompanied by other changes. S is variable, and is greatly influenced by axis deviation, which will be considered later.

The whole QRS complex should not exceed 0.1 second in duration, and rarely exceeds 0.08 second in normal individuals.

RS–T segment

This refers to that short segment between the QRS complex and the T wave, i.e. between the end of the excitatory and the beginning of the recovery processes. In some cases this is so short as to represent merely the RS–T junction. Any deviation of the RS–T segment from the iso-potential base-line should be regarded with suspicion. Slight deviation, of the order of 0.5 mm., may be within normal limits, yet taken in conjunction with other findings may be highly significant.

It is customary to include the proximal portion of the T wave when describing the shape of the RS–T segment, e.g. whether concave, straight, or convex. Speaking in this way, a normal RS–T segment curves gently from its point of origin in the direction of the T wave; it is neither straight, nor does it deviate in the opposite direction first.

T wave

T represents the recovery process or the regression wave (repolarisation), and is known as the second ventricular deflection. It is normally upright in leads I and II, but may be inverted in lead III. It should measure at least 2 mm. in amplitude in the most favourable lead.

Q–T interval

The interval between the beginning of QRS and the end of T represents the total time occupied by ventricular excitation and recovery. It is inversely proportional to the heart rate, ranging between 0.42 second at a speed of 48 per minute, and 0.28 second at a speed of 110. The formula of Bazett (1920) is $Q–T = K\sqrt{C}$, where C represents the cycle length. The constant K is variously given as 0.38—0.39 plus or minus 0.04, and is a trifle longer in women than in men and children.

Taran and Szilagyi (1947) have made the sensible suggestion that the Q–T interval should be recorded as corrected for rate, i.e. as $Q–T_c$. This should equal Bazett's constant, K, i.e. the actual Q–T interval when the heart rate is 60 per minute or when the cycle length is one second. $Q–T_c$ is easily calculated with the aid of a slide rule when the actual Q–T interval and cycle length are known; for $Q–T_c$ (or $K) = \dfrac{Q–T}{\sqrt{C}}$. The Q–T interval is lengthened by hypocalcæmia (fig. 3.33) and shortened by digitalis (fig. 3.27b). $Q–T_c$ may be prolonged in active rheumatic carditis (Taran and Szilegyi, 1947). There is some evidence that $Q–T_c$ is also lengthened by cardiac enlargement from any cause, and shortened by cardiac compression as in percardial effusion (Van Lingen, 1947).

U wave

Following T, and coinciding with the super-normal recovery phase, a small, rounded, positive deflection, the U wave, may be seen. Its significance is not fully understood; but it appears to be exaggerated in chest leads taken from the right of the interventricular septum and to be flattened or even inverted in leads taken from the left of the septum when there is left ventricular hypertrophy, and vice versa when there is right ventricular hypertrophy. It may also be inverted in left ventricular surface leads during an attack of angina pectoris. It is accentuated by digitalis.

THE CARDIAC VECTOR

Maximum potential differences within the heart at any given moment may be represented in magnitude and direction by a line of appropriate length and spatial direction (drawn from the hypothetical centre of electrical events), which may be called a vector, and its direction a spatial axis. Both magnitude and direction of this vector alter from moment to moment during the phases of ventricular excitation and recovery, but may be resolved into mean values. If such a vector is projected on to the frontal plane of the body, its new momentary or mean manifest value may be calculated by suitable measurements, detailed below, of the electrocardiograms obtained from any two of Einthoven's leads: for the frontal plane or manifest vector may be projected on to the sides of an equilateral triangle, the apices of which are represented by the left and right arms (or shoulders) and by the left leg (or symphysis pubis), the sides of the triangle thus representing the three standard leads. For example, if the line AB (fig. 3.09) represents the maximum momentary manifest QRS vector, i.e. if it

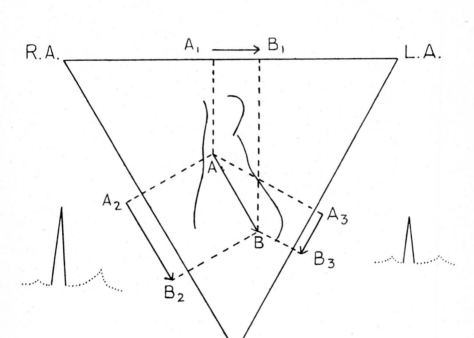

Fig. 3.09—Projection of the frontal plane QRS vector on to the sides of Einthoven's equilateral triangle.

represents the projection on to the frontal plane of the body of a line in space representing the magnitude and direction of maximum potential differences generated within the heart during the period of ventricular excitation, then the lines A_1–B_1, A_2–B_2, and A_3–B_3, obtained by projecting the line AB on to the sides of Einthoven's equilateral triangle, give the magnitude and direction of the maximum QRS deflection in leads I, II and III respectively. Moreover, it can be easily shown that, at any given moment the amplitude of the QRS deflection in lead II equals the algebraic sum of that in leads I and III; or the amplitude of the QRS deflection in any one lead, equals the algebraic sum of that in the other two. The same law applies to atrial activity and to the recovery phase, i.e. to the P, Ta, and T waves, and to mean as well as momentary values. Conversely, if the magnitude and direction of the QRS complex at any given moment is known in any two leads, their resultant drawn from the centre of Einthoven's triangle represents the manifest (frontal plane) vector of QRS at that particular moment, and its direction the manifest electrical axis. In current electrocardiographic nomenclature, the electrical axis refers to this resultant frontal plane axis as obtained from the maximum upright QRS deflection in any two leads, if apparently synchronous; and is expressed in terms of its angle with the horizontal, being plus when rotated clockwise from this base, minus when anti-clockwise. As so expressed, the normal electrical axis lies between 0 and 90 degrees, and has a wider range than the frontal plane anatomical axis.

Triaxial reference system

For convenience Einthoven's triangle may be suitably represented as a triaxial reference system (Bayley, 1943). The lines representing the three sides of the triangle are transposed so that they intersect at a common point, O (fig. 3.10). The horizontal line RL then represents lead I, and the

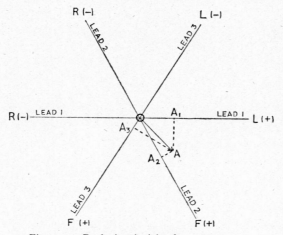

Fig. 3.10—Bayley's triaxial reference system.

lines RF and LF leads II and III respectively. The customary signs are preserved so that R is negative, F positive, and L negative or positive as shown in the diagram. If the vector, OA, is projected on to these lines, its value in the standard leads may at once be determined by the lengths OA_1, OA_2 and OA_3. The converse may be applied with equal simplicity.

By measuring the net area of QRS in any two leads (instead of momentary synchronous points) by means of a planimeter and suitable magnification (or by dividing the amplitude of the wave by half its width), the area below the base-line being subtracted from that above, the resultant mean axis of QRS in the frontal plane can be determined in similar fashion (Wilson *et al.*, 1934). Measurements may be made in millivolt-seconds, microvolt-seconds, or in suitable units based on voltage × time (Ashman and Byer, 1943). Such a resultant, drawn from the centre of Einthoven's triangle, having both magnitude and direction, is called the mean QRS vector in the frontal plane, or the manifest mean QRS vector, and its direction the manifest mean QRS axis. Manifest mean vectors for T and P may be similarly obtained. Bayley (1943) has suggested that the symbol Â might well designate the axis of such vectors, and the symbol A their magnitude: the manifest mean axis of QRS would then be called ÂQRS, and its magnitude AQRS.

If the heart were a simple uniform muscle-block, the algebraic net area occupied by QRS and T would be zero; as it is not, the net area of QRST has a positive or negative value, which if measured in any two leads may be resolved into a vector drawn from the centre of Einthoven's triangle. The axis of this vector, or the manifest mean QRST axis (ÂQRST), has been called the ventricular gradient (Wilson, Macleod, and Barker, 1931) or Ĝ, and its magnitude G. The gradient represents the magnitude and direction of maximum local variations in the speed of the processes of excitation and recovery, whereby the heart differs from a uniform muscle-block.

The manifest mean axis of QRS averages about 60 degrees; that of T about 50 degrees. The ventricular gradient in hearts which are not anatomically rotated ranges between 45 and 65 degrees. On the whole, hearts which are relatively central in position, i.e. rotated clockwise (viewed from the front) about their antero-posterior anatomical axis, are also rotated clockwise (viewed from the apex) about their longitudinal anatomical axis, and show clockwise deviation, i.e. deviation to the right, of all manifest momentary and mean electrical axes; but the greatest shift occurs with the ordinary momentary electrical axis of QRS, and the least with the ventricular gradient. This also applies to transverse hearts with anti-clockwise rotation and deviation of all electrical axes to the left (Ashman and Byer, 1943).

From what has been said it should be clear that the QRS and T vectors in the frontal plane of the body alter in magnitude and direction from moment to moment during the phase of ventricular excitation and recovery. As one end of such a vector is fixed at the centre of Einthoven's triangle, it follows that the other end must describe a continuous curve. Mann (1920) showed how such curves could be reconstructed, and later devised a method of recording them directly (1931). More recently, Wilson and Johnston (1938), employing the cathode-ray oscillograph, published typical curves, and called them vectorcardiograms. Even these, however, are restricted to the behaviour of the vector in the frontal plane of the body, being so limited by use of the standard limb leads. Wire models of spatial vectorcardiograms have been constructed by Duchosal (1949).

ELECTROCARDIOGRAPHIC ABNORMALITIES

ABNORMALITIES OF THE P WAVE

There are four main varieties of P wave deformity: the tall sharp P wave of right atrial hypertrophy (fig. 3.11a); the conspicuous widened P wave of left atrial hypertrophy, which may be bifid, rounded, or flat-topped (fig.

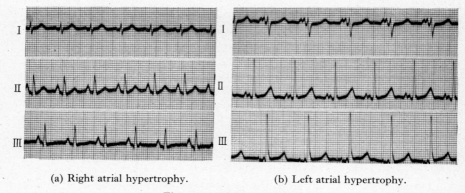

(a) Right atrial hypertrophy.   (b) Left atrial hypertrophy.

Fig. 3.11—Abnormal P waves.

3.11b); the low-voltage widened P wave, which may be also bifid, rounded, or flat-topped (fig. 3.11c); and the inverted P wave (fig. 3.11d).

Tall sharp P waves are characteristic of pulmonary hypertension, pulmonary stenosis, and tricuspid stenosis. The voltage ranges between 2 and 5 mm., and as the wave is not widened, it becomes peculiarly sharp, like an arrowhead. They are usually most evident in leads II and III.

Conspicuous widened P waves, measuring 0.12 second in duration, are almost diagnostic of mitral stenosis. The voltage may be normal or slightly increased, but rarely exceeds 2.5 mm. Most examples are bifid, the first peak representing right atrial activity, the second left atrial activity, so that the P mitrale implies delay in left atrial activation (Reynolds, 1953). They are usually seen best in leads I, II and V_5.

P waves similar in shape and width, but usually of lower voltage, may be seen sometimes in advanced cases of hypertensive heart disease or aortic valve disease. It is uncertain whether they represent left atrial dilatation due to left ventricular failure, as originally suggested by Wood and Selzer (1939), or inter-atrial block (Berconsky and Kloztman, 1945).

Inverted P waves are found in lead I in cases of dextrocardia, in leads II and III in coronary sinus rhythm, and in all leads in many cases of nodal rhythm.

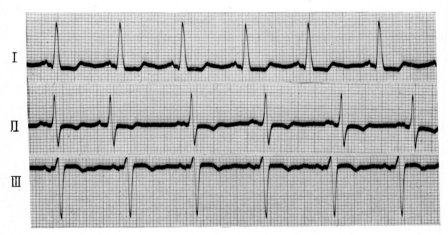

Fig. 3.11 (c)—P waves in hypertensive heart failure.

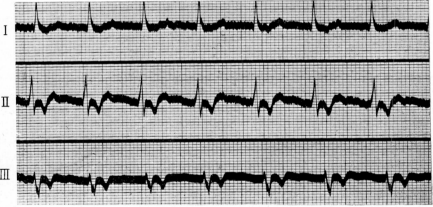

By courtesy of Dr. Hope Goss

Fig. 3.11 (d)—Inverted P waves in nodal rhythm.

ABNORMALITIES OF THE QRS COMPLEX

Axis deviation

It has already been pointed out that the electrical axis of the heart refers to the frontal plane projection of the maximum momentary spatial vector, and usually lies between 0 and 90 degrees, more or less in the anatomical axis. Anti-clockwise rotation of the heart about its antero-posterior axis (viewed from the front), or about its longitudinal axis (viewed from the cardiac apex), causes deviation of the electrical axis to the left, so that the frontal plane vector may make a minus angle with the horizontal; whilst clockwise rotation about similar axes causes right axis deviation, the vector now making an angle of more than 90 degrees with the horizontal. Left or right axis deviation respectively also occurs when the left or right ventricle is disproportionately enlarged. Moreover, left ventricular enlargement is often associated with anti-clockwise rotation about both anatomical axes, and right ventricular enlargement with clockwise rotation.

Reference to Einthoven's triangle will show that if the electrical axis deviates to the left, and approaches or surpasses the horizontal, lead I becomes the axial lead (fig. 3.12). R_I then carries the maximum voltage, R_{II} is smaller, and the maximum QRS deflection in lead III is downwards, i.e. the main deflection is S. In such cases S_{III} is really the electrical counterpart of R_I. Unipolar limb leads commonly show an electrically horizontal heart, R in V_L and S in V_F being unusually conspicuous.

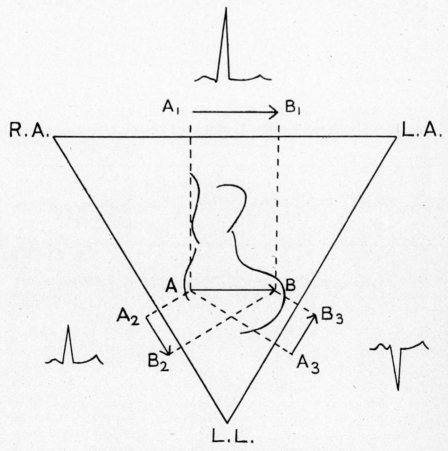

Fig. 3.12—Left axis deviation (Einthoven's triangle).

Left axis deviation occurs in 10 per cent of normal individuals, in any condition in which the left ventricle is disproportionately enlarged, in cardiac displacement to the left from scoliosis or from intrathoracic causes, and when the diaphragm is elevated causing the heart to lie more transversely. It may not be possible from examination of the limb lead QRS complexes alone to decide whether axis deviation is due to displacement or to left

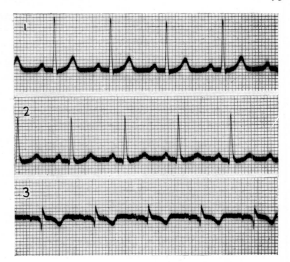

Fig. 3.13—Axis deviation due to elevation of the diaphragm (Q3 S1 type).

ventricular preponderance; but this distinction may often be made by considering the behaviour of the RS-T segment and T wave, and especially by noting the QRS pattern in multiple chest leads (*vide infra*).

A particular form of axis deviation is seen with elevation of the diaphragm, as from obesity, pregnancy, flatulence or ascites. R_I is taller than R_{II}, S_I and Q_{III} are prominent, and T_{III} is inverted (fig. 3.13). In such cases there is no Q wave in lead V_F, and the T wave usually remains inverted in lead V_1.

When the electrical axis is deviated to the right, so that it occupies a more or less vertical position, lead III becomes the axial lead (fig. 3.14). R_{III} then carries the maximum voltage, R_{II} is smaller, whilst the maximum deflection in lead I is S, which is the electrical counterpart of R_{III}. In unipolar limb leads S is conspicuous in V_L and R in V_F. Right axis deviation is the rule in newly born infants, is common in very young children, occurs in 1 per cent of normal children over the age of eight,

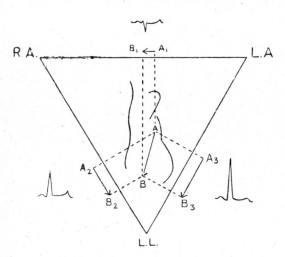

Fig. 3.14—Right axis deviation (Einthoven's triangle).

and is rarely seen in strictly normal adults, It may be caused by appropriate cardiac displacement or rotation, and by right ventricular dominance. As with left axis deviation, it may not be possible from inspection of the limb lead QRS complexes alone to determine whether the axis shift is due to right ventricular dominance or otherwise; but the behaviour of QRS in multiple chest leads may clarify the issue (*vide infra*).

Left ventricular preponderance

When the left ventricle is enlarged, the accession wave takes longer to penetrate that chamber and creates more powerful potential differences. Thus R in leads V_5 and V_6 and S in leads V_1 and V_2 have a larger amplitude (R in $V_{4, 5, or 6} > 25$ mm.; S in $V_1 > 15$ mm.), the intrinsic deflection in left ventricular surface leads is delayed (longer than 0.05 second), and the width of QRS slightly increased (0.1 second). Secondary changes in the T wave occur in advanced cases, the R-T segment being depressed

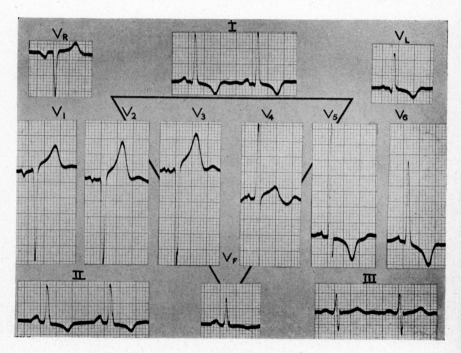

Fig. 3.15—Left ventricular preponderance.

and T inverted in leads V_5 and V_6, and the S-T segment being elevated and T sharply upright in leads V_1 and V_2 (fig. 3.15).

When the heart is horizontal, which is usual, V_L resembles V_5, and V_F resembles V_1 both in respect of QRS and T. The appearances in standard lead I therefore also resemble V_5 or V_6, and those in lead III resemble V_1.

When the heart is more or less vertical, which is less common, left ventricular surface potentials are transmitted more to the left leg. There is then no axis deviation in standard leads (Wilson, 1944), but high voltage and perhaps T wave inversion in all (fig. 3.16). Concordant left ventricular preponderance, as it is called, is best seen in concentric left ventricular hypertrophy, such as may occur in aortic stenosis and malignant hypertension.

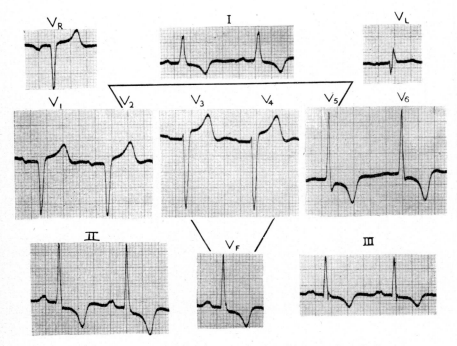

Fig. 3.16—Left ventricular preponderance (heart semi-vertical).

Right ventricular dominance

When there is gross enlargement of the right ventricle the potential differences generated by the wall of that chamber may approach or even surpass those from the left ventricle. Right ventricular surface leads may then truly represent the outward spread of the accession wave beneath the exploring electrode. After a small initial septal R wave a tall secondary R replaces the usual S wave in leads V_1 and V_2, and S is conspicuous in V_5 and V_6 (fig. 3.17). Secondary inversion of the T wave with slight depression of the R-T segment is common in V_1 to V_3. In lesser degrees of right ventricular hypertrophy, clockwise rotation about the longitudinal axis (viewed from below) is usually held responsible for the changes. Thus the occasional appearance of Q in lead V_1, followed by a tall R wave, may be derived from potentials at the back of the heart.

As a rule the heart is also vertical in position; V_L is strongly influenced by negative cavity potentials, and V_F by left or right ventricular surface potentials. In other words, QRS is mainly negative in V_L and strongly positive in V_F. Standard leads therefore show right axis deviation, and

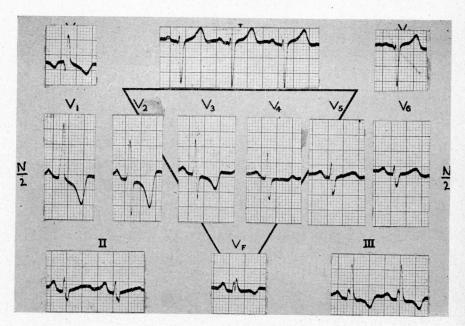

Fig. 3.17—Right ventricular dominance (case of pulmonary stenosis).

there may be inversion of the T wave with depression of the R-T segment in lead III, or in leads II and III. When R is dominant in V_1, and S in V_5, right axis deviation also occurs when the heart is horizontal, for V_L then reflects V_5, and V_F reflects V_1.

Widening of the QRS complex

The accepted maximum normal limit of 0.1 second for the duration of the QRS complex is generous, and includes many instances of abnormal widening due to increased thickness of the ventricular walls. As the accession wave causes almost instantaneous reversal of polarity in the tissue it excites, the width of QRS depends almost entirely on the thickness of the ventricular walls, provided the conducting system is normal, and assuming that the speed of the wave is constant. With extremely hypertrophied hearts it is theoretically possible for QRS to measure as much as 0.12 second in duration; but in fact it rarely exceeds 0.1 second. It is probably wise to regard anything over 0.11 second as intraventricular block. It is found, too, that widening due to ventricular hypertrophy is usually associated with high voltage; whereas in bundle branch block QRS is commonly notched, splintered, or heavily slurred. When the heart is grossly dilated, there may be some delay in the passage of the excitatory impulse down the Purkinje network, causing intraventricular block. Some such mechanism may account for the transient right "bundle branch block" that occurs occasionally in massive pulmonary embolism, and for the right "bundle branch block" so commonly seen with atrial septal defect. A Q wave can nearly always be demonstrated in suitable left ventricular surface leads when widening of the initial ventricular deflection is due to left ventricular hypertrophy, whereas it is ordinarily absent in left bundle branch block.

Widening of the QRS complex is also seen in uræmia, when it is due to a raised blood potassium (figs. 3.33 and 3.34).

Bundle branch block

In *left bundle branch block* the excitatory process spreads through the right ventricle in normal fashion but does not at first reach the left ventricle. As the interventricular septum is excited from the right side, the accession wave spreads through it from right to left. The cavity of the left ventricle therefore becomes initially positive, and this potential is transmitted passively to the surface as an R wave in V_5 or V_6. There can be no Q wave in such leads with a healthy septum. When the accession wave reaches the left side of the septum there is an immediate reversal of polarity, the left ventricular cavity becoming momentarily negative. This negativity is again transmitted passively to the surface, V_5 showing a momentary downward deflection following the initial R wave. Almost immediately, however, the excitatory process spreads throughout the endocardium of the left ventricle, and the accession wave begins to flow outwards in the usual way. The surface of the left ventricle then becomes actively positive and the true R wave is written. When the surface is activated the final intrinsic downward deflection occurs. V_5 or V_6 thus exhibits a large widened R wave interrupted by a relatively early notch representing the arrival of the accession wave at the left side of the septum (fig. 3.18). Right ventricular surface potentials are influenced at first by a normal right ventricular accession wave and later by the delayed negativity of the cavity of the left ventricle which is passively transmitted through the depolarised septum and right ventricle. Thus V_1–V_3 exhibit small R waves, early intrinsic deflections and deep wide S waves. The total duration of QRS commonly measures 0.12 to 0.16 second. As the heart is usually horizontal the V_5–V_6 pattern is seen also in V_L and lead I, and the V_1 pattern in V_F and lead III. Should the heart be vertical, however, the V_5–V_6 pattern is transmitted to the left leg, and the appearances in standard leads may be mistaken for right bundle branch block (fig. 3.18b). Whatever the position of the heart in left bundle branch block deviation of the RS-T segment and the direction of the T wave are usually of opposite sign to the main QRS deflection. Thus, with horizontal hearts the RS-T segment is depressed and the T wave inverted in V_5–V_6, V_L, and standard lead I.

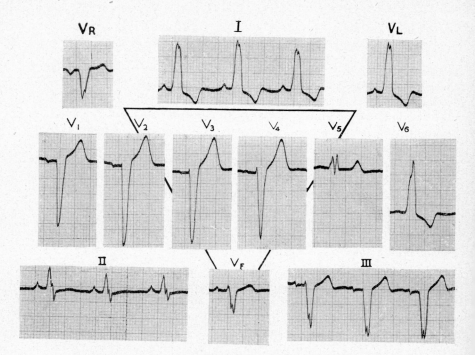

Fig. 3.18 (a)—Left bundle branch block (heart horizontal).

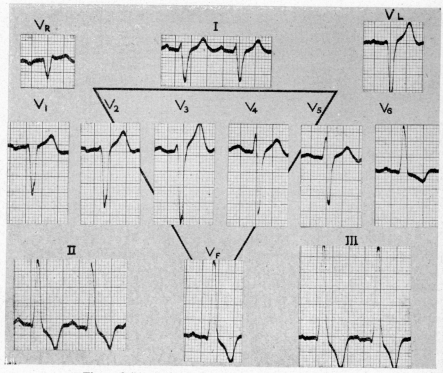

Fig. 3.18 (b)—Left bundle branch block (heart vertical).

Left bundle branch block may occur in diseases chiefly affecting the left ventricle, such as hypertensive heart disease, aortic stenosis, syphilitic aortic incompetence, and ischæmic heart disease; in non-rheumatic myocarditis, cardiac fibrosis, and generalised cardiopathy of almost any type; and occasionally in otherwise clinically normal hearts, although far less commonly than right bundle branch block.

In *right bundle branch block* the septum is activated entirely from the left side. The potential of the right ventricular cavity is therefore initially positive, and is passively transmitted to the surface where it may be recorded as the first part of R. When the accession wave reaches the right side of the septum, the polarity is abruptly reversed, and a pseudo-intrinsic deflection is recorded at the surface. Almost at once, however, the right ventricular wall is invaded, and the surface then becomes actively positive. This results in a second R wave and finally in the true intrinsic deflection. Leads V_1 and V_2 therefore show a widened notched R wave, or a large M complex. T is in the opposite direction (fig. 3.19a). Over the left ventricle in leads

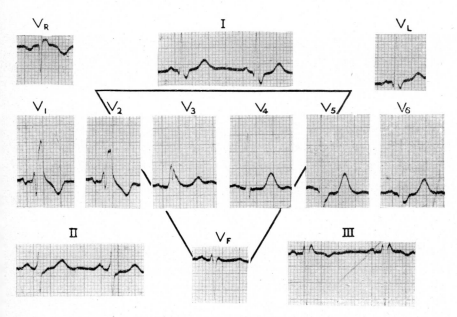

Fig. 3.19 (a)—Right bundle branch block (heart horizontal).

V_5 and V_6 a normal QR wave and intrinsic deflection are followed by a grossly slurred S wave representing delayed negativity of the right ventricular cavity passively transmitted through the depolarised septum and left ventricle. As a rule V_5 and V_6 potentials are transmitted to V_L and form the pattern of standard lead I; the M complex of V_1–V_2 is usually seen in V_F and in standard lead III. When the heart is vertical, however, V_1

potentials may be transmitted to V_L, and standard leads may look like left bundle branch block (fig. 3.19b). Multiple chest leads may be necessary, not only to determine which bundle branch is blocked, but also to detect the lesion at all in some cases: partial right bundle branch block, for instance, is frequently overlooked in standard leads. Right bundle branch

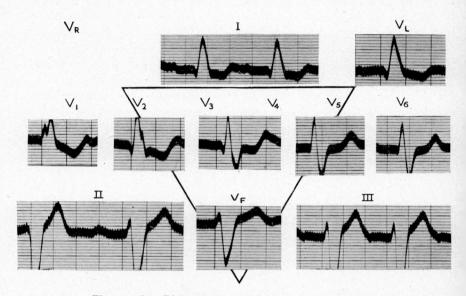

Fig. 3.19 (b)—Right bundle branch block (heart vertical).

block may occur in any of the diseases that may result in great dilatation of the right ventricle, particularly atrial septal defect and Ebstein's disease; in ischæmic heart disease and any of the generalised cardiopathies such as isolated myocarditis; and by no means rarely in otherwise normal hearts.

ABNORMALITIES OF THE RS-T SEGMENT AND T WAVE

It is profitable to consider the RS-T segment and T wave together, and in many cases to consider them also in relationship to the QRS complex, for they are all ventricular events. The various patterns made up by these three variables in limb and multiple chest leads provide a wealth of information concerning the state of the ventricles in health and disease. Secondary inversion of the T wave in relation to QRS changes has already been described.

Myocardial infarction

It is customary to describe two types of electrocardiogram associated with myocardial infarction, T_I and T_{III} types (Parkinson and Bedford, 1927), the first denoting anterior, the second posterior lesions (Barnes and

Whitten, 1929). There is no essential difference in the shape of these two patterns, the difference depending upon the leads in which they are found.

If an infarct involves the whole thickness of the muscle wall, no accession wave can flow through it. The negative cavity potential produced by outward spread of the accession wave through remote healthy muscle is then passively transmitted through the infarct to the surface overlying it. An electrode placed over the infarct therefore registers a monophasic Q wave.

If the infarct involves only the inner third of the myocardium, no electrocardiographic changes occur, for this zone is electrically silent (Prinzmetal et al., 1953).

If the outer layers are patchily involved QR complexes occur at the epicardial surface; the initial Q wave is due to transmission of the negative cavity potential, and the subsequent R wave to spread of the accession wave through patches of live muscle in the outer layers (Prinzmetal et al., 1954). R waves of this kind are usually of reduced voltage. In anterior left ventricular infarcts these QRS changes may be registered in leads V_3, V_4, V_5 and V_6, being more marked in V_3–V_4 in antero-septal infarcts, and in V_5–V_6 in antero-lateral infarcts. They are commonly transmitted to V_L and are therefore seen well in standard lead I (fig. 3.20). Similar QRS changes occur in posterior infarcts but are transmitted to V_F and thus to standard lead III (fig. 3.21). When the heart is vertical, however, typical changes in V_5 from an anterior infarct may be transmitted to lead V_F and hence to standard leads II and III (fig. 3.22).

According to Wilson et al. (1933), partly necrosed muscle sets up a steady current due to the development of potential differences between

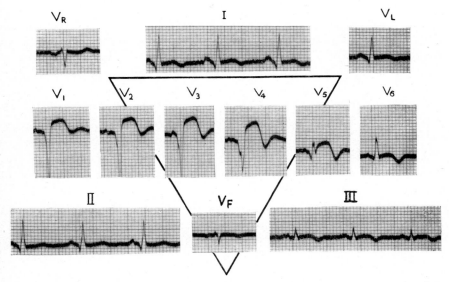

Fig. 3.20—Anterior myocardial infarction showing pathological Q waves and elevation of the RS-T segment in leads V_{1-6}, V_L and standard lead I.

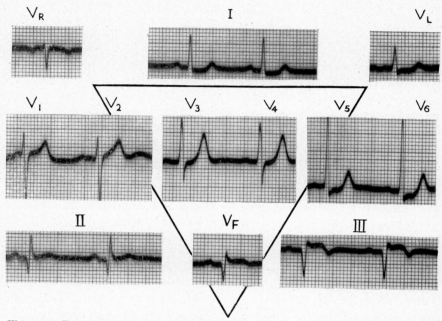

Fig. 3.21—Posterior myocardial infarction showing pathological Q waves and elevation of the RS-T segment in lead V_F and standard leads II and III.

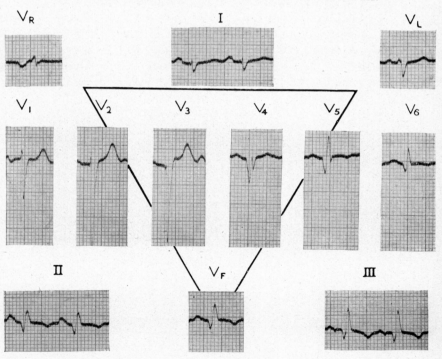

Fig. 3.22—Anterior infarction with vertical heart. Standard leads show changes that simulate those of posterior infarction.

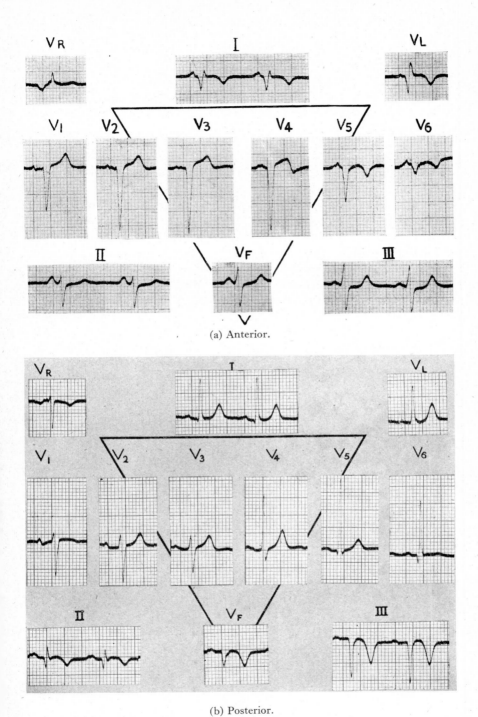

(a) Anterior.

(b) Posterior.

Fig. 3.23—Later stages of anterior (a), and posterior (b), infarction, showing typical Q waves and inversion of the T wave in appropriate leads.

injured and healthy tissue. Injured tissue is electro-negative, healthy tissue
is positive, and completely necrosed tissue electrically inert. When the
injured area involves the outer portion of the ventricular wall, the surface
is therefore negative, the current flowing from without inwards. An electrode placed over the infarct registers this negativity by depressing the
base line. This is shown in the electrocardiogram by abrupt elevation of
the base line when the current of injury is momentarily abolished by
spread of the accession wave through the healthy tissue; for such activation
causes the healthy tissue to take up a negative potential, and so abolishes
the potential differences set up by the injury. In other words, superficial
injury results in elevation of the RS-T segment. In anterior infarcts this
displacement is seen in leads V_3–V_6, and is commonly transmitted to V_L
and hence to standard lead I (fig. 3.20). In posterior infarcts it is seen in
low œsophageal leads, in V_7, and is transmitted to V_F and hence to
standard lead III (fig. 3.21).

This classic theory has been challenged by Prinzmetal (1954) on the
grounds that intramural electrodes from healthy myocardium adjacent to
a fresh infarct do not show depression of the S-T segment as they should
do if there is a current of injury flowing across the boundary zone from the
electrically negative injured tissue to electrically positive healthy muscle;
instead, the S-T segment from adjacent areas is normal. Again, the S-T
segment from surface electrodes overlying a subendocardial infarct is

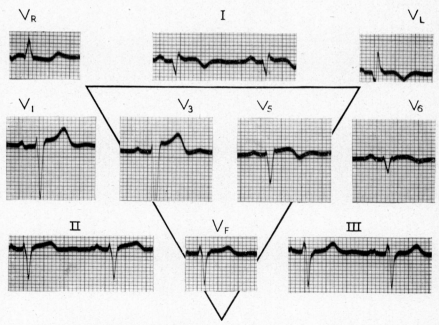

Fig. 3.24—Anterior myocardial infarction showing an R wave which is smaller in V_3 to
V_6 than in V_1.

normal, not depressed. Elevation of the S-T segment is always recorded when the intramural electrode is situated anywhere within the injured zone, and is maximum at the centre. Reciprocal depression occurs over the opposite wall of the ventricle.

Pathological Q waves may be seen in acute cases within a few hours of the onset, and usually outlast all other evidence of infarction, often being permanent. Elevation of the RS-T segment occurs even earlier, but usually subsides within two or three weeks. The shape of the segment is typical, being straight instead of concave when initially elevated, and being convex or cove-shaped (Pardee, 1920) when the RS-T junction approaches or regains the iso-potential level. The T wave itself becomes inverted within a few days of the onset, often profoundly so, reaching its greatest amplitude at about the same time that the RS-T junction first regains the iso-potential level (fig. 3.23 a and b). Further changes are regressive, but the appearances rarely revert to normal.

In T_I patterns reciprocal effects are usually observed in lead III, i.e. the RS-T segment may be depressed at first, and T may be sharply upright later. Again, in posterior infarcts early RS-T depression and later accentuation of the T wave may often be seen in lead 1 and in anterior chest leads. A helpful sign of old anterior infarction is an R wave in V_1–V_2 which is taller than that in V_3–V_4 (fig. 3.24), especially when the appearances in V_5–V_6 are more or less normal. Finally, it is most important to understand that characteristic changes may be found in multiple chest leads or in an œsophageal lead when the standard limb leads are normal, and that a single chest lead may be normal when others show diagnostic features.

Pericarditis. In all types of generalised pericardial disease, except hydropericardium, superficial epicardial involvement may cause a current of injury to flow from the surface towards the underlying healthy muscle: in other words, the surface of the heart develops a negative potential. The situation, therefore, resembles that in superficial myocardial infarction, but the lesion is general instead of local. Thus, in the initial stages, elevation of the RS-T segment may be seen in all chest leads, in both V_L and V_F, and therefore in all standard leads (fig. 3.25a). Unlike most records of acute myocardial infarction, the RS-T segment remains concave. As the underlying muscle is healthy there are no pathological Q waves. After a few days the RS-T segment regains the iso-potential level and the T wave becomes inverted (fig. 3.25b). Upward coving of the RS-T segment does not occur. If pericarditis is localised the changes described may be confined to corresponding leads, but few important forms of pericarditis remain localised for long. Serial records nearly always reveal what may be called the T_{II} pattern in contrast to the T_I or T_{III} types of myocardial infarction. Low voltage QRS complexes usually indicate pericardial effusion. The electrocardiogram returns to normal as the pericarditis recovers.

In *chronic constrictive pericarditis*, flattened or inverted T waves in all

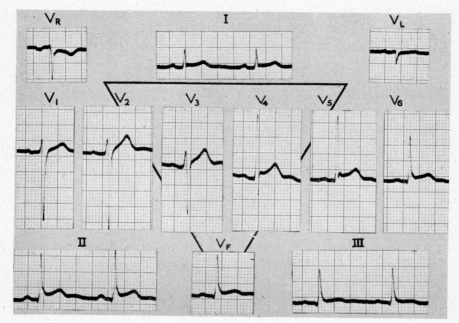

(a) Early stage, showing elevation of the RS-T segment in leads V₄–V₆, V_F, and all standard leads.

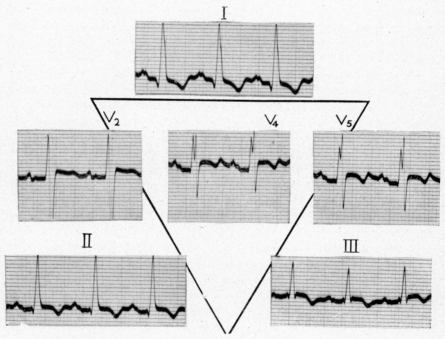

(b) Late stage, showing inversion of the T wave in all standard leads.

Fig. 3.25—Pericarditis.

leads are permanent, and are usually associated with low-voltage QRS complexes (fig. 3.26). Not infrequently the P waves are widened and relatively prominent.

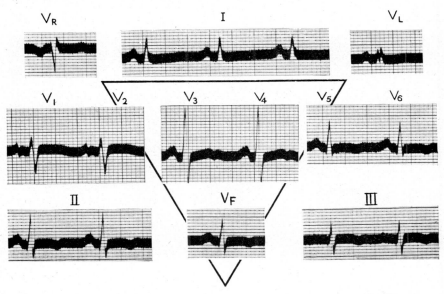

Fig. 3.26—Chronic constrictive pericarditis, showing low voltage and flat T waves.

Digitalis T wave pattern

Digitalis depresses the RS-T segment and shortens the Q-T interval. At first, the RS-T junction is depressed and there is gentle sagging of the RS-T segment, T remaining upright (fig. 3.27a). In the second stage sagging is more marked and the peak of T can no longer be discerned. In extreme digitalisation the RS-T segment becomes a straight line, sloping downwards from its depressed origin to a blunt peak (fig. 3.27b).

In normal hearts these effects are seen in all leads, but especially in lead V_5 and standard lead II. When the heart is electrically horizontal they are seen best in V_5, V_L, and standard lead I; when it is electrically vertical they are best seen in V_5, V_F, and standard lead III. When the left ventricle is enlarged and the heart horizontal the changes occur more markedly in V_5, V_L and standard lead I, and the RS-T segment may be elevated and upwardly convex in V_1, V_F and standard lead III. When the right ventricle is enlarged they may be most conspicuous in V_1, V_F and standard lead III, and the RS-T segment may be elevated and upwardly convex in V_5, V_L and standard lead I.

Anoxic T waves

Electrocardiograms taken from patients during an attack of angina pectoris may show transient depression of the RS-T segment (fig. 3.28)

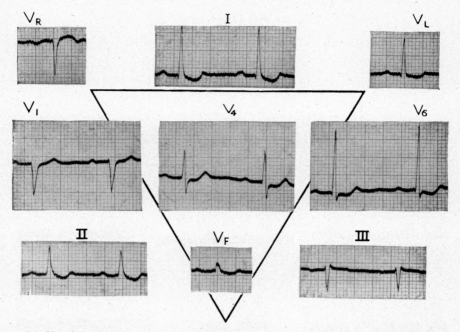

(a) Showing sagging of the RS-T segment and shortening of Q-Tc to 0.33 second.

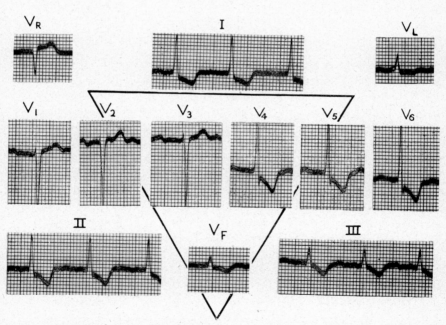

(b) Showing gross depression of the RS-T segment or an inverted T wave with a straight proximal limb; Q-Tc is shortened to 0.36 second.

Fig. 3.27—The affect of digitalis on the electrocardiogram: (a) slight, (b) marked.

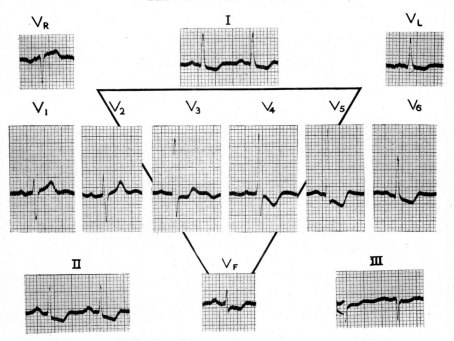

Fig. 3.28—Depression of the RS-T segment during an attack of angina pectoris.

with or without inversion of the U wave (fig. 3.29). Similar records may be associated with carbon monoxide poisoning, vasomotor syncope, asphyxia, and severe hæmorrhage. In all these conditions there is myocardial hypoxia. In carbon monoxide poisoning the changes may last for a week or two, and there may be true T wave inversion (fig. 3.30). Transient depression of the RS-T segment in all leads may be induced in many normal individuals, and especially in those with ischæmic heart disease, by causing them to breathe 10 per cent oxygen (Levy *et al.*, 1938). Exertion may have a similar effect in patients with angina pectoris. The depression has been attributed to a steady current of injury flowing from the inner layers of the myocardium towards the surface, so that the base-line of the electrocardiogram is positively displaced. When the electrical field is momentarily abolished by the spread of the accession wave, the base-line temporarily subsides to its

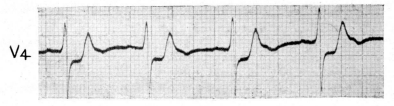

Fig. 3.29—Inversion of the U wave during an attack of angina pectoris.

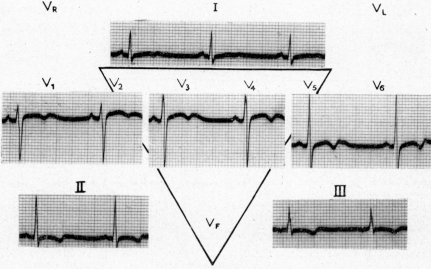

Fig. 3.30—Carbon monoxide poisoning.

normal level, resulting in depression of the S-T segment. Impairment of coronary blood flow leading to anoxic injury is supposed to be maximal in the deeper layers of the myocardium because the intra-myocardial pressure is highest in this situation, so that there is no coronary flow during systole; near the surface coronary flow continues during systole, and so insures a better supply of oxygen to the superficial myocardium.

According to Prinzmetal (1954), however, ischæmic depression of the S-T segment is more likely to be due to functional changes in the outer layers of the myocardium.

Permanent depression of the RS-T segment in left ventricular surface leads or their equivalents may be seen in a minority of cases with severe ischæmic heart disease, and in some cases of severe chronic anæmia. In the latter the QRS voltage is usually lowered.

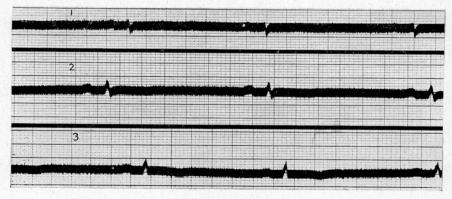

Fig. 3.31—Myxœdema.

Myxœdema pattern. Flat or inverted T waves in all leads are characteristic of myxœdema (fig. 3.31). In such cases the voltage of QRS is usually
below 6 millimetres in the most favourable standard lead, and there is often
bradycardia. Similar appearances may be found in chronic constrictive
pericarditis, in long-standing cases of severe anæmia, particularly pernicious, and in anoxic chronic pulmonary heart disease; but in these there
is commonly tachycardia. In severe cases of ischæmic heart disease with

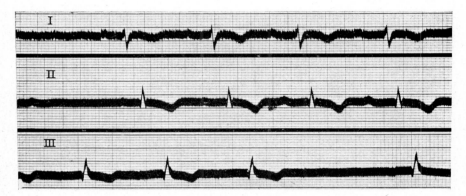

Fig. 3.32—Pneumonic carditis. There is partial heart block with dropped beats and
inversion of the T wave in all leads.

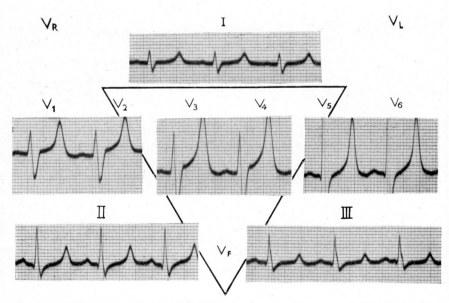

Fig. 3.33—High voltage sharply peaked T waves in uræmia associated with a high blood
potassium. The long Q-T interval is due to hypocalcæmia. Widening of QRS, due to
potassium, is well seen in the chest leads.

repeated myocardial infarction somewhat similar graphs may be encountered. Indeed, when the whole heart is involved in any disease, and when
recurrent heart failure has occurred, the voltage of QRS may be low, and
the T waves flat or slightly inverted in all leads, whatever the etiology.

Carditis pattern

In any form of carditis, but especially in diphtheria and least frequently
in acute rheumatism, simple inversion of the T waves may occur, and may
favour any lead (fig. 3.32). The RS-T segment may be normal or depressed.
The voltage of QRS is usually normal.

Potassium T wave

In uræmia, when the blood potassium is high, unusually sharp T waves
of high voltage are often seen (fig. 3.33). Similar T waves may be produced
in normal subjects by raising the blood potassium to about 25 mg. per
cent by giving 10 to 20 G. of potassium acetate by mouth.* A high blood
potassium also tends to rectify many forms of inverted T wave (fig. 3.34),
but not those due to myocardial infarction, which may be exaggerated

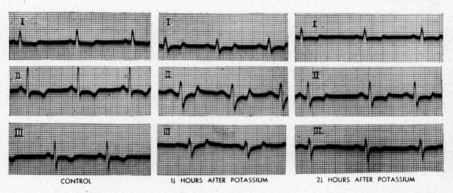

CONTROL   1¼ HOURS AFTER POTASSIUM   2¼ HOURS AFTER POTASSIUM

Fig. 3.34—Effect of potassium on the T waves in a case of concordant left ventricular
preponderance. The QRS complex is also widened.

(Sharpey-Schafer, 1943). Widening of P and QRS is also due to potassium
and is seen in both illustrations.

When the blood potassium is unduly low ($<$12 mg. per cent.) the S-T
segment and T wave may be depressed, and the P-R interval and Q-T$_C$
prolonged (Perelson and Cosby, 1949).

* This procedure is dangerous.

REFERENCES

Ashman, R. (1948): "The physiological and physical aspects of the electro-cardiogram." "The Chest and the Heart"; ed. by Myers, J. A., and McKinlay, C. N.; Vol. II, p. 1421.

—— and Byer, E. (1943): "The normal human ventricular gradient. I. Factors which affect its direction and its relation to the mean QRS axis", *Amer. Heart J.*, **25**, 16.

——, —— (1943): "The normal human ventricular gradient. II. Factors which affect its manifest area and its relationship to the manifest area of the QRS complex", *Ibid.*, **25**, 36.

Barnes, A. R., and Whitten, M. B. (1929): "A study of the R-T interval in myo-cardial infarction", *Ibid.*, **5**, 142.

Bayley, R. H. (1943): "On certain applications of modern electrocardiographic theory to the interpretation of electrocardiograms which indicate myocardial disease", *Ibid.*, **26**, 769.

Bazett, H. C. (1920): "An analysis of the time relations of the electrocardio-gram", *Heart*, 7, 353.

Bell, G. H., Knox, J. A. C., and Small, A. J. (1939): "Electrocardiograph electrolytes", *Brit. Heart J.*, **1**, 229.

Berconsky, I., and Kloztman, M. (1945): "Significado de ciertas alteraciones de la onda P del electrocardiogram: P de bajo voltaje", ancha y bifida, *Medicina*, **5**, 347.

Craib, W. H. (1930): "The electrocardiogram", M.R.C. Special Report Series, No. 147, London.

Curtis, H. J., and Cole, K. S. (1941): "Membrane resting and action potentials of the squid giant axon", *Amer. J. Physiol.*, **133**, 254.

Duchosal, P. W., and Sulzer, R. (1949): "La Vectocardiographie. Méthode d'exploration du champ électrique créé dans le corps humain par les courants d'action du cœur dans les conditions normales et pathologiques", S. Karger, Basle.

Einthoven, W. (1903): "Die galvanometrische Registrirung des menschlichen elektrokardiogramms, zugleich eine Beurtheilung der Anwendung des Capillar-elektrometers in der Physiologie", *Pfluger's Arch.f.d.ges. Physiol.*, **99**, 472.

Goldberger, E. (1942): "A simple indifferent electrocardiographic electrode of zero potential and a technique of obtaining augmented unipolar extremity leads", *Amer. Heart J.*, **23**, 483.

—— (1947): "Unipolar lead electrocardiography", London.

Jenks, J. L., and Graybiel, A. (1935): "Electrode Jelly", *Amer. Heart J.*, **10**, 693.

Kölliker, A., and Müller, H. (1856): "Nachweis der negativen Schwankung des muskelstroms am naturlich sich contrahiranden muskel", *Verhandl. d. phy. med. Gesell. i. Wurzburg*, **6**, 528.

Levy, R. L., Barach, A. L., and Bruenn, H. G. (1938): "Effects of induced oxygen want in patients with cardiac pain", *Amer. Heart J.*, **15**, 187.

Lewis, T. (1925): "The mechanism and graphic registration of the heart beat", London, 3rd ed.

Mann, H. (1920): "Method of analyzing the electrocardiogram", *Arch. intern. Med.*, **25**, 283.

—— (1931): "Interpretation of bundle-branch block by means of monocardio-gram", *Amer. Heart J.*, **6**, 447.

Pardee, H. E. B. (1920): "An electrocardiographic sign of coronary artery ob-struction", *Arch. intern. Med.*, **26**, 244.

Parkinson, J., and Bedford, D. E. (1927): "Successive changes in the electro-cardiogram after cardiac infarction (coronary thrombosis)", *Heart*, **14**, 195.

Perelson, H. N., and Cosby, R. S. (1949): "The electrocardiogram in familial periodic paralysis", *Amer. Heart J.*, **37**, 1126.

Præcordial Leads in Electrocardiography (1938): A joint memorandum of a Committee of the Cardiac Society of Gt. Britain and Ireland, and the Committee of the Amer. Heart Ass., *Brit. med. J.*, i, 187.

Prinzmetal, M., *et al.* (1953): "Intramural depolarization potentials in myocardial infarction. A preliminary report", *Circulation*, 7, 1.

——, *et al.* (1954): "Studies on the mechanism of ventricular activity, XII. Early changes in the RS-T segment and QRS complex following acute coronary artery occlusion", *Amer. Heart J.*, 48, 351.

Reynolds, G. (1953): "The atrial electrogram in mitral stenosis", *Brit. Heart J.*, 15, 250.

Robb, J. S., and Robb, R. C. (1938): "Abnormal distribution of the superficial muscle bundles in the human heart", *Amer. Heart J.*, 15, 597.

Schlamowitz, I. (1946): "An analysis of the time relationships within the cardiac cycle in electrocardiograms of normal man", *Ibid.*, 31, 329.

Sharpey-Schafer, E. P. (1943): "Potassium effects on T-wave inversion in myocardial infarction and preponderance of a ventricle", *Brit. Heart J.*, 5, 80.

Standardisation of Præcordial Leads; Supplementary Report by the Committee of the Amer. Heart Ass. (1938): *Amer. Heart J.*, 15, 235.

Taran, L. M., and Szilagyi, N. (1947): "The duration of the electrical systole (QT) in acute rheumatic carditis in children", *Amer. Heart J.*, 33, 14.

Van Lingen, B. (1947): "Electrocardiographic, radiological, venous pressure, circulation time, and exercise tolerance test studies in the diagnosis of heart disease", being a thesis submitted for the degree of Doctor of Medicine of the University of Witwatersrand, Johannesburg.

Waller, A. D. (1887): "A demonstration on man of electromotive changes accompanying the heart's beat", *J. Physiol.*, 8, 229.

Wilson, F. N. (1930): "The distribution of the potential differences produced by the heart beat within the body and at its surface", *Amer. Heart J.*, 5, 599.

——, and Johnston, F. D. (1938): "The vectorcardiogram", *Ibid.*, 16, 14.

——, ——, Macleod, A. G., and Barker, P. S. (1934): "Electrocardiograms that represent the potential variations of a single electrode", *Ibid.*, 9, 447.

——, ——, Rosenbaum, F. F., and Barker, P. S. (1946): "On Einthoven's triangle, the theory of unipolar electrocardiographic leads, and the interpretation of the precordial electrocardiogram", *Ibid.*, 32, 277.

——, Macleod, A. G., and Barker, P. S. (1931): "The interpretation of the initial deflections of the ventricular complex of the electrocardiogram", *Ibid.*, 6, 637.

——, ——, —— (1931): "The T-deflection of the electrocardiogram", *Tr. Ass. Am. Physicians*, 46, 29.

——, ——, —— (1933): "The distribution of the currents of action and of injury displayed by heart muscle and other excitable tissues", Ann Arbor.

——, ——, ——, Johnston, F. G. (1934): "The determination and the significance of the areas of the ventricular deflections of the electrocardiogram", *Amer Heart J.*, 10, 46.

——, *et al.* (1944): "The precordial electrocardiogram", *Ibid.*, 27, 19.

Wolferth, C. C., and Wood, F. C. (1932): "The electrocardiographic diagnosis of coronary occlusion by the use of chest leads", *Amer. J. med. Sci.*, 183, 30.

——, —— (1932): "Further observations upon the use of chest leads in the electrocardiographic study of coronary occlusion", *M. Clin. North America*, 16, 161.

——, —— (1932): "An electrocardiographic study of experimental coronary occlusion: the inadequacy of the three conventional leads in recording certain characteristic changes in action current", *J. clin. Invest.*, 11, 815.

——, —— (1933): "Experimental coronary occlusion", *Arch. intern. Med.*, 51, 771.

Wood, P. H., and Selzer, A. (1939): "Chest leads in clinical electrocardiography" *Brit. Heart J.*, 1, 49.

——, —— (1939): "A new sign of left ventricular failure", *Ibid.*, 1, 81.

CHAPTER IV

RADIOGRAPHIC DIAGNOSIS

TECHNIQUE

THERE are, at present, six radiological methods applicable to cardiology: fluoroscopy, orthodiagraphy, teleradiography, kymography, tomography, and angiocardiography. Fluoroscopy (screening) is a routine diagnostic procedure; orthodiagraphy is the construction of a simple tracing of the size and shape of the heart in any specified position, as a supplement to fluoroscopy; teleradiography is more accurate and should be preferred when facilities permit; kymography records the character and amplitude of cardiac pulsation; tomography is sectional radiography; angiocardiography is the study of individual cardiac chambers or vessels with the aid of intravascular contrast media.

FLUOROSCOPY

With modern X-ray equipment a remarkably clear view of the heart may be obtained. The patient should be stripped to the waist and pressed close to the viewing screen. The diaphragm, which controls the diameter of the beam emitted from the X-ray tube, is first opened wide, in order to view the thoracic contents as a whole. In this preliminary survey attention is paid to the lungs, to the costophrenic angles, and to the general size and shape of the heart. The diaphragm is then constricted so that only the heart can be seen, and the latter is observed more critically. The size, shape, and pulsation of each part should be noted in regular sequence. On the right side (fig. 4.01), a faint, slightly concave line, representing the superior vena cava, descends from the sterno-clavicular region, close to the shadow of the

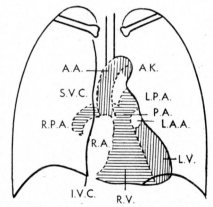

Fig. 4.01—Diagram of postero-anterior view of the heart as seen fluoroscopically.
A.A.   Ascending aorta;
A.K.   Aortic knuckle;
I.V.C. Inferior vena cava;
L.A.A. Left atrial appendage;
L.V.   Left ventricle;
P.A.   Pulmonary artery;
R.A.   Right atrium;
R.V.   Right ventricle;
S.V.C. Superior vena cava.

vertebral column, until it meets the ascending aorta, which both displaces it to the right and causes it to become convex. Below is the border of the right atrium, which usually meets the diaphragm at a slightly acute angle. The left border of the normal heart is made up of three convex curves: from above downwards, these are the aortic knob or knuckle, the pulmonary arc, and the contour of the left ventricle. Between the last two there is a small neutral segment or point of opposing movement which marks the left atrial appendage; above it the pulmonary artery expands during systole, while below the left ventricle contracts. The hilar shadows are chiefly vascular: the right pulmonary artery may be seen dividing early into upper and lower branches, the former being indistinct, the latter sweeping downwards in a well-defined arc; the left limb of the pulmonary artery forms the main pulmonary arc described above.

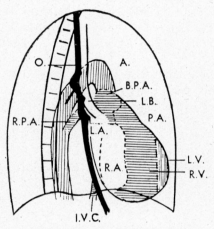

Fig. 4.02 (a)—Diagram of right anterior oblique view of the heart as seen fluoroscopically (1st oblique position).

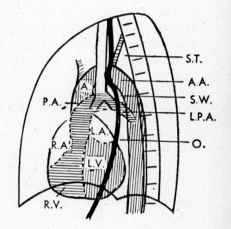

Fig. 4.02 (b)—Diagram of left anterior oblique view of the heart as seen fluoroscopically (2nd oblique position).

A.	Aortic arch;		L.P.A.	Left pulmonary artery;
B.P.A.	Bifurcation of the pulmonary artery;		L.V.	Left ventricle;
			R.A.	Right atrium;
I.V.C.	Inferior vena cava;		R.P.A.	Right pulmonary artery;
L.A.	Left atrium;		R.V.	Right ventricle;
L.B.	Left bronchus;		S.T.	Supra-aortic triangle;
P.A.	Pulmonary arc;		S.W.	Sub-aortic window.
O.	Barium-filled œsophagus.			

The patient is then turned into the first, or right anterior, oblique position. The observer should place his gloved hands on the patient's hips, and manually rotate him (so that the right shoulder is brought to the front) until the position is satisfactory. The arms should be extended; the left forwards and outwards, the right backwards and outwards. In this view (fig. 4.02a) the ventricular shadows are superimposed and the right atrium is rotated towards the front, so that little can be learned about these three chambers; on the other hand, the left atrium is outlined clearly, as it forms the upper part of the posterior border of the heart. Just anterior to the top of the left atrial curve, a rather dense round shadow may be seen, due to the bifurcation of the pulmonary artery; it is connected with the anterior ventricular border by a convex line representing the root of the pulmonary artery and conus of the right ventricle. Above it are the superimposed shadows of the ascending and descending parts of the aortic arch. If the patient is made to swallow a barium emulsion of the consistency of thick cream, the œsophagus is outlined at the back of the heart; under favourable conditions it is indented in turn by the arch of the aorta, by the pulmonary artery and left bronchus, and by the left atrium. The left bronchus may be seen between the œsophagus and the rounded shadow of the dividing pulmonary artery. Between the œsophagus and the vertebral column there should be a translucent space.

In the second, or left anterior, oblique position (fig. 4.02b), the patient is turned to the right through an angle of about 45 degrees, the left shoulder being brought forwards. In this view the two ventricles appear side by side, the left forming the posterior border of the heart shadow and the right the anterior, so that their contours can be readily compared. The shadow of the right atrium overlaps that of the right ventricle; the shadow of the left atrium lies posteriorly above the left ventricle. Cranially, the aorta and pulmonary artery may be seen as two arches, one above the other, separated by a light-space known as the sub-aortic window, and crossed by the translucent trachea and left bronchus. The aortic arch and descending aorta are well defined and shaped like an inverted J; but the pulmonary artery is less distinct. Above the aorta is another light-space, the supra-aortic triangle, bounded by the vertebral column posteriorly, by the left subclavian artery anteriorly, and by the aortic arch below. The barium-filled œsophagus is deflected to the patient's right as it crosses the aortic arch, then lies in close relation to a short segment of the descending aorta, leaves that vessel at about the level of the pulmonary artery, and courses downwards and to the subject's right across the shadow of the left ventricle.

ORTHODIAGRAPHY

Clips should be fitted to the viewing screen to enable tracing paper to be held firmly in position. To make an accurate tracing of the heart shadow, or orthodiagram, special attention should be paid to five points. First, the position of the patient must be properly adjusted to the view required; he must be pressed firmly against the screen; and he should hold on to some support so that he can remain still. Second, the tracing should be made in mid-inspiration, and as it cannot be completed in one period of breath-holding, lines which move with respiration should be checked more than once. Third, to avoid distortion the cardiac outline must be traced by means of parallel rays: this is accomplished by constricting the diaphragm to the smallest aperture consistent with adequate visualisation. Fourth, the greatest accuracy must be maintained when tracing the interior thoracic wall at its widest point, and the lateral borders of the cardiac shadow, so that the cardio-thoracic ratio is reliable. Fifth, the finished orthodiagram should be checked against the shadows traced to make sure the patient has not moved during the procedure.

Fluoroscopes suitable for cardioscopy are so constructed that the X-ray tube may be moved easily in any direction by the lever which operates the diaphragm. In making the tracing, the small light-spot is run swiftly over the contours of the heart, great vessels, clavicles, interior thoracic wall, and diaphragm. With experience it may be completed very quickly, without danger of over-exposing the patient or over-heating the tube; nevertheless, a good technician switches off the current whenever momentarily disengaged. Fluoroscopy and orthodiagraphy are usually carried out with a power of 60 kilovolts and a current of 3 to 4 milliamps.; but with obese subjects it may be necessary to step-up the kilovolts to 65 or 70, in order to obtain sufficient penetration. Tracings are made with a wax pencil; and it is helpful to add signs denoting the degree and direction of pulsation of important chambers and vessels.

TELERADIOGRAPHY

Skiagrams of the heart are always taken at a tube-screen distance of at least 6 feet, preferably 7 feet, to avoid distortion by diverging rays. The duration of exposure used to be half a second, to ensure a diastolic record; nowdays, however, it is commonly 0.1 second, and this has introduced a source of error in interpreting serial skiagrams, for one may be taken in systole, another in diastole, and the difference between the two may be appreciable. The difficulty may be overcome by using a device whereby one of the electrocardiographic complexes, such as R, determines the moment of exposure. Skiagrams of the oblique views are best taken when the most informative degree of rotation has been ascertained by previous fluoroscopy. The normal appearances are illustrated in figure 4.03.

KYMOGRAPHY

A specially constructed kymograph may be attached to a teleradiograph for the purpose of recording cardiac pulsation (Stumpf, 1931). A lead screen, containing horizontal slits 11 mm. apart, is interposed between the film and the patient's chest, and made to descend 1 cm. during one complete cardiac cycle. The timing of the exposure is adjusted to synchronise with the descent of the grid. In kymograms so obtained, the lateral borders of the heart and great vessels appear toothed, like the edge of a saw (fig. 4.04), the ventricular crests representing diastole, the troughs systole. Pulsation is recorded in only one dimension, i.e. in a plane parallel to the film; but if the three standard views are photographed, the records are sufficiently comprehensive.

The electrokymograph is a device for securing an accurate graphic record of pulsation at any point on the cardiac border (Henny and Boone, 1947). A photosensitive pick-up unit is placed between the patient and the screen so that the lead slit aperture lies across the border of the

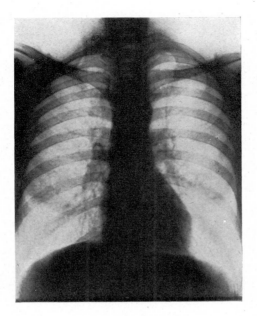

(a) Postero-anterior view.

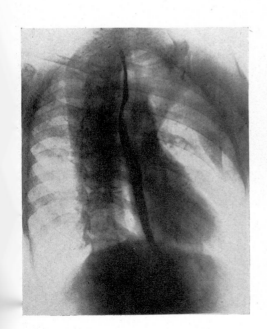

(b) 1st oblique position (right anterior).

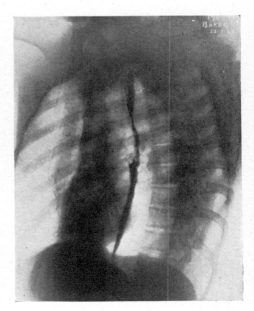

(c) 2nd oblique position (left anterior).

Fig. 4.03—Teleradiogram of a normal subject.

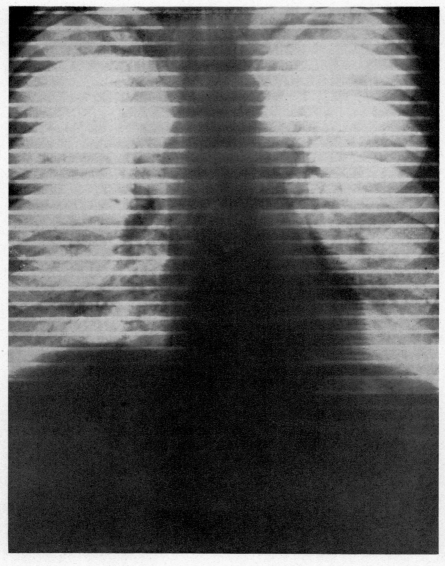

Fig. 4.04—Normal kymogram (P.A. view).

(By courtesy of Dr. Jenner Hoskin.)

122

heart at the point where it is desired to record pulsation. The amount of light transmitted through the aperture varies with the movements of the cardiac border, and is recorded graphically by means of a galvanometer operated by the photo-electric cell (fig. 4.05). The interpretation of the graph is assisted by a simultaneous jugular phlebogram or electrocardiogram.

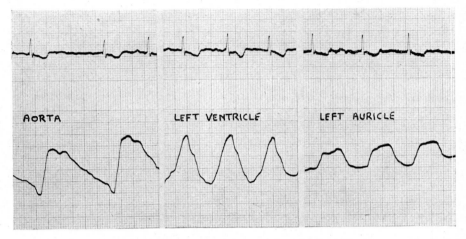

Fig. 4.05—Electrokymogram from aorta, left ventricle and left atrium in a case of mitral stenosis and incompetence with auricular fibrillation.

Neither kymography nor electrokymography have fulfilled earlier expectations. The former is too crude to be helpful, and the latter too dependent upon the precise position of the slit in relation to the cardiac border being studied, so that minor variations in the relationship may alter the graph profoundly.

TOMOGRAPHY

Body section radiography was introduced by Ziedses Des Plantes (1932), and others working independently, to give radiological information about the lung and major bronchi when these were obscured by thoracoplasty, pleural effusion or other large space-filling lesion. The technique was developed in Berlin by Chaoul and Grossmann (1935) and consists essentially of an arrangement whereby the X-ray tube and film move through an arc in opposite directions during the period of exposure. Only the plane focused is seen sharply, structures anterior or posterior to it being blurred.

Although tomography has been used very little in cardiology, it may be helpful in demonstrating coarctation of the aorta (Twining, 1937), calcified valves (Davies and Steiner, 1949), metallic foreign bodies in the heart, arteriovenous aneurysm of the lung, and anomalous pulmonary veins. It is also helpful in distinguishing dilatation or aneurysm of the pulmonary artery or aorta from other mediastinal masses.

Horizontal body section radiography has been used effectively by Stevenson (1950) to demonstrate a double aortic arch and other lesions or anomalies of the aorta.

ANGIOCARDIOGRAPHY

If a sufficient quantity of a radio-opaque solution is introduced rapidly into the venous circulation, its consecutive passage through the right heart, pulmonary circulation, left heart, aorta and major arteries may be recorded by means of serial skiagrams (Castellanos *et al.*, 1938). The technique was elaborated by Robb and Steinberg (1938, 1939), who used 20 to 60 ml. of 70 per cent aqueous solution of diodrast. A mechanical rapid casette changer enabled serial skiagrams to be taken at a rate of two per second (Sussman, Steinberg and Grishman, 1941); others preferred serial fluoro-photographs obtained by means of a special camera or cinematograph (Stewart, Breimer and Maier, 1941).

At the time of writing the best contrast medium is a 70 per cent solution of diaginol, the sodium salt of 3-acetylamino-2 : 4 : 6-triiodobenzoic acid, which contains 66 per cent of iodine. Patients are best lying down, and should be given a preliminary dose of 1 ml. to test for hypersensitivity; if there is no urticarial reaction within half an hour serious hypersensitivity to iodine is unlikely. Premedication varies in different clinics, but a combination of omnopon gr. 1/6 to 1/3, or pethidine 50 to 100 mg. and the

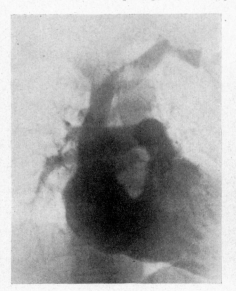

Fig. 4.06—Normal angiocardiogram of right heart, postero-anterior view.

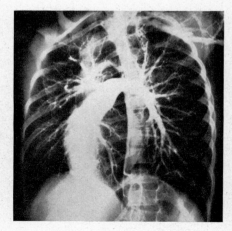

Fig. 4.07—Normal angiocardiogram of the right side of the heart, second oblique position.

anti-histaminic phenergan 25 to 50 mg. has proved satisfactory; the latter is an additional sedative and combats both hypersensitivity reactions to iodine and vomiting from omnopon or pethidine. Chlorpromazine is too strong a vasodilator. An anæsthetic apparatus for delivering oxygen under positive pressure should always be available in cyanotic cases of congenital heart disease, and adrenalin should be handy in cases of serious hypersensitivity.

A good cannula, 6 to 9 inches long, may be made from wide bore polythene tubing. This is inserted into the antecubital vein and tied in position, the proximal end being connected temporarily with a saline

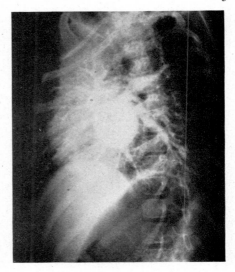

Fig. 4.08—Angiocardiogram showing pulmonary veins and left atrium.

drip or simple syringe. When all is ready 30 to 50 ml. of diaginol, warmed to blood heat, is drawn into a strong 50 ml. syringe and injected through the cannula as rapidly as possible, preferably in about two seconds.

Modern angriocardiographs are designed to take serial films at a rate of about four per second in postero-anterior and lateral views simultaneously. The right atrium is usually well filled 1.5 seconds after the start of the

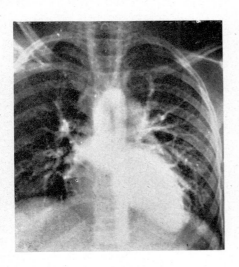

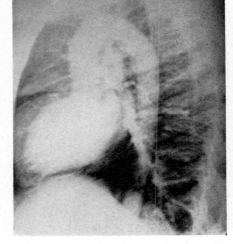

(a) Postero-anterior.   (b) Second oblique.

Fig. 4.09—Normal angiocardiograms of the left side of the heart.

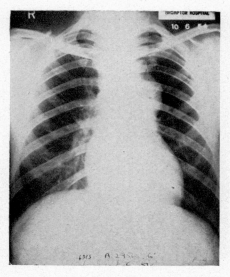

(a) Skiagram showing a mass between the aortic knuckle and the pulmonary artery.

injection, the right ventricle and pulmonary artery in 2 to 3 seconds, the left atrium in about 5 seconds, and the left ventricle and aorta in 6 to 9 seconds (figs. 4.06 to 4.09).

The patient experiences a sensation of extreme heat, but it passes rapidly. The arrival of contrast medium in the lungs may excite a cough, and nausea may follow. The chief dangers, however, apart from hypersensitivity to iodine, are syncope, due to a sharp fall in blood pressure resulting from general vasodilatation, as recorded by Howarth (1950), sudden respiratory arrest, and bronchospasm. The combination of these adverse reactions may prove rapidly fatal in cyanotic cases of congenital heart disease, for they may result in profound anoxia and secondary collapse of the basal centres. Dangerous interference with the coronary circulation may also result from the sharp fall in blood pressure (Lawson, 1945). The

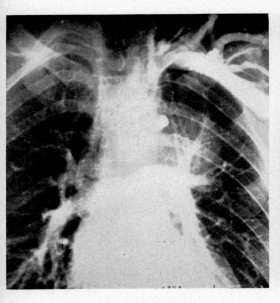

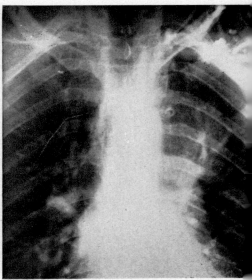

(b) Angiocardiogram showing normal pulmonary arteries, distinct from the mass.

(c) Angiocardiogram showing normal aorta disti from the mass.

Fig. 4.10—Angiocardiographic proof that a mediastinal shadow was extra vascular.

total mortality rate amongst 6,824 angiocardiographic examinations collected from the main investigatory clinics of the U.S.A., Canada, Great Britain and Sweden by Dotter and Jackson (1950) was 0.38 per cent. The best treatment for acute pulmonary œdema due to iodine sensitivity is intravenous hydrocortisone.

The amount of skin irradiation received by the patient during angio-cardiography may be calculated when it is known that about 100 roentgen units are delivered by an X-ray tube with the anode set at 90 cm. from the skin and operating at 75 kV. for 3000 mA. second. For example, at this distance and power 100 r units would be delivered if the patient were exposed for 10 seconds at 300 mA. Thus in angiocardiography, if each film is exposed for 0.04 second, and the tube is operated at 75 kV., 450 mA. and at a distance of 90 cm. from the skin, a series of 40 films would result in the patient receiving a skin dose of 25 r units. When patients are screened, X-rayed frequently, catheterised, and angiocardiographed in two planes simultaneously, considerable care must be taken to make sure they are not over-exposed. The maximum safe dose is 100 r in a week, 200 r in a month and 300 r in a year, but is *not repeatable*.

Angiocardiography has proved especially helpful in establishing the diagnosis of congenital heart disease with right to left shunt, e.g. Fallot's tetralogy, pulmonary stenosis with reversed inter-atrial shunt, pulmonary hypertension with reversed shunt, tricuspid atresia, and transposition of the great vessels; in demonstrating coarctation of the aorta; in distinguish-ing aneurysm of the aorta or pulmonary artery from other mediastinal masses (fig. 4.10), and pericardial effusion from cardiac dilatation; and in showing the site of superior vena cava obstruction. The subject has been well reviewed by Dotter and Steinberg (1951).

SELECTIVE ANGIOCARDIOGRAPHY

Diaginol may be introduced directly into any part of the circulation that can be reached with a relatively wide bore catheter or needle. As a rule complete angiocardiograms are more informative, but under certain cir-cumstances there may be great advantage in the selective technique; for example, if diaginol is introduced into the right ventricle and arrives immediately in the aorta, it must have done so via a ventricular septal defect or because of transposition, not via an atrial septal defect or foramen ovale.

RETROGRADE AORTOGRAPHY

Diaginol may also be introduced directly into the aorta via a catheter passed up the radial artery. To overcome the resistance of the catheter, which cannot be of very wide bore, a special crusher has been designed; by means of a long lever great force can be applied to the plunger of the syringe. Retrograde aortography has been of value in demonstrating coarctation of the aorta (fig. 4.11). Good aortograms may be obtained in infants by forcibly injecting 5 ml. of contrast medium into the brachial artery through a No. 18 needle (Keith and Forsyth, 1950). Diaginol may also be introduced into the aorta via a catheter inserted into the femoral artery or directly by needle puncture from behind (Dos Santos, 1933 and 1937).

Some risk is attached to these procedures. Thus temporary hemiplegia has resulted when diodrast has been injected inadvertently into the common carotid artery (Peirce, 1953); intermittent claudication in the hand and forearm has followed occlusion of the brachial artery; and coronary occlusion is an obvious

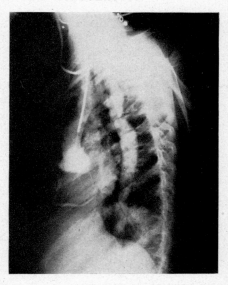

Fig. 4.11—Retrograde aortogram showing coarctation of the aorta.

risk if a catheter is threaded too far down the ascending aorta. Nevertheless, relatively few complications have been reported, and aortography may be helpful at times.

CARDIAC MEASUREMENTS

Numerous measurements have been elaborated to serve as indices of enlargement of the heart, or of one or more of its chambers, but they do not compare with expert opinion based on the methods already outlined. The most reliable is the cardio-thoracic ratio, which is the transverse diameter of the heart (fig. 4.12) over the widest internal diameter of the thorax, and which should not exceed 0.5. In normal adults the transverse diameter of the heart averages 12.2 cm. in the male, and 11 cm. in the female, the range being 8 to 14.5 cm. (Roesler, 1937).

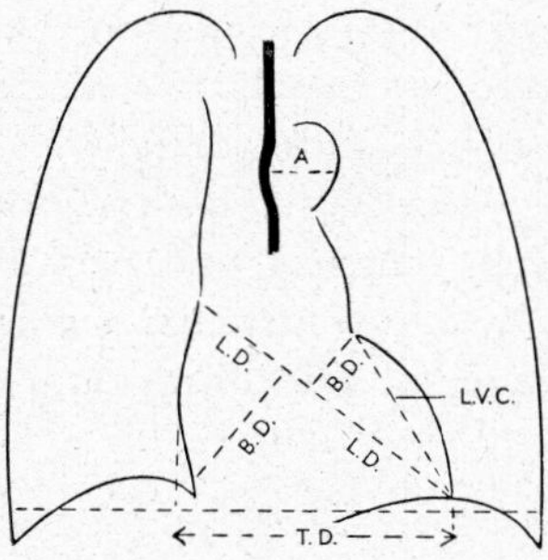

The long diameter is measured from the junction of the superior vena cava and right atrium to the apex of the left ventricle, and lies between 10 and 15.5 cm., averaging 13 cm. (Roesler, 1937). It is especially increased in cases of left ventricular enlargement; but it is also relatively increased in the long narrow heart of asthenic subjects.

The broad diameter is the sum of two

Fig. 4.12—Diagram showing the common cardiac measurements.

A.   Widt h of aorta;
B.D.   Broad diameter;
L.D.   Long diameter;
L.V.C. Left ventricular chord;
T.D.   Tran sverse diameter.

perpendiculars drawn from the long diameter to the right cardio-phrenic angle below, and to the point of opposing movement on the left border of the heart above, and measures 7 to 11 cm. in normal adults, with an average of 9 cm. (Roesler, 1937). It may be increased in cases of mitral stenosis and pulmonary heart disease when the transverse and long diameters are normal.

The location of the point of opposing movement is important; for it tends to be raised or lowered according to whether enlargement is mainly left or right ventricular respectively. Similar significance is attached to the length of the chord which subtends the arc of the left ventricle, measured from the point of opposing movement to the left cardio-phrenic angle: this line is normally 6 to 12.5 cm. long, and averages 9 cm. (Roesler, 1937).

The antero-posterior diameter of the heart is measured from teleradiograms taken in the lateral position, and varies between 7 and 11 cm., with an average of 9 cm. It is a useful check on the significance of an increased transverse diameter; for if this is due to cardiac enlargement, the antero-posterior diameter should be increased proportionately; whereas if it is due to depression of the sternum, the depth of the heart is decreased. The antero-posterior diameter is especially increased in mitral stenosis.

The width of the aorta (2 to 3 cm.) may be measured in the antero-posterior or oblique positions, whichever presents the clearest view of two sides of the vessel. In the anterior view, the measurement should be made from the left side of the barium-filled œsophagus to the left border of the aortic knuckle; but it is only valid when the posterior part of the aortic arch passes directly backwards, i.e. in a direction perpendicular to the frontal plane. In the oblique views barium in the œsophagus may also be helpful: in the second oblique position, for example, the œsophagus may be deflected abruptly as it crosses the aorta, so that the width of the vessel is seen clearly. In practice, a normal aorta is most easily measured in the postero-anterior view; a syphilitic, atheromatous, or unfolded aorta in the second oblique view.

NORMAL VARIATIONS

Both the size and shape of the heart vary greatly in normal individuals: thus in children and adolescents the pulmonary artery may be relatively prominent (fig. 4.13); in lean asthenic subjects the heart may be elongated and central in position (fig. 4.14); in short stocky individuals it is apt to lie transversely (fig. 4.15); rarely, the left atrium can be seen in the P.A. view (fig. 4.16).

Displacement or rotation of the heart to left or right is often due to scoliosis, the common finding being displacement of the heart to the left, the spinal curvature being convex to the right. Rotation of the spine without conspicuous lateral curvature may cause considerable displacement or rotation of the heart. When cardiac displacement is due to partial collapse

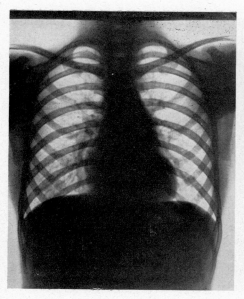

Fig. 4.13—Teleradiogram of a child, showing relative prominence of the pulmonary artery.

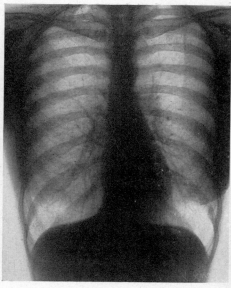

Fig. 4.14—The elongated, centrally placed heart of a lean asthenic subject.

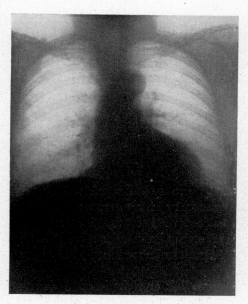

Fig. 4.15—Transversely placed heart of a short stocky subject.

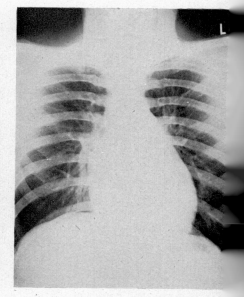

Fig. 4.16—Skiagram of a normal heart in which the border of the left atrium is seen on the right side, between the superior vena cava and the right atrium.

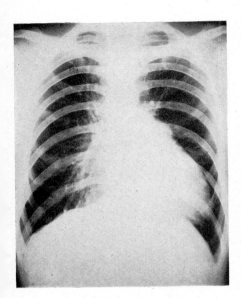

Fig. 4.17—Displacement of the heart to the left without obvious cause.

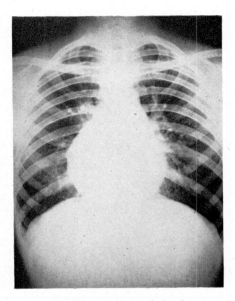

Fig. 4.18—Displacement of the heart to the right, attributed to old mediastinal pleurisy.

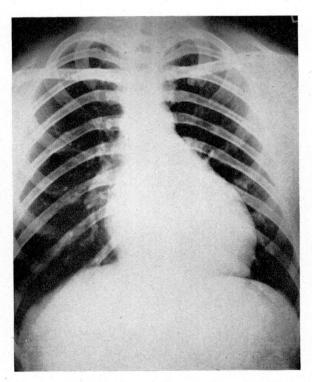

Fig. 4.19—Enlargement of the heart due to sinus brady-cardia.

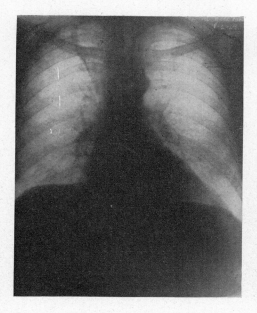

Fig. 4.20—Teleradiogram of an obese subject, showing a triangular opacity at the
apex of the heart (pericardial fat).

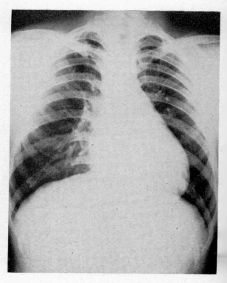

Fig. 4.21—Apparent enlargement of the
heart in a case of depressed sternum.

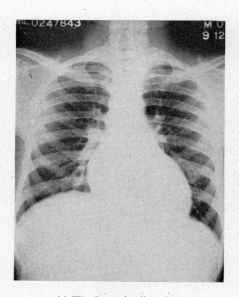

(a) The heart in diastole.

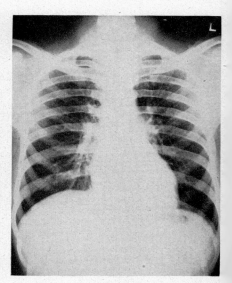

(b) The heart in systole.

Fig. 4.22—Teleradiograms of the same patient taken with short exposures, showing
difference in size of heart shadow in diastole and systole.

of the lung, increased translucency of the over-expanded normal lung on the same side is usually observed, and is a valuable sign when the collapsed part cannot be seen. Occasionally, the heart may be displaced to left or right without obvious cause (figs. 4.17 and 4.18). Mediastinal pleural adhesions can be demonstrated in some of these cases (Kerley, 1954).

Slight enlargement, particularly of the left ventricle and of the transverse diameter, is often seen in patients with slow heart rates, whether due to sinus bradycardia, sino-auricular block, or to heart block. The enlargement depends upon increased diastolic filling, the slow rate being compensated by a large stroke-volume (fig. 4.19). Slight enlargement of similar type may be encountered in athletes; in some it may be explained by sinus bradycardia, which is common in these subjects; but in others it may be due to the extra demands which have been made on the heart.

In obese subjects the left cardio-phrenic angle may be filled out by a triangular pad of fat (fig. 4.20); this must not be confused with left ventricular enlargement. In cases of depressed sternum the postero-anterior skiagram may reveal general enlargement of the heart shadow; but in the oblique views the depth of the heart is seen to be correspondingly reduced (fig. 4.21).

When such causes can be excluded, and unsuspected enlargement of the cardiac silhouette is revealed by a skiagram, it is wise to check the technique employed. Portable X-rays, or pictures taken with the patient lying or sitting, may be misleading owing to distortion. Short exposures may catch the heart in systole and a skiagram so obtained may be appreciably smaller than one photographed in diastole (fig. 4.22).

The heart may be smaller than normal in many wasting diseases, when atrophy takes place, but this is of little practical importance.

RADIOGRAPHIC ABNORMALITIES

Some of the illustrations referable to this section may be found in other chapters, but for the sake of convenience are reproduced here.

ABNORMALITIES OF THE AORTA

Saccular aneurysm (fig. 4.23, a and b) is pathognomonic of syphilis. It may be distinguished from other space-filling lesions by its intimate connexion with the aorta in all views, by calcification of its walls, and by its pulsation; a thrombosed sac, however, may not pulsate. Angiocardiography is helpful in doubtful cases. Fusiform aneurysm (fig. 4.24) usually means syphilitic aortic incompetence, but may also be due to dissection, and when confined to the ascending aorta to congenital hypoplasia; both these conditions may also be complicated by aortic incompetence. Fusiform aneurysm should be distinguished from prominence of the ascending aorta due to aortic stenosis or incompetence of any etiology (fig. 4.25). Syphilitic aortitis without aneurysm or fusiform dilatation can only be diagnosed

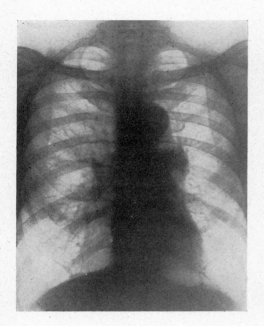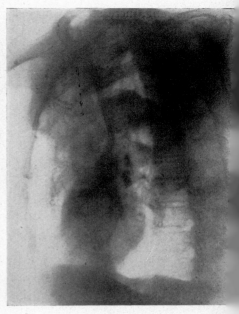

(a) Anterior view.   (b) Second oblique position.

Fig. 4.23—Saccular aneurysm of the aorta.

(By courtesy of Sir John Parkinson)

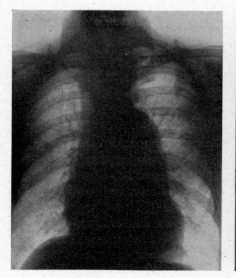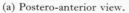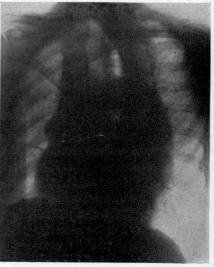

(a) Postero-anterior view.   (b) 2nd oblique position.

Fig. 4.24—Fusiform aneurysm of aorta.

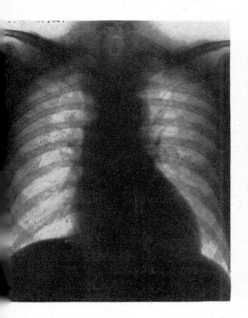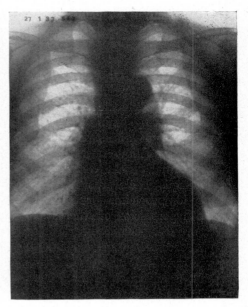

Fig. 4.25—Prominence of the aorta due to rheumatic aortic incompetence.

Fig. 4.26—Unfolding of the aorta in hypertensive heart disease.

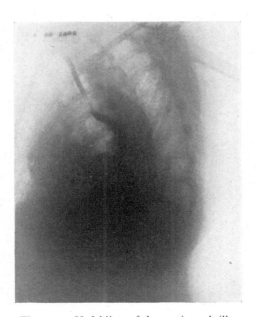

Fig. 4.27—Unfolding of the aortic arch illustrated by barium in the œsophagus.

radiologically if inequalities of outline can be clearly demonstrated, e.g. by means of angio-cardiography.

Unfolding of the aorta may occur in aortic valve disease, in hypertensive heart disease, and in atherosclerosis. The ascending limb is conspicuous, the knuckle is unduly prominent, and the descending limb appears to the patient's left in the posterio-anterior view (fig. 4.26). In the second oblique position the arch is wider than normal, and its posterior part may pull the œsophagus backwards (fig. 4.27). Vigorous pulsation proclaims aortic incompetence rather than hypertension or atherosclerosis.

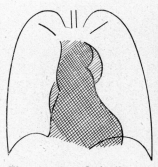

Fig. 4.28 — Orthodiagram illustrating tortuosity of the aorta.

Tortuosity of the aorta is characteristic of atherosclerosis; it is best seen in the second oblique view, but may be so marked that the descending limb appears to the right of the heart shadow in the postero-anterior view (fig. 4.28). Calcification of the aorta is of four main types: (1) calcification of the ascending aorta is practically diagnostic of syphilis; (2) a comma-shaped calcified plaque in the aortic knuckle is characteristic of atherosclerosis; (3) calcification outlining irregularities in the wall of the thoracic aorta in any position means syphilis (fig. 4.29); (4) calcium is frequently laid down in the wall of a saccular aneurysm.

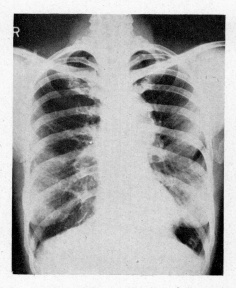

Fig. 4.29—Irregular calcification of the aortic arch in a case of syphilitic cortitis.

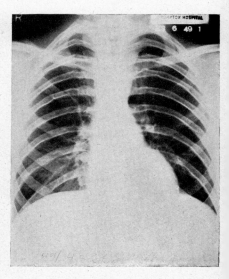

Fig. 4.30—Coarctation of the aorta showing a prominent left subclavian artery, elongated aortic knuckle, post-stenotic dilatation of a short segment of the descending aorta above the pulmonary arc, rib notching and fullness of the left ventricle.

Coarctation of the aorta may be recognised by the prominent left sub-clavian artery, elongated aortic knuckle, and post-stenotic dilatation of a short segment of the descending aorta (fig. 4.30); the diagnosis is confirmed by rib notching and enlargement of the left ventricle, and denied by appearances indicating unfolding of the aorta.

A right-sided aortic arch is seen occasionally as an isolated congenital anomaly, but more often it is associated with Fallot's tetralogy or Eisenmenger's complex. The aortic knuckle projects to the patient's right, and the barium-filled œsophagus is deflected to the left (fig. 4.31).

Hypoplasia of the aorta is rare as a solitary congenital abnormality, but is common in association with certain other congenital or acquired lesions, especially atrial septal defect and mitral stenosis. The aortic knuckle is small and its pulsation diminished.

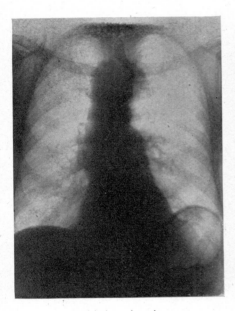 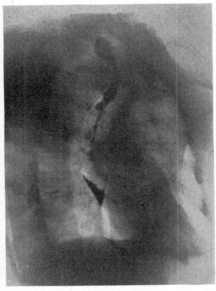

(a) Anterior view.   (b) First oblique position.

Fig. 4.31—Right-sided aortic arch illustrated by means of barium in the œsophagus.

(*By courtesy of Sir John Parkinson*)

ABNORMALITIES OF THE LEFT VENTRICLE

Left ventricular enlargement is encountered chiefly in hypertensive heart disease, aortic valve disease, patent ductus arteriosus, and organic mitral incompetence, but may occur in various conditions as part of general enlargement. It is easily recognised by the density and bulk of the left ventricular shadow in the postero-anterior and second oblique positions, by increase in the transverse and long diameters of the heart and of the

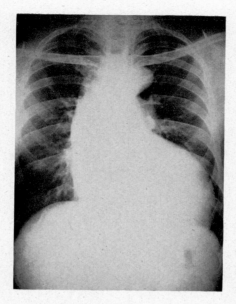

Fig. 4.32—Enlargement of the left ventricle
due to aortic stenosis.

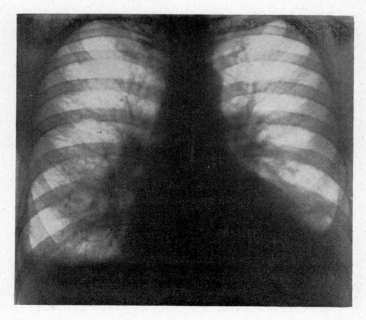

Fig. 4.33—"Pulmonary venous congestion" and bilateral hydrothorax
from left ventricle failure.

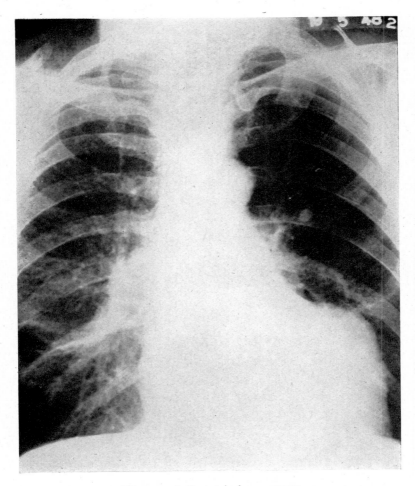

Fig. 4.34—Left ventricular aneurysm.

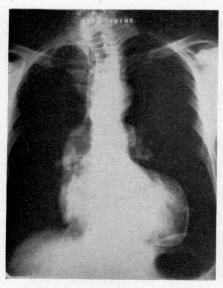

Fig. 4.35—Calcified left ventricular
aneurysm.
(*With acknowledgments to Dr. G. B. Hollings*)

left ventricular chord, and by elevation of the point of opposing movement. In hypertension and aortic valve disease the shadows of the unfolded aorta and of the heart itself may be compared either to two ovals, set at right angles, or to the shape of a boot (fig. 4.32).

When there is left ventricular failure (fig. 4.33), the hilar shadows are exaggerated, a fan-shaped opacity appears at the hilum, representing interstitial œdema, and softer mottling spreads outward towards the periphery when there is pulmonary œdema. Hydrothorax may be present, and if unilateral is usually left sided (Bedford and Lovibond, 1941).

Left ventricular aneurysm may present as a bulge on the left border of the heart, usually towards the apex (fig. 4.34), and may exhibit paradoxical pulsation; occasionally the wall of the aneurysm is calcified (fig. 4.35). Myocardial infarction may be located with precision in some cases by the fluoroscopic demonstration of an area with absent or paradoxical pulsation.

DILATATION OF THE LEFT ATRIUM

Conspicuous dilatation of the left atrium invariably means organic mitral valve disease; but the chamber may be unduly full in cases of left ventricular failure. In the postero-anterior view it may appear as a bump on the left border of the heart between the pulmonary artery and left ventricle (fig. 4.36). The proof that this bump represents the left atrium or left atrial appendage rather than the conus of the right ventricle is as follows: (1) it is only seen in cases of mitral valve disease, when it is related to the size of the left atrium, not to the pulmonary vascular resistance; (2) in angiocardiograms it opacifies with the left atrium, not with the right ventricle (Grishman, Sussman and Steinberg, 1944); (3) it contracts with the atria in cases of complete heart block, and expands with the rest of the left atrium in cases of severe mitral incompetence; (4) it disappears after appendicular resection (fig. 4.37); (5) if a catheter is introduced into the left atrium via an atrial septal defect or foramen ovale, its tip can nearly always be passed to the very edge of the cardiac border at the site in question, whereas in the conus of the right ventricle it is always well medial.

On the right border of the heart an enlarged left atrium appears as a

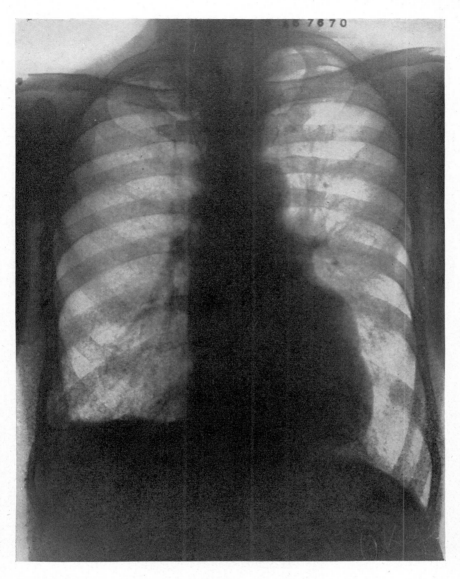

Fig. 4.36—Dilatation of the left atrium forming a bump between the pulmonary arc and left ventricle in a case of organic mitral incompetence.

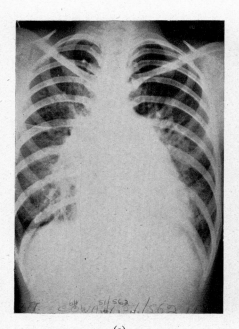
(a)

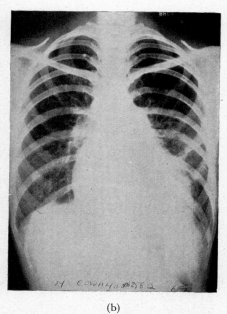
(b)

Fig. 4.37—Skiagram of a case of mitral stenosis showing: (a) intense "pulmonary venous congestion", dilatation of the pulmonary artery and left atrium before operation, and (b) disappearance of both the congestion and the left atrial appendage after mitral valvotomy and appendicular resection.

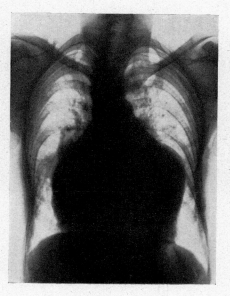

Fig. 4.38—Dilatation of the left atrium seen on both borders of the heart in the postero-anterior view in a case of mitral incompetence.

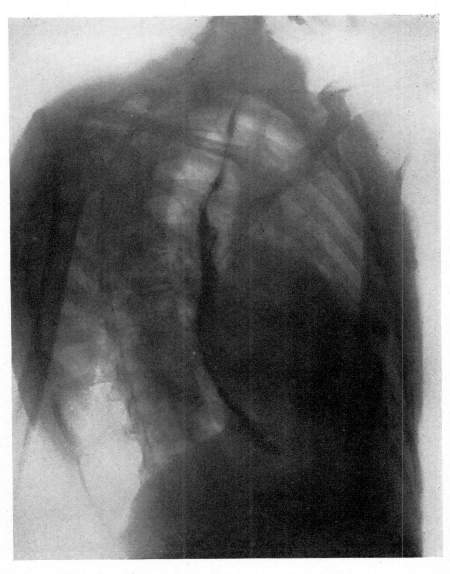

Fig. 4.39—Dilatation of the left atrium illustrated by means of barium in the œsophagus. Case of mitral stenosis. Note the sharp curves produced by the aortic arch and the left bronchus and pulmonary artery.

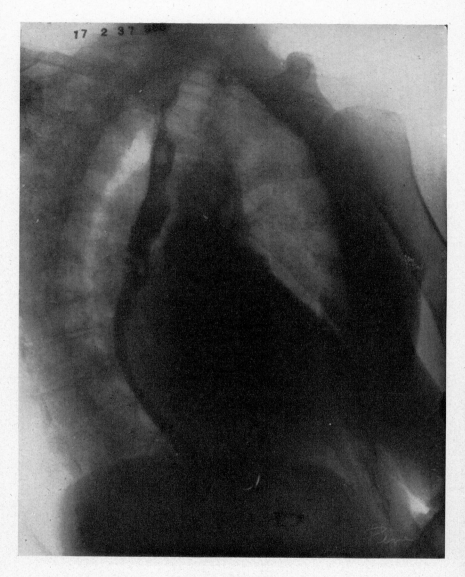

Fig. 4.40—Dilatation of the left atrium in a case of hypertensive heart disease (necropsy proof).

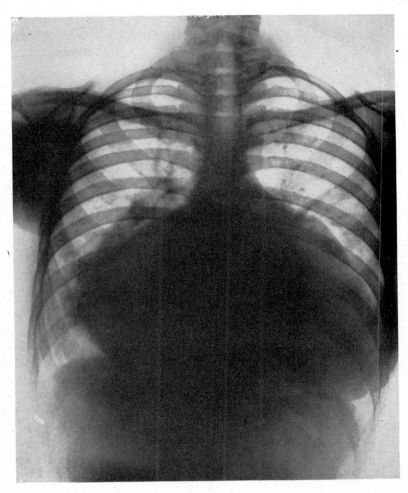

Fig. 4.41—Aneurysmal dilatation of the left atrium in a case of mitral valve disease.

convex shadow above, but overlapping, that of the right atrium (fig. 4.38). The barium-filled œsophagus is usually deflected to the patient's right in the postero-anterior view.

In the right anterior oblique position the œsophagus is displaced backwards in an abrupt manner immediately below the left bronchus and pulmonary artery (fig. 4.39), the antero-posterior diameter of the heart being increased, and the retrocardiac space decreased, correspondingly. Backward displacement of the œsophagus from an enlarged left ventricle is rarely so abrupt or so high; but on occasions it may be indistinguishable (fig. 4.40). In the left anterior oblique position an enlarged left atrium causes the œsophagus to be deflected backwards above the shadow of the left ventricle.

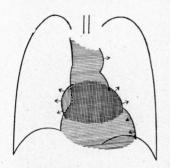

Aneurysmal dilatation of the left atrium (fig. 4.41) may be caused by rheumatic mitral incompetence or stenosis, but it is probable that a high degree of atrial muscle damage is an important contributory factor.

Systolic expansile pulsation of the left atrium is pathognomonic of mitral incompetence, usually organic. It is especially convincing when seen on both borders of the heart in the postero-anterior view (fig. 4.42). In the first oblique position, backward pulsation of the left atrium is often seen in mitral stenosis, but the quality and amplitude of the movement in organic mitral incompetence are most impressive and are easily recognised with experience.

Fig. 4.42—Orthodiagram illustrating expansile pulsation of the left atrium during ventricular systole in a case of organic mitral incompetence.

A rare complication of mitral stenosis is calcification of the left atrial endocardium.

ABNORMALITIES OF THE PULMONARY ARTERY

DILATATION OF THE PULMONARY ARTERY may be associated with congenital or acquired heart disease, and is due to hypoplasia, an increased pulmonary blood flow, or pulmonary hypertension. Congenital causes include idiopathic dilatation of the pulmonary artery, pulmonary valve stenosis with normal aortic root, patent ductus arteriosus, ventricular septal defect, atrial septal defect, and Eisenmenger's syndrome; acquired causes include primary pulmonary hypertension, subacute thromboembolic pulmonary hypertension, hypertensive cor pulmonale, pulmonary hypertensive mitral stenosis, and other varieties of secondary pulmonary hypertension such as schistosomiasis, periarteritis and disseminated lupus. Slight dilatation of the pulmonary artery may occur in any of the hyperkinetic circulatory states and in passive pulmonary hypertension secondary to chronic left ventricular failure or mitral valve disease.

In *idiopathic dilatation* the peripheral pulmonary vessels and the heart

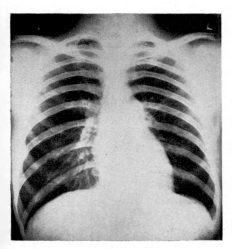

Fig. 4.43—Idiopathic dilatation of the pulmonary artery.

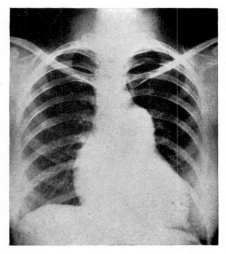

Fig. 4.44—Dilatation of the pulmonary artery in a case of pure pulmonary stenosis.

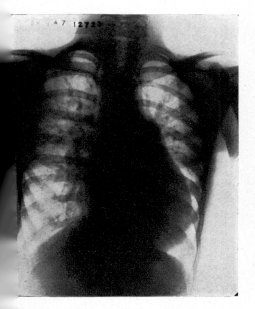

Fig. 4.45—Dilatation of the pulmonary artery and its branches, associated with left ventricular enlargement due to patent ductus.

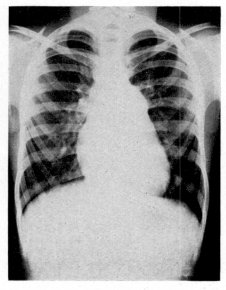

Fig 4.46—Dilatation of the pulmonary artery in a case of Eisenmenger's complex.

147

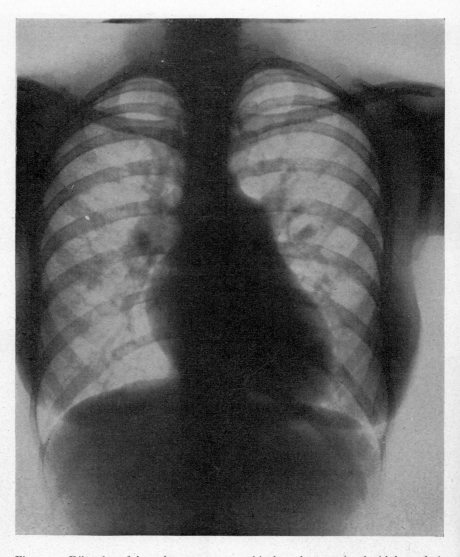

Fig. 4.47—Dilatation of the pulmonary artery and its branches associated with hypoplasia of the aorta and right sided enlargement in a case of atrial septal defect.

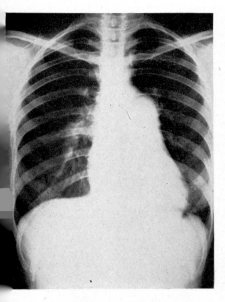

Fig. 4.48—Dilatation of the pulmonary artery due to primary or idiopathic pulmonary hypertension.

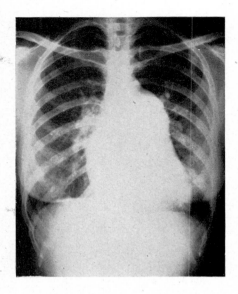

Fig. 4.49—Dilatation of the pulmonary artery due to extreme pulmonary hypertension in a case of mitral stenosis.

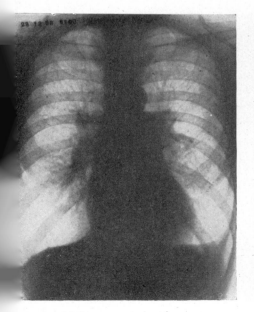

(a) Postero-anterior view.

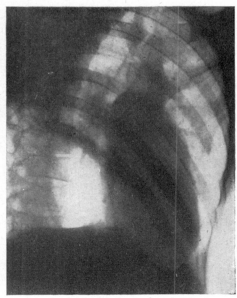

(b) First oblique position.

Fig. 4.50—Dilatation of the pulmonary artery and its main branches in a case of chronic cor pulmonale due to emphysema.

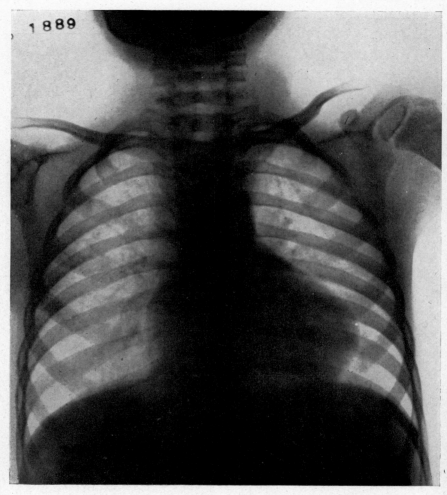

Fig. 4.51—The Cœur en sabot due to Fallot's tetralogy.

itself are normal (fig. 4.43), unless there is secondary pulmonary incompetence when the right ventricle is dilated.

In *pulmonary valve stenosis* (fig. 4.44) the peripheral vascular markings may be diminished and the right ventricle and atrium enlarged, according to the degree of stricture.

In *patent ductus* dilatation of the pulmonary artery is due to an increased pulmonary blood flow and is associated with heavy pulmonary vascular markings and enlargement of the left ventricle (fig. 4.45); the appearances in *ventricular septal defect* are similar, except that the right ventricle is enlarged as well; the appearances are also similar in *atrial septal defect*, but here only the right ventricle and right atrium are enlarged (fig. 4.47).

In *Eisenmenger's syndrome* dilatation of the pulmonary artery is due to pulmonary hypertension; the peripheral vascular shadows are normal or light. The right ventricle is hypertrophied but not dilated, so that the transverse diameter of the heart may be normal (fig. 4.46), as in Fallot's tetralogy.

Primary pulmonary hypertension is characterised by dilatation of the pulmonary artery with diminished peripheral vascular markings due to pulmonary vasoconstriction and a low cardiac output (fig. 4.48). The right ventricle and atrium are enlarged, the left ventricle small. Appearances are similar in subacute cor pulmonale from thrombo-embolism.

The degree of dilatation of the pulmonary artery in mitral stenosis is closely related to the pulmonary vascular resistance; when this is extreme the radiological appearances may resemble those of primary pulmonary hypertension (fig. 4.49).

In hypertensive cor pulmonale radiological evidence of emphysema, polycystic lung or diffuse pulmonary fibrosis are added to the picture (fig. 4.50).

HYPOPLASIA OF THE PULMONARY ARTERY is characteristic of Fallot's tetralogy (fig. 4.51). There may be a distinct gap between the aortic knuckle and the curve of the left ventricle, the vascular shadows at the hilum are reduced on both sides, and the lung fields are remarkably clear.

ENLARGEMENT OF THE RIGHT VENTRICLE

Right ventricular enlargement is more difficult to recognise than left. In the postero-anterior view there is usually some increase in the transverse and broad diameters, the right atrium being pushed a little to the right, and the interventricular septum to the left.

When hypertrophy of the right ventricle is associated with clockwise rotation of the heart, the anterior edge of the septum forms most of the left border of the heart, only the tip of the left ventricle being visible beyond it: the effect produced is that of increased angularity of the cardiac apex and a more acute left cardiophrenic angle, the general shape resembling the Dutch peasant's wooden shoe with turned-up toe. This

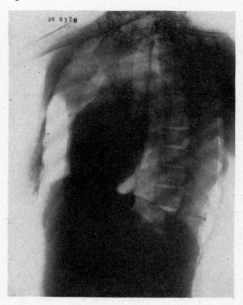

Fig. 4.52—Right ventricular enlargement in a case of mitral stenosis (2nd oblique position).

is the "cœur en sabot", and is especially characteristic of Fallot's tetralogy (fig. 4.51).

When the right ventricle is dilated as well as hypertrophied, as in atrial septal defect, it may occupy the whole of the left border of the heart and form the apex beat proper; in the postero-anterior skiagram it is often impossible to be sure which ventricle is responsible for the enlargement, and experience has proved over and over again that the electrocardiogram is a far more reliable guide.

In the left anterior oblique position, right ventricular enlargement is recognised by the increased curvature of the anterior border of the heart shadow. Instead of the lobsided appearance resulting from normal left ventricular bias, the heart shadow is more globular, the anterior and posterior ventricular curves being more equal (fig. 4.52). If the right atrium is enlarged, however, as may be determined from the postero-anterior view, interpretation is more difficult, for its shadow is superimposed on that of the right ventricle in the second oblique position, and it may be entirely responsible for the increased curvature of the anterior border.

The right ventricle is enlarged particularly in pulmonary hypertension, pulmonary stenosis, pulmonary incompetence and atrial septal defect. Hypertrophy rather than dilatation is characteristic of Fallot's tetralogy and Eisenmenger's complex; dilatation usually means failure from pulmonary hypertension or simple pulmonary stenosis, or an increased stroke volume as in atrial septal defect.

ENLARGEMENT OF THE RIGHT ATRIUM

Dilatation of the right atrium, usually associated with fullness of the superior vena cava is seen in congestive heart failure, atrial septal defect, severe pulmonary hypertension or stenosis, tricuspid stenosis or incompetence and Bernheim's syndrome.

As a rule, a dilated right atrium is recognised by its relatively low position on the right cardiac border and by the blunt angle it makes with the diaphragm (fig. 4.53). When the left atrium appears on the right border of the heart, it is higher, more rounded, and forms a zone of

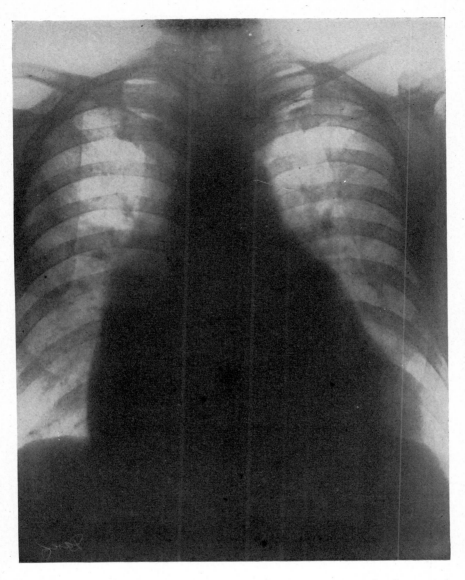

Fig. 4.53—Gross enlargement of the right atrium due to tricuspid valve disease.

increased density where it overlaps the right atrium (fig. 4.38). Pericardial effusion tends to form an acute right cardiophrenic angle (fig. 4.54). A grossly tortuous aorta occasionally gives rise to confusion, for its descending limb may appear to the right of the spine (fig. 4.28). The best way to prove that a shadow on the right cardiac border belongs to the right atrium is to pass a catheter into that chamber and run the tip down its lateral border.

In differential diagnosis particular attention should be paid to the pulmonary vascular shadows, pulmonary artery and left ventricle. Thus in pulmonary hypertension and pulmonary stenosis the pulmonary artery is usually dilated and the peripheral pulmonary vascular markings are light; in atrial septal defect dilatation of the pulmonary artery is associated with pulmonary plethora; in tricuspid stenosis and Bernheim's syndrome the pulmonary artery is not dilated, and in the latter the left ventricle is greatly enlarged.

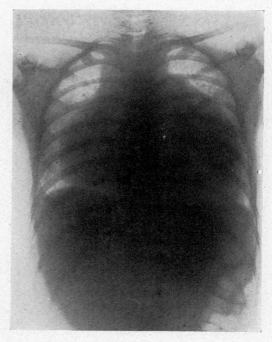

Fig. 4.54—Pericardial effusion showing acute right cardiophrenic angle.

GENERAL ENLARGEMENT OF THE HEART

General enlargement of the heart shadow, involving all diameters, is seen in rheumatic, diphtheritic, and other forms of myocarditis (fig. 4.55); in hyperkinetic circulatory states such as thyrotoxicosis (fig. 4.56), anæmia, arterio-venous fistula, beri-beri, Paget's disease of bone and anoxic cor pulmonale; in certain metabolic disorders such as myxœdema, von Gierke's disease and primary cardiac amyloidosis; in cardiac fibrosis of unknown etiology, including fibro-elastosis; in active pulmonary hypertension with or without congestive failure, secondary to left ventricular failure; in ventricular septal defect, complete heart block, and rheumatic heart disease with multiple valve lesions.

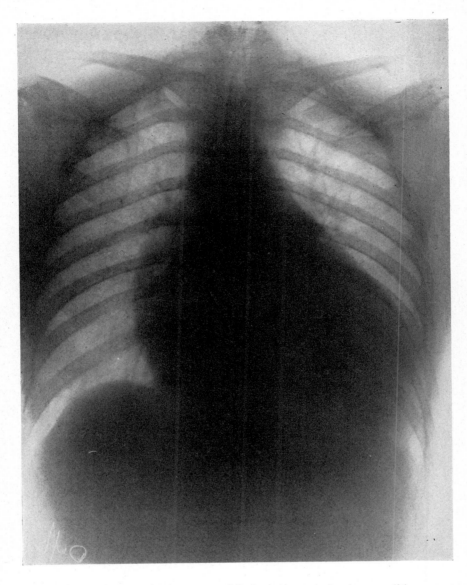

Fig. 4.55—General enlargement of the heart due to isolated myocarditis.

PERICARDIAL EFFUSION

When effusion is considerable, the natural contours of the heart in the anterior view are replaced by single bold curves, and pulsation is absent or greatly reduced. The right cardio-phrenic angle is unusually acute (fig. 4.54). In the first oblique position, the posterior border of the heart shadow may bulge beyond the barium-filled œsophagus. When effusion is slight or moderate, however, radiological diagnosis may be difficult; for pulsation may be clearly visible, and may, indeed, be greater than that often seen in some of the conditions most likely to cause confusion; the natural contours of the heart, on one or other border, may not be entirely lost, and may closely imitate the indefinite demarcations of the chambers which may be

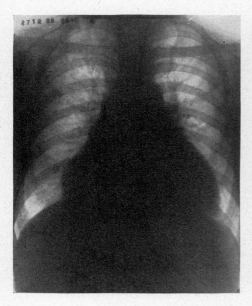

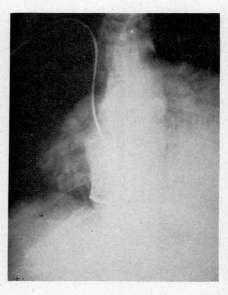

Fig. 4.56—General enlargement of the heart due to thyrotoxic heart failure with auricular fibrillation.

Fig. 4.57—Diagnosis of pericardial effusion by means of cardiac catheterisation: the tip of the catheter is lying against the right atrial wall, which is outlined by a small quantity of diodone; the opacity to the right of the atrial border is all effusion.

seen in acute carditis and myxœdema, for example. Moreover, little reliance can be placed in change of shape with change of posture, diverging vascular shadows beneath the clavicles, or bulging of the posterior inferior angle of the heart shadow in the first oblique position (instead of the normal concavity of the inferior vena cava). Rapid and considerable changes in the size of the heart shadow from week to week provide good evidence of effusion, but proof may only be obtained by means of acupuncture, angiocardiography or cardiac catheterisation (fig. 4.57).

CONSTRICTIVE PERICARDITIS

The most important radiological evidence of constrictive pericarditis is loss of pulsation without cardiac enlargement; but calcification of the pericardium is common and helpful, and is usually best seen in the left anterior oblique position (fig. 4.58). Slight to moderate enlargement of the heart shadow may occur if the pericardium is sufficiently thick (1 to 2 cm.), but the triangular appearance given by the obliquely set straight right and left borders should suggest the correct diagnosis (fig. 4.59).

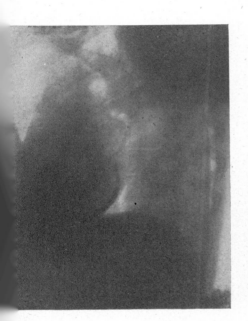

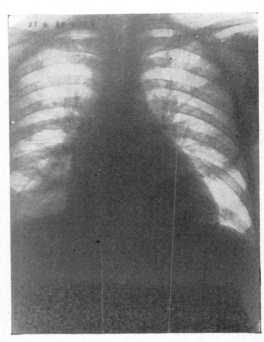

g. 4.58—Case of chronic constrictive peri-rditis showing extensive calcification of the pericardium (2nd oblique position).

Fig. 4.59—Chronic constrictive pericarditis showing triangular shaped heart in the anterior view.

CALCIFIED VALVES

Calcified valves are best seen fluoroscopically; they may be recorded by means of tomography. The patient should be turned 15 degrees to the left, and an imaginary line drawn from the point of opposing movement on the left border of the heart, downwards and to the patient's right, at an angle of 45 degrees with the horizontal (fig. 4.60). The aortic valve is situated just above this line in the centre of the heart shadow, the mitral just below it and a little to the patient's left. Calcification may be recognised by linear or anti-clockwise elliptical movement of dense crescentic opacities, in the direction of the anatomical axis of the heart, synchronous with the heart beat. The technique requires proper accommodation and maximum constriction of the diaphragm so that only a square inch or so of the screen is visible. Calcified aortic valves are sometimes better seen in the second oblique position where they lie at the intersection of a vertical line through

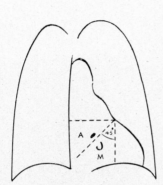

Fig. 4.60—Orthodiagram showing the position of calcified valves. The patient has been turned fifteen degrees to his left.

A. Aortic valve.
M. Mitral valve.

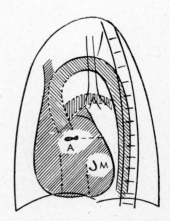

Fig. 4.61—Orthodiagram showing the position of calcified valves in the 2nd oblique position.

A. Aortic valve.
M. Mitral valve.

the centre of the heart shadow and a horizontal line through the top of the left ventricular arc (fig. 4.61). This view may be helpful in valve differentiation, for the mitral valve lies in the posterior third of the heart shadow and at a lower level (Sosman, 1939).

PULMONARY VASCULAR SHADOWS

Radiological examination of the heart is incomplete without careful inspection of the pulmonary vascular shadows. The normal lung markings are practically all vascular. The heavier shadows are arterial and taper evenly to the periphery.

In severe pulmonary hypertension due to a high pulmonary vascular resistance normal tapering disappears, and is replaced by an abrupt change of calibre at a fairly proximal level; the main left and right pulmonary arteries are dense and dilated, but the peripheral vessels are spidery and the outer lung fields unduly translucent (fig. 4.48).

Pulmonary ischæmia (or oligæmia) associated with a dilated pulmonary artery is characteristic of severe pulmonary valve stenosis, the diminished pulmonary blood flow being due to a low cardiac output or to reversed interatrial shunt (fig. 4.44).

Pulmonary ischæmia with a hypoplasic pulmonary artery is seen especially in Fallot's tetralogy (fig. 4.51) and tricuspid atresia.

Clear lung fields due to a diminished pulmonary blood flow are also seen in pericardial effusion, Ebstein's disease (fig. 4.62), and certain other low-output states.

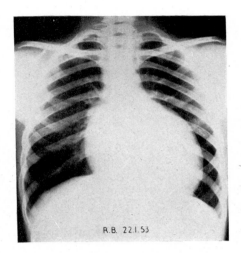

R.B. 22.1.53

Fig. 4.62—Pulmonary ischæmia associated with a low cardiac output in a case of Ebstein's disease; the enlarged heart shadow is due to dilatation of the right ventricle and atrium.

Pulmonary plethora may be defined as heavy pulmonary vascular markings due to an increased pulmonary blood flow; the shadows are peripheral as well as central and are chiefly arterial. Pulmonary plethora is seen in patent ductus arteriosus (fig. 4.45), aorto-pulmonary septal defect, ventricular septal defect, atrial septal defect (fig. 4.46), anomalous pulmonary venous drainage, transposition of the great vessels and persistent truncus arteriosus. Heavy tapering vascular shadows spread far out into the lungs, and in cross section form unusually dense round opacities.

Other arterial abnormalities, such as arterio-venous fistula, absence or occlusion of a major pulmonary artery, and broncho-pulmonary anastamoses are described elsewhere.

"Pulmonary venous congestion" presents as fan-shaped mottling spreading out from the hilum on each side (fig. 4.37a), and is characteristic of mitral stenosis and left ventricular failure. Heavy woolly shadows are superimposed in cases of pulmonary œdema. Fine horizontal lines, best seen near the right costophrenic angle, represent engorged lymphatics (Kerley, 1933).

Anomalous pulmonary venous drainage and anomalies of the venæ cavæ are described in Chapter VIII.

REFERENCES

Bedford, D. E., and Lovibond, J. L. (1941): "Hydrothorax in heart failure", *Brit. Heart J.*, **3**, 93.

Castellanos, A., Pereiras, R., and Garcia, A. (1938): "L'angiocardiography chez l'enfant", *Pr. méd.*, **46**, 1474.

Davies, C. E., and Steiner, R. E. (1949): "Calcified aortic valve: clinical and radiological features", *Brit. Heart J.*, **11**, 126.
Dos Santos, R. (1933): "L'arteriographie en série", *Bull. et mém. Soc. Nat. de Chir.*, **59**, 1.
—— (1937): "Technique de l'aortographie", *J. Internat. Chir.*, **2**, 1.

Evans, William (1952): *Cardioscopy*, Butterworth and Co., London.

Dotter, C. T., and Jackson, F. S. (1950): "Death following angiocardiography", *Radiology*, **54**, 527.
——, and Steinberg, I. (1951): "Angiocardiography", *Annals of Roentgenol.*, XX, Cassell, London.

Grishman, A., Sussman, M. L., and Steinberg, M. F. (1944): "Angiocardiographic analysis of the cardiac configuration in rheumatic mitral disease", *Amer. J. Roentgenol.*, **51**, 33.
Grossman, G. (1935): "Lung Tomography", *Brit. J. Radiol.*, **8**, 733.

Henny, G. C., Boone, B. R., and Chamberlain, W. E. (1947): "Electrokymograph for recording heart motion, improved type", *Amer. J. Roentgenol*, **57**, 409.
Howarth, S. (1950): "Blood-pressure changes during angiocardiography", *Brit. Med. J.*, ii, 1090.

Keith, J. D., and Forsyth, C. (1950): "Aortography in infants", *Circulation*, **2**, 907.
Kerley, P. J. (1933): "Radiology in heart desease", *Brit. med. J. ii*, 594.

Lawson, F. E. (1945): "Gall bladder dye (iodophthalein sodium). Effect of intravenous injections on coronary flow, blood pressure and blood coagulation", *Arch. Intern. Med.*, **76**, 143.

Peirce, E. C. (1953): "Temporary hemiplegia from cerebral injection of diodrast during catheter aortography—report of two cases", *Circulation*, **7**, 385.

Robb, G. P., and Steinberg, I. (1938): "A practical method of visualisation of the chambers of the heart, the pulmonary circulation, and the great vessels in man", *J. clin. Invest.*, **17**, 507.
——, —— (1939): "Visualisation of the chambers of the heart", *Amer. J. Roentgenol.* **42**, 14.
Roesler, H. (1928): "Beitrage zur Lehre von den angeforenen Herzfehlern IV. Untersuchungen an zwei Fallen von Isthmus-Stenose der Aorta", *Weiner, Arch. inn. Med.*, **15**, 521.
—— (1937): "Clinical roentgenology of the cardiovascular system", London.

Sosman, M. C. (1939): "Roentgenological aspects of acquired valvular heart disease", *Amer. J. Roentgenol.*, **42**, 47.
Steinberg, M. F., Grishman, A., and Sussman, M. L. (1943): "Angiocardiography in congenital heart disease." II. "Intracardiac shunts", *Ibid.*, **49**, 766.
Stevenson, J. J. (1950): "Horizontal body section radiography", *Brit. J. Radiol.*, **23**, 319.
Stewart, W. H., Breimer, C. W., and Maier, H. C. (1941): "Cineroentgenographic diagnosis of congenital and acquired heart disease", *Amer. J. Roentgenol.*, **46**, 636.

Stumpf, P. (1931): "Archiv und Atlas der normalen und pathologischen Anatomie in typischen Rontgenbildern. Das rontgenographische Bewegungsbild und seine Anwendung (Flachenkymographie und Kymoskopie)." Fortschr. a.d.Geb. d. Rongenstrahlen [Erganzungsband 41, Georg Thieme, Leipzig].

Sussman, M. L., Steinberg, M. F., and Grishman, A. (1941): "Multiple exposure technique in contrast visualisation of the cardiac chambers and great vessels", *Amer. J. Roentgenol.*, 46, 745.

Twining, E. W. (1937): "Discussion on the clinical value of the tomograph", *Proc. Royal Soc. Med.*, 31, 386.

Ziedses des Plantes, B. G. (1932): "Eine neue methode zur ditterenzierung in der röntgenographie (planigraphie)", *Acta Radiol.*, 13, 182.

CHAPTER V

SPECIAL INVESTIGATIONS

STETHOSCOPIC auscultation, sphygmomanometry, ophthalmoscopy, electrocardiography and radiology have become routine technical methods of investigation which are used by the cardiologist before he arrives at his initial clinical diagnosis. The techniques described in this chapter have not yet become routine in this country and are unlikely to do so, for a precise etiological, anatomical and functional diagnosis can usually be made without them, and they infrequently reveal anything totally unexpected. For the most part they are refinements of simpler techniques— accurate methods of measuring quantity when the quality of something is already known. Occasionally they are used to solve a particular qualititative problem.

DIRECT MEASUREMENT OF THE VENOUS PRESSURE

Whilst elevation of the venous pressure is usually detected clinically with little difficulty, there are occasions when it is valuable to check it by direct measurement (Moritz and Tabora, 1910). The subject should be propped up at an angle of 30 to 45 degrees, because patients with orthopnœa cannot lie flat, and the technique should be the same for all cases. The right arm, bared to the shoulder, is abducted to a right angle and supported on pillows so that the antecubital fossa is roughly at heart level. An infusion needle, connected to a spinal manometer or similar graduated glass tube, is then inserted into the antecubital vein, the zero mark on the manometer being placed at the level of the fourth costal cartilage by means of a spirit-level; the height to which blood rises above this mark represents the venous pressure. Alternatively, the zero mark may be placed at the level of the sternal angle or of some other reference point. To avoid clotting, a saline reservoir containing a drop of heparin should be attached to the system by means of a T-shaped glass connexion, as shown in figure 5.01, a few ml. of the solution being

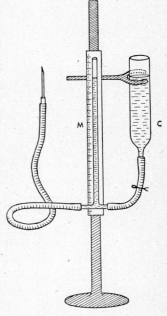

Fig. 5.01—Apparatus for measuring the venous pressure.

M. Manometer graduated in cm.
C. Citrate or saline reservoir.

allowed to flow through from time to time. With this modification the manometer contains saline instead of blood. The result should be expressed in cm. of water (a horizontal line through the fourth costal cartilage with the patient at 45 degrees cuts the superior vena cava just above its junction with the right atrium), or in cm. of water above or below the sternal angle. If the technique is satisfactory, the saline column should rise and fall gently with respiration, and should rise sharply when the arm is constricted above the needle. The normal venous pressure, as so measured, ranges between 2 and 10 cm. of water and averages 5.76 cm. (Wood, 1936); expressed with reference to the sternal angle, it may be plus or minus 0 to 3 cm. in relatively horizontal positions.

In the *phlebomanometer* described by Burch (1950) a 12-cm. glass observation tube with a bore of 1.00 mm. is attached to the veni-puncture needle and is connected by means of rubber tubing to the saline manometer through a three-way tap which is also connected to a pneumatic pressure bulb. Immediately before use 2 per cent sodium citrate is drawn up through the needle into the observation tube until the meniscus reaches a set mark. When the needle is inserted into the vein the positive venous pressure tends to force the meniscus up the observation tube, but this tendency is corrected by increasing the pressure in the pneumatic system connecting the tube with the saline manometer (by means of the pressure bulb). The pressure required to keep the meniscus at the mark is the venous pressure.

THE JUGULAR PHLEBOGRAM

The polygraph is an instrument for making simultaneous graphic records of two or more vascular pulsations. Mackenzie (1902) concentrated on the jugular phlebogram as a means of analysing abnormalities of rhythm. The instrument consists essentially of some sort of receiver which is placed over the internal jugular vein to pick up changes in volume or pressure, connections to transmit these changes to the recorder, an amplifying system to increase the magnitude of the changes, and the recorder itself. In Mackenzie's *clinical polygraph*, which was made by Shaw, the receiver was an open shallow cup, and was connected pneumatically by means of a rubber tube to a tambour. Amplification depended on the length of the lever (usually 6 inches) fixed to the membrane of the tambour. The moving end of the lever was arranged to write on smoked paper covering a revolving drum. Two or more such systems operated together so that the jugular pulse could be timed against the carotid or radial pulse and against the apex beat. The disadvantages of this simple arrangement were the mechanical inertia of the levers, the primitive method of recording, and the pneumatic time lag.

By cementing a small mirror to the membrane of the tambour in an eccentric position Frank (1903) overcame the problem of mechanical inertia. *Optical records* were obtained by photographing the movements of a beam of light reflected from the mirror, the length of the beam providing excellent amplification. But the *mirror capsule* was still operated by volume displacement in an air system and suffered from the same time lag as Mackenzie's instrument.

To overcome this defect the receiver had to be some sort of transducer, i.e. a device which converts a pressure or volume change into a proportional electrical voltage. A *carbon granule microphone*, similar to that used in commercial telephony, answers the purpose fairly well, although it suffers from non-linear distortion. It consists of two electrodes between which are packed the carbon granules; one of the electrodes is movable, and is attached to a diaphragm which is displaced by changes in external pressure. When the diaphragm is pushed inwards the carbon granules are compressed, decreasing the resistance between the two electrodes. A current flowing through the chamber is thus altered by any movement of the diaphragm. The current can be led to a suitable galvanometer the movements of which can be recorded as in an electrocardiograph.

Piezo-electric ($\pi\iota\epsilon\zeta\epsilon\iota\nu$, to press) *crystal microphones* have also been used with some success (Gomez and Langevin, 1937; Miller and White, 1941). They depend on the property of certain crystals, such as quartz and Rochelle salt (sodium potassium tartrate), to develop electrical charges when subjected to mechanical strain. The crystal must be cut in a special way, for it will only respond electrically when pressure is applied to it in a particular direction. It is mounted between two electrodes, one of them being fixed to a projecting button which can be placed on the jugular vein. When the button is pushed in by the jugular pulse, the crystal is compressed, and electrical charges of equal amplitude and opposite sign, proportionate to the stress, develop on each side of the crystal; these are picked up by the electrodes, amplified and led to a suitable galvanometer and recorder.

Microphone receivers are designed to be used in conjunction with multi-channel recorders, so that thermionic valve amplification, galvanometer and recording device are already available. The transducers themselves have a high frequency response, linear in the case of the piezo-electric type, and eliminate time-lag. Unfortunately, the changes that develop are so small that no insulator is sufficiently perfect to preserve them for long, so that these crystals cannot be used as transducers for electromanometers which are required to measure static and mean pressures.

The *jugular phlebogram* is a good qualitative graphic record of what the clinician actually sees at the bedside; it is not quantitative and cannot be standardised. The venous pulse is said to travel at a rate of 1 to 3 metres per second (Morrow, 1900); this means that the delay between right atrial and internal jugular events should lie between 0.15 and 0.05 sec., which is rather longer than that found with modern techniques (about 0.05 sec. in our own laboratories). In using the phlebogram to help identify phono-cardiographic events this venous time lag must be borne in mind.

The chief waves of the venous pulse have already been described in detail and are illustrated again in figure 5.02. The onset of *a* is 0.07 sec. after the peak of the electrocardiographic P wave, which signals the onset of right atrial contraction. The prominent *c* wave is typical of jugular

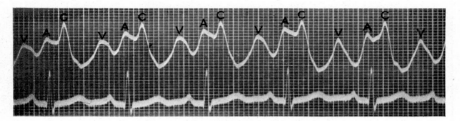

Fig. 5.02—Jugular phlebogram.

A. Atrial contraction.
C. Carotid pulse.
V. The summit signals the opening of the tricuspid valve.

phlebograms and is due to carotid pulsation. The peak of *v* signals the opening of the tricuspid valve when allowance is made for time lag. The two troughs are *x* and *y*.

THE ARTERIOGRAM

A *sphygmogram* (σφυγμός, pulse) is a tracing or graphic record of any kind of pulse, and although the original sphymographs were designed for obtaining arterial pulse tracings, and the word pulse customarily means an arterial pulse unless otherwise specified, it is better to describe an arterial pulse record as an arteriogram, and the procedure arteriography.

Arteriograms may be recorded indirectly by placing a receiver over an arterial pulse, or directly by inserting a needle into the artery. *Indirect arterial sphygmographs* were in common use in the nineteenth century: Marey (1863) designed, and used, an instrument which was of great help to Potain (1867), and in 1902 Mackenzie stated that the construction of these instruments was familiar to all medical men. The receiver had a steel spring, the foot of which was placed directly over the radial or other arterial pulse; a long lever was attached to the spring so that movements were magnified, and the lever was made to write on smoked paper. The Dudgeon type was perhaps best known in this country. Subsequent development has been the same as that described for jugular phlebographs, and carbon microphones or piezo-electric crystals, electrical transmission, thermionic valve amplification and electrocardiographic type of galvanometer and recording are now used.

In the *direct method* a needle (18 to 20 gauge) is inserted into the brachial or femoral artery and is connected to a suitable manometer by a non-elastic plastic or lead tube containing heparinised saline.

Manometers

OPTICAL MANOMETERS use the principle of Frank's mirror capsule (q.v.). In the instrument designed by Hamilton (1934), a 5-mm. square 0.5 dioptre plano-convex mirror, silvered on the plane side, was cemented eccentrically to a membrane made of brass 0.06 mm. thick, or coin silver 0.0015 inches thick, which formed the terminal face of a metal chamber fitted with citrate solution, which was connected hydraulically by means of a lead tube to an 18-gauge Luer needle used for arterial puncture. A slit lamp was arranged so that a beam of light up to 5 metres long was reflected from the mirror on to moving photographic film or paper. The manometer could be standardised by recording the response to known changes of pressure, the length of the beam of light being adjusted to the amplification required. The response of the manometer was linear, and of reasonably high frequency.

This type of apparatus can also be used in conjunction with a *photo-electric cell* which is influenced by the beam of light reflected from the mirror (Rein *et al.*, 1940). There are several kinds of photo-electric cell, the principles of which may play an increasing part in medical recording devices. In the *photo-emission cell* a semi-cylindrical silver cathode coated on the inside with a photo-emitter (such as cæsium and cæsium oxide) faces an anode rod in a vacuum bulb. When light falls on the photo-sensitive surface of the cathode electrons are emitted in linear proportion to the quantity of light falling. If a current is passed through the bulb it is increased by the additional number of electrons emitted by the light-sensitive cathode. The variations in current so produced are directly proportional to the amount of light received and can be recorded by means of a galvanometer with suitable valve amplification.

The *photo-conductive* cell depends on the increased electrical conductivity of certain semi-conductors such as selenium when exposed to light. The response is again linear. The cell is made in the form of a selenium-coated grid through which a current can be passed. The electrical resistance of the cell varies inversely with the amount of light to which it is exposed, and this variation can be recorded in the usual way.

The *photo-voltaic cell* depends on the fact that an electromotive force is generated when light falls on the interface between a layer of copper and a layer of copper oxide, or between layers of iron and iron selenide. The layer of cuprous oxide or iron selenide must be very thin (less than 0.01 mm.) to allow the light to penetrate to the interface. When the two layers are connected current flows in direct proportion to the quantity of light falling on the interface.

ELECTROMANOMETERS transform pressures in the fluid system to equivalent electrical potentials directly, and these are amplified sufficiently to operate suitable galvanometers. A wide range of sensitivity allows pressure changes of 5, 10, 25, 50 or 100 mm. Hg to be represented by a deflection of 1 cm. on the tracing. *Transducers* for converting pressure changes into equivalent variations in electrical potential are of various types according to the basic principle employed. In practically all the fluid pressure acts on a membrane, as with mechanical and optical manometers.

The strain gauge makes use of the principle that wire increases its electrical resistance in proportion to the tension to which it is subjected. Four strain sensitive wires are used and are attached to the membrane by cantilever suspension in such a way that movement in one direction increases the strain on one pair of wires and reduces it on the other, movement in the reverse direction having the opposite effect. When the membrane is at rest the resistances of the two pairs of wires are balanced on a Wheatstone bridge circuit. When the resistances alter as a result of strain the bridge is thrown out of balance and current flows in the output or galvanometer circuit (Lambert and Wood, 1947). If the bridge is powered by a 6 to 20 volt battery no amplification is necessary. The frequency response is low at about 10 cycles per second. The magnitude of the current is directly proportional to the movement of the membrane.

Inductance transducers are based on Faraday's discovery in 1831 that an electrical current could be induced in a circuit by changing a magnetic field in the immediate vicinity of the circuit. The induced current is increased if the coil is wound round a soft iron core. If a battery current is flowing through the coil a magnetic field is set up around it which changes if the soft iron core is moved; this change at once influences the current in the coil by setting up a secondary induced current. Electromanometers have been designed in which the soft iron core of such a system is moved by a membrane influenced by changes of pressure (Wetterer, 1944).

Condenser or *capacitance manometers* are based on the fact that if a condenser is incorporated in an alternating current circuit, it acts like a resistance, and since this resistance varies directly with the distance between the two plates the condenser can serve as a transducer if one of the plates is designed as a membrane which moves in response to changes of pressure. Modern capacitance manometers are relatively complex (Hansen, 1949).

Clinical arteriogram

Arteriograms are of limited clinical value, because they reveal little that cannot be discerned with the trained finger. A normal arteriogram (fig. 5.03) usually exhibits two waves, P and D. The former is the percussion wave and represents the rapidly transmitted shock of left ventricular contraction; it is a pressure wave and must not be confused with blood flow. Its velocity is 5 to 8 metres per second and is inversely proportional to the elasticity of the artery. The length of the wave is 3.5 to 5 metres. The time-lag between aortic and carotid events is about 0.03 second, and between carotid and radial 0.10 second (Lewis, 1925). The sharp upstroke of a brachial arteriogram usually measures about 0.08 second, and the rounded summit of the tracing occupies a similar period. D is the dicrotic wave, and

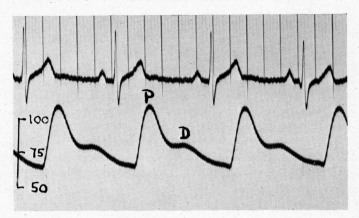

Fig. 5.03—Normal arteriogram.

is produced by the shock of aortic valve closure. The latter synchronises with the incisura (dicrotic or aortic notch) which precedes the dicrotic wave. Under certain circumstances, e.g. in combined aortic stenosis and incompetence, a second systolic wave T follows the percussion wave (fig. 5.04).

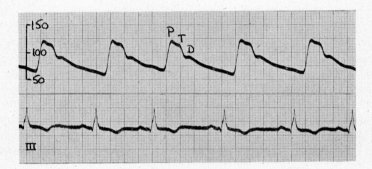

Fig. 5.04—Direct arterial tracing showing a tidal wave T.

Classical types of arteriogram have already been described in the clinical section on the pulse. Direct arterial tracings are apt to be a little different and rather less like what one feels than the indirect. The best example of this is the absence of a trough between percussion and tidal waves in the pulsus bisferiens in direct tracings (fig. 2.04). The difference is attributed to the fact that a certain amount of external pressure is applied to the artery in indirect arteriograms, just as it is when a clinician feels the pulse. Direct tracings are similarly modified when external pressure is applied to the artery.

The peak of the percussion wave of a direct arteriogram is the maximum systolic blood pressure; the diastolic pressure is represented by the gentle downward slope that succeeds the dicrotic wave. The clinical diastolic pressure is the end of this slope, i.e. the arterial pressure immediately preceding systole, or the end-diastolic pressure.

A direct arteriogram may be recorded continuously over a long period if desirable, e.g. when a continuous record of the blood pressure is required. A special needle such as Riley's is then used and must be slipped well up the artery, or a fine plastic catheter is threaded through the needle and the latter withdrawn. Clotting may be prevented by including a slow high-pressure saline drip in the system. This does not influence the tracing.

Arteriograms recorded simultaneously or consecutively with right ventricular pressures help to distinguish Fallot's tetralogy from pulmonary stenosis with normal aortic root; in the former the systolic pressures are equal, in the latter they are not. The same principle serves to distinguish Eisenmenger's complex and pulmonary hypertension with reversed shunt through a patent ductus from other forms of pulmonary hypertension.

Although the form of the arteriogram alone provides good evidence of the severity of aortic stenosis, simultaneous brachial and left ventricular pressure tracings are better, especially if the cardiac output at the time is known. The left ventricular pressure is not easily measured, but can be obtained by passing a fine nylon catheter through a needle inserted into the left atrium via the left bronchus or posterior chest wall (Bjork *et al.*, 1954). Direct puncture, however, is proving less traumatic.

Simultaneous or immediately consecutive direct arteriograms from the brachial and femoral arteries help to confirm or refute the presence of coarctation of the aorta when the diagnosis is in doubt. In coarctation the femoral arteriogram shows a lower systolic pressure and a smaller pulse pressure than the brachial, while the percussion wave is more prolonged and has a delayed summit.

Continuous arteriograms have also proved helpful in the investigation of syncope and in studying the effects of the Valsalva manœuvre.

The Valsalva manœuvre

The Valsalva manœuvre consists of forced expiration against a closed glottis (Valsalva, 1707; Dawson, 1943). It is a simple way of greatly raising the intrathoracic pressure. The effect is more conveniently achieved by blowing up a column of mercury and maintaining the pressure at 50 mm. Hg or as near to this level as possible. This is then the intra-oral pressure and may be assumed to be also the intrabronchial and intrapleural pressure. Alternatively, the intrathoracic pressure may be measured by passing a thin water-filled polythene tube down the œsophagus (Dornhorst and Leathart, 1952); the tube has an internal diameter of 0.5 mm., and should have two or three lateral holes cut near the distal end. The obstruction at the thoracic inlet tends to prevent cardiac filling and the heart shrinks; at the same time the venous pressure rises sharply until it exceeds the intrathoracic pressure. Direct arterial pressure tracings show characteristic changes in blood pressure, pulse pressure and heart rate (fig. 5.05): there is a sharp initial rise of blood pressure equivalent to the rise in intrathoracic pressure during the phase of forced expiration (phase 1);

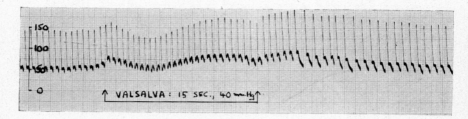

Fig. 5.05—Response of the arterial pressure pulse to the Valsalva manœuvre (see text).

thereafter the blood pressure falls gradually, the pulse pressure diminishes and the heart rate quickens (phase 2), due to a fall in stroke output; on release of strain there is a sudden further drop of blood pressure equivalent to the fall in intrathoracic pressure, and for a few beats the pulse pressure may become very small owing to the sucking of most of the available blood into the near empty pulmonary venous reservoir (phase 3); with restoration of normal conditions the heart fills properly again and the cardiac output increases, but before the physiology of the circulation returns to normal the blood pressure rises well above the original level, the pulse pressure widens, and the heart rate slows (phase 4 or the overshoot), due chiefly to reflex vasoconstriction initiated by the small pulse pressure stimulating aortic and carotid baroreceptors during the period of strain, although the stroke output also rises in response to an increased filling pressure, the right and left atrial pressures being temporarily above normal (Hamilton *et al.*, 1936, 1939; Elisberg *et al.*, 1953). If the period of strain is sufficiently prolonged this reflex vasoconstriction, with its attendant rise of blood pressure, can be seen to develop during phase 2, as in figure 5.05. The net pulmonary artery pressure (P.A.P. minus intrathoracic pressure) behaves like the systemic pressure, but the overshoot is less conspicuous, being attributed only to a rise in stroke output due to the temporarily raised right atrial pressure, there being no evidence of reflex pulmonary vasoconstriction (Lea, Matthews and Sharpey-Schafer, 1954).

The test has some clinical value in distinguishing cases of genuine heart failure from other conditions which may resemble it, for in heart failure (q.v.) there is no overshoot. The presence or absence of the overshoot can be determined easily enough at the bedside by noting whether or not there is bradycardia, for the slowing is secondary to the raised pressure (Elisberg *et al.*, 1953).

THE CIRCULATION TIME

The circulation time may be measured from the antecubital fossa to the head and neck, via the heart and lungs (Blumgart, 1931). Numerous substances may be used for the purpose, and fall chiefly into four groups, illustrated by sodium cyanide, histamine, sodium dehydrocholate and fluorescein.

If 0.25 to 0.5 ml. of 2 per cent *sodium cyanide* is injected into the antecubital vein, the patient takes a sudden deep breath when the substance reaches the carotid sinus, the respiratory reflex being initiated by direct chemical action (Robb and Weiss, 1934). At the same time the sinus node is depressed, so that the objective end-point is also signalled by a sinus pause which can be recorded and timed exactly on the electrocardiogram (Wexler *et al.*, 1947). Sodium cyanide is rapidly rendered inert by oxidation, so that the test may be repeated almost immediately, if necessary. Unfortunately, patients vary considerably in their susceptibility to the drug, and as this cannot be predicted the minimum dose must be tried first: the sensation of choking and strangling which may follow too large a dose in sensitive individuals may be very unpleasant. *Lobeline* in doses of 2.5 to 5 mg. acts similarly on carotid chemoreceptors, and any record of respiration will signal the end-point objectively. It is safer and less unpleasant than cyanide (Berliner, 1940).

Histamine phosphate (Weiss, Robb and Blumgart, 1928), in doses of 0.001 mg. per kg. of body weight in 1 : 5,000 solution, induces a sudden facial flush when it reaches the capillaries of the head and neck. It is not recommended owing to the uncertain end-point and subsequent headache; recorded times are too long.

A 20 per cent solution of *sodium dehydrocholate* (decholin, suprachol) has been used extensively and has given satisfactory results, but sometimes causes vomiting (Winternitz *et al.*, 1931). A dose of 3 to 5 ml. is injected rapidly through a wide-bore needle, the patient having been warned to raise the other hand smartly the instant he should notice a strange taste in or under the tongue. This taste is peculiarly intense and bitter, so that it is difficult for the patient to be mistaken about the moment of its arrival, and objective confirmation may be obtained by the involuntary grimace that accompanies it. The time should be measured from the beginning of the injection to the end-point described. A concentrated solution of *saccharin* (2.5 G. in 4 ml. of water), which produces a sweet taste when it reaches the tongue, is less unpleasant, does not cause vomiting and may be repeated if serial observations are required (Fishberg, Hitzig and King, 1933); but it is apt to cause local venous thrombosis. *Calcium gluconate*, 2.5 to 5 ml. of a 20 per cent solution, causes a hot sensation in the back of the tongue and throat (Goldberg, 1936), and *magnesium sulphate*, 6 ml. of a 10 per cent aqueous solution, has a similar end-point (Neurath, 1937; Bernstein and Simkins, 1939); these substances may be alternated with advantage if the test is repeated, for they are physiological antidotes. In this group the end-points are all subjective, but should not be despised on that account, for they are usually sharp and clear.

The fourth class comprises substances that give an objective end-point wherever desired. In their original papers Blumgart and Weiss (1927) used *radium C* and a special detector which, operating at any given point in the circulation, would signal the arrival of the test dose. The same principle has been employed by Prinzmetal (1948), using *radiosodium* (Na^{24}) and a Geiger-Müller counter, for constructing time concentration curves of the test dose as it passes through the right and left side of the heart. If within a minute of raising a histamine wheal (using 0.1 ml. of a mixture of equal parts of 1 : 1,000 histamine phosphate and 2 per cent procaine) on any part of the skin, a fluorescent substance is injected intravenously, fluorescence develops at the periphery of the wheal as soon as the substance reaches it; a suitable ultraviolet lamp is required. The best substances for this test are *fluorescein* (Lian and Barras, 1930) and *riboflavine*, the dose of the former being 5.4 mg. per kilogram of body weight, and of the latter 0.8 mg. per kilogram (Winsor *et al.*, 1947).

The *normal arm to tongue circulation time* averages 13.5 seconds with extremes of 9 to 18 seconds (Wood, 1936). *The time is fast* (6 to 9 sec.) in all the hyperkinetic circulatory states, and may be very fast (3 to 5 sec.) in congenital heart disease with large right to left shunt. *The time is greatly prolonged* in cases of left ventricular failure, when it averages 28 seconds; it is variable in mitral stenosis according to the physiological situation, and only slightly prolonged, if at all, in pure right ventricular failure. The circulation time is also related to the size of the heart, particularly to the residual stroke volume (Gernandt and Nylin, 1946), and is prolonged in myxœdema.

The *arm-to-lung time* may be measured by injecting 0.25 ml. of ether into the antecubital vein, its arrival in the capillaries of the lung being signalled by a sudden cough or deep dreath, and by the smell of ether in the expired air. Amyl acetate may also be used, the smell of pear-drops being unmistakable when it reaches the lungs. The normal time averages 6 seconds, and ranges between 3.5 and 8 seconds (Hitzig, 1935). The test has a limited value, as explained on page 278.

DYE DILUTION CURVES

The injection method of measuring the cardiac output (Stewart, 1897) was taken up in 1929 by Kinsman, Moore and Hamilton, who studied the behaviour of a small quantity of dye when injected rapidly into models of the circulation. The dye diffused uniformly in the turbulent stream and moved forwards in an ever widening band. If samples of the fluid stream were taken at frequent intervals from a point well away from the site of injection, and the quantity of dye in each sample measured colorimetrically against known standards, a curve could be constructed in which the concentration of dye in mg. per litre was plotted against the time (in

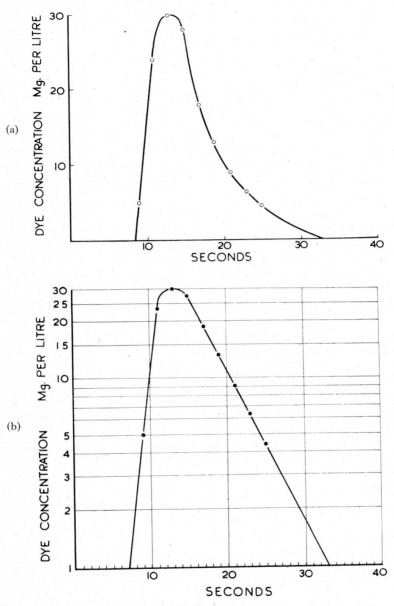

Fig. 5.06—Time concentration curves
(a) Plotted in a linear manner on both scales.
(b) Concentration plotted logarithmically (see text).

seconds) at which the sample was obtained after the onset of the injection. Such time-concentration curves had a characteristic shape, as shown in figure 5.06a. The build-up of concentration, second by second, was rapid, the disappearance of dye more gradual and fading off towards infinity. If recirculation was arranged to make the model more realistic, the down-stroke of the curve was interrupted by a sudden increase of concentration as the dye entered its second circuit. This made it impossible to estimate the time at which the dye would have disappeared from samples had it not recirculated. The difficulty was overcome when it was recognised that the down-stroke of the curve had a logarithmic shape, and when the concentration of dye was plotted logarithmically, the time scale remaining linear, the downstroke became a straight line (fig. 5.06b). By extending the top part of the slope until it met the time scale it was then possible to tell when the dye would have disappeared had it not recirculated.

Suppose now the duration of such a time-concentration curve is 30 seconds, and the mean concentration of dye over that period is 10 mg. per litre, then if the amount of dye injected was 20 mg., it is clear that this must have been diluted by 2 litres of blood in 30 seconds, i.e. by a blood flow or cardiac output of 4 litres per minute.

$$\text{Thus F or C.O.} = \frac{i \times 60}{ct}$$

where F is the blood flow in litres per minute

   i is the quantity of dye injected in mg.

   c is the mean concentration of dye in mg. per litre

   t is the duration of the time-concentration curve in seconds.

The mean concentration of dye is the average of all the samples taken, second by second, over the period of the time-concentration curve. In the hypothetical curve plotted in fig. 5.06, the mean concentration of dye works out at 12 mg. per litre over a period of 24 seconds. Had 24 mg. of dye been injected, the cardiac output per minute would have been $\dfrac{24 \times 60}{12 \times 24} = 5$ litres.

When compared with the Fick principle for measuring cardiac output in animals, results obtained by the dye injection method tallied remarkably closely, the average difference between the two being only 0.2 per cent (Moore *et al.*, 1929). Nearly twenty years later Hamilton and his colleagues (1948) compared the two methods in man and again average results were almost identical.

The dye commonly used now is Evans blue in a dose of 10 to 20 mg. (2 to 4 ml. of a 0.5 per cent solution). An ear oximeter of the photo-electric cell type designed by Millikan (1942) and modified by Wood and Geraci (1949) may be used instead of direct arterial sampling at two-second intervals. Time concentration curves can be recorded directly by means of a galvanometer with this oximeter (Beard and Wood, 1951).

Dye dilution curves may also be used in the study of intracardiac shunts and other cardiovascular abnormalities (Nicholson, Burchell and Wood, 1951). With left to right shunts, as in atrial septal defect, ventricular septal defect and patent ductus, the initial part of the curve is more or less normal in that dye arrives at the ear in normal time, builds up quickly and starts disappearing quickly, although its mean concentration is diminished; but recirculation occurs early and may be repeated once or twice, producing a series of irregular bumps during the return of the graph to normal. With right to left shunts, as in Fallot's tetralogy, dye arrives at the ear well ahead of normal time, giving rise to a premature hump on the upstroke of the normal curve (Swan *et al.*, 1953).

Pulmonary blood volume

Dye dilution curves offer an objective method of measuring the mean pulmonary circulation time (Hamilton *et al.*, 1932), and since the cardiac output at the time can be estimated by the same technique, the amount of blood in the lungs can be calculated from Stewart's formula, which states that

$$Q = \frac{VT}{60} \text{ (Stewart, 1921)}$$

where Q is the quantity of blood in the lungs in litres,
V is the pulmonary blood flow in litres per minute, and
T is the mean pulmonary circulation time in seconds.

In the hypothetical example illustrated in figure 5.06:

$$Q = \frac{5 \times 12 \text{ (say)}}{60} = 1 \text{ litre}$$

When measuring the pulmonary circulation time by means of radium C, Blumgart and Weiss (1928) calculated that the average quantity of blood in the lungs of normal subjects was 984 ml. or 21 per cent of the total blood volume.

Total blood volume

The circulating blood volume is normally around 5 to 6 litres; it is about 3 to 3.5 litres per square metre of body surface, or about 75 to 85 ml. per kilogram of body weight, and averages a little more in men than in women, owing to a rather higher red cell content in men. Plasma constitutes about 55 per cent and cells about 45 per cent of the volume of whole blood.

It may be estimated by injecting intravenously a known quantity of a substance with suitable characteristics and measuring its concentration in the blood after complete mixing has occurred. Evans blue dye (Gregersen *et al.*, 1935) has proved satisfactory, and may be given in a dose of 5 ml. of a 0.5 per cent solution, its concentration in the plasma being determined colorimetrically. The dye technique, originally introduced by Keith, Rowntree and Geraghty in 1915, has largely replaced the older carbon monoxide method of Haldane and Smith (1900), in which a known quantity of the gas was inhaled and its concentration in the blood measured by means of a colorimeter or by blood gas analysis. The injection of radio-active substances, such as tagged red cells, is now challenging the dye method, or is being employed as a supplement to it, for tagged red cells are used for measuring the total circulating red cell volume, whereas dyes measure plasma volume. Of course, the relative quantities of red cells and plasma in whole blood can be determined easily by the hæmatocrit.

CARDIAC CATHETERISATION

Although first performed by Forssmann (1929) on himself, the introduction of cardiac catheterisation as an aid to clinical diagnosis is largely due to the work of Cournand (1941) in the U.S.A. and of McMichael and Sharpey-Schafer (1944) in England.

Cardiac output

Up till then measurement of cardiac output in man depended on methods which could not directly utilise the important principle first enunciated by Fick (1870):

$$\text{C.O. (L./min.)} = \frac{\text{oxygen consumption (ml./min.)}}{\text{A—V oxygen difference (ml./L.)}}$$

For example, if an individual extracts 250 ml. of oxygen from the atmosphere per minute, and the difference in oxygen content between samples of blood from the pulmonary artery and samples from the pulmonary veins (arterio-venous oxygen difference) is 50 ml. per litre, then clearly 5 litres of blood must have passed through the lungs per minute. It was easy enough to measure the oxygen consumption and the oxygen content of arterial samples, but short of direct puncture there was no means of obtaining a mixed venous sample from the right side of the heart. Cardiac catheterisation, however, at once made this possible, and since its introduction a vast amount of accurate work on the cardiac output in health and disease has been carried out.

Pressures in the lesser circulation

At the same time cardiac catheterisation supplied another great need, for it offered a direct and relatively safe method of measuring *pressures in the right side of the heart* and pulmonary artery—a previously inaccessible part of the circulation. Hamilton's optical manometer, already in use for measuring arterial pressure (q.v.), allowed systolic and diastolic pressure to be measured accurately, and soon a number of electromanometers were adapted or designed for the same purpose.

It was discovered later that if the catheter was passed down a branch of the pulmonary artery as far as it would go, the tip usually became wedged in such a manner that a little force was required to withdraw it. The pressure recorded when the catheter was so wedged was called the *pulmonary capillary venous pressure*, for it was believed to represent just that

(Hellems *et al.*, 1948; Lagerlöf and Werkö, 1949). Samples withdrawn from such a site are always near 100 per cent oxygenated and must not be used as an indication of the oxygen saturation of pulmonary venous blood. In fact, however, the pressure obtained when a catheter is wedged in a pulmonary artery branch is the left atrial pressure (fig. 5.07) and the wave

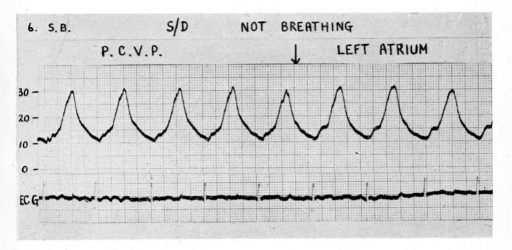

Fig. 5.07—Immediately consecutive tracings from a wedged pulmonary artery and from the left atrium (via the left bronchus) in a case of mitral incompetence, showing an identical pressure pulse in the two situations (from the paper by Epps and Adler from the Cardiac Department of the Brompton Hospital).

form is identical with the left atrial pressure pulse (Epps and Adler, 1953).

If the left atrial pressure pulse cannot be obtained indirectly in this way, it can be recorded directly by inserting a needle into the left atrium via the left bronchus (Facquet, Lemoin *et al.*, 1952), or by paravertebral puncture (Björk *et al.*, 1953). Even left ventricular pressures can be recorded via similar routes (Björk *et al.*, 1954).

The pulmonary vascular resistance can be calculated when the cardiac output, mean pulmonary artery pressure, and mean left atrial pressure are known, according to Poiseuille's equation:

$$\text{Resistance (R)} = \frac{\text{pressure gradient}}{\text{flow}}$$

which adapted becomes:

$$R = \frac{\text{P.A.P.} - \text{L.A.P. (mm. Hg)}}{\text{pulmonary blood flow (L./min.)}}$$

The result may be expressed in simple units of resistance. If it is desired to express resistance in fundamental units of force, as described by Gorlin and Gorlin (1951), pressures in mm. Hg must be converted into dynes/cm.^{2}, and flows expressed in litres per minute must be converted in cm.^{3}/sec. The equation thus becomes:

$$R = U \times \frac{0.1 \times 13.59 \times 981.17 \text{ dynes/cm.}^2}{1,000 \text{ cm.}^3/60 \text{ sec.}}$$

where U stands for the simple unit already described. The figure 13.59 is the specific gravity of mercury, and 981.17 cm. per second per second is the g factor—that is, the acceleration force of gravity. The dividend thus becomes 1,333.4 dynes/cm.^{2}. The equation may now be rewritten:

$$R = U \times \frac{1,333.4 \text{ dynes} \times 60 \text{ sec.}}{1.000 \text{ cm.}^5}$$

$$= U \times 80.004 \text{ dynes sec./cm.}^5$$

Thus it is only necessary to multiply the unit by 80 to express the resistance in dynes sec./cm.^{5}.

Shunts

As cardiac surgery advanced, accurate methods of diagnosing the various forms of congenital heart disease became imperative, and in this new field cardiac catheterisation helped enormously. In left to right shunts samples from chambers beyond and including that which receives the shunt contain more oxygen than samples taken from chambers proximal to the shunt. For example, in ventricular septal defect samples from the venæ cavæ and right atrium may be 70 per cent saturated with oxygen when samples from the right ventricle and pulmonary artery are 80 per cent saturated, proving that arterialised blood has entered the right ventricle from the left side of the heart. Since the pulmonary blood flow and the systemic blood flow can be measured separately, the size of the shunt can be calculated:

$$\text{Pulmonary flow (L./min.)} = \frac{\text{oxygen consumption (ml./min.)}}{\text{P.V.—P.A. oxygen content (ml./L.)}}$$

$$= \text{(say)} \frac{240}{190-160} = 8 \text{ L./min.}$$

$$\text{Systemic flow (L./min.)} = \frac{\text{oxygen consumption (ml./min.)}}{\text{Art.—R.A. oxygen content (ml./L.)}}$$

$$= \frac{240}{190-140} = 4.8 \text{ L./min.}$$

Thus in this example the interventricular shunt is 3.2 L./min. Pulmonary venous blood can only be obtained if the catheter passes through a foramen ovale, but for practical purposes may be assumed to be the same as arterial blood, provided there is no right to left shunt.

In cases of right to left shunt, samples from all chambers in the right side of the heart are similar, but the arterial oxygen saturation is reduced. In such cases:

$$\text{Pulmonary flow} = \frac{\text{oxygen consumption}}{\text{P.V.} - \text{P.A. oxygen content}}$$

$$= \text{(say)} \frac{210}{190 - 120} = 3 \text{ L./min.}$$

$$\text{Systemic flow} = \frac{\text{oxygen consumption}}{\text{arterial} - \text{R.A. oxygen content}}$$

$$= \text{(say)} \frac{210}{160 - 120} = 5.2 \text{ L./min.}$$

giving in this instance a right to left shunt of 2.2 L./min. In making the calculation it has been assumed that the pulmonary venous blood is 95 per cent saturated, i.e. having an oxygen content of 190 ml./L. (oxygen capacity with normal hæmoglobin 200 ml./L.). It should perhaps be explained that in calculating the systemic blood flow the arterial oxygen content, from which the arterio-venous oxygen difference is partly derived, is made up of two components, the content of blood which has passed through the lungs and picked up all the oxygen consumed, and the content of the shunted blood which has picked up no oxygen at all. It is as if the full 5.2 litres passed through the lungs, but 2.2 of them failed to pick up any oxygen.

Further information in congenital heart disease may be obtained if the catheter passes through a septal defect into the left side of the heart, or into anomalous veins.

TECHNIQUE

Radio-opaque nylon catheters, 100 to 125 cm. long, are made in seven sizes (nos. 4 to 10), the smallest (no. 4) having an internal diameter of 0.5 mm. and an external diameter of about 1.3 mm., and the largest (no. 10) having an internal diameter of about 1.8 mm. and an external diameter of 3.2 mm.; when filled they contain from 0.3 to 3.9 ml. of saline, the common sizes (nos. 6, 7 and 8) containing 0.8, 1.2, and 1.5 ml. respectively. They are sufficiently pliable to loop easily inside the heart or blood vessels, yet not so soft as to lose their elasticity as soon as they are warmed in the blood stream. The distal end is bent at about 4 cm. from the tip, so that awkward angles can be negotiated. After use, the catheters are washed out with tap water, and then with a hydrogen peroxide drip for several hours to remove any particles of blood enmeshed in the weave with which the catheters are lined; if this is neglected rigors may arise from pyrogens washed out of the lining of the catheter when it is next used, and can be very dangerous in certain types of heart disease. The catheters are then sterilised in hot formalin vapour and may also be stored in formalin vapour. They should not be boiled or autoclaved.

The patient is prepared with omnopon gr. 1/6 to 1/4 or pethidine 50 to 100 mg., and phenergan 25 mg. The latter acts as an additional sedative and tends to prevent vomiting. Pentothal may be necessary in children under six. Neither quinidine nor procaine amide are now given as a routine beforehand, because they did not prevent or diminish the frequency of ectopic beats or other changes of rhythm, and they are undesirable for three other reasons: (1) they may diminish the peripheral resistance; (2) they encourage cardiac standstill in the rare event of transient heart block during catheterisation; (3) they may turn pre-existing or a paroxysm of atrial fibrillation into flutter with a faster ventricular rate. Procaine amide, however, is always kept handy so that 0.5 to 1 G. may be given through the catheter immediately in the event of paroxysmal ventricular tachycardia or fibrillation. Noradrenalin, 100 μg. in 10 ml. of sterile water, is also kept ready in a second syringe in hazardous cases, for restoration of normal rhythm by means of heavy doses of procaine amide may not restore the blood pressure. Penicillin, 1 million units, is given as a routine to help prevent infection.

The patient is laid flat on a foam rubber mattress overlying an X-ray couch; a window is cut out of the mattress to facilitate fluoroscopy. The couch should be constructed so that it can be tilted easily and should be freely accessible from either side.

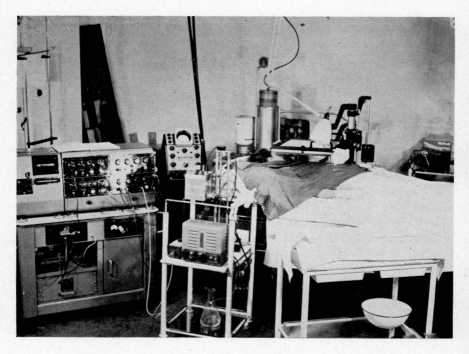

Fig. 5.08—Photograph of the N.E.P. multichannelled recorder, Sanborn electromanometer and cathode-ray monitor used for cardiac catheterisation at the Institute of Cardiology.

The right median cubital vein or the right basilic vein below or above its junction with the cubital vein is exposed, after liberal dermal anæsthesia with 1 per cent procaine. *The right arm* is preferred because the catheter is easier to manipulate from this side (especially if the operator is right handed), because the route is a little shorter (important in large adults if an indirect left atrial pressure tracing is required), and to avoid a left-sided superior vena cava entering the right atrium via the coronary sinus, a very difficult route from which to catheterise the pulmonary artery (encountered in 6 per cent of cases, especially in Fallot's tetralogy). *The median vein* is always chosen because it offers no obstruction to the passage of a catheter, whereas the cephalic route proved impossible in 19 out of 30 cases in which it was tried. *Liberal dermal anæsthesia* means raising an extensive wheal in the skin overlying the vein, using about 10 ml. of 1 per cent procaine; subcutaneous anæsthesia wears off too quickly, and stronger solutions of procaine are initially more painful and may upset previously good sedation in a small child. Efficient dermal anæsthesia has made venospasm very rare.

A catheter should be chosen which fits the vein snugly: if too large it will be difficult to move freely and will excite venospasm; if too small, bleeding will be troublesome. As a rule size 8 is best for adults with good veins, no. 7 for children and adults with small veins, and no. 6 for smaller children. The larger the catheter the easier it is to see, a point of some importance when the heart is large. A no. 6 catheter is also advised for cases of severe pulmonary stenosis with normal aortic root, when there is some danger of a large catheter blocking the pulmonary outflow.

When all is ready the vein is opened and the catheter, which has been previously washed inside and out with saline to remove all traces of formalin, and to the hilt of which is attached a 5 or 10 ml. syringe loaded with saline, is inserted in the manner of introducing a cannula, and pushed up the vein, its curved tip being directed medially, and care being taken to avoid introducing air. Any obstruction can usually be overcome by rotating the catheter a little one way or the other. When the tip is judged to be in the neighbourhood of the superior vena cava, the lights are turned out, 5,000 units of heparin are given through the catheter, and the inelastic sterile tube which will connect the catheter with the electromanometer is set up ready for use, while the operator is accommodating, the rest of the procedure being under fluoroscopic control. Kinks at the thoracic inlet may be passed during deep inspiration; abducting the arm or altering the position of the head and neck are usually a waste of time. If the obstruction appears insuperable it can be overcome by allowing the tip of the catheter to enter the jugular and to rotate it this way or that until some resistance is felt; if then the catheter is pushed gently forwards, a loop will form near the tip and this is encouraged until the bend itself passes down the superior vena cava. In over 1,000 pulmonary artery catheterisations the right superior vena cava has never been absent, and if there was no clinical

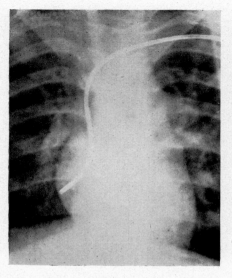

(a) Catheter allowed to impinge on the lateral wall of the right atrium.

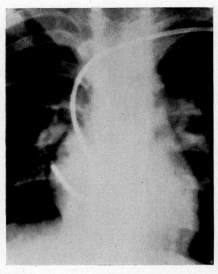

(b) A loop is formed in this situation.

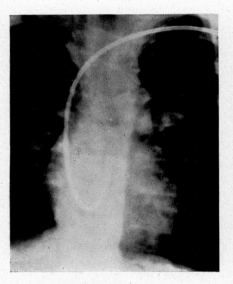

(c) The loop is rotated medially.

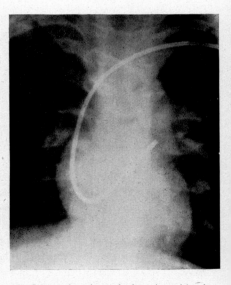

(d) On passing through the tricuspid valve the tip enters the pulmonary artery.

Fig 5.09—Loop technique for introducing a catheter into the right ventricle so that it passes into the pulmonary artery.

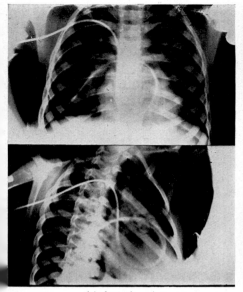
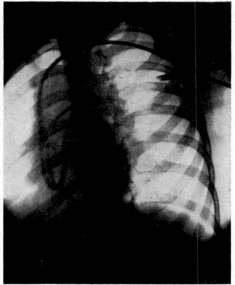

(a) Anterior view.
(b) First oblique position.

(c) Second oblique position.

Fig. 5.10—Catheter in right pulmonary artery.

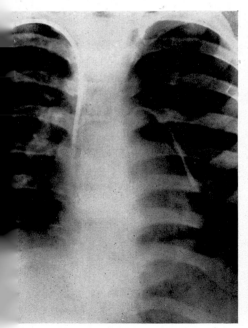
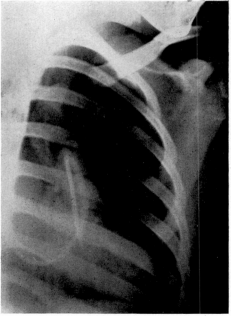

(a) Anterior view.

(b) First oblique position.

Fig. 5.11—Catheter in the left pulmonary artery.

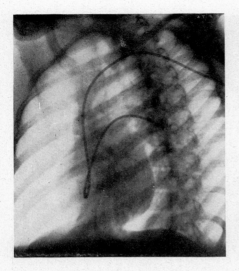

Fig. 5.11(c)—Catheter in left branch of the pulmonary artery (2nd oblique position).

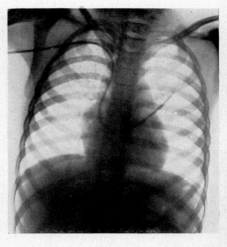

Fig. 5.12—Showing a catheter in the left upper pulmonary vein after passing through a foramen ovale in a normal subject.

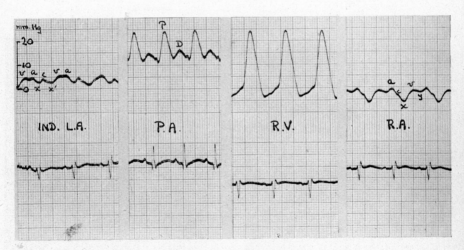

Fig. 5.13—Normal pressure pulses from the left atrium (indirect), pulmonary artery, right ventricle and right atrium.

evidence of thrombosis the vessel has never been blocked. With the aid of deep inspiration and this easily formed loop, difficulty in entering the superior vena cava has been overcome in all cases.

As soon as the catheter lies in the right atrium, its hilt should be connected to the electromanometer, and the right atrial pressure pulse recorded simultaneously with the electrocardiogram. The variable hydraulic damper is then adjusted and the recording system tested while the operator accommodates more thoroughly. Direct writing multichannel recorders have proved very satisfactory for routine diagnostic work; if a photographic recording system is used it is imperative to have a cathode ray monitor as well, so that tracings can be inspected continually. The zero reference point to which the manometer is adjusted may be the sternal angle or a measured distance such as 10 cm. above the surface of the couch, which represents the expected level of the heart itself. There is some advantage in incorporating a high pressure very slow heparinised saline drip in the hydraulic system to combat any possibility of clotting in the lumen of the catheter, but with due care thrombosis can be avoided without it. Blood should never be allowed to enter the catheter inadvertently, and when deliberately withdrawn (as in sampling), or when assumed to have entered (as when advancing into a high pressure zone with the hilt of the catheter attached to an unattended syringe), it should be cleared as soon as possible by injecting saline from the syringe. This is not only to avoid clotting, but also to prevent particles of blood becoming enmeshed in the weave with which the catheter is lined—a fruitful source of future pyrogens and rigors.

The best way to enter the right ventricle from the right arm is to allow the tip of the catheter to impinge against the lateral wall of the right atrium, and by pushing on to form a loop there; when rotated medially this loop ensures that the tip of the catheter is directed upwards when it passes through the tricuspid valve and so passes on readily into the pulmonary artery (fig. 5.09). The position of the catheter is determined by fluoroscopy, by the pressure pulse recorded, and if necessary by sampling. For example, if the tip of the catheter locks as if it were in the outflow tract of the right ventricle, but will not pass onwards, the pressure pulse will probably be atrial in form, and a blood sample may be bright red from the left atrial appendix, or almost black from the coronary sinus.

Typical positions are illustrated in figures 5.10 to 5.12, and a normal series of pressure pulses in figure 5.13. As previously mentioned, an indirect left atrial pressure pulse may be obtained by wedging the tip of the catheter in a distal branch of the pulmonary artery, so that a little force is required to withdraw it. If the catheter can be passed through a patent foramen ovale or atrial septal defect, an indirect pulmonary artery pressure tracing may also be recorded by wedging the catheter in a pulmonary vein (fig. 5.14).

Samples of blood (5 ml.) are withdrawn under paraffin from all important positions which the catheter has entered, preferably in quick succession,

P.A.   Wedged pul. vein

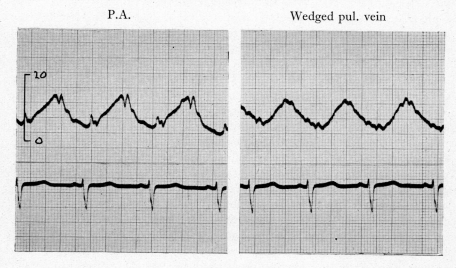

Fig. 5.14—Pulmonary artery pressure pulse recorded indirectly by wedging a catheter in a pulmonary vein.

and an arterial sample is obtained simultaneously with that from the pulmonary artery. The samples are expelled from the syringe by means of a long needle or cannula into the bottom of small glass vessels containing a bead of heparin under a layer of liquid paraffin. In both the syringe and container the paraffin keeps the samples free from contact with air. They should be analysed for oxygen content or unsaturation by means of Van Slyke's or Haldane's method respectively as soon as possible; if blood gas analysis is delayed for several hours, the samples should be stored in a refrigerator.

The *total screening time* should not exceed 30 minutes at 1 m.a.

On withdrawing the catheter the vein is usually ligated; attempts to save its lumen by passing skin sutures under the vein above and below the opening in its wall have been none too successful, and occasionally appreciable hæmorrhage has occurred.

Complications

VENOSPASM often proved troublesome in the early days; it has been practically abolished by efficient local anæsthesia and by selecting a catheter that is not too large for the vein. Its present 2 per cent incidence seems to be associated with inadequate sedation in unduly nervous individuals or improper washing of the catheter so that traces of formalin still remain on its surface.

ECTOPIC BEATS are extremely common and may be disregarded. They occur especially when the tip of the catheter lies in the body of the right ventricle.

PAROXYSMAL SUPRAVENTRICULAR TACHYCARDIA, usually 2–1 auricular flutter, occurred in 3.3 per cent of 1,000 cases catheterised at the National Heart Hospital or Brompton Hospital. It occurred in 11.4 per cent of 88 cases of atrial septal defect, in 9 per cent of 45 cases of ventricular septal defect, but not more frequently than in normal subjects (4 per cent of 50 cases) in any other condition. For example, it occurred in 2.4 per cent of 335 cases of mitral valve disease and in 2 per cent of 145 cases of pulmonary stenosis with normal aortic root. It did not occur at all in 60 cases of patent ductus, in 75 cases of Fallot's tetralogy, nor in 48 cases of pulmonary hypertension with reversed shunt.

PAROXYSMAL VENTRICULAR TACHYCARDIA is fortunately rare (1 per cent) although short bursts of ventricular ectopics are common enough.

VENTRICULAR FIBRILLATION occurred in three cases, once in Ebstein's disease, once in advanced atrial septal defect, and once in primary pulmonary hypertension; it resulted in immediate death in two of them, giving a mortality rate of 0.2 per cent for the whole series.

TRANSIENT RIGHT BUNDLE BRANCH BLOCK occurred in 5 per cent. In one such instance in which permanent left bundle branch block was already present, this resulted in 2–1 heart block and might well have been serious. Since then left bundle branch block has been considered a contraindication to catheterisation.

TRANSIENT NODAL RHYTHM developed in 1.5 per cent and was inconsequential.

AIR EMBOLISM could occur if the operator was careless, and might have dire consequences in cases with right to left shunt. None was recognised in this series, however, but particular care has always been taken to keep the hilt of the catheter below right atrial level when sampling.

THROMBO-EMBOLISM was also totally avoided, although clotting in the catheter occurred in 1 per cent. This was nearly always the fault of the operator and should have been prevented. Subsequent phlebothrombosis was not uncommon, but pulmonary embolism was very rare (0.05 per cent) and never serious. Such cases, however, were treated with heparin and dindevan.

CEREBRAL ABSCESS, which may have been due to paradoxical embolism occurred in two cases of Fallot's tetralogy, one just before catheterisation was about to be undertaken, the other a month afterwards.

RIGORS due to pyrogens washed out of improperly cleaned catheters in which blood had been allowed to lie too long on a previous occasion were very troublesome indeed before the catheters were treated with a hydrogen peroxide drip after use. There have been only two in the last 500 cases.

SYNCOPE due to blocking the outflow tract of the right ventricle with the catheter at valve or infundibular level occurred in three cases of severe pulmonary stenosis with normal aortic root, two with reversed interatrial shunt, an incidence of about 6 per cent, but in no other condition. Vasomotor syncope associated with anxiety occurred twice in the series.

WOUND SEPSIS has never been serious, but can be a nuisance to both patient and staff; its frequency is naturally inversely related to the amount of care and trouble spent on proper aseptic precautions.

Contra-indications

1. Cases of known *ischæmic heart disease* should not be catheterised at all under any circumstances. Three instances are known to the author: one died immediately from ventricular fibrillation; the other two both developed paroxysmal ventricular tachycardia, and the procedure was abandoned.

2. *Ebstein's disease* is dangerous. Out of six I have personally catheterised, one died immediately from ventricular fibrillation, and one developed paroxysmal tachycardia which could have been ventricular. I know of two other deaths amongst the relatively few cases of Ebstein's disease in the world that have been catheterised.

3. Cases with *left bundle branch block* run a 5 per cent risk of developing transient bilateral branch block, which could well result in complete heart block.

4. Cases of *advanced atrial septal defect* with gross dilatation of the right side of the heart need very careful handling; one of the two deaths in the series here analysed occurred in such a case, and another is known to the author.

5. Advanced *anoxic cor pulmonale* has been responsible for at least one death from cardiac catheterisation.

In a review of 973 catheterised cases Hebert, Scebat and Lenegre found the mortality was 0.7 per cent. Two of the deaths were due to cardiac hæmorrhage from trauma, two to severe rigors, one to acute pulmonary œdema, and three to subsequent pulmonary embolism. *Acute pulmonary œdema* occurred in 14 of their series: cases of mitral stenosis in which the pulmonary vascular resistance is judged to be low should be treated with great respect; preliminary dehydration is important, and the X-ray couch should be tiltable foot down.

A mortality rate of 0.2 per cent in 1,000 cases was reported by Zimdahl (1951), and of 0.1 per cent in 5,691 cases by Cournand *et al.* (1953).

Normal pressures

There were 50 normal subjects amongst the 1,000 catheterised. The figures given here are based on these. The reference point to which the pressures are related is the sternal angle, so that they are all 3 to 5 mm. Hg lower than those generally reported.

The right atrial pressure averaged -0.5, -4, -1.5, -1 mm. Hg for *a*, *x*, *v*, and *y* respectively, the average mean pressure being -1.3 mm. Hg with reference to the sternal angle. The range of the mean pressure was $+2$ to -5. The significance of *a*, *x*, *v* and *y* has already been discussed (p. 47).

The indirect left atrial pressure averaged 4 mm. Hg higher, with little to choose between *a* and *v* or *ac* and *v* in good tracings; sound artifacts made precise measurements difficult at these low pressures.

The *right ventricular pressure* averaged 16/—1, with a mean of 4 mm. Hg. The highest systolic pressure recorded was 25 mm. Hg, very few being over 20, and only one under 10.

The *pulmonary artery pressure* averaged 16/7 mm. Hg, and the mean 11.

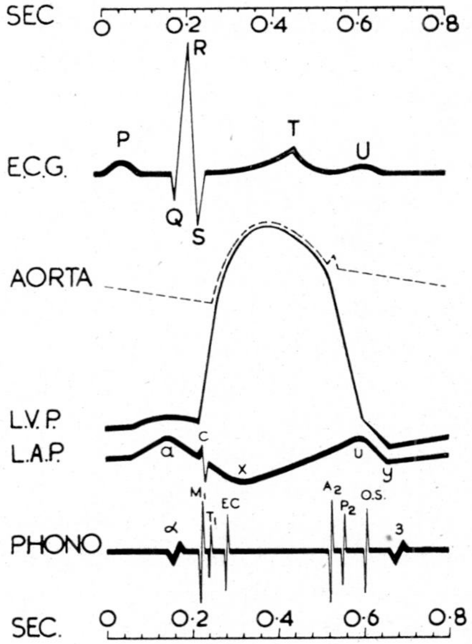

Time relationships of central pressure -pulses (fig. 5.15)

The first recordable event in the cardiac cycle is the right atrial or first half of the P wave of the electrocardiogram. The *a* wave of the right atrial pressure pulse begins at the peak of P, and reaches the jugular pulse about 0.1 second later.

The *x* descent due to atrial relaxation begins before ventricular systole and is interrupted by a notch or deformity representing closure of the tricuspid valve: this is the right atrial *c* wave. It is rarely large enough to be seen in the jugular pulse.

The left atrial *c* wave is synchronous with the onset of left ventricular systole, with the mitral element of the first heart sound, and with the S wave of the electro-

Fig. 5.15—Time relationships between electrocardiogram, aortic, left ventricular and left atrial pressure pulses, and the phonocardiogram (see text).

cardiogram. The right atrial *c* wave probably occurs 0.02 to 0.03 second later and is synchronous with the onset of right ventricular systole and with the tricuspid component of the first sound.

The *x* descent of the right atrial pressure pulse continues after the *c* interruption, the systolic part of the trough being partly attributed to descent of the base, the atrio-ventricular septum moving downwards and to the left towards the apex of the heart as the ventricles contract, so creating negative pressures in the atria.

Isometric ventricular contraction is that part of ventricular systole that occupies the time interval between closure of the tricuspid and mitral valves and the opening of the pulmonary and aortic valves respectively, a matter of 0.04 to 0.05 second.

The opening of the semi-lunar valves, which signals the end of the isometric contraction phase, occurs about 0.03 second before the vascular components of the first heart sound. These are normally inaudible, but under certain circumstances they can be heard as systolic ejection clicks.

Thus the time interval between the mitral component of the first heart sound and an aortic ejection click is a measure of the duration of left ventricular isometric contraction, if 0.03 second delay is allowed (Leatham, 1954).

The ejection phase then begins and lasts about 0.25 second; two-thirds of the ventricular stroke volume are pumped into the great vessels during the first half of this period (Wiggers, 1921). The carotid pulse and the carotid *c* wave of the jugular phlebogram follow left ventricular ejection by about 0.03 second, and the radial pulse is some 0.10 second later (Lewis, 1925).

Protodiastole is the short period of ventricular relaxation between the end of the ejection phase and closure of the semilunar valves. The aortic valve normally closes before the pulmonary and synchronises with the first component of the second heart sound, and more or less with the end of the T wave of the electrocardiogram.

The isometric relaxation phase is the time occupied by the ventricles between closure of the semilunar valves and the opening of the atrio-ventricular valves (0.06 to 0.10 sec.). The two components of the second heart sound signal its onset in respect of each ventricle (P_2 falling 0.02 to 0.05 second after A_2), and the top of the *v* waves of right and left atrial pressure tracings signal its end in respect of each ventricle. The opening snap of mitral stenosis also synchronises with the end of left ventricular isometric relaxation in that disease.

After the opening of the mitral and tricuspid valves, atrial and ventricular diastolic pressures fall together: this is the *y* descent or downstroke of *v* seen in atrial pressure pulses. The subsequent rise of diastolic pressure in both atria and ventricles depends on the venous pressure gradient and the tone of the ventricles. As used here, ventricular tone may be defined as resistance to diastolic filling. Since the left atrial pressure averages 4 mm. Hg higher than the right, it must be assumed that the left ventricular diastolic pressure is also 4 mm. Hg higher than the right, and this may be a function of tone.

From these time relationships it may be observed that if the heart rate is 60 beats per minute, allowing 1 second for the length of each cycle, the ventricles are allotted 0.62 second in which to fill, and 0.28 second in which to contract, 0.10 second being expended in protodiastolic and isometric relaxation.

Normal samples

The oxygen capacity is the total amount of oxygen held by a litre of blood when fully saturated. Since 1 G. of hæmoglobin will hold 1.34 ml. of oxygen at normal temperature and pressure, a litre of normal blood will hold $15 \times 1.34 \times 10 = 201$ ml. of oxygen when fully saturated.

The arterial oxygen saturation is normally 95 per cent of its oxygen capacity. This means that a litre of normal arterial blood holds $\dfrac{95}{100}$ of 201 = 191 ml. of oxygen.

Samples of arterial blood may be obtained from the brachial or femoral artery by direct puncture. A sharp short bevelled 18 gauge needle attached to an all-glass syringe containing a little paraffin should be plunged into the vessel. The arterial blood pressure then lifts the barrel of the syringe spontaneously, little aspiration being necessary. On withdrawing the needle the site of puncture should be compressed digitally for at least a minute.

The oxygen content of a sample is the actual amount of oxygen it contains and may be measured by means of Van Slyke's apparatus. Thus the oxygen content of normal arterial blood in the example given above is 191 ml. per litre. This is sometimes expressed as 19.1 volumes per cent.

The oxygen unsaturation of a sample is its oxygen capacity less its oxygen content, and may be measured by means of Haldane's apparatus. Thus the normal arterial oxygen unsaturation is around 10 ml. per litre or 1 volume per cent.

The arterio-venous oxygen difference averaged 34 ml. per litre in our series of 50 normal subjects, the range being 21 to 48.

The cardiac output calculated from Fick's formula (q.v.) averaged 8.6 litres per minute, the range being 5.8 to 12.8. These figures are not basal, but they certainly represent what is actually found under the conditions inevitably associated with cardiac catheterisation. The "*basal cardiac output*" is said to be around 4 to 5 litres per minute and is about a litre higher in the horizontal than in the erect position (McMichael and Sharpey-Schafer, 1944). The *cardiac index* is the cardiac minute output per square metre of body surface and should be around 3.

Samples from the right side of the heart (superior vena cava, right atrium, right ventricle and pulmonary artery) should not differ by more than 5 per cent in oxygen saturation, the scatter being centred around a mean difference of 3 per cent in our series. The *average oxygen saturation* of all these samples was 75 per cent, the vast majority being between 70 and 80 per cent.

The *pulmonary vascular resistance* (q.v.) averaged 1 unit or 80 dynes sec./cm.^{5}, commonly ranging between 0.5 and 1.5 units. The maximum normal resistance was 2.5 units.

OXIMETRY

Photovoltaic iron-selenium ear oximeters are based on the principle that oxyhæmoglobin and reduced hæmoglobin absorb light differently. Two cells are used. One is covered by a green wratten 61 N filter, which responds to light with wave lengths of 480 to 600 millimicrons and 750 to 800 millimicrons, the intermediate part of the spectrum being filtered out. Both oxy and reduced hæmoglobin transmit light of these wave lengths equally, so that the output of this cell depends on the thickness of the ear and the amount of blood in it. The second cell is covered by a red wratten 29 F filter which transmits light with wave lengths of 600 millimicrons and above. Since this red portion of the spectrum is absorbed in much greater degree by reduced hæmoglobin than oxyhæmoglobin, the amount of light activating this cell is proportional to the percentage of oxyhæmoglobin present in the blood through which the light passes, the first cell balancing the second in respect of other variables (Millikan, 1942).

RESPIRATORY FUNCTION TESTS

An elementary knowledge of respiratory physiology is essential to a proper understanding of the circulation.

CHEMICAL AND NERVOUS CONTROL OF BREATHING

When discussing the causes of dyspnœa it was observed that the respiratory centre reacted to several independent stimuli and that the total response depended on the algebraic sum of these stimuli (Gray, 1950).

ANOXIA (as diminished oxygen tension in the plasma) is a relatively weak stimulus which acts on chemoreceptors in the carotid sinus and aortic bodies (like sodium cyanide, lobeline and coramine); alone it is barely capable of doubling ventilation. An increased oxygen tension in the plasma (p O_2) does not inhibit respiration. Oxygen tension, of course, is an expression of the amount of oxygen dissolved in the plasma, and in arterial blood is nearly equal to the partial pressure of oxygen to which the plasma has been exposed in its journey through the lungs, i.e. to the partial pressure of oxygen in alveolar air. The partial pressure of oxygen in the atmosphere is about 21 per cent of the barometric pressure = 21 per cent of 760 mm. Hg = 159 mm. Hg. In alveolar air the gas mixture is not the same as in the atmosphere, for it is almost fully saturated with water vapour, contains about 5.6 per cent of carbon dioxide which it has collected from the plasma, and is left with only 14.2 per cent of oxygen. The partial pressure of oxygen in alveolar air should therefore be 14.2 per cent of 760 mm. Hg, or allowing for water vapour 14.2 per cent of (760−47) = 101.2 mm. Hg. That the arterial oxygen tension (90 to 95 mm. Hg) is not the same is due to slight perfusion of unventilated alveoli. The oxygen tension of venous blood is only about 40 mm. Hg, so that there is a strong oxygen pressure gradient across the interface between the alveolar wall and the proximal end of the pulmonary capillary, favouring rapid diffusion. The plasma oxygen tension determines whether hæmoglobin takes up oxygen or releases it. The familiar oxygen dissociation curve of hæmoglobin shows the changing affinity that hæmoglobin has for oxygen according to the oxygen tension of the plasma: at high tensions around 100 mm. Hg, hæmoglobin is 95 per cent saturated with oxygen; as the tension falls towards 70 mm. Hg, the proportion of oxyhæmoglobin declines very little to about 90 per cent; as the oxygen tension falls below 70 mm. Hg, however, hæmoglobin appears more and more in its reduced form, so that at an oxygen tension of 40 mm. Hg, which is average for venous blood, hæmoglobin is only about 70 per cent saturated, and at a tension of 30, only about 50 per cent saturated: this behaviour makes hæmoglobin an ideal vehicle for transporting oxygen, storing it when plentiful and releasing it where it is most wanted.

CARBON DIOXIDE stimulates the respiratory centre directly and is capable of increasing ventilation tenfold. Again, it is the tension of carbon dioxide in the arterial blood (p CO_2) that matters, and this is equal to the partial pressure of carbon dioxide in alveolar air, for this gas diffuses far more rapidly in fluid media than oxygen. The partial pressure of alveolar CO_2 is normally about 5.6 per cent of (760—47) mm. Hg = 40 mm. Hg approximately. Thus the arterial CO_2 tension is also 40 mm. Hg. A rise of only 2.5 mm. Hg in arterial CO_2 tension is enough to double ventilation (Gray, 1950); a fall in p CO_2 depresses the respiratory centre.

Like oxygen, carbon dioxide is formed in too great a quantity to be transported as a simple solution in plasma, and so it too has a special means of conveyance. Hæmoglobin is again made use of. Carbon dioxide from the tissues diffuses into the venous blood at a tension around 46 mm. Hg and readily enters the red corpuscles. Here, with the aid of an enzyme carbonic anhydrase, it joins with water to form carbonic acid, H_2CO_3. This combines with potassium base obtained from reduced hæmoglobin, thus:

$$H_2CO_3 + KHb = HHb + KHCO_3$$

because carbonic acid is a stronger acid than reduced hæmoglobin. Dissociation allows bicarbonate anions (HCO_3) so formed in the cells to diffuse out into the plasma, leaving unattached potassium kations (which cannot pass the cell membrane) within the corpuscles. Equilibrium is restored by the well-known chloride shift, dissociation of sodium chloride in the plasma allowing sodium+ to combine with HCO_3 to form plasma bicarbonate, while chloride anions pass into the red cells to combine with potassium:

$$K^+ \ HCO_3^- \qquad Na^+ \ Cl^-$$
$$KCl \qquad\qquad NaHCO_3$$

When the red cells reach the lungs, the chloride shift is reversed, because oxyhæmoglobin is a much stronger acid and promptly re-acquires the potassium base, thus releasing chloride from the cells; the chloride combines with the sodium of the plasma bicarbonate to form the weaker acid H_2CO_3 from which carbon dioxide is finally excreted through the lungs, thus:

$$HHb + KCl = KHb + HCl$$
$$HCl + NaHCO_3 = NaCl + H_2CO_3$$
$$H_2CO_3 \ \geqslant \ H_2O + CO_2$$

It follows that *an increase of carbon dioxide in the blood results in an increase of plasma bicarbonate.* When the carbon dioxide of the body is depleted, as by forced breathing, the plasma bicarbonate falls. In other words, *carbon dioxide is carried as bicarbonate* in the plasma.

Since the plasma bicarbonate is the most important buffer substance available for neutralising fixed acid, such as lactic acid, it has been called the *alkali reserve.* This may be measured by finding out how much carbon dioxide is liberated from the plasma under controlled conditions when exposed to an acid, the answer being expressed in volumes (ml.) per cent. The normal *carbon dioxide content* of plasma is 53 to 75 volumes per cent, when measured in this way. This is often called the *carbon dioxide combining power* or *carbon dioxide capacity* of the plasma. The terms *acidosis* and *alkalosis* refer to states in which the carbon dioxide content of the plasma is below 53 or above 75 volumes per cent respectively. This has caused much confusion, for every clinician knows that forced breathing, which results in CO_2 washout, causes a transient slight rise in pH (alkalæmia), yet the reduction in alkali reserve (carbon dioxide content), to which it also gives rise, entitles it to be called a state of acidosis. Again, in advanced cor pulmonale, particularly if ventilation is depressed by any means, a high CO_2 tension may be associated with a lowered pH (acidæmia) and increased alkali reserve (alkalosis). The confusion would be avoided if the terms acidæmia and alkalæmia were used (as now) to denote a fall or rise of pH, and the terms acidosis and alkalosis were dropped altogether in favour of more precise designations for the plasma bicarbonate.

A less variable and more informative figure is the carbon dioxide content of arterial blood, which in health is 45 to 53 ml. per cent.

A final very important point about the carbon dioxide tension as a respiratory stimulant is the narcotic effect produced when the tension exceeds 60 mm. Hg. At such levels carbon dioxide may not only cause unconsciousness, but actually depresses the respiratory centre. As will be seen later, the treatment of cor pulmonale with oxygen is much influenced by this consideration.

THE HYDROGEN ION CONCENTRATION or pH value is the third important respiratory stimulant, and like carbon dioxide acts directly on chemo-receptors in the respiratory centre. The normal pH is given as 7.41; it remains remarkably constant in health and is one of the last things to alter in disease. It is maintained largely by the buffer systems of the blood, by removal of an ever varying quantity of carbon dioxide by the lungs, and by excretion of acid or alkaline substances in the urine. The chief effect of the buffer systems, such as the plasma bicarbonate, is to ensure as far as possible that no acid stronger than H_2CO_3 can exist in the blood. For example, lactic acid derived from working muscle is at once converted by sodium bicarbonate into sodium lactate and carbonic acid. Any increase of CO_2 tension resulting from the exchange at once stimulates the respiratory centre and excess CO_2 is removed via the lungs. Nevertheless, metabolic disturbances do occur, in diabetes mellitus for example, in which a reduced pH causes hyperventilation; in such cases the carbon dioxide tension will also be reduced (as a result of increased CO_2 washout). An increased CO_2 tension itself also causes slight reduction of the pH.

MUSCULAR EXERCISE is a respiratory stimulant independent of secondary changes in CO_2 tension.

HEAT is also an important respiratory stimulant. Thermoreceptors in the hypothalamus react to changes in body temperature and explain the hyperventilation of high fever. Thermoreceptors in the skin react to change in the temperature of the environment.

The *inter-relationships* between these various respiratory stimuli are complicated and cannot be discussed here; but when considering the effect of any one of them it is most important to consider at the same time what is happening to the others. For example, with very high CO_2 tensions in advanced cor pulmonale, the respiratory centre may be responding only to oxygen lack, as previously explained. If the patient is nursed in an oxygen tent the only stimulant to respiration may be abolished and ventilation may greatly decline. This reduces excretion of carbon dioxide and the patient may become unconscious from CO_2 narcosis.

So much then for the central control of respiration. We now have to consider the physiology of ventilation itself, i.e. the events that take place in the lungs to ensure proper oxygenation of perfusing blood and elimination of carbon dioxide.

VENTILATION

In what is called a *steady state* the amount of oxygen taken up by the lungs exactly equals the amount utilised by the tissues, minute by minute, and the amount of carbon dioxide eliminated by the lungs exactly equals that formed in the tissues. The amount of oxygen consumed varies with the surface area of the body, which can be obtained from tables of height and weight, and is called the metabolic rate. It is usually around 250 ml. per minute, and if measured under basal conditions is called the *basal metabolic rate*, being expressed as a percentage of normal. To every 250 ml. of oxygen consumed, about 200 ml. of carbon dioxide is eliminated. The ratio, in this example $\dfrac{200}{250} = 0.80$, is called the *respiratory quotient*.

Resting ventilation

For each 100 ml. of oxygen consumed about 2.5 litres of air must be breathed. This ratio is the *ventilation equivalent for oxygen*. If 250 ml. of oxygen have to be absorbed per minute, then at this equivalent 6.25 litres of air must be breathed. This is the resting ventilation, and is the *tidal volume* (about 500 ml.) multiplied by the number of inspirations per minute (in this case 12.5), and can be measured very simply with any spirometer. It is the respiratory analogy of the cardiac output at rest.

Reserves

From a state of quiet breathing it is always possible to inspire much more deeply; this extra depth of a single maximum inspiration is the *inspiratory reserve* (2 to 2.5 litres). The term *inspiratory capacity* (or complemental air) refers to the sum of the tidal volume and the inspiratory reserve; it is the maximum inspiration after quiet expiration. The *expiratory reserve* (or supplemental air) is the maximum volume of air that can be expelled after quiet expiration (usually 1 to 1½ litres).

Vital capacity

The sum of the tidal, inspiratory reserve, and expiratory reserve volumes is the vital capacity. It should measure around 3.5 to 4.5 litres.

Total lung volume (or capacity)

After maximum expiration there is still a good deal of air in the bronchial tubes and trachea; this is known as the dead space or *residual volume*, and in disease may include parts of the lung that cannot be deflated. It is possible to measure the dead space plus the expiratory reserve volume during quiet breathing, the sum of the two being called the *functional residual capacity* (air or volume), by finding out how much a known quantity of an inert gas such as helium is diluted when introduced into a closed circuit comprising the air in the spirometer and the space to be measured. The residual volume, of course, is the functional residual capacity so determined, less the expiratory reserve volume as measured directly with a spirometer. The *total lung volume* is the residual volume plus the vital capacity, or the functional residual capacity plus the inspiratory capacity. In health the residual volume measures 1 to 1½ litres, and the total lung volume about 5 litres. The various divisions of the lung volume are shown diagramatically in figure 5.16. A useful ratio is the residual volume expressed as a percentage of the total lung capacity (normal 20 to 25 per cent). According to Motley (1950) this measurement correlates well with the degree of emphysema present.

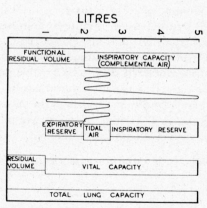

Fig. 5.16—Subdivisions of the lung volume

Maximum breathing capacity

One of the most important measurements of lung function is the maximum breathing capacity, which is the maximum volume of air that can be ventilated per minute. It can be measured with a spirometer provided sufficient attention is paid to eliminating resistance. Maximum forced breathing is continued for 15 seconds, and the result expressed in litres per minute. There is a wide normal range scattering around 75 to 100 litres per minute.

The *breathing reserve* is the maximum breathing capacity less the resting ventilation per minute. As pointed out by Donald (1953), much of this so-called reserve can never be used, for even normal subjects are uncomfortably dyspnœic when using 50 to 60 per cent of their maximum breathing capacity. It may be better simply to express the actual ventilation per minute as a percentage of the maximum breathing capacity.

Mixing efficiency

In normal lungs all functioning alveoli are ideally supplied with an equal quantity of inspired air, and each is perfused with blood from the pulmonary arteries; non-functioning alveoli are collapsed and are not perfused, related capillaries temporarily shutting down. In disease, however, this is not necessarily so; unperfused alveoli may be supplied with air, and perfused alveoli may not be so supplied. When all parts of the lung are properly ventilated, an inert gas like helium, when introduced to a closed spirometer-lung circuit, quickly attains uniform distribution, after which no further dilution occurs. If parts of the lung contain stale air which is not moved to and fro, however, efficient mixing is delayed, and dilution of helium takes longer to reach a static level. The speed at which an inert gas attains maximum dilution is therefore a measure of mixing efficiency, but allowance must be made for a number of variables which influence the rate of mixing, such as the minute volume of respiration at the time (Bates and Christie, 1950).

Unventilated perfused alveoli necessarily lead to a fall in oxygen tension and content of arterial blood. But a similar degree of oxygen unsaturation of arterial blood may result from difficulty in oxygen diffusion across the interface between alveolus and capillary, as in diffuse fibrosis of the lung. In this group of cases, however, mixing efficiency is normal.

Poorly ventilated space

When the concentration of helium is plotted against time in normal subjects, a smooth dilution curve is constructed which at first falls away rapidly and then gradually straightens out until horizontal. When mixing is inefficient owing to parts of the lung being underventilated, rapid dilution is checked early, the initial steep slope suddenly assuming a more gentle gradient. This point signals complete mixing in all properly ventilated parts of the lung, the rest of the curve representing slower mixing in poorly ventilated spaces. From the concentration of helium at the moment its dilution is checked, the volume of properly ventilated lung can be calculated; this subtracted from the total lung volume gives the volume of poorly ventilated space.

Diffusion gradients

Owing to the extremely high rate of carbon dioxide diffusion in fluids, the arterial p CO_2 is always virtually the same as that in the alveoli (Riley and Cournand, 1951). The oxygen tension in the alveoli and the p O_2 of blood leaving the pulmonary capillaries, however, is not necessarily the same, although it has been shown to be so in health (Lilienthal *et al.*, 1946), minor differences between alveolar and arterial p O_2 being due to slight *venous admixture*, i.e. to a little perfusion of unventilated alveoli.

The alveolar oxygen tension may be calculated from the formula:

$$\text{Alveolar p } O_2 = \text{p } O_2 \text{ in inspired air} - \frac{\text{alveolar p } CO_2}{\text{resp. quotient}}$$

as quoted by Donald (1953). This formula is based on two important observations: (1) the differences in partial pressure between O_2 and CO_2 in the inspired air and alveolar air are proportional to the quantities of these gases consumed and excreted; so that

$$\text{R.Q. or } \frac{CO_2 \text{ eliminated}}{O_2 \text{ absorbed}} = \frac{\text{alv. p } CO_2 - \text{insp. p } CO_2}{\text{insp. p } O_2 - \text{alv. p } O_2}$$

and since the partial pressure of CO_2 in inspired air is negligible,

$$\text{R.Q.} = \frac{\text{alv. p } CO_2}{\text{insp. p } O_2 - \text{alv. p } O_2}$$

and (2) the alveolar CO_2 tension is the same as that in arterial blood as previously stated, so that

$$\text{R.Q.} = \frac{\text{arterial p } CO_2}{\text{insp. p } O_2 - \text{alv. p } O_2}$$

$$\therefore \text{Alv. p } O_2 = \text{insp. p } O_2 - \frac{\text{art. p } CO_2}{\text{R.Q.}}$$

Now the partial pressure of oxygen in the inspired air, which is fully saturated with water vapour, is about 21 per cent of $(760-47) = 150$ mm. Hg. Thus in normal subjects

$$\text{the alveolar oxygen tension} = \text{(say) } 150 - \frac{40}{0.8} \text{ mm. Hg}$$

$$= 100 \text{ mm. Hg}$$

Assuming the arterial oxygen tension is 95 mm. Hg, this gives an alveolar-arterial oxygen tension gradient of 5 mm. Hg, which represents the admixture of a small quantity of unventilated perfused venous blood.

The technique of these measurements of lung function must be sought in standard works on lung physiology. The basic principles involved and the terminology employed have been described here in some detail in order to help clinicians understand what the respiratory physiologist is about, and what the various respiratory tests to which his patients may be subjected really mean.

APPLICATIONS

Briefly, *emphysema* is as a rule characterised by a normal or even increased total lung volume, increased residual volume, diminished vital capacity, diminished inspiratory reserve, greatly diminished maximum breathing capacity, increased resting ventilation, poor mixing efficiency, large poorly ventilated space, and in advanced cases by reduction of arterial oxygen tension and saturation, and an increase of arterial carbon dioxide tension and content.

Pulmonary fibrosis in various forms is characterised especially by a raised alveolar-arterial oxygen tension gradient, and in advanced cases by a reduced arterial oxygen saturation, ventilation being more or less normal, and the arterial CO_2 content normal or low.

"*Pulmonary venous congestion*" from left heart failure or mitral stenosis behaves rather like pulmonary fibrosis in respect of its effect on lung function.

Bronchospasm, pneumonia, atelectasis, large pleural effusion, spontaneous pneumothorax and other space-filling lesions interfere chiefly with ventilation.

RENAL FUNCTION TESTS

Testing the urine for albumin and sugar, microscopic examination of the urinary sediment (particularly for red cells and casts), bacteriology when indicated, urine concentration tests, blood urea, urea concentration and clearance, and intravenous pyelography usually give sufficient information to satisfy the cardiologist, but the glomerular filtration rate as measured by inulin or creatinine clearance and the plasma blood flow as measured by diodone or para-amino-hippuric acid clearances are useful refinements. Renal function is particularly important in all hypertensive states, congestive heart failure, bacterial endocarditis and certain collagen diseases.

The *water concentration test* consists simply of withholding all fluids for a maximum of 36 hours (starting at 6 p.m.), or until the specific gravity of the urine is 1027 at room temperature. This is a very simple yet sensitive test of the power of the tubules to reabsorb water. The more damaged the kidney in hypertension, the more nearly does the urine resemble the glomerular filtrate, and in the end its specific gravity is the same as that of the plasma, being fixed at 1010.

Urea concentration is another test of tubular function. After ingesting 15 G. of urea a normal individual should pass urine having a urea concentration of at least 2 G. per cent. The dose is taken immediately after emptying the bladder, and urine is then voided after one and again after two hours, the second specimen being the more important, since diuresis may interfere with concentration during the first hour.

A *blood urea* higher than 45 mg. per cent indicates considerable impairment of glomerular filtration. In uræmia, of course, it may rise as high as 500 mg. per cent. The *blood creatinine*, normally 0.7 to 2 mg. per cent, also rises sharply in uræmia, and may reach 5 or even 10 mg. per cent. Creatinine is normally concentrated to about 75 mg. per cent in the urine.

A *clearance test* measures the amount of blood or plasma passing through the glomeruli or tubules which is cleared of a particular substance per minute. In the familiar urea clearance test of Van Slyke the concentration of urea in the blood and urine, and the volume of urine formed each minute, are measured: suppose the urine flows at a rate of 2 ml. per minute, and each ml. contains 20 mg. of urea (concentration 2 G. per cent), then the quotient 40 mg. per minute represents the quantity of urea filtered from the blood. If the blood urea at the time was 0.4 mg. per ml. (40 mg. per cent), then the amount of blood filtered of urea must have been

$$\frac{40}{0.4} = 100 \text{ ml.} \quad \text{Thus we have the simple formula clearance} = \frac{UV}{B}$$

where U is the concentration of the substance in the urine
V is the volume of urine formed per minute
and B is the concentration of the substance in the blood.

In the case of urea there are two important considerations: (1) blood passing through the glomeruli is not completely cleared of urea, so that the test does not measure the actual amount of blood passing through the glomeruli, but the amount that would have passed had it been totally cleared; (2) urea is partly reabsorbed by the tubules, particularly when its concentration there is high, as it is likely to be when the urine flow is reduced, and under these circumstances Van Slyke found more consistent results were obtained when the formula was changed to

$$\text{urea clearance} = \frac{U\sqrt{V}}{B}$$

The result is expressed as a percentage of normal. Average normal urea clearances were found to be 75 ml. per minute when the urine flow was 2 ml. or more per minute, and 54 (using the square root of V in the formula) when the urine flow was less than 2 ml. per minute. Thus when the *standard* urea clearance is reported as 50 per cent of normal it means that the actual clearance was one-half of 54 or 26 ml. per minute; if the word *maximum* is added it means that the flow was 2 ml. per minute or more and that the actual clearance was one-half of 75 or 37.5 ml. per minute.

Inulin has the advantage of being filtered freely by the glomeruli, but not reabsorbed by the tubules at all (Smith, 1939–40). The plasma inulin

$$\text{clearance is measured in exactly the same way, the formula being } C = \frac{UV}{P};$$

plasma concentration is substituted for blood concentration because inulin does not penetrate the red cell. The average normal plasma inulin clearance is 120 ml. per minute. This test has another meaning, however, for since inulin is filtered freely its concentration in the glomerular filtrate is precisely the same as its concentration in the plasma, and since it is not reabsorbed by the tubules the clearance figure determines the amount of filtrate actually formed, and may be justly called the *glomerular filtration rate*.

Endogenous creatinine clearance is also a good test of filtration, but not so reliable as inulin (Brod and Sirota, 1948). Typical figures are:

$$\text{Creatinine clearance} = \frac{UV}{B} = \frac{80 \text{ mg. per cent} \times 1.5 \text{ ml. per minute}}{1 \text{ mg. per cent}}$$

$$= 120 \text{ ml. per minute.}$$

The *total renal blood flow* may be estimated in two ways. If the urea content of blood samples from the renal artery and vein are known, and the amount of urea excreted in the urine per minute is known, then since the amount lost from the blood must equal the amount in the urine

$$\text{renal blood flow} = \frac{UV}{\text{arterio-venous urea difference}}$$

$$= (\text{say}) \frac{2,000 \text{ mg. per cent} \times 2 \text{ ml. per minute}}{30\text{–}26 \text{ mg. per cent}}$$

$$= 1,000 \text{ ml. per minute.}$$

Renal vein samples may be obtained by means of venous catheterisation and any substance excreted by the kidney may be used instead of urea. In fact urea is not very suitable because of its variable rate of excretion; creatinine serves very well.

The second method is based on the fact that certain substances like diodone and para-amino-hippuric acid are totally excreted by the tubules when their blood concentration is sufficiently low, so that their clearance rates then genuinely represent the *renal plasma flow* itself (Smith, 1939–40).

Milli-equivalents

The quantity of any substance in whole blood, plasma or serum is usually reported in mg. per cent or milli-equivalents. The latter term is used in respect of electrolytes such as sodium, potassium, and chloride, which occur in an ionic form in the plasma. The equivalent weight of a substance is that weight of it which will combine with or displace one gramme-atom of hydrogen, and a milli-equivalent is this weight divided by a thousand. The equivalent weights of monovalent ions like sodium are the same as their atomic weights, e.g. 23 for sodium, so that one *milli-equivalent* of sodium weighs 23 mg. Thus if the serum sodium is 320 mg. per cent it may be expressed as $\dfrac{320 \times 10}{23} = 139$ milli-equivalent per litres.

The advantage of this system is that the unit of any substance is chemically equivalent to the unit of any other substance, a statement that would not be true if applied to a unit of metric weight like a milligram.

Electrolytes

An electrolyte is any substance which in greater or less degree dissociates into its constituent ions when dissolved in water. Thus sodium chloride dissociates into sodium cations (positive) and chloride anions (negative) or Na^+ Cl^-, potassium chloride into K^+ Cl^-, sodium bicarbonate into Na^+ HCO_3^-, and so on. The most important substances of this kind are sodium, potassium, chloride and bicarbonate, and their normal concentrations in the serum are given below:

	Mg. per cent (unless otherwise stated)	M.eq. per litre
Serum sodium	310 to 345	135 to 150
Serum potassium	15 to 21	4 to 5
Plasma chlorides	340 to 390	95 to 110
Plasma bicarbonate	53 to 77 vols. of CO_2 per cent	25 to 35

PHONOCARDIOGRAPHY

Special techniques fall into two major groups, those that give information of a kind that cannot be obtained otherwise, such as radiology, electrocardiography and cardiac catheterisation, and those that offer a more accurate or standardised means of measuring or recording phenomena which can be recognised qualitatively in other and usually simpler ways, such as sphygmomanometry, polygraphy and kymography. Although phonocardiography belongs to the second group, it has contributed much to our knowledge and understanding of heart sounds and murmurs and has provided us with a practical tool with which to solve difficult auscultatory problems.

The heart sounds were first visually recorded by Frank (1904), using a stethoscopic chest piece, pneumatic connection, mirror capsule (q.v.) and optical recording, a relatively simple method perfected by Orias and Braun-Menendez (1939). Einthoven (1907) substituted a carbon microphone (q.v.) for the capsule and let it actuate a string galvanometer. More recently the stethoscopic chest piece has been replaced by a Rochelle salt-crystal microphone (q.v.), which converts sound pressure waves into proportionate electrical charges; these are amplified and led to a suitable string or mirror galvanometer (Leatham, 1949).

Picked up in this way the intensity of heart sounds and murmurs bears little relation to what is actually heard through a stethoscope, low-frequency sounds having a very much higher amplitude than high-frequency sounds. This means that with linear recordings and amplification adjusted so that a high-pitched murmur would show suitably in the tracing, a low-pitched third heart sound would throw the galvanometer beam off the record. The human ear is nicely adjusted to this phenomenon and while being remarkably sensitive to sound frequencies around 2,000 to 3,000 cycles per second it is logarithmically less sensitive to sounds of decreasing frequency, until at 15 cycles per second it does not respond at all; at the other end of the scale the highest frequency that can be heard is 20,000 to 30,000 cycles per second, varying with the individual. In phonocardiography it is usually desirable to record not only what is actually heard, but also what is on the threshold of hearing. Records having a linear response to sound intensity at all frequencies are impracticable, as already explained. The intensity of low-pitched sounds must be attenuated to bring them more into line with the weaker high-pitched sounds, so that both may be recorded in the same tracing. This is achieved by incorporating filters (condensers and resistances) in the amplifying circuit. Three degrees of low-frequency attenuations have been found most useful: in the first or low-frequency response, damping of low-frequency sounds is minimal and

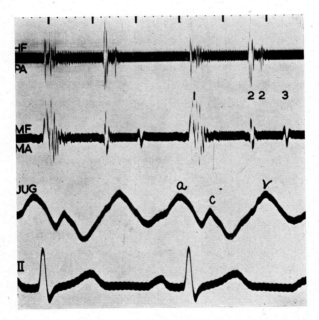

Fig. 5.17*—Normal phonocardiogram taken from apex and base recorded simultaneously with the electrocardiogram and the jugular phlebogram. Time marking 0.04 and 0.2 sec. Split first and second heart sounds best seen in high-frequency tracing from the pulmonary area (top graph).

* With acknowledgements to Dr. Aubrey Leatham.

amplification has to be reduced, so that low-pitched sounds such as the third heart sound and "soft" mitral diastolic murmurs are well seen at the expense of high-pitched sounds which may be insufficiently amplified to appear at all; in the second or medium-frequency record, moderate attenuation of low-pitched sounds allows greater amplification of high-pitched sounds and murmurs, so that these also can be seen; in the third or high-frequency response, sounds of low frequency are greatly weakened, allowing greater amplification and recording of high-pitched murmurs. This last kind of record is similar to the logarithmic curve of Rappaport and Sprague (1941, 1942), and may be called ear-like, for it closely resembles what is actually heard (Leatham, 1949).

The galvanometer must be sensitive to frequencies of at least 1,000 cycles per second, preferably to 2,000 if the highest pitched aortic diastolic murmurs are to be recorded faithfully. Most systolic murmurs have a frequency around 200 to 400 cycles per second, mitral diastolic murmurs 50 to 200 cycles per second, and the lower pitched heart sounds 16 to 50 cycles per second (Leatham, 1949). Theoretically the cathode ray oscillograph would seem the most suitable instrument for recording heart sounds in view of its almost unlimited frequency response, but in practice it has been found less satisfactory, partly on account of base-line wobble and rather hazy photography.

Phonocardiograms should be recorded simultaneously with an electro-cardiogram, jugular phlebogram or some other reference tracing, so that sounds and murmurs may be accurately timed against recognisable events in the cardiac cycle; one of the best reference tracings is actually a second phonocardiogram from a different site (fig. 5.17).

The various heart sounds and murmurs that may be recorded in health and disease, together with their timing and pitch, have already been described in detail in Chapter II, and time relationships with other events in the cardiac cycle are illustrated in figure 5.15.

BALLISTOCARDIOGRAPHY

When a gun is fired it recoils. This illustrates Newton's third law of motion which states that for every action on a body there is an equal and opposite reaction. When a patient with gross aortic incompetence is lying in bed, every clinician knows that the bed may rock—footwards during initial systolic ejection and headwards as blood courses down the descending aorta. As early as 1877 Gordon recorded the movements of a suspended platform on which a man was lying—the first ballistocardiogram. Henderson (1905) suggested that there should be a relationship between such recoil movements of the body and the stroke output of the heart. The principle was introduced into clinical medicine in 1939 by Starr and his associates. Since one of the basic principles of all forms of manometry is that the natural oscillating frequency of a manometer should be well outside the frequency range of the phenomenon being recorded, Starr developed a couch with a natural frequency of 12 to 14 cycles per second when suitably loaded (Starr, 1941, 1946), which is two and a half times the natural frequency of the human body (3 to 7 cycles per sec.). The bed moves with body recoil, such movements being suitably amplified and recorded. Nickerson and Curtis (1944) designed a low-frequency bed with a natural oscillation of 1.5 cycles per second; critical damping is employed to keep the natural frequency at 1.5 whatever the weight of the patient. In the ballistocardiograph designed by Dock and Taubman (1949) the body is allowed to move on its own cushion of fat, the movements of a bar laid across the shins being amplified and recorded. A great deal of work, particularly in the U.S.A., has been done on the ballistocardiograph in recent years, and has been well reviewed by Scarborough *et al.* (1952) and Gubner (1953). An important aspect of this basic research has been the realisation that the forces of acceleration and deceleration are primarily responsible for the ballistic effect.

Clinical ballistocardiogram

The chief waves of the ballistocardiograms are H, I, J, and K (fig. 5.18). H is a relatively small initial headward deflection probably due to venous

deceleration at the end of diastole. I is the first strong downward deflection and is due to recoil from acceleration of blood in the ascending aorta and pulmonary arteries, being synchronous with the rapid ejection phase. J is the maximum deflection and is upright; it is associated with acceleration of blood in the descending aorta, the body recoiling headwards; it is synchronous with the main pulse wave of the body. K is a fairly strong downward movement and has been attributed to deceleration of blood in the descending aorta due to the impact of the pulse wave at the periphery; it disappears in coarctation of the aorta and is augmented in aortic incompetence. It must be admitted, however, that there is no universal agreement about the true origins of these waves.

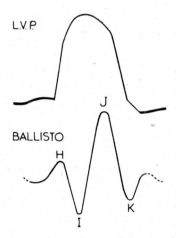

Fig. 5.18—Diagram of a normal ballistocardiogram to show approximate time relationship to the left ventricular pressure pulse (see text).

Various formulæ for estimating the stroke output by measuring the height or area occupied by I and J have been devised by Starr and others, and modified to give results comparable to those found by methods employing the Fick principle (Scarborough *et al.*, 1952).

REFERENCES

Amsterdam, B., and Amsterdam, A. L. (1943): "Disparity in blood pressures in both arms in normals and hypertensives, and its clinical significance: a study of 1,000 normals and 272 hypertensives", *N.Y. State J. Med.*, **43**, 2294.

Bates, D. V., and Christie, R. V. (1950): "Intrapulmonary mixing of helium in health and in emphysema", *Clin. Sci.*, **9**, 17.

Berliner, K. (1940): "Use of alpha lobeline for measurement of velocity of blood flow", *Arch. intern. Med.*, **65**, 896.

Bernstein, M., and Simkins, S. (1939): "The use of magnesium sulphate in the measurement of circulation time", *Amer. Heart J.*, **17**, 39.

Best, C. H., and Taylor, N. B. (1945): "The physiological basis of medical practice", 4th ed., Baillière, Tindall & Cox, London.

Björk, V. O., Blakemore, W. S., and Malmström, G. (1954): "Left ventricular pressure measurement in man", *Amer. Heart J.*, **48**, 197.

——, Malmström, G., and Uggla, L. G. (1953): "Left auricular pressure measurements in man", *Ann. Surg.*, **138**, 718.

Bland, E. F., and Wood, E. H. (1951): "Estimation of cardiac output by the dye dilution method with an ear oximeter", *J. appl. Physiol.*, **4**, 177.

Bloomfield, R. A., Lauson, H. D., Cournand, A., Breed, E. S., and Richards, D. W. (1946): "Recording of right heart pressures in normal subjects and in patients with chronic pulmonary disease and various types of cardiocirculatory disease", *J. clin. Invest.*, **25**, 639.

Blumgart, H. L. (1931): "Velocity of blood flow in health and disease", *Medicine*, **10**, 1.

——, and Weiss, S. (1927): "Studies on the velocity of blood flow. II. The velocity of blood flow in normal resting individuals, and a critique of the method used", *J. Clin. Invest.*, **4**, 15.

——, —— (1928): "Clinical studies on the velocity of blood flow. XI. The pulmonary circulation time, the minute volume blood flow through the lungs, and the quantity of blood in the lungs", *J. Clin. Invest.*, **6**, 103.

Bramwell, C. (1937): "The arterial pulse in health and disease", *Lancet*, ii, 239.

Broadbent, W. (1895): "An unpublished physical sign", *Ibid.*, ii, 200.

Brod, J., and Sirota, J. H. (1948): "The renal clearance of endogenous 'creatinine' in man", *J. Clin. Invest.*, **27**, 645.

Burch, G. E. (1950): "A primer of venous pressure", 2nd ed., Henry Kimpton, London.

Cournand, A., *et al.* (1953): "Report of the committee on cardiac catheterisation and angiocardiography of the American Heart Association", *Circulation*, **7**, 769.

——, and Ranges, H. A. (1941): "Catheterisation of the right auricle in man", *Proc. Soc. exp. Biol., N.Y.*, **46**, 462.

Currens, J. H. (1948): "A comparison of the blood pressure in the lying and standing positions; a study of five hundred men and five hundred women", *Amer. Heart J.*, **35**, 646.

Dawson, P. M. (1943): "An historical sketch of the Valsalva experiment", *Bull. Hist. Med.*, **14**, 295.

Dock, W. (1933): "Mode of production of the first heart sound", *Arch. Int. Med.*, **51**, 737.

——, and Taubman, F. (1949): "Some techniques for recording the ballistocardiogram directly from the body", *Am. J. Med.*, **7**, 751.

Donald, K. W. (1953): "The definition and assessment of respiratory function", *Brit. med. J.*, **1**, 415, 473.

Dornhorst, A. C., and Leathart, G. L. (1952): "A method of assessing the mechanical properties of lungs and air-passages", *Lancet*, **2**, 109.

Einthoven, W. (1907): "Die Registrierung der menschlichen Herztöne mittels des Saiten galvanometers", *Pfügers. Arch. ges. Physiol.*, **117**, 461.

Elisberg, E., *et al.* (1953): "The effect of the Valsalva manœuvre on the circulation. III. The influence of heart disease on the expected poststraining overshoot", *Circulation*, **7**, 880.

——, Goldberg, H., and Snider, G. L. (1951): "Value of intraoral pressure as a measure of intrapleural pressure", *J. appl. Physiol.*, **4**, 171.

——, Miller, G., Weinberg, S. L., and Katz, L. (1953): "The effect of the Valsalva manœuvre on the circulation. II. The role of the autonomic nervous system in the production of the overshoot", *Amer. Heart J.*, **45**, 227.

Epps, R. G., and Adler, R. H. (1953): "Left atrial and pulmonary capillary venous pressures in mitral stenosis", *Brit. Heart J.*, 15, 298.

Facquet, J., Lemoin, J. M., Alhomme, P., and Lefeboic, J. (1952): "La mesure de la pression auriculaire gauche par voie transbronchique", *Arch. Mal. Cœur*, 8, 741.

Fick, A. (1870): "Ueber die Messung des Blutquantums in den Herzventrikeln", Sitzungsberichte der phys.-med. Gesellsch. zu Wurzburg, p. 16.

Fishberg, A. M., Hitzig, W. H., and King, F. H. (1933): "Measurement of circulation time with saccharin", *Proc. Soc. exp. Biol.*, N.Y., 30, 651.

Forssmann, W. (1929):" Die Sondierung des rechten Herzens", *Klin. Wchnschr.*, 8, 2085.

Frank, O. (1903): "Kritik der elastichen Membranmanometer", *Ztschr. f. Biologie*, 44, 445.

Frank, O. (1904): "Die unmittelbare Registrierung der Herztone", *Munch. med. Wschr.*, 51, 953.

Friedberg, C. K. (1949): "Diseases of the Heart", W. B. Saunders Co., Philadelphia and London.

Gernandt, B., and Nylin, G. (1946): "The relation between circulation time and the amount of the residual blood of the heart", *Amer. Heart J.*, 32, 411.

Gibson, J. G., and Evans, W. A. (Jr.) (1937): "Clinical studies of the blood volume. 1. Clinical application of a method employing the azo dye 'Evans Blue' and the spectrophotometer", *J. clin. Invest.*, 16, 301, 317, 851.

Goldberg, S. J. (1936): "Use of calcium gluconate as a circulation time test", *Amer. J. Med. Sci.*, 192, 36.

Gomez, D. M., and Langevin, A. (1937): "Recherches d'hémodynamique et de cardiologie. II. La piézographic directe et instantanée", *Actualités Scientifiques et Industrielles*, 512, 1.

Gordon, J. W. (1877): "On certain molar movements of the human body produced by the circulation of the blood", *J. Anat. and Physiol.*, 11, 533.

Gorlin, R., Haynes, F. W., Goodale, W. T., Sawyer, C. G., Dow, J. W., and Dexter, L. (1951): "Studies of the circulatory dynamics in mitral stenosis. II. Altered dynamics at rest", *Amer. Heart J.*, 41, 30.

Gray, J. S. (1950): "Pulmonary ventilation and its physiological regulation", Charles C. Thomas, Springfield, Illinois, U.S.A.

Gregersen, M. I., Gibson, J. J., and Stead, E. A. (1935): "Plasma volume determination with dyes: errors in colorimetry; use of the blue dye T-1824", *Amer. J. Physiol.*, 113, 54.

Gubner, R. S., et al. (1953): "Clinical Progress. Ballistocardiography. An appraisal of technic, physiologic principles, and clinical value", *Circulation*, 7, 268.

Haldane, J. S., and Smith, J. L. (1900): "The mass and oxygen capacity of the blood in man", *J. Physiol.*, 25, 331.

Hamilton, W. F., Brewer, G., and Brotman, I. (1934): "Pressure pulse contours in the intact animal. I.—Analytical description of a new high-frequency hypodermic manometer with illustrative curves of simultaneous arterial and intracardiac pressures", *Amer. J. Physiol.*, 107, 427.

——, Moore, J. M., Kinsman, J. M., and Spurling, R. G. (1932): "Studies on the circulation. IV. Further analysis of the injection method, and of changes in hæmodynamics under physiological and pathological conditions", *Am. J. Physiol.*, 99, 534.

——, Woodbury, R. A., and Harper, H. T. (Jr.) (1936): "Physiologic relations between intrathoracic, intraspinal and arterial pressures", *J.A.M.A.*, 107, 853.

——, and Vogt, E. (1939): "Differential pressures in the lesser circulation of the unanæsthetised dog", *Amer. J. Physiol.*, 125, 130.

——, et al. (1948): "Comparison of the Fick and dye injection methods of measuring the cardiac output in man", *Amer. J. Physiol.*, 153, 309.

Hansen, A. T. (1949): "Pressure measurements in the human organisms", *Acta physiol. Scand.*, 19, Suppl. 68.

Hellems, H. K., Haynes, F. W., Gowdy, J. F., and Dexter, L. (1948): "The pulmonary capillary pressure in man", *J. Clin. Invest.*, **27**, 540.

Henderson, Y. (1905): "The mass movements of the circulation as shown by recoil curves", *Amer. J. Physiol.*, **14**, 277.

Herbert, J., Scebat, L., and Lenegre, J. (1953): "Incidents and Accidents in Right Heart Catheterisation", *Arch. mal. cœur*, **46**, 324.

Hitzig, W. M. (1935): "The use of ether in measuring the circulation time from the antecubital veins to the pulmonary capillaries", *Amer. Heart J.*, *10*, 1080.

Joint Report of the Committees Appointed by the Cardiac Society of Great Britain and Ireland, and the American Heart Association (1939): "Standardisation of methods of measuring the arterial blood pressure", *Brit. Heart J.*, **1**, 261.

Keith, N. M., Rowntree, L. G., and Geraghty, J. T. (1915): "A method for the determination of plasma and blood volume", *Arch. intern. Med.*, **16**, 547.

Kerr, W. T., Althausen, T. L., Bassett, A. M., and Goldman, M. J. (1937): "The symballophone: a modified stethoscope for the lateralisation and comparison of sounds", *Amer. Heart J.*, **14**, 594.

Kinsman, J. M., Moore, J. W., and Hamilton, W. F. (1929): "Studies on the circulation. 1. Injection method: physical and mathematical considerations", *Amer. J. Physiol.*, **89**, 322.

Lagerlöf, H., and Werkö, L. (1949): "Studies on the circulation of blood in man. VI. The pulmonary capillary venous pressure pulse in man", *Scand. J. clin. Lab. Invest.*, **1**, 147.

Lambert, E. H., and Wood, E. H. (1947): "The use of a resistance wire, strain gauge manometer to measure intra-arterial pressure", *Proc. Soc. Exp. Biol. and Med.*, **64**, 186.

Leatham, A. (1949): "Phonocardiography", *Postgrad. med. J.*, **25**, 568.

—— (1954): "Splitting of the first and second heart sounds", *Lancet*, *ii*, 607.

Lee, G. de J., Matthews, M. B., and Sharpey-Schafer, E. P. (1954): "The effect of the Valsalva manœuvre on the systemic and pulmonary arterial pressure in man", *Brit. Heart J.*, **16**, 311.

Lewis, Sir Thomas (1925): "The mechanism and graphic registration of the heart beat", 3rd ed., Shaw & Sons, London.

Lewis, W. H., Jr. (1938): "Changes in age in the blood pressure of adult men", *J. Physiol.*, **122**, 491.

Lian, M. C., and Barras, E. (1930): "Circulation time determined by use of fluorescein", *Bull. et mém. Soc. méd. d'hôp. de Paris*, **54**, 175.

Lilienthal, J. L. (Jr.), Riley, R. L., Proemmel, D. D., and Franke, R. E. (1946): "Experimental analysis in man of oxygen pressure gradient for alveolar air to arterial blood during rest and exercise at sea level and at altitude", *Amer. J. Physiol.*, **147**, 199.

Loman, J., Dameshek, W., Myerson, A., and Goldman, D. (1936): "Effect of alterations in posture on the intra-arterial blood pressure in man. I. Pressure in the carotid, brachial and femoral arteries in normal subjects", *Arch. Neurol. Psychiat.*, **35**, 1216.

Mackenzie, J. (1902): "The study of the pulse", Edinburgh.

Marey, E. J. (1863): "Physiologie médicale de la Circulation du Sang", Paris.

McMichael, J. (1939): "A rapid method of determining the lung capacity", *Clin. Sc.*, **4**, 167.

——, Sharpey-Schafer, E. P. (1944): "Cardiac output in man by a direct Fick method", *Brit. Heart J.*, **6**, 33.

Miller, A., and White, P. D. (1941): "Crystal microphone for pulse-wave recording", *Amer. Heart J.*, **21**, 504.

Millikan, G. A. (1942): "The oximeter, an instrument for measuring continuously the oxygen saturation of arterial blood in man", *Rev. Scient. Instruments*, **13**, 434.

Moore, J. W., Kinsman, J. M., Hamilton, W. F., and Spurling, R. G. (1929): "Studies on the circulation. II. Cardiac output determinations; comparisons of the injection method with the direct Fick procedure", *Amer. J. Physiol.*, **89**, 331.

Moritz, F., and Tabora, D. (1910): "Ueber eine Methode, beim Menschen den Druck in Oberflächlichen Venen exakt zu bestimmen", *Dtsch. Arch. klin. Med.*, **98**, 475.

Morrow, W. S. (1900): "Ueber die Fortpflanzungsfeschwindigkeit des Venenpulses", *Archiv. f.d. ges physiol.*, **79**, 442.

Motley, H. L. (1950): "Evaluation of function in pulmonary disease by physiologic tests", *Penn. med. J.*, **53**, 119.

Neurath, O. (1937): "The determination of circulation times with magnesium sulphate", *Z. klin. Med.*, **132**, 134.

Nickerson, J. L., and Curtis, H. J. (1944): "The design of the ballistocardiograph", *Amer. J. Physiol.*, **142**, 1.

Nicholson, J. W., Burchell, H. B., and Wood, E. H. (1951): "A method for the continuous recording of Evans' blue dye curves in arterial blood, and its application to the diagnosis of cardiovascular abnormalities", *J. Lab. and Clin. Med.*, **37**, 353.

Orias, O., and Braun-Menendez, E. (1939): "The heart sounds in normal and pathological conditions", London.

Potain, P. C. E. (1867): "On the movements and sounds that take place in the jugular veins", *Bull. et Mem. de la Soc. med. des Hôp. de Paris*, **4**, 3.

Prinzmetal, M., Corday, E., Bergman, H. C., Schwartz, L., and Spritzler, R. J. (1948): "Radiocardiography: A new method for studying the blood flow through the chambers of the heart in human beings", *Science*, **108**, 340.

——, ——, Spritzler, R. J., and Flieg, W. (1949): "Radiocardiography and its clinical applications", *J.A.M.A.*, **139**, 617.

Rappaport, M. B., and Sprague, H. B. (1941): "Physiologic and physical laws that govern auscultation, and their clinical application", *Amer. Heart J.*, **21**, 257.

Rein, H., Hampel, A., and Heinemann, W. A. (1940): "Photoelecktrisches Transmissionsmanometer", *Arch. f.d. ges. Physiol.*, **243**, 329.

Riley, R. L., and Cournand, A. (1951): " 'Ideal' alveolar air and the analysis of ventilation-perfusion relationships in the lungs", *J. appl. Physiol.*, **1**, 825.

Robb, G. P., and Weiss, S. (1934): "The velocity of pulmonary and peripheral venous blood flow and related aspects of the circulation in cardiovascular disease", *Amer. Heart J.*, **9**, 742.

Scarborough, W. R., et al. (1952): "A review of ballistocardiography", *Amer. Heart J.*, **44**, 910.

Smith, H. W. (1939–40): "Physiology of the renal circulation", *Harvey Lectures*, **35**, 166.

Starr, I. (1946–7): "The ballistocardiograph, an instrument for clinical research and for routine clinical diagnosis", *Harvey Lectures*, Series 42, Springfield, Illinois, Charles C. Thomas, 194.

—— (1941): "Clinical studies with the ballistocardiograph; in congestive failure, on digitalis action, on changes in ballistic form, and in certain acute experiments", *Amer. J. med. Sci.*, **202**, 469.

——, Rawson, A. J., Schroeder, H. A., and Joseph, N. K. (1939): "Studies in the estimation of cardiac output in man; of abnormalities in cardiac function from the heart's recoil and the blood's impact", *Amer. J. Physiol.*, **127**, 1.

——, and Mayock, R. L. (1948): "On the significance of abnormal forms of the ballistocardiogram. A study of 234 cases with 40 necropsies", *Ibid.*, **215**, 631.

Stewart, G. N. (1897): "Researches on the circulation time and on the influences which affect it. IV. The output of the heart", *J. Physiol.*, **22**, 159.

—— (1921): "The pulmonary circulation time, the quantity of blood in the lungs and the output of the heart", *Amer. J. Physiol.*, **58**, 20.

Swan, H. J. C., Zapata-Siaz, J., and Wood, E. H. (1953): "Dye dilution curves in cyanotic congenital heart disease", *Circulation*, **8**, 70.

Valsalva, A. M. (1707): "De Aure Humana", *Traj. ad Rhenum* (Utrecht), G. Vande Water, 84.

Weiss, S., Robb, G. P., and Blumgart, H. L. (1928): "The velocity of blood flow in health and disease as measured by the effect of histamine on the minute vessels", *Amer. Heart J.*, 4, 664.

Wetterer, E. (1944): "Eine neue manometrische Sonde mit elektrischer Transmission", *Z. Biol.*, 101, 332.

Wexler, J., Whittenberger, J. L., and Dumke, P. R. (1947): "The effect of cyanide on the electrocardiogram of man", *Amer. Heart J.*, 34, 163.

Wiggers, C. J. (1921): "Studies on the consecutive phases of the cardiac cycle. I. The duration of the consecutive phases of the cardiac cycle and the criteria for their precise determination. II. The Laws governing the relative durations of ventricular systole and diastole", *Amer. J. Physiol.*, 56, 415, 439.

—— (1928): "Pressure pulses in the cardiovascular system", Longmans, Green, New York and London.

—— (1952): "The Henry Jackson memorial lecture. Dynamics of ventricular contraction under abnormal conditions", *Circulation*, 5, 321.

Winsor, T., Adolph, W., Ralston, W., and Leiby, G. M. (1947): "Fractional circulation times using fluorescent tracer substances", *Amer. Heart J.*, 34, 80.

Winternitz, M., Deutsch, J., and Brull, Z. (1931): "Eine klinische brauchbare Bestimmungsmethode der Blutemlaufszeit mittels Decholinijektion", *Med. Klin.*, 27, 986.

Wood, E. H., and Gerachi, J. E. (1949): "Photoelectric determination of arterial oxygen saturation in man", *J. Lab. Clin. Med.*, 34, 387.

Wood, P. H. (1936): "The erythrocyte sedimentation rate in diseases of the heart", *Quart. J. Med.*, 29, 1.

—— (1936): "Right and left ventricular failure; a study of circulation time and venous blood pressure", *Lancet*, ii, 15.

Zimdahl, W. T. (1951): "Disorders of the cardiovascular system occurring with catheterisation of the right side of the heart", *Amer. Heart J.*, 41, 204.

CHAPTER VI

DISORDERS OF CARDIAC RHYTHM

T HE speed and regularity of the heart beat are controlled by the sino-atrial node of Keith and Flack (1907) situated in the upper part of the sulcus terminalis, anterior to, and to the right of, the mouth of the superior vena cava (fig. 6.01). Approximately 70 times per minute this node discharges itself and initiates an excitation wave which spreads in all directions over both atria. Close to the opening of the coronary sinus, above the base of the tricuspid valve, on the right side of the atrial

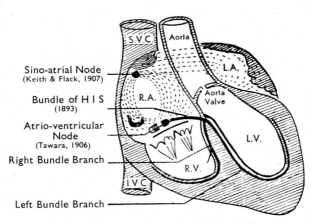

Fig. 6.01—Anatomy of the conducting system.

septum is situated the atrio-ventricular node of Tawara (1906). This also forms impulses, but at a slower rate, so that normally it is prematurely discharged by the excitation wave initiated by the S-A node. The impulse then spreads down the Bundle of His which passes horizontally to the left, to penetrate the membranous interventricular septum, where it divides into left and right bundle branches. These pass down each side of the muscular septum just beneath the endocardium. The bundle branches then break up into a network of Purkinje fibres which carry the excitatory process to the sub-endocardial myocardium.

Physiology of conduction. From the "pace-maker" in the sino-atrial node the excitation wave spreads through atrial muscle at a speed of about 1,000 mm. per second. Passage through the A-V nodal tissue is believed to be relatively slow, and is estimated at 200 mm. per second. Spread down the bundle branches and the Purkinje fibres is rapid and is probably as fast as 400 mm. per second. Conduction through the ventricles, which is believed to proceed directly outwards, is put at 400 mm. per second (Lewis, 1925).

Both the S-A and A-V nodes are under direct autonomic control, being stimulated by sympathetic activity and depressed by vagal activity. Cardiac accelerator nerves arise from the lateral horns of the upper 4th or 5th dorsal segments of the spinal cord, enter the sympathetic chain and pass cranially to the cervical ganglia. Post-ganglionic fibres form the superior, middle and inferior cardiac nerves which terminate in the S-A and A-V nodes.

IRREGULARITIES AND ALTERATION OF HEART-RATE INITIATED OR GOVERNED BY THE SINO-ATRIAL NODE

SINUS ARRHYTHMIA

There is probably no such thing as an absolutely regular heart. Slight irregularity, the heart quickening with inspiration and slowing with expiration, is normal, and depends upon variations in vagal tone governed by a reflex which is thought to be initiated by receptors in the lungs. Another form of sinus arrhythmia occurs independently of respiration. Both are more common in the young and when the heart rate is slow, tend to be exaggerated by drugs that increase vagal tone (such as digitalis), and may be abolished by exercise or atropine.

Other varieties of sinus arrhythmia are not essentially different, but owe their recognition to some particular associated feature: thus there is a form

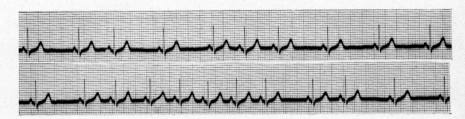

Fig. 6.02—Sinus arrhythmia.

associated with sino-atrial block; another with sinus bradycardia and paroxysmal auricular fibrillation or flutter; a third with convalescence from certain infectious fevers, especially influenza; and so on. Increased vagal tone is common to all these types.

Diagnosis is usually easy, or doubt is soon resolved by means of exercise, atropine, or amyl nitrite. An electrocardiogram provides conclusive evidence (fig. 6.02).

Although sinus arrhythmia is normal, it should not be regarded as a positive sign of a normal cardiovascular system, for it may occur in any form of heart disease.

SINUS TACHYCARDIA

The heart rate varies markedly in different mammals. In the elephant, for example, it is about 30 beats per minute; in the rat it is close on 600. It is considerably slower in the hare than in the rabbit. On the whole, the speed is inversely proportional both to the size and to the athletic endurance of the animal. In man the average heart rate is 72 beats per minute; but there are wide limits of normality ranging between 40 and 100. The pulse is faster in children, averaging 120 to 130 at birth, and slowing gradually during childhood to reach about 80 at puberty. The more athletic the individual the slower the pulse as a rule, and in well-trained athletes resting figures of 45 to 50 are common. It follows that tachycardia may mean a heart rate faster than average, faster than the upper limit of normality, or faster than what is known to be normal for a particular individual.

Applied physiology. Tachycardia has always played an impressive part as a physical sign in general medicine. It has received weighty consideration in fevers, in all forms of heart disease, in shock and hæmorrhage, in various chronic diseases such as pulmonary tuberculosis, and indeed in almost every condition; yet it can mean little unless its immediate cause is understood. This is not to decry tachycardia as a valuable sign, but to emphasise that its significance depends upon its mechanism.

The speed of the sino-atrial pace-maker is strongly influenced by the autonomic nervous system. Complete "paralysis" of the vagus may be produced within a minute by giving 2 to 3 mg. of atropine sulphate intravenously, whereupon the heart accelerates to a speed of 130 to 160 per minute. The cardiac output per minute rises simultaneously; but the fall in venous filling-pressure that accompanies the tachycardia may counteract this effect (McMichael and Sharpey-Schafer, 1944). The ventricular stroke-volume is diminished, even in those with higher outputs. Emotional tachycardia, as in the anxiety states, and the tachycardia of convalescence appear to be due to diminished vagal tone.

Tachycardia may be due to a rise in pressure within the great veins and right atrium, venous receptors initiating the Bainbridge reflex by which vagal tone is reduced. Under these circumstances the stroke-volume may be maintained or increased, the cardiac output per minute rising in proportion to the tachycardia or even higher. This mechanism operates during effort, and in anæmia, beri-beri, arteriovenous shunt, anoxic pulmonary heart disease, generalised active Paget's disease, and pregnancy. The Bainbridge reflex is also partly responsible for the tachycardia so frequently seen in congestive failure.

The speed of the heart is also controlled by reflexes initiated by baro-receptors in the aorta and carotid sinuses. When the blood pressure rises, vagal tone is increased, and the heart slows; when it falls, vagal tone is diminished, and the heart quickens (Marey's Law). This is the mechanism of the bradycardia associated with conditions causing a transient rise of blood pressure, such as acute nephritis, and it is part of the mechanism controlling the tachycardia of low blood-pressure states.

Anoxia may cause tachycardia by direct action on the central nuclei, or possibly reflexly through the carotid sinus. Just what part it plays in the production of tachycardia in anæmia and cor pulmonale is uncertain. Thyroxin and fever have a direct stimulating action on the pace-maker, and so has adrenaline; but the latter may also excite the carotid sinus slowing reflex by raising the blood pressure, so that the heart rate may change but little. The elevated cardiac output that accompanies the tachycardia is also probably due in part to a direct action on the heart. In the case of adrenaline the cardiac output may rise when there is no change in heart rate or blood pressure (McMichael and Sharpey-Schafer, 1944).

Differential diagnosis. From the clinical point of view, sinus tachycardia must be distinguished from auricular flutter and from paroxysmal tachycardia. This is usually possible at the bedside. Sinus tachycardia varies in rate from minute to minute, or at least from hour to hour; and it varies with emotion, effort, and change of posture. Carotid sinus or eyeball compression and release result in gradual rather than abrupt slowing and quickening of the pulse respectively, although changes may be difficult to detect with fast rates. In auricular flutter (and sometimes in paroxysmal auricular tachycardia) the rate is usually fixed, neither varying spon-

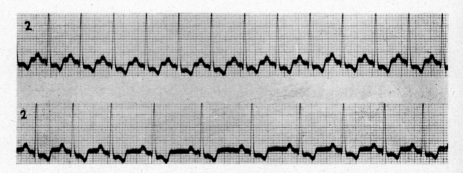

Fig. 6.03—Sinus tachycardia slowed by carotid sinus compression.

taneously nor with emotion, effort, or change of posture; whilst on carotid sinus pressure slowing is abrupt, often to half the rate, 2 : 1 physiological atrio-ventricular block being converted into a 4 : 1 relationship; and on release, reversion to the original rhythm is again abrupt, and may not take place for several seconds. Even without so precise a clinical analysis, the degree of slowing may yet be too gross for sinus tachycardia. In paroxysmal nodal and ventricular tachycardia the rate is also fixed, and carotid sinus pressure either stops the attack abruptly, as in 50 per cent. of the nodal cases, or has no effect whatever. If it is impossible to interpret the results of carotid sinus pressure clinically, the problem may be solved by combining the manœuvre with an electrocardiogram (fig. 6.03). It should be explained that an electrocardiogram *per se* may not afford certain distinction between these three rhythms, although lead V_1 or CR_7 greatly facilitates analysis.

Effect on the heart. Sinus tachycardia presents an important problem in relation to heart failure. Is it a causal factor or merely a reflection of cardiac embarrassment? Or is it part of a compensatory adjustment, beneficial under the circumstances? Such questions are difficult to answer directly, but the presentation of some of the relevant facts may help to clarify the issue. A normal heart tolerates any natural degree and duration of sinus tachycardia, rates approaching 200, for example, being common during violent exertion, and persistent rates of 120 or so being endured for over 20 years in certain cases of Da Costa's syndrome without harmful results. On the other hand, diseased hearts frequently develop congestive failure with heart rates of 150 to 200 in auricular flutter or paroxysmal tachycardia, the effect being attributed to overwork and fatigue resulting from insufficient diastolic rest. The tachycardia of the hyperkinetic forms of cardiovascular disorder (thyrotoxicosis, anæmia, anoxic cor pulmonale, beri-beri, arterio-venous aneurysm, and generalised Paget's disease) is part of the physiological mechanism maintaining a high cardiac output, and therefore performs a useful function; but when the heart fails, i.e. when it is overloaded, the cardiac output falls and the tachycardia is wasted. Under such circumstances tachycardia reflects cardiac embarrassment, and deprives the heart of diastolic rest. In the hypokinetic forms of heart failure, such as those which may be seen in cases of hypertension and mitral stenosis, tachycardia due to the Bainbridge or carotid sinus reflex is a reflection of cardiac distress from the start, and serves no useful purpose. In chronic constrictive pericarditis, and to a lesser extent in high-pressure pericardial effusion, tachycardia may provide the only means of maintaining an adequate cardiac output, for the stroke-volume is strictly limited. In the active forms of carditis (rheumatic, diphtheritic, and Fiedler's), and in bacterial endocarditis, the heart rate may be disturbed by local pathology, fever, toxæmia, or (in diphtheria) by circulatory collapse, and probably adversely affects the heart. On the whole it may be said that the heart tolerates sinus tachycardia, which tends to deprive it of rest, better than a high cardiac output, and much better than a raised blood pressure, both of which increase its work.

There is no treatment for sinus tachycardia itself; but attention should be paid to its cause.

SINUS BRADYCARDIA

As already stated, heart rates of 45 to 50 per minute are common in athletes. Some individuals, irrespective of their physical training, have a naturally slow pulse. Sinus bradycardia is a feature of certain diseases, notably myxœdema and obstructive jaundice, and is not uncommon during convalescence from certain fevers, especially influenza. It also occurs when the blood pressure is raised rather suddenly, as in acute nephritis, the slowing being reflex, through the sino-aortic afferents and vagus. It is a familiar sign of lesions that increase the intracranial pressure, when it may be due to direct stimulation of central nuclei. Slowing of the pulse may be induced temporarily by carotid sinus or eyeball pressure; as a transient event it occurs naturally in vaso-vagal syncope.

The differential diagnosis between sinus bradycardia, sino-atrial block, and heart block, can usually be made at the bedside; but electro-cardiographic confirmation is advised. In sinus bradycardia the pulse quickens gradually with effort, atropine, or amyl nitrite; in sino-atrial block and sometimes in 2 : 1 heart block, the rate doubles abruptly; whilst in complete heart block the degree of acceleration is barely perceptible. Heart block may also be recognised by studying jugular pulsation and heart sounds (q.v.).

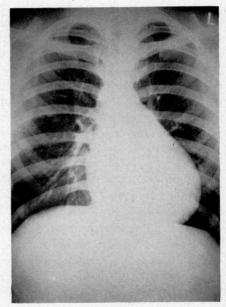

Fig. 6.04—Relative cardiac enlargement due to sinus bradycardia.

One of the consequences of sinus bradycardia is an increased ventricular stroke-volume of sufficient degree to maintain a normal cardiac output per minute. When the heart rate is 40, the stroke-volume approaches double the average normal; the diastolic heart size is larger than usual (fig. 6.04), and in time hypertrophy may occur. Such enlargement is physiological.

When the speed of the pace-maker approaches 40 per minute, it may become slower than the natural speed of impulse-formation in the atrio-ventricular node, in which event nodal rhythm occurs. As sinus arrhythmia is often associated with bradycardia it is more usual to see irregular examples of ventricular escape, the A-V node taking over whenever a pause is unusually long (fig. 6.05). Nodal rhythm would supervene more frequently if the influences that retarded the sinus node did not also depress the A-V node.

Sinus bradycardia is often associated with sinus arrhythmia, sometimes with auricular ectopic beats, and rarely with paroxysmal auricular fibrillation or flutter in elderly subjects. Vagal influences appear to be responsible.

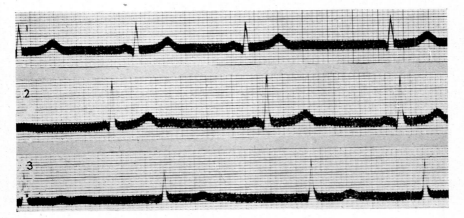

Fig. 6.05—Nodal escape in sinus bradycardia.

SINO-ATRIAL BLOCK

There are three types of sino-atrial block, corresponding to similar varieties of A-V block. First, beats may be dropped irregularly, the pauses being roughly equal to two normal intervals (fig. 6.06), like the dropped beats of partial A-V block with fixed prolonged P-R interval. Second, beats may be dropped more or less regularly, the pauses being always less than two normal intervals, like partial A-V block with progressive lengthening of the P-R interval until conduction fails – the Wenckebach type. Third, there may be 2 : 1 sino-atrial block, every second beat being dropped; this gives rise to a slow regular heart rate which doubles on effort or with atropine (fig. 6.07). It should be understood that there is no electrocardiographic representation of the formation and discharge of the excitatory

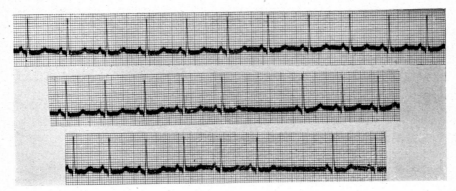

Fig. 6.06—Sino-atrial block, showing irregular dropped beats.

impulse at the sinus node, the first wave (P) of the electrocardiogram
recording the passage of the impulse through the atria, so that failure of
conduction between the S-A node and the atria can only be inferred.

Sino-atrial block is usually encountered in normal individuals, the first
two types being commonly associated with sinus bradycardia. It is a
manifestation of increased vagal tone, and may be abolished with atropine.
When there is 2 : 1 block, and a pulse rate of about 40 per minute, fluoroscopy may reveal cardiac enlargement due to the large stroke-volume

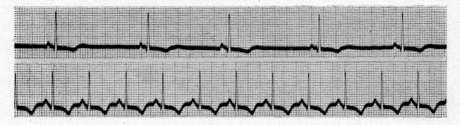

Fig. 6.07—Sino-atrial block: the rate doubles on effort.

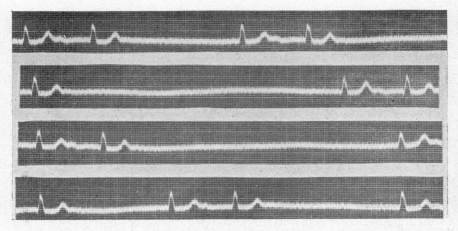

Fig. 6.08—Cardiac standstill occurring spontaneously in sino-atrial block.
(By courtesy of Dr. Raymond Daley)

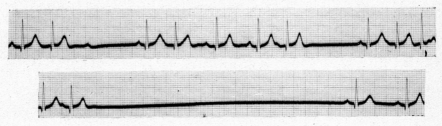

Fig. 6.09—Cardiac standstill due to carotid sinus compression.

necessary to maintain a normal cardiac output. As with sinus bradycardia, ventricular escape may occur, and would probably be more common if the A-V node were not also depressed.

There are no symptoms of sino-atrial block *per se*; but occasionally short periods of cardiac standstill, with dizziness or syncope, may occur, and appear to be due to bursts of extreme vagal activity (fig. 6.08). They may be prevented by atropine. Attacks of this kind may be readily induced in susceptible individuals by carotid sinus pressure (fig. 6.09).

NODAL RHYTHM

The sinus node is the pace-maker of the heart only because its inherent rate of impulse-formation and discharge is quicker than that of any other focus endowed with a similar property; but if it is sufficiently depressed, as by cooling, some other focus may form its impulses at a faster rate, and so become the temporary pace-maker, and in fact this function usually falls upon the atrio-ventricular node. Under such circumstances atrial excitation is retrograde, and the electrocardiogram usually shows an inverted (or deformed) P wave just after the QRS complex, and a heart rate of 40 to 60 per minute (fig. 6.10a). Sometimes, however, the P wave may precede (fig. 6.10b) or coincide with the QRS complex, or it may be absent altogether owing to retrograde block (fig. 6.10c). Occasionally, it may shift its position from moment to moment (shifting or sliding nodal rhythm; fig. 6.11); if such graphs are examined critically, however, they are seen to be examples of sinus bradycardia with normally formed P waves and frequent ventricular escape (so-called wandering or shifting pace-maker). This terminology is misleading, for a 'wandering pace-maker' is simply dual rhythm, both S-A and A-V nodes discharging spontaneously with variable asynchronism.

Clinically, nodal rhythm may be recognised by its effect on the jugular venous pulse, for whenever the right atrium contracts against a closed tricuspid valve, sharp cannon waves occur (fig. 6.12).

Nodal rhythm may be discovered by chance in healthy individuals; it may occur in active rheumatic, diphtheritic, and Fiedler's carditis; it may be momentarily induced by carotid sinus pressure; and it may follow thrombosis of the right coronary artery above the origin of the branch to the sinus node (this branch arises from the left coronary artery in 40 per cent. of cases): but its only common cause is digitalis therapy.

Nodal rhythm is under autonomic control, the heart rate being slowed by vagal stimulation and accelerated by atropine and exercise (White, 1915). It is a harmless rhythm change, gives rise to no symptoms, and requires no treatment. When due to digitalis, there is no need to stop the drug.

Coronary sinus rhythm

The position of the P wave in relation to QRS depends chiefly on the exact site of the pace-maker in the A-V node: when situated in the proximal

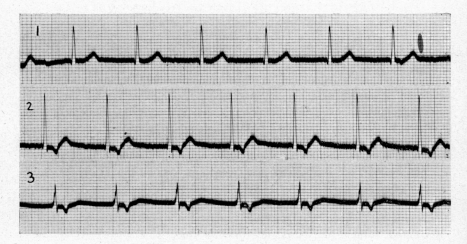

(a) An inverted P wave occurs after QRS.

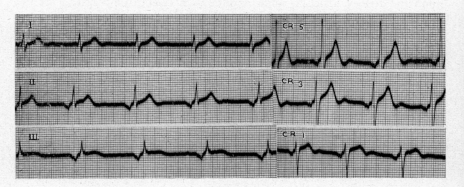

(b) An inverted P wave precedes QRS ("Coronary sinus rhythm").

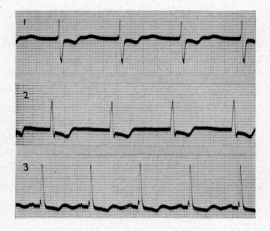

(c)—The P wave is invisible, possibly buried in QRS
(leads 1 and 2; lead 3 shows normal rhythm).

Fig. 6.10—Nodal rhythm.

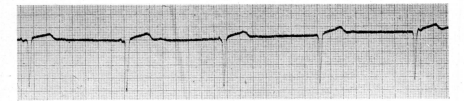

Fig. 6.11—Asynchronous dual rhythm.

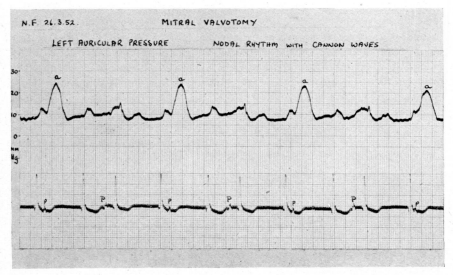

N.F. 26.3.52.   MITRAL VALVOTOMY

LEFT AURICULAR PRESSURE   NODAL RHYTHM WITH CANNON WAVES

Fig. 6.12 (a)—Nodal rhythm with partial retrograde block (Wenckebach type) showing reciprocal beats when the RP interval is sufficiently prolonged, and cannon waves in the left atrial pressure pulse whenever the atria contract during ventricular systole.

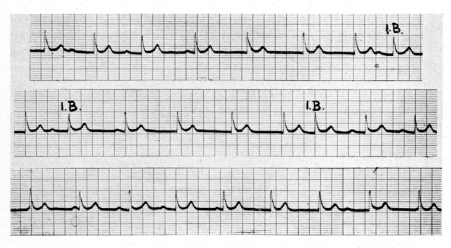

Fig. 6.12 (b)—Interference dissociation. The interference beats are labelled I.B.

or coronary sinus position of the node, the pace-maker is functionally nearer the atria than the ventricles, and P falls just before QRS (fig. 6.10b). This is called coronary sinus rhythm and is the most innocent and common type of nodal rhythm. The P wave is nearly always inverted in standard leads II and III. In view of the short P-R interval the first heart sound may be accentuated.

RECIPROCAL RHYTHM

When retrograde conduction to the atria is delayed in nodal rhythm, the R-P interval may exceed 0.2 second; by then the ventricles may be no longer refractory and may be re-activated by a return of the excitation wave from the atria, so that a *reciprocal* beat, as it is called, follows the P wave. A form of coupling, known as *reciprocal rhythm*, may be brought about in this way, each pair of ventricular beats having an abnormal P wave between them (White, 1921); or if retrograde R-P conduction shows progressive lengthening, reciprocal beats may occur only at intervals when R-P is sufficiently prolonged (fig. 6.12a).

INTERFERENCE DISSOCIATION

If retrograde conduction is completely blocked in nodal rhythm, forward conduction remaining unimpaired, *atrioventricular* dissociation occurs in which the ventricles beat faster than the atria, the rate of discharge of the sinus node being necessarily slower than that of the A-V node. From time to time in such a rhythm atrial activation from the sinus node discharges the A-V node prematurely and causes an *interference beat*, the slightly irregular rhythm so produced being called *interference dissociation* (fig. 6.12b).

HEART BLOCK

When any organic lesion or functional disturbance impedes conduction through the bundle of His, or through both its main branches, we may speak of heart block. There are four grades: prolonged P-R interval, dropped beats, partial block with fixed atrio-ventricular relationship, and complete heart block.

PROLONGED P-R INTERVAL

As discussed elsewhere the upper limit of the normal P-R interval should not exceed 0.22 second. In partial heart block it frequently measures 0.28 to 0.32 second. In extreme cases, or when there is associated tachycardia, electrocardiograms may show P coinciding with, or even preceding, the previous T wave (fig. 6.13).

Prolongation of the P-R interval may be transient or permanent, or it may develop into a higher grade of block. As a transient phenomenon it is especially characteristic of any form of active carditis; but it may also be due to digitalis, to coronary thrombosis, or to temporary nutritional

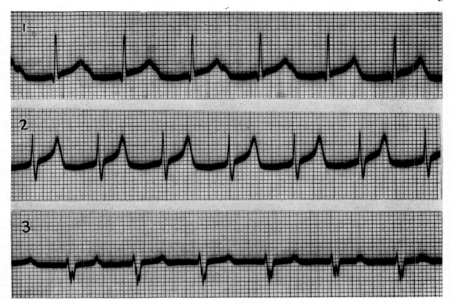

Fig. 6.13—Prolonged P-R interval, with P coinciding with the previous T wave.

changes from other causes, and it may be induced by carotid sinus pressure. Permanent delay in conduction may result from an inflammatory scar involving the bundle of His, as in old rheumatic heart disease, or from ischæmic fibrosis. When the block is not permanent it may be relieved immediately by the intravenous injection of 1 to 3 mg. of atropine sulphate (Bruenn, 1937). A prolonged P-R interval may also be shortened when the subject stands upright (Scherf and Dix, 1952).

Although partial heart block of this kind is usually an electrocardiographic diagnosis, it may be recognised clinically by noting delay between

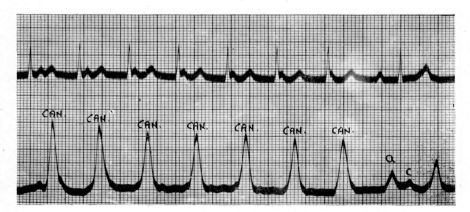

Fig. 6.14—Partial heart block showing jugular cannon waves.

the atrial and ventricular components of cervical venous pulsation or presystolic gallop rhythm, by observing a gap between a presystolic murmur and the first heart sound in cases with mitral stenosis, by hearing an unusually faint first heart sound, or by detecting cannon waves in the neck when the P-R interval is so prolonged that P falls between QRS and T in the previous cycle (fig. 6.14). Its practical importance lies in its value as a sign of active rheumatic carditis.

PARTIAL HEART BLOCK WITH DROPPED BEATS

In a slightly higher grade of partial heart block, conduction through the bundle of His fails altogether from time to time so that ventricular beats are dropped. In the type first recognised by Wenckebach (1899) the P-R interval shortens considerably after a beat is dropped, but subsequently lengthens progressively from cycle to cycle until conduction again fails (fig. 6.15). In another type (Hay, 1906) the P-R interval is fixed and beats are dropped irregularly and unpredictably.

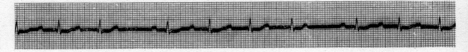

Fig. 6.15—Partial heart block with dropped beats (Wenckebach type).

The condition may be detected clinically by noting a changing a-c interval in the neck, variations in the intensity of the first heart sound, and occasional cannon waves (fig. 6.14). It is commonly transient and recovers spontaneously, but occasionally progresses to complete heart block.

PARTIAL HEART BLOCK WITH FIXED A-V RELATIONSHIP

Relatively stable forms of partial heart block may be encountered, usually with a 2 : 1 atrio-ventricular relationship (fig. 6.16), but occasionally with

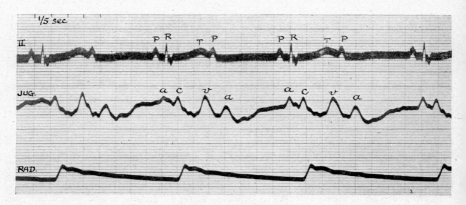

Fig. 6.16—2-1 heart block.
(*By courtesy of Sir John Parkinson*)

3 : 1 or even 4 : 1 A-V ratios. These usually progress to complete heart block; they are much less common in active carditis than in ischæmic cases.

Clinically, 2 : 1 heart block has to be distinguished from sino-atrial block, from sinus bradycardia with a heart rate of about 40 beats per minute, from nodal rhythm, and from complete A-V dissociation. Failure to quicken appreciably with effort or atropine excludes sino-atrial block and sinus bradycardia (and usually nodal rhythm). The absence of both irregular cannon waves and varying intensity of the first heart sound distinguish it from complete heart block.

COMPLETE HEART BLOCK

Etiology. Complete atrio-ventricular dissociation is very rare in active rheumatic carditis, but less so in diphtheritic carditis; it may be induced by digitalis, especially in cases of auricular fibrillation, and has been caused by hæmorrhage into the bundle of His from trauma or asphyxia, and by primary or secondary neoplasm. About 10 per cent of cases are congenital (q.v.). As a rule, however, complete heart block is associated with ischæmic or hypertensive heart disease, with syphilitic aortitis, or with extensive calcification of the aortic cusps or mitral ring in elderly atherosclerotic subjects, and is due to a fibrotic or calcified lesion in the bundle of His, or in both its main branches. Occasionally no cause can be found.

Clinical features. Complete A-V dissociation is four times more common in males than in females, and 84 per cent of cases occur in patients over 50 years of age (Campbell, 1944). It is usually permanent, but under special circumstances may be transient or even paroxysmal (Lawrence and Forbes, 1944). It is characterised by an extremely slow heart rate, a water-hammer or collapsing pulse, elevation of the venous pressure, cervical venous pulsation unrelated to ventricular contraction, audible independent atrial sounds, the occurrence of cannon waves in the neck and varying intensity of the first heart sound, general enlargement of the heart, and syncopal attacks of a special kind. It is proved electrocardiographically (fig. 6.17).

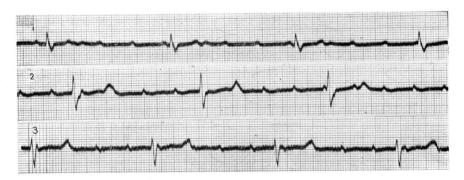

Fig. 6.17—Complete heart block. Ventricular rate 18 beats per minute.

Whilst the pulse rate is usually about 28 to 36 beats per minute, based on the inherent rate of impulse-formation of the idio-ventricular pace-maker distal to the block in the bundle of His, it may be so slow as to induce a state of continual faintness (fig. 6.18), as in the case originally described by Spens (1793) in which it fell to 9 beats per minute. At the other extreme, complete A-V dissociation may be seen with a ventricular rate of over 100, the ventricles sometimes beating more rapidly than the atria (fig. 6.19).

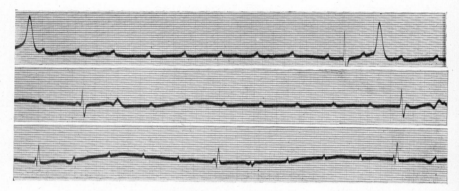

Fig. 6.18—Complete heart block. Ventricular rate 10 beats per minute.

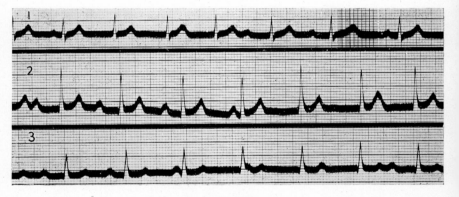

Fig. 6.19—Complete A-V dissociation with the ventricles beating faster than the atria.

On the whole, rates are faster when QRS is normal in width, slower when the QRS resembles left or right bundle branch block (Kay, 1948). Idio-ventricular pace-makers are little affected by stimuli that influence the S-A and A-V nodes, so that the pulse rate usually remains remarkably constant in complete heart block. In transient or paroxysmal cases, however, in which a functional element may be present, temporary restoration of sinus rhythm may accompany fever, as in the case described by Ger-bezius in 1719 (Major, 1932).

A high systolic blood pressure is usual, and is due to the large ventricular stroke-volume. Owing to associated vasodilatation, however, the pressure is not well maintained, but tends to fall away rapidly in diastole, giving rise to a collapsing pulse and to a rather low diastolic blood pressure.

Under favourable circumstances inspection of cervical venous pulsation may reveal atrial waves (*a* waves) independent of ventricular events (*c* and *v* waves), as noted by Stokes (1846). Simultaneously may be heard the faint sounds of isolated atrial contractions (the semi-beats of Stokes), either at the apex beat or down the left border of the sternum.

Venous cannon waves occur when the P wave falls between QRS and T, i.e. when the right atrium contracts against a closed tricuspid valve, and are easily recognised by their abrupt quality, high amplitude and variability. Changing intensity of the first heart sound is equally characteristic: the loudest sounds are heard when the P-R interval is around 0.10 to 0.12 second, left atrial contraction then forcing the mitral cusps wide open just before ventricular systole (Levine, 1948). When the atria contract during the period of rapid ventricular filling a loud third sound or short functional mitral diastolic murmur may be heard; the variability of this summation effect from beat to beat is as characteristic of complete heart block as the varying intensity of the first heart sound.

Cardiac enlargement is usually more conspicuous than that seen in sino-atrial block or in sinus bradycardia, but is of the same quality, unless the size and shape of the heart are altered by other effects of the underlying disease process.

The cardiac output can only be maintained by a large stroke-volume propelled with great force. Diastolic distension is favoured by a compensatory rise in venous pressure, and this must be very considerable during effort. The early development of congestive failure is readily understood.

Stokes-Adams attacks. Syncope due to ventricular asystole (Stokes-Adams attacks) occurs in about 50 per cent. of cases, and is especially common when partial block becomes complete. Loss of consciousness is abrupt, without warning. If standing, the patient collapses, and lies limp, still, pale and pulseless, with fixed, dilated pupils – as if dead; breathing, however, continues. If the attack lasts long enough, i.e. for more than 10 seconds or so, twitchings commence, and may progress to convulsions; and if ventricular asystole continues for more than 2 or 3 minutes, recovery is rare. As a rule, however, ventricular beating is resumed after a few seconds, consciousness returns abruptly, and a vivid flush ensues. When an attack occurs in bed, the lack of warning, short duration of unconsciousness, and abrupt return of full possession of the faculties, may prevent a dull patient from being aware of the fit, and he may only notice the flush. The sequence of events, both symptomatically and objectively, is so characteristic as to make the diagnosis probable on the history alone – a point of some importance in patients with paroxysmal block who may present themselves with normal sinus rhythm. In such cases carotid sinus pressure may provoke an attack or induce paroxysmal heart block (fig. 6.20).

Physiologically, Stokes-Adams attacks are due to depression of a potential or established idio-ventricular pace-maker in cases of complete heart

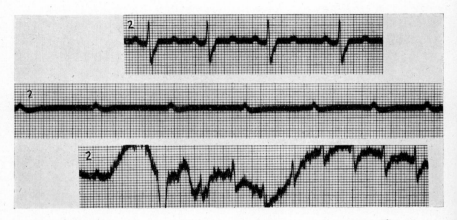

Fig. 6.20—Stokes-Adams fit provoked by carotid sinus pressure in a patient with paroxysmal complete heart block.

block; the ventricles stand still while the atria continue to beat. They are apt to occur when partial block becomes complete either because such an event is usually associated with some depressive influence on conduction which may also depress ventricular pace-makers (even though considered beyond vagal control), or because idio-ventricular pace-makers are by nature initially sluggish. When complete block is well established, attacks may still occur, but are less common. The abrupt loss of consciousness depends upon sudden total failure of cardiac output. Twitching is due to cerebral anoxia, and is not seen in short attacks. Convulsions are of two types, one being an exaggeration of anoxic twitching, the other occurring after restoration of ventricular action and synchronising with the flush (Formijne, 1938). In the second type, convulsions and flushing appear to be due to carbon dioxide depletion in the blood stagnant in the lungs during the phase of asystole with continued respiration, and to vasodilatation resulting from accumulation of tissue metabolites, so that when ventricular beating is resumed, blood rich in oxygen but containing practically no carbon dioxide, is thrown abruptly into a widely dilated vascular bed. More often a period of apnœa follows the attack, with or without subsequent Cheyne-Stokes breathing (Griffith, 1921). Apnœa, of course, may also occur towards the end of long periods of ventricular asystole, when it is due to failure of the respiratory centre resulting from profound cerebral anoxia.

An important complication of Stokes-Adams attacks is paroxysmal ventricular tachycardia or fibrillation (Parkinson, Papp and Evans, 1941). In

such cases it may be impossible to determine clinically whether unconsciousness is due to asystole or to ventricular fibrillation. It is probable that
many deaths are due to the supervention of such rhythm changes rather
than to asystole.

Prognosis. Congenital and transient cases do relatively well, unless the
disease responsible is serious for other reasons. The outlook in paroxysmal
and acquired permanent cases, however, is poor, life expectancy averaging
$4\frac{1}{2}$ years (Graybiel and White, 1936; Campbell, 1944). Those with a history
of Stokes-Adams fits have a much worse prognosis than those without, the
majority of them dying suddenly. Those without fits usually die from
congestive heart failure.

Treatment. The most effective prophylactic treatment for faintness or
syncope is the oral administration of ephedrine, $\frac{1}{2}$ grain (32 mg.) t.d.s. If
attacks are frequent and the patient bedridden, adrenalin, 0.5 mg. (8 minims
or 0.5 ml. of a 1 : 1,000 solution) should be injected subcutaneously, and
repeated every two to six hours. Sublingual isoprenaline, 20 mg., is also
helpful (Nathanson and Miller, 1949); but noradrenalin has very little
stimulating action on ventricular rhythm (Nathanson and Miller, 1950).
Both ephedrine and adrenalin prevent undue depression of the ventricular
pace-maker, and encourage the heart to beat a trifle faster. It is sometimes
said that idio-ventricular rhythm cannot be influenced by any of the drugs
or manœuvres that are known to affect the sinus node. This is not always
strictly true, but changes are admittedly slight. Effort, for example, may
quicken the ventricular rate in complete heart block; the adrenergic drugs,
fever, and even atropine may also do so. In treatment, however, atropine
is valueless alone, although it may enhance the effect of adrenaline. Barium
chloride had a vogue, its action depending upon its power to excite ventricular ectopic beats and so to prevent ventricular standstill; but this is a
poor substitute for the physiological benefit provided by ephedrine. In
paroxysmal cases, when some functional disturbance must be postulated,
inhalations of amyl nitrite may abort attacks (Lawrence and Forbes, 1944).

A problem arises when repeated seizures are partly due to paroxysmal
ventricular tachycardia or fibrillation; for if it is uncertain whether unconsciousness is due to asystole or to fibrillation, the administration of adrenaline may be hazardous, since the drug encourages the latter rhythm-change.
If paroxysmal ventricular tachycardia is demonstrated, neither quinidine
nor procaine amide should be given, for both depress conduction and
may cause ventricular standstill (Miller *et al.*, 1952; Schwartz *et al.*, 1952,
1953). Sublingual isoprenaline, 20 mg., has been recommended in these
cases (Schumacher and Schmock, 1954).

Very slow heart rates may be accelerated by means of intravenous infusions
of sodium lactate in doses of 5 to 15 ml. per minute of a molar (11.2 G.
per 100 ml.) or half molar solution (Bellet, Wesserman, and Brody,
1955). Lactate may serve as a myocardial fuel or the rise in pH (increased
blood bicarbonate) that results from the treatment may accelerate the heart.

Treatment of the primary cardiac condition may help. This applies especially to the rare transient cases associated with active carditis or myocardial infarction, and to permanent cases associated with syphilitic aortitis. Very rarely a small gumma may interrupt the conducting pathway, and the resulting block may be cured with iodides (Major, 1923).

If congestive heart failure calls for digitalis therapy, the drug should not be withheld on account of coincident heart block, but should be administered with caution. Massive and intravenous doses should be avoided; but digitalis leaf, 3 grains (0.2 G) t.d.s. on the first day, 2 grains (0.13 G.) t.d.s. on the second, and 1 grain (65 mg.) thereafter, twice daily, is usually safe. Should a Stokes-Adams fit appear to be provoked, the drug must be discontinued.

In special clinics external electrical pace-makers may be available to tide a heart over a critical period. The machine is designed to deliver an electrical shock of 75 to 150 milliamps, at 45 to 100 volts, for two to three milliseconds, 60 to 90 times per minute; the negative electrode is placed over the region of the apex beat, the positive on the opposite side of the chest posteriorly (Zoll, Linenthal and Norman, 1954).

BUNDLE BRANCH BLOCK

Although bundle branch block is not strictly a disorder of rhythm, it may be discussed here conveniently on account of its close pathological relationship to other forms of conduction defect.

Anatomy. Bundle branch block occurs when some organic lesion interferes with conduction through one or other of the two main branches of the bundle of His. As may be seen from figure 6.01, the main bundle, after piercing the membranous septum, divides into two, one branch passing down each side of the muscular interventricular septum just beneath the endocardium, and spreading out fan-wise distally; the left branch may subdivide into anterior and posterior divisions in the lower half of the septum (Mahaim, 1931). The A-V node, bundle of His, and posterior division of the left bundle branch receive their blood supply from perforating septal arteries arising from the posterior descending branch of the right coronary artery; the right bundle branch and the anterior division of the left are supplied by perforating septal branches of the left anterior descending coronary artery (Gross, 1921). Considerable variations occur, however, especially as vital reactions to ischæmia.

Nomenclature. When the left bundle branch is interrupted, the excitatory process reaches the right ventricle first, through the relatively normal right bundle branch, and spreads throughout that chamber before passing across to the left. The right ventricle therefore contracts first. The electrocardiogram, described and illustrated in Chapter III, shows a wide QRS complex, measuring from 0.11 to 0.18 second, the main deflection of which is usually upright in lead 1 and downward in lead 3, with marked slurring or notching, and followed by a conspicuous T wave, usually in the opposite direction. Right bundle branch block (Wilson *et al.*, 1934) is characterised by widening of the initial ventricular deflection to 0.11 to 0.14 second, by late slurring of QRS – usually best seen in S_1 – and by an upright T wave in lead 1. That the first type of graph described represents left bundle branch block has been proved by the reconstructed vectorcardiograms (monocardiograms) of Mann (1931), by the electrocardiographic discoveries of Wilson and his colleagues (1932), by kymographic and polygraphic studies revealing delayed left ventricular events (Wolferth and Margolies, 1935), by experiments on revived human hearts in normal position in which one or other bundle branch has been cut (Kountz, 1936), and by simultaneous electrocardiographic, phonocardiographic, and polygraphic records demonstrating and analysing ventricular asynchronism (Braun-Menendez and Solari, 1939). The detailed histological work of Mahaim (1931), which at first appeared to support the original view in which the nomenclature for left and right bundle branch block was reversed, has been ably reviewed by Yater (1938), who presented extensive histopathological evidence of his own, and concluded that the bilateral lesions invariably demonstrable rendered reliable interpretation difficult, but that on the whole the findings supported the new terminology. Finally, the clinical facts cannot be disregarded: left bundle branch block is commonly seen in lesions involving the left side of the heart; whereas right bundle branch block is usually associated with enlargement of the right ventricle. This general principle was recognised by Tung and Cheer (1933) and by Bayley (1934).

Etiology. Left bundle branch block is usually due to hypertensive heart disease, ischæmic heart disease, or aortic valve disease; right bundle branch block to mitral stenosis, atrial septal defect, or massive pulmonary embolism. Either form may occur in active rheumatic, diphtheritic or other form of carditis; in any disease affecting the heart as a whole, such as thyrotoxicosis and fibrosis of the myocardium of known or unknown etiology; and as a result of any local lesion such as neoplasm. Partial forms are common and tend to progress; on the other hand, both left and right bundle branch block may be transient, paroxysmal, or even alternating (fig. 6.21), sometimes in association with paroxysmal tachycardia, auricular flutter, or fibrillation; sometimes during an episode such as acute myocardial infarction, congestive heart failure, or massive pulmonary embolism; but also spontaneously. Right bundle branch block is sometimes found in otherwise healthy individuals, even in youth, left bundle branch block very rarely so.

Clinical features. Clinically, left bundle branch block may be suggested by presystolic gallop rhythm in the absence of ventricular distress, and by reversed splitting of the second heart sound, A_2 falling after P_2 so that the split closes on inspiration and widens on expiration. Right bundle branch block is suggested by wide splitting of the second sound, P_2 falling later than usual. When the heart is enlarged and it is uncertain which chamber is mainly involved, the presence of left or right bundle branch block points strongly to the homolateral ventricle. Left bundle branch block provides convincing proof of serious heart disease; but right bundle branch block must be interpreted more cautiously. Neither form is influenced by digitalis, atropine, or by any of the adrenergic or cholinergic drugs.

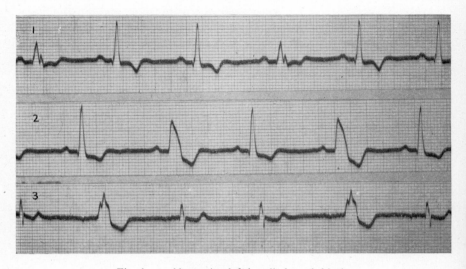

Fig. 6.21—Alternating left bundle branch block.

Prognosis. The average life expectancy for cases of bundle branch block in general has been estimated at 3 years (Campbell, 1944); but it should be clearly understood that in any given patient the prognosis is that of the underlying heart disease, and is not influenced by the conduction defect. Again, if right bundle branch block is found in an otherwise normal individual, the outlook does not differ from normal controls (Wood, Jeffers and Wolferth, 1935).

ECTOPIC BEATS

Ectopic beats are premature systoles induced by the discharge of some ectopic impulse-forming focus situated anywhere in atrial, nodal, or ventricular tissue. They are necessarily premature because all potential impulse-forming foci are otherwise discharged by the excitation which reaches them from the sinus node.

Physiology. In the atrial type (fig. 6.22) the P wave is abnormal in shape or direction according to the site of the ectopic focus and to the direction in which the impulse flows over the atria. In these cases, the partially charged sinus node is discharged when the impulse reaches it, so that the compensatory pause following the ectopic beat is slight, being equal to a normal cycle plus the interval between the onset of the ectopic and the arrival of the retrograde excitatory process at the S-A node. The timing of the heart beat is permanently altered. The ventricular complex is usually normal, but may be slightly deformed as a result of a functional defect in conduction. If an atrial ectopic beat is very premature it may be blocked altogether.

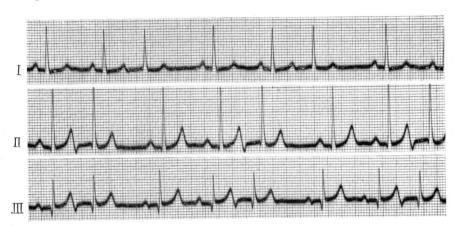

Fig. 6.22—Atrial ectopic beats.

Nodal ectopic beats (fig. 6.23) are premature beats arising in any part of the atrio-ventricular junctional tissue. The QRS complex is normal or slightly deformed as described above; but the P wave is inverted, and occurs just before, during, or just after the QRS complex, according to the more proximal or more distal site of the ectopic focus, and to the degree of resistance opposed to retrograde conduction. Discharge of the sinus node (unless there is retrograde block) again prevents a full compensatory pause.

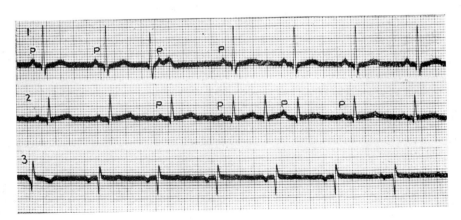

Fig. 6.23—Nodal ectopic beats. Slight deformity of QRS is due to fatigue block. In lead 1 the P wave immediately after the ectopic is blocked. In lead 2 the nodal ectopic is interpolated. In both there is retrograde block.

Ventricular ectopic beats are characterised by a full compensatory pause, for the sinus node is not discharged by the premature impulse, owing to retrograde block (physiological) in the bundle of His, or to natural delay in retrograde conduction, and so continues to function at its usual time. Its first discharge after the ectopic, however, is blocked by the refractory state of the ventricles, and so there is a pause until its second discharge. The final timing of the heart beat therefore remains unchanged. Electrocardiographically, a ventricular ectopic beat resembles a bundle branch block

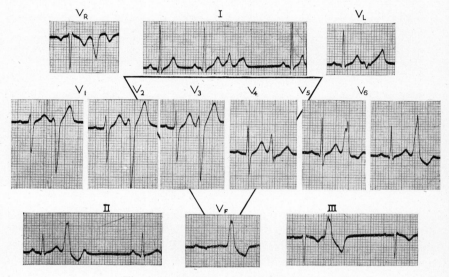

Fig. 6.24—Right ventricular ectopic beats.

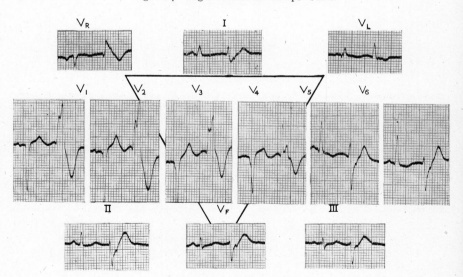

Fig. 6.25—Left ventricular ectopic beats causing coupling.

complex, QRS being widened and notched, and T being prominent and usually in the opposite direction. When the deflection is like left bundle branch block, the ectopic focus lies in the right ventricle (fig. 6.24); when QRS is like right bundle branch block, the ectopic focus lies in the left ventricle (fig. 6.25). There are many variations, however, depending upon the exact site of the irritable focus (Barker *et al.*, 1930; Kountz, 1936). Ventricular ectopic beats may also be interpolated (fig. 6.26).

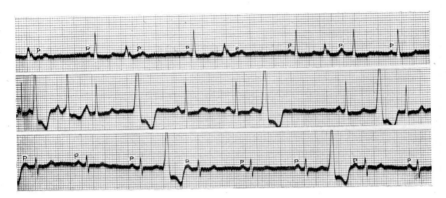

Fig. 6.26—Interpolated ventricular ectopic beats.

Premature beats have a smaller stroke-volume than normal, and if very premature may not be perceptible at the wrist, or audible with a stethoscope. The beat that follows is fuller than usual, and is appreciated by the patient as a hard thump. This is a matter of cardiac filling: the earlier the ectopic beat, the emptier the heart; the longer the compensatory pause, the fuller the heart. The blood pressure varies directly with the stroke output.

Clinical diagnosis. Clinically, ectopic beats must be distinguished from other irregularities, especially from auricular fibrillation and from partial heart block with dropped beats. Whilst this may be easy in the majority of cases, confusion arises with multiple atrial ectopic beats which may be indistinguishable from auricular fibrillation, and with inaudible imperceptible or blocked ectopic beats which mimic partial heart block with dropped beats. Alternate ectopic beats or coupled beats may be confused with S-A block when very premature, with a dicrotic or bisferiens pulse, or even with pulsus alternans. If there is any doubt, the effect of effort, amyl nitrite, or of 1 mg. of atropine sulphate should be determined: ectopic beats usually disappear as the heart quickens, and may be exaggerated as it slows down again. Ectopic beats often cause cannon waves in the neck, whereas auricular fibrillation cannot do so.

Etiology. Experimentally, ectopic beats may be produced by electrical stimulation of any part of the heart. Certain drugs, notably digitalis, barium chloride, and adrenaline, may produce them. Excessive use of tobacco occasionally seems responsible. They are common in pregnancy. Whilst almost any state of ill-health may be blamed for their occurrence, no common factor has been discovered, and in the majority of cases there is no evidence of structural disease of the cardiovascular or other systems. Occasionally, however, atrial ectopic beats may herald auricular fibrillation, especially in mitral stenosis and thyrotoxicosis. Under certain circumstances, also, ectopic beats are probably due to organic disease: for example, their occurrence during the course of diphtheria may be due to toxic carditis; but as innocent ectopic beats are common enough after simple streptococcal tonsillitis, and indeed during convalescence from any fever, it is impossible to draw any conclusion from their presence. Again, ectopic beats following coronary thrombosis are probably significant, and to be explained by irritable foci set up by ischæmia, but are equally common in conditions that may simulate myocardial infarction. On the whole, therefore, it is wise to assume the innocence of ectopic beats under any conditions, and to judge organic disease on other grounds.

Treatment. Many patients are unaware of premature systoles; others may seek relief from palpitations. Treatment includes fresh air, exercise, and a healthy physiological life. Of drugs, potassium bromide 10 grains (0.65 G.) t.d.s., phenobarbitone ½ grain (32 mg.) t.d.s., or quinidine 5 grains (0.32 G.) t.d.s. may prove effective. Alternate ectopic beats (coupling) due to digitalis provide good grounds for stopping the drug or reducing its dose. Potassium salts are efficient (Sampson and Anderson, 1932; Castleden, 1941), but the large dose usually required is not without danger of sudden death, and may provoke symptoms as unpleasant as the palpitations, chiefly nausea and vomiting; the chloride or acetate is employed as a 10 to 20 per cent aqueous solution, and may be given by mouth in safe doses of 2 to 4 G., three or four times a day. Larger doses are not advised. Pronestyl, 0.25 to 0.5 G., four to six hourly by mouth, usually abolishes ventricular ectopic beats. Reassurance is important, and should be unconditional and convincing, for ectopic beats rarely constitute a complaint except in those prone to morbid anxiety.

PARASYSTOLE

Parasystolic rhythm is said to occur when an ectopic focus releases an excitatory impulse at regular intervals, independent of the pace-maker. The ventricles respond to this impulse whenever it reaches them outside their refractory phase.

PAROXYSMAL TACHYCARDIA

When ectopic beats occur in rapid and regular succession from the same focus, one may speak of paroxysmal tachycardia. The name was introduced by Bouveret in 1889. The ectopic focus may be supraventricular (atrial or nodal), or ventricular. The electrocardiographic complexes in the three types are precisely the same as those in the three types of ectopic beat.

The patient usually complains of attacks of palpitations characterised by the abruptness of their beginning and end, by the rapidity and regularity of the beats, and by the relative well-being of the patient (Cotton, 1867). Until an attack is witnessed, the diagnosis rests upon an accurate history. Experience shows that most careful cross-examination is required to establish the true sequence of events. It is not enough to determine that the onset is sudden, it is necessary to be sure it is abrupt: that the full velocity of the attack is reached immediately in the space of one beat; that from no sensation whatever, maximum palpitation develops within one second. To assess the rate and rhythm it is helpful to ask the patient to represent them by tapping with his finger. The manner in which the attack ends may be more difficult to establish: some patients become accustomed to the palpitations and gradually fail to perceive them; others pass from a true paroxysm to sinus tachycardia without appreciating the change, and their description of the end refers to the gradual slowing down of the sinus rhythm.

Attacks may last from a few seconds to several weeks, but are usually measured in hours, and rarely exceed three days. The speed ranges between 110 and 250 beats per minute, but is between 140 and 240 in 90 per cent of cases, and between 150 and 200 in 50 per cent (Campbell, 1947). Occasionally, however, much faster rates have been recorded. For instance, in one of Bouveret's cases the heart rate was 300 per minute, If the heart is normal, as it is in 62 per cent of the supraventricular variety, there is usually a remarkable degree of polyuria *during* the attack, at least in cases with heart rates up to 180 beats per minute; there are usually no other symptoms apart from those provoked by anxiety; but if the attack is unduly prolonged, or the heart rate exceptionally rapid, congestive failure or angina pectoris may occur. If the heart is abnormal, however, as it is in 80 per cent of the ventricular variety, the rapid development of congestive heart failure is common. With very rapid rates syncope may occur, and, in ischæmic heart disease, status anginosus. Physiologically, the effects depend upon the functional capacity of the heart to increase its output with tachycardia, and on its ability to stand up to the extra work imposed with minimal rest. In any given case there must be a critical rate above which the cardiac output falls.

SUPRAVENTRICULAR PAROXYSMS

As just indicated, both paroxysmal atrial and nodal tachycardia are most commonly encountered in healthy individuals, and have little more significance than ectopic beats or spontaneous fluttering of somatic muscle. They are fifteen times more common than ventricular paroxysms. When attacks occur in patients with heart disease, the prognosis is not so good, and depends upon the nature and severity of the cardiac lesion, and the speed and duration of the paroxysm. Even so, the mortality rate is only about 1 per cent.

A clinical diagnosis may be accepted if the spontaneous or induced beginning or end of an attack is proved to be abrupt; if the heart rate during a paroxysm exceeds 150 per minute and does not vary with effort, change of posture, atropine, amyl nitrite, carotid sinus (or eyeball) pressure, prostigmine, or mecholin; if any such measure terminates the paroxysm; if the duration of attacks is a matter of hours rather than one of minutes, days or weeks; if the patient is relatively young, i.e. under 40 years of age, or was so when he had his first attack; if paroxysms have continued with variable frequency for more than five years; and if there is no evidence of organic heart disease or thyrotoxicosis. Electrocardiographic proof, however, which may require a record of the beginning or end of an attack, should be obtained whenever possible. Although only a rare chance will enable the onset to be registered, the end may be recorded in over half the cases by means of a continuous tracing while the attack is terminated by carotid sinus pressure or mecholin (fig. 6.27). If the attack is not terminated, such measures may yet serve to differentiate paroxysmal tachycardia from sinus tachycardia and from auricular flutter; for in paroxysmal tachycardia the heart rate is rarely altered, whereas in sinus tachycardia it is slowed, and in auricular flutter it is often abruptly halved. Occasionally, however, carotid sinus pressure may block paroxysmal atrial tachycardia (fig. 6.28).

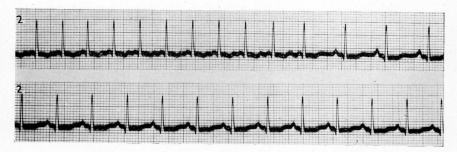

Fig. 6.27—Paroxysmal atrial tachycardia terminated by means of mecholin.

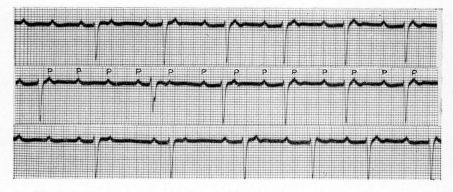

Fig. 6.28—Paroxysmal atrial tachycardia blocked by carotid sinus compression.

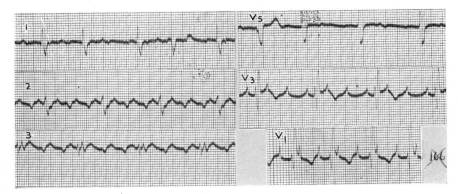

Fig. 6.29—Paroxysmal atrial tachycardia showing varying degrees of spontaneous A-V block.

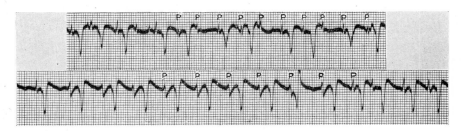

Fig. 6.30—Paroxysmal atrial tachycardia slowed by means of quinidine.

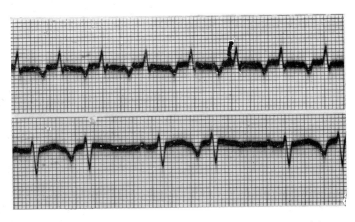

Fig. 6.31—Paroxysmal atrial tachycardia followed by atrial ectopic beats.

Evans (1944) first presented evidence, based on lead CR1, suggesting that many cases that would ordinarily be interpreted as 2 : 1 atrial flutter might really be examples of paroxysmal atrial tachycardia with 2 : 1 A-V block, and that these two conditions were essentially the same. Certainly, paroxysmal atrial tachycardia may show varying degrees of A-V block (figs. 6.28 and 6.29), and the atrial waves may be slowed by means of quinidine (fig. 6.30) in the same way as flutter; there is also no doubt that the same patient may show all varieties of atrial rhythm, suggesting that they all depend upon a similar mechanism, and that the occurrence of atrial ectopics before or after a major attack (fig. 6.31) offers an obvious clue as to their essential nature. Indeed, Prinzmetal (1950) has now provided convincing evidence not only of the unity of paroxysmal atrial tachycardia and flutter, but also of atrial ectopic beats and auricular fibrillation, all four disturbances of rhythm depending upon the presence and behaviour of an ectopic irritable focus. Nevertheless, the clinical differences between paroxysmal tachycardia and flutter (not to mention auricular fibrillation and ectopic beats) are considerable (Campbell, 1945) and their separate identities should be preserved. Similarly, there can be no thought of not maintaining the separate identities of ventricular ectopics, ventricular tachycardia, and ventricular fibrillation, yet all three must depend on a similar physiological mechanism.

PAROXYSMAL NODAL TACHYCARDIA

Nodal paroxysms may be difficult to distinguish from atrial tachycardia when the rate is fast, unless the beginning of an attack can be recorded (fig. 6.32). At slower rates the electrocardiogram resembles fast nodal rhythm. Clinically, nodal tachycardia may often be recognised by the large regular cannon waves which dominate the jugular venous pulse (fig. 6.33).

Nodal tachycardia is commonly innocent and responds particularly well to carotid sinus pressure and cholinergic drugs.

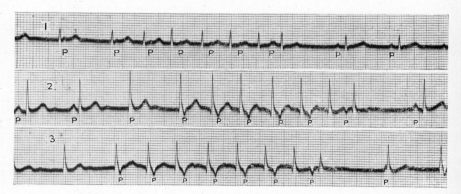

Fig. 6.32—Paroxysmal nodal tachycardia beginning with a nodal ectopic beat.

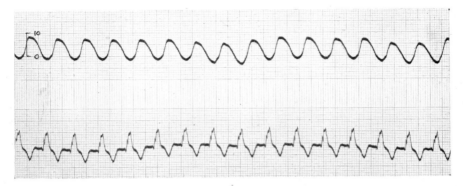

Fig. 6.33—Paroxysmal nodal tachycardia showing regular cannon waves in the right atrial pressure pulse in a case of Ebstein's disease with right branch block.

VENTRICULAR PAROXYSMS

Paroxysmal ventricular tachycardia is relatively rare, is usually associated with organic heart disease in patients between the ages of 40 and 70, and is twice as common in men as in women. It tends to arise in a badly damaged heart, as in heart failure from hypertension or from aortic valve disease; it may follow myocardial infarction, or succeed a Stokes-Adams fit; occasionally it is due to digitalis; in about 20 per cent of cases it is innocent.

It has the same clinical features as the supraventricular variety, apart from the circumstances in which it occurs and its lack of response to carotid sinus pressure and cholinergic drugs; moreover, it is more frequently followed by congestive heart failure, and sometimes by ventricular fibrillation and sudden death. The prognosis is correspondingly grave.

Ventricular tachycardia may be recognised at the bedside if there are

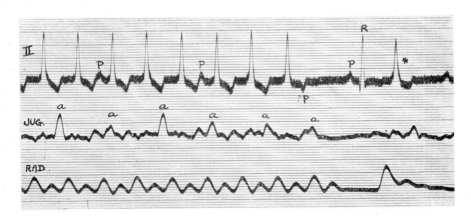

Fig. 6.34—Paroxysmal ventricular tachycardia showing independent P waves at a slower rate. Note the *a* waves and variable cannon waves in the jugular tracing.

(*By courtesy of Sir John Parkinson*)

occasional cannon waves in the jugular pulse or if the first heart sound is occasionally extra loud, for both these phenomena indicate a varying atrioventricular relationship.

Proof of the nature of the attack is obtained by electrocardiography (fig. 6.34); but difficulty may arise when supraventricular paroxysms or auricular flutter are complicated by previously established or functional bundle

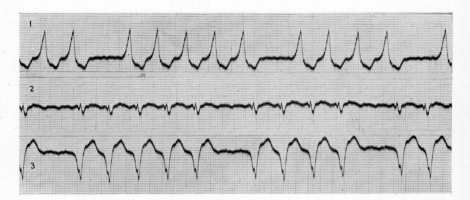

Fig. 6.35—Auricular flutter with left bundle branch block.

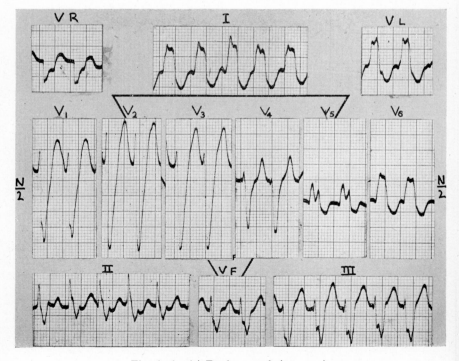

Fig. 6.36—(a) During attack (rate 150).

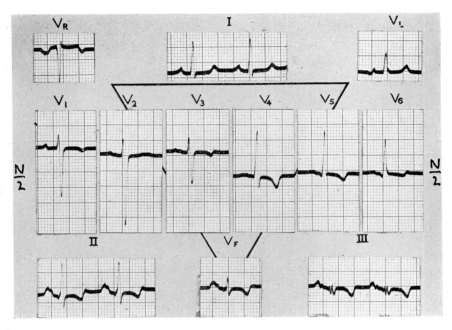

(b) After resumption of normal rhythm showing inverted T waves over a wide area.

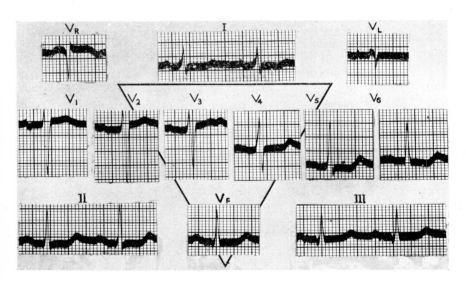

(c) After normal rhythm has been maintained for three months.

Fig. 6.36—Serial electrocardiograms from a case of paroxysmal ventricular tachycardia.

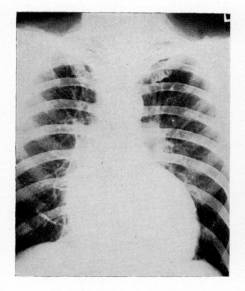 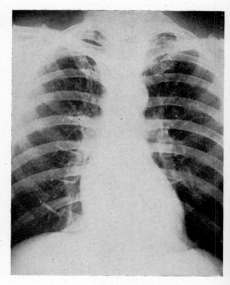

(a) Acute cardiac dilatation.

(b) Normal heart shadow after resumption of normal rhythm and recovery from congestive failure.

Fig. 6.37—Heart failure in primary paroxysmal tachycardia.

branch block (fig. 6.35). The diagnosis is more certain if independent P waves can be made out at a much slower rate, but even then nodal tachycardia with bundle branch block and retrograde A-V block is possible.

Gross heart failure from prolonged paroxysmal ventricular tachycardia does not necessarily signify organic heart disease. When the rhythm is restored to normal, widespread inversion of the T wave points to nutritional changes in the myocardium, but these are always reversible if the rhythm change is primary (fig. 6.36). Cardiac enlargement, due to failure, is also reversible (fig. 6.37).

TREATMENT

Supraventricular paroxysms, *when of nodal origin*, may be terminated by some mechanical trick already known to the patient, such as holding the breath; by carotid sinus or eyeball pressure in about 50 per cent of cases; and by the cholinergic drugs in 75 per cent. Devices discovered by the patient include the adoption of some particular posture, drinking iced water, forced breathing or breath-holding, compression of the abdomen, and self-induced vomiting.

The carotid sinus is located at the bifurcation of the common carotid artery at the level of the superior border of the thyroid cartilage. It should be firmly compressed for several seconds against the bodies of the cervical vertebræ by means of the observer's thumb, first on one side, then on the other; but never together. Bilateral eyeball compression is also carried out with the thumbs, should be sufficiently forceful to cause pain, and should be maintained for 3 to 5 seconds. A depressor response of the same kind may be elicited by stimulating the baroreceptors in both carotid sinuses and in the aortic bodies by injecting some pressor agent, such as phenylephrine (neosynephrine), 0.25 to 0.5 mg., intravenously (Youmans *et al.*, 1949).

Of the cholinergic drugs, mecholin (acetyl-beta-methylcholine) is the most successful (Starr, 1933), and prostigmine the least unpleasant, in the doses employed; doryl (carbo-amino-acetylcholine) is less effective, and acetylcholine itself too drastic, besides being technically difficult owing to its rapid destruction in the bloodstream. Mecholin should be given intra-muscularly or subcutaneously in a dose of 10 to 20 mg., and may be expected to work in about five minutes; prostigmine may be administered intravenously or intramuscularly in a dose of 1 to 2 mg., and has its maxi-mum effect in about half an hour. Side-effects include urgent micturition and defæcation, colic, vomiting, sweating, flushing and faintness; but these are absent or slight with 1 to 1.5 mg. of prostigmine, and rarely severe with 10 mg. of mecholin. Should they prove too unpleasant and the object of the drug has not been achieved, they may be abolished at once by injecting 1 to 2 mg. of atropine sulphate intravenously; but this is obviously not advised unless absolutely necessary. Cholinergic drugs should not be given to patients who are prone to bronchial asthma, for they may then excite violent bronchospasm.

Paroxysmal atrial tachycardia does not usually respond to any of these measures, the drug of choice in these cases being digitalis. It was used originally to slow the ventricular rate by causing partial heart block, as it does in flutter, and also to treat heart failure when that was present; while these objects were being achieved normal rhythm was resumed so fre-quently that digitalis had to be given the credit for that too. For a quick response digoxin should be given intravenously in a dose of 1.0 to 1.25 mg., and repeated in doses of 0.25 to 0.5 mg., four to six hourly until some effect is observed, or until 2.25 mg. have been administered, when subsequent doses must not exceed 0.25 mg. Intravenous digoxin achieves its maximum effect in half to one hour; if injections are given two hourly the dose should not exceed 0.25 mg. after a total of 1.5 mg. has been reached. *An overdose of any digitalis preparation given intravenously may be fatal.*

Ventricular paroxysms may be terminated by injecting intravenously 3 grains (0.2 G.) of quinidine, 0.2 to 1 G. of procaine amide, or 10 to 20 ml. of a 20 per cent solution of magnesium sulphate (Boyd and Scherf, 1943). Both quinidine in doses of 5 to 10 grains (0.3 to 0.6 G.) and procaine amide, 0.25 to 0.5 G., may be given by mouth at two-hourly intervals for four or five doses if the matter seems less urgent. Armbrust and Levine (1950) found quinidine was successful when given by mouth in 81 per cent of cases—mostly ischæmic. Procaine amide has a greater margin of safety than quinidine when given intravenously in the customary doses.

The treatment of resistant cases of all forms of paroxysmal tachycardia may be very difficult. It is essential first to establish the nature of the tachycardia beyond question, a common error being to mistake supra-ventricular tachycardia with functional bundle branch block for ventricular tachycardia and hence to press home the wrong treatment. Next, heart failure must be treated vigorously, if present, by all the usual remedies, for when this is controlled normal rhythm may often be restored and maintained more easily. Any underlying cardiovascular disease amenable to treatment, such as hypertension, thyrotoxicosis, mitral stenosis and cor pulmonale, should not be neglected. Other contributory causes should also be recognised and dealt with, if possible: these include anxiety, insomnia, pregnancy, alcohol, bronchial carcinoma, and other intrathoracic diseases. If, despite attention to such details, the attack cannot be terminated or normal rhythm cannot be maintained for long, the situation may be very serious. Propyl thiouracil, starting with 300 mg. daily, is worth trying. Bilateral stellate and upper dorsal ganglionectomy abolished paroxysmal atrial tachycardia in several difficult cases reported by White and Bland (1950), but proved valueless in a case of the author's.

When standard methods of treatment fail, it is usually more profitable to review what has already been done in the hope of finding some fault in management that can be corrected, than to resort to generally less effective methods of treatment, such as syrup of ipecacuanha, half an ounce (15 ml.), as an emetic (Weiss and Sprague, 1937), or atebrin 0.1 G. intravenously, 0.5 G. in 10 ml. of 1 per cent novocaine intramuscularly, or 0.1 G. three times daily orally (Gertler and Yohalem, 1947).

Maintenance therapy

To prevent attacks of all kinds the best treatment is undoubtedly quinidine sulphate, gr. 3 to 15 (0.2 to 1.0 G.), three times daily. Heavy doses may not be tolerated, but should be tried boldly if necessary (Gold, 1950). Procaine amide, 0.25 to 0.5 G. three times daily, is also very useful, particularly to prevent ventricular tachycardia. A maintenance dose of digitalis may be best for atrial tachycardia, and oral prostigmin, 5 mg. t.d.s., if tolerated, for nodal tachycardia.

When attacks are infrequent, short lived, easily stopped, and not disabling, maintenance therapy is not advised, for all the drugs mentioned may have undesirable effects on the patient's health and well-being. Procaine amide, for example, may cause agranulocytosis.

PAROXYSMAL TACHYCARDIA ASSOCIATED WITH PRE-EXCITATION

The condition first described as physiological bundle branch block with short P-R interval (Wolff, Parkinson and White, 1930) is due to premature excitation of one or other ventricle, usually the right, resulting from an anomalous connexion between the A-V node or right atrium and the right ventricle (Holzman and Scherf, 1932), or to accelerated conduction of a portion of the excitatory process at the A-V node (Prinzmetal *et al.*, 1952), probably the latter. Electrocardiography shows widening of the QRS complex, as in bundle branch block, but at the expense of the P-R interval which is shortened proportionally, the P-S interval, as measured from the beginning of P to the end of the QRS complex, remaining unchanged (fig. 6.38). The appearances usually resemble left rather than right bundle branch block. The anomalous pathway may be through the bundle of Kent (Wood, Wolferth and Geckeler, 1943; Kent, 1914), or through abnormal conducting fibres arising from the upper part of the bundle of His (Wolferth and Wood, 1933), such as those described by Mahaim (1931). The passage of the excitatory impulse down such an alternative pathway might well account for premature right ventricular stimulation. Experimental short circuits of the kind envisaged were devised by Butterworth and Poindexter (1942); the classical appearances of the Wolff-Parkinson-White syndrome resulted. On the other hand, Prinzmetal *et al.* (1952) found that experimental W.P.W. complexes, produced by

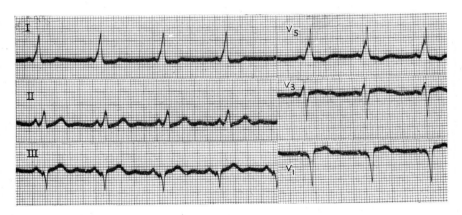

Fig. 6.38—Pre-excitation.

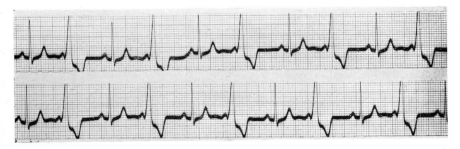

Fig. 6.39—Alternating pre-excitation.

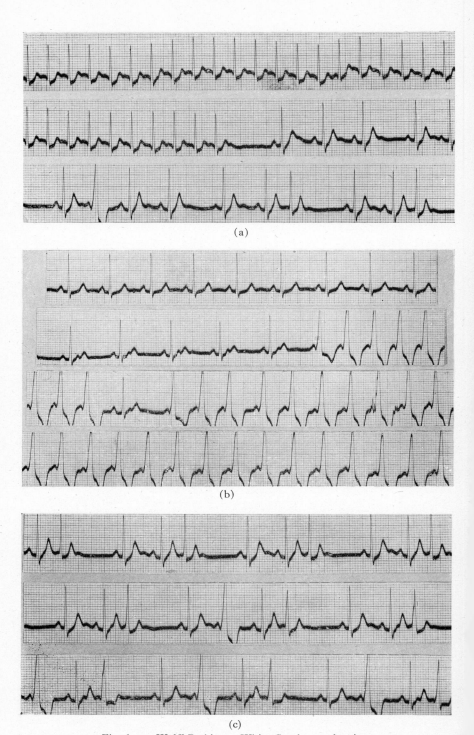

(a)

(b)

(c)

Fig. 6.40—Wolff-Parkinson-White Syndrome showing:
(a) Paroxysmal tachycardia with normal QRS complexes.   (b) Paroxysmal tachycardia
with widened QRS complexes.   (c) Atrial re-entry following the major attack.

248

continuous subthreshold electrical stimulation of the A-V node, would not arise if the bundle of His was cut; that W.P.W. complexes sometimes occurred during cardiac catheterisation when the nodal tissue might be injured, and after posterior cardiac infarction when the nodal tissue was proved to be injured at subsequent necropsy; and that a ventricular form of W.P.W. syndrome existed both clinically and experimentally in which pre-excitation was due to an irritable focus in the ventricle. Prinzmetal points out that one of the major functions of the A-V node is to hold up the excitation wave sufficiently long to allow the atria to contract well ahead of the ventricles, and that impairment of nodal function should therefore lead to accelerated conduction (Borduas *et al.*, 1955). Experimental damage to the A-V node may certainly have this effect.

The condition is usually congenital, occurs in both sexes equally, and is often unstable as shown by serial electrocardiograms; indeed, normal and abnormal complexes may alternate (fig. 6.39). On the whole, normal conduction is encouraged by atropine, abnormal conduction by cholinergic activity (Duthie, 1946). The heart is otherwise normal in at least 70 per cent of cases. Pre-excitation is clinically and academically important on account of its association with paroxysmal tachycardia, and is easily overlooked because casual electrocardiograms may be normal. Paroxysmal tachycardia occurs in 50 to 70 per cent of cases (Willius and Carryer, 1946; Wolff, 1954), and is often closely related to effort. Electrocardiograms obtained during attacks suggest that their mechanism may depend upon a circus movement, the impulse travelling down the bundle of His and back through the short circuit (fig. 6.40a), or down the short circuit and back through the bundle of His (fig. 6.40b), the former being more common. Both types of paroxysm may occur in the same patient, as in the illustrations. In this particular case the second type of paroxysm was provoked by mecholin, and before normal rhythm was resumed there was a period of transition in which abnormal P waves appeared immediately after certain QRS complexes (fig. 6.40c), causing a single premature ventricular beat, and suggesting circus movement due to retrograde conduction through the bundle of Kent or similar structure, initial excitation having passed through the bundle of His. Similar P waves may be seen in the upper half of figure 6.40b, but these fail to excite the ventricles. If Prinzmetal's hypothesis is correct, paroxysmal tachycardia is presumably nodal, and may be regarded as another manifestation of disordered nodal function. Occasionally, attacks resemble auricular flutter or fibrillation, and the ventricular rate may be exceptionally fast. A case described by Littmann and Tarnower (1946) had an irregular ventricular rate of 340 per minute. Paroxysmal tachycardia may also occur in patients with a short P-R interval and without the W.P.W. syndrome. Thus Lows *et al.* (1952) found it in 9.5 per cent of 200 such cases. When all cases with short P-R interval and paroxysmal tachycardia were considered, only 18 per cent had the Wolff-Parkinson-White syndrome.

AURICULAR FLUTTER

Physiology. Auricular flutter in man was so named by Jolly and Ritchie (1910) after obtaining the first electrocardiographic records of the condition, and was attributed to a circus movement by Lewis (1918–20). The excitatory impulse was believed to travel round a ring of atrial tissue, such as the mouths of the venæ cavæ, as proved possible by the physiological researches of Mines (1913). Rosenblueth and Ramos (1947) apparently confirm Lewis' views. Using a high-speed cinematograph technique, however, Prinzmetal (1950) has disproved this thesis, and has shown that auricular flutter and fibrillation, like atrial ectopic beats and paroxysmal atrial tachycardia, depend upon the presence and behaviour of an irritable focus in atrial muscle. The speed of the auricular beats ranges between 260 and 340 per minute, and its rhythm is regular. As the A-V node can rarely transmit impulses faster than 210 to 220 per minute, physiological heart block results, the ventricles usually responding to every second impulse. If the auricular rate is slower, however, and approaches 200 per minute, as it may under the influence of quinidine, the ventricles may be able to keep pace (Lewis, 1925). If vagal tone is increased, as by carotid sinus pressure, a greater degree of physiological block results, and an A-V ratio of 4 : 1 or so may be established, the speed of the "f" waves remaining unaltered. Sometimes the ventricular response is irregular.

Clinical features, incidence, and etiology. Clinically, flutter should be suspected in any patient presenting a regular heart rate of 120 to 170 per minute, uninfluenced by effort, emotion, or change of posture, whether there are other indications of heart disease or not. When the ventricular response is irregular the first heart sound varies in intensity according to the time relationship between atrial and ventricular contractions (Harvey and Levine, 1948).

Flutter is a relatively uncommon but capricious rhythm, and may occur when least expected. It is twice as common in men as in women, and its incidence increases with age, being rare under 30, and most frequent (88 per cent) between the ages of 40 and 70. It is very rare in otherwise normal individuals; it may complicate such diverse conditions as meningitis, pneumonia, cholecystitis, or carcinoma of the colon. In 90 per cent of cases, however, it is associated with organic heart disease, especially rheumatic, hypertensive, ischæmic or pulmonary, and may then precipitate or complicate congestive heart failure. According to Campbell (1947), angina pectoris develops in 25 per cent of paroxysms. Attacks are commonly transient, and have the same abrupt onset as paroxysmal tachycardia; but they tend to last longer, being measured in weeks rather than hours, and may occasionally persist for years. Lewis (1937) described a case in a parson which had continued for 24 years.

Diagnosis is facilitated by carotid sinus pressure, which often causes abrupt temporary slowing of the ventricular rate, as described previously, whereas in sinus tachycardia slowing is commonly slight, and in paroxysmal tachycardia it is usually absent unless the attack is terminated. Electro-cardiography is advised in all suspected cases, however, and reveals a continuous series of rapid regular atrial "f" waves (fig. 6.41) without intervening iso-potential periods. When there is 2 : 1 block, one "f" wave is more or less obscured by the QRS complex, so that the nature of the

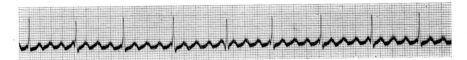

Fig. 6.41—Auricular flutter with 4–1 A-V block.

tachycardia may remain uncertain (fig. 6.42). Carotid sinus pressure aids analysis by increasing the degree of block and so unmasking such hidden "f" waves (fig. 6.43).

Treatment. The patient should be put to bed and treated with adequate doses of digitalis, beginning with 8 grains (0.5 G.) of the powdered leaf, followed by 4 grains (0.25 G.), and then by 2 grains (0.13 G.), at six-hourly intervals, and continuing with 2 grains (0.13 G.) t.d.s., until serial electro-cardiograms show that auricular fibrillation has been established. The drug is then withheld in the hope that normal rhythm may be resumed spon-taneously (fig. 6.44). Electrocardiographic control is necessary because the slow irregular ventricular response that results from such doses of digitalis is no proof of auricular fibrillation under the circumstances. Adequate supervision is important owing to the heavy dose of digitalis usually required to induce fibrillation; and if toxic symptoms appear dangerous before this result is achieved, the attempt may have to be abandoned. The effect of digitalis is twofold, as already indicated: it encourages the irritable focus to assume the properties associated with auricular fibrillation; and by depressing conduction in the bundle of His, it slows the ventricular rate. It was hitherto believed that normal rhythm was resumed when the circus movement was broken by the head of the wave meeting a refractory tail (Lewis, 1925); for circus movement could not occur unless there was a gap of responsive tissue just ahead of the wave. Digitalis, either during its administration or when it was suspended, was thought to close the gap by having an unequal and favourable effect on conduction and on the refractory period. Obviously, if conduction were quickened and the refractory period prolonged in atrial tissue, the hypothetical gap would close. Naturally, no drug has this effect, those quickening conduction also shortening the refractory period (like the cholinergic bodies), and *vice versa* (like quinidine). The action of digitalis is complicated by its cholin-ergic effect: the "f" waves are never retarded, but they may be accelerated, especially in those cases that are made to fibrillate (Wedd, 1924).

Quinidine should not be given alone to cases of flutter in the first instance, for by depressing the irritable focus and slowing the atrial rate, it may

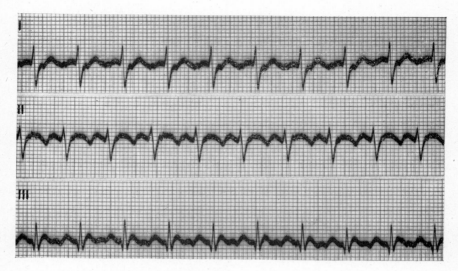

Fig. 6.42—Auricular flutter with 2–1 A-V block.

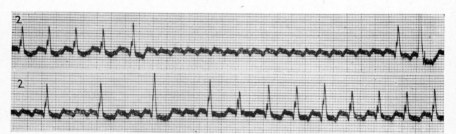

Fig. 6.43—Auricular flutter clarified by means of carotid sinus compression.

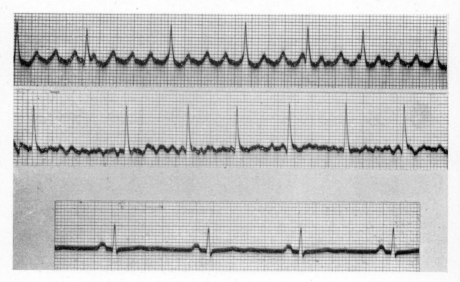

Fig. 6.44—Auricular flutter treated with digitalis. Auricular fibrillation is induced first: on withholding the drug normal rhythm is resumed.

allow the ventricles to keep pace, rapid tachycardia resulting. When auricular fibrillation has been established, however, the resumption of normal rhythm may be encouraged by quinidine in doses of 5 to 10 grains (0.32 to 0.65 G.) two-hourly, to a maximum of 40 to 45 grains (2.5 to 3 G.) in one day. Quinidine may be given safely to resistant cases of flutter so long as the ventricular response is blocked by digitalis.

If flutter continues despite all efforts to break it, the patient should be kept on a maintenance dose of digitalis sufficient to control the ventricular rate; but the result is rarely satisfactory, for short of digitalis intoxication, tachycardia due to 2 : 1 ventricular response is apt to develop on little provocation.

In all cases attention should be paid to any associated disease, cardiac or otherwise, and to combating congestive heart failure.

AURICULAR FIBRILLATION

Physiology. According to Prinzmetal (1950, 1952), two types of atrial contractions may be seen by means of a high-speed cinematograph in experimental auricular fibrillation induced by means of aconitine or electrical stimulation: (1) minute irregular contractions, which he has called M contractions, involving a small area of atrial wall (0.03 × 3 mm.); and (2) large rhythmic wave-like contractions (L contractions), which sweep across the atria 400 to 600 times per minute, without pursuing a circus pathway. Blocking a hypothetical circuit round the mouths of the venæ cavæ had no effect on these waves. Direct atrial leads recorded by means of a cathode ray oscillograph showed very small M waves at 10,000 to 40,000 per minute, and large f waves corresponding to the L contractions. The M waves did not occur in flutter. Lewis's theory of circus movement appears to be untenable.

At "f" wave speeds of 320 to 380, electrocardiograms from chest leads placed over the right atrium show "f" waves which at times are regular and even as in flutter, and which at other times are irregular and uneven as in fibrillation (fig. 6.45). At faster rates the "f" waves are always irregular in time and shape, and the ventricular response is commonly rapid and chaotic, varying between 100 and 200 per minute (fig. 6.46). Sometimes, and of course in treated cases, when there is partial atrio-ventricular block, the ventricular rate is relatively slow. Occasionally there is complete heart block (usually in cases treated with digitalis over a long period of time) and the ventricular rate is not only slow but regular (fig. 6.47).

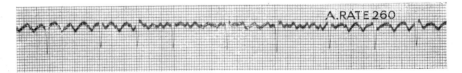

Fig. 6.45—Lead CR1 showing coarse auricular fibrillation or impure flutter.

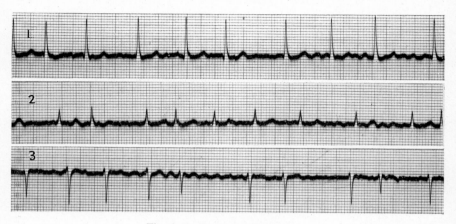

Fig. 6.46—Auricular fibrillation.

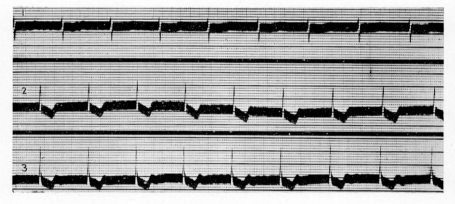

Fig. 6.47—Auricular fibrillation with complete A-V dissociation due to digitalis.

The physiology of the circulation is disturbed by auricular fibrillation in several ways. First, the lack of atrial help deprives the heart of one of its reserves, for powerful atrial contraction can increase the diastolic volume of the ventricles and so augment the force of their contraction; second, the ventricular rate is often fast enough to prevent proper cardiac filling, so that the cardiac output falls—left ventricular filling is especially impaired with fast rates in mitral stenosis; third, the chaotic rhythm interferes with the mechanical efficiency of the heart, many of the beats being wasted; fourth, the nutrition of the myocardium may suffer owing to reduced coronary flow. Physiological studies have shown that when normal rhythm is restored the cardiac output rises immediately, *even when the ventricular rate was previously controlled* by means of digitalis (Hansen *et al.*, 1952).

Etiology. Auricular fibrillation is characteristically associated with mitral stenosis and toxic nodular goitre, and is usually permanent with the former and paroxysmal with the latter. It is not uncommon, however, in the later stages of hypertensive and ischæmic heart disease. On the other hand, it is rare in congenital heart disease, in bacterial endocarditis (2 per cent), in any form of active carditis in young people, in aortic valve disease (unless there is stenosis of the coronary ostia), in pulmonary heart disease, in the high output group (apart from thryotoxicosis), and in pericarditis (although it occurs in 33 per cent of cases of Pick's disease). Like flutter, more-over, auricular fibrillation may occur in patients with no other evidence of heart disease: it may complicate head injuries, meningitis, pneumonia, and other infections in rare instances; and it may even be found in apparently healthy persons. The most important single factor determining the inci-dence of auricular fibrillation in those diseases that favour its occurrence is the advancing age of the patient.

Clinical features. Symptoms may be absent or negligible, or the patient may complain of palpitations. If the ventricular rate is very rapid, syncope or angina pectoris may result, as with flutter and paroxysmal tachycardia. The mechanical inefficiency and nutritional hazards resulting from the rapid irregularity of the heart beat often lead to congestive failure when there is underlying heart disease; on the other hand, auricular fibrillation may be precipitated by congestive failure from other causes.

Diagnosis. The clinical diagnosis rests upon the recognition of a chaotic cardiac rhythm, i.e. one without any semblance of order, and must be dis-tinguished from sinus arrhythmia, from ectopic beats, and from auricular flutter with an irregular ventricular response. Sinus arrhythmia should be recognised by its relation to respiration, and ectopic beats by the perception of some fundamental order; but multiple atrial ectopic beats may be most confusing. The cervical venous pulse should be carefully inspected: the presence of *a* waves, cannon waves, or a convincing *x* descent excludes auricular fibrillation. Electrocardiography, however, is advised in all sus-pected cases.

Treatment. All cases in which the ventricular rate is accelerated should be treated with digitalis. When there is no urgency, a simple and safe method is to give powdered digitalis leaf, 3 grains (0.2 G.) t.d.s. on the first day, 2 grains (0.13 G.) t.d.s. on the second, and 1 grain (65 mg.) t.d.s. there-after, until the ventricular rate is controlled. Subsequently a maintenance dose of 1 grain (65 mg.) twice daily is usually sufficient. When a quicker effect is desired, the method described for cases of auricular flutter is advised. If digoxin is preferred to digitalis folia, equivalent doses may be used for the slow method of digitalising a patient, and 1.5 mg., 1 mg., and 0.5 mg., six-hourly, for the rapid method. In urgent cases with very rapid ventricular rates and severe congestive heart failure, digoxin by the intravenous route may be preferable, but is not without danger, and should never be given in full doses to any patient who may have had digitalis within the previous six weeks, or who still shows a digitalis effect in the electrocardiogram. The initial maximum dose is 1.5 mg., but 1 mg. is safer, and this may be followed by 0.5 mg., and then by 0.25 mg., at intervals of not less than two hours and not more than six hours. In favourable circumstances the ventricular rate may be controlled within half an hour; an oral maintenance dose should then replace the later intravenous doses just recommended. Strophanthin may be used instead of digoxin; as Ouabain it may be given in an initial dose of 1.0 mg. intravenously, followed by 0.5 mg., and then by 0.25 mg., two to six hourly until the desired effect is obtained. As strophanthin is all excreted within forty-eight hours, it is preferable to digoxin when a cumulative effect is not desired.

Other preparations of digitalis may be given by mouth, the dose being calculated according to the following table of equivalent strengths:

Powdered digitalis leaf .   .   . 1 grain (65 mg.)
Tincture of digitalis   .   .   . 10 minims (0.6 ml.)
Digoxin   .   .   .   .   . 0.25 mg.
Digitoxin (Nativelle's Digitaline) . 0.075 mg.

The practitioner is advised to become thoroughly familiar with a few reliable preparations. Digoxin and digitoxin have the advantage of being pure crystalloids of fixed potency. Digoxin is excreted more quickly than digitoxin. The tincture loses strength with the passage of time and when mixed with other drugs, and is therefore least reliable. The powdered leaf has been the standard preparation in this country for many years, but is being gradually displaced by digoxin.

Toxic symptoms include anorexia, nausea, vomiting, diarrhœa, ectopic beats, nodal rhythm, heart block, paroxysmal tachycardia, and sudden death from ventricular fibrillation. Nausea and coupling due to ectopic beats are the best indications that the accumulated dose of digitalis is approaching dangerous concentration. Unfortunately, the worse the heart, the closer the therapeutic dose becomes to the toxic; the margin is never great. The vagal effects may be relieved by atropine.

The correct maintenance dose must be worked out for each individual receiving the drug; but it averages 0.5 mg. of digoxin daily, ranging between 0.25 and 0.75 mg. The average maintenance dose of digitoxin is 0.1 mg. daily, and is very well tolerated by patients prone to nausea and vomiting because it does not irritate the gastric mucosa.

Attempts to restore normal rhythm with quinidine should be made in all cases in which there is no evidence of intrinsic heart disease, and especially in cases of successfully treated mitral stenosis or thyrotoxicosis; also, perhaps, when auricular fibrillation is thought to have occurred prematurely or unexpectedly, having been precipitated by some passing infection, such as tonsillitis or pneumonia, or by some other factor which either no longer operates, such as pregnancy, or which is itself controllable, such as dental sepsis. When fibrillation develops in the natural course of heart disease, however, e.g. in cases of mitral valve disease which are unsuitable for surgical treatment, attempts to restore normal rhythm end in immediate or remote failure, and should therefore be avoided as the procedure is not without risk.

Quinidine should be given by mouth in doses of 5 grains (0.3 G.), two-hourly, on the first day, followed by 10 grains (0.6 G.), two-hourly, on the second, and by 15 grains (1 G.), two-hourly, on the third, to a maximum of 40 to 45 grains (3 G.) per day, the course being terminated immediately the rhythm returns to normal. A maintenance dose of 5 grains (0.3 G.) t.d.s. is continued for a month in successful cases.

Quinidine depresses the activity of the irritable focus, retarding its periodicity and often abolishing it altogether (about 75 per cent of cases). As the "f" waves slow down (fig. 6.48), they may assume the regularity

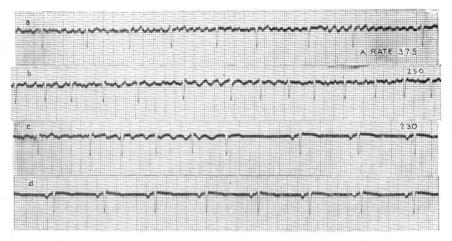

Fig. 6.48—Auricular fibrillation treated with quinidine. The f waves slow down from 375 to 230 per minute before normal rhythm is restored.

of flutter, and if their speed approaches 200 per minute there is danger of a 1 : 1 ventricular response. Tachycardia so provoked by quinidine may be prevented by preliminary digitalis therapy, and a maintenance dose of digitalis is advised throughout the quinidine course. The theoretical consideration that digitalis and quinidine have partly opposing actions does not prejudice successful practical results.

Other complications of quinidine therapy include hypersensitivity and embolism. Hypersensitivity may result in generalised œdema, urticaria, purpura, fever, vomiting and collapse; although such symptoms are rare, it is customary to give an initial trial dose of 3 grains (0.2 G.). Less important symptoms of quinidine intolerance include epigastric pain, nausea, diarrhœa, tinnitus and diplopia. Quinidine lowers the peripheral vascular resistance, and when given intravenously may cause syncope.

To restore normal rhythm quinidine must usually reach a blood concentration of 4 to 10 mgm. per litre (Sokolow and Edgar, 1950). The maximum blood level is achieved about two hours after an oral dose and then declines gradually over 12 to 24 hours. The necessary blood concentration can be obtained when quinidine is given in the manner described above, but Sokolow (1951) showed that it could also be reached with doses of 5 to 15 gr. (0.3 to 1 G.) t.d.s., the drug being cumulative for a period of three days. Yount, Rosenblum and McMillan (1952) agree with Sokolow that there are no contraindications to quinidine except hypersensitivity, and that there is no relation between inability to revert to normal rhythm and age, cardiac failure or duration of fibrillation. British schools are reserved about accepting this conclusion.

Important systemic emboli occur in about 5 per cent of all cases in which normal rhythm is restored, and are due to the expulsion of left atrial thrombi. There is reason to believe that only fresh thrombi are liable to be dislodged, and that these are most likely to form when the ventricular rate is rapid, i.e. at the onset of the attack before digitalis has been given, especially in cases of mitral stenosis, when the left atrium and its appendage are dilated. Since normal rhythm is more likely to be resumed spontaneously or as a result of medical treatment at this time than at any other, and since in fact systemic embolism is known to be a not uncommon complication of auricular fibrillation at this crucial time, *whether normal rhythm is resumed or not*, there are good grounds for treating all such cases with anti-coagulants until the ventricular rate is properly controlled or normal rhythm is resumed, and for withholding quinidine until the clotting mechanism has been depressed for at least five days—at any rate in cases of mitral valve disease. Intracardiac thrombi are rare in thyrotoxic heart disease, even under the most unfavourable circumstances, owing to the rapid circulation associated with it.

Lone auricular fibrillation, also increasingly frequent as age advances, may be paroxysmal or permanent. In about 10 per cent of cases it causes congestive heart failure (Phillips and Levine, 1949), and even in favourable cases it causes palpitations and reduces effort tolerance. Since normal rhythm can be restored with very little risk in about 85 per cent, for an average period of about two years in those that relapse, and permanently in 10 or 20 per cent of cases, the general tendency to treat conservatively with or without digitalis is open to criticism. Heart failure, when it occurs, is reversible.

Auricular fibrillation, flutter and sinus bradycardia, alternating in the same patient, usually middle-aged or elderly and otherwise normal, can be very troublesome. Short periods of cardiac standstill may result in syncope, or very slow rates may give rise to weakness and dizziness; when atrial flutter or fibrillation supervenes, some patients actually feel better, but complain of palpitations. Treatment with atropine in the belief that both the abnormal atrial rhythm and the sinus bradycardia were due to increased vagal tone has proved disappointing.

VENTRICULAR FIBRILLATION

Faradic stimulation of the ventricles invariably induces incoordinated fibrillation of the muscle which usually persists after cessation of the exciting cause. The heart muscle is unable to expel its contents and syncope occurs abruptly. Spontaneous recovery may occur, especially in young healthy animals, but sudden death is the rule. When the heart is unduly excitable, as in asphyxia, digital pressure or gently scratching the surface

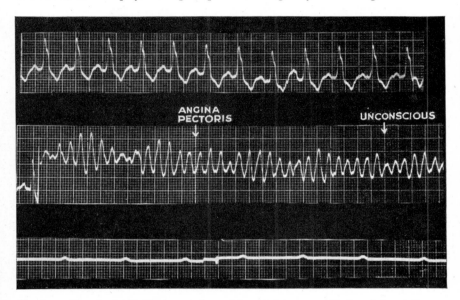

Fig. 6.49—Ventricular fibrillation causing sudden death in a case of ischæmic heart disease.

of the ventricle with a pin may be sufficient to induce ventricular fibrillation (MacWilliam, 1887). Certain drugs may initiate the phenomenon, notably adrenaline, chloroform, and digitalis. Coronary occlusion is also known to be an exciting cause.

Clinically, ventricular fibrillation is often responsible for sudden death, especially in ischæmic heart disease (fig. 6.49), aortic stenosis, syphilitic aortic incompetence, diphtheritic carditis, and complete heart block. It also explains sudden death following intravenous injections of digitalis, mercurial diuretics, adrenaline, and other drugs. It is a rare complication of cardiac catheterisation, and it occurs occasionally during or shortly after operations on the heart.

Treatment is of little avail. The intracardiac injection of quinidine sulphate, 3 to 5 grains (0.2 to 0.3 G.), or of 500 mg. of pronestyl, may be tried if circumstances are favourable. Quinidine or pronestyl may also be given by mouth as a prophylactic agent when the risk of ventricular fibrillation is great. A special electric defibrillator has been developed for surgical use, and with cardiac massage may be life-saving.

REFERENCES

Armbrust, C. A., and Levine, S. A. (1950): "Paroxysmal ventricular tachycardia. A study of one hundred and seven cases", *Circulation*, 1, 28.

Barker, P. S., MacLeod, A. G., and Alexander, J. (1930): "The excitatory process observed in the exposed human heart", *Amer. Heart J.*, 5, 720.
Bayley, R. H. (1934): "The frequency and significance of right bundle branch block", *Amer. J. med. Sc.*, 188, 236.
Bellet, S., Wasserman, F., and Brody, J. I. (1955): "Treatment of cardiac arrest and slow ventricular rates in complete A-V heart block", *Circulation*, 11, 685.
Borduas, J. L., Rakita, L., Kennamer, R., and Prinzmetal, M. (1955): "Studies on the mechanism of ventricular activity. XIV. Clinical and experimental studies of accelerated auriculoventricular conduction", *Ibid.*, 11, 69.
Bouveret, L. (1889): "Concerning essential paroxysmal tachycardia", *Rev. de Méd.*, 9, 753.
Boyd, L. J., and Scherf, D. (1943): "Magnesium sulphate in paroxysmal tachycardia", *Amer. J. Med. Sci.*, 206, 43.
Braun-Menendez, E., and Solari, L. A. (1939): "Ventricular asynchronism in bundle branch block", *Arch. intern. Med.*, 63, 830.
Bruenn, H. G. (1937): "The mechanism of impaired auriculoventricular conduction in acute rheumatic fever", *Amer. Heart J.*, 13, 413.
Butterworth, J. S., and Poindexter, C. A. (1942): "Short PR interval associated with prolonged QRS complex; clinical and experimental study", *Arch. intern. Med.*, 69, 437.

Campbell, M. (1944): "Complete heart block", *Brit. Heart J.*, 6, 69.
—— (1945): "Paroxysmal tachycardia and 2 : 1 heart block", *Ibid.*, 7, 183.
—— (1947): "The paroxysmal tachycardias", *Lancet*, ii, 681.
Castleden, L. I. M. (1941): "The effect of potassium salts on cardiac irregularities", *Brit. med. J.*, i, 7.
Cotton, R. P. (1867): "Notes and observations upon a case of unusually rapid action of the heart (232 per minute)", *Ibid.*, i, 629.

Duthie, R. J. (1946): "Mechanism of the Wolff-Parkinson-White syndrome", *Brit. Heart J.*, 8, 96.

Evans, W. (1944): "The unity of paroxysmal tachycardia and auricular flutter", *Ibid.*, 6, 221.

Formijne, P. (1938): "Apnœa or convulsions following standstill of the heart", *Amer. Heart J.*, 15, 129.

Gertler, M. M., and Yohalem, S. B. (1947): "The effect of atabrine on auricular fibrillation and supraventricular tachycardia in man", *J. Mount Sinai Hosp.*, Baltimore, 13, 323.
Gold, H. (1950): "Quinidine in disorders of the heart", Cassell & Co., London.
Graybiel, A., and White, P. D. (1936): "Complete auriculo-ventricular dissociation. A clinical study of seventy-two cases with a note on a curious form of auricular arrhythmia frequently observed", *Amer. J. med. Sc.*, 192, 334.
Griffith, T. W. (1921): "A clinical study of three cases of heart block", *Brit. med. J.*, i, 763.
Gross, L. (1921): "The blood supply to the heart", New York.

Hansen, W. R., et al. (1952): "Auricular fibrillation", *Amer. Heart J.*, 44, 499.
Hay, J. (1906): "Bradycardia and cardiac arrhythmia produced by depression of certain functions of the heart", *Lancet*, 1, 139.
Holzmann, M., and Scherf, D. (1932): "Uber Elektrokardiogramme mit verkurzter Vorhof-Kammer-Distanz und positiven P-Zacken", *Ztschr. f. klin. Med.*, 121, 404.

Jolly, W. A., and Ritchie, W. R. (1910): "Auricular flutter and fibrillation", *Heart*, 2, 177.

Kay, H. B. (1948): "Ventricular complexes in heart block", *Brit. Heart J.*, 10, 177.

Keith, A., and Flack, M. (1907): "The form and nature of the muscular connexions between the primary divisions of the vertebrate heart", *J. of Anat. and Physiol.*, 41, 172.

Kent, A. F. S. (1914): "Observations on the auriculo-ventricular junction of the mammalian heart", *Quart. J. exper. Physiol.*, 7, 193.

Kountz, W. B. (1936): "Revival of human hearts", *Ann. intern. Med.*, 10, 330.

Lawrence, J. S., and Forbes, G. W. (1944): "Paroxysmal heart block and ventricular standstill", *Brit. Heart J.*, 6, 53.

Levine, S. A. (1948): "Auscultation of the Heart", *Ibid.*, 10, 213.

Lewis, T. (1925): "The mechanism and graphic registration of the heart beat", London.

—— (1937): "Auricular flutter continuing for twenty-four years", *Brit. med. J.*, i, 1248.

——, Feil, H. S., and Stroud, W. D. (1918–20): "Observations upon flutter and fibrillation". Part II. "The nature of auricular flutter", *Heart*, 7, 191.

Littmann, D., and Tarnower, H. (1946): "Wolff-Parkinson-White syndrome. A clinical study with report of nine cases", *Amer. Heart J.*, 32, 100.

Lown, B., *et al.* (1952): "The syndrome of short P-R interval, normal QRS complex and paroxysmal rapid heart action", *Circulation*, 5, 693.

McMichael, J., and Sharpey-Schafer, E. P. (1944): "Cardiac output in man by a direct Fick method", *Brit. Heart J.*, 6, 33.

McWilliam, J. A. (1887): "Fibrillar contraction of the heart", *J. Physiol.*, 8, 296.

Mahaim, I. (1931): "Les maladies organiques du faisceau de His-Tawara", Paris.

Major R. H. (1923): "Stokes-Adams' disease due to gumma of the heart", *Arch. intern. Med.*, 31, 857.

—— (1932): "Classic descriptions of disease", Springfield, Illinois, U.S.A.

Mann, H. (1931): "Interpretation of bundle branch block by means of monocardiogram", *Amer. Heart J.*, 6, 447.

Miller, H., *et al.* (1952): "The action of procaine amide in complete heart block", *Amer. Heart J.*, 44, 432.

Mines, G. R. (1913): "On dynamic equilibrium in the heart", *J. Physiol.*, 46, 349.

Nathanson, M. H., and Miller, H. (1949): "Effect of 1-(3, 4, dihydroxyphenyl)-2-isopropylaminoethanol (isopropylepinephrine) on the rhythmic property of the human heart", *Proc. Soc. exp. Biol. and Med.*, 70, 633.

——, —— (1950): "The action of nor-epinephrine and of epinephrine on the ventricular rate of heart block", *Amer. Heart J.*, 40, 374.

Parkinson, J., Papp, F., and Evans, W. (1941): "The electrocardiogram of the Stokes-Adams' attack", *Brit. Heart J.*, 3, 171.

Phillips, E., and Levine, S. A. (1949): "Auricular fibrillation without other evidence of heart disease", *Amer. J. Med.*, 7, 478.

——, Corday, E., Brill, I. C., Oblath, R. W., and Kruger, H. E. (1952): "The auricular arrhythmias", Charles C. Thomas, Springfield, Illinois.

—— *et al.* (1952): "Accelerated conduction. The Wolff-Parkinson-White syndrome and related conditions", *Modern Medical Monographs*, No. 3, Grune & Stratton, New York.

Prinzmetal, M., et al. (1950): "Mechanism of the auricular arrhythmias", *Circulation*, 1, 241.

Rosenblueth, A., and Ramos, J. G. (1947): "Studies on flutter and fibrillation. II. The influence of artificial obstacles on experimental auricular flutter", *Amer. Heart J.*, 33, 677.

Sampson, J. J., and Anderson, E. M. (1932): "The treatment of certain cardiac arrhythmias with potassium salts", *J. Amer. med. Ass.*, 99, 2257.

Scherf, D., and Dix, J. H. (1952): "The effects of posture on A-V conduction", *Amer. Heart J.*, 43, 494.

Schumacher, E. E., and Schmock, C. L. (1954): "The control of certain cardiac arrhythmias with isopropylnorepinephrine", *Ibid.*, 48, 933.

Schwartz, S. P., *et al.* (1952): "Transient ventricular fibrillation. IV. The effects of procaine amide on patients with transient ventricular fibrillation during established auriculoventricular dissociation", *Circulation*, 6, 193.

———, ——— (1953): "Transient ventricular fibrillation. The effects of the oral administration of quinidine sulphate on patients with transient ventricular fibrillation during established atrioventricular dissociation", *Amer. Heart J.*, 45, 404.

Sokolow, M. (1951): "The present status of therapy of the cardiac arrhythmias with quinidine", *Amer. Heart J.*, 42, 771.

———, and Edgar, A. L. (1950): "Blood quinidine concentrations as a guide in the treatment of cardiac arrhythmias", *Circulation*, 1, 576.

Spens, T. (1793): "History of a case in which there took place a remarkable slowness of the pulse", Medical Commentaries (Edinburgh), 7, 463.

Starr, I. (Jr.) (1933): "Acetyl-B-Methylcholine—its action on paroxysmal tachycardia and peripheral vascular disease", *Amer. J. Med. Sci.*, 186, 330.

Stokes, W. (1846): "Observations on some cases of a permanently slow pulse", *Dublin quart. J. med. Sc.*, 2, 73.

Tawara, S. (1906): "Das Reizleitungssystem des Saugetierherzens", Jena.

Tung, C. L., and Cheer, S. N. (1933): "A correlation of clinical and electrocardiographic findings in human bundle branch block", *Chinese med. J.*, 47, 15.

Wedd, A. M. (1924): "Notes on the action of certain drugs in clinical flutter", *Heart*, 11, 87.

Weiss, S., and Sprague, H. B. (1937): "Vagal reflex irritability and the treatment of paroxysmal auricular tachycardia with ipecac", *Amer. J. med. Sci.*, 194, 53.

—— (1921): "The bigeminal pulse in atrioventricular rhythm", *Arch. Intern. Med.*, 28, 213.

Wenckebach, K. F. (1899): "Zur Analyse des unregelmassigen pulses. II. Ueber den regelmassig intermitterenden Puls", *Zeitschr. f. klin. Med.*, 37, 475.

White, J. C., and Bland, E. F. (1950): "Refractory paroxysmal tachycardias checked by sympathectomy (seven cases)", *Lyon Chir.*, 45, 395.

White, P. D. (1915): "A study of atrio-ventricular rhythm following auricular flutter", *Arch. intern. Med.*, 16, 517.

Willius, F. A., and Carryer, H. V. (1946): "Electrocardiograms displaying short PR intervals with prolonged QRS complexes: an analysis of 65 cases", *Proc.* Mayo Clin., 21, 438.

Wilson, F. N., MacLeod, A. G., and Barker, P. S. (1932): "The order of ventricular excitation in human bundle branch block", *Amer. Heart J.*, 7, 305.

———, Johnston, F. D., Hill, I. G. W., MacLeod, A. and G., Barker, P. S. (1934): "The significance of electrocardiograms characterised by an abnormally long QRS interval and by broad S. deflections in lead 1", *Ibid.*, 9, 459.

Wolferth, C. C., and Margolies, A. (1935): "Asynchronism in contraction of the ventricles in the so-called common type of bundle branch block: its bearing on the determination of the side of the significant lesion and on the mechanism of split first and second heart sounds", *Ibid.*, 10, 425.

———, and Wood, F. C. (1933): "The mechanism of production of short P-R intervals and prolonged QRS complexes in patients with presumably undamaged hearts: hypothesis of an accessory pathway of auriculo-ventricular conduction (Bundle of Kent)", *Ibid.*, 8, 297.

Wolff, L. (1954): "Clinical progress. Syndrome of short P-R interval with abnormal QRS complexes and paroxysmal tachycardia (Wolff-Parkinson-White syndrome)", *Circulation*, 10, 282.

———, Parkinson, J., and White, P. D. (1930): "Bundle branch block with short P-R interval in healthy young people prone to paroxysmal tachycardia", *Amer. Heart J.*, 5, 685.

Wood, F. C., Jeffers, W. A., and Wolferth, C. C. (1935): "Follow-up study of sixty-four patients with right bundle branch conduction defect", *Ibid.*, **10**, 1056.

——, Wolferth, C. C., and Geckeler, G. D. (1943): "Histologic demonstration of accessory muscular connexions between auricle and ventricle in a case of short P-R interval and prolonged QRS complex", *Ibid.*, **25**, 454.

Yater, W. M. (1938): "Pathogenesis of bundle branch block: review of the literature: report of sixteen cases with necropsy and of six cases with detailed histologic study of the conduction system", *Arch. intern. Med.*, **62**, 1.

Youmans, W. B., Goodman, M. J., and Gould, J. (1949): "Neosynephrine in treatment of paroxysmal supraventricular tachycardia", *Amer. Heart J.*, **37**, 359.

Yount, E. H., Rosenblum, M., and McMillan, R. L. (1952): "Use of quinidine in treatment of chronic auricular fibrillation. Results obtained in a series of one hundred and fifty-five patients", *Arch. intern. Med.*, **89**, 63.

Zoll, P. M., Linenthal, A. J., and Norman, L. R. (1954): "Treatment of Stokes-Adams disease by external electric stimulation of the heart", *Circulation*, **9**, 482.

CHAPTER VII

HEART FAILURE

HEART failure has been defined as a condition in which the heart fails to discharge its contents adequately (Lewis, 1933). The words may be applied logically to the heart as a whole or to one or other ventricle. The increased residual stroke volume of the failing human heart implied by Lewis' definition has been confirmed by modern work (e.g. Nylin, 1943, 1945; Friedman, 1950). Normally, there are said to be about 90 ml. of blood left in the right ventricle at the end of systole, the ratio $\frac{\text{residual volume}}{\text{stroke volume}}$ being around 1.75 (probably nearer 1.5); in advanced right ventricular failure the residual stroke volume may average as much as 500 ml., and the ratio 13.6 (Bing *et al.*, 1951).

Alternatively, heart failure may be defined as a state in which the heart fails to maintain an adequate circulation for the needs of the body despite a satisfactory venous filling pressure (the condition excludes extracardiac circulatory failure from hæmorrhage, vasovagal syncope or shock).

MECHANISM

The mechanism, and even the definition, of heart failure have been debated for over a century, and are still a source of controversy. The back-pressure theory, so well expressed by James Hope in 1832, which incorporates the idea of independent ventricular failure, maintains that when a ventricle fails to discharge its contents adequately, blood accumulates behind it, and the pressure rises in the respective atrium and venous system. After holding sway for nearly a century, this conception was replaced by the forward-failure hypothesis of Mackenzie (1913), who believed that congestion depended upon failure of sufficient propulsion from behind, and who insisted that the heart failed as a whole. Before the second world war opinion reverted sharply to Hope's view, the arguments in its favour being well marshalled by Harrison (1935) and by Fishberg (1939); but the newer methods of investigation which provided much of the data upon which these arguments were based were crude, and subsequent technical refinements have disproved many of them. The introduction of cardiac catheterisation to the U.S.A. by Cournand and Ranges (1941) and to Great Britain by McMichael and Sharpey-Schafer (1944) provided a new tool for studying the circulation in man, and modern hypotheses concerning the mechanism of heart failure have been much influenced by the pioneer work of these investigators (Cournand, 1952; McMichael, 1947, 1948).

The clinical facts are superficially simple enough. In predominantly left-sided lesions, such as hypertension and aortic valve disease, certain compensatory mechanisms are brought into play which help the left ventricle to shoulder its additional burden without embarrassing the organism as a whole. Sooner or later, and for one reason or another, these adjustments no longer suffice and dyspnœa develops, at first only on effort and then even at rest, while orthopnœa and paroxysmal cardiac dyspnœa colour the clinical picture. X-rays show "pulmonary venous congestion", but the jugular venous pressure may be normal, and there may be no œdema. This syndrome is called *left ventricular failure*. In purely right-sided lesions, such as primary pulmonary hypertension and isolated pulmonary stenosis, the breakdown of compensatory adjustments (decompensation) results chiefly in fatigue, elevation of the systemic venous pressure, distension of the liver and dropsy, while the lungs remain dry and radiologically clear. This syndrome is called *right ventricular failure*. Not infrequently cases of hypertensive heart disease or aortic valve disease start with left ventricular failure and later develop a rise of systemic venous pressure, enlargement of the liver and dropsy; this is called *congestive heart failure*. A number of conditions that affect the heart as a whole, such as isolated myocarditis, may develop characteristic features of both left and right ventricular failure more or less simultaneously; this, too, is called congestive heart failure. In all the conditions so far mentioned there are usually signs of an impaired peripheral circulation as well, due to a low cardiac output. In the hyperkinetic circulatory states, however, such as thyrotoxicosis, anæmia, arteriovenous fistula, beri-beri, Paget's disease of bone, advanced hepatic disease, and anoxic cor pulmonale, signs of congestive heart failure (both pulmonary and systemic) may be associated with warm hands, throbbing digital vessels, distended forearm veins and other evidence of an increased peripheral blood flow and raised cardiac output. To distinguish these two types of failure McMichael introduced the terms low and high output failure. The question at issue is just how all these manifestations of heart failure are brought about, and what unifying principles underly them?

CARDIAC RESERVES

The terms compensation and decompensation are intended to define the physiological situation in respect of the cardiac reserves. In compensated cases reserve mechanisms come into play which enable the diseased heart to carry on its prime function of maintaining an adequate circulation to all parts of the body without disturbing the function of any organ. In mitral stenosis, for example, a rise of left atrial pressure may compensate for the obstruction, but if this rise is too great pulmonary œdema interferes with the function of the lungs and endangers life, even though the cardiac output is maintained. Decompensation means that the heart can no longer maintain an adequate circulation for the needs of the body, all reserves having been used. At first this occurs only on effort (limited effort tolerance), but finally even at rest (heart failure proper). To understand heart failure, therefore, it is necessary to know just what these reserves are, and how they may break down.

The strength of cardiac contraction

The most obvious way for the heart to meet an extra load would be for the muscle to contract more strongly, in the manner of voluntary muscle. It has long been known, however, that heart muscle always responds in precisely the same fashion to any strength of stimulus, provided its intrinsic state is unaltered. This is the all or none law (Bowditch, 1871). It means that all fibres contract fully every heart beat, so that at first sight there appears to be no room for a reserve mechanism here. The proviso, however, is important, for the intrinsic state of the muscle may well change, not only from day to day, but even from beat to beat. There is good evidence, for example, that increased sympathetic tone augments the strength of cardiac contraction (Wiggers and Katz, 1920) and that increased vagal tone weakens it (Peterson, 1950). Stead, Hickman and Warren (1947) believe that minor changes of cardiac output from minute to minute may well be a function of varying sympathetic tone. Increased adrenergic activity may thus be regarded as the first reserve, and one that can be called upon almost instantaneously. Artificial help of the same kind can be given by injecting adrenergic drugs.

The strength of cardiac contraction must also be greatly influenced by any factor that alters or interferes with the natural biochemistry of heart muscle (Olson and Schwartz, 1951). Digitalis may supply artificial biochemical aid.

Hypertrophy of the heart

Hypertrophy of the heart muscle is the natural long-term method of increasing the strength of cardiac contraction. Heart muscle fibres cannot multiply, but they can increase in length and bulk. This reserve is limited by nutritional difficulties, for the nutritional needs of each muscle fibre depend on its cubic volume, whereas its nutritional supply is proportional to its surface area; thus as the fibre grows in volume there is an increasing disparity between demand and supply, the former increasing by the cube, the latter by the square. Moreover, the capillaries upon which the nutrition of the heart muscle depends do not increase as the heart hypertrophies (Katz, 1954). Thus there may come a time when the heart is too big to be properly nourished.

Increased filling pressure and cardiac dilatation

In 1884 Howell and Donaldson showed that the dog's heart increased its stroke output in response to an increased venous input. More precisely, the strength of cardiac contraction depended on the presystolic volume and tension of the ventricles; it was these which determined the magnitude of the all or none response (Frank, 1895). In a series of papers, Starling and his associates showed that the increase of stroke output that followed an increased filling pressure depended on the degree to which the ventricular muscle fibres were stretched at the end of diastole, rather than upon the diastolic pressure itself; also that a critical point was reached sooner or later beyond which further dilatation of the ventricles resulted in a fall of output (Starling, 1918). In Starling's curve (fig. 7.01), in which the cardiac

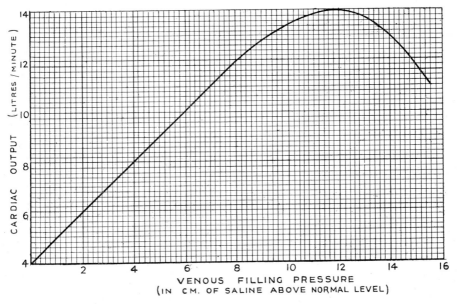

Fig. 7.01—Relationship of cardiac output to venous filling pressure (Starling's curve).

output is plotted against the venous filling pressure (right atrial pressure minus the negative intrathoracic pressure), the ascent represents a compensated situation, the descent a decompensated or overloaded state. It is important to understand that the response of any particular heart to an increased filling pressure varies considerably according to the influence of other factors, particularly those affecting the property of myocardial muscle fibres to stretch in response to a rise in diastolic tension (myocardial tone).

The venous pressure may rise primarily as a result of active or passive venoconstriction, which reduces the capacity of the venous reservoir, or because of an increase in blood volume secondary to sodium and water retention. In either event the cardiac output rises, and the elevated venous filling pressure is physiological (as on effort), compensatory (as in anæmia) or independent (as in acute nephritis). If the heart is flagging, however, and fails to empty itself properly, its diastolic volume and pressure rises and the elevated venous pressure that results represents a state of de-compensation. This overloaded situation may be precipitated by an increase of blood volume resulting from sodium and water retention secondary to impairment of renal blood flow due to reduction of the cardiac output.

A particular form of elevated venous filling pressure results from aug-mented atrial systole. A good example of this is seen in severe pulmonary hypertension or stenosis, when powerful right atrial contraction, causing a giant *a* wave in the venous pulse, increases the diastolic stretch of the right ventricular muscle and so enhances the force of its contraction (fig. 2.22).

The heart rate

If the venous filling pressure is maintained the cardiac output rises with increasing heart rates until a critical speed is reached, beyond which the output falls rapidly (Henderson, 1906). In man the critical rate is around 180, but varies greatly with the state of health of the heart. When the venous filling pressure is maintained tachycardia increases the output because the major part of ventricular filling occurs early in diastole; even at rates of 180 the ventricles may fill almost completely (Rushmer and Thal, 1952).

It is not easy to investigate the effect of tachycardia alone on the cardiac output in man, because other factors are difficult to keep constant: for instance, tachycardia produced by atropine usually results in a fall of venous filling pressure; adrenalin cannot be used because it augments the force of cardiac contraction; tachycardia produced by exercise is associated with a rise of venous filling pressure and with an increased force of cardiac contraction resulting from release of adrenergic tone.

Certain observations on the effects of paroxysmal tachycardia are per-tinent to this subject. When the heart is healthy rates up to 180 are well tolerated and usually give rise to remarkable polyuria, suggesting greatly increased renal filtration. At rates between 200 and 250 polyuria is rare, but angina, breathlessness, and fatigue are common. At rates over 260 syncope is the rule. Another point of importance is the duration of the tachycardia; bouts lasting a few hours may have features suggesting a raised output such as polyuria, hot extremities and distended forearm veins; if the attack continues for several days, however, these signs may be replaced by those of a reduced output—vasoconstriction, a rise of venous pressure, oliguria, œdema and fatigue, suggesting that the nutrition of the myocardium has become impaired; inversion of the T waves of the electro-cardiogram after a prolonged attack confirms this supposition.

In fact, it has long been established that the benefits to be derived from tachycardia are limited by four factors: (1) since the duration of systole varies with the square root of the cycle length, diastole shortens dis-proportionately as the rate increases, until proper recovery can no longer take place; (2) at rates above 180 diastole is so short that proper filling is interfered with; (3) as the rate increases the mechanical efficiency of the heart $\left(\dfrac{\text{work done}}{\text{oxygen consumed}}\right)$ declines; (4) the coronary flow, which is chiefly diastolic, gradually becomes insufficient as the rate increases.

Physiologically, tachycardia is certainly used as a natural means of increasing the cardiac output and usually accompanies an increased filling pressure and greater adrenergic activity. As a cardiac reserve in disease tachycardia is used especially in chronic constrictive pericarditis, when it may be almost the sole means of raising the cardiac output, and in the hyperkinetic circulatory states, such as thyrotoxicosis, anæmia, and beri-beri.

HEART FAILURE

Of these four cardiac reserves, the most important in relation to ordinary clinical heart failure is the combination of a raised venous filling pressure and dilatation of the ventricles; hypertrophy is a long-term matter, autonomic influences of relatively fleeting importance, and tachycardia rarely fast enough to be disadvantageous (except in paroxysmal tachycardia and uncontrolled atrial fibrillation). Heart failure means that the cardiac reserves no longer suffice to enable the heart to maintain an adequate circulation at rest and that increasing elevation of the venous pressure has distended the labouring ventricle beyond the point of critical diastolic stretch, so that further dilatation results in a fall in output.

It is still not entirely clear just what causes the rise of venous pressure. McMichael and Sharpey-Schafer (1944) suggested that it might be a primary compensating mechanism presumably due to reflex veno-constriction somehow excited by an inadequate output, but there is no direct evidence in favour of this hypothesis. There is no doubt that when a ventricle fails its diastolic pressure rises; this must result in an increased pressure in the venous system behind the failing chamber. There is also no doubt that heart failure results in diminution of renal filtration and total renal blood flow, and that retention of sodium and water, which is closely correlated with this, increases the blood volume and causes œdema (Merrill, 1946); the increased blood volume also raises the venous pressure. Perhaps all three mechanisms come into play in greater or less degree.

Forward failure

In the great majority of cases of heart failure the arterio-venous oxygen difference is increased, being over 50 ml. per litre, and the cardiac output reduced, being less than 4.5 litres per minute at rest (Stead, Warren and Brannon, 1948). On effort the cardiac output does not rise, but the arterio-venous oxygen difference increases greatly (Hickam and Cargill, 1948). An exception to this general rule is the clinical syndrome of heart failure (raised venous pressure, hepatic enlargement and dropsy) associated with a raised cardiac output at rest which is found in anæmia, beri-beri, arterio-venous fistula and other hyperkinetic circulatory states. In these cases forward failure is relative.

The effect of the lowered total output on the various territories of the body has been measured with reasonable accuracy.

The cerebral circulation, as might be expected, is usually maintained at or near the normal level of 45 to 50 ml. per 100 Gm. per minute (Novack *et al.*, 1953)—about 0.8 litre per minute. Disturbance of cerebral function in heart failure is therefore more likely to be due to hepatic or renal factors than to cerebral hypoxia.

The renal blood flow, normally about 1.3 to 1.5 litres per minute (Smith, 1951) is notably reduced to about 0.5 litre per minute, while the glomerular filtration rate declines from around 120 ml. per minute to 70 or 80 ml. per minute (Merrill and Cargill, 1948). This is associated with salt and water retention, an increased blood volume, oliguria, œdema, and sometimes with a slight rise of blood urea. The low renal blood flow is due to efferent arteriolar constriction; diuresis is always preceded by an increase of renal blood flow, which may be independent of any change in cardiac output and which occurs spontaneously at night (Brod and Fejfar, 1950).

The total hepatic blood flow averages around 1,500 ml. per minute (Bradley *et al.*, 1945), about 25 per cent of which is carried by the hepatic artery, the rest by the portal vein. In heart failure the flow is reduced in proportion to the reduction in cardiac output (Myers and Hickam, 1948), and centrilobular necrosis is attributed to anoxia.

The blood flow to the extremeties, normally about 1.8 litres per minute (Abramson, 1944), is reduced and further peripheral vasoconstriction occurs at once when patients are tilted head-down, even in left ventricular failure (Brigden and Sharpey-Schafer, 1950).

The coronary blood flow is said to be about 5 per cent of the cardiac output or around 75 ml. per 100 Gm. of heart muscle per minute, i.e. 225 ml. per minute for a 300-Gm. heart. Using the nitrous oxide method and coronary sinus catheterisation in man, Bing *et al.* (1949) found the normal left ventricular coronary blood flow averaged 65 ml. per 100 Gm. of left ventricular muscle per minute. In congestive heart failure (from rheumatic heart disease) the coronary flow was much the same.

Back-pressure

Elevated ventricular diastolic pressure undoubtedly causes the rise in left atrial and pulmonary venous pressures in left ventricular failure. Kopelman and Lee (1951) found that the intrathoracic blood volume was increased from an average normal of 1.8 litres to 2.7 litres. All divisions of the lung volume are reduced except the residual air, the total lung volume averaging about 1.5 litres less than the predicted normal (Richards *et al.*, 1951). The discrepancy between the two sets of figures may be due to an increased amount of extravascular fluid in the lung parenchyma and lymphatics.

Elevation of the right ventricular diastolic pressure (aided by an increased blood volume) raises the systemic venous pressure and distends the liver. It is still uncertain to what secondary effects the raised venous pressure may give rise, but it is not directly responsible for œdema.

CAUSES OF HEART FAILURE

The heart may fail because it is overburdened by a raised ventricular pressure or by a raised cardiac output, or because the health of the myocardium is impaired by inadequate or faulty nutrition, metabolic disorder, intoxication, or intrinsic disease. High outputs are tolerated better than high pressures; but myocardial ill health is probably even more important. Contributory factors include physical effort, anxiety, disturbances of rate or rhythm, infection, and pregnancy; but all these are better expressed in more fundamental terms: for example, infection may increase the cardiac output and impair the health of the myocardium; anxiety may raise the blood pressure in hypertensive heart disease; and so forth. Precipitating causes of this sort are found in 50 per cent of cases of heart failure (Sodeman and Burch, 1938).

Viewing the subject in this way, it should be clear that a high cardiac output is no more incompatible with heart failure than is hypertension; that a heart capable of pumping ten litres of blood per minute is not necessarily better than one capable of maintaining a diastolic blood pressure of 140 mm. of Hg. Each is a measure of part of the total cardiac work performed; neither alone is a sufficient measure of cardiac efficiency, although their behaviour under certain experimental conditions may be. Moreover, the signs and symptoms of heart failure are largely due to alterations of pressure and volume in the pulmonary or systemic venous systems. In left ventricular failure, for example, the redistribution of volume is the result of a short-lived discrepancy between left and right ventricular outputs. Although the balance must be restored quickly, the consequences cannot be rectified until the process is reversed. It should again be clear that such disturbances cannot be detected by casual estimations of the right ventricular output.

LEFT VENTRICULAR FAILURE

When the left ventricle fails to discharge its contents adequately, the pressure rises in the left atrium and pulmonary veins, and blood accumulates in the pulmonary circulation.

ETIOLOGY

Left ventricular failure may result from any disease which imposes an undue burden on the left ventricle or which interferes with its health. These diseases include systemic hypertension from any cause, aortic valve disease, mitral incompetence, myocardial infarction, and a number of rare cardiopathies which may affect mainly the left ventricle. In systemic hypertension, the left ventricle may fail either because it is unable to meet the stress imposed upon it, or because it is enlarged so greatly that it cannot obtain sufficient nourishment. As the nutritional demands of an individual muscle fibre depend upon its cubic volume, and the nutritional supply is limited by its surface area, there is an increasing disparity between the two as the muscle enlarges, which sooner or later becomes critical (Gross and Spark, 1937). In acute nephritis and malignant hypertension, a rapid rise of blood pressure may cause left ventricular failure before there has been appreciable hypertrophy of muscle; on the other hand, in long-standing cases of essential hypertension with gross enlargement of the left ventricle, failure may occur even though the blood pressure has fallen to within normal limits, failure then being attributed to nutritional breakdown. In aortic valve disease, in addition to these two factors, there may be further interference with nutrition as a result of poor coronary filling, due to a low mean blood pressure in aortic stenosis, and to obstruction of the mouths of the coronary vessels in syphilitic aortic incompetence. The cause of failure in uncomplicated ischæmic heart disease with myocardial infarction is due entirely to interference with ventricular nutrition resulting from coronary occlusion.

PHYSIOLOGY

When the left ventricle fails to discharge its contents adequately its output falls, its residual stroke volume increases, its diastolic pressure rises and the pulmonary venous pressure rises; if the right ventricle is healthy it continues to pump its normal quota and within a few minutes the total blood volume is redistributed, more being held in the lungs and less in the greater circulation than before. With increased diastolic stretch the left ventricle may be able to cope with the situation and the balance between ventricular outputs is restored. In other words, in pure left ventricular failure the cardiac output is at first maintained at the expense of a dilated left ventricle, a raised pulmonary venous pressure and an increased quantity of blood in the lungs. Symptoms are due to "pulmonary venous congestion", and in a sense this is still a compensated state, although a none too happy one. If the left ventricle becomes overloaded, any further rise of pulmonary venous pressure results in a fall of left ventricular output, and a vicious circle is established. Several things may prevent disaster: (1) a high pulmonary venous pressure passively raises the pulmonary artery pressure and so loads the right ventricle; (2) sometimes active pulmonary vasoconstriction adds greatly to this load; (3) the redistribution of the blood volume may lower the right ventricular output which can only pump what it receives; (4) bulging of the interventricular septum into the cavity of the right ventricle may reduce the diastolic capacity of that chamber (Bernheim effect); and (5) the pericardium, which tends to limit ventricular distension, must exert some increased pressure on the right ventricle if greatly stretched by enlargement of the left. If the pulmonary venous pressure rises beyond 35 mm. Hg the patient is in danger of losing his life from pulmonary œdema.

CLINICAL FEATURES

The symptoms of left ventricular failure are undue breathlessness on effort, orthopnœa, paroxysmal cardiac dyspnœa, and acute pulmonary œdema. The findings include bilateral basal pulmonary râles, radiological evidence of "pulmonary congestion" and hydrothorax, diminution of all fractions of the lung volume except the residual air, an increased quantity of blood in the lungs, increased intrapleural respiratory pressure swings, a raised left atrial pressure with steep *y* descent, and prolongation of the pulmonary circulation-time. The diagnosis is supported by gallop rhythm, pulsus alternans and Cheyne-Stokes breathing, and is confirmed by the demonstration of a suitable cardiovascular disease, e.g. systemic hypertension, aortic valve disease, mitral incompetence or myocardial infarction.

Undue breathlessness on effort. Breathlessness due to left ventricular failure depends upon "pulmonary venous congestion", which both reduces ventilation and increases the work of breathing (Christie and Meakins, 1934). It is not due to anoxia, to an increased CO_2 tension or to a fall in pH.

Orthopnœa, paroxysmal cardiac dyspnœa, and pulmonary œdema. As these three conditions depend on variations of the same fundamental mechanism, they are considered together. When a patient adopts the upright or sitting position in order to breathe comfortably, he may be said to have *orthopnœa*. Although an almost constant sign of left ventricular failure, it is by no means pathognomonic, for it may be found in severe mitral stenosis, bronchial asthma, and in pericardial effusion. The vital capacity is reduced in all these conditions, and is greater in the upright than in the horizontal position; but its relationship to orthopnœa is not necessarily direct. Moreover, its increase in the erect position is greater than can be explained by descent of the diaphragm. The discrepancy is due to concomitant changes in the pulmonary circulation, the amount of blood in the lungs being greater, perhaps by as much as 500 ml., in the horizontal than in the erect position (McMichael, 1939). The redistribution of blood depends upon the geographical relationship of the atria to their respective venous systems. As the right atrium is nearer the head than the feet, the pressure within it rises when the body is tilted head down, owing to the influence of gravity. The right ventricle responds according to Starling's law and pumps more blood into the lungs in the horizontal than in the vertical position (McMichael, 1937). The pressure within the left atrium, however, which is situated more or less in the centre of the lungs, is not directly influenced by gravity, and the left ventricular output does not, therefore, immediately keep pace with the right. Only when the left atrial pressure rises proportionately, owing to an increased volume of blood in the pulmonary venous system, will the balance be restored. As patients with left ventricular failure already have pulmonary congestion, the extra engorgement which results from adopting the horizontal position may prove critical; moreover, if the left ventricle is already overloaded it will not respond to the rise in the left atrial pressure, but will fail the more.

Paroxysmal cardiac dyspnœa usually occurs at night. The patient awakes with a feeling of suffocation, and sits bolt upright gasping for breath; he may climb out of bed and open a window, or walk about in an agitated way.

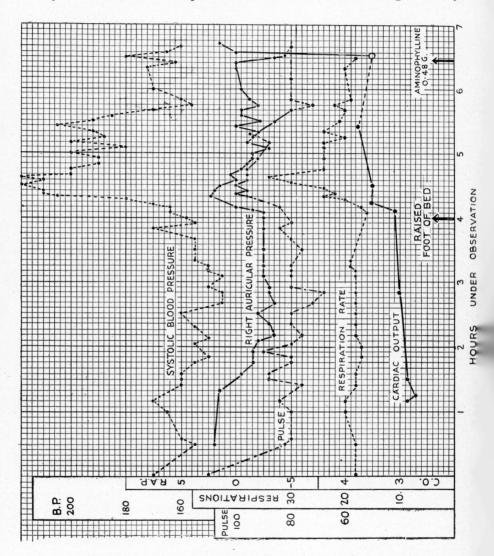

Fig. 7.02—Graph illustrating typical changes in blood pressure, right auricular pressure, pulse rate, respiration rate, and cardiac output in an attack of paroxysmal cardiac dyspnœa initiated in a patient with left ventricular failure by raising the foot of the bed. The effect of aminophylline is shown at the end.

In cases of simple orthopnœa this behaviour brings immediate relief; but in paroxysmal cardiac dyspnœa the feeling of suffocation increases, and the struggle for breath lasts for ten to twenty minutes. Coughing and wheezing are commonly associated (*cardiac asthma*), and the patient may complain of palpitations, faintness, or substernal tightness. The skin is pale, cyanosed and cold, indicating profound vasoconstriction, and sweating may be profuse. The blood pressure and venous pressure are both raised. Attacks usually subside spontaneously, but may be repeated nightly or at intervals of days or weeks. In more severe cases *pulmonary œdema* develops. Widespread crepitations are then heard over the lungs and quantities of frothy pink or white watery fluid are expectorated.

Such attacks may sometimes be provoked by effort or by a rigor. They are easily induced experimentally in susceptible subjects by raising either the venous pressure or the blood pressure by artificial means (fig. 7.02). The mechanism probably depends upon acute discrepancy between right and left ventricular outputs, so that both the pressure and volume of blood in the pulmonary circulation reach critical levels. Measurements of pressure changes by means of an indwelling cardiac catheter in spontaneous nocturnal attacks indicate that the venous pressure may rise before the blood pressure. When attacks are induced by raising the venous pressure, the cardiac output may rise. Thus, although the heart is said to be failing, it may in fact be performing more work than usual, both with respect to blood pressure and output. The laboured breathing may be due in part to the extra effort required to inflate and deflate a turgid lung, the intrapleural pressure showing greatly increased fluctuations (Heyer *et al.*, 1948). In frank pulmonary œdema, however, ventilation is seriously impaired and dyspnœa is partly due to anoxia.

Certain difficulties in our understanding of these attacks must be faced. It is by no means clear just why they occur at night or during sleep: it has been suggested that depression of the nervous system during sleep allows too great a degree of "pulmonary venous congestion" to take place before hyperventilation wakes the patient and forces him to lower the right ventricular output by adopting a more upright posture, so that relief comes too late to prevent a major attack; also that reabsorption into the blood stream of tissue fluid formed during the daytime owing to disturbed renal physiology results in a rise of blood volume and venous pressure which augment right ventricular output and so increase pulmonary venous congestion (Perera and Berliner, 1943). But the physical inactivity and muscular relaxation during sleep lower the systemic venous pressure by providing a larger effective venous reservoir, and this should help to relieve pulmonary venous congestion; again, reabsorption of tissue fluid is due to the spontaneous diuresis that takes place during the night in cases of heart failure, an event which should also relieve pulmonary venous congestion. According to Brod and Fejfar (1950), the increased renal blood flow responsible for nocturnal diuresis is independent of any change in cardiac output or right atrial pressure. Another difficulty is the variable relationship between left atrial pressure and transudation of fluid from the pulmonary capillaries into the alveoli: theoretically this should occur whenever the left atrial pressure exceeds the osmotic pressure of the plasma (about 30 mm. Hg), but in practice much higher hydrostatic pressures may be recorded in the pulmonary capillaries without pulmonary œdema developing. The state of the connective tissue between the alveolar membrane and the capillary may partly explain this, for if collagen is much increased here it may serve as a barrier which tends to prevent fluid passing from the capillaries into the alveolar spaces (Hayward, 1955). The efficiency of the pulmonary lymphatics in removing protein containing fluid from the walls of the alveoli must also be important. Capillary permeability is increased by infection and by anoxia (Maurer, 1940), both of which may encourage pulmonary œdema. The high protein content of pulmonary œdema fluid (2 to 4 per cent) certainly proves that the capillaries are allowing much protein to escape during the attack (Drinker, 1945), and this must greatly reduce the differential osmotic pressure across the capillary membrane. Then, the part played by bronchospasm must not be overlooked. This is a variable complicating factor which increases ventilatory difficulty and the labour of breathing, encourages hypoxia, and favours the small hours; it occurs in about half the cases and is presumably a reaction to congested bronchial mucosa. Finally, it is by no means clear why the attacks usually terminate spontaneously. The great respiratory struggle, the mental anguish that goes with it, the increasing anoxia and bronchospasm, all tend directly or indirectly to encourage the transudate; only the natural adoption of the upright position works in the right direction. Since acute hypoxia causes pulmonary vasoconstriction (Liljestrand, 1948), active pulmonary hypertension might be expected to terminate the attack by reducing the output of the right ventricle, but there is no evidence so far that acute pulmonary œdema increases the pulmonary vascular resistance.

Bilateral basal pulmonary râles and hydrothorax. Basal râles, diminished air entry into the lower lobes, and some impairment of the percussion note at the bases are said to be usual in left ventricular failure, but in the author's experience such auscultatory signs are more likely to be absent or misleading. Crepitations, when due to pulmonary œdema, are widespread, rather than basal, and when there is no pulmonary œdema râles can only be bronchial. *A raised pulmonary venous pressure* per se *gives rise to no auscultatory signs whatever.* If the bronchial mucosa is congested, bronchial secretions may be excessive or there may be broncho-spasm, but these bronchial râles and rhonci are inconstant and unreliable signs of left ventricular failure, and are much more commonly due to chronic bronchitis. Thus the oft-repeated comment concerning the discrepancy between the site of "pulmonary venous congestion" as viewed radiologically, when it is perihilar, and as heard clinically, when it is basal, is explained by the simple fact that what is heard is not pulmonary venous congestion. Bedford and Lovibond (1941) found that hydrothorax was a common complication of pulmonary congestion from left ventricular failure, and that, although often bilateral, tended to be more marked on the left side. Its occurrence may depend upon the fact that the visceral pleura is drained by the pulmonary rather than by the bronchial veins (Miller, 1937), but its precise mechanism is not yet fully understood.

Radiological signs of pulmonary congestion. The increased opacity seen in skiagrams is hilar, and probably due to chronic interstitial œdema (fig. 7.03). During attacks of acute pulmonary œdema a fleecy mottling spreads out from the hilum on both sides (figs. 7.04 and 7.05). Hydrothorax may also be revealed by X-rays, perhaps when unsuspected clinically. Interlobar effusion may be responsible for a rounded, transient, sometimes migratory opacity—the so-called vanishing tumour of the lung. Confirmatory evidence of left ventricular failure may be obtained by noting the size and shape of the heart shadow.

Reduction of the vital capacity and lung volume. The vital capacity is reduced by an amount equivalent to the extra quantity of blood and interstitial fluid in the lungs; it is reduced much more if there is pulmonary œdema or a large hydrothorax as well, and by a further few hundred ml. according to the degree of cardiac enlargement. Readings of 1,000 to 1,500 ml. are common, and may be as low as 500 ml. when there is pulmonary œdema or hydrothorax.

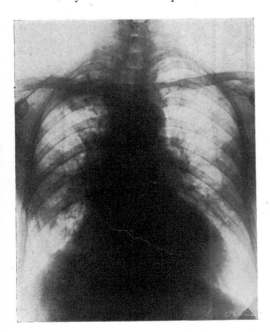

Fig. 7.03—Pulmonary "congestion" in left ventricular failure (case of syphilitic aortic incompetence).

The lung volume is reduced proportionately, the residual air remaining unchanged. This at once distinguishes the condition from emphysema in which a low vital capacity is associated with a normal lung volume and increased residual air.

As stated previously, intrapleural respiratory pressure swings are excessive owing to increased resistance on the part of the turgid lung to both inflation and deflation.

Prolongation of the pulmonary circulation time. The normal arm-to-tongue circulation time, as measured by decholin or saccharin (q.v.), averages 13.5 seconds, ranging between 9 and 18 seconds. Since the time taken by the substance to travel from the left ventricle to the tongue may be neglected, and the journey from the antecubital vein to the right atrium takes only two or three seconds (Blumgart and Weiss, 1927), the total arm-to-tongue time is governed chiefly by passage through the lungs. Using

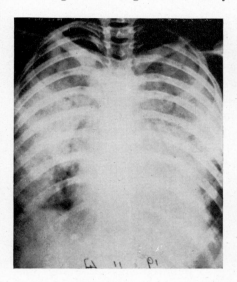

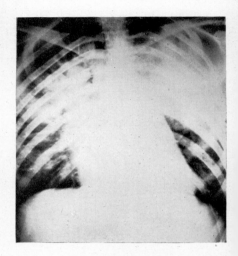

Fig. 7.04—Acute pulmonary œdema from left ventricular failure.

Fig. 7.05—Acute pulmonary œdema in mitral stenosis.

(*Acknowledgments to Dr. Graham Hayward.*)

radium C intravenously, which can be detected at any given point in the circulation by means of a special radio-sensitive instrument, Blumgart and Weiss also showed that when the systemic venous pressure is raised in congestive heart failure, the delay between the antecubital vein and the right atrium does not exceed five seconds, even in gross cases. It follows that with pure right ventricular failure the arm-to-tongue circulation time should not exceed 23 seconds and should often be within normal limits; in fact this is so. On the other hand, in left ventricular failure the average time is 30 seconds (Wood, 1936), and may be much longer. The delay is due to pulmonary congestion and occurs presumably on the venous side.

The arm-to-lung time. The arm-to-lung time, as measured by ether or amyl acetate (q.v.), is said to be helpful in distinguishing primary left from pure right ventricular failure, if the total arm-to-tongue time is also known. When the delay is proximal to the heart, as in pure right ventricular failure, the arm-to-lung time is delayed as much as the arm-to-tongue time; on the other hand, if there is further delay in the pulmonary veins, as in primary left ventricular failure, the arm-to-tongue time is disproportionately prolonged. Although theoretically this test might seem helpful, in fact it is rarely so for two reasons: first, because the end-point in the lung, both with ether and amyl acetate, is often unreliable and indefinite; and second, because it is easier and no less accurate to allow 1 to 5 seconds for delay proximal to the heart according to the degree of systemic venous engorgement.

Raised left atrial pressure with steep y descent

Cardiac catheterisation in cases of left ventricular failure has revealed mean indirect left atrial pressures in the expected range between 10 and 30 mm. Hg above the sternal angle. Unlike the tracings in mitral stenosis, however, the pressure drops rapidly after the opening of the mitral valve, the down-stroke of v or the y descent being remarkably steep; the trough y may be followed by a fairly sharp rise of pressure back to the z point (fig. 7.06); left ventricular and left atrial diastolic pressures are essentially

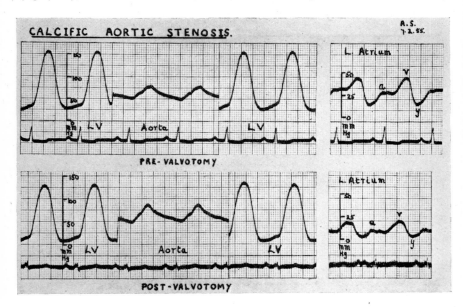

Fig. 7.06—Pressure pulses from aorta, left ventricle and left atrium in a case of aortic stenosis with left ventricular failure before and after aortic valvotomy, showing a typical steep y descent in the left atrial tracing.

the same, potential differences being offset by unobstructed flow. The appearances are similar to those seen in mitral incompetence (Owen and Wood, 1955). In the tracing illustrated, which was obtained from a case of aortic stenosis with left ventricular failure and recorded during aortic valvotomy, the Ry/v ratio (q.v.) was 5.4 before and 6 after the operation.

GALLOP RHYTHM

When the rhythm of the heart sounds has three instead of two beats per cycle, one may properly speak of triple rhythm. The term covers all varieties of cadence in which three heart sounds are heard. Gallop rhythm, on the other hand, should have a stricter meaning, and should be applied only to specified forms of triple rhythm as explained subsequently.

Mechanism. Phonocardiography proves that there are really four normal heart sounds: the atrial or presystolic sound associated with atrial systole and late ventricular distension, the first heart sound due to mitral and tricuspid valve closure, the second heart sound due to closure of the aortic and pulmonary valves, and the third heart sound which is attributed to sudden distension of the ventricles in the phase of rapid filling. Each of these sounds is thus composed of at least two elements. Although these elements may not be strictly synchronous, they are sufficiently so, as a rule, to produce but one obvious sound to the untrained human ear. On more careful analysis, however, they may often be separated sufficiently to be detected individually by auscultation, and we may then speak of split sounds. The word "split" describes the sound well, and also indicates the mechanism of its production. The term "reduplication" is often used instead, but has less to recommend it; for it bears an accidental onomato-pœtic resemblance to the sound of presystolic gallop, and it is illogical to apply a word that means doubling to an act of division. Split sounds do not give the cadence of triple rhythm because of the close proximity of the separated elements.

The "extra" sound that is responsible for triple rhythm is usually an exaggerated atrial sound, the third heart sound, or a summation of the two. Occasionally it is an additional systolic sound of unknown origin.

Presystolic (atrial) gallop. An audible atrial sound associated with a normal or slightly prolonged P-R interval gives rise to triple rhythm with an amphibrachic metre (u — u). As it may be felt as well as heard it is best appreciated by means of a rigid wooden stethoscope or with the naked ear, so that tactile and aural senses may be allied. The presystolic sound is soft and dull, and is usually localised to the region of the apex beat, where it is pathognomonic of left ventricular stress; occasionally it is heard best at the left border of the sternum, when it may denote right ventricular stress. The extra sound occurs about 0.15 second after the onset of the P wave, and about 0.07 second after the onset of atrial systole (Weitzman, 1955); it is attributed to extra-forceful ventricular distension. If the P-R interval is sufficiently prolonged, the atrial sound may fall in mid or early diastole; if the heart rate is fast, its true relation to the first or second heart sound cannot be determined clinically, unless transient slowing is induced by means of carotid sinus compression. Presystolic gallop is never heard when there is atrial fibrillation.

Presystolic gallop is a sign of ventricular stress. That the atrial reserve is being used means that the handicapped ventricle has asked for (and is receiving) extra presystolic stretch to enable it to meet its commitments. The sign does not therefore denote failure, but a particular form of compensated state.

Left atrial gallop is heard chiefly in essential hypertension and following cardiac infarction; right atrial gallop in severe pulmonary hypertension or stenosis.

Normal third heart sound. When the "extra" sound occurs shortly after the second heart sound, giving the metre of a dactyl (— u u), it may represent a normal or abnormal third heart sound (fig. 7.07). The normal third heart

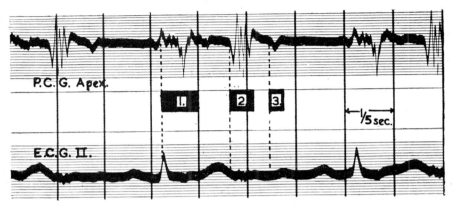

Fig. 7.07—Phonocardiogram showing a normal third heart sound.
(By courtesy of Dr. E. D. H. Cowen)

sound was well described by Gibson (1907). It is soft, low pitched, and usually accompanied by a palpable shock; it is more or less localised to the apex beat, varies in intensity with respiration, and is accentuated when the subject lies on the left side, especially if the venous pressure is raised by pressing on the abdomen. It may be heard in the great majority of children (but not in infants), in about 50 per cent of young adults, occasionally in the middle-aged, and rarely in the elderly. Phonocardiography shows that the third heart sound synchronises with the latter half of the descending limb of the *v* wave of the jugular phlebogram, and therefore with the period of rapid ventricular filling (Ohm, 1913). It is attributed to sudden distension of the left ventricle at this time—about 0.15 second after aortic valve closure.

Protodiastolic gallop. Abnormal third heart sounds are common in mitral incompetence, constrictive pericarditis and in advanced heart failure from any cause, especially when there is atrial fibrillation. The age and clinical condition of the patient emphasise their significance. The term proto-diastolic applied to this form of gallop is unfortunate, for physiologically protodiastole is the first part of ventricular relaxation, immediately before and incorporating the second heart sound; the second phase in diastole is isometric relaxation with all valves closed; the third is the rapid filling phase with atrial pressures chasing ventricular pressures to the *y* trough, and it is towards the end of this third diastolic period that the extra sound occurs: *diastolic gallop* would describe it more simply and without this inaccuracy, and would still be sufficiently descriptive to distinguish it from other forms of gallop.

Left ventricular diastolic gallop implies a raised left atrial pressure and rapid left ventricular filling, and therefore denies mitral stenosis; it also implies absence of those conditions which accentuate the third heart sound without failure, e.g. organic mitral incompetence and Pick's disease; thus by common use the term has come to mean triple rhythm due to an abnormal third heart sound resulting from left ventricular failure or near failure. Whether or not it can be due to some alteration of myocardial tone independent of overloading is still uncertain.

Right ventricular diastolic gallop has a similar meaning in relation to right ventricular physiology and at once denies tricuspid stenosis.

Summation gallop. Summation of atrial and third heart sounds can only occur when there is tachycardia or when the P-R interval is sufficiently prolonged. With tachycardia the metre may seem to be anapaestic (u u —), dactylic (— u u), or amphibrachic (u — u), according to the fancy of the listener, for the "extra" sound occurs in mid-diastole. Summation sounds have no clinical significance if they disappear when the heart is slowed by carotid sinus compression (summation gallop); on the other hand, such slowing may reveal an atrial sound or a normal or abnormal third heart sound.

Extra systolic sounds. It is not uncommon for an extra sound to occur during ventricular systole. Excluding vascular ejection clicks (q.v.), there are three varieties—the systolic click of left-sided pneumothorax, "lesser systolic clicks" possibly associated with pleuro-pericardial adhesions, and a third type in which the extra sound is dull and muffled, and in no way like a click. Patients with partial left-sided pneumothorax may complain of a loud clicking or bubbling noise synchronous with the heart beat. It may be so loud that it can be heard at a distance of several feet from the patient; it varies markedly with respiration and with change of posture, and is always transient. It is occasioned by the activities of bubbles of air between the heart and surrounding structures, and only occurs when the pneumothorax is small, so that clinically it is a late development, appearing when most of the air has been absorbed (Scadding and Wood, 1939). Lesser systolic clicks are heard from time to time in subjects who are perfectly well, and according to Gallavardin (1913) may depend upon pleuro-pericardial adhesions. In these cases the extra sound resembles a click, but is not so impressive, nor so variable, as that associated with left-sided pneumothorax. It may last for weeks, months or years, and may come and go without apparent reason. The third type (systolic gallop) is distinguished from greater and lesser systolic click by the character of the extra sound, which is dull and muffled. Its mechanism is not yet understood. It is uncommon, and when heard may be disregarded, for it occurs in apparently healthy persons.

Note on nomenclature. Introduced by Professor Bouillaud, analysed and popularized by Potain (1876), the term gallop rhythm originally referred to that variety of triple rhythm which denoted impending or actual left ventricular failure, and in the presence of tachycardia is "marvellously adapted to the sound it designates". But by 1900 Potain had extended the meaning of the bruit de galop to include presystolic, protodiastolic, and systolic varieties, attributing these different metres to the same factors that are to-day held responsible. Thus historically it is not incorrect to regard gallop rhythm and triple rhythm as synonyms; but there is an advantage in excluding certain types of triple rhythm from the cadences embraced by the bruit de galop. Thus it is preferable and customary to speak of pre-systolic (atrial), diastolic, systolic, and summation gallops on the one hand; and of systolic clicks, the third heart sound, and the opening snap of mitral stenosis, on the other.

PULSUS ALTERNANS

Pulsus alternans (Traube, 1872) is characterised by a regular rhythm in which the pulse beats are stronger and weaker alternately. It may be detected by palpation or more easily by sphygmomanometry, there being a difference of 5 to 20 mm. of mercury in the systolic pressure between alternate beats. It may be found in association with left ventricular failure, toxic carditis, paroxysmal tachycardia or auricular flutter. Clinically, alternation may be maintained as long as the heart is labouring, occasionally for as long as two or three years. Latent alternation may become manifest when the heart beats faster. Experimentally, under favourable conditions, e.g. when the heart is poisoned by certain drugs including digitalis, when it is made to beat very fast, or when its blood supply is curtailed, short periods of alternation may follow a premature ectopic beat (Mackenzie, 1907–8) or a dropped beat (Hering, 1908). Sphygmograms show that pulsus alternans may begin abruptly, either with an unusually large beat or with a small beat (Lewis, 1925), and that the sum of a large and small beat equals the sum of two normal beats (Gaskell, 1882). Pulsus alternans is exaggerated by any agent or manœuvre that lowers the venous filling pressure, and diminished by any procedure that raises the venous filling pressure (Friedman *et al.*, 1953).

No thoroughly satisfactory hypothesis has been evolved to explain pulsus alternans. It is generally believed that fewer muscle fibres contract with the weaker beats than with the stronger, owing to the development of a state of partial refractoriness (Lewis, 1925): fibres which do not contract with one beat, recover in time for the next; other fibres which contract with the first beat are still refractory and therefore unready for the second. In other words, there is a state of 2 : 1 partial ventricular response. But if this were true, all the beats should be weaker than normal; the hypothesis does not explain the stronger beats. Another suggestion is that pulsus alternans depends upon a disorder of ventricular relaxation, for the ventricles hold

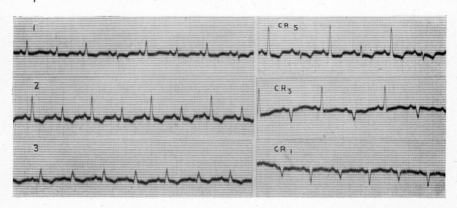

Fig. 7.08—Electrical alternation in a case of malignant disease involving the pericardium: pulsus alternans was present.

more blood with the stronger beats and less with the weaker (Straub, 1917).

Pulsus alternans should not be confused with electrical alternation (fig. 7.08), nor with coupled beats due to premature systoles. Electrical alternation is sometimes associated with pulsus alternans, however, as in the case illustrated.

CHEYNE-STOKES BREATHING

Periodic breathing was described by Cheyne (1818) in what was probably a case of hypertensive heart failure with right hemiplegia: "For several days his breathing was irregular; it would entirely cease for a quarter of a minute, then it would become perceptible, though very low, then by degrees it became heaving and quick, and then it would gradually cease again: this revolution in the state of his breathing occupied about a minute." Stokes (1854) connected the phenomenon with serious heart disease.

Mechanism. In spontaneous Cheyne-Stokes breathing, the respiratory centre is depressed and appears to be insensitive to a normal carbon dioxide tension, but still responds to a raised pCO_2 and reflexly to sufficient anoxia. With normal arterial oxygen and CO_2 tensions, breathing therefore stops: during the apnœic phase the arterial pO_2 falls and the arterial pCO_2 rises, and sooner or later this powerful combination excites the sluggish respiratory centre; during the dyspnœic phase, however, the abnormal blood gas tensions are soon corrected and breathing again stops. The crescendo character of the dyspnœic phase may be due to time-lag: when respiration starts, and carbon dioxide in the blood entering the lungs is blown off, blood which has already passed the pulmonary capillaries must have a higher carbon dioxide tension and lower oxygen tension than that which galvanised the respiratory centre into action; this takes 5 to 10 seconds to reach the respiratory centre in normal subjects, and an average of about 20 to 25 seconds in patients with left ventricular failure.

The administration of carbon dioxide abolishes Cheyne-Stokes breathing by maintaining an arterial pCO_2 high enough to excite the respiratory centre. The inhalation of oxygen prolongs the period of apnœa because it then takes longer for an effective anoxic stimulus to develop. Voluntary hyperventilation precipitates periodic breathing by ensuring an initial period during which the blood gas tensions are such that the respiratory centre must lie idle. Natural sleep, barbiturates, and morphine aggravate Cheyne-Stokes breathing by further depressing the respiratory centre.

Clinical features. Periodic breathing may result from a cerebral lesion, e.g. a head injury or a cerebral vascular accident, or from left ventricular failure, usually in patients with hypertensive or ischæmic heart disease, when sclerosis of cerebral vessels may be associated.

The cerebral type is characterised by a rise of blood pressure and pulse rate during the dyspnœic phase (Eyster, 1906); in patients with left ventricular failure, the central venous pressure and blood pressure rise during dyspnœa, the pulse rate and fore-arm blood flow during apnœa (Sharpey-Schafer, 1948). Rhythmic variation in the size of the pupils may also be observed: they dilate during dyspnœa and contract during apnœa.

Cheyne-Stokes breathing may cause insomnia by waking the patient at the height of the dyspnœic phase.

RIGHT VENTRICULAR FAILURE; CONGESTIVE HEART FAILURE

When the right ventricle fails to discharge its contents adequately, the pressure in the right atrium and venæ cavæ rises, the liver becomes enlarged and tender, and dependent œdema usually develops.

ETIOLOGY

Right ventricular failure in its purest form results from pulmonary hypertension, massive pulmonary embolism, pulmonary stenosis, or atrial septal defect.

The term congestive heart failure is preferable when systemic congestion complicates mitral stenosis, left ventricular failure, rheumatic or other forms of carditis, thyrotoxicosis or other hyperkinetic circulatory states, serious abnormalities of rhythm, ventricular septal defect, or other diseases affecting the heart as a whole.

CLINICAL FEATURES

Elevation of the venous pressure. By far the most important sign of right ventricular failure is a rise of systemic venous blood pressure. Its detection depends essentially upon clinical observation, especially upon inspection of the internal jugular pulse (q.v.).

In untreated heart failure the venous pressure averages about 10 cm. above the sternal angle at 45 degrees, but the range is considerable (3 to 25 cm.). The chief venous pulse wave may be *v* or *y* or the return of *y* to the *z* point. When there is auricular fibrillation and no *x* descent it is difficult to distinguish the venous pulse of heart failure from tricuspid incompetence, but on the whole *v* is bigger in tricuspid incompetence, and is transmitted more obviously to the liver. Clinically, the distinction rarely matters much, for tricuspid incompetence is nearly always functional and secondary to right ventricular dilatation and failure.

When the venous pressure is within normal limits at rest, it may yet rise unduly on slight exertion, and may take several minutes to regain its resting level. This is a manifestation of limited cardiac reserve. The jugular venous pressure normally falls on exertion, because increased ventilation lowers the mean intrathoracic pressure: the true filling pressure tends to rise.

The cause of the elevated venous pressure in congestive heart failure has already been discussed (page 267).

Enlargement and tenderness of the liver. Hepatic distension may cause spontaneous pain in the right hypochondrium, especially when it develops quickly as in failure from paroxysmal tachycardia. Sometimes the pain is related to effort.

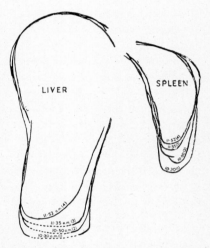

Fig. 7.09—Tracings of serial skiagrams of liver and spleen, opacified by means of thorotrast, demonstrating the rapid shrinkage of the liver and spleen which occurs when 1.5 mg. of digoxin is administered to a case of congestive failure.

Palpation of the liver should be preceded by inspection and percussion. Epigastric fullness and dullness to percussion are characteristic of hepatic engorgement; on the other hand, epigastric flattening or concavity, with resonance to percussion, is incompatible with it. Percussion of the right hypochondrium during the different phases of respiration often reveals the size of the liver with as much precision as palpation. The latter is best carried out with the left hand, the physician standing to the patient's left. It may be helpful to place the right hand high up under the right lower ribs, and to exert forward pressure in order to push the liver towards the anterior abdominal wall; if the organ is distended, its edge can be felt with the forefinger of the left hand as it moves downwards during inspiration. Pressure over an engorged liver is painful. Hepatic pulsation may be felt in cases of tricuspid incompetence, expansion coinciding with ventricular systole. If there is ascites, an enlarged liver may be recognised by "dipping", a repeated sudden pressure of the hand over the region of the liver, when a sensation like that of a patella-tap, or like that of ballotting a fœtus in utero may be appreciated. The liver shrinks as engorgement is relieved (fig. 7.09), and this may be demonstrated within half an hour of giving 1.5 mg. of digoxin intravenously (Wood, 1940).

Anatomically, the liver almost invariably shows centrilobular hepatic necrosis in cases of congestive heart failure. Hepatic function is disturbed to the extent of a raised serum bilirubin (usually short of frank jaundice), increased urobilinogen in the urine, and diminished excretion of brom-sulphalein; alkaline phosphatase, total and differential serum proteins, and the serum colloidal gold precipitation test are all usually normal (Sherlock, 1951).

After repeated attacks of failure, or after years of persistent distension, cirrhotic changes may occur; but they are usually unimportant and rarely interfere seriously with hepatic function or with portal drainage. The most important clinical sign of seriously impaired hepatic function appears to be the bright palmar flush, often associated with warm hands and digital throbbing, despite obviously advanced heart failure and evidence of a low cardiac output.

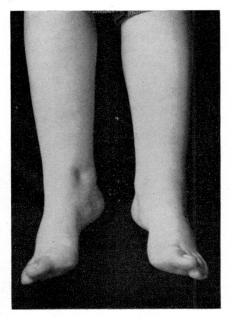

Fig. 7.10—Dependent œdema in congestive heart failure.

Œdema. Of the three classic signs of congestive heart failure, œdema is the least reliable. It may be absent when the venous pressure is high, and gross when it is not so high. It is frequently absent in acute cases, especially in children. Cardiac œdema is essentially dependent (fig. 7.10), but is occasionally observed in the face, and is not infrequent in the arms. It is, of course, accompanied or preceded by oliguria and by a gain in body weight; in fact as much as six litres of fluid may collect in the tissue spaces before pitting œdema is necessarily demonstrable.

The mechanism of the two most important forms of œdema, cardiac and nephritic, is not yet fully understood. In both, as a rule, the protein content of fluid samples is low (less than 1 G. per cent), the venous pressure is raised, and the blood volume is increased (Warren and Stead, 1944); but there are exceptions. Thus in chronic anæmia with congestive heart failure the blood volume is much diminished (Sharpey-Schafer, 1944). Increased capillary permeability is excluded by the low protein content of the œdema fluid; moreover, the theory that anoxia might be the cause of such capillary dysfunction is unlikely in that cardiac œdema may be associated with a high cardiac output and normal arterial oxygen saturation, as in arterio-venous aneurysm. Elevation of the hydrostatic pressure at the venous end of the capillaries must play a part, but not necessarily a major part. In partial superior vena cava obstruction, for example, œdema does not occur until the venous pressure is very much higher than it is in heart failure; and ligation of the inferior vena cava below the renal veins in cases of heart failure relieves œdema in the legs (Cossio and Perratta, 1949). Reduction of renal blood flow to about 25 per cent of normal in most cases of congestive failure has been demonstrated (Merrill, 1946), and there is a considerable degree of sodium retention; according to Merrill and Cargill (1948), œdema occurs when the filtration rate falls below 70 to 80 ml./litre, tubular reabsorption being almost complete. Merrill and Cargill (1947) demonstrated similar impairment of renal blood flow and filtration rate in a case of thyrotoxic heart failure with high cardiac output.

There is also evidence that patients with congestive heart failure excrete an anti-diuretic substance in the urine, and that this is not pitressin (Bercu, Rokaw and Massie, 1950). This opens up yet another line of approach to this fascinating problem.

OTHER MANIFESTATIONS OF CONGESTIVE HEART FAILURE

General symptoms. Owing to the absence of pulmonary venous congestion breathlessness is far less pronounced than in left heart failure, and there is no orthopnœa. The low cardiac output is reflected by fatigue or by a sense of heaviness in the limbs, and on effort there may be dizziness or blurring of vision. In severe cases vomiting may be troublesome, and it is sometimes difficult to know whether heart failure or digitalis therapy is responsible.

Urinary findings. Oliguria, of course, is associated with œdema. The urine, which is rich in colour and of high specific gravity, often contains albumin, leucocytes, red cells, and both hyaline and granular casts.

Hydrothorax may occur from left or right ventricular failure, and though usually bilateral, tends to be left-sided with the former and right-sided with the latter (Bedford and Lovibond, 1941). It should be remembered that the visceral pleura is drained by a venous plexus which is composed of both bronchial and pulmonary venous radicles. In typical instances, the fluid is a transudate with a specific gravity ranging between 1,015 and 1,020; protein is often between two and three per cent, and there may be moderate numbers of leucocytes and red cells. Unsuspected pulmonary infarction may further complicate the picture, increasing the specific gravity, the protein content, the leucocyte count and especially the number of red cells, the overlying pleurisy giving rise to an exudate. If the fluid is frankly hæmorrhagic, associated pulmonary infarction may be diagnosed with confidence.

Ascites is less common than hydrothorax and usually implies long-standing failure. It is a special feature of tricuspid lesions and of chronic constrictive pericarditis.

Hydropericardium is usually of little significance; cardiac compression does not occur, the electrocardiogram is uninfluenced, and there are no symptoms. It is only important in that it alters the size and shape of the heart shadow and so may confuse radiographic observations.

Cerebral symptoms. Difficulty in concentration, impairment of memory, mental confusion, change of character, and manic-depressive, paranoid, or other psychotic states are by no means rare accompaniments of heart failure. They may be due to hypoxia or occasionally to hepatic failure, and are encountered particularly in hypertensive of ischæmic heart failure, when cerebral arteriosclerosis may be partly responsible, and in severe anoxic pulmonary heart disease, especially when complicated by bronchopneumonia.

Cardiac cachexia. Patients with chronic heart failure usually lose flesh, although loss of weight may be prevented by fluid retention; thus wasting may only be noticed after diuresis; sometimes it is so great as to warrant the term cachexia. Elevation of the basal metabolic rate, anorexia, impairment of intestinal function, and enforced muscular inactivity may be partly responsible.

Venous thromboses are common in congestive heart failure, especially when the cardiac output is low. They are responsible for the frequency of pulmonary infarction.

Jaundice may develop in severe cases, and may be mainly obstructive (McMichael and Sherlock, 1945) or mainly hæmolytic, the former depending perhaps upon the raised intra-hepatic pressure, the latter upon the

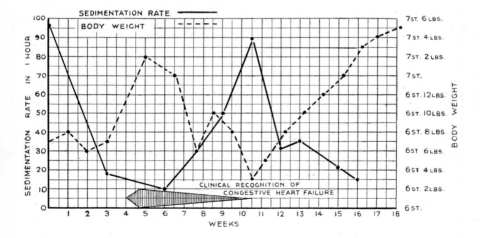

Fig. 7.11—Fall in erythrocyte sedimentation rate resulting from the development of congestive failure in a case of active rheumatic carditis.

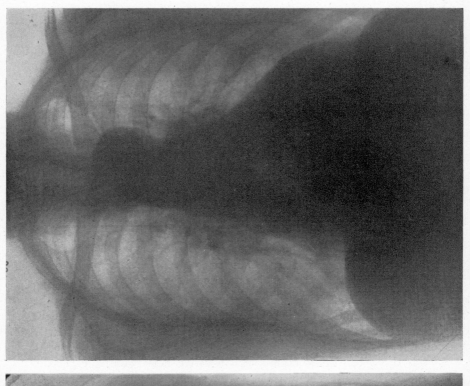

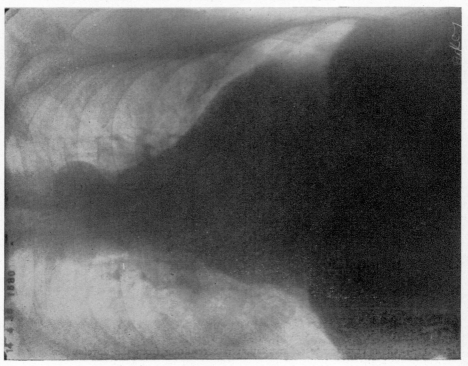

(b) May 19, 1936 (after treatment).

290

destruction of red cells in hæmorrhagic pulmonary infarcts. The serum bilirubin is often in the region of 2 mg. per cent. Itching may occur.

Immature red cells are common, and may be due to stimulation of the bone marrow by anoxia. Polycythæmia may be masked by hydræmia.

The erythrocyte sedimentation rate is often retarded by congestive failure (Wood, 1936). Figures of 50 to 100 in one hour, obtained by the Westergren method in cases of rheumatic carditis, myocardial infarction, and syphilitic aortic incompetence, may drop below 10 with the onset of failure, and rise to their former level with recovery (fig. 7.11).

The basal metabolic rate is usually raised by about 20 per cent in heart failure, as first pointed out by Peabody *et al.* (1916). A 10 per cent increase could be due to a great increase of heart weight, for a 300 Gm. heart consumes about 20 to 25 ml. of oxygen per minute, and a failing 600 Gm. heart about 50 ml. of oxygen per minute (Bing *et al.*, 1949). The discrepancy has been attributed to extra work performed by the muscles of respiration (Resnik and Friedman, 1935).

Radiographic appearances. The transverse diameter of the heart is increased by 1 to 2 cm. during failure (figs. 7.12a and b). In making such measurements care must be taken to exclude apparent enlargement due to raising of the diaphragm by an enlarged liver so that the heart takes up a more horizontal position. The superior vena cava throws a denser shadow than usual, and the right atrium is more prominent. The lesser fissure on the right side may be clearly marked owing to pleural congestion, or hydrothorax may be evident.

Behaviour of the blood pressure. The blood pressure might be expected to fall in congestive heart failure; but in fact it may rise, fall or remain stationary; in the majority of cases it rises. There are only two conditions in which heart failure is characteristically associated with a sharp drop of blood pressure: acute myocardial infarction and massive pulmonary embolism. Conspicuous lowering of the blood pressure associated with heart failure in other diseases is commonly a terminal event. The vasoconstriction that maintains the blood pressure when the cardiac output falls is partly reflex and perhaps partly renal in origin. It may be recognised clinically by cold extremities and peripheral cyanosis. An increased concentration of renin has been found in blood samples obtained from the renal vein in cases of congestive heart failure (Merrill, Morrison and Brannon, 1946). A powerful pressor agent must be at work to raise the blood pressure in the face of a cardiac output that may be only half the normal resting level. In advanced heart failure impairment of hepatic function may lower the blood pressure (Raaschou, 1954).

Character of the heart sounds. Current terminology still includes such expressions as weak, faint, or distant heart sounds, and tic-tac or fœtal rhythms which have been supposed to signify failure or threatened failure. Apart from cases of coronary thrombosis, pulmonary embolism, and pericardial effusion, weak, faint, or distant heart sounds are commonly due to obesity, emphysema, or well-developed thoracic muscles. It is doubtful whether tic-tac or fœtal rhythm is in any way associated with central heart failure; on the other hand, it is heard in patients suffering from shock, and may be associated with diminution of the blood volume. A weak first heart sound associated with a normal second sound is usually due to a P-R interval around 0.21 to 0.22 second, the mitral cusps then having time to float into apposition before the ventricles contract (Levine, 1948).

PHYSIOLOGICAL TESTS FOR CONGESTIVE HEART FAILURE

Although as a rule there are good clinical grounds for being confident whether heart failure is present or not, difficulties arise occasionally; the following tests may then be enlisted.

Valsalva manœuvre

The diastolic hypertension and secondary bradycardia that follow strain in normal individuals are attributed to reflex vasoconstriction from stimulation of carotid and aortic baroreceptors by the diminished stroke output and pulse pressure that follow reduction of the effective filling pressure (fig. 5.06). In heart failure, however, the overloaded ventricle maintains a normal or even increased stroke volume and pulse pressure when its filling pressure is reduced, so that the baroreceptors are either not stimulated at all or respond to the increased pulse pressure by causing vasodilatation and a corresponding fall in diastolic pressure (Sharpey-Schafer, 1955). The square wave in figure 7.13 is due simply to the rise in all

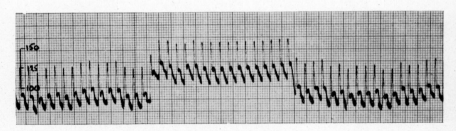

Fig. 7.13—Arterial pressure pulse during Valsalva's manœuvre in a case of congestive heart failure, showing a "square wave" effect (see text).

pressures (venous, intracardiac, pulmonary, systemic and, of course, intrathoracic) that occurs during the period of strain; there is no decrease of pulse pressure, no diastolic hypertension, no overshoot and no secondary bradycardia. It is easy enough to note the effect of strain on the pulse pressure and pulse rate at the bedside, so the test should have considerable clinical value.

Forearm blood flow

A second indirect method of determining whether or not the cardiac output rises in response to an increased or decreased venous filling

pressure is to measure the forearm blood flow when the body is horizontal
and when it is tilted legs down at an angle of 45 degrees or so. In normal
subjects the cardiac output rises in the horizontal position and falls in the
tilted (legs down) position, in response to well-known postural changes in
venous filling pressure, and there are corresponding changes in forearm
blood flow which receives its share of the output. In other words, when the
subject lies flat the forearm flow rises, and when he is tilted legs down, it
falls. In patients with heart failure, however, the forearm blood flow
responds paradoxically to changes of posture, in view of the changed
relationship of venous pressure to output when either ventricle is overloaded (Brigden and Sharpey-Schafer, 1950). This test might have clinical
value if the changes in forearm flow could be detected by means of a skin
temperature thermometer or photoelectric cell (recording digital pulsation).

Direct measurement of intracardiac pressures and cardiac output

Cardiac catheterisation makes it possible to measure both atrial pressures,
right ventricular diastolic pressure and cardiac output more or less at the
same time. In congestive heart failure all these pressures are raised
(fig. 7.14), the arterio-venous oxygen difference is over 50 ml. per litre,

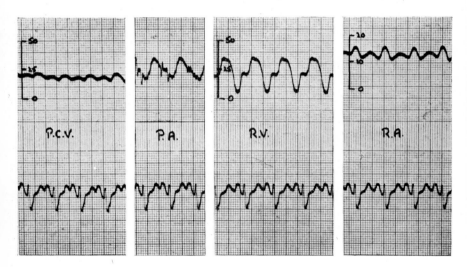

Fig. 7.14—Elevated pressures in both atria in a case of congestive heart failure involving
both ventricles.

the cardiac output less than 4.5 litres per minute at rest, and the cardiac
index (C.O. per square metre of body surface) below 3. In pure right
ventricular failure the findings are similar, except that the left atrial
pressure is normal. If the patient is tilted about 45 degrees legs down, or if
venous tourniquets are applied to the thighs, the right atrial pressure falls
and the cardiac output rises in accordance with Starling's law. On effort

the A-V difference increases greatly, the output little if at all, despite a considerable rise of right atrial pressure and tachycardia.

PROGNOSIS OF HEART FAILURE

When left ventricular failure develops in the natural course of hypertensive or aortic valve disease, the prognosis in untreated cases is poor, patients seldom living more than eighteen months after the onset of orthopnœa or paroxysmal cardiac dyspnœa; but few die before clinical signs of chronic systemic congestion become apparent. Modern treatment, however, has greatly improved the prognosis of left ventricular failure, particularly in hypertensive heart disease and aortic stenosis, and life may be prolonged for years.

The natural prognosis may be less unfavourable when acute myocardial infarction is responsible; because if the patient survives the acute phase, he may make a good recovery, and although the average life expectancy is still only about 5 years, the chances of much longer survival are not remote.

The outlook is entirely different when left ventricular failure complicates acute nephritis; here complete recovery may be anticipated. The ultimate prognosis depends upon the subsequent course of the nephritis. Similar remarks apply to other forms of hypertension which are transient or which can be treated successfully .

The prognosis of right ventricular failure or congestive heart failure depends very much upon its cause. When associated with diseases that can be cured or improved, such as mitral stenosis or thyrotoxicosis, the outlook is excellent. On the other hand, when it occurs in the natural course of chronic and incurable heart disease, few patients survive more than a year or two. Between these extremes are cases of incurable heart disease in which failure is precipitated by some adverse factor which is either transient or which can be improved or cured. Undue physical work, pregnancy, infection, disturbances of rhythm, and pulmonary embolism provide examples of such factors.

TREATMENT

Since the measures used in the treatment of left and right ventricular failure are practically the same they will be considered together.

Rest in bed or in a comfortable armchair is essential and should be continued for a minimum period of three weeks. If signs of failure do not disappear within a few days of instituting adequate therapy, the period of rest should be extended to six weeks. The patient should be nursed against a back rest at an angle of about 60 degrees, whether orthopnœic or not, for there is no easier way of lowering the right atrial pressure and so unloading the overburdened heart; if the legs are lowered, so much the better —hence the value of an armchair or cardiac bed. *Meals* should be small in quantity and fluids limited to about two pints daily. If the *sodium intake*

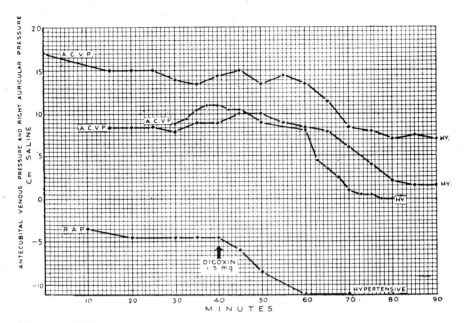

Fig. 7.15—Typical effect of digitalis on the venous pressure or right atrial pressure in four cases of congestive heart failure.

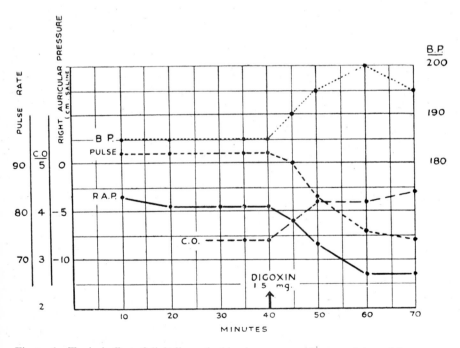

Fig. 7.16—Typical effect of digitalis on the blood pressure, pulse rate, right atrial pressure and cardiac output in a case of hypertensive heart failure with normal rhythm.

295

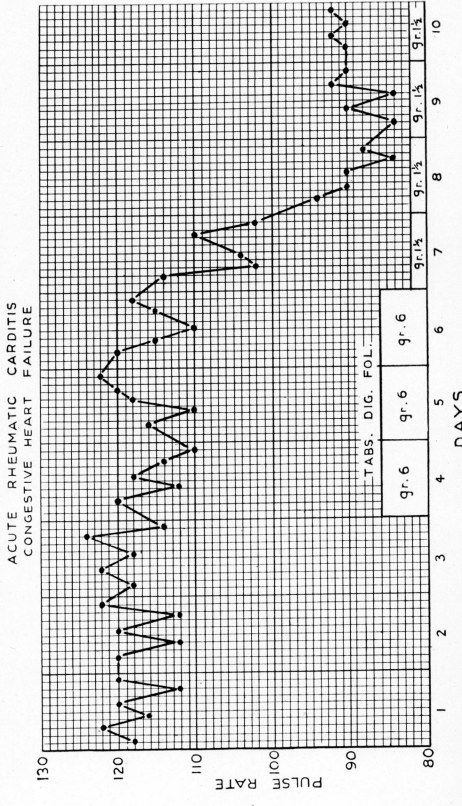

ACUTE RHEUMATIC CARDITIS
CONGESTIVE HEART FAILURE

A clinic in a case of congestive failure with normal rhythm due to active rheumatic carditis.

can be limited to 0.5 G. daily, however, there is no need to restrict fluids. Correct treatment of heart failure usually serves as the best hypnotic; but if insomnia is troublesome at first there should be no hesitation in using powerful sedatives.

Venesection deserves a better reputation. It has fallen out of favour because similar results may be obtained by means of certain drugs; but it offers a quick and sure way of lowering the venous pressure and should not be abandoned. About 600 to 750 ml. of blood may be withdrawn.

Digitalis, obtained from the common foxglove and discovered to be a cure for cardiac dropsy by William Withering in 1785, is beneficial whether there is auricular fibrillation or normal rhythm and whether the pulse rate is fast or slow. It lowers the venous pressure (fig. 7.15), raises the blood pressure (fig. 7.16), slows the heart rate (fig. 7.17), relieves hepatic distension (fig. 7.09), increases the vital capacity, shortens the pulmonary circulation time (fig. 7.18), increases the cardiac output (fig. 7.16) and encourages diuresis (fig. 7.19). Its good effects cannot be attributed to a direct venous-pressure-lowering action as suggested by McMichael and Sharpey-Schafer (1944), for digitalis does not lower a raised venous pressure in the absence of heart failure (fig. 7.20, from Wood and Paulett, 1949), and in cases of left ventricular failure it raises the output, reduces

DIGITALIS IN LEFT VENTRICULAR FAILURE

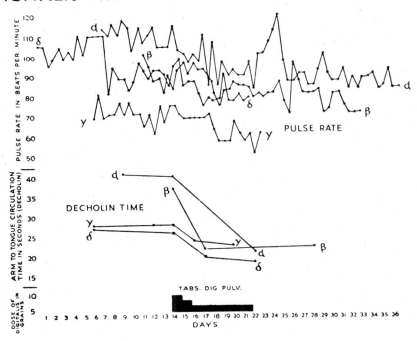

Fig. 7.18—The action of digitalis on the arm-to-tongue circulation time and on the pulse rate in four cases of left ventricular failure with normal rhythm.

passive pulmonary hypertension, and therefore lowers left atrial pressure, without altering the normal right ventricular diastolic pressure (Harvey *et al.*, 1949). The original belief that digitalis improves the function of the heart by virtue of its direct action on the myocardium is probably correct. In normal controls increase of myocardial tone may make the heart smaller and may reduce its output (Stewart *et al.*, 1938).

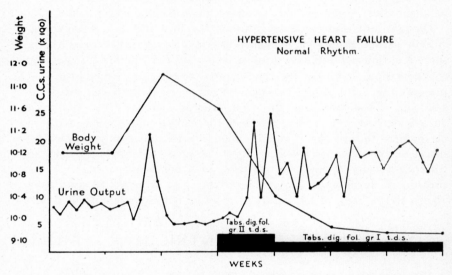

Fig. 7.19—Chart showing considerable diuresis resulting from the administration of digitalis to a case of hypertensive heart failure with normal rhythm.

Digitalis should not be withheld when heart failure is due to cardiac ischæmia, cor pulmonale or heart block.

In ischæmic heart disease digitalis was believed to be dangerous because it was shown to encourage ventricular tachycardia or fibrillation in cats subjected to experimental cardiac infarction (e.g. Travell, Gold and Modell, 1938), and because the microscopic myocardial lesions caused by digitalis in cats (Büchner, 1934), closely resembling those produced by acetylcholine and prolonged vagal stimulation (Hall *et al.*, 1937), were likewise attributed to coronary vasoconstriction because they could be prevented by means of coronary vasodilators such as aminophylline (Kyser, Ginsberg and Gilbert, 1946), and because digitalis is known to have a cholinergic action (Danielopolu, 1946). But in clinical practice digitalis in therapeutic doses has no effect whatever on the severity, duration, or frequency of attacks of angina pectoris (Gold *et al.*, 1938), and both digitalis and ouabain have proved efficient treatment for cardiogenic shock following acute cardiac infarction (Gorlin and Robin, 1955), as well as for ordinary ischæmic heart failure. Finally, Bing *et al.* (1950) have proved that strophanthus has no effect on coronary blood flow.

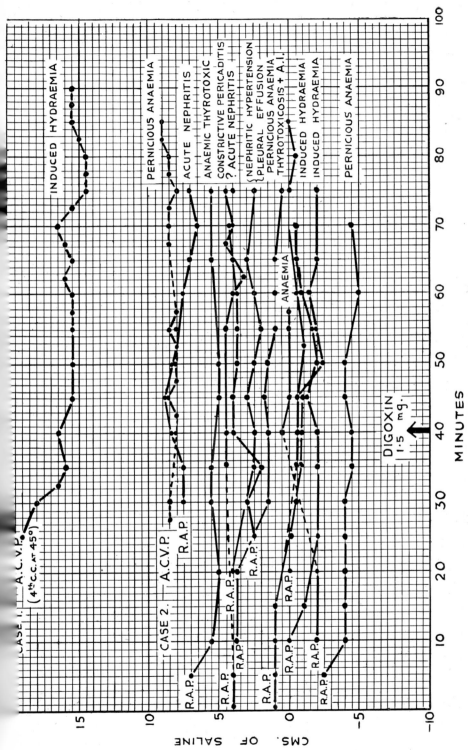

Fig. 7.20—Chart illustrating the failure of digitalis to lower the right atrial pressure in twelve cases in which it was raised from causes other than congestive failure.

299

Digitalis tended to be withheld in cases of cor pulmonale when a raised venous pressure was associated with signs of a raised cardiac output, because Howarth, McMichael and Sharpey-Schafer (1947) had shown that the high output (which was compensatory and beneficial) fell if the venous pressure was lowered (by venesection, for example), and at that time these workers believed that digitalis was a primary venous-pressure-lowering agent; moreover, digitalis seemed to be of little value clinically, unless the cardiac output was obviously low. The hypothesis that digitalis is a primary venous-pressure-lowering agent has since been abandoned (McMichael, 1952), and it is now generally believed that digitalis is beneficial in cor pulmonale if there is true heart failure, but not otherwise; it may certainly be tried, however, without fear of harming the patient.

It is doubtful if there are any real contra-indications to digitalis in therapeutic doses. The suggestion that it encouraged thrombosis has been refuted (Cathcart and Blood, 1950). Potassium depletion appears to make the heart hypersensitive to digitalis (Friedman and Bine, 1948; Lown et al., 1951). Peptic ulcers and other disorders of the gut that react unfavourably to cholinergic agents may be aggravated by digitalis.

For routine purposes the dose of digitalis should be 3 grains (0.2 G.) of the powdered leaf t.d.s. on the first day, 2 grains (0.13 G.) t.d.s. on the second, and 1 grain (65 mg.) t.d.s. thereafter, until demonstrable improvement or evidence of intoxication occurs, when it may be reduced to 1 grain (65 mg.) b.i.d. Heavy loading doses should only be given when it is known that the patient has received no digitalis for at least one month. Other methods of administering digitalis are described on page 255.

Strophanthin may be preferred when a quick action is desired, especially if a cumulative effect is not wanted. A single dose of Ouabain, 1.0 mg. intravenously, may raise the cardiac output in cases of heart failure without affecting the venous pressure (McMichael, 1948), and so presumably acts directly on the heart. Like intravenous digoxin it also has a conspicuous pressor effect and slows the pulse rate. Strophanthin may be the drug of choice in collapsed cases of cor pulmonale.

Mercurial diuretics were discovered more or less by accident at the Wenckebach clinic in Vienna in 1919, when it was noticed that a new anti-syphilitic mercurial substance, novasurol, when injected into a dehydrated young girl with congenital syphilis provoked unexpected diuresis (Vogl, 1950). Novasurol, however, was painful and toxic, and was soon replaced by the more potent yet more benign salyrgan (Bernheim, 1924). Theophylline was combined with the organic mercurial component in 1928 (von Issekutz and von Végh) in the hope that a summation effect would increase the diuresis; but the combination, introduced as novurit, proved less painful and more effective than expected, being better absorbed and more efficiently excreted owing to a fundamental change in the structure of the substance when theophylline was incorporated (de Graff, Batterman and Lehman, 1938). This is the basis of mersalyl (B.P.), modern salyrgan

(Bayer), neptal (M. & B.), esidrone (Ciba), and the American mercuro-phylline and mercuhydrin. All these substances contain about 40 per cent of metallic mercury: ampoules for injection contain 10 per cent of the drug and 5 per cent of theophylline. The usual dose is 2 ml. intramuscularly, which contains 80 mg. of metallic mercury and 0.1 Gm. of theophylline. It may be repeated every third or fourth day, preferably with ammonium chloride gr. 30 t.d.s. on the day of the injection to replace chloride loss.

In mercaptomerin (thiomerin) the organic mercurial substance is com-bined with a mercaptide group instead of theophylline: this has greatly decreased toxicity while preserving full diuretic potency; moreover, thiomerin may be given subcutaneously, for it causes very little local irritation and is therefore practically painless (Batterman et al., 1949).

From time to time attempts have been made to encourage oral mercurial diuretics, but in the past they have never withstood prolonged clinical trials, being too irritating to the gastric mucosa and too inefficient. The latest is merchloran (chlormerodrin) in a dose of 2 tablets, each equivalent to 10 mg. of mercury, three or four times a day (Moyer et al., 1952). With these doses, however, gastro-intestinal symptoms are frequent, and as a rule only 1 tablet is given, three or four times daily at the start and once or twice daily for maintenance.

Mersalyl rectal suppositories, which contain 0.4 Gm. of mersalyl and 0.2 Gm. of theophylline, usually provoke severe local burning pain and cannot be recommended.

Mercurial diuretics act by discouraging tubular reabsorption of sodium, potassium and chloride (Blumgart et al., 1934), and so remove œdema in water-logged patients and cause dehydration in those without œdema (De Vries, 1946). The blood volume declines and the venous pressure falls secondarily. If the heart is overloaded the cardiac output rises, and the whole functional state of the circulation improves. These effects are gradual, beginning an hour or two after the injection, and depend upon the degree of diuresis (Volini and Levitt, 1939). A much earlier and more rapid fall of venous pressure may result from the incorporated theophylline (Pugh and Wyndham, 1949). If the right ventricle is not overloaded, its output probably falls and this helps to decongest the lungs in cases of left ventricular failure or mitral stenosis (Friedman et al., 1935). Thus mersalyl has proved an excellent drug for preventing paroxysmal cardiac dyspnœa (fig. 7.21).

Toxic reactions are rare, but high fever and rigors have been en-countered (Foster and Naylor, 1951).

Sudden death has been reported after intravenous injections. This is a direct toxic effect of a relatively high concentration of mercury on the heart, death occurring from ventricular fibrillation or asystole within 1 to 3 minutes of the injection. It may occur after the first injection, when previous injections seem to have been well tolerated, or after warnings of disaster have been noted on previous occasions (Kaufman, 1948). Sudden death of this kind is very rare after intramuscular or subcutaneous injections. Ventricular fibrillation or asystole, however, may also occur after a massive diuresis; it has been suggested that the combination of potassium depletion (which sensitises the heart to digitalis) and digitalis concentration may be responsible.

Considerable weakness and fatigue may follow the use of mercurial diuretics and have been attributed to sodium, potassium and chloride depletion; the feeling of exhaustion occurs especially the day after the

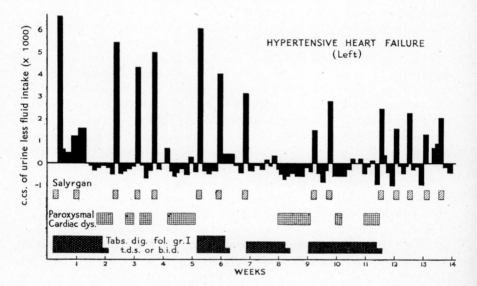

Fig. 7.21—Chart illustrating the beneficial effect of mercurial diuretics in preventing paroxysmal cardiac dypsnœa. Digitalis was less effective.

injection and is only partly relieved by potassium and chloride. Nausea and vomiting, colic, or diarrhœa may be due to digitalis concentration. An attack of gout may be precipitated by the dehydration in susceptible individuals. Patients with prostatic symptoms may develop acute retention as a result of distension of the bladder and should be warned to void urine hourly after an injection without waiting for the desire. Abdominal cramps are due to sodium depletion. Hiccough and drowsiness suggest uræmia, and usually mean that treatment has been too intense, and that the blood sodium and chloride are too low. This is rare unless the patient is also on a low sodium diet.

Toxic nephrosis, characterised by tubular degeneration and calcification, is encountered occasionally, usually after prolonged administration (Waife and Pratt, 1946).

The drug should not be stopped owing to a poor initial response, for the result of the second or third dose, coinciding perhaps with the beneficial effect of rest and digitalis, may exceed expectations. The only contra-indications are known hypersensitivity and acute nephritis.

Other diuretics. Mictine, in doses of 200 to 600 mg. t.d.s. for two consecutive days each week is the most powerful oral diuretic now available, and is usually well tolerated. Of the xanthines, *theobromine* 0.5 G. is the most potent; it is best given in the form of 1.0 G. of diuretin (theobromine and sodium salicylate) which is more soluble.

A low sodium diet has proved a most effective way of relieving obstinate œdema (Schroeder, 1941) and preventing paroxysmal cardiac dyspnœa. The object is to reduce the sodium intake to the order of 0.5 G. daily, so that it is impossible for the tissues to hold much fluid. The blood volume is thus reduced and the venous pressure lowered. The function of the overloaded heart improves as it does after venesection. Both the milk diet of Karell (1866) and the rice diet of Kempner (1944, 1946) owe their diuretic effects to their low sodium content.

The following diet has been constructed from tables giving the composition of numerous foods, compiled by McCance and Widdowson (1946). The first figure after each substance gives the amount of sodium in mgs. per 100 G. of foodstuff. The second figure gives the approximate calorific value of the food per mg. of sodium content. Obviously the best foods are those with a low first figure and a high second figure. For the first 48 hours it is a good plan to give nothing but fruit in any form, fruit juice drinks, sugar, rice and diluted milk. Mercurial diuretics should not, as a rule, be given more than two or three times with this diet, the combination causing too much sodium and chloride depletion; uræmia, which may prove fatal, may then develop (Shroeder, 1949; Black and Litchfield, 1951).

LOW SODIUM DIET

CEREALS

Permitted			Doubtful			Forbidden		
Arrowroot ·	4.8	72	Currant bread ·	164	2	Bread · · ·	393	0.7
Barley · ·	0.8	150	Sweet biscuits ·	216	3	Biscuits · ·	400	0.8
Cornflour ·	52	7	Rusks · · ·	200	2	Cornflakes· ·	1,050	0.3
Flour· · ·	2.5	170				Grapenuts· ·	658	0.5
Macaroni ·	7.9	15				Post-Toasties ·	810	0.5
Oatmeal · ·	33	11				Ryvita · · ·	615	0.5
Rice · · ·	2.2	60				Vita-weat · ·	615	0.5
Sago · · ·	3.4	100						
Semolina ·	12	30						
Shredded								
Wheat ·	16	22						
Tapioca ·	4	86						

NOTE

Biscuits. Water biscuits and cream crackers contain the most sodium. Oatmeal biscuits made without salt and with lard instead of margarine are recommended.

Breakfast cereals. Oatmeal porridge should be made without salt and with equal parts of milk and water. Shredded wheat with diluted milk and plenty of sugar is recommended.

Milk puddings. Milk should be diluted with equal parts of water; margarine must not be used.

Flour sauces. Make without salt and with equal parts of milk and vegetable water. Use dripping instead of margarine.

Bread. Home-made bread made with yeast, flour, lard and milk, without salt, is allowed.

DAIRY PRODUCE AND FATS

Permitted			Doubtful			Forbidden		
Butter (fresh)	223	3.5	Milk (fresh) ·	50	1.2	Cheese · · ·	600	0.5
Cream cheese			Milk (sweet			Egg white · ·	192	0.2
(home made)	110	8	condensed) ·	143	2	Margarine · ·	318	0.5
Cream · ·	31	13				Butter (salted)		
Egg yolk · ·	50	7						
Olive oil · ·	0.1	9,290						
Lard · ·	2	450						
Dripping ·	5	200						
Suet · ·	25	44						

NOTE

Butter may be kneaded in water to reduce its salt content.

Home-made cream cheese must be made without salt.

Dilute milk with half its volume of water.

Use olive oil, dripping, lard or suet in cooking instead of butter or margarine, whenever precisely possible.

MEAT, POULTRY AND GAME

Permitted			Doubtful			Forbidden		
Roast beef · ·	62	6	Chicken · ·	80	2	Bacon · ·	1,200	0.3
Grilled steak ·	67	5	Duck · · ·	195	1.5	Beef		
Stewed steak ·	38	5.5	Goose · · ·	145	2	(silverside)	1,470	0.2
Hare (roast or)			Guinea fowl ·	136	1.5	Brains · ·	150	0.7
stewed) ·	45	4.5	Heart · · ·	153	1.5	Ham · · ·	1,500	0.3
Mutton chop			Liver · · ·	100	2.5	Kidney · ·	250	0.4
(grilled or			Partridge · ⎫			Meat paste ·	940	0.25
fried) · ·	90	6	Pheasant · ⎬	100	2	Smoked pork	1,800	0.15
Mutton, leg, etc.			Pigeon · · ⎭			Sausage · ·	1,000	0.25
(roast, boiled			Turkey · ·	130	1.5	Tongue · ·		
or stewed) ·	68	4	Tripe · · ·	72	1.5	(preserved)	1,870	0.15
Pork, roast · ·	66	5	Veal · · ·	100	2			
Pork chops ·	60	9	Venison · ·	86	2			
Rabbit · · ·	32	6						
Sweetbread ·	69	3						
Tongue (fresh)	79	4						
Topside (beef) ·	50	4						

NOTE

All salted and preserved meats are forbidden.

Roasts are best since they contain more calories per mg. of sodium content.

Meat extracts like Bovril and Oxo are forbidden.

The simple meats – beef, mutton, lamb, pork, hare and rabbit – are the best. Next comes game. Of offal, sweetbread, fresh tongue and liver are best.

FISH

Permitted			Doubtful			Forbidden		
Bass . . .	75	1.7	Bream (sea) .	113	0.88	Bloaters . .	703	0.36
Brill (steamed)	94	1.2	Cod, fried .	161	0.87	Cockles . .	3,520	0.01
Dabs (fried) .	127	2.0	grilled .	110	1.5	Crab (boiled)	366	0.35
Eels (stewed)	73	5.1	steamed	100	0.82	Fish paste .	1,480	0.12
Herring			Cod's roe			Haddock		
(fried) . .	101	2.3	(fried) . .	127	1.6	(smoked) .	1,220	0.08
Herring's roe,			Flounder			Kippers . .	990	0.08
fresh (fried)	87	3.0	(steamed) .	115	0.83	Lobster . .	325	0.36
Mullet . .	94	1.3	Haddock			Mussels		
Plaice (fried) .	124	1.9	(steamed) .	121	0.80	(boiled) .	210	0.41
Salmon			Hake			Oysters . .	505	0.10
(fresh) . .	107	1.9	(steamed) .	118	0.90	Prawns . .	1,590	0.06
Sprats (fried)	132	3.4	Hake (fried) .	153	1.3	Scallops . .	265	0.4
Trout,			Halibut . .	110	1.2	Shrimps . .	3,840	0.03
fresh water	88	1.5	Mackerel			Trout (sea) .	207	0.63
Turbot . .	90	1.1	(fried) . .	153	1.2	Whelks . .	265	0.34
			Plaice			Winkles		
			(steamed) .	120	0.77	(boiled) .	266	0.37
			Pollack					
			(steamed) .	95	0.91			
			Pollack (fried)	162	0.96			
			Skate (fried) .	182	1.3			
			Sole, Dover					
			(fried) . .	192	1.2			
			Sole, Dover					
			(steamed) .	110	0.76			
			Sole, lemon					
			(fried) . .	136	1.6			
			Sole, lemon					
			(steamed) .	115	0.78			
			Whitebait					
			(fried) . .	225	2.4			
			Whiting . .	127	0.71			

NOTE

Fish cakes made with any but forbidden fish, without salt, and fried in olive oil are recommended.

FRUIT

Permitted				Permitted		
Apples · · ·	2	20		Greengages · ·	1.4	34
Apricots · · ·	1	30		Oranges · · ·	2.9	9
Bananas · · ·	1.2	70		Peaches · · ·	2.7	13
Blackberries · ·	3.7	8		Pears · · ·	2.3	18
Cherries · · ·	2.8	16		Pineapple · ·	1.7	29
Currants · · ·	2.7	10		Plums · · ·	1.7	22
Dates · · ·	4.7	27		Quinces · · ·	3.2	8
Figs · · ·	1.6	26		Raspberries · ·	2.5	10
Gooseberry · ·	1.2	31		Rhubarb · · ·	1.5	2.5
Grapes · · ·	1.6	40		Strawberries · ·	1.5	17
Grape-fruit · ·	1.4	16				

NOTE

These are average samples of fresh fruits.

Doubtful fruits are melon (19.5/1) and passion fruit (30/1).

Stewed fruit is best, because of its higher calorific value, e.g. stewed apples (0.1/170).

Tinned fruits in syrup are also good.

Dried fruits are less beneficial, e.g. tinned apricots (0.9/62), dried apricots (56/3). Raisins and sultanas at 52/4.7 may be allowed occasionally.

Preserved olives (2,250/0.05) are forbidden.

NUTS

Almonds ·	· · ·	5.8	100
Brazils	· · ·	1.5	430
Chestnuts	· ·	10.9	16
Coconut .	. . .	16.5	22
Hazelnuts	· · ·	1.4	280
Walnuts ·	· · ·	2.7	200

NOTE

All these fresh nuts are excellent, with their low sodium content and high calorific value.

Obviously salted almonds and peanuts are forbidden.

VEGETABLES

Permitted			Forbidden		
Artichokes,			Beetroot . .	64	0.7
root . . .	2.6	7.3	Carrots . .	50	0.3
Artichokes,			Celery . . .	137	0.07
globe . . .	6.4	1.1	Radishes . .	59	0.25
Asparagus . .	0.9	10	Spinach . .	123	0.2
Broad beans .	19.6	2	Turnips . .	28	0.5
Butter beans .	16.2	6	Watercress . .	60	0.25
French beans .	3.4	2			
Haricot beans .	15	6			
Runner beans .	3.3	2			
Broccoli tops .	6.8	2.1			
Brussels sprouts	7.7	2			
Cabbage . .	10	0.6			
Cauliflower .	11	1			
Chicory . .	7.3	1.2			
Cucumber . .	13	0.7			
Leeks . . .	6.4	4			
Lentils . . .	9.4	10			
Lettuce . . .	3.1	3.5			
Marrow . .	1.2	6			
Mushrooms,					
fried . . .	11	20			
Mustard and					
cress . . .	10	0.5			
Onions, boiled .	6.6	2			
raw .	10.2	2			
fried .	20	18			
Parsnips . .	4.1	14			
Parsnips, dried .	12.6	8			
Potatoes, boiled	3.4	25			
roast .	8.6	14			
Sea kale . .	3.9	2.1			
Spring greens .	10.3	1.0			
Swedes . . .	14.4	1			
Tomatoes . .	2.8	5			
Tomatoes, fried	3.3	21			
Turnip tops .	6.7	1.6			

NOTE

Vegetables must be cooked free from salt. They must not be mashed with margarine or salted butter.

Tinned, or otherwise preserved, vegetables, e.g. tinned peas (260/0.3), are banned.

SWEETS

Sugar (0.4/984) adds a low sodium high calorific value to most sweets.

Plain chocolate (18.6/29) is better than milk chocolate (93.4/6).

Honey (10.7/26) and jam (15.9/16) are recommended.

Golden syrup (270/1), chutney (150/1) and mincemeat (200/0.5) are prohibited.

Toffee (115/3.5) and black treacle (96/2.5) should be avoided.

BEVERAGES

Permitted			Prohibited		
Coffee	0.3	15	Bournvita	360	1
Lemonade	0.5	100	Bovril	5,580	0.02
Tea	0.4	2	Cocoa	650	0.7
Beer	15	3	Horlicks	690	0.6
Wine			Marmite	6,130	0.01
Spirits			Ovaltine	249	1.5
			Oxo Cubes	10,600	0.02
			Virol	374	1

CONDIMENTS

Permitted			Prohibited		
Ginger	34	7.5	Curry	450	0.5
Mustard	5	90	Salt	38,500	0
Pepper	7	45			
Vinegar	20	0.2			

NOTE

Since so small a quantity of curry is required to flavour a dish it may be allowed despite the adverse figures shown.

CAKES, PASTRIES AND PUDDINGS

Permitted			Doubtful			Forbidden		
Apple dishes	50	4	Biscuits	150	3	Cakes	150–	2–3
Blancmange	45	2.5	Buns	120	3		500	
Cereal puddings			Cheese-cake	138	3	Dumplings	488	0.5
(rice, etc.)	50	3	Jam roll	151	2.5	Gingerbread	336	1
Custard	50	2	Rock cakes	150	3	Mince pies	225	1.5
Doughnuts	60	6	Tarts	150	3	Pastries	250	2
Fruit custard	30	3				Puddings	100–	1–3
Fruit tarts	76	3					250	
Jelly	8	9.5				Scones	170	2
Milk jelly	33	3				Swiss roll	650	0.4
Pancake	88	4				Yorkshire		
Shortbread	86	6				pudding	412	0.5
Sponge cake	79	4						
Trifle	50	3						

NOTE

Oatmeal biscuits are allowed if made without salt and with lard instead of butter or margarine.

Cereal puddings should be made with diluted milk and without margarine.

Yorkshire pudding is permissible if made without salt.

GENERAL RULES

No free salt or ordinary salt substitutes; no salt in cooking. Sodium free salt substitutes, usually made with potassium, such as neo-seleron, are permitted.

No foods made with baking powder.

No medicines containing sodium.

No preserved, salted, smoked or tinned foods (except dried and tinned fruit)

Dilute milk with half its volume of water.

Use dripping, lard, olive oil or suet instead of butter or margarine, wherever possible.

Supply calories chiefly with selected cereals, cream, fat, fresh meat, potatoes, sugar, sweets, fruit, and nuts.

Avoid bread, biscuits, certain cereals, margarine, salted butter, cheese, bacon, ham, tongue, sausages, meat extracts, shell-fish, fish paste, milk beverages, cakes and pastries.

Fluid should be encouraged, but few patients feel like drinking much if they are adhering to the diet faithfully.

Cation-exchange resins are synthetic insoluble macromolecular organic compounds in powder form which, when suspended in a solution, behave like electrolytes; acid resins exchange hydrogen ions for any other cation in the solution, but prefer calcium, potassium or sodium in that order. In 1946 Dock pointed out that such resins would absorb sodium from the gut, and since then they have gradually found their place as adjuncts to the mercurial diuretics and the low sodium diet (Dock and Frank, 1950). At the present time the most effective and readily available cation-exchange resin for therapeutic purposes is probably carbo-resin (Lilly). Two-thirds of the 88 per cent cation-exchange fraction of this resin is in the carboxylic acid form, one-third in the form of its potassium salt. In the human gut each gramme of carbo-resin is capable of absorbing 1 meq. (23 mg.) of sodium and passing it out in the fæces when the patient is taking about 1.5 Gm. of sodium per day. If the dose is 15 Gm. suspended in water three times a day, 1 Gm. of sodium should be removed daily in this way. The amount of sodium absorbed by the resin is proportional to the quantity of sodium in the diet. Thus with a 0.5 Gm. low sodium diet, 1 Gm. of resin absorbs only 0.3 meq. of sodium; on a 3 Gm. low sodium diet it may absorb as much as 2 meq. Undue loss of potassium presents no problem with this resin, but calcium deficiency may arise if treatment is prolonged. As a rule, however, patients do not like taking resins, and they are mostly used intermittently as a protection against unavoidable or wilful dietetic indiscretions or liberties—e.g. while on holiday. Neither potassium nor calcium should be given at the same time as the resin, or it will absorb less sodium; and if there is constipation, which is a common complication of resin therapy, it should not be relieved by magnesium salts for the same reason.

Carbonic anhydrase inhibitors

Conservation of body base and excretion of acid is partly achieved by the distal tubules where sodium alkaline phosphate interacts with carbonic acid to form acid phosphate and bicarbonate:

$$Na_2HPO_4 + H_2CO_3 = NaH_2PO_4 + NaHCO_3$$

The acid phosphate is excreted and the bicarbonate reabsorbed, so that half the sodium is saved. This reaction is helped by an anzyme, carbonic anhydrase, which accelerates the formation of carbonic acid from CO_2 and water.

$$H_2O + CO_2 \rightarrow H_2CO_3$$

If the formation of H_2CO_3 were to be suppressed, alkaline phosphate would be excreted as such and sodium would be no longer conserved.

In 1940 Mann and Keilin identified sulphanilamide as a specific inhibitor of carbonic anhydrase, and after further research Roblin and his colleagues found that of all the active heterocyclid sulphonamides diamox was the most promising in this respect (Miller *et al.*, 1950). It is rapidly absorbed and is excreted unchanged by the kidney in 6 to 12 hours. A single oral dose of 250 mg. is sufficient to interfere with the chain of events outlined above, so that the tubules experience difficulty in reabsorbing sodium.

In clinical practice, however, diamox in doses of 250 mg. daily has so far proved disappointing, and certainly the weakest of the four methods of relieving the body of sodium.

Combined low sodium regime

With these four weapons, adequate control of the sodium balance is not at all difficult. The art is to find the best combination for each particular patient, and the danger is the low salt syndrome first described by Shroeder (1949). The most powerful of the four is the diet, and if patients will only abide by it absolutely, the other three methods may usually be withheld altogether; moreover, patients tend to lose their taste for salt if they resolutely refuse to titillate it. If patients prefer a 2- or 3-Gm. sodium diet they will certainly need weekly injections of mersalyl or thiomerin, daily merchloran if they can tolerate it, or fairly heavy doses of a potent cation-exchange resin; diamox alone is rarely strong enough to hold the situation in check. Patients who do not mind the diet for the most part, but who insist on occasional breaks, can have these lapses adequately covered by a mercurial diuretic or resin.

The low sodium regime has revolutionised the treatment of heart failure, and is a great deal more effective than digitalis except in cases of auricular fibrillation with rapid ventricular rate. It is also just as successful in isolated left ventricular failure as in congestive heart failure or pure right ventricular failure. It has the triple value of combatting œdema itself, reducing the blood volume and venous pressure and so improving the function of the overloaded heart, and relieving "pulmonary venous congestion" whether due to heart failure or mitral stenosis.

Aminophylline

Aminophylline (theophylline-ethylenediamine) benefits cases of heart failure in four different ways: (1) it lowers the venous pressure promptly and thereby relieves both left and right ventricular failure; (2) it is an excellent bronchial antispasmodic and therefore particularly helpful in cor pulmonale; (3) it is a powerful respiratory stimulant acting reflexly by way of carotid sinus chemoreceptors, and abolishes Cheyne-Stokes breathing as first recognised by Vogl (1927, 1942); (4) to some extent it appears to be a cardiac tonic, for it makes the heart beat more strongly. There is no evidence that it improves the cerebral circulation (Wechsler, Kleiss and Kety, 1950), and direct measurements of coronary blood flow in man by means of coronary sinus catheterisation do not support the belief that aminophylline is a coronary vaso-dilator (Foltz *et al.*, 1950).

The drug may be given intravenously in doses of 0.25 to 0.5 Gm. in cases of paroxysmal cardiac dyspnœa or pulmonary œdema with dramatic results; it should be injected slowly in order to avoid overstimulating respiration. Unfortunately, aminophylline is often very painful when given intramuscularly owing to its high pH, although preparations are on the market for use by this route.

Orally, aminophylline causes severe dyspepsia if given in effective doses, the usual 0.1-Gm. tablet three times daily after meals being far too small. Some attempts have been made to overcome this difficulty, perhaps the best preparation so far being theodrox (Riker), in which 0.2 Gm. of aminophylline is combined with 4 gr. of dried aluminium hydroxide gel; taken four-hourly, 0.2 Gm. of aminophylline is an adequate dose, and theodrox is relatively well tolerated.

An aminophylline suppository of 0.4 Gm. at night will prevent both Cheyne-Stokes breathing and paroxysmal nocturnal dyspnœa, and in doing so may earn the patient's thanks for a good night's sleep.

Etophylate, a preparation in which theophylline-ethanoic acid is combined with diethylenediamin (piperazine), has the great advantage of having a pH around 7, and is therefore non-irritant; moreover it is freely soluble and stable, while retaining the therapeutic properties of theophylline. It may be given orally in doses of 0.5 Gm. three times daily, and is painless if injected intramuscularly in similar dosage.

Choline theophyllinate may also be taken by mouth in doses of 0.3 to 0.5 G. t.d.s., without fear of gastric disturbance, but since the pH of a 0.8 per cent aqueous solution is 9.7, it is unsuitable for intramuscular injection.

Oxygen is of little value in heart failure except in the following circumstances: (1) in anoxic cor pulmonale, (2) when acute bronchitis or bronchopneumonia has precipitated or complicated heart failure from other causes, (3) in massive pulmonary embolism, (4) in acute pulmonary œdema, (5) in rare cases of heart failure occurring in cyanotic forms of congenital heart disease, and (6) in acute cardiogenic shock from cardiac infarction.

Acupuncture. When œdema is gross and fails to respond to the measures previously outlined, it may be necessary to resort to acupuncture. A triangular cutting needle is used and about a dozen punctures are made in each leg; the patient is then seated in a chair with his legs in a tub. To facilitate drainage, the legs may be swabbed down with warm citrate solution from time to time. Due antiseptic precautions must be maintained. Fluid may continue to exude for twenty-four to forty-eight hours, and it is not uncommon for the total quantity to be measured in gallons. Southey's tubes constitute a cleaner way of removing fluid on the same principle. Several large-bore needles are inserted into the subcutaneous tissues of the thighs or calves, and fluid is allowed to drain away through attached rubber tubes into a container.

Relatively little protein but a lot of sodium is lost by this method, and the good effect is not merely cosmetic; on the contrary, the blood volume diminishes, the venous pressure falls, the cardiac output may pick up, and spontaneous diuresis may follow.

Attacks of paroxysmal cardiac dyspnœa or of acute pulmonary œdema are treated by methods designed to lower the venous filling pressure as quickly as possible and so to reduce the output of the right ventricle. The sitting position will usually have been adopted already by the patient. Morphine, $\frac{1}{4}$ to $\frac{1}{3}$ of a grain (15 to 20 mg.) intramuscularly, or $\frac{1}{6}$ of a grain (10 mg.) intravenously, depresses the excited respiratory reflexes and soothes the patient. Pethidine, 50 to 100 mg. intramuscularly, may be equally effective. Venous tourniquets may be applied round the thighs, to trap blood in the legs, or venesection may be preferred. Theophylline-ethylene-diamine (aminophylline), 0.24 to 0.48 G. intravenously, lowers the venous pressure immediately, relieves bronchial spasm, and may have a direct stimulating action on the heart (fig. 7.02). Tetraethylammonium bromide, 200 to 300 mg. intravenously, is a useful agent for lowering venous pressure, and may relieve attacks quickly (Hayward, 1948). Hexamethonium bromide, 20 to 30 mg., or pentapyrrolidinium bitartrate (ansolysen), 5 mg. subcutaneously, may be equally effective.

Digoxin and strophanthin are probably best avoided in view of their pressor actions; indeed, paroxysmal cardiac dyspnœa may occasionally be initiated by intravenous digoxin.

Oxygen is of little value in paroxysmal cardiac dyspnœa, for the arterial oxygen saturation is normal, but may be given with advantage in acute pulmonary œdema. Nikethamide is contraindicated, for the aim is to depress respiration, not to stimulate it. Adrenaline is dangerous in ischæmic cases because it may provoke angina pectoris, paroxysmal ventricular tachycardia or ventricular fibrillation; but it may be given in doses of 0.5 mg. subcutaneously to relieve bronchial spasm in hypertensive cases (Platz, 1947). Atropine should be avoided, for it has no therapeutic value and causes unnecessary tachycardia.

Dramatic results may follow treatment directed against *the cause of the underlying heart disease*. This applies particularly to cases of thyrotoxicosis, anæmia, beri-beri, arterio-venous aneurysm, severe pulmonary stenosis, large patent ductus, atrial septal defect, mitral or aortic stenosis, and primary abnormalities of rhythm; and to a lesser extent to bronchitis and asthma, active syphilitic aortitis, bacterial endocarditis, and any form of systemic hypertension.

If, in spite of all these measures, heart failure continues, an attempt may be made to reduce the oxygen requirement and therefore the work of the heart by means of antithyroid drugs *or total ablation of the thyroid gland* (Blumgart, Levine and Berlin, 1933). The former is preferable because the treatment can be abandoned if unsuccessful (Bedford, 1949). Relatively large doses are necessary, usually 0.2 to 0.3 Gm. of propyl thiouracil daily. It must be admitted, however, that results are far from satisfactory. Radioactive iodine offers another means of inducing artificial myxoedema (Blumgart *et al.*, 1950).

Ligation of the inferior vena cava below the renal veins may be tried in obstinate cases (Cossio, 1952). The surgical mortality is about 6 per cent, and in at least half the cases initial improvement has been maintained for months or years. The operation lowers the central venous pressure. Œdema tends to clear rather than increase. The chief complication is recurrent phlebothrombosis in the legs.

REFERENCES

Abramson, D. I. (1944): "Vascular responses in the extremeties of man in health and disease", Chicago, University of Chicago Press.

Batterman, R. C., Unterman, D., and De Graff, A. C. (1949): "The subcutaneous administration of mercaptomerin (Thiomerin). Effective mercurial diuretic for the treatment of congestive heart failure", *J. Amer. med. Ass.*, 140, 1268.

Bedford, D. E. (1949): "Obstinate heart failure", *Brit. med. J.*, ii, 172.

——, and Lovibond, J. L. (1941): "Hydrothorax in heart failure", *Brit. Heart J.*, 3, 93.

Bercu, B. A., Rokaw, S. N., and Massie, E. (1950): "Antidiuretic action of the urine of patients in cardiac failure", *Circulation*, 2, 409.

Bernheim, E. (1924): "Ueber das neues Quecksilberpraparat Salyrgan, als Diuretikum", *Therap. d. Gegenw.*, 65, 538.

Bing, R. J., Hammond, M. M., Handelsman, J. C., Powers, S. R., and Spencer, F. C. (1949): "Coronary blood flow, cardiac oxygen consumption and cardiac efficiency in man", *Bull. Johns Hopkins Hispital*, Baltimore, 84, 396.

——, ——, ——, ——, ——, Eckenhoff, J. E., Goodale, W. T., Hafkensheil, J. H., and Kety, S. S. (1949): "The measurement of coronary blood flow, oxygen consumption, and efficiency of the left ventricle in man", *Amer. Heart J.*, 38, 1.

——, *et al.* (1950): "The effect of strophanthus on coronary blood flow and cardiac oxygen consumption of normal and failing human hearts", *Circulation*, 2, 513.

——, Heimbecker, R., and Falholt, W. (1951): "An estimation of the residual volume of blood in the right ventricle of normal and diseased human hearts in vivo", *Amer. Heart J.*, 42, 483.

Black, A. B., and Litchfield, J. A. (1951): "Uræmia complicating low salt treatment of heart failure", *Quart. J. Med.*, 20, 149.

Blumgart, H. L., Freedberg, A. S., and Kurland G. S. (1950): "Hypothyroidism produced by radioactive iodine", *Circulation*, 1, 1105.

——, Gilligan, D. R., Levy, R. C., Brown, M. G., and Volk, M. C. (1934): "Action of diuretic drugs: 1. Action of diuretics in normal persons", *Arch. intern. Med.*, 54, 40.

——, Levine, S. A., and Berlin, D. D. (1933): "Congestive heart failure and angina pectoris. The therapeutic effect of thyroidectomy on patients without clinical or pathological evidence of thyroid toxicity", *Arch. intern. Med.*, 51, 866.

——, and Weiss, S. (1927): "Studies on the velocity of blood flow. The velocity of blood flow in the systemic and pulmonary circulations in health and disease", *J. clin. Invest.*, 4, 15, 149, 173, 199, 389, 399; (1928): 5, 343, 379.

Bowditch, H. P. (1871): "Ueber die Eigenthümlichkeiten der Reizbarkeit, welche die Muskelfasern des Herzens zeigen", *Berichte d. math.-phys. säch. Gesellsch. d. Wissensch., Leipzig*, p. 662.

Bradley, S. E., Ingelfinger, F. J., Bradley, G. P., and Curry, J. J. (1945): "The estimation of hepatic blood flow in man", *J. clin. Invest.*, **24**, 890.

Brigden, W., and Sharpey-Schafer, E. P. (1950): "Postural changes in peripheral blood flow in cases with left heart failure", *Clin. Sc.*, **9**, 3.

Brod, J., and Fejfar, Z. (1950): "The origin of œdema in heart failure", *Quart. J. Med.*, **19**, 187.

Büchner, R. (1934): "Herzmuskelnekrosen durch hohe Dosen von Digitalis- glykosiden", *Arch. f. exper. Path. u. Pharmakol.*, **176**, 59.

Cathcart, R. T., and Blood, D. W. (1950): "Effect of digitalis on the clotting of the blood in normal subjects and in patients with congestive heart failure", *Circulation*, **1**, 1176.

Cheyne, J. (1818): "A case of apoplexy, in which the fleshy part of the heart was converted into fat", *Dublin Hosp. Rep.*, **2**, 216.

Christie, R. V., and Meakins, J. C. (1934): "The intrapleural pressure in congestive heart failure and its clinical significance", *J. clin. Invest.*, **13**, 323.

Cossio, P. (1952): "Ligation of the vena cava in the treatment of heart failure", *Amer. Heart J.*, **43**, 97.

——, and Perretta, A. (1949): "Inferior cava ligation and edema of the legs", *Rev. argent. de cardiol*, **16**, 293.

Cournand, A. (1952): "A discussion of the concept of cardiac failure in the light of recent physiologic studies in man", *Ann. intern. Med.*, **37**, 649.

——, and Ranges, H. A. (1941): "Catheterisation of the right auricle in man", *Proc. Soc. exp. Biol. and Med.*, **46**, 462.

Danielopolu, D. (1946): "La digitale et les strophantines", Paris, Masson et Cie.

De Graff, A. D., Batterman, R. C., and Lehman, R. A. (1938): "The influence of theophylline upon the absorption of mercupurin and salyrgan from the site of intramuscular injection", *J. Pharmacol. exp. Therap.*, **62**, 26.

De Vries, A. (1946): "Changes in hemoglobin and total plasma protein after injection of mercurophylline", *Arch. intern. Med.*, **78**, 181.

Dock, W. (1946): "Sodium depletion as a therapeutic procedure: the value of ion-exchange resins in withdrawing sodium from the body", *Tran. Ass. Amer. Phys.*, **59**, 282.

——, and Frank, N. R. (1950): "Cation exchanges: their use and hazards as aids in managing edema", *Amer. Heart J.*, **40**, 638.

Drinker, C. K. (1945): "Pulmonary edema and inflammation", Harvard University Press, Cambridge.

Eyster, J. A. E. (1906): "Clinical and experimental observations on Cheyne- Stoke's respiration", *Johns Hopk. Hos. Bull.*, **8**, 232.

Fishberg, A. M. (1939): "Hypertension and nephritis", 4th ed., London.

Foltz, E. L., Rubin, A., Steiger, W. A., and Gazes, P. C. (1950): "The effects of intravenous aminophylline upon the coronary blood oxygen exchange", *Circulation*, **2**, 215.

Foster, C. A., and Naylor, P. F. D. (1951): "Sensitivity to mercurial diuretics", *Lancet*, **i**, 614.

Frank, O. (1895): "Zur Dynamik des Herzmuskels", *Zrschr. f. Biol.*, **32**, 370.

Friedman, B., Resmik, H. Jr., Calhoun, J. A., and Harrison, T. R. (1935): "Effect of diuretics on the cardiac output of patients with congestive heart failure", *Arch. intern. Med.*, **56**, 341.

——, Daily, W. M., and Sheffield, R. (1953): "Orthostatic factors in pulsus alternans", *Circulation*, **8**, 864.

Friedman, C. E. (1950): "The residual blood of the heart", *Amer. Heart J.*, **39**, 397.

Friedman, M., and Bine, R. (1948): "Observations concerning the influence of potassium upon the action of a digitalis glycoside (lanatoside C)", *Amer. J. med. Sc.*, **214**, 633.

Gallavardin, L. (1913): "Pseudo-deboublement du deuxième bruit du coeur simulant de doublement mitral", *Lyons Méd.*, **121**, 409.

Gaskell, W. H. (1882): "On the rhythm of the heart of the frog, and on the nature of the action of the vagus nerve", *Phil. Trans. Roy. Soc.*, **173**, 993.

Gibson, A. G. (1907): "The significance of a hitherto undescribed wave in the jugular pulse", *Lancet*, ii, 1380.

Gold, H., Otto, H., Kwit, N. T., and Satchwell, H. (1938): "Does digitalis influence the course of cardiac pain? A study of 120 selected cases of angina pectoris", *J. Amer. med. Ass.*, **110**, 859.

Goldberg, H., Elisberg, E. I., and Katz, L. N. (1952): "The effects of the Valsalva-like maneuver upon the circulation in normal individuals and patients with mitral stenosis", *Circulation*, **5**, 38.

Gorlin, R., and Robin, E. D. (1955): "Cardiac glycosides in the treatment of cardiogenic shock", *Brit. med. J.*, i, 937.

Gross, H., and Spark, C. (1937): "Coronary and extra-coronary factors in hypertensive heart failure", *Amer. Heart J.*, **14**, 160.

Hall, G. E., Ettinger, G. H., and Banting, F. G. (1936): "An experimental production of coronary thrombosis and myocardial failure", *Canad. med. Ass. J.*, **34**, 9.

——, Manning, G. W., and Banting, F. G. (1937): "Vagus stimulation and the production of myocardial damage", *Canad. med. Ass. J.*, **37**, 314.

Harrison, T. R. (1935): "Failure of the circulation", Baltimore.

——, (1935): "The pathogenesis of congestive heart failure", *Medicine*, **14**, 255.

Harvey, R. M., Ferrer, M. I., Cathcart, R. T., Richards, D. W. Jr., and Cournand, A. (1949): "Some effects of digoxin upon the heart and circulation in man", *Amer. J. Med.*, **7**, 439.

Hayward, G. W. (1948): "Tetraethyl ammonium bromide in hypertension and hypertensive heart failure", *Lancet*, i, 18.

—— (1955): "Pulmonary œdema", *Brit. med. J.*, i, 1361.

Henderson, Y. (1906): "Volume curve of the ventricles of the mammalian heart and the significance of the curve in respect to the mechanics of the heart beat and the filling of the ventricles", *Amer. J. Physiol.*, **16**, 325.

Hering, H. E. (1908): "Das Wesen des Herzalternans", *Munch. med. Wschr.*, **55**, ii, 1417.

Heyer, H. E., Holman, J., and Shires, G. T. (1948): "The diminished efficiency and altered dynamics of respiration in experimental pulmonary congestion", *Amer. Heart J.*, **35**, 463.

Hickam, J. B., and Cargill, W. H. (1948): "Effect of exercise on cardiac output and pulmonary arterial pressure in normal persons and in patients with cardiovascular disease and pulmonary emphysema", *J. clin. Invest.*, **27**, 10.

Hope, J. (1832): "A treatise on the diseases of the heart", London.

Howarth, S., McMichael, J., and Sharpey-Schafer, E. P. (1947): "Effects of oxygen, venesection and digitalis in chronic heart failure from disease of the lungs", *Clin. Sc.*, **6**, 187.

Howell, W. H., and Donaldson, F. (1884): "Experiments upon the heart of the dog with reference to the maximum volume of blood sent out by the left ventricle in a single beat", *Philosophical Tr. London*, part 1, 154.

Karell, P. (1866): "De la cure de lait", *Arch. gén. Méd.* (6th series), **8**, 513.

Katz, L. (1954): "The mechanism of cardiac failure", *Circulation*, **10**, 663.

Kaufman, R. E. (1948): "Immediate fatalities after intravenous mercurial diuretics", *Ann. intern. Med.*, **28**, 1040.

Kempner, W. (1944): "Treatment of kidney disease and hypertensive vascular disease with rice diet", *North Carolina med. J.*, **5**, 125.

——, (1946): "Some effects of the rice diet treatment of kidney disease and hypertension", *Bull. N.Y. Acad. Med.*, **22**, 358.

Kopelman, H., and Lee, G. de J. (1951): "The intrathoracic blood volume in mitral stenosis and left ventricular failure", *Clin. Sc.*, 10, 383.

Kyser, F. A., Ginsberg, H., and Gilbert, N.C. (1946): "The effect of certain drugs upon the cardiotoxic lesions of digitalis in the dog", *Amer. Heart J.*, 31, 451.

Levine, S. A. (1948): "Auscultation of the heart", *Brit. Heart J.*, 10, 213.

Lewis, T. (1925): "The mechanism and graphic registration of the heart beat", London.

—— (1933): "Diseases of the heart", 1st ed., London and New York, The Macmillan Co.

Liljestrand, G. (1948): "Regulation of pulmonary arterial blood pressure", *Arch. intern. Med.*, 81, 162.

Lown, B., Salzberg, H., Enselberg, C. D., and Weston, R. E. (1951): "Interrelation between potassium metabolism and digitalis toxicity in heart failure", *Proc. Soc. exper. Biol. and Med.*, 76, 797.

Mackenzie, J. (1907–8): "The extrasystole; a contribution to the functional pathology of the primitive cardiac tissue", *Quart. J. Med.*, 1, 481.

—— (1913): "Diseases of the heart", 3rd ed., London, Henry Frowde and Hodder & Stoughton.

Mann, T., and Keilin, D. (1940): "Sulphanilamide as a specific inhibitor of carbonic anhydrase", *Nature*, 146, 164.

McCance, R. A., and Widdowson, E. M. (1946): "The chemical composition of foods", London.

McMichael, J. (1937): "Postural changes in cardiac output and respiration in man", *Quart. J. Exper. Physiol.*, 27, 55.

—— (1939): "Hyperpnœa in heart failure", *Clin. Sc.*, 4, 19.

—— (1947): "Circulatory failure studied by means of venous catheterisation", *Advances in Internal Medicine*, 2, 64.

—— (1948): "Pharmacology of the failing human heart", *Brit. med. J.*, 1, 927.

—— (1952): "Dynamics of heart failure", *Brit. med. J.*, ii, 525.

——, and Sharpey-Schafer, E. P. (1944): "The action of intravenous digoxin in man", *Quart. J. Med.*, 13, 123.

——, —— (1944): "Cardiac output in man by a direct Fick method", *Brit. Heart J.*, 6, 33.

——, and Sherlock, S. P. V. (1945): "Jaundice in heart failure", *Quart. J. Med.*, 14, 222.

Maurer, F. W. (1940): "Effects of decreased blood oxygen and increased blood carbon dioxide on flow and composition of cervical and cardiac lymph", *Amer. J. Physiol.*, 131, 331.

Merrill, A. J. (1946): "Œdema and decreased renal blood flow in patients with chronic congestive heart failure. Evidence of forward failure as primary cause of œdema", *J. clin. Invest.*, 25, 389.

——, and Cargill, W. H. (1947): "Forward failure: the mechanism of cardiac œdema formation in subjects with normal or high cardiac outputs", *J. clin. Invest.*, 26, 1190.

——, —— (1948): "The effect of exercise on the renal plasma flow and filtration rate of normal and cardiac subjects", *Ibid.*, 27, 272.

——, Morrison, J. L., and Brannon, E. S. (1946): "Concentration of renin in renal venous blood in patients with chronic heart failure", *Amer. J. Med.*, 1, 468.

Miller, W. H., Dessert, A. M., and Roblin, R. O. Jr. (1950): "Heterocyclid sulphonamides as carbonic anhydrase inhibitors", *J. Amer. Chem. Soc.*, 72, 4893.

Miller, W. S. (1937): "The Lung", London.

Moyer, J. H., Handley, C. A., and Wilford, I. (1952): "Results over a two-year period on three experimental diuretics administered orally to patients with cardiac failure", *Amer. Heart J.*, 44, 608.

Myers, J. D., and Hickam, J. B. (1948): "An estimation of the hepatic blood flow and splanchnic oxygen consumption in heart failure", *J. clin. Invest.*, 27, 620.

Novack, P., et al. (1953): "Studies of the cerebral circulation and metabolism in congestive heart failure", *Circulation*, 7, 724.

Nylin, G. (1943): "On the amount of and changes in the residual blood of the heart", *Amer. Heart J.*, **25**, 598.

—— (1945): "The dilution curve of activity in arterial blood after intravenous injection of labeled corpuscles", *Amer. Heart J.*, **30**, 1.

Ohm, R. (1913): "Venenpuls und Herztone", *Dtsch. Med. Wsch.*, **39**, 1493.

Olson, R. E., and Schwartz, W. B. (1951): "Myocardial metabolism in congestive heart failure", *Medicine*, **30**, 21.

Owen, S. G., and Wood, P. (1955): "A new method of determining the degree or absence of mitral obstruction", *Brit. Heart J.*, **17**, 41.

Peabody, F. W., Meyer, A. L., and Dubois, E. F. (1916): "Clinical calorimetry. XVI. The basal metabolism of patients with cardiac and renal disease", *Arch. intern. Med.*, **17**, 980.

Perera, G. A., and Berliner, R. W. (1943): "Postural hemodilution and paroxysmal dyspnœa", *J. clin. Invest.*, **22**, 25.

Peterson, L. H. (1950): "Some characteristics of certain reflexes which modify the circulation", *Circulation*, **2**, 351.

Plotz, M. (1947): "Bronchial spasm in cardiac asthma", *Ann. intern. Med.*, **26**, 521.

Potain, P. C. (1876): "Concerning the cardiac rhythm called gallop rhythm", *Bull. et mém. soc. méd.d.Hôp. de Paris*, **12**, 137.

Pugh, L. G. C., and Wyndham, C. L. (1949): "The circulatory effects of mercurial diuretics in congestive heart failure", *Clin. Sc.*, **8**, 11.

Raaschou, F. (1954): "Liver function and hypertension. Blood pressure and heart weight in chronic hepatitis", *Circulation*, **10**, 511.

Resnik, H. Jr., and Friedman, B. (1935): "Studies on the mechanism of the increased oxygen consumption in patients with cardiac disease", *J. clin. Invest.*, **14**, 551.

Richards, D. G. B., Whitfield, A. G. W., Arnott, W. M., and Waterhouse, J. A. H. (1951): "The lung volume in low output cardiac syndromes", *Brit. Heart J.*, **13**, 381.

Rushmer, R. F., and Thal, N. (1952): "Changes in configuration of the ventricular chambers during the cardiac cycle", *Circulation*, **4**, 211.

Scadding, J. G., and Wood, P. H. (1939): "Systolic clicks due to left-sided pneumothorax", *Lancet, ii*, 1208.

Schroeder, H. A. (1941): "Studies on congestive heart failure", *Am. Heart J.*, **22**, 141.

—— (1949): "Renal failure associated with low extracellular sodium chloride; low salt syndrome", *J. Amer. med. Ass.*, **141**, 117.

Sharpey-Schafer, E. P. (1944): "Cardiac output in severe anæmia", *Clin. Sc.*, **5**, 125.

—— (1948): Personal communication.

—— (1955): "Effects of Valsalva's manœuvre on the normal and failing circulation", *Brit. med. J.*, *i*, 693.

Sherlock, S. (1951): "The liver in heart failure. Relation of anatomical, functional and circulatory changes", *Brit. Heart J.*, **13**, 273.

Smith, F. M., Rathe, H. W., and Paul, W. D. (1935): "Theophylline in treatment of disease of coronary arteries", *Arch. intern. Med.*, **56**, 1250.

Smith, H. W. (1951): "The kidney; structure and function in health and disease", New York, Oxford University Press.

Sodeman, W. A., and Burch, G. E. (1938): "The precipitating causes of congestive heart failure", *Amer. Heart J.*, **15**, 22.

Starling, E. H. (1918): "The law of the heart beat" (Linacre lecture), Longman's, London.

Stead, E. A., Hickman, J. B., and Warren, J. V. (1947): "Mechanism for changing the cardiac output in man", *Tr. A. Amer. Phys.*, **60**, 74.

——, Warren, J. V., and Brannon, E. S. (1948): "Cardiac output in congestive heart failure", *Amer. Heart J.*, **35**, 529.

Stewart, H. J., Deitrick, J. E., Crane, N. F., and Wheeler, C. F. (1938): "Action of digitalis in uncomplicated heart disease", *Arch. intern. Med.*, **62**, 569.

——, ——, ——, and Thompson, W. P. (1938): "Action of digitalis in compensated heart disease", *Arch. intern. Med.*, **62**, 547.

Stokes, W. (1854): "The diseases of the heart and aorta", 1st ed., Dublin.

Straub, H. (1917): "Dynamik des Herzalternans", *Deutsch. Archiv. klin. Med.*, **123**, 403.

Traube, L. (1872): "Ein Fall von Pulses Bigeminus nebst Bermerkungen uber die Leberschwellungen bei Klapperfehlern und uber acute Leberatrophie", *Berl. klin. Wochenschr.*, **9**, 185.

Travell, J., Gold, H., and Modell, W. (1938): "Effect of experimental cardiac infarction on response to digitalis", *Arch. intern. Med.*, **61**, 184.

Vogl, A. (1932): "Erfahrungen über Euphyllin bei Cheyne-Stokes und anderon Formen Zentraler Atemstörung", *Med. Klinik*, **28**, 9.

——, (1950): "The discovery of the organic mercurial diuretics", *Amer. Heart. J.*, **39**, 881.

Volini, I. F., and Levitt, R. O. (1939): "Studies on mercurial diuretics: II. The immediate effect on the venous blood pressure", *Amer. Heart J.*, **17**, 187.

Von Issekutz, B., and Von Végh, F. (1928): "Ueber die diuretische Wirkung Organischer Quecksilberverbindungen", *Arch. f. exper. Path. u. Pharmakol.*, **138**, 245.

Waife, S. O., and Pratt, P. T. (1946): "Fatal mercurial poisoning following prolonged administration of mercurophylline", *Arch. intern. Med.*, **78**, 42.

Warren, J. V., and Stead, E. A., Jr. (1944): "Fluid dynamics in chronic congestive heart failure; interpretation of mechanisms producing œdema, increased plasma volume and elevated venous pressure in certain patients with prolonged congestive failure", *Arch. intern. Med.*, **73**, 138.

Wechsler, R. L., Kleiss, L. M., and Kety, S. S. (1950): "The effects of intravenously administered aminophylline on cerebral circulation and metabolism in man", *J. clin. Invest.*, **29**, 28.

Weitzman, D. (1955): "The mechanism and significance of the auricular sound", *Brit. Heart J.*, **17**, 70.

Wiggers, C. J., and Katz, L. N. (1920): "The selective effect of the accelerator nerves on ventricular systole", *Proc. Soc. exper. Biol. and Med.*, **17**, 94.

Withering, W. (1785): "An account of the foxglove and some of its medicinal uses: with practical remarks on dropsy and other diseases", Swinney, Birmingham.

Wood, P. H. (1936): "The erythrocyte sedimentation rate in diseases of the heart", *Quart. J. Med.*, **5**, 1.

—— (1936): "Right and left ventricular failure. A study of circulation time and venous blood pressure", *Lancet*, ii, 15.

—— (1940): "The action of digitalis in heart failure with normal rhythm", *Brit. Heart J.*, **2**, 132.

——, and Paulett, J. (1949): "The action of digitalis on the venous pressure", *Ibid.*, **11**, 83.

CHAPTER VIII

CONGENITAL HEART DISEASE

CONGENITAL heart disease is found in about 0.35 per cent of all live births, and in 0.1 per cent of all who survive infancy (MacMahon *et al.*, 1953); it accounts for 1 to 2 per cent of all cases of organic heart disease (Brown, 1939).

It is very rarely hereditary, although dextrocardia, familial cardiomegaly, coarctation of the aorta and atrial septal defect occasionally provide exceptions to this rule. Twins, whether dizygotic or identical, are rarely both affected. A familial factor is perhaps less uncommon, especially in relation to atrial septal defect (Courter *et al.*, 1948) and patent ductus.

The commonest known cause of congenital heart disease is undoubtedly some maternal illness or metabolic upset during the first three months of pregnancy. Rubella at this time, for example, was clearly implicated by Gregg (1941) and Swan (1943); it has been said to account for about 4 per cent of all cases of congenital heart disease (Conte *et al.*, 1945), especially ventricular septal defect and patent ductus (Wesselhoeft, 1949). Cataract, deafness, and mental deficiency from microcephaly are often associated. According to Swan (1949) a woman contracting rubella during the first four months of pregnancy has a three to one chance of giving birth to a congenitally defective infant. The period from the fifth to the eighth week is most critical with regard to the development of the heart. Other maternal virus infections at this time may also be culpable, e.g. mumps (Grönvall and Selander, 1948) and influenza (Landtman, 1948).

Other congenital abnormalities are found in 10 to 20 per cent of cases (the higher figures being reported from autopsy series, the lower from clinical series), especially arachnodactyly, mongolism, hyperteleorism, deformities of the chest and accessory nipples.

About one third of all cases of *arachnodactyly* (fig. 8.01) have congenital heart disease (Rados, 1942), especially atrial septal defect and hypoplasia of the aorta (Reynolds, 1950). From Brown's study of the literature some 20 per cent of *mongols* have congenital heart disease (Brown, 1950), chiefly ventricular septal defect (Silvy, 1934; Evans, 1950) and atrial septal defect due to persistent ostium primum (Abbott, 1927).

Hyperteleorism (fig. 8.02) is being noted with increasing frequency (Bonham-Carter, 1955), especially, perhaps, in association with fibroelastosis and pulmonary stenosis with reversed interatrial shunt.

Deformities of the chest were recorded by Campbell and Reynolds (1949) in no less than 40 per cent of 332 cases of congenital heart disease, mainly cyanotic. Pigeon chest, Harrison's sulcus, and prominence of the ribs usually on the left side but sometimes on the right or bilateral, occurred with equal frequency.

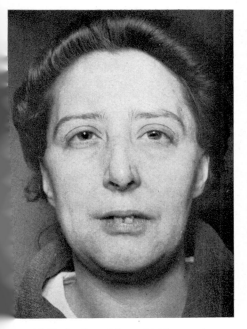

(a) Facies (note bilateral iridectomy).

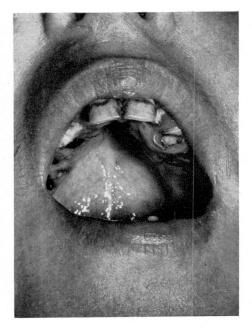

(b) Showing high arched palate and deformed teeth.

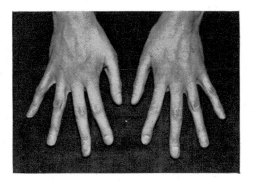

(c) Spider fingers.

Fig. 8.01—A case of arachnodactyly.
This patient was 6 ft. high and also showed hypotonia, scoliosis, and flat feet.

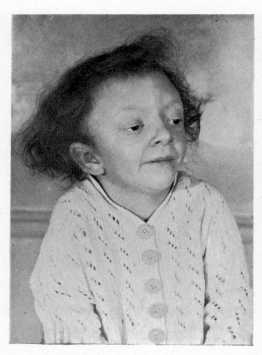

Fig. 8.02—Hyperteleorism in a case of pulmonary stenosis with reversed interatrial shunt.

CLASSIFICATION

It has been customary to divide congenital heart disease into acyanotic and cyanotic forms, and to subdivide the latter into types with permanent cyanosis (morbus cœruleus or blue babies) and types with late, terminal or transient cyanosis (cyanose tardive). This has never proved entirely satisfactory, and a new classification is therefore offered. It was based originally on a series of 200 proved clinical cases (Wood, 1950), and takes function into account. The series has since increased to 900 and the relative incidence of each type is now given in the table. These figures do not apply to infants, many of whom die during the first year of life.

NO SHUNT					
GENERAL		LEFT-SIDED		RIGHT-SIDED	
	per cent		per cent		per cent
Dextrocardia . .	0.5	Aortic atresia . .	rare	Ebstein's anomaly of the tricuspid valve* . . .	1.0
Familial cardio-megaly . .	rare	Aortic hypoplasia .	0.5		
		Aortic incompetence	0.5		
Friedreich's disease	rare	Aortic rings . .	rare	Idiopathic dilatation of the pulmonary artery . . .	1.0
Gargoylism . .	rare	Aortic stenosis . .	3.0		
Heart block . .	1.5	Coarctation of the aorta . . .	9.0	Pulmonary stenosis (isolated):	
Von Gierke's disease	rare	Cor triatriatum .	rare	infundibular .	2.0
		Fibroelastosis . .	rare	valvular . .	10.0
		Left coronary artery arising from pulmonary artery	rare		
		Mitral stenosis . .	rare		
		Right-sided aortic arch (isolated) .	rare		
Total . . .	2.0	Total . . .	13.0	Total . . .	14.0

* Some cases are cyanotic.

WITH SHUNT	
ACYANOTIC LEFT TO RIGHT SHUNT (pulmonary plethora)	CYANOTIC RIGHT TO LEFT SHUNT

	per cent		per cent
Left ventricular enlargement		DIMINISHED PULMONARY BLOOD FLOW	
Patent ductus	13.0	NORMAL OR LOW P.A. PRESSURE	
Aorto-pulmonary septal defect	0.3	*Left ventricular enlargement*	
		Tricuspid atresia . . .	1.5
Right ventricular enlargement		Anomalous drainage of S.V.C.	
Atrial septal defect . . .	18.0	or I.V.C. into left atrium .	rare
A.S.D. with pulmonary steno-		Single ventricle with pulmo-	
sis	2.0	nary stenosis . . .	rare
Anomalous pulmonary venous		*Right ventricular enlargement*	
drainage (partial) . .		Fallot's tetralogy . .	11.0
		Pulmonary atresia . .	1.7
Enlargement of both ventricles		Pulmonary stenosis with re-	
Ventricular septal defect .	8.0	versed interatrial shunt .	3.0
V.S.D. with pulmonary steno-		HIGH P.A. PRESSURE	
sis	1.3	Pulmonary hypertension with	
		reversed shunt:	
		i. Patent ductus . .	2.0
		ii. Ventricular septal defect	
		(Eisenmenger's com-	
		plex)	3.0
		iii. Atrial septal defect .	1.5
		Cor triloculare biatriatum* .	rare
		INCREASED PULMONARY BLOOD FLOW	
		Transposition of the great	
		vessels	1.0
		Persistent truncus . . .	rare
		Total anomalous pulmonary	
		venous drainage into S.V.C.	
		or R.A.	rare
Miscellaneous . 3.7 per cent		Cor biventriculare triloculare .	rare
Total	42.6	Total	24.7

* Some cases may have pulmonary plethora.

DEXTROCARDIA

Mirror image dextrocardia is usually but not invariably associated with complete transposition of the viscera. The heart is functionally and structurally healthy. The electrocardiogram, for obvious reasons, shows reversal of all complexes in lead 1 with leads 2 and 3 interchanged (fig. 8.03).

The diaphragm is always lower on the cardiac side of the chest, its position not being influenced by the location of the liver or stomach.

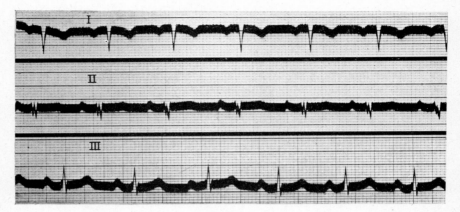

Fig. 8.03—Electrocardiogram showing reversal of all complexes in lead I, while leads II and III are interchanged.

IDIOPATHIC HYPERTROPHY OF THE HEART

Under this heading in the past were grouped a heterogenous collection of cardiopathies in infancy which bore little or no relationship to one another, and which for the most part have since been defined in more precise terms. The group included examples of von Gierke's disease, anomalous left coronary artery arising from the pulmonary artery, isolated myocarditis, thyroid deficiency, nutritional cardiopathy in infants born of diabetic mothers, and fibroelastosis. Nothing would be gained by discussing "idiopathic hypertrophy" as an entity in itself.

FAMILIAL CARDIOMEGALY

From time to time, cases of cardiac enlargement are encountered in young subjects, for which there is as yet no adequate explanation. They are prone to paroxysmal tachycardia and atrial fibrillation, and on examination there is often diastolic gallop. X-rays show considerable cardiac enlargement, particularly of the left ventricle (fig. 8.04). Left bundle branch block is usually found. These patients are apt to die suddenly, presumably from ventricular fibrillation, or by degrees from congestive heart failure when still relatively young.

Some of these cases appear to have a familial basis (Addarii *et al.*, 1946; Evans, 1947 and 1949). Necropsy reveals myocardial fibrosis and compensatory hypertrophy of muscle. Von Gierke's disease, isolated myocarditis, nutritional cardiopathies, Friedreich's disease, and abnormal coronary vessels must be excluded.

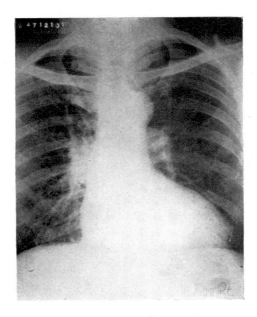

Fig. 8.04—Unexplained cardiac enlargement in a relatively young man (there was also left bundle branch block).

FRIEDREICH'S ATAXIA

Cardiac manifestations associated with Friedreich's ataxia were first noted in five of six cases reported by Friedreich himself in 1863. Degeneration of muscle fibres, interstitial fibrosis and compensatory hypertrophy of remaining muscle are the usual pathological findings, the left ventricle being chiefly involved, and the picture being not unlike that of familial cardiomegaly.

In the majority there are no cardiac symptoms, but the electrocardiogram may show flat or inverted T waves chiefly in antero-lateral left ventricular surface leads or their equivalents or bundle branch block (Evans and Wright, 1942). In a minority there are paroxysmal rhythm changes, usually atrial tachycardia or fibrillation, and occasionally there is fatal congestive heart failure (Russell, 1946).

CONGENITAL HEART BLOCK

It has long been thought that congenital heart block was related to ventricular septal defect, the association being accepted in 30 out of 44 cases reviewed by Yater, Lyon and McNabb (1933), four of them proved at necropsy. At that time, however, ventricular septal defect was diagnosed far too readily (Wood *et al.*, 1954), and there is little doubt that the relationship has been over-emphasised. Thus routine electrocardiography in 200 cases of ventricular septal defect seen by Brown (1950) did not reveal heart block in a single instance. In a personal series of 72 cases of isolated ventricular septal defect proved by modern methods, heart block occurred only once, and in 162 cases in which ventricular septal defect was associated with other anomalies, it also occurred only once. Conversely, ventricular septal defect was not present in 13 out of a consecutive series of 15 cases of congenital complete heart block, although it had been diagnosed previously in several of them.

Congenital heart block is complete and permanent twice as often as it is partial or variable (Aitken, 1932). Although congenital complete heart block does not differ radically from acquired heart block (q.v.), it has several characteristic features of its own.

1. It is present from birth and rarely may be familial (Wendkos and Study, 1947).
2. The resting ventricular rate is usually faster, averaging 50 beats per minute (range 36 to 80).
3. The rate commonly increases by about 33 per cent after a sub-cutaneous injection of atropine gr. 1/75 (Aitken, 1932), or on effort (Campbell and Suzman, 1934).
4. In view of the faster rate and its increase on exercise effort tolerance may be almost normal and the heart but little enlarged.
5. Stokes-Adams fits are rare according to Brown (1950), although Janet Aitken (1932) tabulated syncopal attacks of unspecified nature in 18 per cent of the 39 cases she reviewed. None of my own series of 15 cases has had a Stokes-Adams seizure, and only one of the eight described by Campbell and Suzman (1934) had genuine attacks. It should be remembered that heart block may be acquired in cases of congenital heart disease, including ventricular septal defect, and Stokes-Adams fits may certainly occur then, as in the case reported by Rogers and Rudolph (1951).
6. A functional mitral diastolic murmur due to the large mitral stroke blood-flow was heard in over three-quarters of the present series, particularly when the rate was under 50, and was accentuated when the atria contracted synchronously with the period of rapid ventricular filling; it should not be misinterpreted as evidence of active rheumatic valvulitis.
7. The QRS complex of the electrocardiogram is normal, bundle branch block complexes at once suggesting an acquired lesion. Inverted T waves in antero-lateral chest leads over the left ventricle are not necessarily sinister in congenital heart block and may become upright on exertion (fig. 8.05).

The prognosis of uncomplicated cases of congenital complete heart block is believed to be good if the ventricular rate is over 50, and still fairly

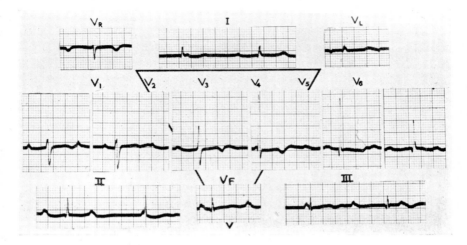

(a) At rest, showing inverted T waves in chest leads.

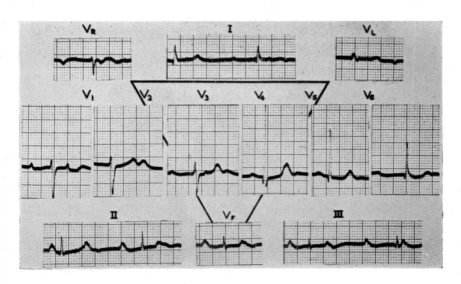

(b) After effort: the rate is unchanged, but the T waves are now upright.

Fig. 8.05—Congenital heart block with a ventricular rate of 48 beats per minute.

good if the rate is between 40 and 50. The oldest in the present series was 39, and two of the others were over 30. Sudden unexpected deaths have occurred, however, and perhaps one should be a little guarded.

Treatment, when necessary, is the same as for acquired cases, but is rarely indicated.

VON GIERKE'S DISEASE

General enlargement of the heart, sooner or later resulting in sudden death or congestive failure, may be due to glycogen storage in the myocardial muscle fibres as well as in the liver, kidneys, and other organs (Von Gierke, 1929). Although few cases survive childhood, Von Gierke's disease has been reported occasionally in adults, even as late as the fifth decade. It is characterised by hepatomegaly, retardation of growth and sexual development, persistent ketosis with acetonuria, hypercholesterolæmia, raised blood glycogen (normal 12–20 mg. per cent), low fasting blood sugar, and a flat blood sugar curve following the subcutaneous injection of 0.25 to 0.5 mg. of adrenalin, due to failure of mobilisation of glycogen (Ellis and Payne, 1936; Crawford, 1946). Some cases are familial. When the heart is involved, microscopy reveals heavily vacuolated muscle fibres, which when specially stained are seen to be filled with glycogen. It is believed that Von Gierke's disease is due to deficiency of one or more of the enzymes, such as liver phosphatase, that are indispensable to the breakdown of glycogen to glucose (Cori, 1952).

GARGOYLISM

Another rare congenital metabolic disorder involving the heart is gargoylism. Here there is a widely distributed abnormal storage of a macromolecular glycoprotein in parenchymal, fibroblastic and other connective tissue cells (Lindsay, 1950). Gargoyles are mentally retarded, large-headed, pot-bellied dwarfs with deep guttural voices, deafness, coarse heavy features, large tongues, abundant hair and other skeletal peculiarities. Of 26 cases in the literature the heart was involved in 85 per cent (Emanuel, 1954). There was usually interstitial myocardial fibrosis and thickening of the valves—chiefly the mitral, less frequently the aortic, sometimes the tricuspid, and rarely the pulmonary (as in rheumatic heart disease). Many of the cases died from heart failure.

FIBROELASTOSIS

One of the relatively common causes of sudden death or rapidly fatal congestive heart failure in infancy is what is now termed fibroelastosis. Affected infants may appear to be normal at birth, but within a few weeks or months suddenly develop attacks of dyspnœa and cyanosis due to acute left ventricular failure, and either die suddenly in an attack or more gradually in a state of congestive failure (Adams and Katz, 1952). The condition may occur alone or in conjunction with coarctation of the aorta, aortic stenosis, aortic atresia, or mitral stenosis, and is characterised by enlargement of the left ventricle overlying a uniformly thick dense white endocardium. Bonham-Carter (1955) has stressed its association with

aortic system by the aorto-pulmonary septum which divides the truncus into anterior and posterior halves: the anterior half becomes the ascending aorta, the posterior the pulmonary artery. The division of the truncus extends cranially to a point just beyond the anterior ends of the sixth pair of arches, the mouths of which are included in the posterior section and therefore in the pulmonary system. On the right side the sixth arch becomes the right pulmonary artery and loses its connexion with the right dorsal aorta; on the left it becomes the left pulmonary artery and preserves its connexion with the left dorsal aorta in the form of the ductus arteriosus. While these changes are going on, harmonious alterations take place in the ventral and dorsal aortas. In front the two ventral aortas fuse into a single ascending aorta, as already indicated. Behind, the dorsal aortas undergo considerable modification: the upper part forms a portion of the internal carotid artery, as previously described; the segment between the third and fourth arches disappears; caudal to the fourth arch the dorsal aorta disappears on the right side, except for that part of it which is incorporated in the right subclavian artery, and forms the posterior part of the aortic arch on the left side. The left subclavian artery links up with the left dorsal aorta just below the junction of the sixth arch, i.e. just below the ductus.

Many anomalies may result from faulty development of this aortic system. Thus, the caudal part of the right dorsal aorta may persist, so that there are two aortic arches; or the caudal part of the left dorsal aorta may disappear in favour of the right, so that the final aortic arch is right-sided. The most important, however, is partial obliteration of that part of the left dorsal aorta which lies between the fourth and sixth arches, i.e. just above the ductus, or between the sixth arch and the point of fusion of the two dorsal aortas, i.e. just below the ductus. This short segment of the aorta is often called the isthmus on account of the frequency with which it is narrowed; but in coarctation or isthmus stenosis narrowing is extreme and often remarkably abrupt. There are said to be two main types, infantile and adult (Bonnet, 1903). In the former (fig. 8.07a) the constriction is above the ductus, which remains patent and carries venous blood to the descending aorta: it is incompatible with more than a few years of life. In the latter (fig. 8.07b)

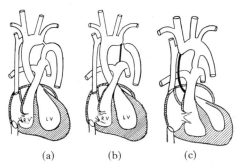

(a)   (b)   (c)

Fig. 8.07—Diagrams illustrating the three main types of coarctation of the aorta.
(a) Infantile type with patent ductus feeding the descending aorta.
(b) Common adult type.
(c) Aortic atresia with patent ductus feeding the whole systemic circulation.

the ductus is closed, or if patent the constriction is below it, so that it plays no part in compensating for the defect. Aortic atresia with a patent ductus feeding the whole systemic circulation (fig. 8.07c) constitutes a third type (Bramwell, 1947), but such cases all die in infancy. Other variants of these three main types have been described by Evans (1933).

This simple anatomical classification, however, is no longer satisfactory, for it does not tally with the physiological facts and is of little practical help to the surgeon. In the first place, the pressure in the descending aorta is maintained by blood flowing into the aorta from collateral channels and by the peripheral vascular resistance, not by the small quantity of blood passing through the stricture; thus, it is not altered by obliterating the coarctation altogether. Secondly, if a patent ductus joins the aorta below the stricture, blood ordinarily flows from aorta to pulmonary artery, as in the adult type with patent ductus, for the pressure in the descending aorta is far higher than that in the pulmonary artery, even when the stricture is totally occluded. In a typical case of this sort investigated by the author the pressure was 150/90 in the brachial artery, 95/80 in the descending aorta, and 45/27 in the pulmonary artery. The catheter was passed through the ductus and emerged into the descending aorta below the coarctation. The shunt was undirectional from aorta to pulmonary artery, samples from the right brachial artery and descending aorta were 95 and 93 per cent saturated with oxygen respectively; the pulmonary blood flow was 12 litres per minute, or about twice the systemic flow. When a patent ductus, joining the aorta below the stricture, actually supplies the descending aorta with venous blood, it can only do so because the pulmonary vascular resistance is equal to or greater than the systemic resistance, i.e. about eight times higher than normal. This occurs in 10 to 15 per cent of all cases of patent ductus, and is an essential part of the Eisenmenger syndrome (q.v.), but it is not due to the coarctation. Bonnet's infantile type of coarctation therefore becomes pulmonary hypertension with reversed aorto-pulmonary shunt with coincidental coarctation of the aorta above the ductus. It is also undesirable and unhelpful to include aortic atresia in any classification of coarctation of the aorta, for it is an entirely separate entity. On the other hand, the site of the stricture is of the greatest importance. It is proximal to the left subclavian artery in about 2 per cent of cases (Abbott, 1928; Reifenstein et al., 1947), and low, usually below the diaphragm, in about 2 per cent (vide infra).

In presubclavian coarctation the left arm may be under-developed; palpable collateral vessels and rib notching, if present, occur only on the right side; and X-rays do not show the elongated shadow of a dilated left subclavian artery above the aortic knuckle. The anatomical arrangement can be seen clearly with the aid of angiocardiography or retrograde aortography via the right radial artery. Such cases have so far been considered unsuitable for surgical repair.

Low coarctation comprises a small group of cases in which the stricture is in the descending thoracic aorta, well below the usual site, or in the abdominal aorta, above or below the renal arteries. The group probably includes cases of local arteritis, including periarteritis, and that form which has been described in young women usually under the title "pulseless disease" or Takayasu's disease (Caccamise and Whitman, 1952). A short segment of the aorta is thickened and indurated, and its lumen greatly reduced. The history and subsequent course, with the development of similar lesions in major peripheral arteries, especially the subclavians, reveal the true nature of such cases. At least one of the two cases described by Bahnson *et al.* (1949) seemed to be of this type, and one of four abdominal "coarctations" in my own series is probably inflammatory (also in a young woman). But true congenital coarctation of the abrupt type can certainly occur below the diaphragm, as in the 12-year-old girl with hypertensive heart failure described by Kondo and his colleagues (1950). The distinguishing clinical features of low coarctation include a coarctation murmur best heard over the lumbar spine or anteriorly through the abdominal wall, no palpable collateral vessels, rib notching which is either absent or limited to the last two or three ribs, and a normal or unfolded aortic arch radiologically. Hypertension has been present in nearly all cases reported, but the lesion has usually been above or has involved the renal arteries. Surgical repair should be undertaken if technically feasible.

A second anatomical point of practical importance is whether the coarctation is elongated or abrupt, for this may determine whether or not a graft is necessary.

Then, if associated congenital anomalies are to be taken into account, mitral stenosis, fibroelastosis, bicuspid aortic valve, aortic incompetence, and aortic stenosis each deserves as much consideration as patent ductus (*vide infra*). The commonest cause of death from coarctation in infancy, for example, is left ventricular failure from fibroelastosis (Bonham-Carter, 1955): this combination, therefore, has more justification to be entitled the infantile type of coarctation than Bonnet's type with a patent ductus.

On the whole, therefore, coarctation of the aorta might be better classified quite simply, according to its site, nature, and associated anomalies, thus:

CLASSIFICATION

SITE	NATURE	ASSOCIATED ANOMALIES

1. Presubclavian.
2. Isthmus.
3. Lower dorsal.
4. Subphrenic.
	Abrupt.
	Elongated.
	Hooked.
		1. Fibroelastosis.
		2. Bicuspid aortic valve
		   (Aortic incompetence).
		3. Aortic stenosis.
		4. Patent ductus (with):
		   i. Direct shunt.
		   ii. Reversed shunt.
		5. Mitral stenosis.

Hæmodynamics. The clinical features of the adult form of coarctation depend upon the mechanical effect of the constriction and upon the development of an extensive collateral circulation. Much use is made of the branches of the subclavian artery, e.g. the superior intercostal, and the internal mammary, with its intercostal, superior epigastric, and musculo-phrenic rami; also of the thoracic and subscapular branches of the axillary artery. These vessels link up with the intercostal branches of the descending aorta, and with the inferior epigastric branches of the femoral arteries, and so by-pass the constriction. The blood pressure is elevated in vessels arising from the aorta above the isthmus; below it the pulse pressure is much reduced, systolic and diastolic pressures oscillating gently around a mean which is nearly always well below the mean brachial pressure (fig. 8.08), but which may be slightly raised, normal or low compared with

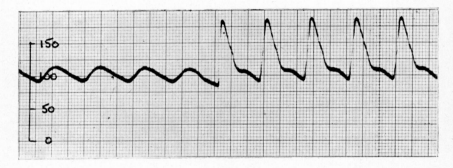

Fig. 8.08—Femoral and brachial pressure pulses in a case of coarctation of the aorta.

average normal controls. The cause of the hypertension is uncertain. A raised mean pressure in the legs does not support the mechanical hypothesis. Renal ischæmia was blamed by Rytand (1938) on the grounds that hypertension was only produced experimentally when the aorta was constricted above the origin of the renal arteries; according to Friedman, Selzer and Rosenblum (1941), the renal blood flow is appreciably reduced in coarctation, although glomerular filtration is normal. In acute experiments in dogs the mean pressure in the legs is always reduced (Gupta and Wiggers, 1951).

Incidence

Coarctation occurred in 9 per cent of a personal series of 900 cases of congenital heart disease. It is said to be 4 to 5 times more frequent in men than in women (Abbott, 1928; Reifenstein *et al.*, 1947), but the ratio was only 2 to 1 in the author's series, and also in the 270 cases seen by Gross (1953). The oldest case in the literature died at the age of 92 years (quoted by Abbott, 1928). Most cases seen are young adults, the anomaly being discovered as a result of mass radiography. About 1 per cent of cases appear to be hereditary or familial, although very few such instances have been published (Taylor and Pollock, 1953). One of my patients, for example, a married woman of 34 (now 37), had a brother with coarctation who died from cerebral hæmorrhage at the age of 17, and a male cousin with coarctation who died from dissecting aneurysm or aortic rupture at the age of 37.

CLINICAL FEATURES

Symptoms

Two-thirds of clinical cases are free from all symptoms when first seen. They are commonly well-developed young men who have experienced no discomfort even on strenuous exercise. Minor symptoms include *epistaxis* (6 per cent), *headaches* (6 per cent), or discomfort from *throbbing in the neck*. *Migraine* occurs in only 2 per cent despite the frequency of mal-formed cerebral vessels. "*Rheumatism*", especially round the shoulder girdle, attributed to pressure effects from dilated collateral arteries, was mentioned in no less than eight of Bramwell's 26 cases, but occurred in only 3 per cent of the author's series, despite a routine leading question. A history of rheumatic fever was obtained in 5 per cent, which is the same as in controls. *Intermittent claudication* in the legs occurred in 5 per cent of 212 cases, combining the reports of Bramwell (1947), Christensen and Hines (1948) with my own. In one instance it interfered seriously with the career of a dancer. Although the measured blood flow in the legs is within normal limits at rest (Wakim, Slaughter and Clagett, 1948), it may not be so on effort, and it usually rises after surgical treatment (Bing *et al.*, 1948). The blood flow in the arms is usually elevated at rest and falls post-operatively.

Major symptoms are always due to complications, and will be discussed later.

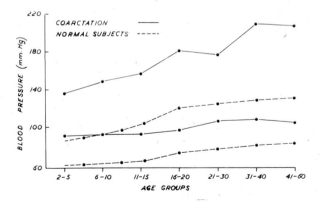

Fig. 8.09—Chart showing the relationship between blood pressure and age in cases of coarctation of the aorta compared with normal controls.

Physical signs

Excessive pulsation of the carotid arteries may be visible on inspection.

The blood pressure in the arms is raised moderately, and both systolic and diastolic levels rise gradually with the years, much as they do in normal subjects (fig. 8.09). There is no vicious circle mechanism because the renal vessels are protected. The blood pressure rises sharply on exercise, at least during the first few minutes, but probably no more than in patients with essential hypertension of similar degree. Diminished pulsation in the left subclavian artery may be due to presubclavian coarctation, an anomalous vessel, or compression from an aortic aneurysm. Diminished pulsation in the right subclavian is nearly always due to its having an anomalous origin.

The blood pressure in the legs is lower than in the arms in all but the mildest cases. Femoral pulsation is poor and at times impalpable (20 per cent). The small pulse is obviously delayed in 95 per cent of cases in which it can be felt. Direct arterial tracings reveal a wave form that looks grossly overdamped or not unlike the pattern of a mean arterial pressure (fig. 8.08).

In 21 cases investigated by Brown *et al.* (1948) at the Mayo Clinic, the pressure in the radial artery averaged 196/96, and in the femoral 113/81, whereas in controls they were identical; the onset of the femoral pulse was delayed by an average of 0.03 second, and the peak by 0.08 second. The mean pressure in the femoral artery is usually within normal limits, or may be a little low, but it is rarely raised. If the femoral arteries were palpated as a routine, very few cases of coarctation would be overlooked.

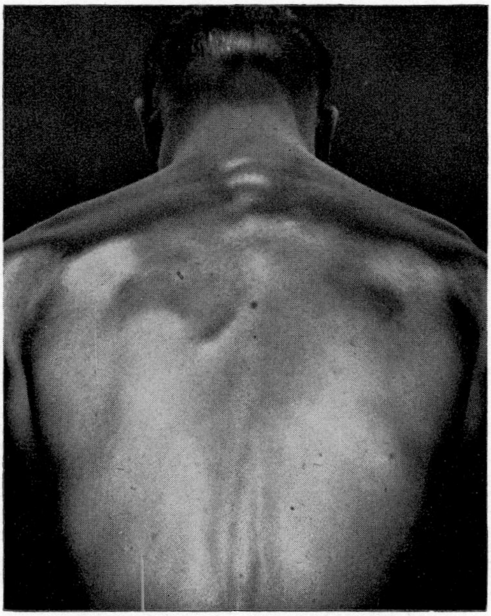

Fig. 8.10—A visible collateral anastomotic intercostal artery in a case of coarctation of the aorta.

Visible or palpable pulsation of collateral vessels, particularly in the interscapular region posteriorly (fig. 8.10), can be demonstrated in about 80 per cent of cases in the age groups usually seen (Christensen and Hines, 1949), but is unusual in small children. Tortuous and dilated intercostal vessels show up better if the patient bends forward with the arms hanging down—Suzman's sign (Campbell and Suzman, 1947).

The retinal arteries may be normal, tortuous or somewhat constricted, but serious hypertensive retinopathy does not occur.

Retinal hæmorrhages are seen occasionally, however, and subhyaloid hæmorrhage may accompany a subarachnoid bleed. Papillœdema at once points to a different etiology, as was substantiated in two of my cases.

The heart itself has all the usual features associated with moderate hypertension (q.v.). It is hypertrophied rather than dilated, and rarely fails in the absence of complications, at least under the age of 50 (Reifenstein *et al.*, 1947). The cardiac output in uncomplicated cases is normal (Bing *et al.*, 1948). Left ventricular failure in infancy is commonly due to associated fibroelastosis, and in older children or relatively young adults to aortic stenosis or incompetence, mitral valve disease, other congenital anomalies such as ventricular septal defect and patent ductus, or bacterial endocarditis (*vide infra*).

Auscultation

In uncomplicated cases an *aortic systolic murmur*, often initiated by an ejection click, is usually heard at the apex and base.

In practically one-third of my cases a *mitral diastolic murmur* was heard at the apex, indistinguishable in timing, pitch, intensity and duration from the Carey Coombs murmur of active rheumatic carditis (Wood, 1950). In arriving at this figure of 33 per cent, three cases of rheumatic mitral stenosis and five cases in which turbulence could have been due to an excessive mitral blood flow (three with patent ductus and two with ventricular septal defect) were excluded. It is inconceivable that a murmur heard so frequently could have been due to active rheumatic valvulitis, although this was believed to be the explanation in one instance: the erythrocyte sedimentation rate was practically never raised; subacute rheumatism, rheumatic fever, or chorea, past or present, was no more frequent than in controls (5 per cent); and the incidence of rheumatic mitral stenosis in adults with coarctation was only 2 per cent. A similar murmur may be heard in congenital aortic stenosis, and in both conditions slight thickening of the mitral cusps, due to minor fibroelastotic changes, provide a possible though purely speculative explanation. The murmur may or may not disappear after successful surgical treatment.

The third important murmur of uncomplicated coarctation is heard posteriorly between the scapulæ, and is due to the jet produced by the stricture. It may spill into diastole, as demonstrated phonocardiographically by Wells, Rappaport and Sprague (1949). It was heard high up in the typical situation in 85 per cent of the present series, and in four cases in which aortic stricture was proved to be subphrenic (only one of them thought to be congenital) the murmur was only heard posteriorly in the lumbar region and anteriorly through the abdominal wall. There is therefore strong evidence that the site of the posterior murmur at once distinguishes classical coarctation from the subphrenic variety. According to both Abbott (1928) and Reifenstein *et al.* (1947) there is complete occlusion of the aorta at the site of coarctation in about one-quarter of all cases that come to necropsy. It is not unlikely, therefore, that the 15 per cent of my series that did not have the murmur had complete occlusion. It is admitted that large collateral vessels may sometimes cause a murmur, for digital compression of such a vessel may abolish it; but this is exceptional, and as a rule the murmur cannot be influenced by digital compression of any of the palpable collateral arteries. That a coarctation jet may cause a murmur (and thrill) has been verified at operation.

Electrocardiogram

In the present series the electrocardiogram was strictly normal in 46 per cent, and showed slight left ventricular preponderance, as judged by the voltage of QRS, in 23 per cent. Marked left ventricular preponderance with inverted T waves in leads V_5 and V_6 occurred in 20 per cent, and three-quarters of these cases had well-developed aortic valve disease, usually stenosis. Thus in uncomplicated coarctation only 5 per cent of cases showed electrocardiographic evidence of serious left ventricular strain.

Right bundle branch block occurred in 11 per cent; only a quarter of this small group had a patent ductus, the other cases being straightforward. Ziegler (1954) suggested that right bundle branch block might represent a residual change from strong right ventricular preponderance in utero when the fœtal ductus joined the aorta above the stricture.

X-ray appearances

There are three virtually diagnostic X-ray signs of coarctation of the aorta: elongation of the aortic knuckle due to dilatation of the left subclavian artery (64 per cent), post-stenotic dilatation of a short segment of the descending aorta which can be seen clearly in the postero-anterior view (61 per cent), and notching of the inferior margin of the ribs (51 per cent). The figures given are from my own series.

Dilatation of the left subclavian artery also obliterates the supraaortic triangle in the second oblique position (Evans, 1952). Even when not distinguished clearly in the anterior view, it seems to change the outline of the aortic knob so that the latter rarely looks normal.

Post-stenotic dilatation of the proximal end of the descending aorta immediately below the stricture was described by Bramwell (1947) as a double aortic knuckle (fig. 8.11). It is a most important sign, for it shows the presence and site of the stricture itself.

Notching of the inferior margins of the ribs (fig. 8.12), known as Dock's sign, is due to pressure erosion from dilated intercostal arteries (Railsbach and Dock, 1929; Dock, 1948). In my series it was seen in only one fifth of children under 12 years of age; the youngest with notching was six. Its higher incidence in past literature (about 80 per cent) may be due to the fact that coarctation was frequently overlooked in children, and that notching of the ribs *per se* was perhaps the chief means of detecting it.

Enlargement of the left ventricle was relatively slight or radiologically absent in 85 per cent of the cases. Considerable enlargement was present

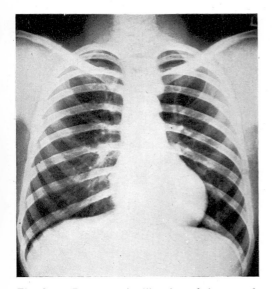

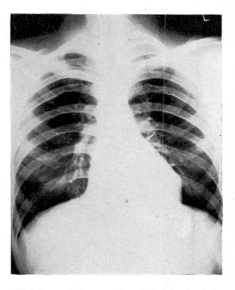

Fig. 8.11—Post-stenotic dilatation of the top of the dorsal aorta in a case of coarctation.

Fig. 8.12—Rib notching (Dock's sign) in coarctation of the aorta.

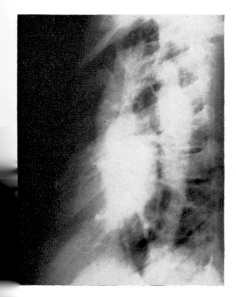

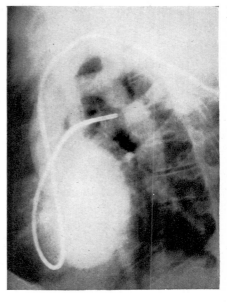

Fig. 8.13—Mild coarctation of the aorta demonstrated by means of angiocardio-graphy; there is post-stenotic dilatation of the proximal segment of the dorsal aorta and overlapping of proximal and distal segments owing to the plane in which the picture has been taken.

Fig. 8.14—The abrupt type of coarctation of the aorta demonstrated by selective angiocardiography, diaginol having been injected directly into the pulmonary artery through a wide-bore catheter.

337

in 15 per cent, but nearly all of these cases had serious aortic valve disease or were otherwise complicated.

Entirely normal X-ray appearances were seen in only 5 per cent of cases. Aortic aneurysm, usually mycotic and very close to the stricture, was seen in two instances.

The constriction itself (figs. 8.13–8.16) may be demonstrated clearly by means of angiocardiography (Grishman, Steinberg and Sussman, 1941), or retrograde aortography (Broden, Hanson and Karnell, 1948).

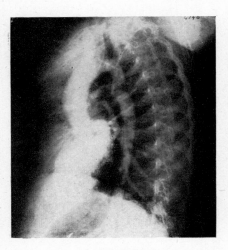

Fig. 8.15—Angiocardiogram demonstrating the hooked type of coarctation.

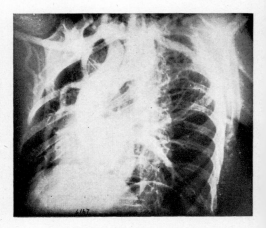

Fig. 8.16—Angiocardiogram in a case of coarctation of the aorta with complete occlusion, showing marked dilatation and tortuosity of collateral channels.

ASSOCIATED ANOMALIES

Bicuspid aortic valve occurred in 23.5 per cent of 200 autopsied cases reviewed by Abbott (1928), and in 42.3 per cent of 104 autopsied cases reviewed by Reifenstein, Levine and Gross (1947). It is the usual cause of the aortic diastolic murmur that has been heard so frequently—in 20 per cent of 96 cases reported by Christensen and Hines (1948), and in 10 per cent of the author's series. It was recorded phonocardiographically by Wills, Rappaport and Sprague (1949) in 5 out of 15 cases of coarctation. Aortic incompetence is rarely severe, however, unless bacterial endocarditis supervenes.

Significant aortic stenosis, presumably congenital, occurred in 7.5 per cent of the author's series, and calcific aortic stenosis was reported at necropsy in 11 per cent of the fatal cases collected from the literature by Reifenstein *et al.* (1947). The presence of calcium, however, does not invalidate a congenital etiology (Campbell and Kauntze, 1953). The stenosed valve is usually bicuspid (Smith and Matthews, 1955). It is by no means easy to be sure whether aortic stenosis is present or not in cases of coarctation with a basal systolic thrill and large left ventricle. A convincing anacrotic pulse is exceptional, the blood pressure is still raised, and the aortic second sound may be loud. An aortic systolic thrill without any other evidence of stenosis was appreciated in only three per cent of the series. Two other cases thought to have some degree of aortic stenosis, on account of considerable left ventricular enlargement and strong left ventricular preponderance electrocardiographically, in addition to the thrill, did not have a pressure gradient across the aortic valve at operation, although in one of them the central aortic tracing looked stenotic in form. Although the significance of a systolic thrill over the root of the aorta in cases of coarctation must remain in doubt, the fact remains that judged on other grounds, particularly on the size of the left ventricle and electrocardiographic evidence of left ventricular strain, 75 to 85 per cent of such cases have aortic stenosis.

The lesion is important because it increases the risk of surgical repair, and because such repair may be valueless unless aortic valvotomy is also undertaken.

Patent ductus arteriosus, with most of the usual clinical features, occurred in 7 per cent of my series. The shunt was always from left to right, whether the ductus joined the aorta above or below the stricture. Rib erosion and a demonstrable collateral circulation were evident in only one instance, their absence in the presence of patent ductus being noted by Bramwell (1947) in his three cases.

Four remarkably illustrative cases were published by Edwards *et al.* (1949): judged by the clinical features, the microscopical appearances of the small pulmonary vessels, and the relative sizes of the two ventricles at necropsy, there was pulmonary hypertension with reversed shunt in two of them, and a direct aorto-pulmonary shunt in the other two; the ductus joined the aorta above the coarctation in one of those with reversed shunt and in one with direct shunt, and it joined below the coarctation in one each of these two functionally different types also.

Patent ductus presents no special problem when complicating coarctation of the aorta in children or adults. It should be ligated or divided at the same time as the stricture is repaired, provided the shunt is from aorta to pulmonary artery; if the shunt is reversed both the ductus and the coarctation should be left alone.

Ventricular septal defect complicating coarctation of the aorta occurred in 2 per cent of this series and presents a rather similar physiological picture, the raised pressure in the left ventricle tending to increase the left to right shunt.

In a case investigated by the author and subsequently proved at necropsy, the mean pulmonary arterial pressure was 95 mm. Hg, whilst that in the right ventricle was 55 mm. Hg. Samples from the pulmonary artery were 86 per cent saturated with oxygen, from the middle of the right ventricle 70 per cent, and from the right atrium and superior vena cava 60 per cent. Clinically, coarctation of the aorta was recognised by the presence of high blood pressure in the carotid

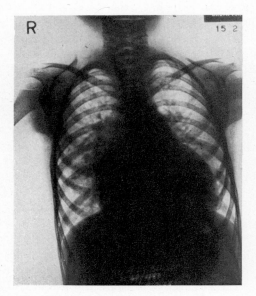

Fig. 8.17—Coarctation of the aorta associated with patent interventricular septum
proved at necropsy.

and subclavian arteries (160/100 mm. Hg in a boy of six) with an immeasurable
pressure in the legs, but there was little evidence of a collateral circulation. The
pulmonary arteries were grossly engorged radiologically (fig. 8.17), there was a
pulmonary diastolic murmur at the base, and a mitral diastolic murmur with
triple rhythm at the apex. Despite the absence of a machinery murmur, patent
ductus arteriosus was believed to be responsible for the shunt, and seemed to be
confirmed by the catheter findings, the raised oxygen content of the right
ventricular sample being attributed to pulmonary incompetence. At necropsy,
coarctation of the aorta of the adult type was associated with a large defect of the
membranous interventricular septum. The aortic cusps were normal, the aortic
ring admitted only the little finger, and the ascending aorta was small. The defect
in the septum admitted the middle finger, whilst the pulmonary ring admitted
both middle and fore-fingers. A very small patent ductus joined the aorta below
the isthmus. Although the huge pulmonary artery did not sit astride the septal
defect, there could be no doubt that the major portion of the left ventricular
contents was expelled into that vessel. The mitral diastolic murmur was clearly
functional, for there was no sign of mitral stenosis. Both ventricles were greatly
enlarged, the left retaining its natural dominance.

Fibroelastosis (q.v.) appears to be the chief cause of heart failure and
death in infants with coarctation of the aorta, and usually makes surgical
repair at that age pointless (Bonham-Carter, 1955). It seems to be rare in
the large number of cases that survive infancy. Whether a minor degree of
fibroelastosis is responsible for an unusual degree of left ventricular

enlargement in children, or for any of the aortic or mitral anomalies sometimes associated with coarctation, is unknown.

Variations in one or other subclavian artery, rarely both, occur in about 5 per cent of cases (King, 1937), and may be due to its anomalous or stenotic origin (East, 1932; Love and Holms, 1939). Presubclavian coarctation is a rare cause of a small pulse in the left arm.

COMPLICATIONS

Since practically all the important complications of coarctation of the aorta used to be fatal, their relative frequencies are known from previous necropsy studies. The figures from two carefully documented series in the literature, those by Abbott (1928) and by Reifenstein, Levine and Gross (1947) are tabulated below:

FREQUENCY OF COMPLICATIONS

CAUSE OF DEATH	ABBOTT (per cent)	REIFENSTEIN et al. (per cent)	AVERAGE AGE (years)
Aortic rupture (or dissection) . . .	20	23	25
Bacterial endocarditis (or endarteritis) .	16	22	29
Cerebral vascular accident . . .	12.5	11	28
Congestive heart failure	29	18	39
Incidental	22.5	26	47

Aortic rupture is through the ascending aorta in 80 per cent of the cases and just distal to the coarctation in the remainder. The ascending aorta is thin walled and "rupture" usually means dissection into the pericardium (Reifenstein *et al.*, 1947).

Bacterial endocarditis infecting a bicuspid aortic valve is three times more common than bacterial endarteritis involving the aorta immediately adjacent to the coarctation, usually just below it (Reifenstein *et al.*, 1947).

Saccular aneurysm of the descending aorta in the immediate neighbourhood of the stricture, usually just below it, is seen in about 3 per cent of cases (Abbott, 1928; Gross, 1953), and is nearly always secondary to bacterial endarteritis. There were two instances in the present series of 90 cases, both of which were due to previous bacterial endarteritis. Calcification in the wall of the aneurysm is the rule and occurred in each of the two mentioned. One of them had the coarctation and the aneurysm excised and successfully replaced with a graft by Sir Russell Brock.

Cerebral vascular accidents, usually subarachnoid hæmorrhage, may be due to rupture of a berry aneurysm or of a vessel weakened by defective or degenerative elastic tissue (Glynn, 1940). Similar defects may be found in other vessels, including the aorta (Davies and Fisher, 1943). Hypertension presumably encourages the disaster.

Heart failure is rare in uncomplicated cases under 40 years of age, but takes an increasing toll as age advances; even then some new complication may be responsible, as in two of three cases that were observed over a period of 25 to 30 years when the development of heart block precipitated the breakdown (Newman, 1948). As previously stated, heart failure in infancy is usually due to associated fibroelastosis, and in children or relatively young adults to aortic stenosis or incompetence, bacterial endo-carditis, other congenital anomalies such as patent ductus and ventricular septal defect, or coincidental rheumatic heart disease.

Mitral valve disease may complicate coarctation of the aorta, but probably not more often than would be expected from its known frequency of 2 per cent in the general population. Unquestionable rheumatic mitral stenosis occurred in only two of the series reported here, and in one of them Sir Russell Brock undertook mitral valvotomy at the same time as he successfully repaired the coarctation. Relatively mild organic mitral in-competence may be aggravated by the hypertension associated with coarctation, but this was only witnessed in one instance. Amongst the children there was only one convincing case of rheumatic valvulitis, in which a soft mitral diastolic murmur was heard for the first time after an attack of rheumatic fever. Congenital mitral stenosis was not observed in this particular series, but is a real, although rare, association.

Pregnancy in cases of coarctation deserves a note. The raised blood pressure may be discovered for the first time in an ante-natal clinic, and this is one of the standard ways in which the presence of coarctation comes to be recognised. Of 96 instances collected from the literature by Rosenthal (1955), including 5 of his own, 11 died during pregnancy, chiefly from aortic rupture just before or during labour.

PROGNOSIS AND TREATMENT

Although many patients live well into middle life without serious handi-cap, some even to the eighth decade, the majority succumb between the ages of 20 and 40 to one of the complications mentioned above (Abbott, 1928). The average age of death is 35 (Reifenstein, Levine and Gross, 1947). Surgical repair (Crafoord and Nylin, 1945; Crafoord, 1948) should therefore be offered. The physiological results of such an operation are usually good: the blood pressure falls, symptoms disappear, the heart becomes smaller, and it may be assumed that the risks of intracranial hæmorrhage, aortic rupture and late heart failure are diminished. Bacterial endocarditis on bicuspid aortic valves should not be prevented.

The constriction is excised and the two ends joined together by direct suture or by means of an aortic homograft (Gross, 1951). A patent ductus may be ligated or a post-stenotic mycotic aneurysm removed at the same time. The mortality rate attending the resection has fallen from 16 per cent in 1949 (Shapiro) to under 5 per cent. A series of papers by Gross (1949, 1950, 1953) illustrates this very well: by 1953 he had operated on 270 cases; in the first hundred of these (reported in 1950) there were eleven deaths, in the last hundred only two. Over the last five years our total surgical mortality rate at the Brompton hospital has been 8 per cent. According to Gross (1953), the optimum time for the operation is between the ages of 10 and 20 years, but 11 per cent of his cases were between 30 and 40 years old, and the blood pressure may fall to normal even at this age. Grafts become endothelialised, but remain inert. They seem capable of withstanding the blood pressure indefinitely.

Selection of cases for surgery

Now that the operative mortality rate is under 5 per cent, it is probably right to advise all patients with uncomplicated coarctation of the aorta to have it repaired between the ages of 7 and 30, the earlier the better. An exception should be made if the stricture is trivial, judged by a normal or near-normal blood pressure, good femoral pulsation without clinically detectable delay, and no collateral circulation clinically or radiologically. The diagnosis in these rare cases is made on the presence of a coarctation murmur posteriorly, and post-stenotic dilatation of the aorta radiologically; it may be confirmed by means of angiocardiography.

The effect of complications on the question of surgical treatment has already been discussed.

RIGHT-SIDED AORTA

As an isolated anomaly a right-sided aortic arch joining a right dorsal aorta is rare, and is discovered radiologically by chance (fig. 4.31). Its radiological features (Bedford and Parkinson, 1936) have already been described in Chapter IV. Clinically it is of no significance.

It may be important, however, when associated with other congenital anomalies, because its presence may help their identification. For example, a right-sided aorta occurs in some 20 per cent of cases of Fallot's tetralogy, but not in pulmonary stenosis with normal aortic root; again, it may occur in Eisenmenger's complex proper, but not in pulmonary hypertension with reversed shunt through a patent ductus or atrial septal defect.

AORTIC RINGS

During the development of the aortic system certain anomalies may arise which may compress the œsophagus or trachea and cause dysphagia or distressing attacks of wheezing and choking in infancy. Bronchopneumonia is a common complication and not infrequently fatal. If the infant survives, symptoms usually disappear as the vessels lengthen (Apley,

1949), but may return again with middle age owing to the development of arteriosclerosis (Sprague *et al.*, 1933). The chief anomalies responsible for this clinical syndrome are double aortic arch, aberrant right subclavian artery, and a ligamentum arteriosum joining a right aortic arch to the left pulmonary artery (Gross and Neuhauser, 1951). The vascular arrangements are varied (Edwards, 1948), but the three most common varieties may be described here.

In *double aortic arch* the primitive fourth right arch, which normally involutes distal to the innominate artery, persists and joins the primitive *left* dorsal aorta. Beyond the origins of the right subclavian and right common carotid arteries anteriorly, the anomalous vessel courses posteriorly behind the trachea and œsophagus and links up with the normal anterior arch below the origin of the left subclavian artery, where they join to become a left dorsal aorta. The effect is to encircle the trachea and œsophagus.

A *right-sided aortic arch crossing behind the œsophagus* to join a left dorsal aorta may constrict the œsophagus and trachea by being pulled forward by a patent ductus or ligamentum arteriosum connecting it to the left pulmonary artery (Neuhauser, 1949). It should be understood that an ordinary right-sided aortic arch joins the *right* dorsal aorta, the left dorsal root involuting, so that the completed aorta courses down the right side of the thorax and causes no trouble.

An *aberrant right subclavian artery* arises from the aorta distal to the left subclavian artery and passes across to the right and upwards behind the œsophagus, which it indents obliquely. The filling defect of the barium-filled œsophagus can be seen radiologically (Brean and Neuhauser, 1947). Lifelong dysphagia has been caused by this anomaly (Bayford, 1789).

All three anomalies may be modified surgically in such a way as to relieve the pressure on the trachea and œsophagus. In double aortic arch the anterior channel can be divided between the left common carotid and left subclavian arteries, a patent ductus or ligamentum arteriosum completing a vascular ring can be divided, and an aberrant subclavian artery can be divided, collateral pathways ensuring an adequate blood supply to the limb (Gross and Neuhauser, 1951).

The whole rather complicated subject has been well reviewed by Brown (1950).

AORTIC HYPOPLASIA

Hypoplasia of the aorta is a common manifestation of Marfan's syndrome (q.v.), as pointed out by Baer, Taussig and Oppenheimer (1942). Only the ascending aorta is usually involved, especially at its root within the pericardium. Pathologically, it presents initially with features indistinguishable from cystic medial necrosis, and later with degeneration and disruption of the elastic lamellæ, disorganised masses of hypertrophic and hyperplasic smooth muscle, and numerous dilated vascular channels penetrating the media from the adventitia (McKusick, 1955). At first it is clinically unrecognisable, unless the ascending aorta looks peculiarly small. Sooner or later, however, dilatation of the aortic ring may lead to free aortic incompetence, the ascending aorta may become obviously dilated, or the aorta may rupture or dissect without warning, usually into the pericardial sac.

Coarctation of the aorta is rarely associated with arachnodactyly, but the pathological appearances of the ascending aorta in cases of aortic rupture or dissection secondary to coarctation are similar to those described above.

Occasionally, hypoplasia of the aorta is seen without any such associations, and in rare instances hypoplasia and dilatation of the pulmonary artery accompany it (fig. 8.18). The case illustrated was in a man of 33 with no symptoms and no abnormal physical signs; cardiac catheterisation also revealed nothing abnormal.

In these days of mass radiography, difficulty may be experienced in trying to interpret the significance of an unusually prominent aorta as an isolated finding in a young individual. The attitude advised is to take a serious view of any such anomaly if there is any trace of Marfan's syndrome in the family, or if the apparent dilatation ceases abruptly at the origin of the innominate artery; if neither condition applies the peculiarity may be better disregarded for the time being and treated as a normal variation.

CONGENITAL AORTIC INCOMPETENCE

Aortic incompetence may be due to a bicuspid or quadricuspid aortic valve (*vide infra*), especially under the stress of hypertension, whether acquired or due to associated coarctation of the aorta; anomalous aortic valve cusps, however, may leak without any complication, sometimes quite freely.

The second important cause of congenital aortic incompetence is dilatation of the root of the ascending aorta, as seen characteristically in Marfan's syndrome (q.v.). The leak in these cases is usually considerable, and may be already well advanced at a time when the radiologically visible part of the ascending aorta still looks normal. The prognosis in such cases is poor, the risks being aortic rupture or dissection and heart failure.

A third and rare cause of congenital aortic incompetence is ventricular septal defect (q.v.).

BICUSPID AORTIC VALVE

Abbott (1932) estimated the incidence of bicuspid aortic valve at 1.3 to 1.4 per cent. Owing to the frequency of superimposed infection or sclerosis it is often difficult to be sure microscopically whether a disorganised valve is congenitally bicuspid or not, but Lewis and Grant (1923) put its microscopic recognition on a firm basis.

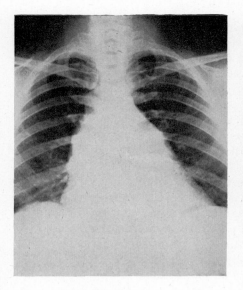

(a) Anterior view.

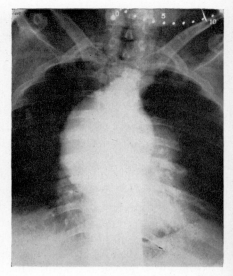

(b) Angiocardiogram demonstrating dilatation of the aorta.

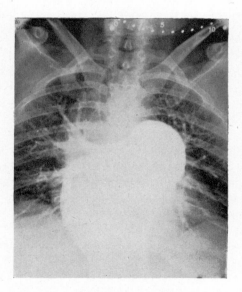

(c) Angiocardiogram showing dilatation of
the pulmonary artery.

Fig. 8.18—Idiopathic dilatation of both the aorta and pulmonary artery resulting from
hypoplasia of these vessels.

At the time of Abbott's review 46 per cent of 147 proved cases and 21 per cent of 316 proved or probable cases of bicuspid aortic valve had coarctation of the aorta. Conversely, she calculated that 28.5 per cent of cases of coarctation had a bicuspid aortic valve. Its significance in this condition has already been described.

Apart from its association with coarctation, bicuspid aortic valve is clinically important for three main reasons: (1) it may leak spontaneously or as a result of acquired hypertension, an insidious sclerosing process increasing this tendency; (2) about one-quarter of all cases become infected sooner or later; (3) an associated weakness of the sinuses of Valsalva may lead to aneurysmal dilatation or rupture.

AORTIC ATRESIA

Clinically this is unimportant since it is rarely compatible with more than a few days of life (Roberts, 1936); it is also very uncommon (Brown, 1950). Pulmonary hypertension with reversed shunt through a patent ductus allows venous blood to be transported to the systemic circulation. Oxygenated blood can only escape from the lungs via broncho-pulmonary anastomotic venous channels unless there is an atrial septal defect or anomalous pulmonary venous drainage. Even with a large atrial septal defect the situation is wholly unsatisfactory, for if a proper systemic output is to be maintained, the pulmonary vascular resistance must be very high, and this must prevent an adequate pulmonary blood flow. According to Horley (1955) all reported cases have had fibroelastosis of the left ventricle unless the interventricular septum has been patent. He suggests that both the complete fusion of the aortic cusps and the fibroelastosis may be due to anoxia resulting from the temporary formation of a complete impenetrable interatrial septum during some period of its development.

AORTIC STENOSIS

Pathology

Congenital aortic stenosis may be valvular due to fusion of the cusps, or subvalvular due to defective absorption of the primitive bulbus cordis; in the latter type a perforated membrane lies proximal to the valve (Keith, 1924). Although in Abbott's necropsy series of 1,000 cases of congenital heart disease, aortic valve stenosis was present in 11 and subaortic stenosis in 12 (Abbott, 1931 and 1951), it is now generally believed that the great majority of cases are valvular. All degrees of severity are encountered, and it is probable that some of the relatively mild cases end up with calcific stenosis when they may be mistaken for rheumatic strictures (Campbell and Kauntz, 1953). Even at necropsy it may be very difficult, if not impossible, to make certain of the etiology when infective or sclerosing processes have grossly distorted the whole structure of the valve. It is not possible clinically to distinguish the two types of congenital aortic stenosis.

Incidence

Aortic stenosis accounted for 3 per cent of the 900 cases of congenital heart disease in this series. There were three males to one female, as in Campbell's series. A congenital etiology was accepted if a loud aortic systolic murmur was first heard in infancy, if any other congenital anomaly was present, if there was a strongly suggestive family history such as that described by Davies (1952), or if an obviously tight stricture was found in childhood in the absence of a history of rheumatism or chorea.

Clinical features

Although the clinical features of congenital aortic stenosis are more or less similar to those of acquired rheumatic stenosis (q.v.), there are minor points of difference that deserve emphasis.

Of the 30 patients in the author's series, only five of whom were over 18 years old, symptoms were absent in 18, slight in two and moderate in five. None had frank left ventricular failure. Only one had angina pectoris and only two had syncopal attacks on effort. For the most part, therefore, aortic stenosis is well tolerated in those that survive infancy; infant mortality, however, is high, the average age of death in Abbott's series, for example, being 3.75 years, and this must account for the rarity of severe cases in later childhood and adolescence.

Of the well-known physical signs of aortic stenosis (q.v.), the peripheral pulse was normal in 15, small but not otherwise characteristic in 12, and detectably anacrotic in only three. The left ventricle was a little heaving clinically in two-thirds (but rarely displaced much to the left), normal or a little bulky radiologically (but not dilated) in 86 per cent, and hypertrophied electrocardiographically in two-thirds (considerably so with inverted T waves in leads V_5 and V_6 in a quarter). A loud aortic systolic ejection murmur, usually heard as well at the apex as at the base, and always accompanied by a well-marked thrill, was heard in all; and since our attention was drawn to it by Leatham (1954) an aortic ejection click has also been heard in all but one instance. The second heart sound was split normally in half the cases, A_2 falling before P_2; it was clinically single in a third, however, due to delay in the aortic component, and the split was reversed in two instances. When single, the second sound could usually be well heard over the carotid and over the left ventricle at the apex beat, as well as at the base, from which the presence of the aortic element was inferred. An aortic diastolic murmur was heard in only 10 per cent, which contrasts rather strongly with the 45 per cent incidence of associated aortic incompetence in the series reported by Campbell and Kauntz (1953); but this may be a matter of selection, for we were at first disinclined to accept a diagnosis of congenital aortic stenosis in the presence of obvious incompetence. A soft mitral diastolic murmur, indistinguishable from that heard in many cases of coarctation of the aorta, was detected in one-sixth of this small series.

The electrocardiogram provided the best evidence of the degree of left ventricular hypertrophy and has already been referred to.

The X-ray appearances were very similar to those described by Campbell and Kauntz (1953). The ascending aorta is usually a little prominent and curved out to the right, but the aortic knuckle is normal or inconspicuous. The left ventricle looks dense and hypertrophied rather than dilated, so that the cardiothoracic ratio is not much increased.

Cardiac catheterisation in six relatively mild cases revealed normal pulmonary artery pressures, normal arteriovenous oxygen differences (average 32 ml. per litre), and of course normal cardiac outputs.

Prognosis

Severe cases usually die in infancy. The majority of those seen in childhood are mild or relatively so and have a good prognosis. Precise figures are difficult to arrive at in view of uncertainty concerning etiology in old calcific cases of aortic stenosis. A minority, in which the stenosis is more severe, may die suddenly when young, especially those with a history of angina pectoris or syncope on effort (Marquis and Logan, 1955).

TREATMENT

Aortic valvotomy should be advised when serious symptoms begin to develop in severe cases.

MITRAL STENOSIS

Congenital mitral stenosis is exceptionally rare, being found in only six of Abbott's 1,000 cases. Three examples are included in my own series of 900 clinical cases, one of them confirmed at operation. Out of 43 collected from the literature by Ferencz, Johnson and Wigleworth in 1948 (to which they themselves contributed nine) only eight were isolated; by far the most common association was fibroelastosis (25), next came patent ductus (17), then aortic valvular stenosis (12), coarctation of the aorta (7) and ventricular septal defect (2). The great majority died in infancy.

The clinical features appear to be similar to those of rheumatic mitral stenosis, but are usually modified by the associated lesion. In those who survive infancy the commonest associated lesions are patent ductus and coarctation of the aorta.

Mitral valvotomy is advised if the symptoms warrant it, although it may be awkward technically owing to difficulty in recognising exactly where the commissures should be. D'Abreu undertook the operation in two cases, one of which had a patent ductus (Bower *et al.*, 1953), and Sir Russell Brock operated on one for me, ligating a patent ductus at the same time.

The increased pulmonary blood flow from the patent ductus might be expected to cause death from pulmonary œdema at an early age in these cases, but in the patient mentioned, a girl of 19, the pulmonary vascular resistance was high, and cyanosis from shunt reversal began when she was only 18 months old, and may well have saved her life. Cyanosis on effort increased a little over the years, and was sufficiently differential to cause no clubbing of the fingers, but at least moderate clubbing of the toes; the hæmoglobin was 104 per cent; there was, of course, no Gibson murmur, the physical signs being those of mitral stenosis with moderate pulmonary hypertension, and X-rays showing a combination of pulmonary venous congestion and slight plethora. Cardiac catheterisation (when she was 17 years old) revealed an indirect left atrial pressure of 18 mm. Hg above the sternal angle, a pulmonary artery pressure of 96/58 (rising to 130/90 on effort), a simultaneous right brachial pressure of 120/60, and bidirectional shunt, the pulmonary artery sample being 74 per cent saturated, the right ventricular sample 65 per cent and the right brachial 87 per cent. Unfortunately no femoral sample could be obtained at the time, but from our experience of reversed shunts in patent ductus (confirmed by means of angiocardiography in this case), the femoral sample could hardly have been above 80 per cent saturated. The pulmonary blood flow worked out at 6 litres per minute, and the pulmonary vascular resistance at 10 units. It was argued that although shunt reversal was taking place, the pulmonary blood flow was still above normal, the pulmonary resistance was only borderline between high and extreme, and that if the left atrial pressure were lowered the left to right shunt would increase. It was decided, therefore, to advise ligating the duct as well as mitral valvotomy. At operation the mitral orifice measured 1.25 × 0.75 cm., and the duct 1.5 cm. long and 1.5 cm. wide, both much as predicted.

A year later she was looking and feeling well, there was no cyanosis and no evidence of right ventricular embarrassment, while her effort tolerance had increased considerably. There were still well-marked signs of mitral stenosis, however, for a complete valvotomy had not been achieved owing to the technical difficulty mentioned earlier.

COR TRIATRIATUM

A physiological situation very similar to that produced by congenital mitral stenosis may be caused by the anomalous development of a transverse septum which separates that part of the left atrium joined by the pulmonary veins from the rest of the chamber. In the case reported by Barnes and Finlay (1952), the anomalous septum was perforated by a small hole measuring only 2 mm. in diameter, through which the whole cardiac output had to pass. There was intense pulmonary venous congestion, but no evidence of mitral stenosis. Pedersen and Therkelsen (1954) described a similar case in which cardiac catheterisation revealed typical evidence of mitral stenosis; at operation the mitral valve was normal and the anomalous septum was overlooked.

IDIOPATHIC DILATATION OF THE PULMONARY ARTERY

Mass radiography brings an increasing number of cases for cardiological review on account of real or apparent dilatation of the pulmonary artery as an isolated abnormality. Quite a number of such cases can be dismissed

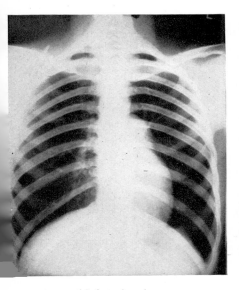 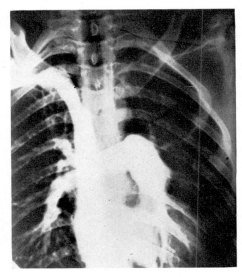

(a) Anterior view.   (b) Angiocardiogram.

Fig. 8.19—Apparent dilatation of the pulmonary artery in a normal subject.

immediately as variants of normal or as rotational effects (fig. 8.19). In the example illustrated the left pulmonary artery is responsible for the left middle arc, and the angiocardiogram proves that the pulmonary artery is not dilated (cf. fig. 8.16c). There remain, however, a small group of cases in which the pulmonary artery is undoubtedly dilated for no apparent reason (Laubry, Routier and de Balsac, 1941).

There are no symptoms and no abnormal physical signs in uncomplicated cases, except a pulmonary ejection click, which is common, and a soft pulmonary systolic murmur, which is perhaps less common. The second heart sound is physiologically split and the pulmonary component of average intensity. The electrocardiogram is normal. Angiocardiography is the only reliable way of proving the existence of true dilatation (fig. 8.16c).

Cardiac catheterisation, whilst demonstrating essentially normal pressures and flows, not infrequently reveals a slight systolic pressure gradient of 5 to 10 mm. Hg across the pulmonary valve; the right ventricular pressure, however, is not above normal. The significance of this phenomenon, which was recorded consistently in four out of eight such cases catheterised, and which was noted by Cournand, Baldwin and Himmelstein (1949), is not yet understood. Trivial pulmonary valve stenosis is difficult to exclude, and in some of the cases the tracings themselves are unsatisfactory and suggest an artefactual gradient.

Functional pulmonary incompetence may complicate cases of idiopathic dilatation, and despite the normal pressure in the pulmonary artery may be considerable in degree. Conspicuous dilatation of the right ventricle results and the electrocardiogram may show prolonged right ventricular activation. Secondary tricuspid incompetence and final overloading of the right ventricle may complete the breakdown. Admittedly such cases are rare, but they may serve to correct an impression that pulmonary incompetence is always harmless in the absence of a high pulmonary vascular resistance.

"Idiopathic" dilatation of the pulmonary artery is occasionally due to the same abiotrophy that affects the ascending aorta in cases of Marfan's syndrome, and in these rare cases has been known to rupture. A good example of the double lesion is illustrated in fig. 8.18.

EBSTEIN'S DISEASE

A rare anomaly, of which there were ten examples in the present series, all diagnosed during life, is malformation and displacement of the tricuspid valve (Ebstein, 1866). With greater precision in diagnosis an increasing number of live cases are coming to light. Helpful reviews are those by Yater and Shapiro (1937), Engle *et al.* (1950), Baker *et al.* (1950) and Medd *et al.* (1954).

Pathology

The anterior cusp always retains some attachment to the annulus fibrosus, but the posterior loses its connection entirely and is attached to the walls of the right ventricle (Brown, 1950). The cusps themselves are also grossly malformed and present a curious basket-like arrangement that is difficult to describe. The right ventricle and atrium are grossly dilated, the infundibulum distal to the valve usually less so. The foramen ovale is patent and functions in varying degree in about two-thirds of the cases.

Clinical features

Males and females are affected equally. There were six males and four females in the present series.

Ages vary greatly according to the severity of the lesion, and range from early childhood to 80. The ages of my patients when first seen were 13, 15, 25, 28, 18 months, 14, 4, 5, 22, and 53.

Symptoms are remarkably mild in relation to the size of the heart shadow radiologically and have been overrated in the literature. Cyanosed cases have gravitated to special clinics in the hope of obtaining relief by means of cardiac surgery, and after an unsuccessful operation or otherwise have tended to find their way into the medical press. Thus the general impression seems to be that Ebstein's disease is a cyanotic form of congenital heart disease; yet of the ten new cases reported here, only one presented as such, although the patient herself denied it, and only one of three other cases that I catheterised for my colleagues was centrally cyanosed clinically. Many of these acyanotic cases are still being overlooked and continue to masquerade under a motley variety of diagnoses.

Effort intolerance was negligible in four of my cases, slight (grade 1) in four, and moderate (grade 2A) in the other two. None were in the least disabled, except during attacks of paroxysmal tachycardia (*vide infra*). In the worse cases dyspnœa and fatigue limit physical activity.

Attacks of faintness accompanied by intense cyanosis are probably due to paroxysmal tachycardia, but they are unusual. Baker *et al.* (1950) found only two examples in some 25 clinical records in the literature. In a case that I observed, intense cyanosis accompanied paroxysmal *nodal* tachycardia that caused giant venous cannon waves and obvious reversed inter-atrial shunt (fig. 6.33). With normal rhythm the venous pressure oscillated gently around sternal angle level (fig. 8.22) and central cyanosis was only just apparent (denied by the patient).

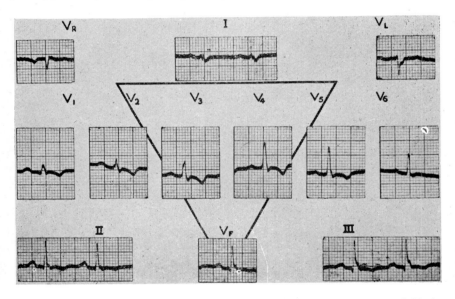

Fig. 8.20—Electrocardiogram in Ebstein's disease showing a right bundle branch block pattern and rather low voltage.

Physical signs

The physical signs are highly characteristic, and together with the electrocardiogram and X-ray appearances usually make the bedside diagnosis obvious.

1. Central cyanosis at rest, clubbing and polycythæmia *are usually absent*. Only one of my ten cases had these features. A second had doubtful cyanosis at rest, but no clubbing. Three had a highly coloured moon facies, peripheral cyanosis, and no clubbing. The other five looked entirely normal. The majority of cases in the literature have been cyanosed from birth or have developed cyanosis in childhood or adolescence. The discrepancy is attributed to selected material.

2. The peripheral pulse is usually small and the blood pressure rather low, figures around 110/80 being typical.

3. The venous pressure and pulse are of two kinds: they are either inconspicuous, the pressure being around or below sternal angle level, with *a*, *c*, and *v* of rather low amplitude (fig. 8.22), or they have the features of tricuspid incompetence (fig. 8.23); giant *a* waves were *not* seen in any of my cases, and a moderate *a* wave, about 3 mm. Hg above *v*, in only two instances. The literature is not at its best in respect of the clinical venous pulse in Ebstein's disease, but on the whole the findings seem to have been similar.

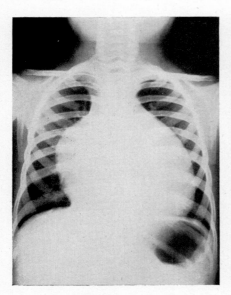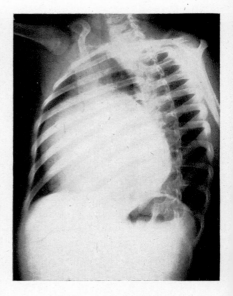

(a) Anterior view.   (b) Second oblique position.

Fig. 8.21—Typical skiagram in a case of Ebstein's disease showing gross dilatation of the right ventricle and atrium and clear lung fields.

4. *The heart is quiet.* On two occasions cases of pulmonary valve stenosis were referred as ? Ebstein's disease when there was a grade 3 right ventricular heave; on another occasion a case of Ebstein's disease was referred as ? severe pulmonary valve stenosis when no cardiac impulse could be felt anywhere. No convincing impulse could be felt over the right ventricle in any of these ten cases; in one there was slight retraction. A gentle localised left ventricular impulse was felt far out towards the axilla in at least three instances; the point was not always recorded, however—there was merely the statement that the heart felt unusually quiet.

5. On auscultation most observers have commented on the frequency of gallop rhythm, the extra sound being a right ventricular third heart sound. Right atrial gallop is very unusual. If the P-R interval is prolonged right atrial contraction may accentuate the third heart sound.

6. The moderately loud—presumably pansystolic—murmur that was heard over a wide area in about 80 per cent of cases in the literature, accompanied by a thrill in three of my patients, may be attributed to tricuspid incompetence.

7. A very characteristic superficial diastolic scratch, giving the cadence of triple rhythm (disregarding the gallop sound) was heard in all but two cases in this series, and has been mentioned in about half the recorded cases in which auscultatory details have been given. It is usually heard best close to the sternum in the third left space, but in two of my cases it was louder *well to the right of the sternum* at the same level. It sounds more like diastolic pericardial friction over the distended right atrium than a true intracardiac murmur, occurring at a time when the right atrial pressure falls steeply: maximal right atrial movement due to volumetric change provide a possible explanation, but its exact mechanism awaits elucidation. In two recent cases this diastolic murmur may well have been tricuspid, for it was much accentuated during inspiration.

Electrocardiogram

All observers have stressed the frequency of partial or complete *right bundle branch block*, which has been recorded in about 90 per cent of all cases. There were no exceptions among the ten reported here. The form of the complexes, however, is often a little bizarre, as in the case illustrated (fig. 8.20), and in eight out of the ten the voltage was low.

Tall sharp P waves have been described in well-nigh 80 per cent of published cases. In the present series, however, P was inconspicuous (as in the illustration) in eight, and prominent (3 or 4 mm. high and 0.08 second wide) in two.

The *P-R interval* has been slightly prolonged (usually 0.24 sec.) in a little over one-third of cases. In the present series it ranged between 0.14 and 0.2 second in eight out of the ten cases, and was 0.24 second in the other two. *WPW is frequent*

X-ray appearances

The radiological features of Ebstein's disease are as characteristic as the physical signs and the electrocardiogram. The aorta is small, and the lung fields clear and translucent. The enormous, relatively still, heart shadow produces a sharp stencilled effect on the skiagram reminiscent of pericardial effusion (fig. 8.21); the bulk of this shadow represents the distended right ventricle and atrium, the former approaching the left lateral wall of the thorax, the latter bulging far to the right.

DIFFERENTIAL DIAGNOSIS

Faced with such a characteristic picture made up of so many striking and unusual features it is difficult to think of any other possible diagnosis. If the history gives no indication of the duration of the condition, pericardial effusion might well be considered in acyanotic cases, and was in fact the way one of my patients presented. Like Ebstein's original case, and five out of 28 reviewed by Baker *et al.* (1950), this patient had pulmonary tuberculosis, and the "effusion" had an all-too-ready explanation. The Ebstein diastolic scratch lends superficial credence to such a diagnosis. But the jugular venous pressure pulse, the curious and unexpected gallop, and the electrocardiogram should prevent error.

In practice the commonest mistake has been confusion between Ebstein's disease and severe pulmonary valve stenosis with or without reversed interatrial shunt. There is rarely much excuse for such an error, for there are at least seven major points of difference (see pulmonary stenosis).

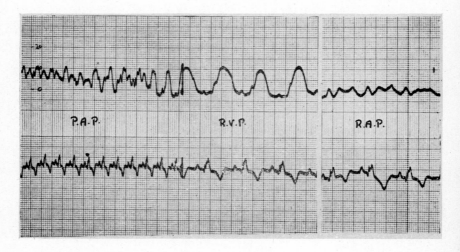

Paper speed 2.5 mm./sec.

Fig. 8.22—Relatively normal intracardiac pressures in a case of Ebstein's disease.

Cardiac catheterisation

I have personally catheterised seven cases of Ebstein's disease, but do not propose to catheterise another wittingly. Three deaths due to catheterisation are known to me, one being in the present series, and paroxysmal tachycardia occurred in another of mine. There need be no hesitation in using the catheter to disprove a case referred as Ebstein's disease, if the real diagnosis is thought to be pulmonary valve stenosis on firm clinical grounds, and the catheter can be used safely in the right atrium to check the possibility of pericardial effusion, if there is any real doubt about the matter; but in the great majority of cases the clinical diagnosis of Ebstein's disease is beyond question, and should be left at that. Of the ten cases in this series, five were confirmed by means of catheterisation (two also at necropsy), and five have not yet been confirmed or catheterised, but are still alive.

The findings at catheterisation are as follows:

1. All pressure pulses may be more or less normal, but of rather low amplitude (fig. 8.22); in the illustration the right atrial *c* wave is unduly prominent and has overcome the *x* descent. This appears to be the rule.

2. Right atrial and right "ventricular" pressure pulses are more or less indistinguishable and resemble right atrial tracings in gross tricuspid incompetence (fig. 8.23).

According to Van Lingen (1952) it may be possible to locate the position of the tricuspid valve by demonstrating two ventricular chambers, that portion proximal to the valve behaving like the right atrium, that distal to the valve like a true ventricle.

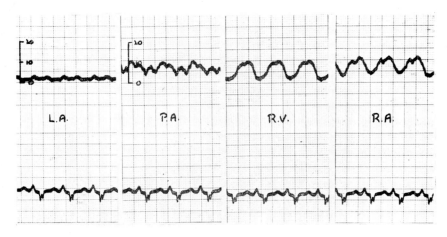

Fig. 8.23—Tricuspid incompetence type of pressure tracing in a case of Ebstein's disease showing an almost identical systolic pressure in the pulmonary artery, right ventricle and right atrium.

3. The pulmonary artery pressure, which was recorded in five of my seven cases, is normal, but low, the systolic level being the same as that in the right ventricle distal to the tricuspid valve.

4. The arterial oxygen saturation varies greatly, according to the degree of reversed interatrial shunt. In the horizontal position it is usually between 70 and 90 per cent saturated. In my five successfully catheterised cases it was 87, 83, 78, 72, and 90 per cent saturated. But it would be interesting to know what it was in the vertical position. One of these cases was clinically cyanosed at rest, and she was the only one with an oxygen capacity above 190 ml. per litre. The pulmonary blood flow in four adults was 6.4, 4.4, 3.1, and 3.3 litres per minute—the fifth patient (aged 4) did not have her oxygen uptake measured.

5. The pulmonary capillary venous pressure, measured in two cases, was normal (fig. 8.23), proving that in these two cases any opening in the atrial septum could have been no more than a small foramen ovale.

Prognosis and treatment

Life expectancy varies with the degree of cyanosis; the average age of death in cases cyanosed from birth is 12 years, whereas in acyanotic cases it is over 28 years (Baker *et al.*, 1950). Patients who are symptom free and wholly acyanotic have a good chance of surviving to middle age or beyond.

No specific treatment is possible.

ATRIAL SEPTAL DEFECT

Embryology. Atrial septal defect refers to a relatively large non-valvular opening in the atrial septum, through which blood may flow either way. Embryologically, the atrial septum is formed in the first place by the sickle-shaped septum primum which grows forwards from the dorsal wall of the common atrium, dividing it into two. For a time, communication exists between the two atria in front of the crescentic edge of the growing septum. If development is arrested at this stage, a septal defect results and is situated in the lower anterior part of the septum just below, and usually including, part of the fossa ovalis. When growth proceeds normally, this hole is obliterated and a new one, the foramen ovale, appears in the upper and dorsal part of the septum primum; arrest at this stage results in a defect just above the site of the fossa ovalis. With further normal development the foramen ovale comes to lie more anteriorly, and is turned into a valve by the growth of the septum secundum on the right side of the septum primum and covering it at all points except over the area known as the fossa ovalis. When the septum secundum develops fully and the septum primum degenerates completely, the defect occurs at the site of the fossa ovalis.

In *patent foramen ovale* the septa are fully developed, but imperfectly fused. When pressure is applied to the right side of the fossa ovalis, the septa are parted, blood penetrates between them and escapes into the left atrium through the patency in the upper part of the septum primum known as the foramen ovale proper. In fœtal life, the relatively high pressure in the right atrium keeps the valve open, and causes blood to be shunted from right to left in order to avoid the pulmonary circulation. At birth the pressure rises in the left atrium and forces the septum primum against the septum secundum, thereby closing the valve. In 80 per cent of all individuals fusion then takes place between the two septa and the foramen ovale is permanently closed. In the remaining 20 per cent fusion fails and valvular patency continues. It is then a potential cause of reversed interatrial shunt, if for any reason the pressure in the right atrium comes to exceed that in the left. This may happen in such conditions as pulmonary hypertension, pulmonary stenosis, and pulmonary embolism.

A cardiac catheter may slip through a patent foramen ovale into the left atrium without difficulty, and may enter the left ventricle (fig. 8.24), or any of the pulmonary veins (fig. 8.25), or the left atrial appendage (fig. 8.26). The pressures and electrical potentials in these chambers may thus be

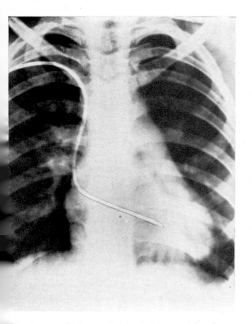

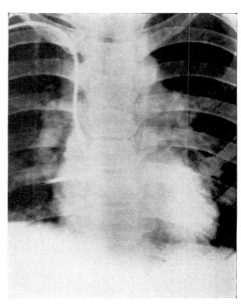

Fig. 8.24—Catheter in the left ventricle via a patent foramen ovale.

Fig. 8.25—Catheter in a pulmonary vein via a patent foramen ovale.

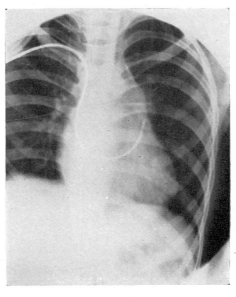

Fig. 8.26—Catheter in left atrial appendage.

obtained in favourable cases, including otherwise normal hearts. The mean left atrial pressure is about 4 mm. Hg higher than the right. Pulmonary venous samples have usually been around 96 per cent saturated with oxygen. Uncomplicated patent foramen ovale is easily distinguished from atrial septal defect because of the absence of any appreciable inter-atrial shunt, as judged by samples from both atria and their respective venous systems.

Hæmodynamics. An atrial septal defect is usually 1 to 3 cm. in diameter and carries a considerable shunt from left to right atrium, the right ventricle offering less resistance to filling than the left. Oxygenated blood is thus added to the normal intake of the right ventricle, the stroke output of which is correspondingly increased. The shunt results in enlargement of the right atrium and ventricle, dilatation of the pulmonary artery, and pulmonary plethora. Left atrial leakage deprives the left ventricle of its full intake; the left ventricular stroke output is diminished, the left ventricle and aorta hypoplasic, and the pulse small. Progressive right ventricular enlargement eventually leads to failure: the pressure in the right atrium then rises, and if it exceeds that in the left, the shunt is reversed and cyanosis develops. As a rule, however, the left atrial pressure also rises with heart failure and shunt reversal is prevented; this may be due to a reversed Bernheim effect or to the pressure-equalising influence of a stretched pericardium. According to some authorities a high jugular venous pressure in A.S.D. means left ventricular failure. Cyanosis in A.S.D. nearly always means an extreme pulmonary vascular resistance (see Eisenmenger's syndrome).

Incidence. A.S.D. accounted for 18 per cent of the author's series of 900 cases of congenital heart disease. It shows a slight preference for females, the sex ratio being 3 : 2 in their favour. The average age for the whole group was 23 years. The number per cent in each decade was as follows:

Age .	.	1–10	11–20	21–30	31–40	41–50	51–60	61–70
No. per cent	19	38	15	12.5	7	5	3.5

The oldest was 68 and the oldest on record 82 (Ellis, Greaves and Hecht, 1950).

Associated lesions. Arachnodactyly, high arched palate alone, or obvious thoracic deformity alone (usually Kyphoscoliosis or pigeon chest) occurred with equal frequency in one quarter of the cases. Coincident mitral stenosis (Lutembacher, 1916), whether congenital or acquired, was recognised clinically in only two instances and discovered at operation in another; it is difficult to understand the high incidence of Lutembacher's syndrome in past necropsies: Bedford, Papp and Parkinson (1941), for instance, put it at 25 per cent. Current opinion has swung sharply away from this concept and finds support in modern figures concerning its frequency at post-mortem, e.g. 6 per cent in the series reported by Nadas and Alimurung (1952).

CLINICAL FEATURES

Symptoms

The majority of uncomplicated cases of atrial septal defect have no symptoms. This statement applied to 57 per cent of the author's series. Effort intolerance was slight in 12.5 per cent, moderate in 12.5 per cent, considerable in 6 per cent and gross (total incapacity) in 12 per cent. Of those with grade 3 or 4 effort intolerance, 55 per cent were between the ages of 43 and 68 (average 55.5); of the remainder, one-third were infants,

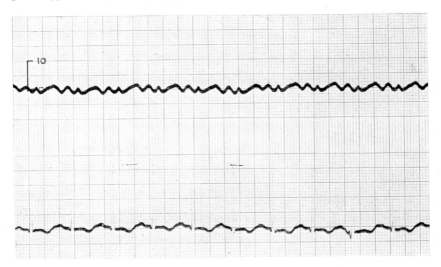

Fig. 8.27—Normal right atrial pressure oscillating gently around zero in a case of A.S.D.

one-third ordinary severe cases in younger adults, and one-third owed much of their disability to other lesions such as emphysema, polycystic kidney or mitral stenosis. It follows that symptomless uncomplicated atrial septal defect in young adults is a relatively benign anomaly.

Recurrent bronchitis or bronchopneumonia occurred in 10 per cent of all cases, and was attributed to the tendency of already hyperæmic lungs to react excessively to minor respiratory infections.

Hæmoptysis occurred in only 3 per cent, and bronchial tuberculosis was responsible for the hæmorrhage in two of these cases

Physical signs

Patients with atrial septal defect are not infrequently under-developed, frail or gracile in build, and any of the associated congenital anomalies mentioned above may be present.

The *peripheral pulse* is characteristically small. The *jugular venous pressure* was strictly normal in 75 per cent of the series reported here (fig. 8.27), slightly raised (about 3 cm. above the sternal angle) with *a* and *v* more or less equal in amplitude in 17 per cent, and high with a wave form suggesting tricuspid incompetence in 8 per cent. The *right atrial pressure pulse* was recorded in 58 cases and confirmed these clinical observations. Neither giant nor dominant *a* waves were seen in uncomplicated cases, nor was *v* in any way remarkable except in those with tricuspid incompetence.

The left ventricle is nearly always impalpable, but a substantial systolic lift over the *hyperdynamic right ventricle* from the left sternal edge to the mid-clavicular line or beyond is almost invariable. *Pulmonary artery pulsation* in the second left space can be felt in 50 per cent of cases.

There are several important auscultatory signs. A *pulmonary ejection murmur* due to an increased pulmonary blood flow was heard in 80 per cent of the series, and was accompanied by a thrill in one-quarter of all cases. When the thrill was very pronounced, catheterisation or other physical signs usually demonstrated coincident pulmonary stenosis, and such cases have been excluded from the group under consideration. A pulmonary ejection click was heard occasionally, but was unusual in the absence of a high pulmonary vascular resistance or slight pulmonary stenosis. A *pulmonary diastolic murmur* due to functional pulmonary incompetence (Graham-Steell murmur) was rare in the absence of pulmonary hypertension, but a soft *mid-diastolic murmur*, usually in the third or fourth left space near the sternal edge or towards the apex of the right ventricle, was heard in 30 per cent. This mid-diastolic murmur, which is accentuated during inspiration, is attributed to turbulence set up at the defect itself, or to a torrential tricuspid blood flow; necropsies have disproved its mitral origin (except in Lutembacher's syndrome). The *second heart sound is widely split*, and varies very little, if at all, with respiration. The second or pulmonary element may be a little accentuated, but is more often normal unless there is pulmonary hypertension. The wide split was attributed by Barber, Magidson and Wood (1950) either to right bundle branch block or to delayed emptying of the overfilled right ventricle, perhaps to both. Earlier closure of the pulmonary valve has been noted after successful repair of atrial septal defect without significant change in the electrocardiogram, and right ventricular pressure curves timed against the electrocardiogram prove that there is no delay in the onset of right ventricular contraction (Leatham and Gray, 1955): it follows that the wide split must be due to prolongation of right ventricular systole (or shortening of left ventricular systole). Failure of the split second heart sound to widen on inspiration was first noticed by Mr. W. W. Dicks, the senior cardiological technician at the London Hospital, and was confirmed by Towers (1952), and by Leatham and Gray (1955); we have assumed that the greatly distended right ventricle is unable to fill much more on inspiration, or that

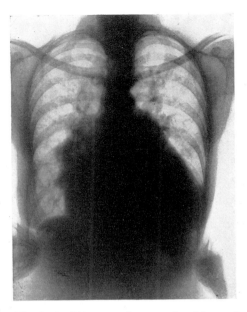

Fig. 8.28—Skiagram of a case of atrial septal
defect, showing dilatation of the pulmonary
artery and its branches, enlargement of the
right ventricle and atrium, and hypoplasia of
the aorta.

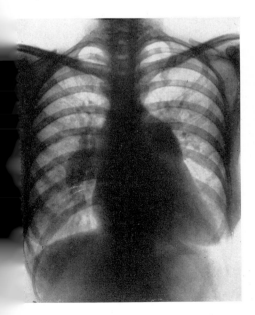

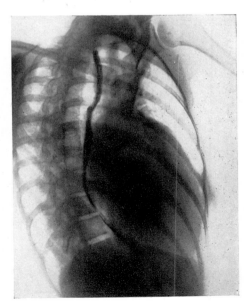

(a) Antero-posterior view.
(b) First oblique position showing dilatation of
the left atrium.

Fig. 8.29—Lutembacher's syndrome.

the increased inspiratory flow from the systemic veins into the right atrium tends to inhibit the shunt proportionally.

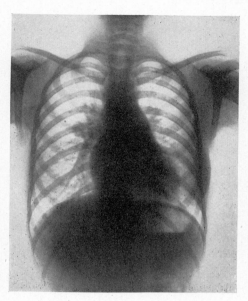

Fig. 8.30—Atrial septal defect in a child aged 10.

Fluoroscopy in well developed cases (fig. 8.28) reveals gross dilatation and conspicuous pulsation (hilar dance) of the pulmonary artery and its branches, peripheral pulmonary plethora, enlargement of the right atrium and ventricle, and hypoplasia of the aorta and left ventricle (Bedford, Papp, and Parkinson, 1941). In Lutembacher's syndrome (fig. 8.29) the left atrium is also enlarged. In less advanced cases, however, and especially in children, the changes described may be much less noticeable (fig. 8.30).

Electrocardiograms show a partial or complete right bundle branch block pattern in 95 per cent of cases (fig. 8.31) (Barber, Magidson and Wood (1950). The prolonged activation of the right ventricle is almost certainly due to dilatation of that chamber and not to any real interruption of the right bundle branch. The secondary R wave in lead V_1 seldom exceeds 10 mm. in height in uncomplicated cases, and is usually well under this. The P wave was normal, under 2 mm. in height, in 90 per cent of the present series; when it is tall and sharp, associated pulmonary stenosis or a high pulmonary vascular resistance should be suspected. A slightly prolonged P-R interval (around 0.24 sec.) was seen in 10 per cent. Atrial fibrillation occurred in 10 per cent of the whole series and was closely related to age: thus it was found in only one patient under 30 years old, in 12.5 per cent of those between 30 and 50, in 50 per cent of those between 51 and 60, and in 80 per cent of those over 60 years.

The diagnosis may be proved by obtaining samples of relatively oxygenated blood from the right atrium, right ventricle, and pulmonary artery, by means of cardiac catheterisation, when samples from the venæ cavæ show ordinary venous blood (Howarth, McMichael and Sharpey-Schafer, 1947). In 86 cases investigated at the Institute of Cardiology, samples obtained from the right atrium, right ventricle and pulmonary artery differed little, and ranged between 75 and 90 per cent saturated with oxygen, caval samples being normal (55 to 75 per cent saturated). Samples from the left atrium, left ventricle and femoral artery were normal (94 to

96 per cent saturated) in about half the cases, and between 84 and 93 per cent saturated in the other half. According to Swan, Burchell and Wood (1954) slight shunt reversal can usually be demonstrated by means of dye concentration curves, especially when the dye is injected into the inferior vena cava, and they think this explains the slightly reduced arterial oxygen saturation not infrequently found. But in 12 cases in the present series pulmonary venous samples* were obtained and proved to be similarly unsaturated in five of them, suggesting that hurry through a widely dilated pulmonary vascular bed may also be responsible. In uncomplicated atrial

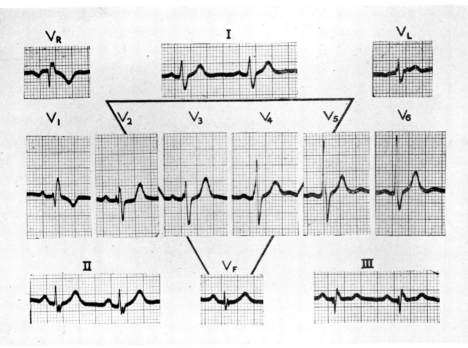

Fig. 8.31—Electrocardiogram in a case of A.S.D. showing a partial right bundle branch block pattern.

septal defect the pulmonary blood flow is usually two to three times the systemic flow, i.e. about 10 to 15 litres per minute. The systemic flow is commonly normal, but may be reduced in severe cases.

Pressure tracings from the two atria usually show little actual difference (fig. 8.32), the potential gradient from left to right being masked by the flow. It is assumed that the normal difference between left and right atrial pressure is due to greater resistance on the part of the left ventricle to

* In taking pulmonary venous samples the vessel must not be blocked by the catheter or the sample is bound to be 99 to 100 per cent saturated. When a pulmonary vein is blocked the distal pressure rises sharply, until it equals the pulmonary artery pressure, and the tracing becomes arterial in form.

diastolic filling, i.e. to a higher diastolic tone in the left ventricle than in the right. The greatest shunt flow may therefore occur during the period of rapid ventricular filling immediately after the opening of the tricuspid valve.

The pulmonary artery pressure was normal or only slightly raised in 90 per cent of these cases and between 60/30 and 100/50 in 10 per cent, excluding 15 cyanotic cases with an extreme pulmonary vascular resistance and reversed inter-atrial shunt which are considered later in relation to Eisenmenger's syndrome. It is clear that the normal long-term reaction of the pulmonary arterial tree to the increased blood flow is vasodilatation. This prevents any serious rise of pressure with flows up to 15 litres per

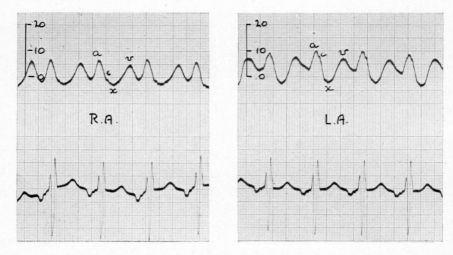

Fig. 8.32—Left and right atrial pressure tracings in a case of A.S.D. showing a slightly higher pressure on the left side although the R.A.P. is raised secondary to heart failure.

minute (in an adult); with flows greater than this, relatively harmless hyperkinetic pulmonary hypertension occurs without an increased pulmonary vascular resistance. Over the years secondary vascular changes may increase the resistance a little, but never seriously. In 20 per cent of cases, however, the reaction is of an entirely different order: in these the pulmonary vascular resistance is high, being 5 to 9 units in the group discussed here (about half of the 20 per cent), and 10 to 20 units in those with reversed shunt. This vasoconstrictive response seems to be determined at birth and is discussed more fully in connexion with Eisenmenger's syndrome.

COMPLICATIONS

Pulmonary hypertension complicating atrial septal defect, as described above, may be recognised by exaggeration of the *a* wave of the jugular pulse, a more sustained left parasternal heave, a pulmonary ejection click, closer splitting of the second heart sound and obvious accentuation of the second or pulmonary element, free pulmonary incompetence, greater dilatation of the pulmonary artery, less pulmonary plethora with loss of peripheral arterial tapering, and the development of a tall sharp P wave in standard leads and of a higher voltage secondary R wave in lead V_1 of the electrocardiogram. If the pressure in the right atrium comes to exceed that in the left, central cyanosis develops and the peripheral pulmonary vascular shadows diminish.

Tricuspid incompetence may result from gross dilatation of the right ventricle, with or without pulmonary hypertension, and is usual when there is *congestive failure.* It is remarkable that the shunt does not usually reverse

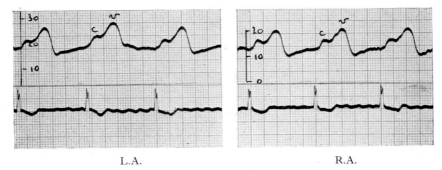

L.A.   R.A.

Fig. 8.33—Pressure tracings from both atria in a case of A.S.D. showing a slightly higher pressure on the left side despite marked tricuspid incompetence and a very high right atrial pressure.

in such cases, despite right atrial pressures of 10 to 20 cm. above the sternal angle. That the left atrial pressure remains higher than the right even under these circumstances (fig. 8.33) demands some special mechanism which increases the resistance to left ventricular filling. Whether this is a reversed Bernheim effect, a manifestation of left ventricular failure, or due to the pressure-equalising influence of a stretched pericardium is as yet uncertain.

Pulmonary stenosis complicates atrial septal defect in about 10 to 15 per cent of cases. It may be very mild and may hardly alter the physical signs or the hæmodynamics; but an impressive systolic thrill over the pulmonary artery is suggestive, and a pulmonary artery pressure at least 10 mm. Hg lower than that in the right ventricle is diagnostic.

Severe pulmonary stenosis associated with atrial septal defect causes reversal of the interatrial shunt and a cyanotic form of congenital heart disease (q.v.).

Partial anomalous pulmonary venous drainage into the right atrium (q.v.) is not uncommon and increases the left to right shunt.

Bacterial endocarditis is very rare in uncomplicated cases of atrial septal defect (about 1 per cent), and its occurrence at once suggests associated pulmonary stenosis.

PROGNOSIS

Of the 167 cases in this series, five died naturally—three (aged 2, 3, and 43) from congestive failure, one from associated cor pulmonale, and one from polycystic kidneys. Five others died from attempted surgical repair, all advanced cases, and one (also in failure) died as the result of cardiac catheterisation. The average age of these 11 patients (6.6 per cent of the series) was 21.

According to McGinn and White (1933) and Roesler (1934), the average age of death in atrial septal defect is 35 to 36.

On the whole, however, it is believed that the prognosis in uncomplicated cases with average shunts is good, congestive failure being a late development and not to be expected before middle life. This must influence selection of cases for surgical treatment.

TREATMENT

Over the past few years a determined attempt has been made to find the best method of closing atrial septal defects. Murray (1948) passed fascia lata sutures through the atrial septum in such a way as to occlude the defect, but the method was too uncertain to be followed up. Bailey (1953) closed many defects by suturing part of the wall of the distended right atrium to the interatrial septum, making sure that free passage was preserved between the mouths of the venæ cavæ and the tricuspid orifice. This technique has been used by many surgeons with considerable success, but lacks the precision of direct suture. Gross (1952, 1953) showed that atrial septal defect could be closed by direct suture if a leak-proof rubber well was first attached to the right atrial wall; when the right atrium is opened, blood rises in the well to a level which represents the central venous pressure, and so maintains normal right ventricular filling and allows the surgeon to perform his task under water as it were. Air embolism is avoided because the tricuspid valve is totally immersed. The introduction of open heart surgery, however, made possible by hypothermia or crossed circulations, has resulted in the modern method of closing the defect by simple suturing under direct vision (Lewis and Taufic, 1953; Swan et al., 1953). Subsequent physiological studies have proved that the defect remains closed (Blount et al., 1954).

Eighteen of the present series were operated on, six by Mr. W. C. Cleland using Bailey's technique, and twelve by Sir Russell Brock with the aid of hypothermia. Although six of these patients died, they were very advanced and the results in the survivors have been most gratifying.

At the present time surgical repair should be recommended if the pulmonary blood flow is more than three times the systemic flow, if the pulmonary vascular resistance is between 6 and 10 units, or if there is obvious tricuspid incompetence or congestive heart failure. Until the mortality rate is under 5 per cent, uncomplicated cases with good effort tolerance and 2 to 1 shunts should certainly be left alone. With bidirectional shunt it is reasonable to advise repair *as long as the pulmonary blood flow is still increased*, even though the pulmonary vascular resistance is above 10 units (800 dynes sec./cm^5), for the resistance may be expected to fall if the flow can be diminished; but it is not reasonable to advise repair when an extreme resistance has resulted in a normal or reduced pulmonary blood flow and reversed shunt.

PERSISTENT COMMON ATRIOVENTRICULAR CANAL

A common atrioventricular opening with deformed mitral and tricuspid valves is always associated with a persistent ostium primum (A.S.D.), usually with a ventricular septal defect, and often with mongolism.

Of 55 cases reviewed by Rogers and Edwards (1948) over half died within the first year of life, and only five survived to the age of 30.

Clinically these cases usually present with all the features of an exceptionally large atrial septal defect complicated by mitral (as well as tricuspid) incompetence; an appreciable number, however, have the Eisenmenger reaction and reverse the shunt.

PARTIAL ANOMALOUS PULMONARY VENOUS DRAINAGE

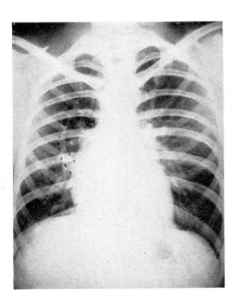

Fig. 8.34—Skiagram showing an anomalous pulmonary vein joining the right atrium.

One or more pulmonary veins may drain directly into the azygos, superior vena cava, right atrium or inferior vena cava. According to Brody (1942) anomalous pulmonary veins are twice as frequent in the right lung as in the left. A left to right shunt at caval or atrial level occurs, and results in a physiological situation similar to that found in atrial septal defect, with which it is not infrequently associated. In isolated cases the shunt is relatively small, and the condition may be only recognised as a result of a routine skiagram (fig. 8.34). The anomalous vessel is commonly dilated and shows up well in tomograms (fig. 8.35). A cardiac catheter may enter such a vessel directly from the superior vena cava (fig. 8.36), inferior vena cava, or right atrium, and may be filled with contrast medium so that its course may be seen more clearly; or

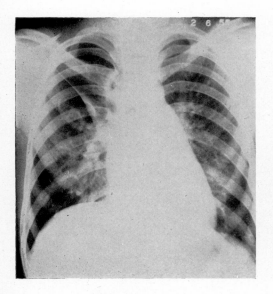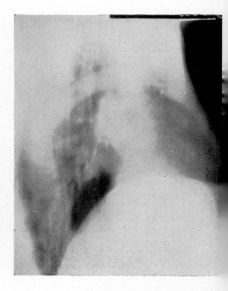

(a) Anterior view. (b) Lateral tomogram.

Fig. 8.35—Anomalous right pulmonary venous drainage into the azygos vein.

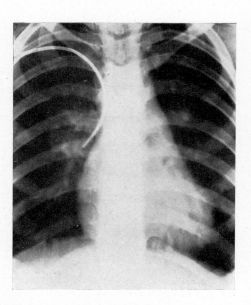

Fig. 8.36—Skiagram showing a catheter lying in an anomalous pulmonary vein joining the superior vena cava.

diaginol may be injected directly into the pulmonary artery through a No. 9 catheter so as to delineate the whole course of the vessel.

When anomalous pulmonary venous drainage is associated with atrial septal defect it may be important to know how much blood is being shunted through each. If the anomalous vein joins the azygos or either vena cava, this can be learned easily enough by analysing samples obtained from the vena cava above and below the entrance of the vessel, and from the right atrium; if it joins the right atrium, however, the shunt is more difficult to estimate, but comparison of time-concentration curves recorded by means of an ear oximeter after the injection of 30 mg. of Evans blue dye, first into one pulmonary artery and then into the other, may help; when the injection is made on the side of the anomalous pulmonary veins the left to right shunt is greater than when it is made on the contralateral side, and the quantitative difference between the two curves represents the magnitude of the venous shunt.

TREATMENT

It is rarely necessary to interfere with partial anomalous pulmonary venous drainage, because the shunt carried is usually too small to cause any trouble, and the prognosis excellent (Smith, 1951). Transplantation may have to be considered, however, in exceptional cases, and if there is a suitable pulmonary vein on the same side direct venous anastomosis can be performed.

VENTRICULAR SEPTAL DEFECT

Ventricular septal defect commonly refers to an isolated defect of the membranous part of the interventricular septum due to failure of the aortic septum to fuse with the ventricular septum. Diagnosed clinically for the first time by Roger (1879), the lesion has been said to account for 35 to 37 per cent of all cases of congenital heart disease recognised at school age (Perry, 1931; Muir and Brown, 1934). Such high figures probably include many instances of aortic stenosis, simple pulmonary stenosis, infundibular stenosis and mitral incompetence.

NOMENCLATURE

The term maladie de Roger, if used at all, should be reserved for those mild cases of ventricular septal defect that conform to Roger's original description, i.e. to about one-third of pure uncomplicated cases (Wood, Magidson and Wilson, 1954). The remainder have so many characteristic features denied by this description that they have no right to the title. Nor is Taussig's classification of ventricular septal defect into high (severe) and low (mild) types justified, for in 90 per cent of cases the defect, whether severe or mild, is located in the anterior part of the membranous septum (Selzer, 1949).

INCIDENCE

In the author's series of 900 virtually proved cases of congenital heart disease, ventricular septal defect occurred in its pure uncomplicated form in 8 per cent, as part of Eisenmenger's complex in 3 per cent, in association with simple pulmonary stenosis in 1.3 per cent, and as part of Fallot's tetralogy or pulmonary atresia in 12.7 per cent; thus in one form or another ventricular septal defect was found in one-quarter of all cases. The present section deals only with uncomplicated ventricular septal defect.

The sex ratio in this series was equal, as it was in the 92 post-mortem cases mostly collected from the literature by Selzer (1949).

The average age of the 72 cases described here was 12.7 years and the percentage in each decade as follows:

0–10	11–20	21–30	31–40	41–50	51–60 years
51	31	10	5	2	1

HÆMODYNAMICS

During systole, from the shutting of the mitral and tricuspid valves to well after aortic valve closure, the high pressure gradient across the ventricular septum ensures a left to right shunt. The extra quantity of blood received by the right ventricle is pumped into the lungs and is received in due course by the left atrium and left ventricle. Thus both ventricles and the left atrium do more than their normal share of work, only the right atrium being spared. As in atrial septal defect the pulmonary vascular resistance usually remains normal, so that the pulmonary blood pressure only rises when the pulmonary blood flow approaches or exceeds 15 litres per minute (hyperkinetic pulmonary hypertension). The systemic output is maintained as near to normal as possible, and the arterial blood is adequately saturated with oxygen.

CLINICAL FEATURES

Symptoms

Cases of mild or moderate severity have no symptoms, but when the shunt is considerable patients are usually under-developed, and may complain of breathlessness, palpitations, and recurrent attacks of bronchitis. In severe cases congestive failure must be expected sooner or later, and is not infrequent in childhood (Marquis, 1950).

Physical signs

The *facies* is normal or lean, never bloated. By definition all uncomplicated cases are acyanotic.

The *peripheral pulse* is small when the shunt is relatively large, normal in the maladie de Roger.

The *jugular venous pressure and pulse* are normal unless there is heart failure.

A *hyperdynamic left ventricular thrust* at the apex beat, and a *lift over the right ventricle* near the left sternal border can both be felt as a rule, and pulsation over the pulmonary artery in the second left space occurs in a quarter of the cases. Only in the maladie de Roger is the cardiac impulse normal.

Roger (1877) accurately described the *characteristic murmur* as "surprisingly loud, extending right through systole covering both heart sounds,

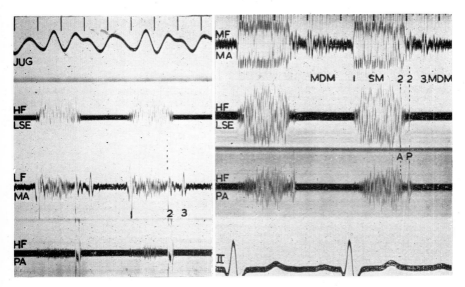

Fig. 8.37—Phonocardiogram illustrating the pan-systolic murmur of V.S.D. with a simultaneous jugular phlebogram.

Fig. 8.38—Phonocardiogram showing a functional mitral diastolic murmur (top tracing) in a case of V.S.D.

H.F., high frequency; M.F., medium frequency; L.F., low frequency; L.S.E., left sternal edge; M.A., mitral area; P.A., pulmonary area.

Acknowledgments to Dr. Aubrey Leatham.

and with its maximal intensity . . . over the upper third of the precordial region and chiefly median." This loud pansystolic murmur (figs. 8.37 and 8.38) was heard in 95 per cent of the present series, usually in the 3rd and 4th left spaces near the sternal edge, and was accompanied by a *thrill* in four-fifths of them. The murmur was soft in 3 per cent and absent altogether in 2 per cent. A functional *mitral diastolic murmur* (fig. 8.38), indistinguishable in timing, quality, intensity and duration from the Carey-Coombs murmur of active rheumatic carditis, was heard in precisely half the cases. This murmur was noted by Laubry and Pezzi (1921) and may be attributed to a torrential mitral blood flow (Wood, 1950). It is present in 90 per cent of severe cases, 60 per cent of those with moderate shunts and 10 per cent of mild cases (Wood *et al.*, 1954). A *Graham Steell murmur* due to functional pulmonary incompetence was heard in 14 per cent, chiefly in those with pulmonary hypertension.

The *second heart sound*, when not obscured by the murmur, is split normally or rather closely; the pulmonary element is only accentuated in those with pulmonary hypertension. The third heart sound is usually accentuated owing to rapid ventricular filling (fig. 8.37).

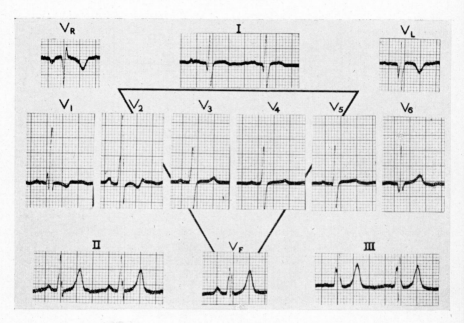

Fig. 8.39—Electrocardiogram in a case of V.S.D. showing an RSR complex in lead V_1 indicating right ventricular dilatation, and a conspicuous Q wave in leads V_6 and V_L, pointing to a powerful left ventricle as well.

Electrocardiogram

The electrocardiogram is normal in the maladie de Roger. In those with moderate or large shunts the appearances vary according to the pulmonary vascular resistance: when this is low good Q waves and large R waves in leads V_5 and V_6, with or without depression or inversion of T or U, and deep S waves in leads V_1 and V_2 confirm the left ventricular enlargement and dominance, the pattern resembling that seen in patent ductus; when the resistance is raised, however, a conspicuous secondary R wave is seen in lead V_1 and a terminal S wave in lead V_6, the graph resembling that seen in atrial septal defect. In the majority of cases, however, a variable mixture of these two types of graph is seen, good Q waves in leads V_5 and V_6, emphasising the presence of a vigorous left ventricle, and secondary R waves in lead V_1 proclaiming right ventricular enlargement as well (fig. 8.39).

Skiagram

In mild cases the appearances are normal (fig. 8.40). In the majority, however, radiology reveals a small aorta, a variable degree of dilatation of the pulmonary artery and its two main branches (with or without hilar dance), pulmonary plethora, hyperdynamic enlargement of both ventricles, and slight dilatation of the left atrium (fig. 8.41).

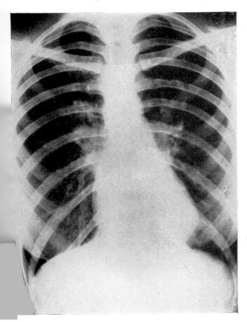

Fig. 8.40—Maladie de Roger—X-ray appearances.

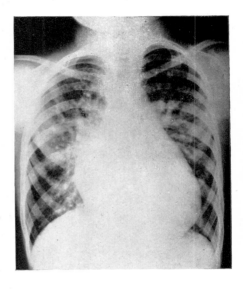

Fig. 8.41—Skiagram of a case of ventricular septal defect with considerable increase of pulmonary blood flow.

Differential diagnosis

The maladie de Roger is frequently confused with mild pulmonary valve stenosis, simple infundibular stenosis, acyanotic Fallot's tatralogy, mild aortic stenosis, and "innocent left parasternal murmur", whatever that may be.

Mild pulmonary valve stenosis should be distinguished by the higher position of the thrill and murmur, wide splitting of the second sound, and post-stenotic dilatation of the pulmonary artery.

Mild infundibular stenosis with its low thrill and murmur and normal pulmonary artery, is very difficult to distinguish from the maladie de Roger, unless delayed pulmonary valve closure can be recognised.

Acyanotic Fallot's tetralogy usually causes moderate effort intolerance, even squatting in some cases, and a clear single second heart sound; in all other respects it may closely resemble maladie de Roger.

Mild aortic stenosis should be recognised by the aortic ejection click, and by the geography and timing of the aortic systolic murmur (q.v.).

Cases of ventricular septal defect with moderate or considerable shunt are apt to be confused with patent ductus without a continuous murmur, atrial septal defect, and mitral incompetence with anticlockwise rotation of the heart.

Patent ductus with a pulmonary systolic thrill and murmur rather than a continuous murmur is rare in the absence of a high pulmonary vascular resistance, but does occur. It may be distinguished from ventricular septal defect by the water hammer pulse and Corrigan sign, reversed splitting of the second heart sound, more conspicuous aorta, and absence of right ventricular enlargement clinically and electrocardiographically.

Atrial septal defect should be recognised by the absence of left ventricular enlargement, wide fixed splitting of the second sound, and uncomplicated partial right bundle branch block pattern in the electrocardiogram.

Mitral incompetence with anticlockwise rotation may cause a pan-systolic murmur and thrill in the Roger area, hyperdynamic left ventricle, accentuated third heart sound and short mitral diastolic murmur—a combination that may well be mistaken for ventricular septal defect. The skiagram, however, shows pulmonary venous congestion instead of plethora, and the left atrium is usually too conspicuous for ventricular septal defect.

PHYSIOLOGICAL FINDINGS

Of the 72 cases in this series, 48 were proved by means of cardiac catheterisation, and the essential findings are given in the accompanying table. From experience gained in investigating small ducts subsequently

PHYSIOLOGICAL DATA IN VENTRICULAR SEPTAL DEFECT

	NO. OF CASES	GAIN IN O₂ SATURATION OF R.V. SAMPLES (per cent)		PULMONARY BLOOD FLOW EXPRESSED AS MULTIPLES OF SYSTEMIC FLOW		USUAL SHUNT (L./min.)	PULMONARY HYPER-TENSION	ESTIMATED SIZE OF DEFECT (diam.)
		Range	Av.	Range	Av.			
Maladie de Roger	17	4 to 13	7.5	1.2 to 1.9	1.5	1.5 to 3	Absent	2 to 4 mm.
Moderate V.S.D.	14	9 to 22	14	2 to 3	2.3	4 to 8	Trivial	5 to 9 mm.
Severe V.S.D. uncomplicated	9	18 to 33	28	3 to 5	4	10 to 15	Hyperkinetic (may approach systemic level)	10 to 15 mm.
Severe V.S.D. with raised pulmonary resistance	8	7 to 18	12.5	1.7 to 2.8	2	3 to 5	Considerable (to systemic level)	10 to 15 mm.

proved at operation, and in consideration of the technical errors involved in sampling, it is clear that defects measuring less than 2 mm. in diameter and passing shunts of less than 1 litre per minute would not be detected with ordinary routine methods of investigation. It must be admitted, therefore, that a pansystolic left parasternal murmur with entirely normal physiological findings could well be due to a minute ventricular septal defect, for necropsies have certainly proved the existence of such minute defects. This does not mean, however, that the maladie de Roger is common after all, because the majority of cases so labelled on traditional evidence have been proved by modern techniques to have a different explanation for the murmur.

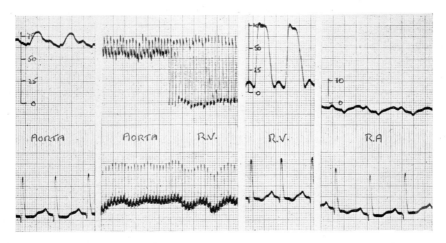

Fig. 8.42—Pressure pulses from a case of ventricular septal defect with hyperkinetic pulmonary hypertension at systemic level; the pulmonary blood flow was 20 L/min. and the resistance 3 units.

In one third of the mild cases there was a significant difference between infundibular and low right ventricular samples, the former resembling samples from the pulmonary artery, the latter samples from the right atrium; this difference was very rarely found in moderate or severe cases.

The pulmonary vascular resistance was raised moderately in half the severe cases. There is good evidence that the size of the defect is not directly responsible for the behaviour of the small pulmonary vessels in these instances (see Eisenmenger's complex), but it was never smaller than the critical 1 cm. in diameter. Severe cases without a raised resistance are apt to die of left ventricular failure or bronchopneumonia in childhood, for there is then little to prevent an intolerable shunt. The pulmonary blood pressure alone gives little indication of the resistance, and may even reach systemic level when the resistance is normal if the shunt is large enough (fig. 8.42). This may be called hyperkinetic pulmonary hypertension.

COMPLICATIONS

Eisenmenger's complex (q.v.), which may be defined as pulmonary hypertension with bidirectional or reversed interventricular shunt, usually occurs when the pulmonary vascular resistance lies between 10 and 20 units.

Complete heart block occurred in only one of the 72 cases recorded here. Conversely, when ventricular septal defect had been diagnosed elsewhere in several cases of congenital heart block, no shunt could be demonstrated by means of cardiac catheterisation, and careful auscultation supported by phonocardiography usually proved that the systolic murmur on which the diagnosis had been based was in fact an aortic or pulmonary ejection murmur. Functional mitral incompetence may also mislead.

Bacterial endocarditis was the cause of death in 22 per cent of the 80 necropsied cases reviewed by Selzer (1949). Its true incidence is difficult to assess, frequency rates as high as 57 per cent being recorded in post-mortem material (Gelfman and Levine, 1942; Welch and Kinney, 1948), and as low as 1 per cent in clinical series (Perry, 1937; Muir and Brown, 1934; Wood *et al.*, 1954); perhaps 10 to 20 per cent would be near the truth. Vegetations form on the right ventricular side of the septum around the defect, and on the opposite wall of the right ventricle where the shunted blood stream impinges. Emboli are confined to the pulmonary circulation and may cause subacute or recurrent hæmorrhagic pulmonary inflammation or infarction.

Pulmonary or infundibular stenosis with normal aortic root and left to right shunt may be associated with ventricular septal defect (Abrahams and Wood, 1950), the combination occurring in 1.5 per cent of all cases of congenital heart disease (Wood *et al.*, 1954). When the stenosis is mild it is usually overlooked until demonstrated by means of cardiac catheterisation; when it is relatively severe, the ventricular septal defect is usually overlooked clinically. Cases with bidirectional or reversed shunt are indistinguishable from Fallot's tetralogy.

Aortic incompetence, the anterior cusp being prolapsed into the defect (fig. 8.43), or tethered towards the defect by a fibrous band (Laubry and Pezzi, 1921), occurs in about 2 per cent of cases (Wood, Magidson and Wilson, 1954). The combination may be mistaken for patent ductus and so lead to fruitless thoracotomy.

PROGNOSIS

During the seven-year period in which these 72 cases of isolated uncomplicated ventricular septal defect have been studied, none have died of the lesion. But there were only three patients over 40 years old, whereas 15.5 per cent of patients with atrial septal defect were over 40. Again, 29 per cent of 88 fatal cases collected by Selzer (1949) died during the first year of life, and another 20 per cent between the ages of 1 and 5. The average age of death in Abbott's series was 14, the oldest being 49. It is clear, therefore, that ventricular septal defect is a serious anomaly, patients often dying from congestive failure in early childhood (Baldwin, Moore and Noble, 1946), and it is only the mild maladie de Roger that has a good prognosis. The only risk in these mild cases is bacterial endocarditis, and with modern treatment this can usually be cured.

There have been some interesting cases in which characteristic signs of a ventricular septal defect discovered in childhood have disappeared with advancing years. Whilst it is difficult to prove that these were not examples of innocent left parasternal murmur, it has been suggested that spontaneous obliteration of small defects may sometimes occur (Parkes Weber, 1918).

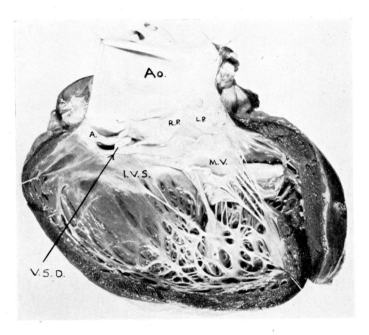

Fig. 8.43—Photograph of a specimen from a case of aortic incompetence complicating V.S.D.; the anterior aortic cusp is prolapsed into the defect.

Acknowledgments to Dr. Reginald Hudson.

TREATMENT

No reparative treatment is yet available, but Murray (1948) first made the attempt. Mild cases should be encouraged to lead normal unrestricted lives, but severe cases need care and should limit their physical activities. Dental treatment, sore throat and other pyogenic infections should be covered by a short course of penicillin to prevent endocarditis.

PATENT DUCTUS ARTERIOSUS
EMBRYOLOGY

In fœtal life the ductus arteriosus joins the root of the left pulmonary artery to the aorta at a point immediately distal to the left subclavian artery, and it is a short muscular vessel, 1 cm. or so in length and about as wide as the great vessels which it joins. In the unærated lung of the fœtus the pulmonary capillaries and arteries are practically shut down and offer a resistance to flow that is much higher than the systemic resistance; mixed venous and placental blood from the right ventricle therefore passes directly from the pulmonary artery into the descending aorta. At the same time mixed venous and placental blood which has passed through the foramen ovale is pumped by the left ventricle into the ascending aorta. Although further mixing undoubtedly takes place in the arch of the aorta, on the whole left ventricular blood passes to the head and upper extremities, while right ventricular blood passes to the trunk and lower extremities. It should be clearly understood that the systolic pressures in the two ventricles and great vessels are identical; the ventricles are subjected to the same filling pressure and work against the same total peripheral resistance.

At birth aeration of the lung is followed by a rapid decline in pulmonary vascular resistance, alveolar oxygenation discouraging pulmonary vaso-constriction. Within three hours of birth blood sent to the right arm is over 90 per cent saturated with oxygen, whereas blood sent to the legs is still partly venous; from the end of the third hour the pulmonary vascular resistance gradually falls below systemic level, the process being completed in normal individuals by the end of the third day, after which arterial samples from the arms and legs are the same (Eldridge, Multgren and Wigmore, 1954). The duct itself normally closes by some inherent process within the first six weeks after birth.

INCIDENCE

Patent ductus was the chief or sole lesion in 9.2 per cent of Abbott's 1,000 collected cases of congenital heart disease, and accounted for 13 per cent of my own 900, an additional 2 per cent having reversed shunt.

The sex ratio is 7 : 3 in favour of females (Gross, 1952); there were 78 females and 37 males in the present series.

In the 115 cases reported here the average age was 17, and the percentage distribution per decade as follows:

Age		0–10	11–20	21–30	31–40	41–50	51–60
No. per cent		36	32	15	9.5	6.5	1

HÆMODYNAMICS

Since the systemic peripheral resistance is normally about eight times the pulmonary, the shunt in uncomplicated patent ductus is from aorta to pulmonary artery. The total systemic resistance is lowered by the leak from the aorta; arterial blood enters the pulmonary circulation, the total pulmonary blood flow is increased, and the left atrium and left ventricle have to deal with the augmented flow; the total blood volume is raised (Cassels and Morse, 1947). Hyperkinetic pulmonary hypertension may occur with large shunts as with atrial septal defect and ventricular septal defect, but the pulmonary vascular resistance is not ordinarily raised. High pulmonary resistances around 15 units (systemic level) occur in 10 to 15 per cent of cases and may result in reversed shunt (see Eisenmenger's syndrome). Included in the present section is a small group (7 per cent) in which the pulmonary resistance is moderately raised, but insufficiently so to prevent a predominant aorto-pulmonary shunt.

CLINICAL FEATURES

There are no symptoms in mild or moderate cases. In severe cases with large shunts recurrent bronchitis and bronchopneumonia are common in childhood as with severe atrial septal defect and ventricular septal defect. Physical development is usually poor, palpitations and throbbing may be troublesome, and there may be symptoms of left ventricular failure.

Physical signs

The *peripheral pulse* is water-hammer in quality, Corrigan's sign may be present in the neck, and the diastolic blood pressure tends to be low, according to the degree of aorto-pulmonary shunt.

The *venous pressure* is normal in uncomplicated cases, but may be raised a little if the pulmonary vascular resistance is high or as a result of an increased blood volume.

The *cardiac impulse* is left ventricular in type and hyperdynamic. Medial retraction over the right ventricle confirms that the left ventricle is alone enlarged. Pulsation in the second left space over the pulmonary artery may be appreciated when the shunt is large or when there is a raised pulmonary vascular resistance.

On *auscultation* the chief sign is the classical "machinery" murmur of Gibson (1900): it is usually heard best in the first or second left interspace, is more or less continuous, waxes towards the end of systole, wanes in mid-diastole, and is accompanied by a thrill in two-thirds of cases. It may be absent in infancy, although it has been recorded as early as the sixth week (Adler, 1953). This typical murmur was heard in 95 per cent of the present series. The murmur was systolic only in two cases with gross shunt, in one trivial case, and in two with a raised pulmonary vascular resistance which was insufficient to prevent an aorto-pulmonary shunt. A continuous murmur was never heard in the pulmonary hypertensive cases with reversed shunt. In difficult cases a doubtful Gibson murmur may be brought out be any device that increases total flow (such as exercise), or that increases the pressure gradient across the duct (such as Müller's experiment).

The *second heart sound* was usually difficult to analyse clinically in view of the loud coincident bruit, but phonocardiography showed that aortic

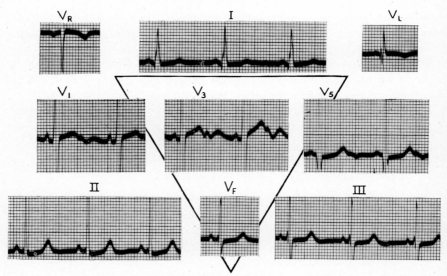

Fig. 8.44—Electrocardiogram in a case of patent ductus showing left ventricular enlargement. There is a strong QR pattern with inverted U waves in lead V_5.

valve closure was delayed in cases with large shunt, A_2 often falling after
P_2, the split being reversed (Gray, 1955). The phenomenon was attributed
to delayed emptying of an overfilled left ventricle.

A *pulmonary diastolic murmur* due to functional pulmonary incompetence
was recognised in 8 per cent. In the group with pulmonary hypertension
and reversed shunt (discussed later) it was heard in 70 per cent.

A *functional mitral diastolic murmur* due to a torrential mitral blood flow
was detected in 39 per cent of all uncomplicated cases: it was present in
87 per cent of those with large shunts and in one-third of those with

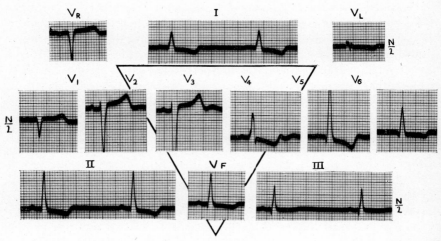

Fig. 8.45—Gross left ventricular preponderance in a case of patent ductus.

moderate shunts, but never in mild or trivial cases. It commonly disappeared after ligation of the duct; this rapid flow murmur was never heard in the true pulmonary hypertensive group.

Electrocardiogram

The electrocardiogram is normal in mild cases, and usually normal in cases of moderate severity; but when the shunt is large, prominent Q waves, unusually tall R waves, and perhaps inverted U waves in leads V_5 and V_6, confirm the enlargement of the left ventricle (fig. 8.44), and in the most florid cases the T waves may be inverted in left ventricular surface leads or their equivalents (fig. 8.45). In striking contrast to atrial septal defect, no case of patent ductus had a partial right bundle branch block pattern.

Radiological appearances

Skiagrams (figs. 8.46 and 8.47) reveal pulmonary plethora, dilatation of the pulmonary artery, enlargement of the left ventricle and slight dilatation of the left atrium (Donovan, Neuhauser and Sosman, 1943). A conspicuous hilar dance is unusual, and the right branch of the pulmonary artery is rarely impressive. The aorta in patent ductus is not so small (fig. 8.48) as in atrial septal defect and ventricular septal defect, and may be more pulsatile. The right ventricle and atrium are strictly normal in uncomplicated cases. Rarely a comma-shaped arc of calcium can be seen in the ductus or in the wall of the left pulmonary artery opposite to the opening of the ductus.

A local bulge in the region of the aortic isthmus can be demonstrated by means of angiocardiography in a limited number of cases, and is thought to represent the widened mouth of the ductus, or possibly a traction aneurysm of the aorta (Steinberg, Grishman and Sussman, 1943). A characteristic filling defect at the top of the left pulmonary artery has been described by Goetz (1951). With suitable technique, angiocardiograms may also show the pulmonary artery filling twice, first from the right ventricle, then from the aorta. Retrograde aortography offers an alternative means of obtaining good angiograms.

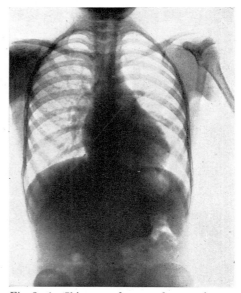

Fig. 8.46—Skiagram of a case of patent ductus showing enlargement of the left ventricle, but little dilatation of the pulmonary artery.

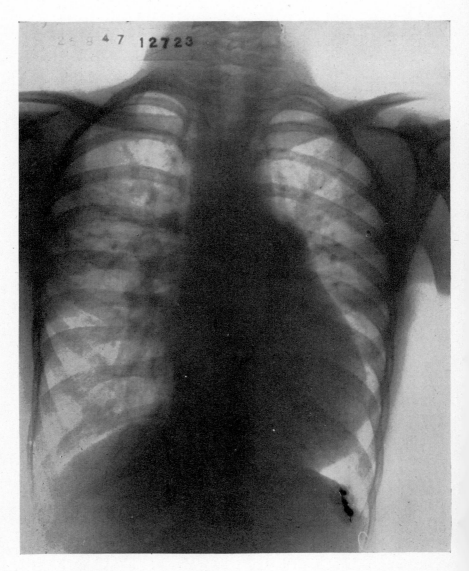

Fig. 8.47—Skiagram of a more advanced case of patent ductus, showing considerable left ventricular enlargement and engorgement of the pulmonary vessels in addition to dilatation of the pulmonary artery.

PHYSIOLOGICAL FINDINGS

The diagnosis may be proved in doubtful cases by means of cardiac catheterisation. Samples of blood from the superior vena cava, right atrium and right ventricle are normal (about 70 per cent saturated), whereas samples from the pulmonary artery are usually 80 to 85 per cent saturated. Slight admixture of arterial blood in right ventricular samples may be found when there is functional pulmonary incompetence.

In the present series 61 cases were catheterised, about a third of them in each group of severity. In mild cases the pulmonary blood flow measured about 1.5 times the systemic flow, and in three instances no shunt at all could be demonstrated, even in one catheterised twice. At operation in these mild cases the duct did not exceed 0.6 cm. in external diameter.

In the moderate group the pulmonary blood flow was 2 to 2½ times the systemic flow, being commonly around 10 to 12 litres per minute.

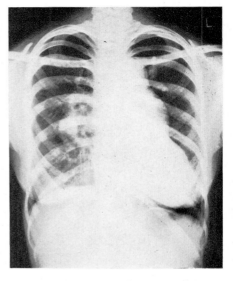

Fig. 8.48—Skiagram of a case of patent ductus showing a prominent aortic knuckle in addition to dilatation of the pulmonary artery and pulmonary plethora.

The pulmonary blood pressure and vascular resistance were normal (fig. 8.49), and at operation the duct usually measured from 7 to 12 mm. in external diameter.

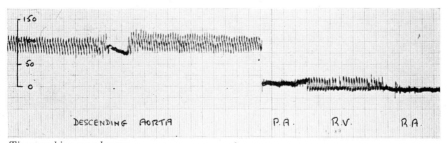

DESCENDING AORTA P. A. R. V. R. A.

Time marking 1 and 5 sec.
Fig. 8.49—Pressure pulses from the descending aorta and pulmonary artery in an uncomplicated case of patent ductus showing a steep pressure gradient between the two.

In the severe cases with normal resistances the pulmonary blood flow averaged 3.5 times the systemic flow, ranging between 12 and 30 litres per minute. Hyperkinetic pulmonary hypertension was demonstrated in all but two of these cases, the average pressure being 55/35 mm. Hg, and the range from 32/15 to 75/55. The pulmonary vascular resistance was normal, averaging 2 units, the range being 0.5 to 4. The pulmonary blood pressure never quite reached systemic level at rest in this group, but approached it very closely in several instances as a result of temporary stress, and would presumably do so also on exercise. At operation the duct was always more than 1 cm. in external diameter.

The arterial oxygen saturation was normal for catheter conditions (90 to 97 per cent) in 88 per cent of all these cases, and between 87 and 89 per cent in the remainder.

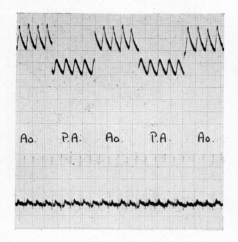 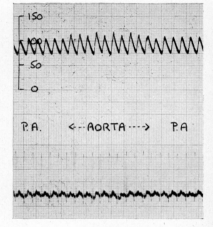

Duct closed · Duct open

Time marking 0.2 *and* 1.0 *sec.*

Fig. 8.50—Case of patent ductus with hyperkinetic pulmonary hypertension, together with a moderately raised pulmonary vascular resistance; when the ductus was open the pulmonary artery pressure was 10 mm. Hg lower than the aortic; when the ductus was closed the aortic pressure rose from 115 to 150 mm. Hg and the pulmonary artery pressure fell from 105 to 83 mm. Hg.

Finally, there was a small group (5 per cent) of severe cases in which the pulmonary vascular resistance was raised (5 to 9 units), but in which the shunt was still unidirectional or predominantly from aorta to pulmonary artery. Although the ductus itself was about 1 cm. in diameter, the raised resistance prevented a large shunt, the average pulmonary blood flow being barely twice the systemic flow. The pulmonary blood pressure was more or less at systemic level (fig. 8.50). These cases are not yet in the Eisenmenger group, but could become so.

By repeatedly guiding the tip of the catheter from the left to the right pulmonary artery and back again the ductus was sooner or later entered in one-third of the last 42 cases catheterised. As it passes through the duct the catheter lies at the level of the left pulmonary artery, with the sub-aortic window above it (fig. 8.51). The tip nearly always passes straight down the descending aorta, very rarely into the left subclavian artery. When a catheter passes through an aorto-pulmonary window its course up the ascending aorta and round the arch is higher, as can be demonstrated by superimposing on the skiagram a second film with the catheter lying in the left pulmonary artery. Again, in the anterior view a catheter passing through a duct and down the descending aorta usually curves backwards in a medial direction (fig. 8.63), whereas a catheter passing up the ascending aorta and round, curves backwards in a left lateral direction (fig. 8.101); in other words, the former tends to loop anticlockwise, the latter clockwise.

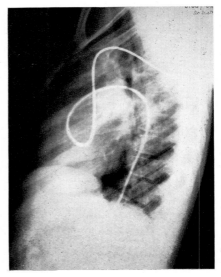

Fig. 8.51—Skiagram in the second oblique position showing a catheter passing through a patent ductus down the descending aorta; the sub-aortic window lies above the catheter.

DIFFERENTIAL DIAGNOSIS

Errors in the diagnosis of patent ductus arteriosus fall into four main groups:

1. *Mistaking other continuous murmurs for Gibson's murmur*

A *jugular venous hum* can be abolished at once by compressing the jugular veins at the root of the neck.

Pulmonary atresia with a broncho-pulmonary anastomosis may cause a continuous murmur on either or both sides; but such cases are cyanotic and patent ductus with reversed shunt causing cyanosis loses the Gibson murmur.

Arterio-venous fistula in the left upper lobe of the lung may cause a continuous murmur under the left clavicle, but the skiagram should reveal the opacity, and if the lesion is of any size there should be central cyanosis. *Coronary arterio-venous fistula* causes a machinery murmur at a lower level, and the skiagram may show a calcified aneurysm. A *congenital arterio-venous angioma* in the thoracic wall is very rare and unlikely to be in the right place to cause confusion.

Perforation of an aortic sinus into the pulmonary artery secondary to bacterial endocarditis, and therefore usually with aortic incompetence as well, may be very confusing. In the only case I have seen, which was presented to me as a recanalised duct (for the patient had had the ligamentum arteriosum ligated), the gross water-hammer pulse (blood pressure 180/40) and greatly enlarged and hyperdynamic left ventricle were out of proportion to the relatively slight degree of pulmonary plethora and the 2 : 1 shunt demonstrated by cardiac catheterisation.

An *aorto-pulmonary septal defect* is clinically indistinguishable from patent ductus, for physiologically it is identical. It is likely to be encountered in 1 to 2 per cent of all cases submitted for ligation. The machinery murmur may be exceptionally loud and perhaps a little low and central, but little confidence can be placed on minor differences of this kind. If a catheter can be passed through the communication its course may settle the question; failing that, retrograde aortography or selective dye concentration curves may solve the problem. But on the whole it may be more economical to accept the slight risk of diagnostic error, and to proceed as if any aorto-pulmonary shunt were due to patent ductus, for such an assumption will save 98 patients out of 100 much discomfort. Aorto-pulmonary septal defects may themselves be repaired, but require the help of hypothermia or some form of temporary artificial circulation.

2. *Mistaking certain combinations of murmurs for Gibson's murmur*

Ventricular septal defect with aortic incompetence has often been mistaken for patent ductus, not only because the combined murmurs have been misinterpreted, but also because of the water-hammer pulse, predominant hyperdynamic left ventricle, functional mitral diastolic murmur and pulmonary plethora. Nevertheless, this is an error that should not be made, for the two or three murmurs present do not make the Gibson murmur, and the degree of water-hammer pulse and left ventricular enlargement are disproportional to the amount of plethora.

Combined mitral and aortic incompetence in children without a rheumatic history may also confuse experienced cardiologists, again because the combination of murmurs superficially resembles the Gibson murmur, and because of the water-hammer pulse, predominant and hyperdynamic left ventricle, and short mitral diastolic murmur. But there is no pulmonary plethora—only pulmonary venous congestion—and the murmurs should not really be mistaken for Gibson's murmur.

3. *Mistaking other members of the plethoric group for patent ductus*

The difficulty here is only encountered in relation to patent ductus without a continuous murmur. The syndrome includes a pulmonary systolic murmur, perhaps a Graham-Steell murmur, a hyperdynamic enlarged left ventricle, a functional mitral diastolic murmur, and pulmonary plethora. Possible causes include ventricular septal defect, patent ductus, and persistent truncus. A small pulse, right ventricular dilatation as well as left, pansystolic murmur, close but normal splitting of the second sound, and diminutive aorta favour ventricular septal defect. Central cyanosis, of course, at once distinguishes persistent truncus, but failing that there is still the loud single second sound, and the prominent aorta. Patent ductus without a continuous murmur is suggested by a water-hammer pulse, pure left ventricular enlargement, and reversed splitting of the second sound.

Despite these considerations, real difficulty in accurate bedside diagnosis often arises, and is not always resolved by means of cardiac catheterisation, although theoretically the physiological data should be conclusive.

4. *Difficulty with the Eisenmenger syndrome*

Cases with pulmonary hypertension due to an extreme pulmonary vascular resistance (average 17 units) and reversed aorto-pulmonary, interventricular or interatrial shunt are very difficult to sort out at the bedside, and will be discussed fully later (see Eisenmenger's syndrome). Fortunately, at the present time, the distinction between these three conditions is purely academic.

ASSOCIATED ANOMALIES AND COMPLICATIONS

Although patent ductus may be associated with almost any other congenital anomaly, in clinical practice it usually occurs alone; the more common associated lesions include *coarctation of the aorta*, as already described, and *tricuspid atresia*. In the latter the ductus serves a useful purpose by providing a natural pathway whereby mixed venous and arterial blood can reach the lungs. Patent ductus is remarkably rare in any form of pulmonary stenosis and I have not so far encountered it in otherwise uncomplicated atrial septal defect.

Patent ductus may be associated by chance with certain acquired conditions such as rheumatic mitral valve disease and essential hypertension. Organic *mitral incompetence* is seriously aggravated by the increased left ventricular stroke volume resulting from the shunt and provides a strong reason for ligating the ductus without delay, although the result may be disappointing if the incompetence is already severe. The effects of *mitral stenosis* are also seriously aggravated by the increased pulmonary blood flow resulting from the shunt, and the combination calls for urgent surgical treatment; mitral valvotomy and ligation of the ductus may be undertaken at the same operation. In view of the serious consequences of coincident patent ductus and mitral valve disease, active rheumatic carditis itself constitutes an important indication for advising early ligation. *Essential hypertension* increases the aorto-pulmonary shunt through a patent ductus and therefore puts a double load on the left ventricle; on the other hand, the aorto-pulmonary communication lowers the total systemic resistance and tends to check the rise of blood pressure. It is probably best to advise ligation of the ductus in these rare cases and to treat the increased hypertension that results by medical means.

True complications of patent ductus include bacterial endarteritis, heart failure, functional mitral incompetence and pulmonary hypertension. These are all discussed elsewhere.

PROGNOSIS

An appreciable number (perhaps 20 to 25 per cent) of cases of patent ductus die from left ventricular failure in infancy (Ziegler, 1952). The average age of death was 24 in Abbott's post-mortem series (1932), and 36 in a group of 60 cases reported by Shapiro and Keys (1943). The lesion is therefore not as benign as might be supposed. The maximum age of survival so far recorded is 75 (Fishman and Silverthorn, 1951). The chief dangers are bacterial endarteritis and congestive heart failure. Bacterial endarteritis occurred in 30 per cent of Abbott's series, and in 37.5 per cent of those who survived early childhood. Vegetations appear first at the pulmonary end of the ductus or on the opposite wall of the left pulmonary artery. Spread to the heart valves (pulmonary, aortic or mitral) occurs in 75 per cent of untreated cases (Vesell and Kross, 1946).

Congestive heart failure occurred in 32 per cent of Abbott's 73 cases that survived infancy, and in 30 per cent of 60 cases reported by Shapiro and Keys (1943). The gloomy prospects suggested by these reports are not entirely valid, however, for cases that come to necropsy are highly selected. Clinical studies on unselected cases of patent ductus indicate a more favourable prognosis. Thus, Wilson and Lubschez (1942) followed 38 cases for an average period of 20 years, during which there were no deaths from bacterial endocarditis or congestive failure. Again, Benn (1947) followed 30 cases for an average period of 8 years, without meeting a single complication.

TREATMENT

Radical cure, first achieved by Gross and Hubbard (1939), consists of ligation of the ductus or of excision of the ductus between ligatures, and has proved very effective (figs. 8.52 and 8.53). The most favourable age is between 6 and 10. Surgical treatment not only prevents bacterial endocarditis, but usually cures this complication after its development (Touroff and Vesell, 1940; Vesell and Kross, 1946). Recanalisation is rare. The total operative mortality is now 2 per cent, and in uncomplicated cases only 0.5 per cent (Gross, 1947; Craafoord, 1948; Gross and Longino, 1951). Of the author's cases, 60 have so far been operated on without a death. Bacterial endocarditis should be cured by means of penicillin, if possible, before submitting the patient to operation.

Selection of cases for surgical treatment

Infants with large shunts should have the ductus ligated and divided if possible without delay, for the risk of early death from heart failure is considerable (Ziegler, 1952). Indeed, *all patients with large shunts* should be operated on without delay, whatever the age, at least up to the sixth decade.

A *moderately raised pulmonary vascular resistance* (5 to 9 units) is a strong indication for surgical treatment, for if the duct is not ligated the resistance

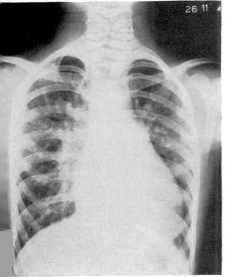

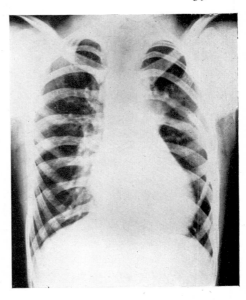

Fig. 8.52—Case of patent ductus with large shunt.

Fig. 8.53—Same case one year after ligation.

may be expected to reach systemic level sooner or later, when it would be too late to help. Surgery is contra-indicated when the shunt is prevented or reversed by a pulmonary vascular resistance over 10 units. Continued disregard for this rule has resulted in many deaths from unrelieved pulmonary hypertension then and there or within a year of the operation, for without the duct there is no safety-valve in the pulmonary circulation and the physiological situation becomes similar to that in primary pulmonary hypertension. It is unreasonable to expect the resistance to fall after ligating the ductus when the pulmonary blood flow is already normal or diminished. Surgery may still be advised, however, in cases of bi-directional shunt, if the pulmonary blood flow is increased.

Bacterial endarteritis, past or present, provides strong grounds for ligation, for infection is likely to be recurrent and on the next occasion may well prove fatal or do untold damage before being brought under control by means of antibiotics. If bacterial endarteritis does not respond to medical treatment the operation should not be delayed, for closure of the ductus alone cures the infection in two-thirds of cases (Tubbs, 1944).

The only remaining question is whether or not to advise ligation in uncomplicated cases of mild or moderate degree. In this group the surgical mortality is 0.5 per cent, and the risk of subsequent bacterial endarteritis not less than 10 per cent at the most conservative estimate. Since at least one-fifth of cases of bacterial endocarditis prove fatal, it follows that the immediate surgical risk is four times less than the ultimate risk of conservative management. It is believed that this is not offset by the significant difference between the words *immediate* and *ultimate*, and that therefore all uncomplicated cases of patent ductus should be operated on, at least up to the age of 50 years.

EISENMENGER'S SYNDROME
OR
PULMONARY HYPERTENSION WITH REVERSED SHUNT

DEFINITION

Eisenmenger's complex is ventricular septal defect with reversed shunt in the absence of pulmonary stenosis (Eisenmenger, 1897). Until quite recently the reversed shunt was attributed to displacement of the root of the aorta to the right, its position astride the defect seeming to favour reception of blood from both ventricles. Eisenmenger himself was not responsible for this misconception and thought that any apparent override demonstrated at necropsy could be the result rather than the cause of the reversed shunt (Eisenmenger, 1898). It is now known that the essential cause of the altered physiology in cyanotic cases of ventricular septal defect without pulmonary stenosis is a pulmonary vascular resistance more or less at systemic level. The definition of Eisenmenger's complex therefore becomes *pulmonary hypertension with reversed interventricular shunt*. Whether the aorta appears to ride over the defect or not is physiologically irrelevant.

At the bedside, and after viewing the electrocardiogram and skiagram, it is usually easy enough to make a diagnosis of pulmonary hypertension with reversed or bidirectional shunt, but often extremely difficult or impossible to determine the level of the shunt. The term Eisenmenger's syndrome has been used to describe this clinical picture (Wood, 1952), reserving the title Eisenmenger's complex to define a reversed shunt at ventricular level, and there is something to be said for this attitude. Alternatively, the group as a whole might be called pulmonary hypertension with reversed shunt, leaving the site of the shunt unspecified.

HÆMODYNAMICS

When the pulmonary vascular resistance is less than the systemic, blood flows through a patent ductus or ventricular septal defect from left to right; when the resistances are the same there may be no shunt at all, and when the pulmonary resistance is higher the shunt is reversed. This general law is not absolute, for a shunt may occur at any time during the cardiac cycle, but it is true enough as a working hypothesis. To some extent it is also true for atrial septal defect, although here there is obviously room for much greater variation, for atrial pressures are only indirectly related to peripheral resistances.

In patent ductus the reversed shunt is directed chiefly down the descending aorta, so that the feet may be blue while the hands and face are pink (differential cyanosis). In ventricular septal defect and atrial septal defect with reversed shunt cyanosis is uniform.

In patent ductus and ventricular septal defect with reversed shunt the systolic pressure in the pulmonary artery and right ventricle is always precisely the same as the systolic pressure in the aorta and left ventricle, any potential pressure gradient between the two circulations being compensated for by the shunt flow. This does not apply to atrial septal defect with reversed shunt, in which the pulmonary artery pressure may be higher, equal to, or lower than the aortic; in atrial septal defect also the pressure relationship between the two circulations may alter with changing conditions, e.g. with exercise.

When the shunt is wholly reversed, the pulmonary blood flow is diminished, the total systemic output remaining about normal.

In patent ductus the left ventricular stroke volume is diminished by an amount equal to the shunt from pulmonary artery to descending aorta, so that the right ventricle does the greater work, the total resistance against which each ventricle is pumping being the same. In ventricular septal defect the work of each ventricle is identical, for although the left still receives a diminished amount from the left atrium, its full quota is made up by the shunt at ventricular level. In atrial septal defect with unidirectional reversed shunt, the right ventricle pumps less blood than the left, but if the pulmonary resistance is higher than the systemic it may have to do more work.

On the whole the physiological situation is not bad. The naturally high systemic resistance tends to prevent too great a right to left shunt at any level and so ensures a fair pulmonary blood flow; at the same time the high pulmonary resistance is prevented from overburdening the right ventricle by the defect acting as a safety valve in the pulmonary circulation.

The defect in Eisenmenger's complex is always 1 cm. or more in diameter, and *the high pulmonary resistance seems to be established at birth*. Cases with ventricular septal defect of similar size, in which the high fœtal pulmonary resistance falls to normal soon after birth, run a serious risk of dying from heart failure in infancy. It may be pointed out, however, that there is a well-defined limit to the size of a left to right shunt when the pulmonary vascular resistance is normal, the ceiling being reached when hyperkinetic pulmonary hypertension reaches systemic level. Unfortunately, the pulmonary blood flow has to be four to six times the systemic flow before this happens, and few ventricles will tolerate such a burden. It follows that in many cases the high pulmonary resistance of Eisenmenger's syndrome is life-saving. The ideal physiological reaction would be a pulmonary resistance of 5 to 6 units, enough to ensure equalisation of pressures in the two circulations with moderate left to right shunts.

Just what causes the high resistance is unknown. Edwards (1950) and

Civin and Edwards (1950 and 1951) originally suggested that it represented persistence of the fœtal type of pulmonary circulation, in which a high resistance is maintained by thick muscular arteries, the object being to divert the blood flow from the lungs to the descending aorta via the ductus arteriosus. Failure of this high resistance to subside when the lungs become aerated may be due to the hyperkinetic pulmonary hypertension that would occur at once if it did so; in other words, pulmonary hypertension itself may be responsible for the vasoconstriction that maintains it. Much the same idea was expressed by Soulié *et al.* (1953), except that these authors blamed the riding aorta for the initial pulmonary hypertension.

INCIDENCE

Pulmonary hypertension with bidirectional or reversed shunt through a patent ductus occurred in 2 per cent, through a V.S.D. in 3 per cent, and through an A.S.D. in 1.5 per cent of the author's series of 900 cases of congenital heart disease. Considering the relative frequencies of these three anomalies when uncomplicated (13 per cent, 8 per cent, and 18 per cent respectively) it may be seen that the Eisenmenger reaction occurred in 13.3 per cent of those with patent ductus, 27.2 per cent of those with V.S.D., and 7.7 per cent of those with A.S.D. These rather startling differences are qualitatively just what might have been expected, for of the three only atrial septal defect can be of unlimited size without necessarily endangering life, and there are stricter limits to the size of a patent ductus than there are to the size of a ventricular septal defect. In other words most cases of large atrial septal defect do not depend on the Eisenmenger reaction for their survival, and there should be relatively more cases of ventricular septal defect of the necessary critical size than cases of patent ductus. Swan *et al.* (1953) found the same qualitative difference between the relative frequencies of raised resistances in these three conditions; with direct left to right shunts still operating and pulmonary flows averaging twice the systemic flows, the mean pulmonary artery pressure was above 40 mm. Hg in 41.5 per cent of cases of patent ductus, 70 per cent of cases of ventricular septal defect, and only 5 per cent of cases of atrial septal defect.

The *sex bias,* when present, was much the same as in uncomplicated cases of patent ductus, V.S.D. and A.S.D. This denies the implication of the strong female sex factor operating in primary pulmonary hypertension.

	SEX RATIO		
	Patent ductus	*V.S.D.*	*A.S.D.*
	M : F	M : F	M : F
Uncomplicated . . .	1 : 2	1 : 1	2 : 3
Eisenmenger syndrome .	6 : 10	14 : 14	3 : 11

The *average age* of the patients with Eisenmenger's syndrome was also much the same as in uncomplicated cases of patent ductus and atrial septal defect, but was older in Eisenmenger's complex proper than in simple ventricular septal defect as shown in the table:

	AVERAGE AGE (years)		
	Patent ductus	V.S.D.	A.S.D.
Uncomplicated . . .	17	12.7	23
Eisenmenger syndrome .	16	22	22

These figures help to show that *the high pulmonary vascular resistance of Eisenmenger's syndrome is not the end result of a direct shunt acting over a long period of time.*

CLINICAL FEATURES

Life-long *effort dyspnœa* had limited physical activity in all but one of these 58 cases, and had changed little through the years. Those with atrial septal defect were most incapacitated, averaging grade 3 (considerable) effort intolerance; those with patent ductus were best, averaging grade 2 effort intolerance, while cases with ventricular septal defect fell midway between the two. A history of *squatting* was obtained in 10 per cent, but in none with patent ductus.

Angina pectoris occurred in 10 per cent and was encountered equally in each group. These six patients were all young adults aged 21 to 36 years, and were no more cyanosed at rest than those without pain.

Syncopal attacks also occurred in 10 per cent, again with examples in each group. They were usually provoked by effort and were associated with increased cyanosis. None were fatal and they seemed neither as frequent nor as dangerous as in Fallot's tetralogy. No opportunity to investigate the mechanism presented itself.

Recurrent hæmoptysis was as frequent as angina pectoris and syncope, but not more so. The best examples were in older patients with either ventricular septal defect or atrial septal defect. The cause of the hæmorrhage is obscure.

Central cyanosis at rest, usually dating from infancy (Donzelot *et al.*, 1949), was almost invariable in those with V.S.D. (95 per cent), usual in those with A.S.D. (75 per cent), and relatively uncommon with patent ductus (27 per cent). Even on effort one third of those with patent ductus remained acyanotic in the head and upper extremeties; over half of them (57 per cent), however, showed differential cyanosis at rest, the face and hands being pink and the toes blue, especially in a hot bath. The idea that the onset of central cyanosis is typically late in Eisenmenger's syndrome, occurring first around the age of puberty, perhaps, could not be substantiated, although minimal cyanosis in childhood may certainly become more marked with advancing years. Indeed, the sudden onset of dyspnœa and cyanosis in adults with a septal defect suggests some special reason for the sudden rise of pulmonary vascular resistance, the two most likely causes being multiple pulmonary embolism (especially in relation to pregnancy), and chronic bronchitis and emphysema. *Clubbing of the fingers* was similarly most common in those with V.S.D. (92 per cent), frequent enough with A.S.D. (60 per cent) and least common in those with patent ductus (20 per cent). Clubbing of the toes alone was seen in two cases with patent ductus. *Polycythæmia* (hæmoglobin over 15 G. per cent) occurred in 85 per cent of the V.S.D. cases, 75 per cent of the A.S.D. cases, and 40 per cent of those with patent ductus. Thus on all three counts in Eisenmenger's syndrome ventricular septal defect was associated with the greatest shunt reversal and patent ductus with the least, while atrial septal defect occupied a middle position. It must be said here, however, that this clinical conclusion was not confirmed by catheter studies, for the arterial oxygen saturation averaged 80 per cent in those with V.S.D. and 79.5 per cent in those with A.S.D.; with patent ductus it averaged 91.4 per cent in the right brachial artery and 81.2 per cent in the descending aorta.

The *peripheral pulse* was usually small in those with A.S.D., more often normal than small in those with V.S.D., and either small or normal with patent ductus. The pulse was normal in quality in all three groups.

The *blood pressure* averaged 110/80 in those with A.S.D. and 120/80 in those with V.S.D. and patent ductus, confirming the clinical impression of a smaller pulse when the shunt was at atrial level.

The *jugular venous pressure* and pulse were normal in 60 per cent of all cases; *a* was dominant, usually measuring 3 mm. Hg above *v* in 30 per cent, and a large high-pressure *v* wave due to heart failure or tricuspid incompetence was seen in 10 per cent. Both conspicuous *a* waves and large *v* waves were relatively more common in cases with A.S.D. than in the other two groups. Giant *a* waves measuring more than 5 mm. Hg were seen in only one instance.

The *cardiac impulse* was impalpable in the region normally occupied by the left ventricle in one-third of those with atrial septal defect and in two-thirds of the other two groups; the right ventricle occupied the apex beat in two-thirds of those with atrial septal defect and in one-third of the other two groups. There was a conspicuous left parasternal heave over the hypertrophied right ventricle in half the atrial cases and in a quarter of the others, while in the remainder the lift over the right ventricle was relatively slight, and was absent altogether in 10 per cent of those with V.S.D. and patent ductus. In other words the right ventricle tended to be largest when the shunt was at atrial level. *Pulsation over the pulmonary artery* itself was felt in three-quarters of all cases.

Auscultation revealed a systolic murmur over the right ventricular outflow tract and pulmonary artery in 82 per cent of all cases. With A.S.D. and patent ductus it was always an ejection murmur and usually followed a loud pulmonary ejection click; with two exceptions it was loudest in the second or third left interspaces. In one-quarter of the cases with Eisenmenger's complex proper, however, the murmur was loudest lower down in the third and fourth spaces and may have been due to turbulence set up at the defect. In two such instances the phonocardiogram showed it to be pansystolic. A thrill accompanied the systolic murmur in one-sixth of those with A.S.D., one-half of those with V.S.D., and one-quarter of those with patent ductus.

The *second heart sound* was single or closely split (0.01 to 0.02 sec.) with equal frequency in three-quarters of the cases with V.S.D., and obviously split (0.03 to 0.05 sec.) in the remainder; with patent ductus it was usually closely split and very rarely single; with A.S.D. it was obviously or even widely split (0.07 sec.) in nearly half the cases, and never single. The pulmonary element of the second sound was nearly always loud unless pulmonary incompetence was severe.

A *Graham-Steell murmur* due to functional pulmonary incompetence was heard in two-thirds of all cases and was equally frequent in each group.

Electrocardiogram

Auricular fibrillation occurred in only two instances, in a woman of 65 with atrial septal defect and a man of 62 with ventricular septal defect.

Complete heart block occurred in two cases, both with V.S.D.

The *P wave* was extra sharp and measured 2 mm. or more in amplitude (average 2.75 mm.) in the most favourable lead in 56 per cent of cases with A.S.D. or V.S.D., but was normal in all but three cases with patent ductus; in these three exceptions it measured only 2 mm. in amplitude.

Considerable right ventricular preponderance (grade 3 or 4) in chest leads was seen in 70 per cent of those with atrial septal defect, and in 37 per cent of those with ventricular septal defect or patent ductus, its frequency being much the same in the last two groups. *Normally balanced QRS-T complexes* were never seen when the shunt was at atrial level, but occurred in 16 per cent of those with V.S.D. *Right bundle branch block* was seen occasionally in each group (total 8 per cent).

X-ray appearances

Conspicuous dilatation of the pulmonary artery was almost invariable: it averaged grade 3 in those with A.S.D., grade 2 in those with V.S.D., and something between the two, but nearer grade 3, in those with patent ductus.

A *clear gap* or obvious concave recess *between the aortic knuckle and pulmonary arc* was rarely seen in cases with patent ductus (fig. 8.54), but was well defined in about a quarter of those with Eisenmenger's complex or atrial septal defect (fig. 8.55). A calcified arc identifying a patent ductus was seen only once. The aortic knuckle was usually inconspicuous in all three groups, but perhaps less so in those with patent ductus; a prominent aortic knuckle was only seen in older subjects and then did not help to determine the site of the shunt.

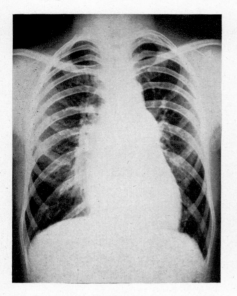

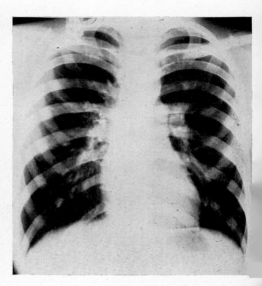

Fig. 8.54—Case of pulmonary hypertension with reversed aorto-pulmonary shunt through a patent ductus, which can be seen as an abnormal convexity between the aortic knuckle and pulmonary arc.

Fig. 8.55—Case of pulmonary hypertension with reversed interatrial shunt showing a concave recess between the aortic knuckle and pulmonary arc.

Dilatation of the right ventricle and atrium was most marked in cases with atrial septal defect, and least evident in Eisenmenger's complex proper. Thus in the former group grade 3 enlargement was recorded in two-thirds of the cases, whereas in the latter it was recorded in only 16 per cent. Again, the heart shadow was rarely normal in size when the shunt was interatrial, whereas it was normal in 45 per cent of cases when the shunt was interventricular. The average size of the heart shadow in cases with patent ductus lay midway between the two.

The *peripheral pulmonary vascular markings* were light in nearly all cases (fig. 8.56); in those with patent ductus or ventricular septal defect even the right main branch of the pulmonary artery was usually unimpressive, only the left branch (left middle arc) being really conspicuous. With atrial septal defect the proximal vessels tended to be heavier (fig. 8.57).

A *right sided aortic arch* joining a right dorsal aorta occurred in 12 per cent of cases of Eisenmenger's complex proper (fig. 8.58), but was never seen with A.S.D or patent ductus.

Angiocardiography

In Eisenmenger's complex the ascending aorta and pulmonary artery opacify simultaneously from the right ventricle (fig. 8.59); with atrial septal defect diaginol enters both atria and both ventricles more or less

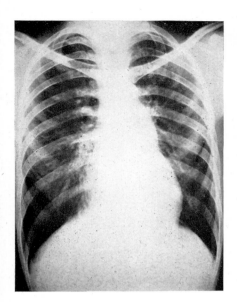

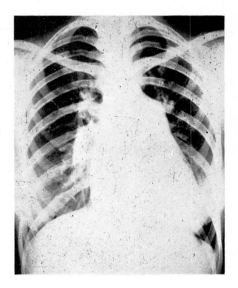

Fig. 8.56—Eisenmenger's complex proper showing dilatation of the pulmonary artery and slight pulmonary ischæmia.

Fig. 8.57—Eisenmenger's syndrome associated with atrial septal defect showing considerable enlargement of the heart and dilatation of the proximal branches of both pulmonary arteries; the peripheral vascular shadows, however, are narrow.

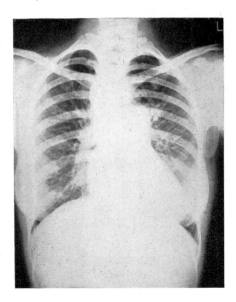

Fig. 8.58—Right-sided dorsal aorta and dilatation of the pulmonary artery in a case of Eisenmenger's complex proper.

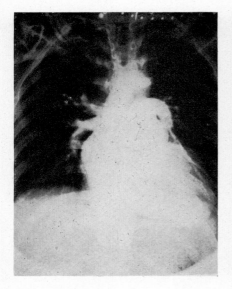

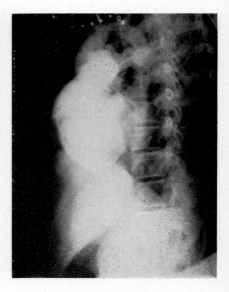

(a) Anterior view.   (b) Second oblique position.

Fig. 8.59—Angiocardiogram in a case of Eisenmenger's complex proper showing simultaneous filling of the whole of the aorta and pulmonary artery mainly from the right ventricle, although diaginol has also entered the left ventricle.

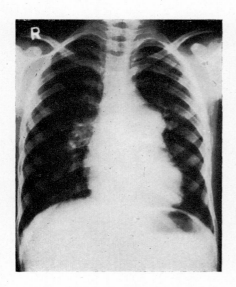

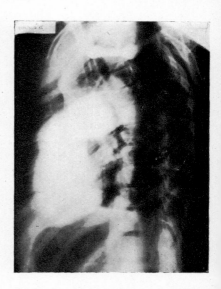

(a) Anterior skiagram.   (b) Angiocardiogram showing opacification of the right side of the heart, pulmonary artery and descending aorta, the ascending aorta remaining translucent.

Fig. 8.60—Case of Eisenmenger's syndrome associated with patent ductus.

simultaneously, becoming much diluted in the process, so that good contrast is more difficult to obtain; with patent ductus the opaque medium enters the descending aorta from the pulmonary artery (fig. 8.60).

Dye concentration curves

Evans blue dye injected selectively into the right ventricle through a cardiac catheter appears in the ear immediately in cases of Eisenmenger's complex, its concentration being strongly fortified a few seconds later by dye that has passed through the lungs. With atrial septal defect the initial hump is only seen when dye is injected into the right atrium, and with patent ductus it is not seen at all in the majority of cases, for little if any

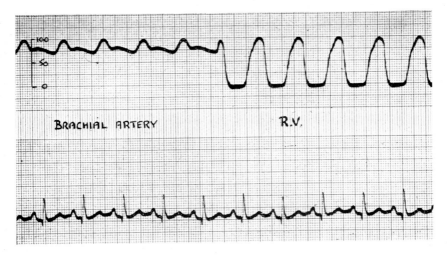

Paper speed 2.5 *mm./sec.*

Fig. 8.61—Immediately consecutive pressure tracings from the brachial artery and right ventricle in a case of Eisenmenger's complex proper.

shunted dye enters the carotids; on the other hand, dye injected directly into the pulmonary artery appears at once in samples obtained from the femoral artery.

Cardiac catheterisation usually reveals a *bidirectional shunt* at atrial, ventricular or pulmonary artery level, according to the site of the communication between the two circulations, as pointed out by Bing *et al.* (1947). In the present series the shunt was bidirectional in half the cases with atrial septal defect, three-quarters of the cases with ventricular septal defect, and one-third of the cases with patent ductus. In three cases with patent ductus (18 per cent) there was *no shunt either way*, but the catheter was passed through the duct and the systemic and pulmonary artery pressures were identical. A perfectly balanced state of this kind was never

encountered with atrial or ventricular septal defect. In the remainder of
each group the *shunt was wholly reversed*. The magnitude of the shunt was
rarely great either way, being usually of the order of 2–3 litres per minute.
The pulmonary blood flow averaged around 4.5 litres per minute in all
groups. With bidirectional shunts there was often very little difference
between net systemic and net pulmonary blood flows, but unidirectional
reversed shunts naturally resulted in reduction of the pulmonary flow,
which in such cases averaged 3.3 litres per minute.

The *systolic pressure* in the two circulations was identical in all cases of
Eisenmenger's complex (fig. 8.61) and in all but one with patent ductus

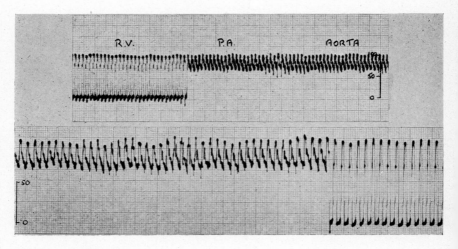

Paper speed 5 mm./sec.

Fig. 8.62—Immediately consecutive pressure tracings from the descending aorta and
pulmonary artery in a case of Eisenmenger's syndrome associated with patent ductus.

(fig. 8.62); the *diastolic pressure* was also identical in nearly half these cases,
but when there was a difference the aortic diastolic pressure was usually
higher than the pulmonary in Eisenmenger's complex and lower with
patent ductus. With atrial septal defect the systolic pressures in the two
circulations were much closer than expected, commonly within 5 mm. Hg
of each other; the diastolic, however, was usually higher on the systemic
side, sometimes considerably so.

The *pulmonary vascular resistance* averaged around 17 units in all groups,
the common range being between 13 and 22 units.

In cases with patent ductus no difficulty was ever experienced in passing
the catheter through it from the pulmonary artery to the descending aorta
(fig. 8.63), failure to do so under technically favourable conditions making
the diagnosis virtually untenable. In Eisenmenger's complex the ascending
aorta was entered from the right ventricle in 40 per cent of cases, and with

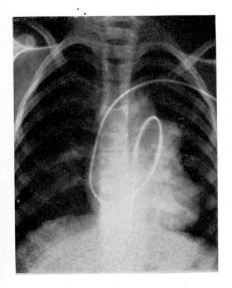 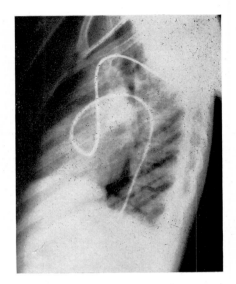

(a) Anterior view. (b) Second oblique position.

Fig. 8.63—Case of Eisenmenger's syndrome showing the usual lie of a catheter when it passes down a patent ductus into the descending aorta.

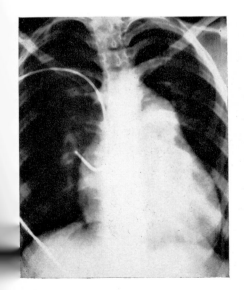 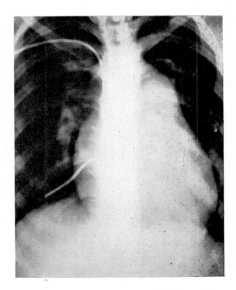

Fig. 8.64—Case of Eisenmenger's syndrome associated with atrial septal defect; the catheter has passed through the defect and is lying in (a) the left upper pulmonary vein, and (b) the left lower pulmonary vein.

atrial septal defect the left side of the heart was entered in 80 per cent (fig. 8.64), including the left ventricle in half of them. The left atrium was entered through a patent foramen ovale in only one case with patent ductus and two of Eisenmenger's complex.

DIFFERENTIAL DIAGNOSIS

It has already been stated that the clinical identification of the site of shunt in cases of Eisenmenger's syndrome is often very difficult, if not impossible, despite the details given and marshalled in the accompanying Table I.

TABLE I

DIFFERENTIAL DIAGNOSIS OF THE EISENMENGER SYNDROME

(Clinical)

	A.S.D.	V.S.D.	PATENT DUCTUS
Frequency (per cent) . . .	1.5	3.0	2.0
Sex ratio (M : F)	1 : 3	1 : 1	1 : 2
Average effort intolerance . .	Grade 3	Grade 2 to 3	Grade 2
Central cyanosis, clubbing and polycythæmia.	Three-quarters	90 per cent	One-third
Differential cyanosis . . .	—	—	One-half
Dominant *a* or large *v* in J.V.P. .	One-third	Rare	Unusual
Right ventricular lift . . .	Considerable (never absent)	Slight or moderate (absent in 10 per cent)	Slight or moderate (absent in 10 per cent)
Roger murmur in addition to pulmonary ejection murmur.	—	One-quarter	—
Second heart sound	Obviously split	Single or close split	Close split
Electrocardiogram:			
Complete heart block . . .	—	10 per cent	—
conspicuous P pulmonale . .	Over 50 per cent	Under 50 per cent	Unusual
Grade 3 or 4 R.V. preponderance	Two-thirds	One-third	One-third
Normal QRS-T	—	15 per cent	Rare
X-ray appearances:			
Right-sided aorta	—	12 per cent	—
Left S.V.C.	—	8 per cent	—
Conspicuous concave aortopulmonary recess.	One-quarter	One-quarter	Rare
Calcified duct or P.A. . . .	—	—	Rare
Considerable dilatation of right atrium.	Two-thirds	One-sixth	One-sixth

By means of special tests, however, an accurate diagnosis can usually be made (Table II).

TABLE II

DIFFERENTIAL DIAGNOSIS OF THE EISENMENGER SYNDROME

(Special tests)

	A.S.D.	V.S.D.	PATENT DUCTUS
Angiocardiography . .	Simultaneous filling of both circulations at atrial level	Simultaneous filling of ascending aorta and P.A. from right ventricle	Simultaneous filling of P.A. and descending aorta (2nd oblique view)
Selective dye concentration curves	Dye reaches ear immediately only when injected proximal to the right ventricle	Dye reaches ear immediately when injected into right ventricle	Dye does not usually reach ear at all, but may be picked up immediately in femoral artery
Differential arterial oxygen saturation	Right brachial and femoral samples similar	Right brachial and femoral samples similar	Femoral samples about 10 per cent lower than right brachial
Cardiac catheterisation: Catheter can be passed through the specified communication	80 per cent	40 per cent	100 per cent
Left to right shunt at specified level (bidirectional shunt)	50 per cent	75 per cent	33 per cent
Systolic pressure in two circulations	Should be dissimilar but often very close	Identical	Identical

It is not, as a rule, difficult to distinguish Eisenmenger's syndrome from other conditions which may simulate it superficially, but it may be as well to specify the lesions with which it is confused.

1. *Atrial septal defect with reversed shunt but without pulmonary hypertension.* As previously stated, slight right to left interatrial shunt, sufficient to drop the arterial oxygen saturation to 85–90 per cent, is by no means uncommon in simple atrial septal defect, but such cases are clinically acyanotic. Occasionally, however, shunt reversal is considerable in the absence of pulmonary hypertension, and the case presents as a cyanotic form of congenital heart disease. There were two instances of this phenomenon amongst the 900 congenital cases analysed here. Neither had congestive failure and in both cyanosis was life-long. The shunt was bidirectional and the cases differed from ordinary atrial septal defect only in the increased right to left component. It was not at all clear why this

happened. Clinically, the physical signs were those of simple atrial septal defect, apart from the cyanosis, clubbing and polycythæmia.

A somewhat similar situation arises in *cases having a common atrium*, and in advanced atrial septal defect with right ventricular failure or tricuspid incompetence, although reversal of the shunt does not occur at all readily in this latter group. At the bedside the tell-tale signs of pulmonary hypertension are missing. With a common atrium blood samples from all chambers and from both systemic and pulmonary arteries are similar. Since the right ventricle offers less resistance to filling than the left, the pulmonary blood flow is increased as in simple atrial septal defect, unless the pulmonary vascular resistance is high.

Total anomalous pulmonary venous drainage into the right atrium also suggests atrial septal defect with reversed shunt but without pulmonary hypertension. This is discussed fully later.

2. *Transposition of the great vessels with patent septa.* If there is a high pulmonary vascular resistance, the physiological situation is very like Eisenmenger's complex, a bidirectional shunt taking place at ventricular level and the systolic pressure in the two circulations being identical; but pulmonary artery samples are more saturated with oxygen than aortic samples, since the former derive chiefly from the left ventricle and the latter from the right.

Persistent truncus arteriosus with the pulmonary arteries arising from the root of the aorta is physiologically like Eisenmenger's complex only when the pulmonary vascular resistance is high. Radiologically the aortic root is unduly prominent, however, and although the left branch of the pulmonary artery may be conspicuous, the main pulmonary trunk is absent. The diagnosis may be proved by angiocardiography or cardiac catheterisation as described later.

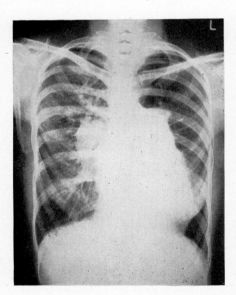

Fig. 8.65—Skiagram of a case of anoxic cor pulmonale due to emphysema complicating atrial septal defect with direct left to right shunt.

3. *Primary pulmonary hypertension* with late reduction of arterial oxygen saturation to around 80 per cent may be distinguished by its relatively short duration (usually less than two years), rapid development of heart failure, marked peripheral cyanosis, giant *a* waves in the jugular pulse, right atrial gallop, frequent absence of a pulmonary systolic murmur

tall P pulmonale and gross right ventricular preponderance electrocardio-graphically; angiocardiography shows no right to left shunt, and cardiac catheterisation no left to right shunt; the pulmonary artery pressure is usually lower than the systemic at rest and higher on effort.

4. *Anoxic cor pulmonale* with secondary pulmonary hypertension and a normal or reduced cardiac output can usually be recognised by the history and the presence of advanced emphysema. When the causal bronchitis and emphysema complicate atrial septal defect, bedside diagnosis can be very difficult (fig. 8.65). Catheterisation, however, then reveals a uni-directional shunt from left to right atrium, and pulmonary venous samples as unsaturated as those from the left atrium, left ventricle and systemic arteries, as in the case illustrated, which was later confirmed at necropsy.

PROGNOSIS

Of 35 fatal cases of Eisenmenger's complex reported in the literature and reviewed by Selzer and Laqueur (1951), 8 died in infancy, 4 between the ages of three and ten, and 5, 7, 7, 1, and 3 in each subsequent decade respectively, the oldest being 60. Figures for pulmonary hypertension with reversed interatrial or aorto-pulmonary shunt should not be dissimilar, and since ages are always younger in necropsy series, it follows that on the whole the prognosis is fair. The ages of the patients in the present series (tabulated earlier) confirm this view.

TREATMENT

Surgical repair of the defect is contra-indicated in all forms of the Eisenmenger syndrome, because it not only fails to relieve the pulmonary hypertension but also removes the safety valve in the pulmonary circula-tion. It must be clearly understood, however, that pulmonary hypertension due to a raised pulmonary vascular resistance is no bar to ligation of a patent ductus or repair of an atrial septal defect if the pulmonary blood flow is still elevated, i.e. if the left to right shunt is still dominant, for the resistance may be expected to fall if the pulmonary blood flow can be reduced to normal. *Surgical correction of central cyanosis is not the thera-peutic objective in Eisenmenger's syndrome, and if performed can only be regarded as a cosmetic operation which endangers life.*

PULMONARY STENOSIS

CLASSIFICATION AND FREQUENCY

ACYANOTIC Normal aortic root		CYANOTIC Dextroposed aortic root	
Simple (with closed septa):		Fallot's tetralogy:	
valvular . . .	10%	chiefly valvular . .	4%
infundibular . .	2%	chiefly infundibular .	7%

With direct left to right shunt via:			(pulmonary atresia, 1.7%) *Normal aortic root*
patent ductus	.	. rare	Pulmonary stenosis with reversed shunt:
V.S.D.	. .	. 1.3%	interventricular . . rare
A.S.D.	. .	. 2%	interatrial . . . 3%

Anatomically and embryologically the fundamental difference between the two main types of pulmonary stenosis depends on the position of the aortic root: in simple stenosis, whether the septa are patent or not, the aortic root is normal and arises wholly from the left ventricle, posteriorly and to the left; in Fallot's tetralogy it is dextroposed and arises partly from the right ventricle, so that it sits astride the interventricular septum, which is necessarily defective. In the former, the pulmonary artery completely covers the root of the aorta, crossing over it anteriorly from right to left; in the latter, the root of the pulmonary artery is displaced to the left and posteriorly, so that it may not cover the aorta at all, the origins of the two vessels tending to lie side by side, the aorta on the right, the pulmonary artery on the left.

In simple stenosis the stricture is valvular in 80 per cent and infundibular in 20 per cent; in Fallot's tetralogy it is mainly valvular in 40 per cent and mainly infundibular in 60 per cent. In valve stenosis the cusps are fused or represented by a conical membrane with a small circular hole in the centre. In fundibular stenosis, a small chamber, the primitive bulbus cordis (Keith, 1909), is separated off from the body of the right ventricle by a fibrous ring, which is the seat of the obstruction.

Physiologically, Fallot's tetralogy is pulmonary stenosis with reversed interventricular shunt, and the only difference between it and simple pulmonary stenosis with ventricular septal defect is the degree of stricture, which is sufficient to reverse the shunt in the former and usually insufficient to do so in the latter. In relatively mild cases of Fallot's tetralogy and in severe cases after infundibular resection, the shunt may be wholly from left to right, despite the over-riding aorta; again, in simple stenosis with ventricular septal defect the shunt may be reversed if the stricture is tight enough.

PULMONARY STENOSIS WITH NORMAL AORTIC ROOT

INCIDENCE

Of all cases of congenital heart disease only atrial septal defect (18 per cent) is more common than pulmonary stenosis with normal aortic root (16 per cent excluding cases in which associated atrial septal defect or ventricular septal defect is dominant).

The sex ratio was unity in the series analysed here.

The age distribution was as follows:

Age . . .	0–10	11–20	21–30	31–40	41–70
No. per cent .	38	35	19	5	3

It was more or less similar in all sub-groups. The oldest patient in the series was 67.

HÆMODYNAMICS

Pulmonary stenosis obviously interferes with the free passage of blood to the lungs, and to overcome the obstruction the right ventricle must contract more powerfully. This is achieved by hypertrophy and increased diastolic stretch. The right atrium helps by contracting more strongly and forcibly distending the right ventricle at the end of diastole (fig. 2.22). A giant *a* wave in the jugular pulse, right atrial gallop, and a tall P pulmonale are manifestations of this atrial contribution.

In mild cases normal pulmonary artery pressures and flows are easily maintained with right ventricular systolic pressures of only 25 to 50 mm. Hg (at rest). When the stricture is moderate, satisfactory pulmonary artery pressures and flows can still be maintained with right ventricular systolic pressures of 50 to 100 mm. Hg. In severe cases, however, the cardiac output is low and fixed and the pressure in the pulmonary artery is low, despite systolic pressures in the right ventricle between 100 and 300 mm. Hg. Peripheral vasoconstriction helps to maintain the systemic blood pressure.

In these severe cases the resistance of the stenosis is greater than the peripheral systemic resistance, so that the right ventricular systolic pressure is higher than the left. If there is an associated ventricular septal defect, the ventricular pressures are equalised, as in Fallot's tetralogy, by a shunt flow from right to left. Without such a safety valve, right ventricular pressures may rise very high indeed, and the right atrial pressure also, owing to the resistance of the thick right ventricle to extra diastolic stretch. If the foramen ovale is patent, or if there is an associated atrial septal defect, shunt reversal then takes place at atrial level, thereby relieving the right ventricle of some of its load.

In cases of mild or moderate severity, pressures in the right side of the heart are lower than in the left, and an associated ventricular septal defect or atrial septal defect results in the usual direct left to right shunt.

CLINICAL FEATURES

In view of the physiological situation described above it is clear that the clinical behaviour of cases of pulmonary stenosis must vary greatly according to the severity of the lesion. In the present series of 170 cases, the stenosis was mild in 38 per cent, moderate in 25 per cent, and severe in 37 per cent. These three groups will be discussed first separately.

Mild uncomplicated cases

There are no symptoms and effort tolerance is normal. All cases are acyanotic.

The only abnormal physical sign is a loud pulmonary systolic murmur, usually initiated by a pulmonary ejection click (Leatham and Vogelpoel, 1954) and accompanied by a thrill in 86 per cent. There is no significant *a* wave in the venous pulse, the cardiac impulse is normal (left ventricular), there is no lift over the right ventricle, and the second heart sound is obviously split, with the pulmonary element quite loud and clear.

The electrocardiogram is normal. Skiagrams show characteristic post-stenotic dilatation of the pulmonary artery, but nothing else abnormal.

Uncomplicated cases of moderate severity

There are still no symptoms and all cases are acyanotic. Effort tolerance is usually normal. Included amongst the 80 patients with uncomplicated pulmonary valve or infundibular stenosis of mild or moderate grade were a New Zealand long-distance swimming champion, a woman athlete, a Cambridge University wing three-quarter, a captain of a regional English hockey XI, and a first-class long-distance runner.

In addition to the thrill and murmur the physical signs now include slight exaggeration of the jugular *a* wave (about 3 mm. Hg), an impalpable left ventricle, and wide splitting of the second heart sound, the pulmonary component being late, none too loud, curiously brief and rather high pitched, even metallic in quality.

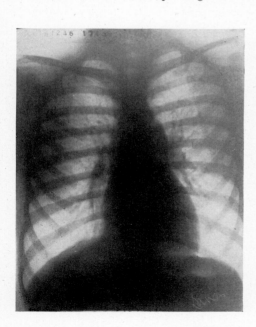

Fig. 8.66—Skiagram of a case of simple pulmonary valve stenosis showing post-stenotic dilatation of the pulmonary artery.

The electrocardiogram always shows some degree of right ventricular preponderance, usually grade 2, sometimes grade 1 or grade 3, but never grade 4. A small P pulmonale (2 mm./0.08 sec.) is seen in about 40 per cent of cases.

Fluoroscopy still reveals no more than post-stenotic dilatation of the pulmonary artery in one-third of the cases (fig. 8.66), but in two-thirds there is now slight enlargement of the right side of the heart, and occasionally (15 per cent) slight pulmonary ischæmia.

Uncomplicated severe cases

When the stricture is severe, *effort dyspnœa* ranges between none (10 per cent), slight (30 per cent), moderate (30 per cent), and considerable or gross (30 per cent together). *Angina pectoris* occurred in 15 per cent of the 32 uncomplicated cases in the present series, and *syncope* in 12 per cent.

The physical signs are highly characteristic and usually pathognomonic. The face is highly coloured, unusually full, even bloated (moon facies), in one-third of the cases, not unlike that in patients treated with A.C.T.H. (fig. 8.67). Cyanosis, when present, is peripheral, unless the foramen ovale is patent (*vide infra*). The pulse

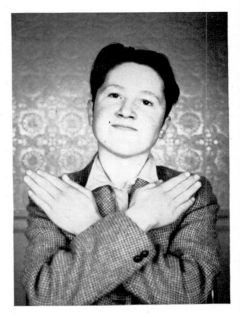

Fig. 8.67—The moon facies in a case of pulmonary valve stenosis.

is usually small, and the blood pressure normal or rather low.

There was a *giant a wave* (fig. 8.68) in the jugular venous pulse reaching 5 to 15 mm. Hg above the sternal angle in half the severe cases, and a smaller but clearly dominant *a* wave measuring about 3 mm. Hg in a quarter. Of the remainder, some had a normal venous pulse and a similar number had gross tricuspid incompetence. The giant *a* wave is, of course, presystolic in timing, peculiarly abrupt and collapsing in quality (like a venous Corrigan's sign), can be felt as well as seen, and is transmitted to the liver; it leaps to the eye, towering above and dwarfing the other waves of the venous pulse (Abrahams and Wood, 1951).

The left ventricle is always impalpable in severe cases, but a conspicuous *right ventricular heave* may be seen and felt from the left sternal edge to the mid-clavicular line or beyond; this parasternal lift should be felt as high as the third space provided the stenosis is valvular.

Right atrial presystolic gallop usually accompanies the giant *a* wave. A pulmonary ejection click does not occur in severe cases (Leatham and Vogelpoel, 1954). A loud and long *pulmonary systolic murmur*, invariably accompanied by a thrill, spills through the aortic second sound, and the *pulmonary second sound* is either inaudible or both very late and very quiet. With only two exceptions the murmur was heard best in the second left space in all these cases of valve stenosis.

The *electrocardiogram* invariably shows considerable or gross right ventricular preponderance (fig. 8.69) apart from rare instances in which

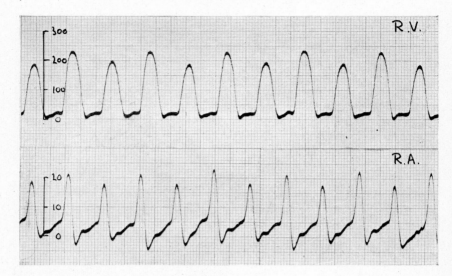

Fig. 8.68—Giant *a* waves measuring 20 mm. Hg in a case of severe pulmonary valve stenosis; note the alternation in both right atrial and ventricular pressures.

there is fully developed right bundle branch block. A tall P pulmonale averaging 3 mm. nearly always accompanies the QRS-T changes.

Skiagrams show a small aorta, post-stenotic dilatation of the pulmonary artery, light pulmonary vascular markings, and a variable degree of right atrial and ventricular enlargement (fig. 8.70); occasionally the latter is so gross that it masks the dilated pulmonary artery.

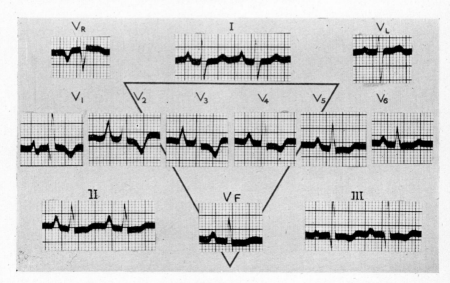

Fig. 8.69—Gross right ventricular preponderance in a case of severe pulmonary stenosis (infundibular).

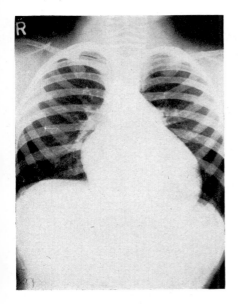

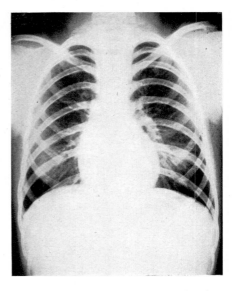

Fig. 8.70—Severe pulmonary valve stenosis showing a small aorta, conspicuous dilatation of the pulmonary artery, pulmonary ischæmia and considerable dilatation of the right side of the heart.

Fig. 8.71—Infundibular stenosis showing no dilatation of the pulmonary artery.

INFUNDIBULAR STENOSIS

Simple infundibular stenosis, whether mild, moderate, or severe, differs from the type described above in three respects only: (1) no right ventricular lift may be felt as high as the third left space; (2) the thrill and murmur are usually maximum low down in the fourth space or even at the apex; (3) there is rarely radiological evidence of post-stenotic dilatation of the pulmonary artery (fig. 8.71). Unfortunately, there are exceptions to all these rules, but the first is true in over half the cases, the second in 80 per cent, and the third in 85 per cent. When mild or moderate, infundibular stenosis is usually mistaken for maladie de Roger.

PULMONARY STENOSIS WITH DIRECT SHUNT

When an atrial or ventricular septal defect complicates pulmonary stenosis with normal aortic root, the shunt is direct from left to right if the stricture offers less resistance to flow than the systemic peripheral resistance. The clinical features vary according to the degree of stricture and the size of the defect, and are determined chiefly by the dominant lesion.

When atrial septal defect is dominant, pulmonary stenosis should be suspected if there is a pulmonary ejection click, a coarse systolic thrill, and unusually wide splitting of the second heart sound. When ventricular septal defect is dominant the stenosis is usually overlooked. When pulmonary valve or infundibular stenosis is dominant, relatively small direct shunts are apt to escape notice, but may be suggested by discrepancy between the size of the right ventricle and the pulmonary vascular shadows.

PULMONARY STENOSIS WITH REVERSED INTERATRIAL OR INTERVENTRICULAR SHUNT

Moderately severe cases of pulmonary stenosis may have a patent foramen ovale that is functionally closed. As life advances, the stricture may tighten; the pressure in the right side of the heart then rises, and the foramen ovale may suddenly begin to function and permit the passage of blood from right to left atrium. Such cases illustrate very well what is meant by late central cyanosis or cyanose tardive. Patients with pulmonary stenosis and A.S.D. or V.S.D. may behave similarly.

The change is apt to occur in adolescence and is accompanied by the development of breathlessness (Allanby and Campbell, 1949). Cyanosis is notably variable and patients may only turn blue on exertion. Pulmonary stenosis with reversed interventricular shunt resembles Fallot's tetralogy, but the aorta is not over-riding.

In most severe cases of pulmonary stenosis, however, the pressure in the right atrium exceeds that in the left from birth, and the foramen ovale cannot close. Under these circumstances patients have permanent central cyanosis and proportionate functional incapacity from birth. In the present series of 30 cases with reversed interatrial shunt breathlessness and cyanosis had been present since birth in 80 per cent; cyanosis had appeared first between the ages of 8 and 16 in 12 per cent, and the remainder were clinically acyanotic at rest. According to Joly *et al.* (1950) the condition was described by Fallot in 1888, and has therefore been called Fallot's trilogy by the French school.

The clinical features are similar to those of severe pulmonary stenosis with closed septa with the addition of *central cyanosis*, *clubbing* and *polycythæmia*, together with certain other modifications. *Effort intolerance*, usually dating from birth, is moderate or considerable with equal frequency in the vast majority; occasionally it is gross (and, of course, must become so in the end), but it is very rarely slight. Since the right ventricle is spared some of the load, and therefore fares better than cases of equal severity without a defect in the atrial septum (Brecher and Opdyke, 1951), the greater effort intolerance must be due to the drop in arterial oxygen saturation, as it is in Fallot's tetralogy. Both angina pectoris and syncope occurred only twice each in the 30 cases comprising this series.

A *moon facies* was seen in a quarter of the cases, *arachnodactyly* in 11 per cent, and hyperteleorism in two instances. A *giant* a *wave*, 5 to 55 mm. Hg in amplitude, was recorded in 60 per cent, and a dominant *a*

3 mm. Hg above *v* in 26 per cent. Two of the cases with giant *a* waves that came to necropsy had large atrial septal defects, so that powerful right atrial contraction does not necessarily mean a small foramen ovale. A *right ventricular heave* was slight (or even absent) in half the cases, moderate in a quarter and considerable in a quarter.

The characteristic *thrill and long murmur*, and their lower position when the stenosis was infundibular, were the same as in acyanotic cases. The thrill was absent in only two instances. The *second heart sound* was single (aortic) in all but three cases, and in these it was very late. A very soft late P_2 could often be demonstrated, however, phonocardiographically. In three instances a soft relatively short mid-diastolic murmur could be heard in the third left space and was attributed to turbulence set up at the atrial septal defect; in two others there was a murmur strongly suggesting slight pulmonary incompetence.

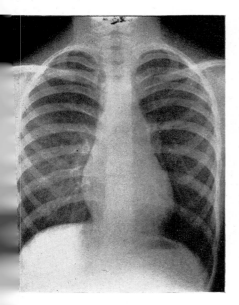 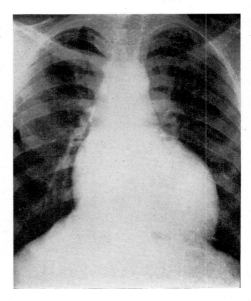

Showing dilatation of the pulmonary arc   (b) Showing considerable cardiac enlargement
and pulmonary ischæmia.   and pulmonary ischæmia.

Fig. 8.72—Pulmonary stenosis with reversed interatrial shunt.

Teleradiograms showed considerable dilatation of the right heart in only a quarter of the cases, moderate enlargement being the rule, and slight or no enlargement occurring in one-third (fig. 8.72). There was usually more pulmonary ischæmia than in acyanotic cases. Post-stenotic dilatation of the pulmonary artery was seen in nearly all those with valve stenosis.

The *electrocardiogram* showed evidence of considerable or gross right atrial and right ventricular hypertrophy in 85 per cent.

DIFFERENTIAL DIAGNOSIS

Mild pulmonary stenosis may be confused with atrial or ventricular septal defect, idiopathic dilatation of the pulmonary artery, mild aortic stenosis, and normality. *Atrial septal defect* should be distinguished by the size and behaviour of the right ventricle, the absence of a pulmonary ejection click, fixed splitting of the second sound, frequent mid-diastolic murmur associated with tricuspid turbulence, partial right branch block pattern of the electrocardiogram, and pulmonary plethora.

Maladie de Roger is easily confused with mild infundibular stenosis, but may be suggested by the closer splitting of the second heart sound. Maladie de Roger should not be mistaken for mild pulmonary valve stenosis in view of the earlier and lower position of the systolic murmur, absence of a pulmonary ejection click, closer splitting of the second sound, and absence of dilatation of the pulmonary artery. The clinical features of pulmonary stenosis and ventricular septal defect diverge more and more widely as their severity increases.

Idiopathic dilatation of the pulmonary artery may give rise to difficulty when the pulmonary ejection click is followed by a grade 2 systolic murmur. In fact in such cases it is often impossible to be sure whether there is trivial stenosis or not, and one may be still in doubt when cardiac catheterisation reveals a 5 to 10 mm. Hg pressure gradient across the pulmonary valve when the right ventricular systolic pressure is still within normal limits.

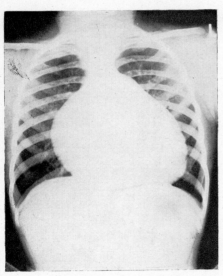

Fig. 8.73—Pulmonary valve stenosis with gross dilatation of the right ventricle and atrium resulting in appearances similar to those of Ebstein's disease except for the dilatation of the pulmonary artery.

In *mild aortic stenosis* the systolic murmur and thrill begin later, and end well before the second heart sound, which is closely split, A_2 being slightly delayed; moreover, the murmur is well heard at the apex beat and over the right carotid.

A *normal heart* with a grade 2 functional pulmonary ejection murmur and prominence of the pulmonary arc radiologically may also be mistaken for mild stenosis.

Pulmonary stenosis of moderate severity is one of the easiest bedside diagnoses and can hardly be mistaken for anything else, whether the stricture is valvular or infundibular.

Severe stenosis is also unmistakable in acyanotic cases unless there is gross failure. In such instances a deep *y* descent or large systolic wave from tricuspid incompetence may replace the giant *a* of the jugular pulse; the overloaded and grossly distended right heart loses its former vigour and may not be recognised by palpation; the electrocardiogram may show right bundle branch block, and X-rays reveal a grossly enlarged stencilled heart shadow (fig. 8.73), which in view of the findings just mentioned is easily mistaken for that of Ebstein's disease. However, the typical thrill and murmur of stenosis are still present and the characteristic diastolic scratch of Ebstein's disease is missing; moreover, it is very rare to meet the full combination of confusing features described above, and as a rule a giant *a* wave, right ventricular heave, high voltage electrocardiogram with gross right ventricular preponderance, or post-stenotic dilatation of the pulmonary artery, makes a diagnosis of Ebstein's disease untenable.

Severe stenosis with reversed shunt may be confused with *Fallot's tetralogy.* Favouring a normal aortic root and atrial septal defect are arachnodactyly, a moon facies, giant *a* wave, considerable right ventricular heave, right atrial gallop, long systolic murmur and thrill, faintly audible late P$_2$, soft mid-diastolic murmur in the third or fourth left space, gross right ventricular preponderance electrocardiographically, considerable enlargement of the right heart radiologically, and post-stenotic dilatation of the pulmonary artery; for all these features are absent in Fallot's tetralogy.

A history of squatting, normal venous pressure and pulse, quiet heart, short systolic thrill and murmur, loud single (aortic) second sound, moderate right ventricular preponderance electrocardiographically, normal transverse diameter of the heart radiologically, a poorly defined pulmonary arc, and a right-sided thoracic aorta all favour Fallot's tetralogy.

PHYSIOLOGICAL FINDINGS (based on 150 cases catheterised)

In *mild cases* of pulmonary stenosis with normal aortic root the right atrial pressure is normal, the right ventricular pressure 30/0 to 50/0, and the pulmonary artery pressure normal (fig. 8.74a); the cardiac output is normal and rises normally with effort with the aid of some elevation in right ventricular pressure. The arterial oxygen saturation is normal.

In *moderate cases* the findings are similar except that a dominant *a* wave measuring about 3 mm. Hg may appear in the right atrial tracing, and the right ventricular systolic pressure lies between 50 and 100 mm. Hg at rest, and may rise well over 100 on effort.

In *severe cases* a giant *a* wave rising 5 to 15 mm. Hg above the zero point is almost invariable. The right ventricular pressure lies between 100/0 and 275/20 at rest, the raised end-diastolic pressure being usually due to the giant *a* rather than to heart failure. The pulmonary artery pressure is usually low (fig. 8.74b). The right ventricular systolic pressure is commonly higher than the systemic blood pressure at rest, and rises well above it on exercise. The cardiac output is low and rises little on exertion; the arterio-venous oxygen difference is nearly always over 50 ml. per litre, and

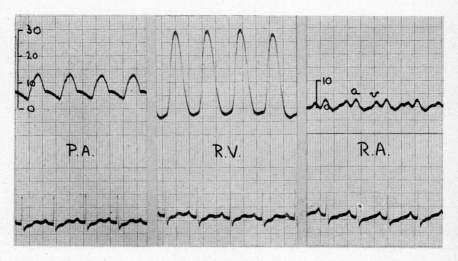

(a) Mild.

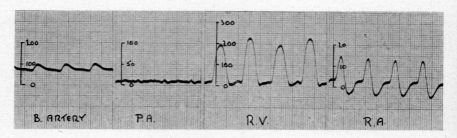

(b) Severe.

Fig. 8.74—Pressure tracings from two cases of pulmonary valve stenosis.

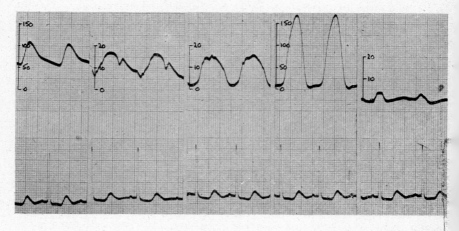

Fig. 8.75—Pressure tracings from a case of infundibular stenosis. The systolic pressure in the infundibular chamber is the same as that in the pulmonary artery, while the diastolic pressure is the same as that in the right ventricle.

increases greatly on effort. The arterial oxygen saturation is normal in cases with closed septa.

When the stenosis is infundibular the systolic pressure in the infundibular chamber is the same as that in the pulmonary artery, while the diastolic pressure is the same as that in the right ventricle (fig. 8.75). The position of the tip of the catheter when the systolic pressure changes provides good evidence concerning the site of the stricture.

Pulmonary stenosis with atrial septal defect or ventricular septal defect, and direct left to right shunt is proved by finding an increased oxygen saturation in samples taken from the right atrium or right ventricle respectively in addition to a significant systolic pressure gradient across the pulmonary valve or infundibulum.

In severe pulmonary stenosis with reversed interatrial shunt it is usually possible to pass the catheter through the defect into the left atrium and left ventricle, or out into a pulmonary vein (fig. 8.76). In the 30 cases catheterised, the right ventricular systolic pressure ranged between 105 and 260, averaging 165 mm. Hg, and was usually well above the left ventricular pressure (fig. 8.77). Giant *a* waves in right atrial pressure tracings were never transmitted to the left atrium in cases with relatively small shunts due to patent foramen ovale (fig. 8.77), but were seen occasionally in left atrial tracings when the shunt was large and due to atrial septal defect proper. The arterial oxygen saturation averaged 75 per cent and arterial samples were similar to those obtained from the left ventricle, but left atrial samples varied considerably according to whether the tip of the catheter was lying in the shunt stream or near the mouth of a pulmonary vein. Pulmonary venous samples were always normally saturated.

In the differential diagnosis between pulmonary stenosis with reversed interatrial shunt and Fallot's tetralogy, there are two points of crucial importance: (1) a catheter may pass through a valve-patent foramen ovale in Fallot's tetralogy, but when it does so left atrial samples are usually fully saturated, the foramen being functionless; (2) when the right ventricular systolic pressure is more or less the same as the systemic blood pressure, simultaneous or immediately consecutive right ventricular and brachial arterial pressures should be recorded both at rest and on exercise, for in Fallot's tetralogy they remain identical, whereas in pulmonary stenosis with reversed interatrial shunt they do not. Slight differences between right ventricular and systemic arterial pressures at rest may be due to artefact or over-damping in one of the systems, or to a slight local build-up of pressure in the femoral artery, if that vessel is used, and do not therefore exclude Fallot's tetralogy.

Selective dye concentration curves may prove the site of a reversed shunt. If Evans blue dye is injected into the right ventricle, for example, it appears immediately in the ear only when the shunt is at ventricular or aorto-pulmonary level.

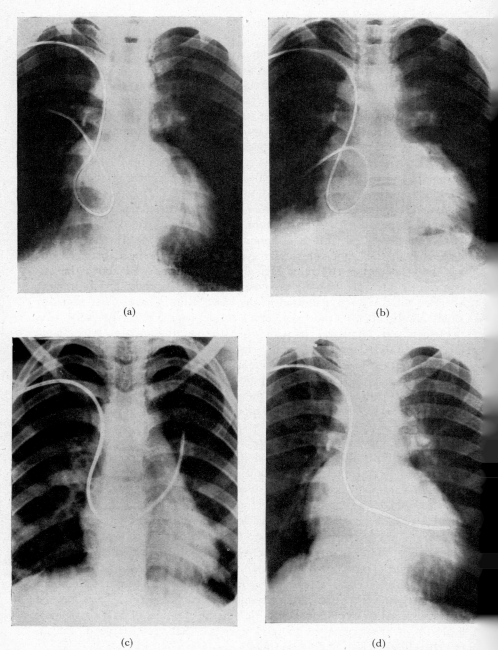

(a)

(b)

(c)

(d)

Fig. 8.76—Pulmonary stenosis with reversed interatrial shunt: the catheter has passed through the defect and is lying (a) in the right upper pulmonary vein, (b) in the right lower pulmonary vein, (c) in the left upper pulmonary vein, and (d) in the left atrium, close to the mitral valve.

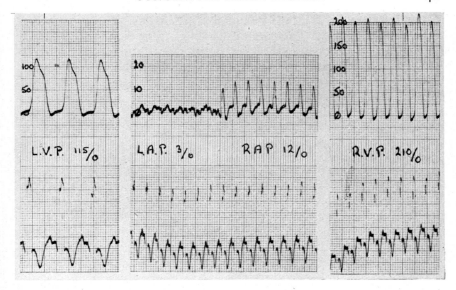

Fig. 8.77—Pressure tracings from a case of pulmonary valve stenosis with reversed interatrial shunt showing giant *a* waves in the right atrium, but not in the left.

ANGIOCARDIOGRAM

Routine intravenous angiocardiograms demonstrate the site of pulmonary stenosis in the majority of cases, but by no means in all; selective

angiocardiograms obtained after injecting diaginol into the right ventricle, preferably through a wide catheter provided with lateral holes near the tip so as to avoid recoil, are more informative (Jönsson, Broden and Karnell, 1953). Whether the stricture can be seen directly or not, angiocardiography may confirm the diagnosis of pulmonary stenosis in three indirect ways: (1) there is a hold-up in the passage of the contrast medium through the right side of the heart which is proportional to the severity of the stricture; (2) during systole in cases of valve stenosis powerful contraction

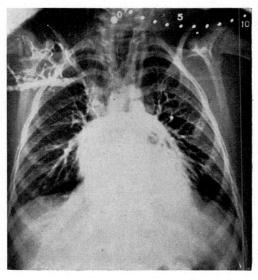

Fig. 8.78—Angiocardiogram in a case of pulmonary stenosis with reversed intra-atrial shunt; the contrast medium is passing through both sides of the heart simultaneously.

of the hypertrophied infundibulum may cause remarkable narrowing of the outflow tract; (3) post-stenotic dilatation of the pulmonary artery is well demonstrated in cases of valve stenosis.

In cases with reversed interatrial shunt there is more or less simultaneous filling of both sides of the heart (fig. 8.78). With selective angiocardiography simultaneous filling of the aorta and pulmonary artery is only seen when diaginol is injected into the right atrium.

COURSE AND PROGNOSIS

The average age of death in cases that have come to necropsy was 20.6 years in Abbott's (1931) series, 22.8 years in the group reported by Bauer and Astbury (1944), and 26 in the series reviewed by Green *et al.* (1949). The usual cause of death was congestive heart failure, which was three times as common as bacterial endocarditis. It follows that these serious mortality figures apply chiefly to severe cases, for mild stenosis does not cause heart failure, and moderate stenosis is unlikely to do so.

The oldest case in Green's series was 75 years, the oldest in my own 67. This was a man still in fairly good health apart from emphysema: the clinical features fulfilled the criteria for mild or moderate stenosis partly masked by emphysema; his right ventricular pressure was 75/3, pulmonary artery pressure 15/3, and right atrial pressure 3, —3, 0, —3, for *a, x, v*, and *y* respectively, the cardiac output at the time being 3.7 litres per minute; the right ventricle was not dilated radiologically, and there were no signs of impending break-down. There can be little doubt, therefore, that the prognosis of mild and moderate cases is good apart from the risk of bacterial endocarditis.

Severe cases, whether acyanotic or with reversed shunt, become progressively incapacitated, but may linger on with chronic congestive failure and ascites. The oldest acyanotic case in this group was 33 when he died, the oldest with central cyanosis 26 years.

Bacterial endocarditis has not yet been witnessed in any case in the present series, but two of the patients gave a convincing history of it. Prior to the infection both had had grade 3 effort intolerance, one of them having had considerable central cyanosis, obviously due to reversed interatrial shunt. Following cure of the infection both improved remarkably, one being now symptom free, the other having only slight effort intolerance. These are the only two cases in the whole series with obvious pulmonary diastolic murmurs, and it seems reasonable to conclude that the infection performed a medical valvotomy.

Pulmonary tuberculosis complicated two severe cases, one of them acyanotic, the other with reversed shunt; it was met in only one other instance in this series, despite the fact that one of the clinics at which patients were seen was at the Brompton hospital. This gives an incidence of about 2 per cent, which is the same as in the general population.

TREATMENT

Mild cases should be encouraged to lead a normal life without any restrictions; cases of moderate severity do not require surgical help and should also be allowed to lead normal lives, although competitive effort is probably best avoided. Patients in all groups should be protected against dental and other sources of infection by means of penicillin or other suitable antibiotics when the occasion arises.

Pulmonary valvotomy (Brock, 1948; Brock and Campbell, 1950) should be undertaken in all severe cases, preferably around the age of 6 to 10. Infundibular resection is better performed under direct vision, either with

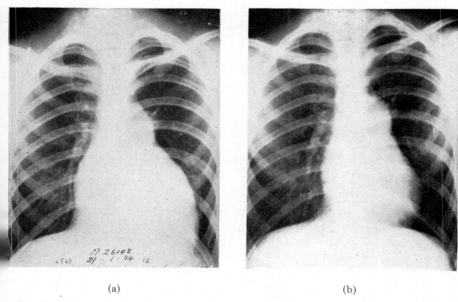

(a) (b)

Fig. 8.79—Case of pulmonary valve stenosis (a) before and (b) after valvotomy, showing considerable reduction in heart size following the operation.

the help of hypothermia or crossed circulation. Anastomotic operations are contraindicated in cyanotic cases, because the increased pulmonary blood flow that results raises the left atrial pressure, and by reducing the reversed shunt increases the load on the right ventricle, which frequently fails. Secondary elevation of the right atrial pressure then restores the right to left interatrial shunt, so that little is gained at considerable cost.

Pulmonary valvotomy was undertaken by Sir Russell Brock in 30 patients in this series, and infundibular resection in four others. The results were excellent or good in a little over half, and fair or poor in a quarter; 20 per cent died. When the result was excellent patients became symptom free and cases with previously reversed shunt lost all trace of cyanosis and clubbing. The right ventricle and atrium diminished considerably in size (fig. 8.79) and the electrocardiogram showed less right ventricular preponderance. At operation effective valvotomy was considered to have been achieved when the pulmonary artery pressure rose to normal and developed a good pulse pressure, while the right ventricular systolic pressure fell to 50 mm. Hg or less (fig. 8.80).

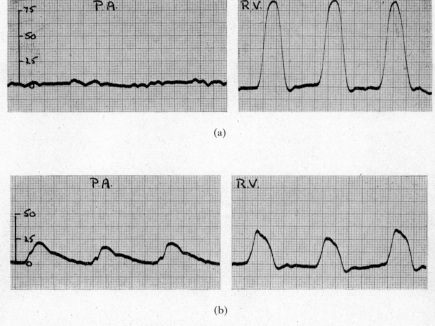

(a)

(b)

Fig. 8.80—Case of severe pulmonary valve stenosis showing pulmonary artery and right ventricular pressure pulse (a) before and (b) after pulmonary valvotomy.

At the present time the operative mortality is nearer 6 than 20 per cent (Campbell and Brock, 1955), and the results from infundibular resection under direct vision are as good as those for valvotomy, apart from the added risk of hypothermia.

Pulmonary incompetence has never caused trouble in this group, although a faint or moderate pulmonary diastolic murmur has been heard following valvotomy in nearly half the cases.

Subsequent cardiac catheterisation a year or two later in a limited number of these cases has revealed physiological findings in harmony with the clinical situation, the right ventricular systolic pressure being under 50 mm. Hg at rest and the pulmonary artery pressure pulse normal in the best of them.

PULMONARY STENOSIS WITH DEXTROPOSED AORTIC ROOT

(FALLOT'S TETRALOGY)

The combination of pulmonary stenosis, patent interventricular septum, "riding" aorta, and enlargement of the right ventricle is known as Fallot's tetralogy (Fallot, 1888), and accounts for 66 per cent of cases of congenital heart disease with clubbing of the fingers, polycythæmia, and permanent central cyanosis. The stenosis is purely infundibular in just over half the cases, purely valvular in about a third, and both infundibular and valvular in the remainder. The defect in the ventricular septum measures 10 to 16 mm. in diameter according to the size of the heart (Brinton and Campbell, 1953). The pulmonary artery, instead of being dilated as in simple pulmonary stenosis, is remarkably small, at least in cases with infundibular stenosis, and may resemble a vein. By "riding" aorta is meant displacement of the root of the aorta to the right (dextroposed aorta), so that it sits astride the septum, and appears to arise as much from the right as from the left ventricle. The association of these three malformations is no accident, but depends upon the same embryological defect, the fault lying with arrested evolution of the bulbus cordis with incomplete torsion. A right-sided aortic arch is found in 20 to 25 per cent of cases (Taussig, 1947), an association not found in cases with normal aortic root. It occurred in 20 per cent of the present series of 100 cases. A left-sided superior vena cava (always with a right S.V.C. as well) was demonstrated by means of cardiac catheterisation or angiocardiography in 20 per cent also; conversely, Fallot's tetralogy was present in just over 50 per cent of all cases in which a left S.V.C. was recognised, no other condition, except perhaps Eisenmenger's complex proper, having any special association with it.

Hæmodynamics. Aortic blood is arterio-venous, being composed of the full output of the left ventricle and part of that from the right. The right ventricle competes with the left ventricle against the systemic peripheral resistance, which is less than that of the stricture. The situation is met by hypertrophy of the right ventricle, the fourth constant finding in the tetralogy. The deficient pulmonary circulation is occasionally improved by extensive development of the bronchial vascular system. Polycythæmia helps to compensate for anoxæmia.

The pressures in the left and right ventricle are always identical, and on effort the right ventricular systolic pressure cannot rise above aortic level. The right ventricle accommodates itself to this situation from birth and is as thick or thicker than its fellow; it is not distended and rarely fails, for it can empty freely and quickly into the aorta if the obstruction increases. Since left and right atrial pressures are also practically identical in Fallot's tetralogy (easily demonstrated when there is a patent foramen ovale), diastolic ventricular tone must also be much the same on the two sides. This explains why there is no detectable interatrial shunt when there is a patent foramen ovale or small atrial septal defect.

Relatively mild cases occur in which the resistance of the stenosis is about the same as the systemic peripheral resistance; there is then a bidirectional shunt as in Eisenmenger's complex, or there may be a perfectly balanced state between the two circulations with no detectable shunt either way, such cases being acyanotic at rest. If the stenosis is milder still, a unidirectional left to right shunt can occur, as it may also after successful valvotomy or infundibular resection. About 10 per cent of all cases of Fallot's tetralogy behave in one of these ways and help to prove that the direction and magnitude of the shunt are determined a great deal more by the total resistances in the two circulations than by the degree of over-ride.

FREQUENCY, AGE AND SEX

Fallot's tetralogy accounted for 11 per cent of the author's series of 900 cases of congenital heart disease. The number per cent in each decade was as follows:

Age group	.	0–10	11–20	21–30	31–40	41–50
No. per cent	.	50	33	15	1	1

The average age was 12 years, the oldest 42. The sex ratio was 7 : 4 in favour of males. This contrasted with the 3 : 4 M/F ratio in pulmonary stenosis with reversed interatrial shunt.

CLINICAL FEATURES

Cyanosis, polycythæmia, and *clubbing* of the fingers may be absent in infants, but develop in early childhood, and tend to be progressive. Central cyanosis means an arterial oxygen saturation below 85 per cent. Of the 100 cases in this series, 15 per cent were acyanotic at rest, as described by Wood, Magidson and Wilson (1954), and had neither polycythæmia nor clubbing. The arterial oxygen saturation ranged between 87 and 97 per cent in this group. Polycythæmia was demonstrated in 82 per cent of cyanosed cases. Growth may be stunted, but mental development is usually normal. The bloated facies of severe pulmonary stenosis with normal aortic root is not seen in the tetralogy. The chief symptom is *breathlessness*, and to obtain maximum comfort children often adopt a characteristic *squatting* posture (Taussig, 1947). Squatting improves the arterial oxygen saturation (Lequime, Callebaut and Denolin, 1950), but the reason for this is not yet clear. Effort intolerance is usually considerable (grade 3), and is rarely less than grade 2B even in acyanotic cases. It is attributed to a fall in arterial oxygen saturation on effort and perhaps to some disturbance of ventilation not yet fully understood; it is not due to right ventricular strain and temporary overloading of that chamber, for nothing of that sort occurs.

Angina pectoris is extremely rare, but *syncope* occurs in 20 per cent of cases, especially in infancy and early childhood. Attacks may be related to effort, crying, breath-holding or some other transient disturbance, but are often capricious and unexpected. Theoretically anoxic syncope might be expected to result from any agent which lowered the systemic resistance sufficiently to cause a critical increase of right to left shunt, as demonstrated by Hamilton, Winslow and Hamilton (1950); in fact, however, the blood pressure has not fallen in any of four cases studied by the author, nor did a powerful pressor agent which raised the blood pressure from 100 to 150 mm. Hg in an infant make any difference to the grossly reduced pulmonary blood flow. It is suggested that syncope in Fallot's tetralogy, which is always associated with gross cyanosis and virtual cessation of the pulmonary blood flow, is due either to pulmonary vasoconstriction or to overactivity of the hypertrophied infundibulum, so that during systole it blocks the circulation to the lungs. Such behaviour on the part of the infundibulum would be no more than an exaggeration of its function in reptiles and amphibia in which it serves as a muscular valve to protect the lungs from the full force of ventricular systole, its late systolic contraction deflecting blood from the common ventricle into the systemic aorta (Keith, 1924). Functional infundibular stenosis has been demonstrated by means of angiocardiography in cases of Fallot's tetralogy (Hilario, Lind and Wegelius, 1954), and has been observed by Brock when operating on cases with valve stenosis. Pulmonary artery pressure pulses that show a late systolic trough are also highly suggestive.

Physical signs

The *pulse* and *venous pressure* are usually normal, but a small dominant *a* wave rising some 3 cm. above *v* is seen in 20 per cent of cases; giant *a* waves do not occur.

The left ventricle is nearly always impalpable at the expected position of the apex beat, and there is very little or no demonstrable lift over the right ventricle in 90 per cent of cases, a moderate lift occurring in the remainder. A strong grade 3 right ventricular heave practically excludes Fallot's tetralogy. Pulsation can never be felt in the second space over the pulmonary artery.

There is always a *systolic murmur* over the outflow tract of the right ventricle, maximum as a rule in the third left space, but occasionally higher or lower. It is loud in 85 per cent, moderate in 12 per cent, and soft in 3 per cent. A *thrill* accompanies 85 per cent of the loud murmurs, but not the others; it is therefore present in nearly three-quarters of all cases. The murmur is caused by turbulence set up at the stricture and is not due to the shunt. It is a pulmonary or infundibular ejection murmur, starting early because the pulmonary diastolic pressure is low, and finishing usually just before the aortic second sound; it does not spill through A_2 like the long murmur of severe pulmonary stenosis with normal aortic root

(Vogelpoel and Shrire, 1955). This may be because the right ventricle empties relatively quickly as previously described or because of total (partly functional) infundibular obstruction in late systole. As might be expected, the intensity and length of the murmur vary inversely with the pulmonary blood flow, and diminish greatly during spontaneous attacks of increased cyanosis; with syncope the murmur usually disappears altogether (functional pulmonary atresia). Conversely, after pulmonary valvotomy or infundibular resection the murmur often becomes explosive.

The *second heart sound* is invariably single and usually fairly loud at the base, because the root of the aorta is uncovered and it is only aortic valve closure that is heard. There is no gallop, no ejection click, no pulmonary diastolic murmur and no mid-diastolic murmur. I have yet to hear a continuous murmur in Fallot's tetralogy, whether due to patent ductus, which must be extremely rare, or to a broncho-pulmonary communication. Indeed, such a murmur occurring in a case which has many features suggesting Fallot's tetralogy makes a diagnosis of pulmonary atresia virtually certain.

Electrocardiogram

The P pulmonale is often said to be typical of Fallot's tetralogy, and has been reported as occurring in 80 per cent of cases (Donzelot *et al.*, 1951). This statement needs tempering, for it is near the margin of truth and is physiologically misleading. The right ventricle is not ordinarily embarrassed in Fallot's tetralogy and needs relatively little atrial help: in the 100 cases analysed here the P wave was normal in 42 per cent, 2 to 2.5 mm. high in the most favourable lead in 26 per cent, 3 to 3.5 mm. high in 25 per cent, and 4 or more mm. high in 7 per cent. Thus in two-thirds of the cases it did not exceed 2.5 mm. While it is agreed, therefore, that a P pulmonale is common in Fallot's tetralogy, its small stature and the frequency of a normal P wave are stressed, for in these respects the P wave differs from its behaviour in pulmonary stenosis with reversed interatrial shunt.

Right ventricular preponderance as customarily interpreted from multiple chest leads was slight in 9 per cent of cases, moderate in 24 per cent, considerable in 57 per cent, and gross in 7 per cent, the graph being normal in 3 per cent. Here again the point that requires emphasis is the relatively minor change found in one-third of all cases (fig. 8.81), in remarkable (but expected) contrast to the findings in severe pulmonary stenosis with normal aortic root. There was no convincing correlation between the grade of right ventricular preponderance and the degree of cyanosis or effort intolerance: for example, when right ventricular preponderance was slight or moderate, one-third of the cases had considerable or gross cyanosis; when it was grade 3 or 4, 41 per cent had considerable or gross cyanosis. This is not surprising because the work of the right ventricle is the same whether cyanosis is absent or gross and whether the

91.4 per cent). Left atrial samples were invariably between 90 and 97 per cent saturated, and averaged 93.4 per cent, proving the absence of reversed interatrial shunt despite the patent foramen ovale. Left ventricular samples ranged between 74 and 92 per cent saturated, averaging 81 per cent; in these cases the arterial oxygen saturation averaged 78 per cent, proving that the shunt in Fallot's tetralogy is chiefly at ventricular level, as it is in Eisenmenger's complex, and not a matter of the right ventricle expelling part of its contents directly into an over-riding aorta; it is unlikely that any appreciable shunt takes place in diastole, for if diastolic ventricular pressures favoured a right to left shunt at ventricular level, they must also do so at atrial level, which has already been proved untrue. Bidirectional shunt was never found in cyanotic cases, and only once in the acyanotic group; but in three of the latter no shunt at all could be demonstrated, and in one there was a unidirectional slight left to right shunt.

The site of the stenosis can be recognised as high, intermediate or low during cardiac catheterisation, but while the last two denote infundibular stenosis it is impossible to be sure whether a high site means valve stenosis or high infundibular stenosis. It is most unusual in Fallot's tetralogy to be able to reproduce the clean type of infundibular tracing obtained in the great majority of cases of infundibular stenosis with normal aortic root.

In calculating the size of the shunt the pulmonary blood flow must be worked out on the assumption that pulmonary venous blood is 95 per cent saturated. In the present series the systemic blood flow averaged 5 L/min., and the pulmonary flow 3 L./min , giving an average shunt of 2 L./min.

Dye Concentration Curves

Evans blue dye reaches the ear well ahead of normal time; as its rapidly built-up concentration levels out or falls off, it is suddenly reinforced by dye that has circulated through the lungs. If the dye is injected directly into the right ventricle its immediate appearance in the ear proves that the reversed shunt is at ventricular or aorto-pulmonary level, not below.

If an oximeter is not available, saccharin or some other test substance may be injected into the right ventricle with similar qualitative results.

DIFFERENTIAL DIAGNOSIS

The chief difficulty is to distinguish Fallot's tetralogy from *pulmonary stenosis with reversed interatrial shunt*. In their characteristic form these two conditions are very different, but when atypical may be remarkably similar (see page 417).

Pulmonary atresia is easily recognised by the absence of a pulmonary ejection murmur, the almost invariable presence of a continuous murmur under one or other or both clavicles, and the more conspicuous ascending aorta.

Eisenmenger's complex proper with a single second heart sound and minimal dilatation of the pulmonary artery may cause real difficulty. Absence of squatting, slight pulsation over the pulmonary artery, a pulmonary ejection click, absence of a pulmonary systolic thrill, the presence of a Roger murmur, and a faint pulmonary diastolic murmur are all strongly in favour of pulmonary hypertension with reversed inter-ventricular shunt.

Acyanotic examples of Fallot's tetralogy are usually confused with *maladie de Roger*. The history alone should prevent any such error, for effort intolerance is at least moderate in the former and invariably absent in the latter. The chief differences in the physical signs are the timing of the murmur and the character of the second heart sound: the murmur is a pulmonary ejection murmur in Fallot's tetralogy, a pansystolic shunt murmur in maladie de Roger; the second heart sound is always single in Fallot's tetralogy, split in maladie de Roger.

COMPLICATIONS

Pulmonary tuberculosis complicated only 2 per cent of the cases in this series, which is similar to its incidence in the general population.

Cerebral abscess, presumably from a small paradoxical embolism, is responsible for death in about 5 per cent of all fatal cases of congenital heart disease (Robbins, 1945; Gates, Rogers and Edwards, 1947). Fallot's tetralogy has been the primary lesion in half the reported cases. The abscess, which is usually solitary, is not secondary to bacterial endocarditis, but to some somatic infection often of a trivial nature. A history of such infection, however, has been obtained in only a third of the cases (Sancetta and Zimmerman, 1950).

Cerebral thrombosis with hemiplegia is not uncommon, especially in infancy, and is attributed to polycythæmia.

Bacterial endocarditis is relatively uncommon, probably because of the high natural mortality of most cyanotic forms of congenital heart disease in childhood and adolescence.

PROGNOSIS

Uncomplicated relatively mild cases may reach middle life, but the majority die young. According to Campbell (1948, 1950), only one patient in ten with congenital cyanotic heart disease reaches the age of 21, only one in five reaches puberty, and only one in two reaches the age of 7. The most common cause of death in infancy and early childhood is undoubtedly *syncope*, the mechanism of which has already been discussed. *Bacterial endocarditis* and *cerebral abscess* each takes its toll of about 10 per cent, and *cerebral thrombosis* may be fatal. *Intercurrent infection* is probably responsible for most of the remainder, not because these children are especially prone to such infections, but because they tolerate them badly *Congestive heart failure* is very unusual, for as stated repeatedly, the right ventricle is not overburdened in Fallot's tetralogy. According to Rich (1948), 90 per cent of fatal cases show widespread thrombotic obstruction of the small pulmonary vessels, possibly due to polycythæmia. Just what part this plays is open to question; an increased pulmonary vascular resistance has yet to be demonstrated at catheterisation.

TREATMENT

Since the operative mortality is around 30 per cent in infants under 3 years old, it is wise to defer operation until the child is 5 or 6, if possible. In severe cases the wait may be trying and not without its own mortality. Attacks of severe dyspnœa and cyanosis with or without syncope are the chief danger. For these Taussig (1948) advised placing the child in the knee-chest position, and if relief was not immediate giving morphine in a dose of 1 mg. per kilogram of body weight, which she found almost specific. An oxygen tent may have to be used in the worst cases to carry the infant through a difficult period. This usually increases the arterial oxygen by about 10 per cent, as noted by Taussig and Blalock (1947) when oxygen was given by the anæsthetist as a preliminary to opening the thorax. Operation should not be delayed after the age of 3, however, if serious attacks continue.

As a result of Taussig's observation that infants with Fallot's tetralogy deteriorated when the ductus arteriosus closed, and that cases complicated by persistent patent ductus fared better than those without, she and Blalock devised the anastomotic operation that proved so successful (Blalock and Taussig, 1945; Blalock, 1946; 1947). One or other subclavian artery is anastomosed to the homolateral branch of the pulmonary artery. Better alignment is obtained, as a rule, with the right subclavian; but the left has a longer intrathoracic course and is therefore easier to bring down. If results are poor, a second anastomosis may be carried out later on the opposite side. Another method of achieving the same object is to make a direct anastomosis between the aortic arch and the left pulmonary artery (Potts et al., 1946; 1948).

The physiological results of technically successful anastomosis are good: cyanosis and clubbing may disappear, breathlessness decreases, the habit of squatting is usually given up, and effort tolerance improves; the arterial oxygen saturation rises to the region of 80 per cent and the blood count returns to normal (Taussig, 1948); a loud machinery murmur and coarse thrill may be detected on the homolateral side immediately after the operation in nearly all cases, and are permanent. Blalock's total mortality rate for this operation is 17 per cent, but this includes infants (mortality rate 25 per cent), cases of tricuspid atresia and other anomalies. His mortality rate for selected cases of Fallot's tetralogy is not more than 10 per cent The results and mortality rate of Potts' operation are much the same (Potts, 1949).

Both Brock (1948) and Sellors (1948), however, proved that pulmonary stenosis was amenable to direct attack, the approach being through the wall of the right ventricle. Valvotomy is undertaken when the stenosis is valvular, infundibular resection (Brock, 1949) when the stricture is below the valve. Campbell, Deuchar and Brock (1954) have reported the results on the first 100 cases of Fallot's tetralogy treated by valvotomy (37 cases), infundibular resection (45 cases) or both (18 cases) at Guy's Hospital and the Brompton Hospital. Two-thirds of them were greatly improved, one-sixth were better but not in the same class, and nearly one-sixth died as a result of the operation; the mortality from pulmonary valvotomy was stated to be 11 per cent and from infundibular resection 18 per cent. Although the risk was greater with infundibular resection the results were better in those who survived. Campbell and Deuchar (1953) also report the results of 200 Blalock-Taussig anastomotic operations, most of which were undertaken for Fallot's tetralogy. A comparison of the results obtained in the two types of operation by the same team is especially valuable. The mortality in the anastomotic operation in Fallot's tetralogy was only 8 per cent, and 75 per cent of the cases "benefited greatly"; but the authors were careful to say that some incapacity usually remained, and that cyanosis, clubbing and polycythæmia were not as a rule abolished, though much reduced. The matter may be summed up by saying that the reports from Guy's indicate that the best immediate results are obtained by infundibular resection at the cost of twice the operative mortality. The physiological results from pulmonary valvotomy were not quite so good, but probably better than from the Blalock-Taussig operation; on the other hand the operative mortality was a little higher.

Personal experience at Brompton and elsewhere has been more or less similar, but enthusiasm for the Blalock-Taussig operation is difficult to maintain. These patients are better than they were, but none of them can be classed as excellent: most of them are still somewhat cyanosed and a little clubbed, and effort tolerance is still limited. At the Brompton Hospital 41 direct operations have been carried out on cases of Fallot's tetralogy, mostly by Sir Russell Brock. There were 15 primary pulmonary valvotomies and 26 primary infundibular resections; seven cases had the combined operation. There were only two deaths in this series, one from valvotomy, the other from infundibular resection. There is no doubt at all that when the operation was technically satisfactory, the results, if judged by effort tolerance and disappearance of cyanosis, far exceeded anything seen following Blalock's operation. Excellent results of this kind were observed in at least 40 per cent, more often from infundibular resection than from pulmonary valvotomy, as in the Guy's group. But half the "excellent" cases produced by infundibular resection have been transformed into cases of ventricular septal defect with left to right shunt, the pulmonary resistance remaining normal. The shunt is quite considerable, there is radiological pulmonary plethora, and the hearts are much enlarged

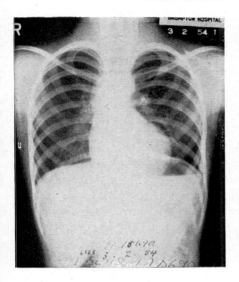
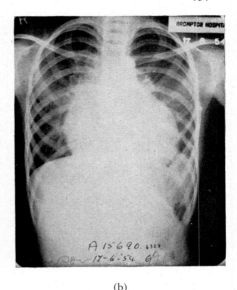

(a) (b)

Fig. 8.88—Skiagrams (a) before and (b) after infundibular resection in a case of Fallot's tetralogy showing post-operative pulmonary plethora and considerable enlargement of both sides of the heart.

(fig. 8.88). Physiological studies in four members of this group a year or two after the operation revealed a pulmonary blood flow of 6.3 to 10.6 litres per minute (average 8.4), which was about twice the systemic flow. In three of them the shunt was purely from left to right, despite the over-riding aorta; in the fourth it may have been bidirectional, for the arterial oxygen saturation was 88 per cent. Right ventricular systolic pressures remained identical with those in the aorta or brachial artery; the systolic pressures in the infundibular chamber and pulmonary artery were normal in two cases and raised in the other two (fig. 8.89). Nothing approaching Eisenmenger's complex was ever seen. The enlargement seems to be due to dilatation of both ventricles, particularly the right, resulting from their increased stroke volume, and is greater than in simple ventricular septal defect with comparable shunt. This is because the right ventricle has to pump double its normal volume at systemic pressure, an uncommon physiological situation. In simple ventricular septal defect with 2 : 1 shunt, the pulmonary artery pressure is usually normal; in Eisenmenger's complex, when the right ventricle is working at systemic pressure, its stroke volume is usually normal.

In the other half of the group with excellent results following infundibular resection, and in all excellent results following valvotomy, the physiological situation is well nigh as perfect as it can be in the presence of a large ventricular septal defect and an over-riding aorta, for the two circulations appear to be delicately balanced. Effort tolerance is practically

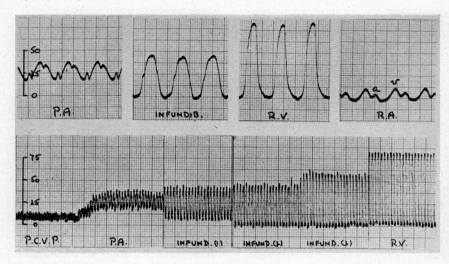

Fig. 8.89—Intracardiac pressure pulse in a case of Fallot's tetralogy one year after infundibular resection.

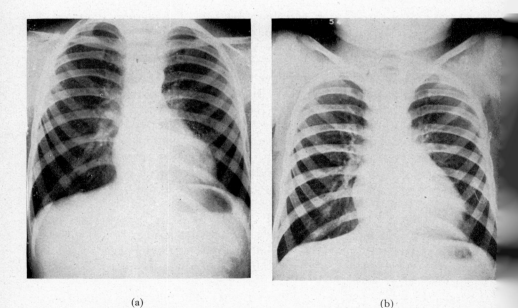

(a)   (b)

Fig. 8.90—Skiagram showing ideal result from infundibular resection in a case of Fallot's tetralogy (a) before and (b) after the operation. The pulmonary vascular shadows are only slightly heavier and the heart has increased only slightly in size.

normal, there is no cyanosis, clubbing or polycythæmia, the arterial oxygen saturation is around 90 per cent, the heart is only slightly if at all larger, and the pulmonary vascular shadows have improved without becoming plethoric (fig. 8.90).

At operation one of the technical difficulties is to know when sufficient infundibular resection has been achieved. The ideal physiological result is to restore the arterial oxygen saturation to normal without increasing the pulmonary blood flow beyond normal or at most beyond a critical safe limit (probably about 6 litres per minute at rest for a child of 10). Under the artificial conditions imposed by anæsthesia, oxygen administration, thoracotomy and cardiotomy, much experience and fine judgment are necessary if the surgeon is to achieve this ideal: he cannot rely on the

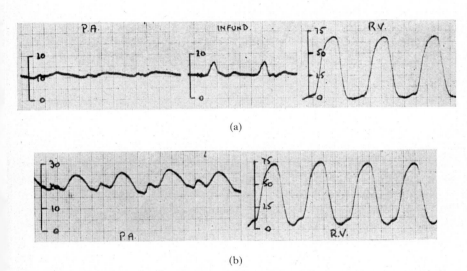

(a)

(b)

Fig. 8.91—Intracardiac pressure pulse (a) before and (b) after infundibular resection in a case of Fallot's tetralogy: in (b) the pressure pulse in the pulmonary artery is much better defined and at a higher level; the right ventricular systolic pressure is unchanged.

oximeter, and can obtain no help from the right ventricular pressure, which remains at systemic level under all circumstances; he can, however, aim at producing a good pressure pulse in the pulmonary artery without an abnormal rise in pressure (fig. 8.91).

There is not the same risk of over-zealous surgery when undertaking pulmonary valvotomy. So far there have been no examples of serious cardiac enlargement resulting from too great a shunt in this group; on the contrary, the difficulty has been to achieve a sufficiently good valvotomy to prevent the right to left shunt and to ensure a good pulmonary blood flow. A determined attempt to split the valve efficiently, however, carries with it a risk of another sort, that of causing serious pulmonary incompetence. A pulmonary diastolic murmur has developed in one-quarter of these cases following valvotomy, and in three instances the leak was by no means trivial; in fact one is very serious and has led to heart failure. Pulmonary incompetence is rarely important unless a left to right shunt has been created by the operation.

Finally, it is hoped that all this work and controversy will prove of historical interest only, for the time is already ripe for repairing the ventricular septal defect, as well as relieving the stricture, under direct vision with the aid of hypothermia or some kind of artificial circulation.

PULMONARY ATRESIA

Complete obliteration of the pulmonary valve and root of the main pulmonary artery accounted for 15 of the 900 cases in this series (1.7 per cent). It was always associated with a ventricular septal defect, marked over-riding of the aortic root, and a well-developed broncho-pulmonary anastomosis.

HÆMODYNAMICS

Life depends on the efficiency of the broncho-pulmonary anastomosis, rarely on the presence of a large patent ductus. In those that survive infancy large bronchial arteries join one or more primary or secondary division branches of the pulmonary artery on one or both sides (Allanby *et al.*, 1950). Mixed venous and arterial blood from the aorta is thus carried to the lungs through the normal pulmonary arterial tree, by-passing only the main pulmonary trunk. A less important peripheral anastomosis between the two circulations also develops. The output of both ventricles is expelled entirely through the ascending aorta, which is enlarged accordingly. The low pulmonary vascular resistance and high feeding pressure ensures a good pulmonary blood flow if the total cross-section of the communicating bronchial arteries is around 0.25 sq. cm.

AGE AND SEX

The average age of the patients in this small series was 11, and the range 3 to 35 years. There were two males to one female.

CLINICAL FEATURES

Pulmonary atresia resembles Fallot's tetralogy in many ways, but it has several distinguishing features which enable it to be recognised at the bedside with ease.

Cyanosis, clubbing and polycythæmia are usually considerable or gross, but not necessarily; clinically acyanotic cases are never seen. Breathlessness is considerable in two-thirds, and mild to moderate in one-third. Squatting occurred in only one-quarter of the present series.

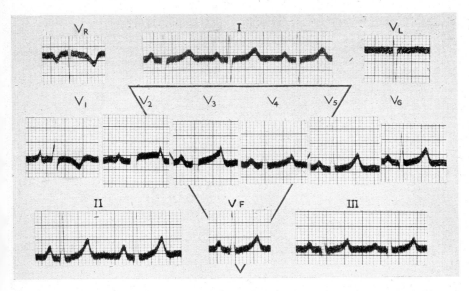

Fig. 8.92—Electrocardiogram in a case of pulmonary atresia showing relatively slight right ventricular preponderance; there is a 3-mm. P pulmonale in standard lead 2.

One quarter also had syncopal attacks, sometimes with convulsions: in pulmonary atresia such attacks obviously cannot be due to transient functional occlusion of the infundibulum during systole, and suggest, therefore, that pulmonary vasoconstriction or a fall in systemic peripheral resistance is responsible. No opportunity to study an attack presented itself.

The *physical signs* were like those of Fallot's tetralogy except that instead of a pulmonary ejection murmur, which of course was absent, there was a continuous murmur in all 15 cases. It was best heard just below the clavicle and was bilateral in two-thirds of the cases; when it was unilateral it was as often on the right side as on the left. There is good reason to believe, therefore, that this murmur is nearly always caused by a proximal broncho-pulmonary anastomosis, and not by a patent ductus.

The electrocardiogram does not differ from that in Fallot's tetralogy (fig. 8.92), but the skiagram usually shows a more prominent ascending aorta (fig. 8.93) or knuckle. Angiocardiography may reveal the broncho-pulmonary anastomosis and shows no main pulmonary artery (fig. 8.94).

The pulmonary blood flow may be measured very easily, for it is only necessary to obtain a sample of blood from the brachial or femoral artery and to measure the oxygen consumption; the mixed blood in the arterial sample is the same as that in the pulmonary arteries, and pulmonary venous blood may be assumed to be 95 per cent saturated. In the few that have been measured, the pulmonary blood flow has ranged between 2.8 and 4 litres per minute.

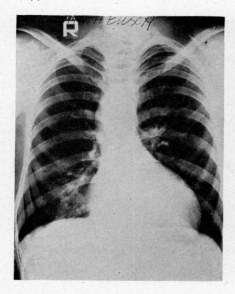 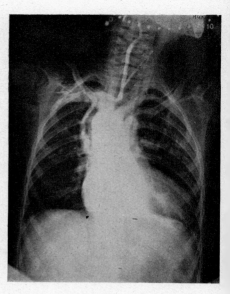

Fig. 8.93—Skiagram from a case of pulmonary atresia showing a prominent
ascending aorta, conspicuous pulmonary
bay and pulmonary ischæmia. Angiocardiography proved that the aortic arch and
dorsal aorta were left sided.

Fig. 8.94—Angiocardiogram from a case of
pulmonary atresia showing dense opacification of the right ventricle and aorta, and a
large broncho-pulmonary anastomotic vessel on the left side.

The *prognosis* in those who survive infancy seems much the same as in
Fallot's tetralogy.

Surgical treatment is not nearly so satisfactory as in Fallot's tetralogy,
and the mortality is higher. Blalock's operation is usually advised if the
pulmonary blood flow is below 4 litres per minute. Considerable care
must be taken not to interfere with the broncho-pulmonary shunt, particularly if unilateral, while constructing the artificial anastomosis.

ABSENT LEFT OR RIGHT BRANCH OF THE PULMONARY
ARTERY

From time to time cases are seen in which the pulmonary vascular
markings are very light on one side and unduly heavy on the other. When
there is no kyphoscoliosis and no evidence of unilateral emphysema this
usually means congenital absence of the left or right pulmonary artery.
The whole of the right ventricular output passes down the normal branch,
as it does following pneumonectomy. There is no rise in resting pulmonary
artery pressure, because the flow is only twice normal, but there is less
reserve and the pressure may well rise on exercise. The ischæmic lung
handles about one-third of the inspired air, but takes up only 6 per cent
of the total oxygen uptake (McKim and Wiglesworth, 1954).

As a rule, the aortic arch is on the side opposite that of the absent pulmonary artery. The deficiency may be associated with other congenital anomalies, such as Fallot's tetralogy (Nadas *et al.*, 1953), when it may have an important bearing on the surgical treatment.

TRICUSPID ATRESIA

Tricuspid atresia accounted for 1.5 per cent of the 900 cases analysed here. Uncomplicated cases (type 1 of Edwards and Burchell, 1949) have an atrial septal defect or patent foramen ovale through which blood escapes from the otherwise closed right atrium into the left atrium; blood reaches the lungs from the left side of the heart through a ventricular septal defect, patent ductus, or broncho-pulmonary anastomosis. In addition there may be pulmonary atresia or stenosis, valvular or infundibular. Complicated cases (type II of Edwards and Burchell, 1949), have transposition of the great vessels with or without pulmonary stenosis; venous blood entering the left atrium via the foramen ovale mixes with blood from the lungs and passes directly into the pulmonary artery and indirectly into the aorta via a ventricular septal defect. In either case the left ventricle does all or most of the work, but the lungs are ischæmic in type I, plethoric in type II.

AGE AND SEX

Of 37 cases mostly collected from the literature, 28 died within the first year, three within the second year, and six between the ages of 2 and 5 (Sommers and Johnston, 1951). The average age of the 13 cases described here, however, was 9.4 years and the range 3 to 17.

The sexes are fairly equally represented, perhaps with a slight bias in favour of females (M/F=4/5).

CLINICAL FEATURES

Effort intolerance, cyanosis, clubbing and polycythæmia are invariably considerable or gross; squatting is the rule, angina occasional, and syncope rare.

The physical signs include a giant *a* wave when there is a foramen ovale rather than an atrial septal defect, a forceful left ventricular cardiac impulse, a systolic murmur usually accompanied by a thrill at the base due to ventricular septal defect in over half the cases, and a single second heart sound owing to absence of the pulmonary element in the majority. Sometimes there is only a trivial aortic flow murmur at the base and a continuous murmur under the left clavicle, which in tricuspid atresia is more likely to be caused by a patent ductus than by a broncho-pulmonary anastomosis. Occasionally, the second heart sound is split, especially when there is a good-sized ventricular septal defect; the pulmonary element can be very late when there is associated pulmonary stenosis.

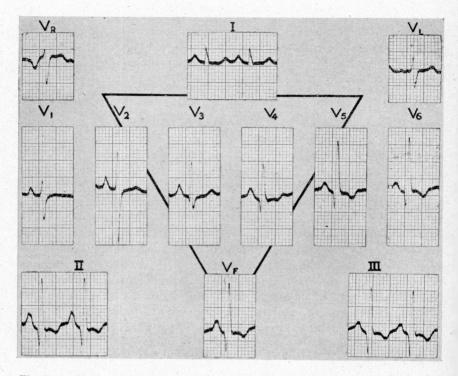

Fig. 8.95—Electrocardiogram in a case of tricuspid atresia showing considerable left ventricular preponderance.

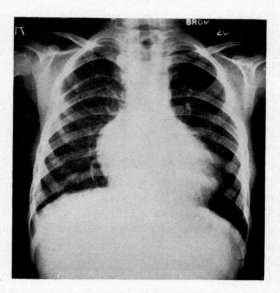

Fig. 8.96—Tricuspid atresia showing pulmonary ischæmia with enlargement of the right atrium and left ventricle.

The *electrocardiogram* is characterised by a conspicuous P pulmonale, averaging 3.5 to 4 mm. in amplitude, and grade 2 to 3 left ventricular preponderance (fig. 8.95).

X-rays show a combination of pulmonary ischæmia, hypoplasic pulmonary artery, left ventricular enlargement and dilatation of the right atrium (fig. 8.96).

Angiocardiography shows diaginol filling the two atria in high concentration almost simultaneously, followed by opacification of the left ventricle and aorta, the pulmonary artery remaining invisible or but faintly delineated (fig. 8.97).

Cardiac catheterisation is not advised because it can only reveal a giant *a* wave in the right atrium and reversed interatrial shunt, findings which do not exclude pulmonary hypertension or stenosis with reversed interatrial shunt. Failure to pass the catheter through the tricuspid orifice is no evidence of atresia.

The *prognosis* is poor, most patients dying in infancy. Blalock's or Pott's operation may greatly improve the pulmonary blood flow and so relieve cyanosis and dyspnœa, but the shunt adds to the burden of the left ventricle and may lead to heart failure. Nevertheless surgical treatment is well worth while, despite a fairly high mortality.

TRANSPOSITION OF THE GREAT VESSELS

Transposition, the aorta rising anteriorly from the right ventricle and the pulmonary artery posteriorly from the left ventricle, occurred in 1 per cent of these 900 congenital cases and in 6.9 per cent of Abbott's series. It is a relatively common form of cyanotic congenital heart disease in infancy (Astley and Parsons, 1952), but few patients survive. Obviously, if the two circuits are closed and independent, life cannot be sustained. Clinical cases, therefore, must have some means whereby blood is transferred from the systemic to the pulmonary circuit and vice versa; ventricular and atrial septal defects usually provide these means, blood entering the pulmonary circulation through a ventricular septal defect and leaving it via an atrial septal defect. Cases may be further complicated by a high pulmonary vascular resistance, pulmonary stenosis, tricuspid atresia or other anomalies.

HÆMODYNAMICS

If the pulmonary vascular resistance is more or less normal, a ventricular septal defect allows venous blood from the right ventricle to enter the left ventricle and pulmonary artery, where it mixes with oxygenated blood from the left atrium. If these is no atrial septal defect the pulmonary circulation is flooded, the only escape being through bronchial anastomotic veins. With an atrial septal defect the pulmonary circulation is still plethoric, but less so, oxygenated blood escaping into the right atrium and

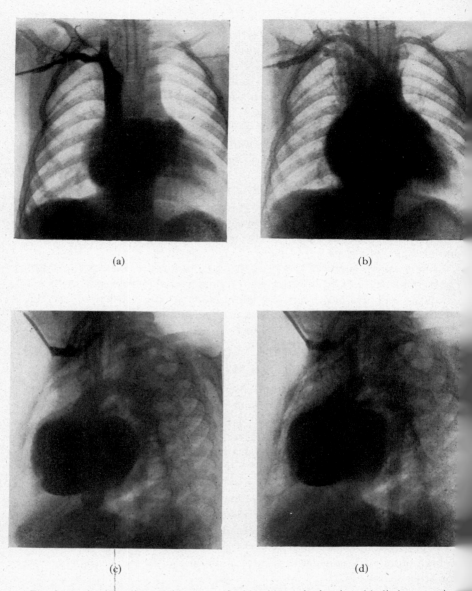

Fig. 8.97—Angiocardiogram in a case of tricuspid atresia showing: (a) diodone passing directly into the left atrium (1 second); (b) early filling of the left ventricle and aorta (2 seconds); (c) in the second oblique position the left side of the heart and aorta are filled in 2 seconds; (d) at 3 seconds a small left pulmonary artery is becoming visible. Note bronchial collaterals in right upper zone in (b).

so to the right ventricle and aorta. In otherwise uncomplicated cases there may be hyperkinetic pulmonary hypertension and samples from the pulmonary artery are always more saturated with oxygen than samples from the aorta.

If the pulmonary vascular resistance is raised, or if there is associated pulmonary stenosis, the right to left interventricular shunt is limited or reversed according to the degree of obstruction to pulmonary flow; the interatrial shunt is adjusted accordingly, being proportionately limited or reversed respectively. When the shunts are reversed, venous blood from the right atrium enters the left atrium through the atrial septal defect, and after mixing with oxygenated blood from the lungs, passes on to the left ventricle; part of this mixed blood then enters the pulmonary artery, and part is shunted into the right ventricle and aorta through the V.S.D. Under these circumstances the pulmonary blood flow is diminished, although samples from the pulmonary artery are still more oxygenated than samples from the aorta. Tricuspid atresia complicating transposition causes similar reversed shunting through both septal defects.

Finally, when the defects are large, bidirectional shunts may occur at atrial or ventricular level.

AGE AND SEX

The average age of the eight patients in this small series was 13 years, and the range 3 to 33 years. The sexes were equally represented.

CLINICAL FEATURES

Effort intolerance, cyanosis, clubbing and polycythæmia were moderate to gross; squatting was noticed in only one instance, and in only four of 25 cases reported by Campbell and Suzman (1951). Neither angina pectoris nor syncope occurred.

The *physical signs* vary according to the chief complication. The pulse and venous pressure are usually normal, but the jugular pulse may show a small dominant *a* wave. The cardiac impulse is usually right ventricular in type, a moderate systolic thrust extending from the left sternal edge towards the mid-clavicular line. In about a quarter of the cases there is no murmur at all; in some there is a Roger murmur and thrill, and in others a pulmonary ejection murmur and thrill, particularly in those with pulmonary stenosis. Continuous murmurs are very rare if they occur at all, even in those with patent ductus. A pulmonary diastolic murmur may be heard when the pulmonary vascular resistance is high, and a functional mitral diastolic murmur when there is marked pulmonary plethora. The second heart sound also varies according to the nature of the chief complication. As a rule it is loud because the root of the aorta is anterior and uncovered by the pulmonary artery. In about a third of the cases it is recognisably split, and when the pulmonary vascular resistance is raised the split may be very close and the pulmonary element also accentuated. When there is pulmonary stenosis P_2 is usually absent, perhaps because the soft pulmonary component originates too far posteriorly to be heard.

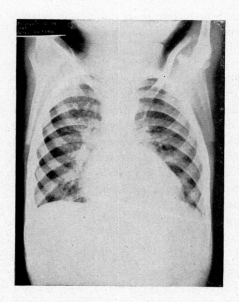

Fig. 8.98—Case of transposition of the great vessels showing pulmonary plethora and a narrow vascular pedicle.

The *electrocardiogram* showed varying grades of right ventricular preponderance, usually considerable. The P waves were bifid and widened in three cases, 3 mm. high and 0.08 second wide in three, and unremarkable in the other two.

Fluoroscopy in the anterior view revealed the narrow vascular pedicle described by Taussig (1938) in two instances, the aorta lying immediately in front of the pulmonary artery (fig. 8.98). Pulmonary plethora (fig. 8.99) was invariable, but was very slight in one case with considerable pulmonary stenosis. Absence of plethora may also be seen when the pulmonary vascular resistance is extreme. Dilatation of the pulmonary arc was rarely convincing radiologically, and in two cases a long convex shadow on the left border of the heart in the region usually occupied by a dilated left pulmonary artery was shown by means of angiocardiography to be the ascending aorta (fig. 8.100), as in the case described by Goodwin, Steiner and Wayne (1949) and as in four out of 14 cases reported by Astley and Parsons (1952). The heart shadow itself was at least moderately enlarged in all cases, sometimes considerably so.

Angiocardiography can be very helpful in showing the exact position of the aortic root, which fills directly from the right ventricle. Opacification of the pulmonary artery varies considerably according to the nature of the associated anomalies, and in some cases may be very difficult to see at all; when visible the root of the pulmonary artery is seen to be posterior in the lateral films, but in the anterior view may be more to the right than expected, the heart being rotated clockwise (viewed from below) so that the left ventricle is twisted round to the right posteriorly.

Cardiac catheterisation always reveals identical aortic and right ventricular samples and systolic pressures, and higher oxygen saturation in samples from the pulmonary artery than from the aorta. The catheter usually passes naturally into the ascending aorta (fig. 8.101), but can often be manœuvred into the pulmonary artery. Other findings vary according

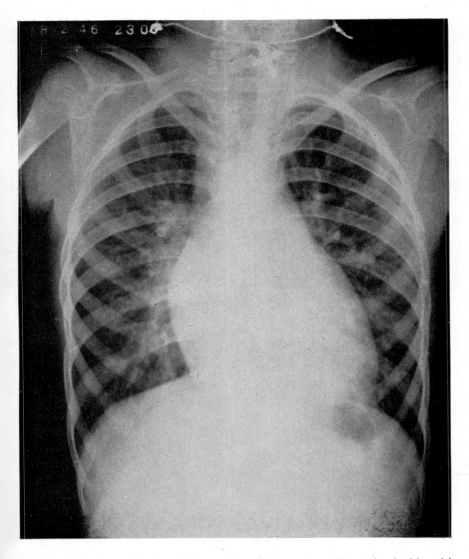

Fig. 8.99—Skiagram of a case of transposition of the great vessels associated with artial and ventricular septal defects.

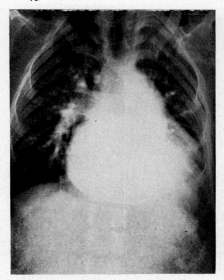

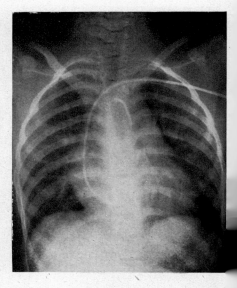

Fig. 8.100—Angiocardiogram in a case of transposition showing a convex arc high up on the left border of the heart; this is the ascending aorta and not the pulmonary artery.

Fig. 8.101—Case of transposition of the great vessels showing the typical position of a catheter which has been passed up the ascending aorta and round the aortic arch.

to the nature of the associated anomalies. As a rule, there is a left to right shunt at atrial level if there is an atrial septal defect, and a right to left shunt at ventricular level with ventricular septal defect; but either shunt may be bidirectional or reversed, particularly if there is a raised pulmonary vascular resistance or pulmonary stenosis; with tricuspid atresia both shunts are entirely reversed. Pressures in the right ventricle and pulmonary artery depend on the pulmonary blood flow, the pulmonary vascular resistance, and the degree of pulmonary stenosis, if present. The pulmonary blood flow is high in relatively uncomplicated cases, even when the shunts are small, for there is a large volume of oxygenated blood permanently trapped in the pulmonary circulation; it may be only slightly in excess of normal, however, when the pulmonary vascular resistance is high or when there is severe pulmonary stenosis.

DIFFERENTIAL DIAGNOSIS

The triad comprising central cyanosis, unquestionable pulmonary plethora, and right ventricular dominance usually means transposition of the great vessels or *total anomalous pulmonary venous drainage* into the right side of the heart, and these two can usually be distinguished radiologically. *Persistent truncus* with cyanosis and pulmonary plethora is at once recognised by the large left ventricle.

When pulmonary plethora is unconvincing because of associated pulmonary stenosis, there may be great clinical difficulty in distinguishing transposition from *Fallot's tetralogy* with a relatively good pulmonary blood flow; in fact the only real differences between them are the degree of cyanosis, which in transposition is considerable and in Fallot's tetralogy of this kind slight, and the size of the heart, which is usually larger in transposition. If angiocardiography shows no filling of the pulmonary artery, *pulmonary atresia* may be diagnosed in error; but this mistake should not be made at the bedside.

When pulmonary plethora is doubtful because the pulmonary vascular resistance is raised, transposition is commonly confused with *Eisenmenger's complex*. Genuine dilatation of the pulmonary artery favours Eisenmenger's complex, but angiocardiography or cardiac catheterisation may be necessary to establish the diagnosis with certainty.

PROGNOSIS

The average duration of life in 123 cases with associated anomalies of the kind described above was 19 months (Hanlon and Blalock, 1948); without such associated anomalies life is impossible. The patients in the present series, however, had already survived infancy, and their ages show that with good communications between the two circulations the immediate outlook is far from hopeless; 9 out of 25 cases of probable transposition reported by Campbell and Suzman (1951) were between 6 and 18 years of age, the rest being under 5.

TREATMENT

So far attempts to improve the efficiency of communications between the two circulations, such as the creation of an artificial atrial septal defect (Blalock and Hanlon, 1950), have proved disappointing. Surgical correction of the transposition itself, with the aid of some form of artificial circulation to the brain, is still in the experimental stage.

PERSISTENT TRUNCUS ARTERIOSUS

Persistent truncus results from failure of development of the aortopulmonary septum, so that a single large vessel arises from both ventricles. The solitary valve usually has four cusps and a ventricular septal defect is inevitable. The pulmonary arteries should arise from the common trunk, and if they fail to do so the probable diagnosis is pulmonary atresia.

Persistent truncus is a very rare anomaly and there was but one proved example amongst the 900 congenital cases reported here.

HÆMODYNAMICS

If the pulmonary vascular resistance is normal, the pulmonary circulation is flooded to its maximum capacity, because the pulmonary arteries are filled at systemic pressure. The left ventricle enlarges greatly to cope with the torrential flow that is received from the lungs, and the right ventricle hypertrophies to adapt itself to systemic conditions. The truncus itself may be very large, not simply because it represents two great vessels, but because it may have to carry an enormous flow. Cyanosis may be minimal, because mixed venous blood from the systemic and pulmonary circulations is about five-sixths pulmonary and therefore likely to be well over 80 per cent saturated.

A normal pulmonary vascular resistance, however, may be unusual in cases that survive infancy, and physiological studies may well reveal a resistance in the Eisenmenger range (around 17 units) in the majority. Pulmonary and systemic blood flows would then be balanced and the two ventricles would perform identical work. Cyanosis should be considerable in this group.

If the pulmonary resistance rose much above systemic level, the pulmonary blood flow would be diminished, and the left ventricle would perform less work than the right. Such cases would be intensely cyanosed and similar physiologically to pulmonary atresia.

CLINICAL FEATURES

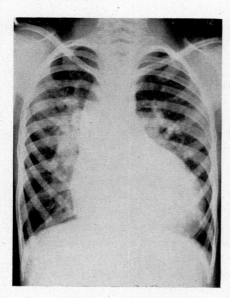

Fig. 8.102—Case of persistent truncus arteriosus showing marked pulmonary plethora, a conspicuous bay in the region of the pulmonary artery, and considerable enlargement of the heart shadow due chiefly to dilatation of the left ventricle.

Persistent truncus with a relatively normal pulmonary vascular resistance is characterised by slight central cyanosis, clubbing and poly-cythæmia, and relatively slight effort intolerance until there is left ventricular failure; the pulse may be water-hammer in quality and there may be a small dominant *a* wave in the jugular venous pulse, but the venous pressure is usually normal until heart failure develops; the left ventricle is thoroughly enlarged and hyperdynamic, the right less so; there is usually a systolic ejection murmur with or without thrill at the base, a loud single second sound, and sometimes a basal diastolic murmur due to a leaking quadricuspid valve, the incompetence affecting both ventricles. A functional mitral diastolic murmur would be expected. A continuous broncho-pulmonary anastomotic murmur means pulmonary atresia, not persistent truncus.

The electrocardiogram shows conspicuous Q waves and tall R waves in leads V_5 and V_6, and perhaps a secondary R wave in leads V_1 and V_2 from right ventricular hypertrophy as well. The P wave may be normal, bifid and widened from left atrial enlargement, or a little tall and sharp from right atrial hypertrophy.

The skiagram shows gross pulmonary plethora, absence of the pulmonary arc, a conspicuous ascending "aorta", and considerable enlargement of the heart shadow, particularly the left ventricle (fig. 8.102).

When the pulmonary vascular resistance is high the clinical features are more like Eisenmenger's complex. Cyanosis and clubbing are much more conspicuous, and dyspnœa more severe. The pulse loses its water-hammer quality. The ventricles are about equal in size, and clinically the right may be dominant. Auscultatory signs are unchanged except that a mitral diastolic murmur would not be expected. The electrocardiogram shows a P pulmonale and considerable right ventricular preponderance. Radiologically there is less pulmonary plethora (if any) and less cardiac enlargement, whilst the left ventricle is no longer hyperdynamic.

DIFFERENTIAL DIAGNOSIS

Many cases of persistent truncus present clinical, electrocardiographic and radiological features that lie somewhere between the two prototypes described above. Essentially the pattern is one of central cyanosis, enlargement of both ventricles, particularly the left, a single second heart sound, absence of the pulmonary arc and pulmonary plethora. This combination admits of no other diagnosis.

Pulmonary atresia with its continuous broncho-pulmonary anastomotic murmur, small quiet left ventricle, and obvious pulmonary ischæmia presents an entirely different picture and should not enter into the differential diagnosis at all.

Eisenmenger's complex can nearly always be distinguished by the dilated pulmonary artery. *Transposition* alone presents any real difficulty. Both it and persistent truncus have central cyanosis, pulmonary plethora, and a hyperdynamic left heart; but in transposition the second heart sound may be split, the ascending aorta is inconspicuous or in its wrong position, and the right ventricle is nearly always dominant.

Angiocardiography should reveal the essential anatomical arrangement in persistent truncus. On *cardiac catheterisation* the pathognomic finding is to enter either pulmonary artery from the "ascending aorta". In the case studied in this series, there was no difficulty in accomplishing this: pulmonary artery, aortic, and right ventricular systolic pressures were identical; the oxygen saturation of samples was 48 per cent in the right atrium, 58 per cent in the right ventricle, and 72 per cent in the truncus, proving the presence of a left to right shunt at ventriculo-aortic level.

PROGNOSIS AND TREATMENT

Cases with a low pulmonary vascular resistance probably die from cardiac failure in infancy. When the pulmonary resistance is raised sufficiently to protect the lungs from over-flooding, and the left ventricle from overwork, but not so much as to diminish the pulmonary blood flow, the outlook is not so bad and may be more like that in Eisenmenger's complex. As a general rule, however, patients who survive infancy die from congestive heart failure in childhood or adolescence. No surgical treatment is possible.

TOTAL ANOMALOUS PULMONARY VENOUS DRAINAGE

Embryologically a single pulmonary vein originally joins the sinus venosus. The superior horns of the sinus, ducts of Cuvier, and lower part of the anterior cardinal veins become the superior vena cava on the right side, and the oblique vein of the left atrium (vein of Marshall) and coronary sinus on the left. A persistent left superior vena cava therefore joins the oblique vein of the left atrium and enters the right atrium via the coronary sinus.

The formation of the interatrial septum separates that part of the sinus venosus that the pulmonary vein joins from the rest of the right atrium. Since there are normally four pulmonary veins joining the left atrium it is clear that the original single pulmonary venous trunk becomes absorbed into the sinus venosus. It is not at all difficult for one or other of the right pulmonary veins to find itself entering the primitive atria on the wrong side of the growing septum. *Partial anomalous pulmonary venous drainage* arising in this way has already been described, and is not infrequently associated with atrial septal defect.

In total anomalous pulmonary venous drainage, the original single pulmonary vein may join up with almost any other part of the sinus venosus system: thus it is found entering the coronary sinus in 19 per cent, left superior vena cava in 43 per cent, right superior vena cava in 12 per cent, right atrium in 14 per cent, and even the inferior vena cava sometimes (Keith *et al.*, 1954). When it enters the coronary sinus there is usually a left superior vena cava as well, and this invariably communicates with the left innominate vein and so with the right superior vena cava, through which the pulmonary venous blood eventually drains into the right atrium.

HÆMODYNAMICS

All the blood from the lungs enters the right atrium by one route or another, and after mixing with blood from the systemic veins passes to the left ventricle via an atrial septal defect or foramen ovale, and to the right ventricle through the tricuspid valve. Samples from all cardiac chambers are therefore identical.

Since the right ventricle offers less resistance to filling than the left, and since the tricuspid valve opening is usually wider than that in the atrial septum, more blood enters the right ventricle than the left. The pulmonary blood flow is therefore increased, and the systemic output tends to be low. This also means that the majority of blood entering the right atrium is already 95 per cent saturated, so that the mixed venous sample arriving in the left ventricle is likely to be around 85 per cent saturated. Central cyanosis is therefore slight or even absent at rest. If the pulmonary vascular resistance is raised, the right ventricular diastolic pressure tends to rise, the right to left interatrial shunt increases, the pulmonary blood flow is reduced, and cyanosis may then be intense, but this is unusual.

There were only two proved examples of this rare anomaly in the present series. But five typical cases were described by Snellen and Albers (1952), four by Gardner and Oram (1953), six by Whitaker (1954), and fourteen by Keith *et al.* (1954), who also reviewed 45 other cases culled from the literature. A good earlier review is that by Brody (1942).

The majority of cases in the literature occurred in infancy, 80 per cent proving fatal within the first year of life.

The sex ratio is three males to two females.

CLINICAL FEATURES

There is a very great discrepancy between the high infant mortality in this condition and the relatively good health of many classical cases described in adolescents and young adults. The explanation, of course, lies with the behaviour of the foramen ovale or with the size of the interatrial communication. Many infants die because the foramen ovale becomes sealed off, despite the higher pressure on the right side of the atrial septum (Taussig, 1947). Others in whom the foramen ovale remains patent have to depend on this small opening for the whole of their systemic blood flow. On the other hand, patients with a good-sized atrial septal defect are likely to have an adequate right to left interatrial shunt and fare relatively well (Snellen and Albers, 1952). The syndrome to be described is that seen in children and young adults with good interatrial shunts.

Effort intolerance is not severe, and cyanosis is minimal unless the pulmonary vascular resistance is high. Recurrent bronchitis may occur as in other cases with plethoric lungs. Physical development is poor.

The peripheral pulse is small and the jugular venous pressure and pulse normal, unless the pulmonary vascular resistance is raised (Eisenmenger reaction) or the right heart fails.

The central cardiac signs are very similar to those of atrial septal defect: the left ventricle is impalpable, the right thrusting and hyperdynamic, and an impulse may be felt over the pulmonary artery; there is nearly always a pulmonary ejection murmur in the third left space, often accompanied by a faint or moderate thrill, and the second heart sound is widely split and presumably unaltered by respiration; the intensity of P_2 no doubt

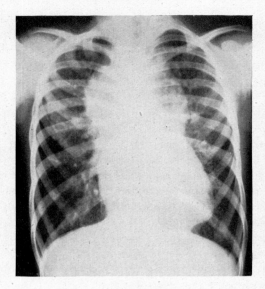

Fig. 8.103—Typical figure-of-eight appearance in
a case of total anomalous pulmonary venous
drainage into the left superior vena cava.

varies with the pulmonary artery pressure; pulmonary incompetence occurs
in a minority. A superior vena caval hum, uninfluenced by posture or
compressing the root of either jugular vein, may be heard in the aortic
area in about a quarter of the cases (Snellen and Albers, 1952). A functional
mid-diastolic murmur caused by interatrial or tricuspid turbulence, was
heard in three out of four cases reported by Gardner and Oram (1953),
and in two out of six cases described by Whitaker (1954).

The *electrocardiogram* shows a partial right bundle branch block pattern,
as in atrial septal defect.

The *skiagram* reveals a figure-of-eight appearance (fig. 8.103), the upper
half of which represents the dilated left superior vena cava, left innominate
vein, and right superior vena cava, as first clearly illustrated by Taussig
(1947), and emphasised by Snellen and Albers (1952). Other features
include a small aorta, pulmonary plethora, and dilatation of the pulmonary
artery, right ventricle and right atrium, as in atrial septal defect.

Routine *angiocardiography* shows more or less simultaneous filling of
both sides of the heart, the reversed shunt being at atrial level; after passing
through the lungs, contrast medium enters the left superior vena cava. A
clearer picture of the anomalous pulmonary venous drainage is obtained
if diaginol is injected directly into the pulmonary artery.

The *physiological findings* are also pathognomonic, for samples from all
intracardiac chambers and from both the aorta and pulmonary artery are
identical, or if the interatrial communication cannot be penetrated, then at

least the arterial sample is the same as those from the right side of the heart. S.V.C. samples are more saturated than those from the right atrium, and much more so than those from the I.V.C. If the catheter is passed up the left subclavian vein it may enter the left superior vena cava, and then fully saturated pulmonary venous blood may be obtained. The pulmonary blood flow is usually over 15 litres per minute, unless the pulmonary vascular resistance is raised, the systemic flow averaging around 4 litres per minute. The pulmonary artery pressure is usually raised moderately owing to the very great flow.

DIFFERENTIAL DIAGNOSIS

The combination of slight central cyanosis, otherwise typical clinical features of a large atrial septal defect with direct shunt, the addition sometimes of a basal venous hum, and the pathognomonic figure-of-eight skiagram, can hardly be mistaken for any other condition. At the bedside, however, atrial septal defect with bidirectional shunt, despite the absence of a high pulmonary vascular resistance, and cases of single atrium, present very similar features. Selective angiocardiography and cardiac catheterisation should establish the diagnosis with certainty.

PROGNOSIS AND TREATMENT

As already stated, if the foramen ovale closes or tends to close, infants necessarily die; but if there is a good-sized atrial septal defect the outlook is fair, most such cases reaching adult life, although very few have been reported over 30 years old.

Surgical transplantation of the misplaced pulmonary vein has yet to be accomplished.

ANOMALOUS DRAINAGE OF THE S.V.C. OR I.V.C. INTO THE LEFT ATRIUM

A rare but interesting anomaly, seen only once in this series, is anomalous drainage of the superior vena cava into the left atrium. The patient was a girl aged 10 with life-long slight central cyanosis and grade I effort intolerance. There were no obviously abnormal physical signs, but the left ventricle was a little thrusting, for it was working harder than the right, and the second heart sound was single, A_2 being slightly later and P_2 earlier than normal. The electrocardiogram showed an S wave in lead V_2 measuring 28 mm., but was otherwise normal. The skiagram looked normal. Angiocardiography, however, revealed anomalous superior vena cava drainage into the left atrium, diaginol passing directly into the left side of the heart without entering the right atrium at all (fig. 8.104a). When diaginol was injected into the saphenous vein, the inferior vena cava was seen to join the right atrium normally (fig. 8.104b). On cardiac

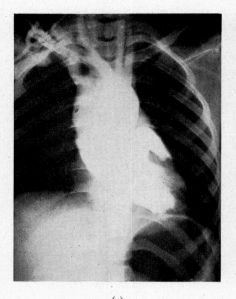 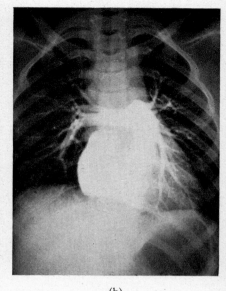

(a)   (b)

Fig. 8.104—Angiocardiogram from a case of anomalous drainage of the superior vena cava
into the left atrium: (a) showing diaginol in the superior vena cava, left atrium, left atrial
appendage, left ventricle and aorta; (b) showing diaginol in the right atrium, right ventricle
and pulmonary arteries after being injected into the saphenous vein; the top of the right
atrium ends blindly.

catheterisation it was not at first realised that the catheter had entered the
left atrium directly, its immediate passage into a pulmonary vein being
attributed to the presence of an atrial septal defect; when a ventricle was
entered the bluish sample obtained (70 per cent saturated) suggested that
it was the right ventricle, although its systolic pressure was at systemic
level, and it was, of course, the left.

Surgical correction should be possible, but the disability was too slight
in this case to warrant interference.

A good example of a case in which the *inferior vena cava drained directly
into the left atrium* was reported by Gardner and Cole (1955). This patient
died suddenly at the age of 32, and necropsy showed an old posterior
cardiac infarct in addition to the anomaly under consideration. The clinical
features of the congenital anomaly were essentially the same as in the case
of anomalous superior vena cava drainage described above, there being
central cyanosis without other abnormal physical signs, and the skiagram
also looked normal. The electrocardiogram was influenced by the old
infarct.

COR TRILOCULARE BIATRIATUM

Hearts with two normal atria and a single ventricle are rare (1.3 per cent
of Abbott's 1,000 cases), but not so rare as two-chambered hearts. Trans-

position of the great vessels, the aorta lying anteriorly and a little to the right, the pulmonary artery posteriorly and a little to the left, without any spiral arrangement, is usually associated. A rudimentary outflow chamber, from which either the aorta or pulmonary artery (or both) may arise, is sometimes found (Taussig, 1947), and pulmonary valve stenosis is not uncommon. The famous Holmes heart was from a moderately cyanosed man of 23, who died after a bout of dissipation for which he had a "turn". The pulmonary artery arose anteriorly from a small rudimentary outflow chamber protected proximally by an "infundibular" stenosis, which clearly limited the blood flow to the lungs; the aorta arose posteriorly from the body of the common ventricle, there being no transposition in this case (Abbott, 1901).

Complete mixing of systemic and pulmonary venous blood takes place in the common ventricle, from which it is ejected at systemic pressure. If the pulmonary vascular resistance were normal, the lungs would be flooded and survival unlikely; as in persistent truncus arteriosus, therefore, fœtal pulmonary vasoconstriction is usually maintained, and this regulates the amount of blood sent to the lungs (Rogers and Edwards, 1951). Pulmonary stenosis, usually valvular, occurs in about a quarter of all cases (Campbell, Reynolds and Trounce, 1953), and performs a similar service. When the lungs are flooded, cyanosis is minimal or absent, but the single ventricle, which has to perform double work under the best conditions, becomes grossly overloaded. When the aorta arises from a rudimentary outflow chamber with proximal stenosis, extreme pulmonary vasoconstriction would be necessary to provide an adequate systemic blood flow and prevent gross flooding of the lungs.

AGE AND SEX

Although the majority die in infancy, probably as a result of other anomalies or because the pulmonary arterioles fail to regulate the pulmonary flow satisfactorily, about 20 per cent reach adult age, the oldest recorded being 56 (Mehta and Hewlett, 1945).

The sex ratio is 3 : 2 in favour of males (Campbell, Reynolds and Trounce, 1953).

CLINICAL FEATURES

The degree of dyspnœa and cyanosis is probably proportional to the pulmonary vascular resistance or to the degree of pulmonary stenosis when that is present. Nevertheless, slight to moderate cyanosis is physiologically desirable, for acyanotic cases are far more likely to die in infancy from heart failure due to overloading of the single ventricle secondary to a flooded pulmonary circulation.

No good descriptions of the physical signs of patients with single ventricle are available in the medical literature, but most have a basal systolic murmur with or without thrill, and this is probably a pulmonary ejection murmur as in Eisenmenger's complex, which these cases imitate closely. When there is associated pulmonary stenosis the physical signs are presumably more like those of Fallot's tetralogy.

The electrocardiogram is variable: normal Q waves are usually seen in antero-lateral chest leads or in one of the left-sided unipolar limb leads, despite the absence of the interventricular septum, as in the univentricular heart of fishes and frogs (Kisch, 1949); otherwise the graph is apt to show changes which might ordinarily be more easily attributed to clockwise or anticlockwise rotation. In cases with pulmonary stenosis, Campbell, Reynolds and Trounce (1953) could not distinguish the graph from that seen in Fallot's tetralogy.

The skiagram resembles that in Eisenmenger's complex when there is pulmonary hypertension and Fallot's tetralogy when there is pulmonary stenosis, but in both types the heart is apt to be larger.

Few physiological studies have yet been reported. In uncomplicated cases the findings are similar to those of Eisenmenger's complex with bidirectional shunt, but there is no difference between samples from the aorta and from the pulmonary artery. When there is pulmonary stenosis the findings are like those in Fallot's tetralogy in respect of the pressures recorded, and like uncomplicated single ventricle in respect of the samples.

Angiocardiography shows simultaneous filling of the aorta and pulmonary artery as in Eisenmenger's complex and Fallot's tetralogy; but with good technique it should be possible to demonstrate complete opacification of the whole ventricular shadow from the right atrium, the left atrium remaining translucent.

PROGNOSIS AND TREATMENT

The outlook is fair in those who survive infancy and depends on how satisfactorily the pulmonary circulation can be regulated by the pulmonary vascular resistance or the pulmonary stenosis.

Surgical treatment is impossible in those with pulmonary hypertension, and usually inadvisable in those with pulmonary stenosis unless the pulmonary blood flow is obviously inadequate.

COR BIVENTRICULARE TRILOCULARE

Hearts with a single atrium and two ventricles are exceptionally rare. They cannot be distinguished clinically from those rare cases of atrial septal defect with bidirectional but predominantly left to right interatrial shunt and a normal pulmonary vascular resistance. Cardiac catheterisation, however, should show identical samples from all cardiac chambers beyond the superior vena cava and inferior vena cava, as if all the pulmonary veins drained directly into the right atrium. The pulmonary blood flow is greatly increased because the right ventricle offers less resistance to filling than the left.

The prognosis is similar to that in cases of gross atrial septal defect, the few examples reported usually dying from heart failure in childhood or adolescence (Brown, 1950).

No surgical treatment is possible unless an artificial septum could be created.

COR BILOCULARE

A two-chambered heart is probably the rarest of all congenital cardio-pathies and practically never occurs without other anomalies (Brown, 1950). Physiologically, the situation should be precisely the same as that in a heart with two atria and a single ventricle, except that mixing of pulmonary and systemic venous blood takes place in the atrium instead of the ventricle.

REFERENCES

Abbott, M. E. (1901): "Unique case of congenital malformation of the heart: cor triloculare biatriatum with pulmonary artery given off from small supplementary cavity. From a case reported in 1824 by Andrew F. Holmes, M.D., Montreal, Lower Canada", *Montreal med. J.*, **30**, 522.

―― (1927): "Congenital heart disease" in Osler and McCrae's system of medicine, Philadelphia, Lea and Febiger, 3rd. ed.

―― (1928): "Coarctation of the aorta of the adult type. II. Statistical and historical retrospect of 200 recorded cases, with autopsy, of stenosis or obliteration of the descending arch", *Amer. Heart J.*, **3**, 392.

―― (1931): "Statistics of congenital cardiac disease (1,000 cases analysed)". Reprinted in *Disorders of the Heart and Circulation*, ed. Robert L. Levy (1951), New York, Thomas Nelson & Sons.

―― (1932): "Congenital heart disease", "Nelson loose-leaf living Medicine", **4**, 207.

―― (1932): "On the relative incidence and clinical significance of a congenitally bicuspid aortic valve. With five illustrative cases", *Emanuel Libman Anniversary Volumes*, p. 1.

Abrahams, D. G., and Wood, P. (1951): "Pulmonary stenosis with normal aortic root", *Brit. Heart J.*, **13**, 519.

Adams, F. H., and Katz, B. (1952): "Endocardial fibroelastosis", *J. Pediat.*, **41**, 141.

Addarii, F., Martini, L., Mahaim, I., and Winston, M. (1946): "Anatomical and clinical data in a case of irreducible cardiac insufficiency of uncertain etiology, occurring in a young man. New investigations on incomplete bilateral block", *Cardiologia*, **11**, 36.

Adler, D. (1953): "Patent ductus arteriosus. A review based on 24 cases", *South African med. J.*, **27**, 367.

Aitken, Janet K. (1932): "Congenital heart-block", *Lancet*, ii, 1375.

Allanby, K. D., Brinton, W. D., Campbell, M., and Gardner, F. (1950): "Pulmonary atresia and the collateral circulation to the lungs", *Guy's Hosp. Rep.*, **99**, 110.

――, and Campbell, M. (1949): "Congenital pulmonary stenosis with closed ventricular septum", *Ibid.*, **98**, 18.

Apley, J. (1949): "Congenital anomalies of the aortic arch and its branches", *Proc. R. Soc. Med.*, **42**, 918.

Astley, R., and Parsons, C. (1952): "Complete transposition of the great vessels", *Brit. Heart J.*, **14**, 13.

Baer, R. W., Taussig, H. B., and Oppenheimer, E. H. (1942): "Congenital aneurysmal dilatation of the aorta associated with arachnodactyly", *Bull. Johns Hopk. Hosp.*, **72**, 309.

Bahnson, H. T., Cooley, R. N., and Sloan, R. D. (1949): "Coarctation of the aorta at unusual sites", *Amer. Heart J.*, **38**, 905.

Bailey, C. P., Boulton, H. E., Jamison, W. L., and Neptune, W. B. (1953): "Atrio-septo-pexy for interatrial septal defects", *J. Thorac. Surg.*, **26**, 184.

Baker, C., Brinton, W. D., and Channell, C. D. (1950): "Ebstein's disease", *Guy's Hosp. Rep.*, **99**, 247.

Baldwin, E. de F., Moore, L. V., and Noble, R. P. (1946): "The demonstration of ventricular septal defect by means of right heart catheterisation", *Amer. Heart J.*, **32**, 152.

Barber, J. M., Magidson, O., and Wood, P. (1950): "Atrial septal defect", *Brit. Heart J.*, **12**, 277.

Barnes, C. G., and Finlay, H. V. L. (1952): "Cor triatriatum", *Ibid.*, **14**, 283.

Bauer, D. de F., and Astbury, E. C. (1944): "Congenital cardiac disease. Bibliography of the 1,000 cases analyzed in Maude Abbott's Atlas", *Amer. Heart J.*, **27**, 688.

Bayford, D. (1789): "An account of a singular case of obstructed deglutition", *Mem. med. Soc. Lond.*, **2**, 275.

Bedford, D. E., and Parkinson, J. (1936): "Right-sided aortic arch (situs inversus arcus aortæ)", *Brit. J. Radiol.*, N.S., **9**, 776.

——, Papp, C., and Parkinson, J. (1941): "Atrial septal defect", *Brit. Heart J.*, **3**, 37.

Benn, J. (1947): "The prognosis of patent ductus arteriosus", *Ibid.*, **9**, 283.

Bing, R. J., Vandam, L. D., and Gray, F. D. (1947): "Physiological studies in congenital heart disease. I. Procedures. II. Results of pre-operative studies in patients with tetralogy of Fallot. III. Results obtained in five cases of Eisenmenger's complex", *Bull. Johns Hopk. Hosp.*, **80**, 107, 121, 323.

——, Handelsman, J. C., Campbell, J. A., Griswold, H. E., and Blalock, A. (1948): "The surgical treatment and the physiopathology of coarctation of the aorta", *Ann. Surg.*, **128**, 803.

Blalock, A. (1946): "Physiopathology and surgical treatment of congenital cardiovascular defects", *Bull. New York Acad. Med.*, **22**, 57.

—— (1947): "The technique of creation of an artificial ductus arteriosus in the treatment of pulmonic stenosis", *J. Thorac. Surg.*, **16**, 244.

—— (1948): "Surgical treatment of pulmonic stenosis". *Brit. Heart J.*, **10**, 68.

——, and Taussig, H. B. (1945): "The surgical treatment of malformations of the heart in which there is pulmonary stenosis or pulmonary atresia", *J. Amer. med. Ass.*, **128**, 189.

——, and Hanlon, R. C. (1950): "The surgical treatment of complete transposition of the aorta and the pulmonary artery", *Surg. Gynec. Obstet.*, **90**, 1.

Bland, E. F., White, P. D., and Garland, J. (1933): "Congenital anomalies of the coronary arteries: report of an unusual case associated with cardiac hypertrophy", *Amer. Heart J.*, **8**, 787.

Blount, S. G., Swan, H., Gensini, G., and McCord, M. C. (1954): "Atrial septal defect. Clinical and physiologic response to complete closure in five patients", *Circulation*, **9**, 801.

Bohn, H. (1938): "Ein wichtiges diagnostisches Phanomen zur Erkennung des offenen ductus art. Botalli", *Klin. Wchnschr.*, **17**, 907.

Bonham-Carter, R. E. (1955): Personal communication.

Bonnet, L. M. (1903): "Sur la lesion Dite Stenose congenitale de l'aorte" *Rev. Med.*, **23**, 108.

Bower, B. D., Gerrard, J. W., D'Abreu, A. L., and Parsons, C. G. (1953): "Two cases of congenital mitral stenosis treated by valvotomy", *Arch. Dis. Childh.*, **28**, 91.

Bramwell, C. (1947): "Coarctation of the aorta: II. Clinical features", *Brit. Heart J.*, **9**, 100.

Brean, H. P., and Neuhauser, E. B. D. (1947): "Syndrome of aberrant right subclavian artery with patent ductus arteriosus", *Amer. J. Roentgenol.*, **58**, 708.

Brecher, G. A., and Opdyke, D. F. (1951): "The relief of acute right ventricular strain by the production of an interatrial septal defect", *Circulation*, **4**, 496.

Brinton, W. D., and Campbell, M. (1953): "Necropsies in some congenital diseases of the heart, mainly Fallot's tetralogy", *Brit. Heart J.*, **15**, 335.

Brock, R. C. (1948): "Pulmonary valvulotomy for the relief of congenital pulmonary stenosis", *Brit. med. J.*, i, 1121.

—— (1949): "The surgery of pulmonary stenosis", *Ibid.*, ii, 399.

——, and Campbell, M. (1950): "Valvulotomy for pulmonary valvular stenosis", *Brit. Heart J.*, **12**, 377.

——, —— (1950): "Infundibular resection or dilatation for infundibular stenosis", *Ibid.*, **12**, 403.

Broden, B., Hanson, H. E., and Karnell, J. (1948): "Thoracic aortography, preliminary report", *Acta Radiol.*, **29**, 181.

Brody, H. (1942): "Drainage of the pulmonary veins into the right side of the heart", *Arch. Path.*, **33**, 221.

Brown, G. E., Clagett, O. T., Burchell, H. B., and Wood, E. H. (1948): "Preoperative and postoperative studies of intraradial and intrafemoral pressures in patients with coarctation of the aorta", *Proc. Mayo Clin.*, **23**, 352.

Brown, J. W. (1939): "Congenital heart disease", London.

—— (1950): "Congenital heart disease", 2nd ed., London, Staples Press.

Caccamise, W. C., and Whitman, J. F. (1952): "Pulseless disease", *Amer. Heart J.*, **44**, 629.

Campbell, M. (1948): "The Blalock-Taussig operation for morbus cœruleus", *Guy's Hosp. Rep.*, **97**, 1.

—— (1948): "Surgery of congenital heart disease", *Brit. med. J.*, ii, 669.

—— (1950): "Congenital heart disease", *Ibid.*, i, 1250

——, and Brock, R. (1955): "The results of valvotomy for simple pulmonary stenosis", *Brit. Heart J.*, **17**, 229.

——, and Deuchar, D. (1953): "Results of the Blalock-Taussig operation in 200 cases of morbus cœruleus", *Brit. med. J.*, i, 349.

——, ——, and Brock, Sir Russell (1954): "Results of pulmonary valvotomy and infundibular resection in 100 cases of Fallot's tetralogy", *Ibid.*, ii, 111.

——, and Kauntze, R. (1953): "Congenital aortic valvular stenosis", *Brit. Heart J.*, **15**, 179.

——, and Reynolds, G. (1949): "The physical and mental development of children with congenital heart disease", *Arch. Dis. Childh.*, **24**, 294.

——, ——, and Trounce, J. R. (1953): "Six cases of single ventricle with pulmonary stenosis", *Guy's Hosp. Rep.*, **102**, 99.

——, and Suzman, S. S. (1934): "Congenital complete heart-block. An account of eight cases", *Amer. Heart J.*, **9**, 304.

——, —— (1947): "Coarctation of the aorta", *Brit. Heart J.*, **9**, 185.

——, —— (1951): "Transposition of the aorta and pulmonary artery", *Circulation*, **4**, 329.

Cassels, D. E., and Morse, M. (1947): "Blood volume in congenital heart disease", *J. Pediat.*, **31**, 485.

Christensen, N. A., and Hines, E. A. (1948): "Clinical features in coarctation of the aorta: A review of 96 cases", *Proc. Mayo Clin.*, **23**, 339.

Civin, W. H., and Edwards, J. E. (1950): "Pathology of the pulmonary vascular tree. I. A comparison of the intrapulmonary arteries in the Eisenmenger complex and in stenosis of ostium infundibuli associated with biventricular origin of the aorta", *Circulation*, **2**, 545.

——, ——, (1951): "The postnatal structural changes in the intrapulmonary arteries and arterioles", *Arch. Path.*, **51**, 192.

Conte, W. R., McCammon, C. S., and Christie, A. (1945): "Congenital defects following maternal rubella", *Am. J. Dis. Child.*, **70**, 301.

Cori, C. F. (1952): *In* Carbohydrate Metabolism, Baltimore.

Cournand, A., Baldwin, J. S., and Himmelstein, A. (1949): "Cardiac catheterization", p. 42. New York, The Commonwealth Fund.

Courter, S. R., Felson, B., and McGuire, J. (1948): "Familial interauricular septal defect with mitral stenosis (Lutembacher's Syndrome)", *Amer. J. med. Sci.*, **216**, 501.

Crafoord, C. (1948): "Coarctation of the aorta", *Brit. Heart J.*, **10**, 71.

—— (1948): "Patent ductus arteriosus", *Ibid.*, **10**, 74.

——, Nylin, G. (1945): "Congenital coarctation of the aorta and its surgical treatment", *J. thor. Surg.*, **14**, 347.

Crawford, T. (1946): "Glycogen disease", *Quart. J. Med.*, **15**, 285.

Cronk, E. S., Sinclair, J. G., and Rigdon, R. H. (1951): "An anomalous coronary artery arising from the pulmonary artery", *Amer. Heart J.*, **42**, 906.

Davies, J. N. P., and Fisher, J. A. (1943): "Coarctation of the aorta, double mitral A-V orifice, and leaking cerebral aneurysm", *Brit. Heart J.*, **5**, 197.

Davies, L. G. (1952): "A familial heart disease", *Brit. Heart J.*, **14**, 206.

Dennis, J. L., Hanser, A. E., and Corpening, T. N. (1953): "Endocardial fibroelastosis", *Pediatrics*, **12**, 130.

Dock, W. (1948): "Erosion of ribs in coarctation of the aorta. A note on the history of a pathognomonic sign", *Brit. Heart J.*, **18**, 148.

Donovan, M. S., Neuhauser, E. B. D., and Sosman, M. C. (1943): "The Roentgen signs of patent ductus arteriosus. A summary of 50 surgically verified cases", *Amer. J. Roentgen*, **50**, 293.

Donzelot, E., Metianu, C., Durand, M., Cherchi, A., and Vlad, P. (1951): "The electrocardiogram in tetralogy of Fallot (a study of 100 cases)", *Arch. mal. du coeur*, **44**, 97.

East, T. (1932): "Coarctation of the aorta", *Proc. Roy. Soc. Med.*, **25**, 796.

Ebstein, W. (1866): "Ueber einen sehr seltenen Fall von Insufficienz der Valvula Tricuspidalis, bedingt durch eine Angeborene hochgradige Missbildung derselben", *Arch. f. Anat. u. Physiol.*, 238.

Edwards, J. E. (1948): "Anomalies of the derivatives of the aortic arch system", *Med. Clin. N. Amer.* (Mayo), **32**, 925.

—— (1950): "Structural changes of pulmonary vascular bed and their functional significance in congenital cardiac disease", *Proc. Inst. Med. Chicago*, **18**, 134.

——, and Burchell, H. B. (1949): "Congenital tricuspid atresia. A classification", *Med. Clin. N. Amer.*, **33**, 1177.

——, Douglas, J. M., Burchell, H. B., and Christensen, N. A. (1949): "Pathology of the intrapulmonary arteries and arterioles in coarctation of the aorta associated with patent ductus arteriosus", *Amer. Heart J.*, **38**, 205.

Eisenmenger, V. (1897): "Die angeborenen Defecte de Kammerscheidewand des Herzens", *Ztschr. f. klin. Med.*, **32**, Suppl. 1.

—— (1898): "Ursprung der Aorta aus Seichen Ventrikeln beim defecte des Septum Ventriculorum", *Wien. Klin. Wschr.*, **11**, 25.

Eldridge, F. L., Multgren, H. N., and Wigmore, M. E. (1954): "The physiologic closure of the ductus arteriosus in newborn infants: A preliminary report", *Science*, **119**, 731.

Ellis, F. R., Greaves, M., and Hecht, H. H. (1950): "Congenital heart disease in old age", *Amer. Heart J.*, **40**, 154.

Ellis, R. W. B., and Payne, W. W. (1936): "Glycogen disease (Von Gierke's disease; hepatonephromegalia glycogenica)", *Quart. J. Med.*, **5**, 31.

Emanuel, R. W. (1954): "Gargoylism with cardiovascular involvement in two brothers", *Brit. Heart J.*, **16**, 417.

Engle, M. Q., Payne, T. B. P., Bruins, C., and Taussig, H. B. (1950): "Ebstein's anomaly of the tricuspid valve. Report of three cases and analysis of clinical syndrome", *Circulation*, **1**, 1246.

Evans, P. R. (1950): "Cardiac anomalies in mongolism", *Brit. Heart J.*, **12**, 258.

Evans, W. (1933): "Congenital stenosis (Coarctation), atresia, and interruption of aortic arch; study of 28 cases", *Quart. J. Med.*, **2**, 1.

Evans, W. (1949): "Familial cardiomegaly", *Brit. Heart J.*, **11**, 68.

—— (1952): "Cardioscopy", Butterworths, London.

——, and Wright, G. (1942): "Electrocardiogram in Friedreich's disease", *Brit. Heart J.*, 4, 91.

Fallot, A. (1888): "Contribution a l'anatomie pathologique de la maladie bleue (cyanose cardiaque)", *Marseille Med.*, 25, 77.

Ferencz, C., Johnson, A. L., and Wigleworth, F. W. (1954): "Congenital mitral stenosis", *Circulation*, 9, 161.

Fishman, L., and Silverthorne, M. C. (1951): "Persistent patent ductus arteriosus in the aged, including the report of the oldest case on record with diagnosis confirmed post mortem", *Amer. Heart J.*, 41, 762.

Friedman, M., Selzer, A., and Rosenblum, H. (1941): "The renal blood flow in coarctation of the aorta", *J. clin. Invest.*, 20, 107.

Friedreich, N. (1863): "Ueber deginerative Atrophie der Spinal en Hinterstränge", *N. Arch. Path. Anat.*, 26, 391, 433.

Gardner, D. L., and Cole, L. (1955): "Long survival with inferior vena cava draining into left atrium", *Brit. Heart J.*, 17, 93.

Gardner, F., and Oram, S. (1953): "Persistent left superior vena cava draining the pulmonary veins", *Ibid.*, 15, 305.

Gates, E. M., Rogers, H. M., and Edwards, J. E. (1947): "The syndrome of cerebral abscess and congenital cardiac disease", *Proc. Mayo Clin.*, 22, 401.

Gibson, G. A. (1900): "Clinical lectures on circulatory affections; Lecture 1, persistence of the arterial duct and its diagnosis", *Edin. med. J.*, 8, 1.

Glynn, L. E. (1940): "Medial defects in circle of Willis and their relation to aneurysm formation", *J. Path. Bact.*, 51, 213.

——, and Reinhold, J. D. L. (1950): "The relationship of idiopathic cardiac hypertrophy to foetal endocarditis", *Arch. Dis. Childhood*, 25, 170.

Goetz., R. H. (1951): "A new angiocardiographic sign of patent ductus arteriosus", *Brit. Heart J.*, 13, 242.

Goodwin, J. F., Steiner, R., and Wayne, E. J. (1949): "Transposition of the aorta and pulmonary artery demonstrated by angiocardiography", *Ibid.*, 11, 279.

Gray, I. R. (1955): in the Press.

Gregg, N. M. (1941): "Congenital cataract following German measles in the mother", *Trans. Ophth. Soc. Australia*, 3, 35.

Green, D. G., Baldwin, E. de F., Baldwin, J. S., Himmelstein, A., Roh, C. E., and Cournand, A. (1949): "Pure congenital pulmonary stenosis and idiopathic congenital dilatation of the pulmonary artery", *Amer. J. Med.*, 6, 24.

Grishman, A., Steinberg, M. F., and Sussman, M. L. (1941): "Contrast roentgen visualisation of coarctation of the aorta", *Amer. Heart J.*, 21, 365.

——, ——, —— (1941): "Tetralogy of Fallot: contrast visualisation of the heart and great vessels", *Radiology*, 37, 178.

Grönvall, H., and Selander, P. (1948): "Nagra virussjukdomar under graviditet och deras verkan pa fostret", *Nord. Med.*, 37, 409.

Gross, P. (1941): "Concept of fetal endocarditis. A general review with report of an illustrative case", *Arch. Path.* (Chicago), 31, 163.

Gross, R. E. (1947): "Complete division for the patent ductus arteriosus", *J. thor. Surg.*, 16, 314.

—— (1949): "Surgical treatment for coarctation of the aorta. Experience from 60 cases", *J. Amer. med. Ass.*, 139, 285.

—— (1950): "Coarctation of the aorta. Surgical treatment on one hundred cases", *Circulation*, 1, 41.

—— (1951): "Treatment of certain aortic coarctations by homologous grafts: a report of nineteen cases", *Ann. Surg.*, 134, 753.

—— (1952): "The patent ductus arteriosus. Observations on diagnosis and therapy in 525 surgically treated cases", *Amer. J. Med.*, 12, 472.

—— (1953): "Surgical closure of interauricular septal defects", *J. Amer. med. Ass.*, 151, 795.

—— (1953): "Clinical progress: Coarctation of the aorta", *Circulation*, 7, 757.

——, and Hubbard, J. P. (1939): "Surgical ligation of a patent ductus arteriosis, *J. Amer. med. Ass.*, 112, 729.

Gross, R. E., and Longino, L. A. (1951): "The patent ductus arteriosus. Observations from 412 surgically treated cases", *Circulation*, III, 125.

——, and Neuhauser, E. (1951): "Compression of the trachea or œsophagus by vascular anomalies", *Pediatrics*, 7, 69.

Gross, R. F., Pomeranz, A. A., Watkins, E., and Goldsmith, E. I. (1952): "Surgical closure of defects of the interauricular septum by the use of an atrial well", *New Eng. J. Med.*, 247, 455.

Gupta, T. C., and Wiggers, C. J. (1951): "Basic hemodynamic changes produced by aortic coarctation of different degrees", *Circulation*, 3, 17.

Hamilton, W. F., Winslow, J. A., and Hamilton, W. F., Jr. (1950): "Notes on a case of congenital heart disease with cyanotic episodes", *J. clin. Invest.*, 29, 20.

Hanlon, C. R., and Blalock, A. (1948): "Complete transposition of the aorta and the pulmonary artery; experimental observation on various shunts after corrective procedures", *Ann. Surg.*, 127, 385.

Hayward, G. W. (1954): "Pulmonary œdema", *Brit. med. J.*, i, 1361.

Hilario, J., Lind, J., and Wegelius, C. (1954): "Rapid biplane angiocardiography in tetralogy of Fallot", *Brit. Heart J.*, 16, 109.

Howarth, S., McMichael, J., and Sharpey-Schafer, E. P. (1947): "Cardiac catheterisation in cases of patent interauricular septum, primary pulmonary hypertension, Fallot's tetralogy, and pulmonary stenosis", *Brit. Heart J.*, 9, 292.

Ingham, D. W., and Willius, F. A. (1938): "Congenital transposition of the great arterial trunks", *Amer. Heart J.*, 15, 482.

Johnson, F. R. (1952): "Anoxia as a cause of endocardial fibroelastosis in infancy", *Arch. Path.*, (Chicago), 54, 237.

Joly, F., Carlotti, T., Sicot, J. R., and Piton, A. (1950): "Congenital cardiopathies. II. The trilogy of Fallot", *Arch. d. mal. du coeur*, 43, 687.

Jönsson, G., Brodén, B., and Karnell, J. (1953): "Angiocardiographic demonstration of pulmonary stenosis", *Acta. Radiol.*, 40, 547.

Kaunitz, P. E. (1947): "Origin of left coronary artery from pulmonary artery", *Amer. Heart J.*, 33, 182.

Keith, A. (1909): "The Hunterian lectures on malformations of the heart", *Lancet*, ii, 359, 433, 519.

—— (1924): "Fate of the bulbus cordis in the human heart", *Ibid.*, ii, 1267.

Keith, J. D., Rowe, R. D., Vlad, P., and O'Hanley, J. H. (1954): "Complete anomalous pulmonary venous drainage", *Amer. J. Med.*, 16, 23.

King, J. T. (1937): "The blood pressure in stenosis at the isthmus of the aorta", *Ann. intern. Med.*, 10, 1802.

Kisch, B. (1949): "The electrical topography of the surface of the univentricular heart (fish and frog)", *Exper. Med. and Surg.*, 7, 1.

Kondo, B., Winsor, T., Raulston, B. O., and Kuroiwa, D. (1950): "Congenital coarctation of the abdominal aorta. A theoretically reversible type of cardiac disease", *Amer. Heart J.*, 39, 306.

Kugel, M. A. (1939): "Enlargement of the heart in infants and young children", *Amer. Heart J.*, 17, 602.

Landtman, B. (1948): "On the relationship between maternal conditions during pregnancy and congenital malformations", *Arch. Dis. Childh.*, 23, 237.

Laubry, C., and Pezzi, C. (1921): "Traité des Maladies Congénitales du Coeur", J. B. Bailliere et Fils, Paris.

——, Routier, D., and de Balsac, R. (1941): "Grosse pulmonaire: petite aorte; affection congenitale", *Bull et mém. Soc. méd. d. hôp. de Paris*, 56, 847.

Leatham, A. (1954): "Splitting of the first and second heart sounds", *Lancet*, ii, 607.

——, and Gray, I. R. (1955): in the Press.

——, and Vogelpoel, L. (1954): "The early systolic sound in dilatation of the pulmonary artery", *Brit. Heart J.*, 16, 21.

Lequime, J., Callebaut, C., and Denolin, H. (1950): "The phenomenon of squatting in patients with congenital heart disease", *Cardiologia*, 15, 175.

Lewis, F. J., and Taufic, M. (1953): "Closure of atrial septal defect with the aid of hypothermia; experimental accomplishments and the report of one successful case", *Surgery*, **33**, 52.

Lewis, T., and Grant, R. T. (1923): "Observations relating to subacute infective endocarditis. Part I. Notes on the normal structure of the aortic valve. Part 2. Bicuspid aortic valves of congenital origin. Part 3. Bicuspid aortic valves in subacute infective endocarditis", *Heart*, **10**, 31.

Lindsay, S. (1950): "The cardiovascular system in gargoylism", *Brit. Heart J.*, **12**, 17.

Love, W. S., and Holms, J. H. (1939): "Coarctation of the aorta with associated stenosis of the right subclavian artery", *Amer. Heart J.*, **17**, 628.

Lowe, J. B. (1953): "The angiocardiogram in Fallot's tetralogy", *Brit. Heart J.*, **15**, 319.

Lutembacher, R. (1916): "De la stenose mitrale avec communication inter-auriculaire", *Arch. d. mal. d. Cœur*, **9**, 237.

McGinn, S., and White, P. D. (1933): "Interauricular septal defect associated with mitral stenosis", *Amer. Heart J.*, **9**, 1.

McGregor, M. (1950): "The genesis of the electrocardiogram of right ventricular hypertrophy", *Brit. Heart J.*, **12**, 351.

McGuire, J., and Goldman, F. (1937): "Apparent increased velocity of blood flow in cases of congenital heart disease with septal defects having right to left shunts", *Amer. Heart J.*, **14**, 230.

McKim, J. S., and Wiglesworth, F. W. (1954): "Absence of the left pulmonary artery. A report of six cases with autopsy findings in three", *Amer. Heart J.*, **47**, 845.

McKusick, V. A. (1955): "The cardiovascular aspects of Marfan's syndrome: a heritable disorder of connective tissue", *Circulation*, **11**, 321.

MacMahon, B., McKeown, T., and Record, R. G. (1953): "The incidence and life expectation of children with congenital heart disease", *Brit. Heart. J.*, **15**, 121.

Marquis, R. M. (1950): "Ventricular septal defect in early childhood", *Brit. Heart J.*, **12**, 265.

——, and Logan, A. (1955): "Congenital aortic stenosis and its surgical treatment", *Brit. Heart J.*, **17**, 373.

Medd, W. E., Matthews, M. B., and Thursfield, W. R. R. (1954): "Ebstein's disease", *Thorax*, **9**, 14.

Mehta, J. B., and Hewlett, R. F. L. (1945): "Cor triloculare Biauriculare; an unusual adult heart", *Brit. Heart J.*, **7**, 41.

Muir, D. C., and Brown, J. W. (1934): "Patent interventricular septum (maladie de Roger)" *Arch. Dis. Child.*, **9**, 27.

Murray, G. (1948): "Closure of defects in cardiac septa", *Ann Surg*, **128**, 843.

Nadas, A. S., and Alimurung, M. M. (1952): "Apical diastolic murmurs in congenital heart disease", *Amer. Heart J.*, **43**, 691.

——, et al. (1953): "Tetralogy of Fallot with unilateral pulmonary atresia. A clinically diagnosable and surgically significant variant", *Circulation*, **8**, 328.

Neuhauser, E. B. D. (1949): "Tracheo-esophageal constriction produced by right aortic arch and left ligamentum arteriosum", *Am. J. Roentgenol.*, **62**, 493.

Newman, M. (1948): "Coarctation of the aorta. Review of 23 service cases", *Brit. Heart J.*, **10**, 150.

Pedersen, A., and Therkelsen, F. (1954): "Cor triatriatum: A rare malformation of the heart, probably amenable to surgery", *Amer. Heart J.*, **47**, 676.

Perry, C. B. (1931): "Congenital heart disease as seen in elementary school children", *Bristol med. chir. J.*, **48**, 41.

Potts, W. J. (1949): "Surgical treatment of congenital pulmonary stenosis", *Ann. Surg.*, **130**, 342.

——, and Gibson, S. (1948): "Aortic pulmonary anastomosis in congenital pulmonary stenosis", *J. Amer. med. Ass.*, **137**, 343.

——, Smith, S., and Gibson, S. (1946): "Anastomosis of the aorta to a pulmonary artery. Certain types in congenital heart disease", *Ibid.*, **132**, 627.

Prior, J. T., and Wyatt, T. C. (1950): "Endocardial fibroelastosis", *Am. J. Path.*, **26**, 969.

Rados, A. (1942): "Marfan's syndrome (arachnodactyly coupled with dislocation of lens)", *Arch. Ophth.*, **27**, 477.

Railsbach, O. C., and Dock, W. (1929): "Erosion of ribs due to stenosis of isthmus (coarctation) of aorta", *Radiol.*, **12**, 58.

Reifenstein, G. H., Levine, S. A., and Gross, R. E. (1947): "Coarctation of the aorta. A review of 104 autopsied cases of the 'adult type', 2 years of age or older", *Amer. Heart J.*, **33**, 146.

Reynolds, G. (1950): "The heart in arachnodactyly", *Guy's Hosp. Rep.*, **99**, 178.

Rich, A. R. (1948): "A hitherto unrecognized tendency to the development of widespread pulmonary vascular obstruction in patients with congenital pulmonary stenosis (tetralogy of Fallot)", *Bull. Johns Hopk. Hosp.*, **82**, 389.

Robbins, S. L. (1945): "Brain abscess associated with congenital heart disease", *Arch. intern. Med.*, **75**, 279.

Roberts, J. T. (1936): "A case of congenital aortic atresia with hypoplasia of ascending aorta, normal origin of coronary arteries, left ventricular hypoplasia and mitral stenosis", *Amer. Heart J.*, **12**, 448.

Roesler, H. (1928): "Beitrage zur Lehre von den angeborenen Herzfehlern. IV. Untersuchungen an zwei Fallen von Isthmus-stenose der Aorta", *Wien. Arch. inn. Med.*, **15**, 521.

—— (1934): "Interatrial septal defect", *Arch. intern. Med.*, **54**, 339.

Roger, H. (1879): "Recherches cliniques sur la communication congenital des deux cœurs, par inocclusion du septum interventriculaire", *Bull. Acad. Med. d. Pari* , **8**, 1074.

Rogers, H. M., and Edwards, J. E. (1948): "Incomplete division of the atrioventricular canal with patent interatrial foramen primum", *Amer. Heart J.*, **36**, 28.

——, —— (1951): "Cor Triloculare Biatriatum: an analysis of the clinical and pathologic features of nine cases", *Amer. Heart J.*, **41**, 299.

——, and Rudolph, C. C. (1951): "Congenital ventricular septal defect with acquired complete heart block", *Ibid.*, **41**, 770.

Rosenthal, L. (1955): "Coarctation of the aorta and pregnancy. Report of five cases", *Brit. med. J.*, **i**, 16.

Russell, Dorothy S. (1946): "Myocarditis in Friedreich's ataxia", *J. Path. and Bact.*, **58**, 739.

Rytand, D. A. (1938): "The renal factor in arterial hypertension with coarctation of the aorta", *J. clin. Invest.*, **17**, 391.

Sancetta, S. M., and Zimmerman, H. A. (1950): "Congenital heart disease with septal defects in which paradoxical brain abscess causes death. Review of the literature and report of two cases", *Circulation*, **1**, 593.

Sellors, T. H. (1948): "Surgery of pulmonary stenosis", *Lancet*, **1**, 988.

Selzer, A. (1949): "Defect of the ventricular septum", *Arch. intern. Med.*, **84**, 798.

——, and Laqueur, G. L. (1951): "The Eisenmenger complex and its relation to the uncomplicated defect of the ventricular septum", *Ibid.*, **87**, 218.

Shapiro, M. J. (1949): "Clinical studies on twenty-one cases of coarctation of the aorta", *Amer. Heart J.*, **37**, 1045.

——, and Keys, A. (1943): "Patency of ductus arteriosus in adults", *Ibid.*, **25**, 158.

Silvy, M. (1934) : "Mongolisme et Malformations Cardiaques", Paris.

Smith, D. E., and Matthews, M. B. (1955): "Aortic valvular stenosis with coarctation of the aorta with special reference to the development of aortic stenosis upon congenital bicuspid valves", *Brit. Heart J.*, **17**, 198.

Smith, J. C. (1950): "Review of single coronary artery with report of two cases", *Circulation*, **1**, 1168.

—— (1951): "Anomalous pulmonary veins", *Amer. Heart J.*, **41**, 561.

Snellen, H. A., and Albers, F. H. (1952): "The clinical diagnosis of anomalous pulmonary venous drainage", *Circulation*, **6**, 801.

Sommers, S. C., and Johnson, J. M. (1951): "Congenital tricuspid atresia", *Amer. Heart J.*, 41, 130.

Soulié, P., Carlotti, J., Voci, G., and Joly, F. (1953): "The physiopathology of Eisenmenger's complex", *Arch. mal. cœur*, 46, 481.

Sprague, H. B., Ernlund, C. H., and Albright, F. (1933): "Clinical aspects of persistent right aortic root", *New England J. Med.*, 209, 679.

Steinberg, M. F., Grishman, A., and Sussman, M. L. (1943): "Angiocardiography in congenital heart disease. III. Patent ductus arteriosus", *Amer. J. Roentgenol.*, 50, 306.

Sussman, M. L., and Grishman, A. (1947): "A study of angiocardiography and angiography", *Advances in internal Medicine*, New York, 2, 102.

Swan, C. (1949): "Rubella in pregnancy as an ætiological factor in congenital malformation. Stillborn, miscarriage and abortion. Part II", *J. Obst. and Gynec. Brit. Emp.*, 56, 591.

——, et al. (1943): "Congenital defects in infants following infectious diseases during pregnancy, with special reference to relationship between German measles and cataract, deaf-mutism, heart disease and microcephaly, and to period of pregnancy in which occurrence of rubella is followed by congenital abnormalities", *Med. J. Australia*, 2, 201.

Swan, H. J. C., Burchell, H. B., and Wood, E. H. (1954): "The presence of venoarterial shunts in patients with interatrial communications", *Circulation*, 10, 705.

——, Zapata-Diaz, J., Burchell, H. B., and Wood, E. H. (1954): "Pulmonary hypertension in congenital heart disease", *Amer. J. Med.*, 16, 12.

——, Zeavin, I., Blount, S. G., Jr., and Virtue, R. W. (1953): "Surgery by direct vision in the open heart during hypothermia", *J. Amer. med. Ass.*, 153, 1081.

Taussig, H. B. (1938): "Complete transposition of great vessels", *Amer. Heart. J.*, 16, 728.

—— (1947): "Diagnosis of the tetralogy of Failot and medical aspects of the Surgical treatment", *Bull. N.Y. Acad. Med.*, 23, 705.

—— (1947): "Congenital malformations of the heart", New York.

—— (1948): "The surgery of congenital heart disease: Diagnosis and treatment of the cyanotic group", *Brit. Heart J.*, 10, 65.

—— (1948): "Tetralogy of Fallot: Especially the care of the cyanotic infant and child", *Pediatrics*, 32, 307.

——, and Blalock, A. (1947): "Observations on the volume of the pulmonary circulation and its importance in the production of cyanosis and polycythæmia", *Amer. Heart J.*, 33, 413.

Taylor, Maj. R. R., and Pollock, Col. B. E. (1953): "Coarctation of the aorta in three members of a family", *Ibid.*, 45, 470.

Touroff, A. S. W., and Vesell, H. (1940). "Subacute streptococcus viridans endarteritis complicating patent ductus arteriosus", *J. Amer. med. Ass.*, 115, 1270.

Towers (1952): personal communication.

Tubbs, O. S. (1944): "The effect of ligation on infection of the patent ductus arteriosus", *Brit. J. Surg.*, 32, 1.

Van Lingen, B., et al. (1952): "Clinical and cardiac catheterization findings compatible with Ebstein's anomaly of the tricuspid valve. A report of two cases", *Amer. Heart J.*, 43, 77.

Vesell, H., and Kross, I. (1946): "Patent ductus arteriosus with subacute bacterial endarteritis; diagnosis and indications for operation", *Arch. intern. Med.*, 77, 659.

Vogelpoel, L., and Shrire, V. (1955): "The role of auscultation in the differentiation of Fallot's tetralogy from severe pulmonary stenosis with intact ventricular septum and right to left interatrial shunt", *Circulation*, 11, 714.

Von Gierke, E. (1929): "Hepato-Nephromegalia glykogenica (Glykogenspeicherkrankheit der heber und Nieren)", *Beitr. Path. Anat.*, 82, 497.

Wakim, K. G., Slaughter, O., and Clagett, O. T. (1948): "Studies on the blood flow in the extremeties in cases of coarctation of the aorta: Determinations before and after excision of the coarctate region", *Proc. Mayo Clin.*, 23, 347.

Weber, F. (1918): "Can the clinical manifestations of congenital heart disease disappear with the general growth and development of the patient?" *Brit. J. child. Dis.*, **15**, 113.

Wells, B. G., Rappaport, M. B., and Sprague, H. B. (1949): "The sounds and murmurs in coarctation of the aorta", *Amer. Heart J.*, **38**, 69.

Wendkos, M. H., and Study, R. S. (1947): "Familial congenital complete A-V heart block", *Ibid.*, **34**, 138.

Wesselhoeft, C. (1949): "Rubella (German measles) and congenital deformities", *New England J. Med.*, **240**, 258.

Whitaker, W. (1954): "Total pulmonary venous drainage through a persistent left superior vena cava", *Brit. Heart J.*, **16**, 177.

Wilson, M. G., and Lubschez, R. (1942): "Prognosis for children with congenital anomalies of the heart and central vessels", *J. Pediat.*, **21**, 23.

Wood, P. (1950): "Congenital Heart Disease", (St. Cyres Lecture), *Brit. med. J.*, ii, 639 and 653.

—— (1952): "Pulmonary hypertension", *Brit. med. Bull.*, **8**, 348.

——, Magidson, O., and Wilson, P. A. O. (1954): "Ventricular septal defect with a note on acyanotic Fallot's tetralogy", *Brit. Heart J.*, **16**, 387.

Yater, W. M., Lyon, J. A., and McNabb, P. E. (1933): "Congenital heart block. Review and report of the second case of complete heart block studied by serial sections through the conduction system", *J. Amer. med. Ass.*, **100**, 1831.

——, and Shapiro, M. J. (1937): "Congenital displacement of the tricuspid valve (Ebstein's disease): review and report of a case with electrocardiographic abnormalities and detailed histologic study of the conducting system", *Ann. intern. Med.*, **11**, 1043.

Ziegler, R. F. (1952): "The importance of patent ductus arteriosus in children", *Amer. Heart J.*, **43**, 553.

—— (1954): "The genesis and importance of the electrocardiogram in coarctation of the aorta", *Circulation*, **9**, 371.

CHAPTER IX

RHEUMATIC FEVER AND ACTIVE RHEUMATIC CARDITIS

RHEUMATIC fever is a particular form of polyarthritis following streptococcal infection: its hall-marks are pancarditis, chorea, subcutaneous nodules and erythema marginatum. It may be acute, subacute or chronic.

INCIDENCE

According to the 1927 report of the Child Life Committee of the Medical Research Council, "Social Conditions and Acute Rheumatism", 10 to 15 per cent of all children at 12 years of age in England are affected by rheumatism. Of 22,800 children under 15 years of age card-indexed by the London County Council, 2.6 per cent had had rheumatic fever (Bach et al., 1939). The crude annual death-rate from rheumatic fever declined from 67 per million persons in 1901 to 22 per million in 1937 (Glover, 1939). During 1937, according to Glover, rheumatic fever accounted for 2.3 per cent of all deaths in children between the ages of 5 and 9 years.

The disease is rare in infancy and in old age, and is most common in childhood and adolescence, attacking the poor rather than the rich, and having an incidence climatically and geographically parallel to streptococcal tonsillitis (Coburn, 1931). The peak incidence is in children between the ages of 6 and 12, particularly during the months of October-November and of January-February. Apart from arachnodactyly there is no evidence that a particular physical type is predisposed to rheumatic fever (Hill and Allan, 1929); but hereditary predisposition is now accepted (Wilson, 1940; Wilson and Schweitzer, 1954).

THE NATURE OF THE RHEUMATIC STATE

There is no evidence, as yet, that rheumatic fever is caused directly by any infective agent. Cultures from blood, joint fluid, pericardial or pleural effusions, and from affected tissues are bacteriologically sterile, and filtrates from similar samples are incapable of transmitting the disease when inoculated into animal or man. There is still, perhaps, a remote possibility that a virus is responsible, but the known facts are against it.

On the other hand, the evidence that rheumatic fever is intimately related to streptococcal infection is beyond dispute. The relationship was first propounded by Poynton and Payne in 1900. They isolated a diplococcus from blood and other cultures and produced polyarthritis and carditis by injecting it into animals; but the lesions were shown later to be infective, not rheumatic. However, they confirmed the observation of Haig-Brown (1886), that rheumatic fever was nearly always preceded by streptococcal sore throat, the latent interval being 10 to 20 days (Poynton and Payne, 1913). The most convincing proof of this was later given by Schlesinger (1930). The responsible organism is always a hæmolytic streptococcus (Collis, 1931). As previously stated, the incidence of rheumatic fever follows closely the geographic, social, and seasonal incidence of streptococcal tonsillitis (Coburn, 1931), and small epidemics of rheumatic fever in closed communities always follow epidemics of streptococcal sore throat (Glover, 1930). Culpable streptococci belong serologically to group A, and may liberate powerful erythrogenic toxins and hæmolysins—in fact they are often scarlatinal strains (Coburn and Pauli, 1935). Serum from the subjects of rheumatic fever agglutinate these strains in high titre, and anti-streptococcal hæmolysins (antibodies excited by the antigenic properties of streptococcal hæmolysins) have been found in high titre in the early stages of practically all cases of active rheumatic fever, whether or not a history of streptococcal infection is obtained (Todd, 1932). Most of these observations have been confirmed independently by other workers, notably Griffith (1935), Sheldon (1931), and Bradley (1932).

It is now generally believed that rheumatic fever is an abnormal tissue reaction to the products of hæmolytic streptococcal infection in a sensitised individual. A number of other observations supports this hypothesis. Thus allergic polyarthritis, with a latent interval of 8 to 9 days, may follow the injection of foreign serum; polyarthritis may similarly follow gonococcal, dysenteric, and other bacterial infections in individuals sensitised by previous attacks; associated skin lesions in rheumatic fever, such as erythema multiforme, strongly suggest allergy. The experimental work of Rich and Gregory (1943, 1944), who succeeded in producing carditis of the rheumatic type in rabbits by injecting horse serum, and of Cavelti (1947), who was equally successful in rats which were injected with an antigen consisting of killed streptococci and heart or connective tissue emulsion, provides convincing evidence of the existence of an allergic form of carditis, which may be related to the streptococcus, and which at least resembles that seen in rheumatic fever. Finally, Murphy and Swift (1949) produced microscopic lesions in the hearts of rabbits, closely resembling those seen in rheumatic carditis, by repeated intradermal injections of group A beta hæmolytic streptococci.

The relationship between rheumatic fever and rheumatoid arthritis is still uncertain. Serum from patients with rheumatoid arthritis commonly agglutinates all strains of hæmolytic streptococci in high dilution (Dawson et al., 1932), but does not, as a rule, contain the high titre anti-hæmolysins characteristic of rheumatic fever (Stuart-Harris, 1935); nevertheless, the anti-streptolysin titre is much higher than in normal controls (Goldie and Griffiths, 1936). Whether there is any essential difference between the pathology of the affected joints and in the structure of subcutaneous nodules in the two conditions, other than those which might be due to the age of the patient or to the chronicity of the lesion, is still a matter of controversy (Goldie, 1938). The incidence of a rheumatic type of cardiac lesion in rheumatoid arthritis is difficult to assess from the literature, but appears to range between 3 and 30 per cent in clinical studies, and between 25 and 66 per cent in post-mortem studies (Rogen, 1947). These figures are probably too high. The subject is well reviewed by Bywaters (1950).

PATHOLOGY

In a fulminating attack which ends fatally within two or three weeks, tissue microscopy reveals only non-specific lesions consisting of œdema, fragmentation of collagen, leucocytic infiltration, hyperæmia and capillary hæmorrhage (Coburn, 1933). Similar lesions may occur in most acute infections, toxæmias and allergic states, and represent the Arthus phenomenon (Werner, 1938). Many tissues are so affected, particularly the synovial membranes of the larger joints, the pericardium, myocardium, and endocardium, the pleura and lung. Petechiæ may be seen clinically in the skin (purpura rheumatica) or in the ocular fundi, and at autopsy they are often most obvious in the pericardium and pleura. Inflammatory œdema of soft tissues may be seen clinically, independent of arthritis. Effusion into the large joints, and sometimes into the pericardial or pleural cavities, is characteristic and is the best example of the exudative type of lesion.

The specific rheumatic lesion, however, is proliferative, and occurs rather later; it is characterised by the Aschoff node (Aschoff, 1904). This is a small collection of large, often multinucleated, reticulo-endothelial cells, mixed with lymphocytes and plasma cells, surrounding a necrotic collagenous centre; there is also fibroblastic proliferation. Whilst it is in no sense perivascular, it lies in close relationship to a vessel. This lesion is particularly well seen in the myocardium. Another example of the proliferative lesion is the subcutaneous nodule, which may be regarded as an aggregation of Aschoff nodes with fibroblastic tissue predominating (fig. 9.01).

Occasionally, vascular lesions are found in the viscera which show all the features of panarteritis. Involvement of the cerebral, pulmonary, coronary, and mesenteric arteries has been described (Ritchie, 1939). Secondary thrombosis may occur, but is uncommon. Later, the media may become calcified.

Rheumatic inflammation of the heart valves is a true valvulitis, the baneful agent entering the valve through the minute vessels which supply it (Shaw, 1929). There has been considerable disagreement concerning the vascularity of normal and diseased heart valves. Langer (1887) first demonstrated the dependence of valvular blood vessels upon the presence of muscle: he showed that vessels and muscle fibres reached the free edge of the valve in the fœtus and new-born child, but soon regressed; also that diseased valves were frequently vascularised whereas normal adult valves were not. Gross and Kugel (1921, 1925–26, 1927–28, 1931), who studied the coronary circulation in detail by means of radiography after injecting a barium sulphate gel, confirmed Langer's observations. They also found that in the fœtus the pulmonary valve was the one best provided with muscle and blood vessels, whereas in children it was the aortic cusp of the mitral valve. The belief that endocarditis *in utero* usually affected the pulmonary valve, whereas in children it usually affected the mitral valve, thus appeared to have a rational basis. The decreasing incidence of valvulitis as age advanced was similarly explained. More recent work based on the

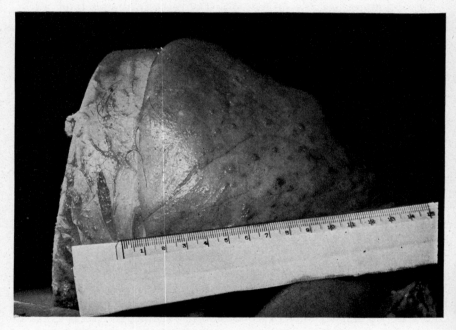

Fig. 9.01—Rheumatic nodules in the occipital aponeurosis.

injection of Indian ink instead of barium gel, however, has thrown doubt on these conclusions. Wearn *et al.* (1936), for instance, found capillaries in the valves of 84 per cent of seventy-four normal hearts, and were unable to correlate the relative incidence of endocarditis of a given valve with the frequency with which it contained blood vessels. Thus the mitral valve was vascularised in 66 per cent, the tricuspid in 64 per cent, the pulmonary in 28 per cent and the aortic in 16 per cent. It is possible that the factor governing the relative frequency with which each valve is involved is simply the degree of natural trauma to which each is exposed. In a child of 10, for example, with a systemic blood pressure of 100/60 mm. Hg and a pulmonary blood pressure of 15/5 mm. Hg, the load supported by the mitral, aortic, tricuspid and pulmonary valves is in the proportion of 100,

60, 15, and 5 mm. Hg respectively. According to Cabot (1926), the mitral valve is involved in 85 per cent of cases, the aortic in 44 per cent, the tricuspid in 10 to 16 per cent, and the pulmonary in 1 to 2 per cent, which is very close to the relative frequencies that would be predicted if the above hypothesis were correct.

In the acute stage of rheumatic inflammation the valve is œdematous, and soon shows signs of damage just proximal to its free edge where the cusps come into apposition, i.e. at the site of maximum natural trauma. Small thrombi form on the valve at this site giving rise to a ridge, or to a row of small pink nodules. As the inflammation subsides, secondary sclerosis follows and results particularly in fusion of the cusps at the critical areas of tendon insertion (Brock, 1952), as described in the next chapter. Sclerosis may affect the cusps themselves, the chordæ tendineæ, the papillary muscles and the mitral ring in varying degree: when the damage is slight, simple fusion of the cusps (mitral stenosis) is the most likely consequence; when the damage is considerable all parts of the valve mechanism become thickened and disorganised, and serious mitral incompetence develops. According to Carey Coombs (1924), mitral stenosis usually takes 2 to 8 years to develop, the stricture increasing very slowly over the years. Mitral incompetence usually begins at once during the stage of active inflammation, and may progress rapidly in severe cases, abetted by dilatation of the mitral ring as the left ventricle dilates in response to its increasing load or as a result of myocarditis; once heavy scarring of the mitral valve is well established, however, the degree of incompetence is unlikely to increase further, perhaps rather to the contrary.

Fusion of the aortic cusps, leading to aortic stenosis, also results from secondary sclerosis and usually takes several years to develop, the stricture then increasing gradually over the years. Aortic incompetence, on the other hand, like mitral incompetence, usually begins during the active stage of the disease, and may progress rapidly in severe cases. Slight or moderate leaks may increase gradually over the years as a result of secondary sclerotic changes, or if the latter cause increasing fusion of the cusps early incompetence may be replaced by dominant stenosis.

CLINICAL FEATURES

In childhood, the heart often bears the brunt of the attack, and indeed the joints may escape entirely. Once the heart has been involved, however, carditis or valvulitis should be assumed in all subsequent attacks; the increased vascularity of a valve which has been subjected to rheumatic inflammation may partly explain this tendency to recurrence. If the first attack occurs over the age of 21, carditis is unlikely, and becomes progressively rare with advancing years, although it may still occur even in old age. Polyarthritis, on the other hand, becomes increasingly common.

Of 588 rheumatic children studied in detail by Ash (1948), 58 per cent presented first with polyarthritis, 8 per cent with subacute rheumatism, 19 per cent with chorea, and 15 per cent with isolated rheumatic carditis. About one-quarter of acute cases have evidence of pre-existing rheumatic heart disease when first seen (joint report, 1955).

The diagnosis of rheumatic carditis is based on three major issues: upon signs of some inflammatory process, upon evidence that this process is rheumatic, and upon proof of cardiac involvement.

SIGNS OF SOME INFLAMMATORY PROCESS

These are fever, leucocytosis, and elevation of the erythrocyte sedimentation rate. Fever may be of any degree, but is usually moderate or high initially in children, and moderate or low grade in adults; it is irregular in type, and inclined to relapse; it may last only a few days, or it may continue for months. The temperature is normal in subacute rheumatism, and may be normal when polyarthritis is still active in acute attacks. Leucocytosis is slight to moderate in the early phase of acute rheumatic fever, figures of 10,000 to 15,000 white cells per c.mm. being the rule. The differential count may show a slight relative increase of polymorphs, but is often normal. In subacute rheumatism the total count is commonly between 7,000 and 10,000 per c.mm. The sedimentation rate is by far the most valuable evidence of some active inflammatory process, and is often remarkably high when there are no other signs. Weekly readings have proved a reliable index of the course of the disease and of the degree of activity. In less than 5 per cent of cases the test is valueless, the E.S.R. remaining normal throughout the illness.

It will be appreciated that these three features are non-specific; they point to some inflammatory process, but they do not determine its nature. Secondary anæmia and loss of weight, or failure to gain weight, may be regarded in a similar light. According to Cochran (1951), the normocytic orthochromic "anæmia" is often apparent rather than real, for it may result from hæmodilution, the plasma volume being increased as originally observed by Bradley (1938).

EVIDENCE THAT THE INFLAMMATORY PROCESS IS RHEUMATIC

1. *Polyarthritis*. Non-suppurative polyarthritis with sterile effusions into the large joints is characteristic. Involved joints may be painful, swollen, hot, flushed, and tender; on the other hand, slight effusion into a knee joint may be detected when there are no other signs or symptoms, or the patient may complain of joint pains when there are no signs, as in subacute rheumatism. The older the patient the more often are the small joints affected, and it becomes increasingly difficult to distinguish rheumatic fever from rheumatoid arthritis. Pains and effusions tend to flit from joint to joint, one recovering as another is involved, but not necessarily. Occasionally, one

ee or other large joint alone is inflamed, especially if previously injured,
1 may remain so for weeks or even for months; but minimal pains else-
ere may suggest its true nature. Other forms of what is thought to be
ergic polyarthritis, such as the dysenteric variety, may be indistinguish-
e except on other grounds. For example, dysenteric polyarthritis is pro-
imed by associated conjunctivitis and urethritis, and by its relation to
sentery.

In subacute rheumatism, recurrent joint pains occur without effusion,
1 usually without fever or leucocytosis; but the sedimentation rate is
sed. "Growing pains" confined to the hips, knees, or ankles, mean sub-
te rheumatism; growing pains described in the muscles, ligaments, or
dons probably do not (Hawksley, 1939).

2. *Relationship to streptococcal infection.* The diagnosis is favoured if the
nptoms follow a streptococcal sore throat, or some other streptococcal
ection, including scarlet fever. There is a latent interval of 1 to 3 weeks,
ially 10 to 14 days. The significance of this relationship cannot be over-
essed. It appears to be fundamentally the same as the relationship be-
een dysenteric polyarthritis and acute bacillary dysentery, or between
nococcal polyarthritis and gonorrhœa. Opportunity to study the dysen-
ic form was afforded by its frequency amongst the troops in North
rica and Italy in the second world war. It was characterised by acute poly-
hritis involving the large joints, by resistance to salicylates, by prolonged
ivity averaging about three months, and by associated conjunctivitis and
ethritis. Joint effusions were sterile and cultures from the conjunctiva
1 urethra yielded no pathogenic organisms. The provocative attack of
sentery was often abortive or very mild, and the latent period 10 to 14
ys. A previous attack of dysentery was invariable, and was usually un-
ated. The evidence suggested that a fairly high degree of immunity was
cessary for the development of the syndrome. Gonococcal polyarthritis
s equally common and behaved similarly, except that tenosynovitis re-
iced conjunctivitis, and urethritis was primary. The facts suggest that
eumatic fever is streptococcal polyarthritis, and bears the same relation-
p to the streptococcus as does dysenteric polyarthritis to the dysentery
cilli, and gonococcal polyarthritis to the gonococcus; but instead of con-
nctivitis, urethritis, or tenosynovitis, there may be carditis, chorea, sub-
aneous nodules, or marginate erythema.

If there is no history of recent sore throat or other streptococcal infection,
dence of such may be afforded by an anti-streptolysin titre in the region
200 Todd units. High titres do not prove that an illness is rheumatic
er, only that there has been recent hæmolytic streptococcal infection.
nilar proof may be obtained by finding that the patient's serum aggluti-
es an emulsion of hæmolytic streptococci at a titre of 1 : 200. It is highly
probable that any case of acute rheumatic fever, whether it be the first
ack or a recurrence, will not show such serological changes.

A positive test for C-reactive protein in the serum provides good

evidence of activity (Anderson and McCarty, 1950), but is far from
specific in the rheumatic state, the abnormal *alpha*-globulin that react
with C-polysaccharide being found in a variety of infections, necroses and
collagen diseases, including uncomplicated streptococcal sore throat
rheumatoid arthritis, and periarteritis.

That continued hæmolytic streptococcal infection is not responsible fo
the disease may be proved by the lack of improvement after treatment with
penicillin.

3. *Response to salicylates.* Joint pains and effusions in rheumatic feve
commonly respond dramatically to sodium salicylate in initial doses of 1
to 20 grains (1 to 1.5 G.), aspirin (or calcium aspirin) 5 to 10 grains (0.3 t
0.6 G.) three- or four-hourly. Only the exudative lesion and the associate
fever respond; no effect is observed on proliferative lesions. Sodium
salicylate is often used as a diagnostic test, but although a good one, it i
not infallible.

4. *Chorea.* Rheumatic or Sydenham's chorea is mysterious in severa
ways. First, it has a solitary nature, preferring to occur alone rather tha
in the company of other rheumatic manifestations. Secondly, it does no
affect the sedimentation rate. Thirdly, there is no specific rheumatic patho
logy in the brain (Shaw, 1929). Nevertheless, it is certainly part of th
rheumatic state. About 20 per cent of patients with chorea alone develo
rheumatic heart disease, about 50 per cent develop other rheumatic mani
festations with or without carditis (Sutton and Dodge, 1938), and most o
the remainder have a familial link. Conversely, about 20 per cent of a
rheumatic cases have chorea (Ash, 1948). Clinical features include spon
taneous, involuntary, inco-ordinated movements, muscular weakness an
alteration of tendon jerks, emotional instability, and some disturbance o
higher cortical function. Occasionally, it is more or less confined to on
side of the body. Movements disappear during sleep.

The diagnosis of chorea must be made from common tics and othe
forms of hysteria. Reliance should be placed on the quality of the move
ments. They are quick, complicated, elaborate, irregular and varied. Th
same movement is rarely repeated exactly. The hands writhe and twis
the patient trying to stop them, or attempting to conceal them by som
volitional act. She often drops things she is holding, especially crockery, o
she is clumsy in other ways. Facial grimaces are odd and varied, unlike th
repeated twitch of a tic. After protruding the tonge for inspection, sh
withdraws it like a lizard, snapping the jaws over it. When the hands ar
held out, the wrist is flexed and the fingers hyper-extended. The knee-jer
may be sustained, the leg being held up at the height of its extension for a
appreciable interval before relaxation occurs.

Hysterical movements are more jerky, and show constant repetitio
Experience and familiarity with both conditions usually makes their dis
tinction easy. The involuntary athetotic movements of encephalitis an
Wilson's disease may be more confusing.

due to pericardial effusion or to a greatly dilated heart. Pulmonary congestion or œdema, and infarcts of the lung, should be recognised without difficulty.

7. *Tolerance to Heparin*. Patients with acute rheumatic fever show a remarkable tolerance to heparin, and possibly to other sulphated polysaccharides. This is at present under investigation and may prove a useful test for the active rheumatic state (Abrahams and Glynn, 1949).

EVIDENCE OF CARDITIS

To establish the diagnosis of rheumatic carditis, at least one of its five chief manifestations must be recognised. It should be clearly understood that while these offer proof of cardiac involvement, they do not by themselves necessarily signify a rheumatic etiology—that must be demonstrated in other ways.

1. *Mitral valvitis*

The development of a *mitral pan-systolic murmur* embracing both heart sounds at the apical area must be taken seriously. Towards the end of the nineteenth century apical systolic murmurs of all kinds were attributed to mitral valve disease and patients were put to bed for long periods unnecessarily: to combat this tendency Mackenzie taught that the apical systolic murmur could be safely disregarded when unaccompanied by other signs of heart disease, and this teaching was perpetuated and emphasised by Lewis and Parkinson. As a result, the original diagnostic fault has been over-corrected, and it is becoming increasingly obvious that an important murmur is not receiving proper attention. The confusion has been caused partly by failure to distinguish the pan-systolic murmur of mitral incompetence from the relatively short mid-systolic aortic ejection murmur transmitted to the apex. The latter is often innocent, as explained elsewhere, but the mitral pan-systolic murmur means mitral incompetence and nothing else, and it is high time this indisputable fact was more widely recognised. The mitral murmur, of course, must be distinguished from the pan-systolic murmur of ventricular septal defect and tricuspid incompetence, both of which may be heard best sometimes at the apex of the heart; but if the apical murmur is mitral, then the only diagnostic problem is whether the mitral incompetence is functional, secondary to ring dilatation, or organic, resulting from a diseased mitral valve. Functional mitral incompetence means left ventricular dilatation, just as functional tricuspid incompetence means right ventricular dilatation, and both are important, for dilatation of either ventricle cannot be viewed with equanimity. In rheumatic carditis, for example, functional mitral incompetence usually means serious aortic incompetence, with or without left ventricular failure, and is far more important than trivial mitral valvulitis, to which an isolated mitral pan-systolic murmur should be ordinarily attributed.

In quality the mitral pan-systolic murmur is usually loud, smooth and blowing; being of fairly high frequency it is better heard with the diaphragm type of chest-piece. A thrill is uncommon in the early stage of active inflammation, and when it occurs usually means considerable permanent damage to the valve. Follow-up studies have shown that chronic rheumatic heart disease develops in 45 per cent of cases in which the original murmur was loud, and in only 9 per cent of those in which it was soft (Boone and Levine, 1938; Kuttner and Markowitz, 1948).

Other evidence of significant mitral incompetence includes a small, slightly water-hammer pulse, an otherwise unexplained rise of venous pressure, a hyperdynamic enlarged left ventricle (clinically, electrocardiographically and radiologically), a loud third heart sound, and radiological evidence of dilatation of the left atrium with or without pulmonary venous congestion. When valvitis is severe, permanent incompetence may be established within a few weeks of the onset of rheumatic carditis.

The development of a *soft short mitral diastolic murmur* (Carey Coombs murmur) in the absence of any other sign of mitral stenosis provides by far the most useful and conclusive evidence of mitral valvitis. At the rheumatic fever centre, Taplow, this murmur has been heard in 75 to 80 per cent of active cases. Although transient in 20 to 25 per cent, it usually proves to be more or less persistent, or reappears on the least provocation, until pre-systolic accentuation and a loud first heart sound proclaim the development of mitral stenosis (Carey Coombs, 1924).

This characteristic and diagnostic murmur is frequently overlooked because it is very low pitched, soft and short; it is best heard with the bell stethoscope when the patient lies on the left side, especially as the heart slows down after effort, and has the typical mid-diastolic timing of all mitral diastolic murmurs. We thought at Taplow that the murmur could be brought out or accentuated by any agent that increased the mitral stroke blood-flow, and that phenylephrine (neosynephrine) was perhaps the best way of achieving this. When given in doses of 0.25 mg. intravenously, the blood pressure rises sharply and the murmur develops as the heart slows down (Besterman, 1951).

Necropsies have confirmed the fact that this murmur may occur in active rheumatic carditis when the mitral valve is scarcely altered (Bland, White and Jones, 1935). It has therefore been suggested that its mechanism depends upon left ventricular dilatation; that it is related to the Austin Flint murmur, and to the soft mitral diastolic murmur that is occasionally heard in thyrotoxic heart failure. But it must be pointed out that the Carey Coombs murmur is usually heard when no enlargement of the heart can be demonstrated, and it is more reasonable to believe that some change in the structure of the mitral valve is responsible. Whatever the explanation, there is no doubt that this murmur occurs early in the course of rheumatic carditis, and may disappear as activity subsides.

2. *Aortic valvitis*

Inflammation of the aortic valve usually leads to immediate and permanent aortic incompetence, which may be recognised at once by the tell-tale aortic diastolic murmur. The initial leak is small so that other evidence is usually lacking. When first heard, the murmur may be remarkably short and high pitched, and its onset is slightly delayed, being inaudible until the diastolic pressure gradient across the aortic valve is approaching its maximum, i.e. towards the end of the period of isometric relaxation, when the left ventricular pressure is approaching zero. The triple rhythm cadence so produced may be disconcerting to the student who is only familiar with the to-and-fro murmurs of well-established aortic valve disease, but it is characteristic of these early cases.

An aortic diastolic murmur was heard in 45 per cent of cases at Taplow, and one in five was transient. Phenylephrine was again helpful in accentuating the murmur or bringing it out when it could not otherwise be heard, for the temporarily raised blood pressure and increased stroke volume encouraged the leak (Besterman, 1951).

An isolated aortic mid-systolic ejection murmur, heard best at apex or base, provides insufficient evidence of aortic valvitis to warrant a diagnosis of active rheumatic carditis, for it is too commonly produced by a simple increase of blood flow associated with any fever, or as a result of other innocent phenomena, such as a depressed sternum. A functional basal systolic bruit may also be pulmonary rather than aortic, and this too is usually a functional flow murmur, turbulence being created by a variety of innocent causes.

3. *Partial heart block*

Transient prolongation of the P-R interval (fig. 9.06) is recorded in about 10 per cent of cases, but may well be more frequent than this. It may be recognised clinically by premature *a* waves in the jugular venous pulse, occasionally by regular venous cannon waves when P falls between the onset of QRS and the end of the T wave of the previous cycle, by premature pre-systolic gallop rhythm, the interval between pre-systolic and first heart sounds being prolonged, and by softening of the first heart sound, the atrioventri-

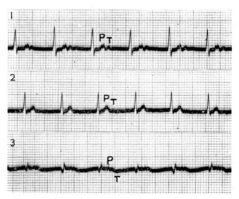

Fig. 9.06—Electrocardiogram showing prolongation of the P-R interval in a case of active rheumatic carditis.

cular valve cusps floating into apposition after atrial contraction is completed so that the atrioventricular valves are already more or less closed when the ventricles contract. Dropped beats are unusual, and more severe grades of heart block rare. Normal conduction can be temporarily restored in 90 per cent of cases by means of 1 to 2 mg. of atropine sulphate intravenously (Bruenn, 1937). Some degree of permanent block is likely in those that do not respond to atropine.

4. *Pericarditis*

Rheumatic pericarditis occurs in about 10 per cent of cases; it is always acute, commonly develops during the first month of the illness, and leaves no clinical sequelæ. In mild cases there is little more than transient pericardial friction with or without pain. Most cases that are recognised, however, are relatively severe, and the inflammation is accompanied by considerable pain, high fever, rapid breathing, and obvious distress; there is usually leucocytosis and the sedimentation rate is always high. A rise of venous pressure and proportionate distension of the liver are usual, for fluid tends to accumulate rapidly; dangerous tamponade, however, is rare, and therapeutic tapping nearly always unnecessary. The electrocardiogram may show characteristic early elevation of the S-T segment followed by flattening or slight inversion of the T waves in most leads as in other forms of pericarditis (fig. 9.07), but these changes are found in only a little over half the cases and are rarely very conspicuous. Rapid changes in the size of the heart shadow provide the most reliable radiological evidence of pericardial effusion (fig. 9.08), changes in shape being less important. Samples of the fluid are straw-coloured, sterile, and have the physical properties of an exudate.

Pericardial effusion is the usual cause of apparent cardiac enlargement in rheumatic carditis in the absence of serious valve damage or heart failure (Wood, 1950; Thomas, Besterman and Hollman, 1953).

5. *Heart failure*

Investigations on cardiac function in rheumatic carditis carried out at Taplow seemed to establish three things: (1) in cases uncomplicated by gross valve damage, pericardial effusion or congestive heart failure, tachycardia is not disproportionate to fever and anxiety, and the relationship between cardiac output and heart rate does not differ from that in normal controls (Hollman, 1950); (2) cardiac dilatation rarely, if ever, occurs in simple rheumatic carditis, enlargement of the heart shadow nearly always being caused by serious permanent valve damage, pericardial effusion, or congestive failure (Wood, 1950; Besterman and Thomas, 1953); (3) the resting cardiac output in uncomplicated cases is probably normal, but the maximum output is strictly limited and frequently reached as a result of anxiety alone (Besterman, 1954). There is no simple bedside way of demonstrating this impairment of cardiac function.

Congestive heart failure proper, with elevation of the venous pressure distension of the liver, and a fall in cardiac output, with or without œdema or ascites, is rare in the absence of advanced aortic or mitral valve disease

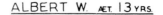

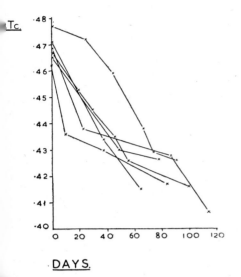

·DAYS.

ig. 9.11—Behaviour of QT$_c$ in six cases of
:ute rheumatic carditis with rapid clinical
recovery.

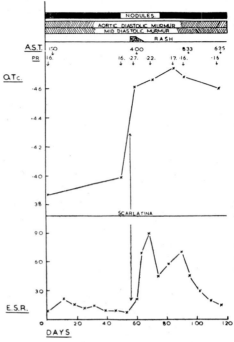

Fig. 9.12—Prolonged QT$_c$ following a recur·
rence of active rheumatic carditis.

(By courtesy of Dr. Derek Abrahams.)

TREATMENT

All cases of acute or subacute rheumatic polyarthritis should be put to
bed and treated with sodium salicylate, 15 to 20 grains (1 to 1.5 G.), combined or not with twice as much sodium bicarbonate, three-hourly (Lees,
1904), until relieved, or until ringing in the ears and deafness proclaim
that the desired therapeutic salicylate blood level of 30 to 35 mg. per cent
has been reached, when the interval between doses may be increased to
four or six hours. Aspirin or calcium aspirin, 10 gr. (0.6 G.), is equally
effective. Fever, pain, and joint effusions usually subside quickly, but
proliferative lesions, including carditis, are resistant. Toxic effects are
minimised by alkalis: this has been attributed to an increased rate of
salicylate excretion in their presence (Parker, 1947, 1948). Toxic effects
include central vomiting, hyperventilation associated with an increased
oxygen consumption (Cochran, 1952) and which sometimes results in
reduction of the plasma CO_2 content (Graham and Parker, 1948), and
petechiæ associated with prolongation of the prothrombin time (Link et al.,
1943). Fatal hæmorrhagic encephalopathy has been reported (Ashworth

and Mckemie, 1944). Circulating prothrombin can usually be restored by means of vitamin K in doses of 10 to 50 mg. (Shapiro, 1944).

When the patient has been free from symptoms for a week, or if he fails to derive benefit, salicylates should be stopped. If clinical relapse follows, no harm is done, for the exudative lesion is relatively innocent, and is soon controlled by another course.

Salicylates were introduced by Bliss (1875) and Maclagan (1876), and their action is still uncertain. It was suggested long ago that they might inhibit antibody formation (Derick, Hitchcock and Swift, 1927–8), a conception that received some support from Jager and Nickerson (1947), who showed that salicylates reduced the amount of H and O antigens produced in response to typhoid vaccine. Salicylates increase the plasma volume (York and Fischer, 1947), there being a profound shift in the distribution of body fluid from intracellular to extracellular compartments (Reid, Watson and Sproull, 1950). Following this line of thought, Copeman and Pugh (1950) reported rapid clinical improvement in 7 cases of acute rheumatic fever following an injection of hypertonic saline, the patients having been dehydrated previously by means of food and fluid starvation for 36 hours. Another way in which salicylates may influence the symptoms of rheumatic fever is by inhibiting hyaluronidase (Guerra, 1946). This enzyme hydrolyses hyaluronic acid, a polysaccharide present in mucoprotein which is a constituent of the ground substance of all connective tissue (Chain and Duthie, 1939). The effect of this is to increase the rapidity with which substances spread through collagen, as may be demonstrated by measuring the rate of spread of a suitable dye when injected intradermally. In rheumatic fever injected dye spreads more rapidly than in normal controls, as if an excess of hyaluronidase were present (Guerra, 1946), and serum from patients with active rheumatic fever has been shown to contain an excess of anti-hyaluronidase (Quinn, 1948). Whether the hyaluronidase factor in rheumatic fever depends on the power of the culpable streptococcus to produce it, or whether it arises from some other source is immaterial in respect of the action of salicylates, although possibly fundamental in relation to the cause of rheumatic fever itself. Another effect of salicylates is to reduce the permeability of damaged capillaries (Swyer, 1948), and this should certainly limit the exudative reaction. Yet another hypothesis is that salicylates have an action like A.C.T.H., for Hetzel and Hine (1951) have shown that therapeutic doses of salicylates diminish the ascorbic acid content of the suprarenal glands in rats (generally regarded as evidence of increased cortical activity), the effect being abolished by hypophysectomy; Van Cauwenberge (1951) found a reduction of circulating eosinophils in rats four to six hours after the ingestion of salicylates, preceded by a significant increase of the urinary uric acid/creatinine ratio, both of which have been attributed to increased activity of the suprarenal cortex. Finally, it must be remembered that a break-down product of sodium salicylate may well be responsible for its therapeutic effects, rather than the drug itself, and in gentisic acid we have a metabolite that seems to fulfil these expectations; sodium gentisate in doses of 1 G. three-hourly relieves the symptoms of rheumatic fever as quickly and completely as salicylates and has the advantage of minimal toxic effects (Meyer and Ragan, 1948; Clarke, 1953).

Recent work at the Mayo Clinic on the beneficial effect of cortisone (17-hydroxy-11-dehydrocorticosterone) on rheumatoid arthritis (Hench *et al.*, 1949) provided a new approach to the treatment of rheumatic states in general; but initial enthusiasm has already abated, and in rheumatic fever both cortisone and A.C.T.H. have been shown to be no more effective than aspirin (joint report, 1955). The usual dose of cortisone is 200 mg. daily for the first week, 100 mg. daily for the second and third weeks, and 75 to 25 mg. thereafter, the daily dose being reduced by 25 mg. at weekly intervals, and the total course lasting six weeks. Cortisone may be given intramuscularly or by mouth. A.C.T.H. (adreno-cortico-trophic hormone or corticotropin) is given intramuscularly in daily doses of 100 units for the first week, 80 units for the second, 60 units for the third, 40 for the fourth, 30 for the fifth and 20 for the sixth.

Both cortisone and corticotropin, like aspirin, relieve fever and joint pains quickly in rheumatic fever, and the sedimentation rate falls in a gratifying manner; but myocarditis, endocarditis, pericarditis, nodules, erythema marginatum and chorea do not seem to be influenced by any of these substances.

Neither sulphonamides nor penicillin have any influence on the course of rheumatic fever if given after the onset of rheumatic symptoms, but both are valuable prophylactic agents. Sulphadiazine in doses of 0.5 G. once or twice daily, oral penicillin or benzathine penicillin in doses of 200,000 to 500,000 units daily, or monthly intramuscular injections of 1.2 to 1.5 mega units of benzathine penicillin, all greatly reduce the frequency with which group A hæmolytic streptococci can be cultured from the throats of rheumatic children or carriers, and reduce the frequency of recurrencies (Stollerman, Rusoff and Hirschfeld, 1954; Perry and Gillespie, 1954). Unfortunately, intramuscular benzathine penicillin is often very painful. There is also good evidence that penicillin lessens the chances of the rheumatic reaction if given early enough to cases of group A hæmolytic streptococcal sore throat (Rammelkamp, 1952), and this may be supported by the demonstration that penicillin therapy suppresses antibody formation as judged by the anti-streptolysin titre, and that the sooner penicillin is given in cases of tonsillitis the greater the suppression of antibody (Brock and Siegel, 1953).

Tonsillectomy is only necessary if there is chronic sepsis, or if there is recurrent tonsillitis; it has little influence on the disease, and does not prevent relapse or recurrence (Ash, 1938). A good nourishing diet, fresh air, vitamins, especially vitamin C, appropriate treatment of secondary anæmia, and high morale are more important.

Chorea usually lasts 6 to 12 weeks. Patients should be put to bed during the active phase, and may need heavy sedation. If there is no evidence of carditis they may be allowed up when recovery begins. They should be kept away from school and from social engagements until well.

Carditis requires absolute rest. Little else is of lasting value. Digitalis is helpful when there is congestive heart failure, and although the therapeutic dose is said to be close to the toxic, ill effects have not been observed at Taplow. Mercurial diuretics and a low sodium diet are rarely necessary.

Absolute rest means that the patient is allowed to do nothing for himself; he is washed and fed, and must use bed-pan and urine bottle. Diet should be light and constipation avoided. In the past it was usual to insist on nursing the patient in the horizontal position, with one low pillow; but it is clear from experience gained in the treatment of angina decubitus and of paroxysmal cardiac dyspnœa, and from certain direct investigations in man, that the cardiac output, and therefore the work of the heart, is greater in the horizontal than in the upright position, owing to the influence of gravity on the venous filling pressure. It is therefore logical to nurse patients with carditis in the sitting posture. The wisest course may be to chose the position of maximum comfort, whether lying or sitting, unless there is failure, when the latter should be insisted upon.

By far the best index of activity is the E.S.R., which should be measured weekly, and as a rule the patient should not be allowed up until it is normal. This applies especially to children, in whom carditis should be assumed *for purposes of early management*. Adults without evidence of previous or present carditis may be treated more leniently, and may be allowed up as soon as they appear well enough on clinical grounds. The duration of bed rest varies between a week or two and several months, according to the severity and persistence of the active process. If patients are allowed up too soon, swift relapse is the rule.

Convalescence from carditis should be extended over several months, the régime being similar to that for pulmonary tuberculosis. Relapse is common and may be due to over-exertion, exposure, emotional upset, cold damp weather, and to almost any infection. Relapse follows the advent of the responsible agent immediately, and must be distinguished from a recurrence or second attack of rheumatic fever, in which streptococcal infection is always to blame, and following which a latent interval can usually be recognised. At least one recurrence occurs in two-thirds of all cases, usually within three years (Roth, Lingg and Whittemore, 1937).

It is as important to prevent cardiac neurosis in patients with organic heart disease as it is in those without. This is a difficult task in susceptible individuals, for reassurance cannot very well be unconditional. Rheumatic carditis may be symptom free, and pass without influencing the subject's activities at all. Thus only about 55 per cent of cases of mitral stenosis give a history of the original attack (Parkinson and Hartley, 1946). Many others are only restricted by subacute rheumatism. Little immediate harm comes to these patients; indeed there is no direct evidence that subsequent development of mitral stenosis could have been prevented by bed rest at the time of active inflammation. It follows that failure to diagnose carditis when it is present in rheumatic fever is not necessarily disastrous. On the other hand, its diagnosis in error may not be far short of it, for the resulting cardiac neurosis, which is so common, may be life-long and may be more incapacitating than organic heart disease. Physicians should be more aware of their responsibility in this respect. Too much emphasis is laid on overlooking a mild lesion; not enough on finding what is not there. The most common mistake is to misinterpret tachycardia. A patient confined strictly to bed for several weeks with rheumatic fever is fully aware that his heart may be involved, and is likely to become nervous on that account. Tachycardia may then be due to anxiety. Again, the autonomic nervous system is frequently disturbed by fever and infections of all kinds: tachycardia, dizziness, headache and fatigue may result, especially during convalescence when activities are resumed. Such findings call for reassurance and rehabilitation, not for alarm and further rest.

In the absence of diagnostic evidence of carditis throughout the active phase of rheumatic fever, subsequent medical management should be based on the assumption that none existed, not upon the fear that it escaped recognition; and patients should be sent for convalescence as after any other fever of equal severity. This attitude is based, not on the belief that carditis does not occur in a certain percentage of children with rheumatic fever, but on the fact that if it does occur in an indetectable degree, it is either of no consequence, or it is not aggravated by this kind of management; and on the fact that the over-cautious attitude breeds neurosis.

COURSE AND PROGNOSIS

Following convalescence from rheumatic fever, between 60 and 65 per cent of cases have evidence of residual valve damage, but 10 to 20 years later 9 to 16 per cent of these seem to have recovered completely; on the other hand, 23 to 44 per cent of those who appear to escape unscathed develop signs of chronic rheumatic heart disease within the same 10- to 20-year period (Ash, 1948; Bland and Jones, 1951). The net result is that at least two-thirds of all cases of rheumatic fever in childhood develop permanent valve damage.

Rheumatic carditis is more likely to be associated with polyarthritis (61 per cent), than with subacute rheumatism (38 per cent), or chorea (20 per cent). Isolated carditis, however, must occur much more frequently than its 15 per cent incidence would imply, because 40 per cent of all cases of chronic rheumatic heart disease in adults give no history of any rheumatic manifestations in childhood. Allowing for this it is estimated that one-third of all rheumatic cases in childhood have isolated carditis and that two-thirds of these are overlooked at the time. No previously published figures concerning early mortality and ultimate prognosis have allowed for these silent cases of primary carditis. For example, according to Ash (1948), about 48 per cent of cases presenting with primary carditis in childhood die within 10 years; but these, of course, are the cases that are recognised because of their severity, and isolated rheumatic carditis must be severe to cause symptoms. If allowance is made for the relatively mild unrecognised cases, practically none of which die within 10 years, Ash's figure changes from 48 to 16 per cent.

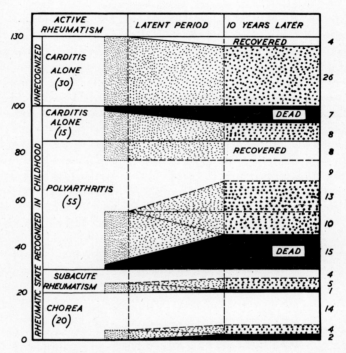

Fig. 9.13—Chart depicting the course of the rheumatic state over the first ten years (modified from figures published by Rachel Ash, 1948).

no carditis.
active carditis.
transition.
permanent valve disease.
dead.

In figure 9.13 an attempt has been made to chart the course of rheumatic fever over the first 10 years, based on the papers by Ash (1948), and Bland and Jones (1951), but modified so as to allow for the unrecognised cases. Taking into consideration the known data, it may be calculated that to every 100 recognised cases of juvenile rheumatism with or without carditis, there must be an additional 30 cases of unrecognised pure rheumatic carditis, assuming that between 10 and 15 per cent of the latter recover completely as in the recognised cases of carditis. The chart shows that 10 years after the onset of the rheumatic state, 25 out of 130 cases are dead (19 per cent), 66 (51 per cent) have chronic rheumatic heart disease, and 39 have recovered completely (30 per cent). It also shows that of the 66 living cases with permanent valve damage, 26 (40 per cent) were not recognised during the stage of active carditis. The relatively good prognosis of subacute rheumatism and chorea will not escape notice.

Of the fatal cases, one-third die within one year of the onset of rheumatic carditis, and two-thirds (Bland and Jones, 1938) to three-quarters (Ash, 1948) within the first five years. Thus the immediate mortality is 6.5 per cent, as reported by Scott (1943). Sudden unexpected death is rare, in contrast to its frequency in diphtheritic and certain other forms of toxic myocarditis: thus there were only three such instances amongst a group of 7,165 cases of active rheumatic fever reported by Griffith and Huntington (1946); coronary angiitis was blamed.

The prognosis is of course greatly influenced by the severity of the active state. Thus in a 20-year follow-up study of 1,000 cases, Bland and Jones (1951) found that 80 per cent of those who had developed heart failure, 63 per cent of those with pericarditis, and 37 per cent of those with nodules had died.

Recurrences or relapses are the rule rather than the exception, 40 per cent of cases having a second attack within 2 years, 58 per cent within 5 years, and 63 per cent within 10 years (Ash, 1948). Thus two-thirds of recurrences might be prevented by adequate antibiotic therapy for a period of two years after the initial attack.

REFERENCES

Abrahams, D. G. (1949): "The Q-T interval in acute rheumatic carditis", *Brit. Heart J.*, **11**, 342.
——, and Glynn, L. E. (1949): "Heparin tolerance in rheumatic fever", *Clin. Sc.*, **8**, 171.
Anderson, H. C., and McCarty, M. (1950): "Determination of C-reactive protein in blood as measure of activity of disease process in acute rheumatic fever", *Amer. J. Med.*, **8**, 445.
Aschoff, L. (1904): "Zur Myocarditisfrage", *Verhandl. d. deutsch. path. Geselsch.*, **8**, 46.
Ash, R. (1938): "Influence of tonsillectomy on rheumatic infection", *Amer. J. Dis. Child*, **55**, 63.
—— (1948): "The first ten years of rheumatic infection in childhood", *Amer. Heart J.*, **36**, 89.
Ashworth, C. T., and McKemie, J. F. (1944): "Hæmorrhagic complications, with death probably from salicylate therapy; report of 2 cases", *J. Amer. med. Ass.*, **126**, 806.
Bach, F., Hill, N. G., Preston, T. W., and Thornton, C. E. (1939): "Juvenile rheumatism in London", *Ann. rheum. Dis.*, **1**, 210.

Barlow, T., and Warner, F. (1881): "On subcutaneous nodules connected with fibrous structures, occurring in children the subjects of rheumatism and chorea", *Trans. internat. Med. Cong.*, 4, 16, London.

Besterman, E. M. M. (1951): "The use of phenylephrine to aid auscultation of early rheumatic diastolic murmurs", *Brit. med. J.*, 2, 205.

—— (1954): "The cardiac output in acute rheumatic carditis", *Brit. Heart J.*, 16, 8.

——, and Thomas, G. T. (1953): "Radiological diagnosis of rheumatic pericardial effusion", *Ibid.*, 15, 113.

Bland, E. F., and Jones, T. D. (1938): "Fatal rheumatic fever", *Arch. int. Med.*, 61, 161.

——, —— (1951): "Rheumatic fever and rheumatic heart disease. A twenty-year report", *Circulation*, 4, 836.

——, White, P. D., and Jones, T. D. (1935): "The development of mitral stenosis in young people with a discussion of the frequent misinterpretation of a mid-diastolic murmur at the cardiac apex", *Amer. Heart J.*, 10, 995.

Boone, J. A., and Levine, S. A. (1938): "The prognosis in potential rheumatic heart disease and rheumatic mitral insufficiency", *Amer. J. med. Sc.*, 195, 764.

Bradley, W. H. (1932): "Epidemic of acute rheumatism in public school", *Quart. J. Med.*, 1, 79.

—— (1938): "The influence of acute streptococcus pyogenes infection on the rheumatic subject", *Proc. Int. Congr. rheum. and hydrol.*, p. 86. Headley Bros., London.

Brock, L. L., and Siegel, A. C. (1953): "Studies on the prevention of rheumatic fever: the effect of time of initiation of treatment of streptococcal infections on the immune response of the host", *J. clin. Invest.*, 32, 630.

Brock, R. C. (1952): "The surgical and pathological anatomy of the mitral valve", *Brit. Heart J.*, 14, 489.

Bruenn, H. G. (1937): "Mechanism of impaired auriculo-ventricular conduction in acute rheumatic fever", *Amer. Heart J.*, 13, 413.

Buss, C. E. (1875): "Ueber die Anwendung der Salicylsäure als Antipyreticum", Leipzig, J. E. Hirschfeld.

Bywaters, E. G. L. (1950), "The relation between heart and joint disease including 'Rheumatoid heart disease' and 'Chronic post-rheumatic arthritis (Type Jaccoud)' ", *Brit. Heart J.*, 12, 101.

Cabot, R. C. (1926): "Facts on the heart", Philadelphia, W. B. Saunders.

Cavelti, P. A. (1947): "Studies on the pathogenesis of rheumatic fever. II. Cardiac lesions produced in rats by means of autoantibodies", *Arch. Path.*, 44, 13.

Chain, E., and Duthie, E. S. (1940): "Identity of hyaluronidase and spreading factor", *Brit. J. exp. Path.*, 21, 324.

Cheadle, W. B. (1889): "Rheumatic state in childhood", London.

Clarke, N. E., Mosher, R. E., and Clarke, C. N. (1953): "Phenolic compounds in the treatment of rheumatic fever. 1. A study of gentisic acid derivatives", *Circulation*, 7, 247.

Coburn, A. F. (1931): "Factor of infection in the rheumatic state", Baltimore, p. 35.

—— (1933): "Hæmorrhagic manifestations of rheumatic fever", *Amer. J. Dis. Child*, 45, 933.

——, and Pauli, R. H. (1935): "Studies on immune response of rheumatic subject and its relationship to activity of rheumatic process; active and passive immunisation to hemolytic streptococcus in relation to rheumatic process", *J. clin. Invest.*, 14, 755.

Cochran, J. B. (1951): "The anæmia of rheumatic fever", *Brit. med. J.*, 2, 637.

—— (1952): "The respiratory effects of salicylate", *Ibid.*, 2, 964.

Collis, W. R. F. (1931): "Acute rheumatism and hemolytic streptococci", *Lancet*, 1, 1341.

Copeman, W. S. C., and Pugh, L. G. C. E. (1950): "Dehydration treatment of rheumatic fever", *Lancet*, 2, 675.

Coombs, C. F. (1924): "Rheumatic heart disease", Bristol, p. 203.

Dawson, M. H., Olmstead, M., and Boots, R. H. (1932): "Agglutination reactions in rheumatoid arthritis. Agglutination reaction with streptococcus hemolyticus", *J. Immunol.*, **23**, 187, 205.

Derick, C. L., Hitchcock, C. H., and Swift, H. F. (1927–8): "The effect of antirheumatic drugs on the arthritis and immune body production in serum disease", *J. clin. Invest.*, **5**, 427.

Eiman, J., and Gouley, B. A. (1928): "Rheumatic pneumonitis", *Arch. Path.*, **5**, 558.

Gairdner, D. (1948): "The Schönlein-Henoch syndrome (anaphylactoid purpura)", *Quart. J. Med.*, **17**, 95.

Glover, J. A. (1930): "Incidence of rheumatic diseases", *Lancet*, i, 499.

—— (1939): "Rheumatic fever", *Ibid.*, i, 465.

Goldie, W. (1938): "The haemolytic streptococcus in the etiology of rheumatic fever and rheumatoid arthritis", *Ibid.*, ii, 246.

——, and Griffiths, G. J. (1936): "Aetiological relation of the streptococcus hæmolyticus to the 'rheumatic diseases' ", *Brit. med. J.*, ii, 755.

Gouley, B. A. (1938): "The rôle of mitral stenosis and of post-rheumatic pulmonary fibrosis in the evolution of chronic rheumatic heart disease", *Amer. J. med. Sc.*, **196**, 11.

—— (1938): "The evolution of the parenchymal lung lesions in rheumatic fever and their relationship to mitral stenosis and passive congestion", *Ibid.*, **196**, 1.

Graham, J. D. P., and Parker, W. A. (1948): "The toxic manifestations of sodium salicylate therapy", *Quart. J. Med.*, **17**, 153.

Griffith, F. (1935): "Serological classification of streptococcus pyogenes", *J. Hygiene*, **34**, 542.

Griffith, G. C., and Huntington, R. W. (1946): "Sudden death in rheumatic fever", *Ann. int. Med.*, **25**, 283.

Gross, L. (1921): "The blood supply to the heart", New York.

——, and Kugel, M. A. (1931): "Topographic anatomy and histology of the valves in the human heart", *Amer. J. Path.*, **7**, 445.

Guerra, F. (1946): "Hyaluronidase inhibition by sodium salicylate in rheumatic fever", *Science*, **103**, 686.

Hadfield, G. (1938): "The rheumatic lung", *St. Bartholomew's Hosp. Rep.*, **71**, 17.

Haig-Brown, C. (1886): "Tonsillitis in adolescents", London.

Hawksley, J. C. (1939): "The nature of growing pains and their relation to rheumatism in children and adolescents", *Brit. med. J.*, i, 155.

Hawthorne, C. O. (1900): "Rheumatism, rheumatoid arthritis and subcutaneous nodules", London.

—— (1938): "On subcutaneous nodules", *Brit. J. Rheum.*, **1**, 109.

Hench, P. S., et al. (1949): "The effect of a hormone of the adrenal cortex and of the pituitary adrenocorticotrophic hormone on rheumatoid arthritis", *Proc. Mayo Clin.*, **24**, 181.

Hetzel, B. S., and Hine, D. C. (1951): "The effect of salicylates on the pituitary and suprarenal glands", *Lancet*, **2**, 94.

Hill, N. G., and Allan, M. (1929): "Rheumatic type", *Brit. med. J.*, ii, 499.

Hollman, A. (1950): Unpublished data from work undertaken at Taplow under the direction of the author.

Jager, B. V., and Nickerson, M. (1947): "Altered response of human beings to intramuscular administration of typhoid vaccine during massive salicylate therapy", *Amer. J. Med.*, **3**, 408.

Joint Report (1955): "Treatment of acute rheumatic fever in children. A co-operative clinical trial of A.C.T.H., Cortisone and aspirin", by the rheumatic fever working party of the M.R.C., Gt. Britain, and the sub-committee of principal investigators of the American council on rheumatic fever and congenital heart disease, Amer. Heart Ass., *Brit. med. J.*, **1**, 555.

Jones, T. D., and Bland, E. F. (1942): "Rheumatic fever and heart disease: completed ten-year observations on 1,000 patients", *Tr. Ass. Amer. Physicians*, 57, 265.

Keil, H. (1938): "The rheumatic subcutaneous nodules and simulating lesions", *Medicine*, 17, 261.

Kugel, M. A. (1927-8): "Anatomical studies on the coronary arteries and their branches: I. Arteria anastomotica auricularis magna", *Amer. Heart J.*, 3, 260.

——, and Epstein, E. Z. (1928): "Lesions in the pulmonary artery and valve associated with rheumatic cardiac disease", *Arch. Path.*, 6, 247.

——, and Gross, L. (1925-6): "Gross and microscopical anatomy of the blood vessels in the valves of the human heart", *Amer. Heart J.*, 1, 304.

Kuttner, A. G., and Markowitz, M. (1948): "The diagnosis of mitral insufficiency in rheumatic children", *Ibid.*, 35, 718.

Langer, L. (1887): "Ueber die Blutgéfasse in den Herzklappen bei Endocarditis valvularis", *Virchows Arch.*, 109, 465.

Lees, D. B. (1904): "The treatment of some acute visceral inflammations; and other papers", London.

Link, K. P., *et al.* (1943): "Studies on hæmorrhagic sweet clover disease; hypoprothrombinemia in rat induced by salicylic acid", *J. biol. Chem.*, 147, 463.

Maclagan, T. (1876): "The treatment of acute rheumatism by salicin", *Lancet*, 1, 342.

Massell, B. F., Coen, W. D., and Jones, T. D. (1950): "Artificially induced subcutaneous nodules in rheumatic fever patients", *Pediatrics*, 5, 909.

Medical Research Council Report (1927): "Social conditions and acute rheumatism", M.R.C. Special Report Series, No. 114.

Meyer, K., and Ragan, C. (1948): "The antirheumatic effect of sodium gentisate", *Science*, 108, 281.

Murphy, G. E., and Swift, H. E. (1949): "Induction of cardiac lesions, closely resembling those of rheumatic fever in rabbits following repeated skin infections with Group A streptococci", *J. exper. Med.*, 89, 687.

Naish, A. E. (1928): "The rheumatic lung", *Lancet*, ii, 10.

Parker, W. A. (1947): "Clinical pharmacology of sodium salicylate", *Quart. J. Med.*, 16, 309.

—— (1948): "Factors influencing plasma concentrations of salicylate", *Ibid.*, 17, 229.

Parkinson, J., and Hartley, R. (1946): "Early diagnosis of rheumatic valvular disease in recruits", *Brit. Heart J.*, 8, 212.

Paul, J. R. (1928): "Pleural and Pulmonary lesions in rheumatic fever", *Medicine*, 7, 383.

Perry, C. B. (1937): "Erythema marginatum (rheumatism)", *Arch. Dis. Child.*, 12, 233.

——, and Gillespie, W. A. (1954): "Intramuscular benzathene penicillin in the prophylaxis of streptococcal infection in rheumatic children", *Brit. med. J.*, 2, 729.

Poynton, F. J., and Payne, A. (1900): "The etiology of rheumatic fever", *Lancet*, ii, 861.

——, —— (1913): "Researches on rheumatism", London.

Quinn, R. W. (1948): "Antihyaluronidase studies of sera from patients with rheumatic fever, streptococcal infections, and miscellaneous non-streptococcal diseases", *J. clin. Invest.*, 27, 471.

Rammelkamp, C. H. (1952): "Prevention of rheumatic fever", *Bull. rheumatic Dis.*, 2, 13.

Reid, J., Watson, R. D., and Sproull, D. H. (1950): "The mode of action of salicylate in acute rheumatic fever", *Quart. J. Med.*, 19, 1.

Rich, A. R., and Gregory, J. E. (1943): "On the anaphylactic nature of rheumatic pneumonitis", *Bull. Johns Hopk. Hosp.*, 73, 465.

——, —— (1943): "Experimental evidence that lesions with the basic characteristics of rheumatic carditis can result from anaphylactic hypersensitivity", *Ibid.*, 73, 239.

Rich, A. R., and Gregory, J. E. (1944): "Further experimental cardiac lesions of the rheumatic type produced by anaphylactic hypersensitivity", *Ibid.*, 75, 115.

Ritchie, W. T. (1939): "Acute rheumatic carditis", *Lancet, ii*, 582.

Ritter, S. A., Gross, L., and Kugel, M. A. (1927–8): "Blood vessels in the valves of normal human hearts", *Amer. Heart J.*, 3, 433.

Rogen, A. S. (1947): "The heart in rheumatoid arthritis", *Brit. med. J., i*, 87.

Roth, I. R., Lingg, C., and Whittemore, A. (1937): "Heart disease in children; rheumatic group; certain aspects of age at onset and of recurrences in 488 cases of juvenile rheumatism ushered in by major clinical manifestations", *Amer. Heart J.*, 13, 36.

Schlesinger, B. (1930): "The relationship of throat infection to acute rheumatism in childhood", *Arch. Dis. Child.*, 5, 411.

Scott, G. E. M. (1943): "Rheumatic infection in childhood: survey from Children's Hospital, Melbourne, with addendum on follow-up system of almoners of the hospital", *Med. J. Australia*, 2, 309.

Shapiro, S. (1944): "Studies on prothrombin; effect of synthetic vitamin K on prothrombinopenia induced by salicylate in man", *J. Amer. med. Ass.*, 125, 546.

Shaw, A. F. B. (1929): "Topography and pathogenesis of lesions in rheumatic fever", *Arch. Dis. Child.*, 4, 155.

Sheldon, W. (1931): "On acute rheumatism following tonsillitis", *Lancet, i*, 1337.

Stollerman, G. H., Rusoff, J. H., and Hirschfeld, I. (1954): "Prophylaxis against Group A streptococci in rheumatic fever patients by the use of single monthly injections of N.N dibenzylethylenediamine dipenicillin G (Bicillin)", Meeting of American Rheumatism Association, 19th June 1954, San Francisco.

Stuart-Harris, C. H. (1935): "A study of hæmolytic streptococcal fibrinolysis in chronic arthritis, rheumatic fever, and scarlet fever", *Lancet, ii*, 1456.

Sutton, L. P., and Dodge, K. G. (1938): "The relationship of Sydenham's chorea to other rheumatic manifestations", *Amer. J. med. Sci.*, 195, 656.

Swyer, G. I. M. (1948): "Antihistamin effect of sodium salicylate and its bearing upon skin-diffusing activity of hyaluronidase", *Biochem. J.*, 42, 28.

Taran, L. M., and Szilagyi, N. (1947): "The duration of the electrical systole (QT) in acute rheumatic carditis in children", *Amer. Heart J.*, 33, 14.

Thomas, G. T. (1954): "Heart failure in children with active rheumatic carditis", *Brit. med. J.*, 2, 205.

——, Besterman, E. M. M., and Hollman, A. (1953): "Rheumatic pericarditis", *Brit. Heart J.*, XV, 29.

Todd, E. W. (1932): "Antihæmolysin titres in hæmolytic streptococcal infections and their significance in rheumatic fever", *Brit. J. exper. Path.*, 13, 248.

Wearn, J. T., Bromer, A. W., and Zschiesche, L. J. (1936): "The incidence of blood vessels in human heart valves", *Amer. Heart J.*, 2, 22.

Weens, H. S., and Heyman, A. (1946): "Cardiac enlargement in fever therapy induced by intravenous injection of typhoid vaccine", *Arch. int. Med.*, 77, 307.

Wells, W. C. (1810): "On rheumatism of the heart", *Tr. Soc. Improv. Med. and Chir. Knowledge*, 3, 373.

Werner, M. (1938): "Uber die Ursachen der Verquellung der Kollagenen Fasern bei hyperergischen Entzüdung (Arthussches Phanomen) (Zugleich ein Beitrag zur Funktion des Bindegewebes)", *Virschows. Arch. f. path. Anat.*, 301, 552.

Wilson, M. G. (1940): "Rheumatic fever", New York.

——, and Schweitzer, M. (1954): "Pattern of hereditary susceptibility in rheumatic fever", *Circulation*, 10, 699.

Wood, P. H. (1949): "Cardiac complications of rheumatic fever", *Proc. Roy. Soc. Med.*, 43, 195.

York, C. L., and Fischer, W. J. H., Jr. (1947): "Plasma volume determinations in rheumatic subjects during oral salicylate therapy", *New England J. Med.*, 237, 477.

CHAPTER X

CHRONIC RHEUMATIC HEART DISEASE

R HEUMATIC carditis refers to active inflammation of the heart. The after-effects, which include valve sclerosis, patchy myocardial fibrosis, and adherent pericardium, are best described under the general heading of rheumatic heart disease, to which the appropriate ana-tomical abnormality may be appended. Thus we may speak of rheumatic heart disease with mitral stenosis.

About 5 per cent of healthy young adults give a previous history of rheumatic fever in childhood (Parkinson and Hartley, 1946). It is clear, therefore, that all patients who have rheumatic fever do not later develop clinical rheumatic heart disease. According to Carey Coombs (1924), 50 per cent of children who have their first attack of rheumatic fever before they are five years old, and 25 per cent of those whose first attack occurs after the age of ten, subsequently develop rheumatic heart disease. As described in the last chapter, recent studies indicate that more accurate figures for these two groups would be 75 and 50 per cent respectively. The frequency of permanent valve damage from primary rheumatic fever after the age of 20 does not seem to be known, but is far from negligible.

From large samples of the younger male population of Great Britain examined for military service between 1939 and 1945, it was calculated that there were about 240,000 cases of rheumatic heart disease of both sexes between the ages of 18 and 44 in Great Britain at that time, or about 2.6 per cent of the population in that age-group (Parkinson, 1945). Rheu-matic heart disease accounts for approximately 20 per cent of all cases of heart disease in temperate climates, and causes about 10,000 deaths annually in Great Britain.

Practically all clinical cases of inactive rheumatic heart disease have one or more valve lesions. The mitral valve is involved in 85 per cent, the aortic in 44 per cent, the tricuspid in 10 to 16 per cent, and the pulmonary in 1 to 2 per cent (Cabot, 1926). The relative frequency with which each valve is affected is proportional to the pressure load against which each normally operates.

The rheumatic process affects the heart muscle as well as the valves, and this may result in a varying degree of permanent interstitial myocardial fibrosis. Moreover, it has long been known that careful microscopy reveals Aschoff nodes in all stages of development, maturity and senescence in about 50 per cent of all fatal cases of chronic rheumatic heart disease, the figure being higher in those that die under the age of 40 years than in older patients (de la Chapelle, Graefe and Rottino, 1934; Werner, 1936).

The more recent frequent discovery of Aschoff nodes in left atrial appendicular biopsies in 45 to 50 per cent of cases of mitral stenosis treated by valvotomy (Decker *et al.*, 1953; McKeown, 1953) should have caused no surprise, and merely confirms what was already well established. Although there is usually no other pathological or clinical evidence of activity in these cases, there is no valid reason for doubting that these Aschoff nodes represent continually relapsing or chronic active carditis. Although the myocardial lesion is certainly less important than the valve damage in at least 95 per cent of cases, it cannot be ignored.

Rheumatic pericarditis leaves no clinical sequelæ. Although the pericardium may become adherent to surrounding structures or its two layers fused and thickened, such changes do not seem to interfere with cardiac function. Chronic constrictive pericarditis is never rheumatic. For the most part then, chronic rheumatic heart disease is mitral, aortic or tricuspid valve disease, or any combination of these three lesions, together with their complications; its course may be modified but very rarely determined by relapsing or chronic myocarditis or by the degree of myocardial fibrosis present.

MITRAL INCOMPETENCE

In the last century this was the most common valve lesion diagnosed. Owing to the exertions of Mackenzie, Lewis, Parkinson, and others, the first half of the twentieth century witnessed a diagnostic revolution, so that a physician who asserted that a patient had organic mitral incompetence had to be very sure of his grounds. The change in outlook saved a host of normal subjects from invalidism. But the pendulum swung much too far, and serious efforts were being made to correct this tendency when the introduction of mitral valve surgery in 1948 forced the pace, so that in a short space of time the whole subject received the concentrated attention of investigators all over the world, and mitral incompetence was quickly seen in its proper perspective.

INCIDENCE

In an unselected series of 300 cases of mitral valve disease studied in detail by the author, mitral incompetence was the major hæmodynamic fault in 34 per cent (Wood, 1954). About half of these cases had no obstructive stenosis, and the other half had mixed stenosis and incompetence with the latter dominant. Mild incompetence complicating dominant stenosis will be considered later. This means that in rheumatic heart disease mitral incompetence is the main valve lesion more often than aortic stenosis or aortic incompetence, but not as often as aortic valve disease as a whole. Approximately 70 per cent of the cases were serious and would have been treated surgically had there been a satisfactory valve repair operation to offer.

AGE AND SEX

The average age of the patients with mitral incompetence was 37.2, which was the same as the average age of the patients with mitral stenosis.

The sex ratio is 3 : 2 in favour of males in cases of pure mitral incompetence, and 1 : 1 in mixed cases in which incompetence is at least as important as the stenosis.

PATHOLOGY

As emphasised by Brock (1952), serious mitral incompetence means greater disorganisation of the mitral valve mechanism than that found in simple mitral stenosis, and implies a more vicious form of active endocarditis in the first instance, a view supported by the previous history actually obtained (Wood, 1954).

The most important causes of mitral incompetence are shortening of the valve cusps, so that they cannot meet in systole, and shortening of the musculo-tendinous control, the papillary muscles and chordæ tendinæ being shortened, matted and densely adherent to the valve, so that the latter cannot close. Brock (1952) graphically described the situation as a "fibrous ankylosis of the valve mechanism", the two chief causes cited being commonly found together. Heavy calcification is not infrequently associated and adds to the rigidity of the system, although its very exuberance may diminish the size of the orifice.

Mitral ring dilatation is a relatively rare cause of incompetence in chronic rheumatic heart disease: in these cases the orifice is very large, and although the cusps may be short and thick there is less fibrous rigidity than in the type previously described. Early left ventricular failure with ring dilatation during the stage of active carditis may be responsible.

HÆMODYNAMICS

During systole the blood that leaks back into the left atrium increases the volume of that chamber and the pressure within it. When the left ventricle relaxes in diastole it is subjected to the high filling pressure built up in the left atrium during systole, and since there is no real obstruction at the mitral orifice, it fills rapidly, and dilates to accommodate the extra blood that leaked back during the previous cycle. The stroke volume of the left ventricle is therefore increased by the amount of regurgitant blood, forward flow being maintained as near to normal as possible, although falling short of the ideal in all serious cases. In the majority of cases with fibrous ankylosis of the mitral valve, left ventricular dilatation is unlikely to exert any influence on the mitral ring or size of the orifice; a vicious circle mechanism, however, is easily established in active rheumatic carditis and in functional mitral incompetence secondary to left ventricular failure from other causes.

Although the left atrial pressure may be very high during ventricular systole, it falls quickly to ventricular level in diastole, so that mean left atrial and pulmonary artery pressures are lower than in mitral stenosis of comparable severity. Short of left ventricular failure, the patient with mitral incompetence is also less embarrassed by tachycardia or sudden increases of right ventricular output than his sister with mitral stenosis, for a shortened diastole does not prevent proper ventricular filling and the hyperdynamic left ventricle may have sufficient reserve to deal with an increased flow. Moreover, peripheral vasodilatation on effort encourages forward flow.

The pulmonary vascular resistance may rise moderately in severe mitral incompetence, but rarely reaches extreme levels, probably because passive pulmonary hypertension is rarely high enough to excite a vasoconstrictor response.

CLINICAL FEATURES

Life-history

Organic mitral incompetence severe enough to shape the medical destiny of the patient is usually well established during the stage of active carditis; unlike mitral stenosis, its detection demands no latent interval. Subsequent sclerosis of valve cusps and chordæ may modify the leak, but as a rule there is little basic change in the physiology of the situation over the years until left ventricular failure sets in or reactive pulmonary hypertension alters the course of events. The date of the initial inflammation and the average age of death are much the same as in mitral stenosis (q.v.), but the symptom-free period is a little longer and the downhill course, once symptoms have started, is a little quicker in mitral incompetence (5.3 years to reach total incapacity against 7.3 years in mitral stenosis).

Symptoms

The symptoms of pure mitral incompetence are usually less spectacular than those of mitral stenosis. Acute pulmonary œdema, for example, is eight times less common, presumably because the mean left atrial pressure is rarely so high as in mitral stenosis of comparable severity, and does not rise so sharply on effort or as a result of tachycardia. Hæmoptysis is half as common as in mitral stenosis, no doubt for the same reason. Angina pectoris is also only half as common, despite the increased work undertaken by the left ventricle; this may be attributed to the rarity of an extreme pulmonary vascular resistance, so that forward flow and therefore coronary filling are not hindered by this additional factor. Systemic embolism is at least one and a half times less frequent than in mitral stenosis, probably because there is less stasis in the left atrium.

In mixed cases in which it is uncertain whether stenosis or incompetence is dominant, even after elaborate investigation and even digital examination of the valve, both hæmoptysis and systemic embolism are at least as common as they are in mitral stenosis, perhaps more so. The mean left atrial pressure is higher in these cases then in pure incompetence, and there is more stasis to encourage thrombosis in the conspicuously dilated left atrium.

According to Brigden and Leatham (1953) the only special symptom of mitral incompetence is palpitation, and they ascribe this to the frequency of ectopic beats. The hyperdynamic action of the left ventricle, however, may also contribute to this symptom.

Effort intolerance is usually due to dyspnœa caused by pulmonary venous congestion, as in mitral stenosis, but sooner or later left ventricular failure adds its own contribution. Some protection may be afforded by the rapid dilatation of the left ventricle early in diastole, so that the inter-ventricular septum bulges into the cavity of the right ventricle, and interferes with proper filling of that chamber (Bernheim effect). "Con-gestive failure" usually occurs without a high pulmonary vascular resist-ance, the œdema being due to the poor renal blood flow secondary to the low output, and the raised venous pressure partly to hydræmia and perhaps partly to a Bernheim effect. The left ventricle is certainly over-loaded, but the right may very well not be. This behaviour is radically different from the congestive failure of mitral stenosis, for which a high pulmonary vascular resistance or uncontrolled atrial fibrillation is nearly always chiefly responsible.

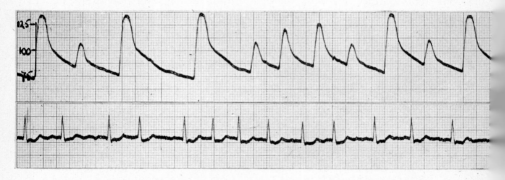

Fig. 10.01—Direct brachial arteriogram from a case of mitral incompetence showing an abrupt percussion wave, ill sustained peak and late systolic collapse.

Physical signs

The patient is usually a man and may look well. Peripheral cyanosis may be seen in mixed cases of stenosis and incompetence with a high pulmonary vascular resistance, but is rare with pure incompetence.

The *peripheral pulse* is small and often slightly water-hammer in quality, for there is a pronounced leak from the arterial system during systole. Arteriograms in well-developed cases show an abrupt upstroke measuring 0.05 to 0.07 second from the onset to the beginning of the blunt peak; the peak itself is relatively brief, occupying another 0.05 to 0.07 second; the down-stroke proper is early, beginning about 0.12 second after the onset of the pulse wave and tends to be precipitous (fig. 10.01).

The *jugular venous pressure* is not infrequently raised in mitral incompetence when the pulmonary vascular resistance and heart rate are normal, and when both pericardial effusion and tricuspid valve disease have been excluded. In cases with normal rhythm *a* and *v* are about equal in amplitude and in those with atrial fibrillation, the large *v* wave is followed by a steep *y* descent and conspicuous *y* trough. In other words, the form of the venous pulse is the same as that seen in congestive heart failure. Under the circumstances mentioned a similar rise of venous pressure is rarely seen in cases of mitral stenosis. Whether myocarditis or myocardial fibrosis is responsible, serious mitral incompetence signifying a more vicious primary rheumatic attack than simple stenosis, or whether the phenomenon should be attributed to a filling defect of the right ventricle (Bernheim's syndrome), awaits solution. In a typical example, necropsy showed a huge dilated left ventricle, a normal pulmonary artery, a small right ventricle, a normal tricuspid valve, and a large distended right atrium, the cavity of the right ventricle being greatly reduced by the bulged interventricular septum (fig. 10.02). In the majority of mixed cases of mitral stenosis and incompetence a high venous pressure is associated with a high pulmonary vascular resistance around 6 to 9 units.

The *cardiac impulse* at the apex beat is hyperdynamic and displaced to the left, and can hardly be confused with the impalpable left ventricle of mitral stenosis. If it is suspected that a very large right ventricle might be occupying the apex beat, the question can be settled at once by consulting the electrocardiogram.

On *auscultation* the characteristic signs of mitral incompetence are absence of a presystolic murmur, a soft or normal first heart sound, a loud apical pan-systolic murmur embracing both first and second heart sounds and often accompanied by a palpable thrill; absence of the opening snap of mitral stenosis, a loud third heart sound, and a short or absent mitral diastolic murmur.

A *presystolic murmur* implies appreciable late ventricular filling and is *incompatible* with serious mitral incompetence.

A loud *mitral first sound* with a normal P-R interval or with atrial fibrillation implies a powerful potential or factual pressure gradient across the valve immediately before the left ventricle contracts, a situation that is also incompatible with serious incompetence.

The *systolic murmur* of mitral incompetence is usually loud and of fairly high frequency, so that it is best heard with the Bowles type of stethoscope; it is maximal at the apex beat over the surface of the left ventricle and outwards towards the axilla; sometimes it is transmitted posteriorly over the surface of a greatly dilated left atrium. The murmur necessarily begins with the mitral component of the first heart sound (fig. 10.03), for the leak must commence as the valve tries to close. This is some 0.05 second before

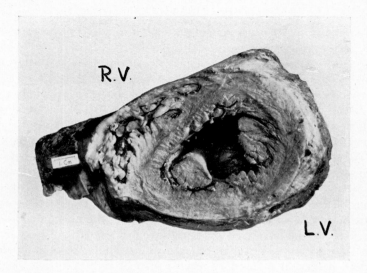

(a) Transverse section showing great enlargement of the left ventricle and a small right ventricle.

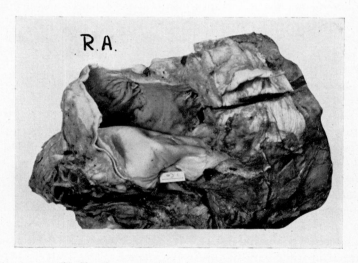

(b) Showing great distension of the right atrium.

Fig. 10.02—Photographs illustrating the Bernheim phenomenon in a fatal case of severe mitral incompetence.

the aortic valve opens. Again, mitral incompetence must continue well into if not beyond the time of aortic valve closure, for there is still a strong pressure gradient across the mitral valve at that moment; only as the rapidly falling left ventricular pressure approaches that in the left atrium should the leak stop (Brigden and Leatham, 1953). Aortic systolic murmurs heard over the left ventricular apex beat start and finish earlier, as described elsewhere (Leatham, 1951). Tricuspid systolic murmurs heard over the right ventricular apex beat are also pan-systolic, but are accentuated during inspiration. The pan-systolic murmur of ventricular septal defect may be clinically identical with the mitral murmur in quality and timing, but ordinarily occurs at the Roger area, well away from the apex beat; when the heart is rotated clockwise in cases of ventricular septal defect, however, or anticlockwise in cases of mitral incompetence, confusion is inevitable.

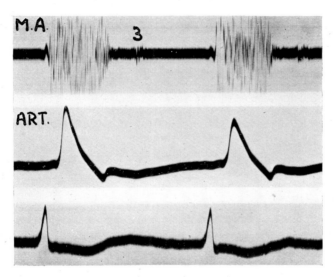

Fig. 10.03—Phonocardiogram in a case of mitral incompetence showing a pan-systolic murmur and accentuated third heart sound (top tracing). The murmur starts with the mitral first sound, well ahead of the arterial pulse (middle tracing); the electrocardiogram is seen below.

The *absence of the opening snap* in serious mitral incompetence is generally attributed to the rigidity of the whole valve mechanism, for there is certainly a sufficiently high pressure built up in the left atrium during ventricular systole to snap back the aortic cusp of the mitral valve as the pressure gradient between ventricle and atrium is abruptly reversed in early diastole. This fibrous ankylosis also ensures a soft first heart sound even when the P-R interval is short, or after brief diastolic periods in cases with atrial fibrillation. Heavy calcification, so common in mixed cases, enhances the effect (Wynn, 1953).

A *third heart sound*, usually loud, was heard in 85 per cent of the author's series, and is attributed to unusually rapid left ventricular filling. Its occurrence in mitral incompetence was noted long ago by Sprague and White (1926).

Not enough attention is paid to the *duration of the mitral diastolic murmur*. A murmur that completely fills diastole at a normal heart rate categorically denies serious mitral incompetence, for a long murmur means prolonged left ventricular filling. Again, a short atrio-ventricular diastolic murmur is characteristic of unusually rapid ventricular filling, whether the relevant atrioventricular valve is diseased or not, as in thyrotoxicosis, anæmia, patent ductus, ventricular septal defect and atrial septal defect. In serious mitral incompetence the short murmur is often loud, because the diseased valve increases the turbulence set up by the torrent of blood that pours through the mitral orifice as soon as it opens; but the flow virtually ceases almost as abruptly as it starts, long before the next ventricular contraction, because the ventricle is rapidly distended and the filling pressure falls off steeply. Thus a short mitral diastolic murmur, far from invalidating a diagnosis of pure mitral incompetence, is characteristic of it. In cases of heavily calcified mitral valve disease with atrial fibrillation, the length of the diastolic murmur and the presence or absence of the third heart sound become the only two auscultatory signs of any diagnostic significance, for the pan-systolic murmur gives no quantitative information, and the absent presystolic murmur, soft first heart sound, and absent opening snap merely confirm the two circumstances mentioned.

The electrocardiogram

In well-developed cases the electrocardiogram shows an unobtrusive P mitrale and left ventricular preponderance (fig. 10.04). In mixed border-line cases of stenosis and incompetence with a pulmonary vascular resistance of 6 to 9 units, slight right ventricular preponderance may be seen.

RADIOLOGICAL APPEARANCES

The chief characteristics of mitral incompetence are an enlarged, hyper-dynamic, rapidly filled left ventricle associated with considerable dilatation and conspicuous pulsation of the left atrium (fig. 10.05). In the anterior view the left atrium may be seen expanding during ventricular systole both to the left and right (fig. 4.42). It has become fashionable to deride this sign, but I have never seen the left atrium behave in this way in mitral stenosis or in any other condition. In the first oblique view systolic expansion of the left atrium is common in mitral stenosis, particularly when there is atrial fibrillation, but even then the movement is not so abrupt nor the excursion so great as it often is with free incompetence. Aneurysmal dilatation of the left atrium is also in favour of incompetence, although it may occur occasionally with pure stenosis. The larger the left

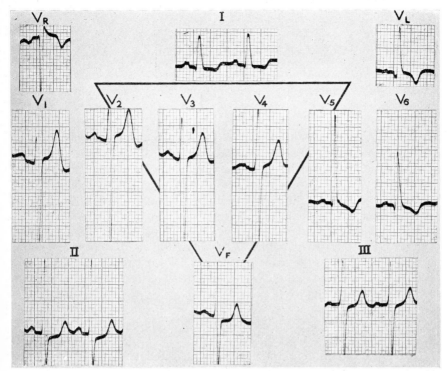

Fig. 10.04—The electrocardiogram in a case of severe mitral incompetence showing considerable left ventricular preponderance.

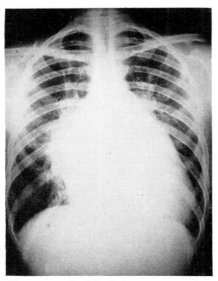

Fig. 10.05—Radiological appearances in a case of severe mitral incompetence showing considerable dilatation of the left atrium and left ventricle and marked "pulmonary venous congestion".

atrium, the less does it pulsate, because the amount of regurgitant blood represents a smaller percentage of the left atrial volume.

The aorta is usually rather small, but less so than in mitral stenosis. The pulmonary artery is rarely dilated except in cases of combined stenosis and incompetence with moderate elevation of the pulmonary vascular resistance. The right atrium may be dilated if the venous pressure is raised, as described previously. "Pulmonary venous congestion" may be marked in severe cases, especially when there is left ventricular failure, but in the average case it is inconspicuous. Heavy calcification of the mitral valve occurs in 50 per cent of cases with combined stenosis and incompetence, but is uncommon with pure incompetence.

Many attempts have been made to record the movements of the left atrium graphically, either by means of electrokymography (e.g. Luisada and Fleischner, 1948), or indirectly by means of an œsophageal pressure pulse tracing (e.g. Lassar and Loewe, 1952; Zoob, 1954). On the whole such methods have proved disappointing and have been discarded in most clinics, perhaps prematurely.

PHYSIOLOGICAL FINDINGS

Cardiac catheterisation usually reveals a raised left atrial pressure, a normal or slightly raised pulmonary vascular resistance and a normal or low cardiac output. The indirect left atrial pressure tracing obtained by the wedged catheter technique rewards careful study. For several years these tracings did not seem to distinguish mitral stenosis from incompetence, but attention had always been directed to the systolic part of the curve. After studying the y descent of the venous and right atrial pressure pulses in a variety of conditions, including tricuspid incompetence and tricuspid stenosis, it was gradually established that the higher the filling pressure the steeper was the y descent and the more conspicuous the y trough, *provided there was no obstruction at the tricuspid orifice*. In tricuspid stenosis, however, the obstruction delayed ventricular filling and prevented rapid equalisation of atrial and ventricular pressures, so that the y descent was relatively slow, and the y trough inconspicuous; indeed, with severe stenosis there was no y trough at all, the right atrial pressure continuing to fall after the v peak until interrupted by the next atrial or ventricular contraction, a pressure gradient being demonstrable across the tricuspid valve throughout the whole of diastole. It seemed virtually certain that obstruction of the mitral orifice would affect the left atrial pressure pulse in the same way, i.e. in mitral stenosis the y descent should be slow and the y trough absent (fig. 10.06), whereas in mitral incompetence or left ventricular failure, the y descent should be rapid and the y trough conspicuous and early (fig. 10.07). Careful analysis of technically satisfactory wedged pressure tracings and direct left atrial pressure tracings obtained at operation confirmed the thesis that obstruction to forward flow retarded the rate of *y* descent, and since the latter (Ry) was directly proportional to the height of *v* in all circumstances, the degree of obstruction to forward flow was expressed as a ratio Ry/v, Ry being measured in mm. Hg per second, and v in mm. Hg above the sternal angle. In mitral stenosis the

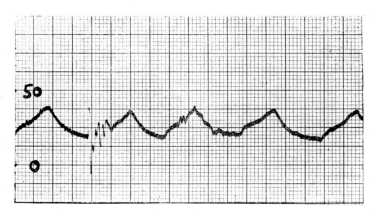

Before valvotomy Ry/v=1.3

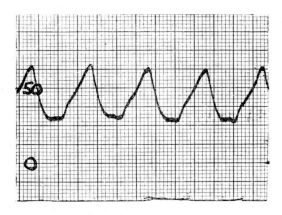

After valvotomy Ry/v=3.3

Fig. 10.06—Left atrial pressure pulses before and after mitral valvotomy showing a change in the Ry/v ratio from 1.3 to 3.3 after relief of the obstruction.

ratio was commonly between 0.6 and 1.0, the extreme upper limit compatible with obstruction to forward flow being 1.6 (Owen and Wood, 1955). In pure mitral incompetence, left ventricular failure and Pick's disease the ratio usually lay between 2 and 6. Difficult borderline cases had ratios close to 1.6. It should be clearly understood that the Ry/v ratio is an index of obstruction to forward flow only, and that a figure demonstrating the absence of such obstruction does not distinguish mitral incompetence from left ventricular failure. It has already proved its value, however, in helping to distinguish between dominant stenosis and dominant incompetence when both are present.

Selective angiocardiography through a needle inserted directly into the left atrium through the posterior chest wall in the eighth intercostal space close to the vertebral column may show mitral incompetence clearly and gives a good idea of the actual size of the mitral aperture in systole and diastole (Biörk *et al.*, 1955).

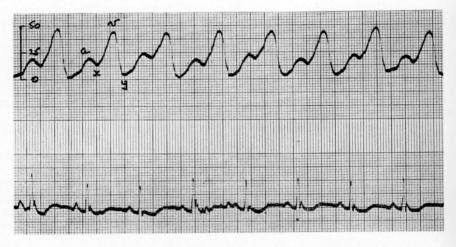

Fig. 10.07—Left atrial pressure pulse in a case of mitral incompetence showing a very rapid *y* descent and conspicuous *y* trough; the Ry/v ratio is 7.

COMPLICATIONS

Pulmonary œdema, hæmoptysis, angina pectoris, and systemic embolism have already been discussed under *symptoms*.

Atrial fibrillation is found in about a third of any average series of cases, and is closely related to the age of the patient. The great majority of patients over 50 years of age fibrillate. Cases of mixed stenosis and incompetence fibrillate more than twice as frequently as cases of pure incompetence, and more than one and a half times as frequently as cases of pure stenosis. This may be a consequence of the greater severity of the original rheumatic onslaught in the mixed group, or because the left atrium tends to be larger in these cases.

The ventricular rate may be difficult to control with digitalis in severe cases of mitral incompetence with atrial fibrillation, possibly because of the hyperdynamic behaviour of the left ventricle. It may be worth pointing out that this difficulty is common to all hyperkinetic circulatory states complicated by atrial fibrillation, whether the left, right or both ventricles are involved; thus it may be encountered in patent ductus, atrial septal defect, and thyrotoxicosis, to give an example from each group.

Bacterial endocarditis seems to have a predilection for cases of mild mitral incompetence, and may offer tragic proof of the organic nature of an apical systolic murmur hitherto regarded as functional. Though the infection may be cured by means of penicillin or other antibiotics, much damage has usually been inflicted by the time it is brought under control, and serious mitral incompetence usually results.

TREATMENT

No operative treatment yet devised has been of the slightest benefit to cases of mitral incompetence, although heroic efforts have been made to repair the leak (e.g. Logan and Turner, 1952). Nevertheless mitral incompetence is a simple mechanical fault and must remain a constant challenge to surgeons until it can be properly dealt with.

Medical treatment and management are essentially the same as for mitral stenosis (q.v.).

MITRAL STENOSIS

INCIDENCE

Mitral stenosis with or without an unimportant leak is four times as common as virtually pure mitral incompetence, and twice as common as combined stenosis and incompetence; it accounts for 64 per cent of all cases of chronic mitral valve disease and for about 54 per cent of all cases of chronic rheumatic heart disease. There are at least 100,000 cases of mitral stenosis in Great Britain between the ages of 18 and 44, and four-fifths of them will require surgical treatment sooner or later (Wood, 1954).

AGE AND SEX

Cowan and Ritchie (1935), who analysed 2,155 cases, found that the frequency of chronic mitral valve disease in each decade up to the fifth was 2, 19, 21, 19, and 16 per cent respectively, a further 23 per cent of cases occurring over the age of 50. The figures seem to be much the same for both stenosis and incompetence, and in my own series the average age of all cases in each group was 37.

The M : F sex ratio for cases with pure mitral stenosis is 4 : 1; when there is trivial incompetence as well it falls to 3 : 1, and when there is serious incompetence to 1 : 1. In pure mitral incompetence males predominate, the M : F sex ratio then being 3 : 2 (Wood, 1954).

LIFE HISTORY

A previous history of rheumatic fever, subacute rheumatism or chorea is obtained in about 60 per cent of cases. On the whole, the more florid recurrent the original rheumatic state the worse the permanent valve damage and the more probable serious mitral incompetence. Mild cases of pure mitral stenosis, for example, are twice as likely to have had isolated chorea as recurrent rheumatic fever, whereas cases of combined stenosis and incompetence, most of which have grossly disorganised valves, are ten times more likely to have had recurrent rheumatic fever than isolated chorea.

In my own series the average age of the initial rheumatic attack was 12 years, the latent symptom-free period 19 years, the average age of onset of symptoms 31 years, and the time spent in each of the first three grades of effort intolerance 2.7, 2.7, and 1.94 years respectively, total incapacity being reached 7.3 years after the onset of symptoms. The average duration of total incapacity was about three years in 644 fatal cases of chronic rheumatic heart disease analysed by de Graff and Lingg (1935), and was the same for mitral stenosis as for other valve lesions. There is, of course, considerable variation in individual cases, but the general trend cannot be ignored.

PATHOLOGY

Brock (1952) has referred to the monotonous regularity with which most cases of mitral stenosis submitted to operation have a small oval orifice measuring 1 × 0.5 cm. In the simplest cases of pure stenosis the chief points of fusion are where the shortest, stoutest and most direct chordæ tendineæ, arising from the very summit of the papillary muscles, join the margins of the cusps on each side of what Brock has called the central pathway of the mitral valve. These two "critical areas of tendon insertion" are about 2 cm. apart, which means that the central pathway through which most of the blood normally enters the left ventricle is only about 3 sq. cm. in cross section, and lateral to this there is relatively little flow, the commissures acting merely as hinges, allowing the central parts of the cusps to open widely. In a mild attack of rheumatic carditis, the only damage to the valve may be along the line of closure of the cusps, just proximal to their free margins, where they receive the maximum natural trauma. Perhaps as the result of deposition of platelets and fibrin on the surface of this damaged zone, a stickiness develops which encourages the two cusps to adhere to one another where they meet most firmly. The strong blood flow through the central pathway prevents fusion at the centre, but there is less resistance to fusion at the critical areas of tendon insertion on each side of the central pathway and there is good reason to believe that this is where the two cusps first stick together. The lateral parts of the valve are usually spared in a mild attack of rheumatic fever and have no reason to adhere of themselves; nor has lateral fusion alone ever been observed. Once the two cusps are held together at the critical areas of tendon insertion, however, their lateral parts necessarily come into permanent apposition, and since there is little or no flow in this zone to prevent it, light lateral adhesions then form. The result is fusion of the two cusps from the ring to the edges of the central pathway. Since the hinge-like action of the lateral parts of the valve can no longer function, the central portion of the two cusps cannot open fully; the aperture thus becomes oval, and cannot measure much more than 2×1 cm. in the mildest cases. Gradual reduction in the size of the lumen between the two critical areas of tendon insertion may result from repeated deposits of fibrin at the edges, the excrescences becoming covered by endothelium and then fibrosed, as described by Magarey (1951).

This attractive hypothesis, so ably presented by Brock (1952), leaves one important question and its corollaries unanswered. When does cross fusion of the critical areas of tendon insertion occur? If it is during the stage of active carditis, which the hypothesis favours, why does the initial 2×1 cm. stenosis give rise to no physical signs? There is ample proof that a presystolic murmur and loud first heart sound occur when stenosis is trivial, the cardiac output normal, and the left atrial pressure around 5 mm. Hg with reference to the sternal angle. If, on the other hand, the stenosis develops when it seems to, i.e. some 5 to 10 years after the initial attack, why should sudden fusion of the critical areas of tendon insertion occur then, at a time when the surface of the cusps should have no cause for stickiness? If the hypothesis is correct, it would seem that initial fusion of the critical zones would have to occur during the active stage, but that this would not result in physiological stenosis. This is quite likely, especially if the initial points of fusion were 2.5 cm. apart, for the central pathway of the mitral valve would then be as large as the aortic orifice, assuming that the central parts of the cusps were able to open widely enough. Physiological stenosis with a pressure gradient across the valve would then develop slowly and variably over the years, according to the speed with which the commissures of the oval orifice gradually silted up. From experience gained at operation, mild physiological stenosis, with typical physical signs but no symptoms, occurs when the oval orifice is between 1.5 and 2 cm. in length, and perhaps half this in width. Critical stenosis requiring valvotomy is associated with an oval orifice averaging 1×0.5 cm., as repeatedly pointed out by Brock. By extreme stenosis is meant an orifice materially smaller than this, in the region of 5×3 mm. Although Brock has criticised the terms mild, average and severe stenosis, when used with the intention of conveying some idea of the degree of stricture present rather than the patient's disability, in the author's view their use with just this meaning is thoroughly justified. A simple mathematical sum will show that a relatively mild stenosis measuring 1.5×0.75 cm. is more than twice as large as an average orifice of 1×0.5 cm., and nearly eight times as large as a severe stricture measuring 5×3 mm.

Whether gradually increasing stenosis results chiefly from the effects of continued smouldering activity, or whether it is a more or less inevitable secondary change due to repeated deposition of fibrin on a damaged area has yet to be settled.

HÆMODYNAMICS

Initial cross-fusion of the critical areas of tendon insertion during the stage of active carditis leaves a sufficiently large central pathway probably measuring 2.5×1.5 cm., through which a normal blood flow can be maintained without any form of compensation. According to the Gorlin formula such an orifice, which would measure about 2.5 sq. cm. in cross section, would allow a blood flow of 6.8 litres per minute with a left ventricular filling pressure of 6 mm. Hg, and a heart rate of 70 to 80 beats per minute. As the commissures of this oval orifice gradually silt up, the size of the aperture dwindles until it begins to obstruct the blood flow. The left atrial pressure then rises a few mm. Hg and wholly compensates for the obstruction. It is calculated that an oval orifice measuring $2–2.25 \times 1$ cm. is small enough to cause this grade 1 physiological stenosis. Physical signs (presystolic murmur and accentuated first heart sound) first develop at this stage, which is ordinarily some 3 to 10 years after the original rheumatic attack. Grade 2 or moderate stenosis implies an oval aperture measuring $1.5–1.75 \times 0.75–0.9$ cm. This, too, is easily compensated for by a further rise of left atrial pressure, which at rest is found to be around 10 mm. Hg above the sternal angle. Under ordinary circumstances there are no symptoms, but the auscultatory physical signs of mitral stenosis are now complete, the opening snap being easily heard, and the mitral diastolic murmur occupying practically the whole of diastole. The elevated left atrial pressure is associated with a similar rise of pulmonary venous pressure, pulmonary capillary pressure, and pulmonary arterial pressure, the pulmonary arterio-venous pressure gradient remaining normal (about 10 mm. Hg).

On strenuous exercise there is some danger of unexpected acute pulmonary œdema in these cases of moderate severity, for no protective mechanisms have yet come into play. It may be calculated, for example, that a cardiac output of 16 litres per minute with a heart rate of 120, would raise the left atrial pressure to 35 mm. Hg above the sternal angle, if the mitral aperture was 1.5 cm.^{2}. With no acquired barrier between pulmonary capillaries and alveoli, a capillary pressure of this level, which is above the osmotic pressure of the plasma, must cause pulmonary œdema. Practical experience supports these statements.

Grade 3 or considerable stenosis is the classic text-book type. According to Brock and other surgeons the valve in these typical dyspnœic cases measures about 1×0.5 cm., but physiological calculations suggest it is more likely to have a cross section of 0.75 sq. cm., which means dimensions nearer 1.5×0.75 cm. Dexter's group puts the critical orifice at 1 cm.^{2}, which implies an oval aperture measuring about 1.75×0.85 cm. (Lewis et al., 1952). [The discrepancy between physiological calculations and surgeons' estimates is consistent with all grades of stenosis. Post-mortem measurements are closer to physiological expectations.] Under these circumstances an adequate cardiac output can only be maintained with a left atrial pressure around 20 to 25 mm. Hg above the sternal angle at rest. This causes "pulmonary venous congestion" and its consequences. Exercise, excitement, pregnancy, or simple tachycardia (which diminishes the ventricular diastolic filling time) results in considerable further elevation of the pulmonary venous pressure, which may rise well above the osmotic pressure of the plasma (30 mm. Hg). At this stage a proportion of patients die from acute pulmonary œdema; but the majority do not, because certain mechanisms come into play which serve to protect the lungs and it is important to understand just what these are.

If the mean left atrial pressure is 30 mm. Hg, the mean pressure in the pulmonary artery must be at least 40 mm. Hg if the necessary gradient between the two is to be preserved. In acute experiments this passive pulmonary hypertension, as it may be called, maintains a linear relationship to the left atrial pressure at all levels (Lasser and Loewe, 1954), and this is the rule in chronic cases (Wood, 1954). In 28 per cent of individuals, however, as soon as the left atrial pressure begins to rise at all seriously, the pulmonary arterioles constrict. This obstructs the circulation proximal to the pulmonary capillaries and so prevents their developing dangerously high pressures. In response to the high pulmonary vascular resistance the pulmonary blood pressure rises considerably, and may reach systemic level. This puts a heavy burden on the right ventricle, which sooner or later fails. Thus by this mechanism early death from acute pulmonary œdema is prevented at the cost of a low cardiac output and ultimate right ventricular failure.

A second change that tends to prevent pulmonary œdema is the development of a physical barrier between the capillaries and alveoli, the capillary wall, interstitial tissue and alveolar basement membrane all becoming thickened, so that it becomes increasingly difficult for fluid to enter the alveoli even though it may pass into the interstitial tissue (Hayward, 1955). This helps to explain why acute pulmonary œdema is usually an early symptom, and why attacks tend to cease spontaneously if life can be preserved long enough for this barrier to be erected. Fluid is removed from the interstitial tissue by the lymphatics, which themselves become engorged.

The very high left atrial pressures that may develop on exercise in these stereotyped cases of mitral stenosis, even as high as 60 mm. Hg, seem to deny the importance of a broncho-pulmonary venous shunt mechanism which theoretically might relieve pulmonary venous congestion. According to Marchand, Gilroy and Wilson (1950) the true bronchial veins within the substance of the lung drain directly into the pulmonary veins, so that the bronchial venous pressure must be the same as the pulmonary venous pressure. This may explain early hæmoptysis in mitral stenosis, but provides no basis for belief in a shunt mechanism that might relieve the pulmonary venous pressure. However, these workers also confirmed that the extrapulmonary bronchial veins, which they called the pleuro-hilar veins, drained into the azygos, hemiazygos and intercostal veins, and communicated freely with the pulmonary veins, as previously described by Miller (1947) and others; in mitral stenosis the pleuro-hilar bronchial veins were dilated and sometimes tortuous and varicose (Gilroy, Marchand and Wilson, 1952). It must be admitted, then, that the pulmonary venous circulation is in fact provided with a safety valve at the root of the lung, and that when well developed this could lower the pulmonary venous pressure at the expense of the cardiac output. Patients relieved of pulmonary congestion in this way should complain of fatigue and perhaps œdema, when the pulmonary venous pressure is only moderately raised, the pulmonary vascular resistance normal, and the estimated cardiac output normal when based on an A-V difference calculated from samples obtained from the pulmonary artery, right ventricle or right atrium. From such physiological data the physician would conclude that stenosis was mild and that the symptoms must have some other explanation. Only unexplained enlargement of the right ventricle might point to the true state of affairs, unless samples obtained from the superior vena cava above and below the junction of the azygos vein proved the existence of a significant broncho-pulmonary shunt, as when an anomalous pulmonary vein joins the azygos. No physiological studies on this point have yet been reported, but two observations may be mentioned: (1) I have not myself been able to detect much difference between high and low superior vena cava samples in several cases of mitral stenosis in which the possibility of a broncho-pulmonary shunt was considered; (2) in the few cases of mitral stenosis in which unexplained enlargement of the right ventricle has been associated with a relatively low pulmonary venous pressure and a normal pulmonary vascular resistance, the cardiac output, based on routine pulmonary artery samples, has been low, and has failed to rise properly on exercise, so that a myocardial fault has been invoked (Harvey et al., 1955). This myocardial dysfunction may be due to active carditis or residual fibrosis, and may be regarded as the fourth factor that tends to protect the lungs.

To sum up, it must be repeated that in the typical case of critical mitral stenosis, the usual problem is not why the pulmonary venous pressure is lower than expected, but why pulmonary œdema does not develop when the pulmonary venous pressure rises well above the osmotic pressure of the plasma, and the answer to this may lie in the development of a physical barrier between the capillaries and alveoli. A high pulmonary vascular resistance explains the behaviour of the vast majority of cases in which elevation of the left atrial pressure is limited, the right ventricle large, and the cardiac output low, and a myocardial fault adequately explains the remainder. There may or may not be a small group of cases that are materially influenced by the development of a broncho-pulmonary venous shunt. This might be best detected by analysing low S.V.C. samples for traces of Evans blue dye a few seconds after injecting a suitable quantity into the pulmonary artery.

SYMPTOMS

The chief symptom of mitral stenosis is *dyspnœa*. This appears to be due to increased rigidity of the lungs so that the intrathoracic pressure swings have to be greater than normal in order to inflate and deflate the lungs (Marshall, McIlroy and Christie, 1954); in other words, respiration becomes laborious, and ventilation on effort readily approaches 50 per cent of the maximum breathing capacity. The increased rigidity is apparently caused by changes in the interstitial tissue, including chronic interstitial œdema (Hayward, 1955), for the pulmonary blood volume is normal (Lagerlöf *et al.*, 1949). The extra space occupied by the interstitial tissue reduces the vital capacity and total lung volume. Œdema of the bronchial mucosa, with or without broncho-spasm, due to the high intrapulmonary bronchial venous pressure (Marchand *et al.*, 1950), adds to the ventilatory difficulty. Except during attacks of acute pulmonary œdema, the arterial pO_2, pCO_2 and pH are usually normal. Whether stretch receptors are stimulated by the changes in the interstitial tissue and excite the Hering-Breuer reflex, inhibiting the depth of inspiration, is uncertain.

The degree of dyspnœa on effort usually determines the clinical grading of effort intolerance in mitral stenosis. Four grades are commonly recognised corresponding to the four adjectives of degree—slight, moderate, considerable and gross. In grade I symptoms are provoked by more than average activity, e.g. running, hurrying, walking up hills, playing games, polishing or scrubbing. Patients in this grade usually undertake the activities that make them breathless, but cannot compete with their fellows. In grade II symptoms occur on ordinary activity such as walking at an average pace or up two flights of stairs, carrying a shopping basket, dancing, and any form of manual labour. Patients in this grade limit their physical activities, but can still lead an almost normal social life. In grade III symptoms develop with less than ordinary physical activity and force patients to walk slowly on the level; shopping and all but the lightest housework is abandoned. Grade IV means total incapacity.

Orthopnœa occurs in 70 per cent of cases in grades III or IV. Sitting up, especially with the legs down, lowers the right atrial pressure and thus diminishes the output of the right ventricle. This in turn lowers the left atrial pressure and therefore the pulmonary venous and capillary pressures. In the horizontal position these effects are reversed so that transudation of fluid from the pulmonary capillaries into the interstitial tissue is encouraged. Although Donald *et al.* (1953) have denied that sitting up in bed lowers the cardiac output sufficiently to be of any importance, they noted that in cases of mitral stenosis it resulted in a marked fall of pulmonary artery pressure, which certainly suggests a drop in output.

Attacks of frank pulmonary œdema occur in about 10 per cent of all cases of mitral stenosis in which the mitral orifice is more or less critically reduced (Wood, 1954). Precipitating agents include effort, emotion, sexual intercourse, pregnancy, respiratory infections, uncontrolled atrial fibrillation, and anæsthesia. Physiologically the most important provocative factors are tachycardia, which reduces the left ventricular diastolic filling time, hydræmia, a rise of cardiac output, and perhaps some neurogenic or chemical disturbance which alters capillary permeability. Physiological data during an attack are necessarily limited, but the left atrial pressure is usually between 30 and 50 mm. Hg and always well above the osmotic pressure of the plasma, the heart rate is nearly always 120 or more beats per minute, the cardiac output is higher than usual, and the pulmonary vascular resistance commonly normal. The transudate is believed to be much the same kind of fluid that normally passes through the capillary walls into the tissue spaces, which in the interstitial tissues of mammalian lung contains 2.5 to 3 G. per cent of protein (Warren and Drinker, 1942; Drinker, 1945). As the attack proceeds the arterial oxygen saturation gradually falls, and in severe cases may become as low as 50 per cent; at the beginning of the attack, however, it is normal, so that anoxia cannot be blamed for initiating events by increasing the permeability of the capillary walls. By having this effect later in the attack, however, anoxia could well establish a vicious circle, were it not for the fact that it also causes a sharp rise of pulmonary vascular resistance (Liljestrand, 1948), which must tend to lower the capillary pressure and terminate the attack. Limited evidence that the pulmonary vascular resistance does not rise during spontaneous attacks of pulmonary œdema should be accepted with considerable reserve, because these cases are very difficult to investigate.

Protective mechanisms or complications tending to prevent acute pulmonary œdema include a high pulmonary vascular resistance, the development of a capillary-alveolar interstitial barrier, atrial fibrillation when controlled by means of digitalis, myocarditis or cardiac fibrosis, associated tricuspid stenosis, and perhaps a broncho-pulmonary venous shunt.

The most important of these is probably a high pulmonary vascular resistance. In my own series, this averaged 2.9 units in cases giving a history of pulmonary œdema and never exceeded 5.2 units, whereas in patients who had never had orthopnœa, paroxysmal dyspnœa, or frank pulmonary œdema, but whose stenosis was no less severe, it averaged 9.2 units.

Clinically, acute pulmonary œdema occurs characteristically in young women with an average grade of stenosis relatively early in its course, before protective mechanisms have had time to develop. Thus the average age of patients with pulmonary œdema in the author's series was 32, compared with 37 for the series as a whole. Normal rhythm is nearly twice as frequent as atrial fibrillation, despite the fact that the onset of the latter may precipitate acute pulmonary œdema. The attack itself may start insidiously with slight dyspnœa, orthopnœa, and a gentle repetitive cough (stage 1), but soon develops strongly, dyspnœa becoming extreme and often accompanied by wheezing (cardiac asthma): the face pales, the heart rate quickens, the blood pressure rises, the extremities turn cold and blue, and the heart pounds (stage 2). The patient becomes greatly distressed and frightened, and as suffocation increases fine crepitations become widespread, and quantities of frothy white or pink fluid may be expectorated (stage 3). Central cyanosis appears late in the attack, and if the arterial oxygen saturation falls sufficiently the vasomotor centre may fail, and a state of collapse sets in: the blood pressure falls, the skin becomes grey, cold and wet, the pulse almost imperceptible, and the respirations shallow (stage 4). If treatment fails the patient finally sinks into a state of unconsciousness and dies.

Paroxysmal cardiac dyspnœa is similar, but transudation of fluid from the capillaries does not enter the alveoli, being prevented from doing so by the physical barrier described earlier. Interstitial œdema makes the lungs very rigid and breathing is laboured, but there are no crepitations, no fluid is expectorated, and the arterial oxygen saturation falls little, if at all.

Thus orthopnœa, paroxysmal cardiac dyspnœa and acute pulmonary œdema are all manifestations of a tendency for fluid to pass out of the pulmonary capillaries into the interstitial tissue of the lung. Although from the patient's point of view the order in which they have just been given represents an increasing grade of severity, the disease as a whole is usually most advanced when there is orthopnœa only, and least advanced when there are attacks of acute pulmonary œdema, cases of paroxysmal cardiac dyspnœa occupying a middle position. The reason for this has already been explained.

Hæmoptysis

There are five kinds of hæmoptysis complicating mitral valve disease: (1) the sudden unexpected profuse hæmorrhage known as pulmonary apoplexy; (2) blood-streaked mucoid sputum associated with winter bronchitis; (3) blood-stained sputum associated with attacks of paroxysmal cardiac dyspnœa; (4) pink frothy sputum accompanying acute pulmonary œdema; (5) frank hæmoptysis due to pulmonary infarction.

A history of *pulmonary apoplexy* is obtained in one-quarter of cases severe enough to warrant valvotomy. It is characteristically an early symptom, often the very first, and although usually recurrent, attacks tend to cease spontaneously after two or three years. The most important precipitating agents are pregnancy and physical effort, but at least half of the attacks occur without warning and for no reason known to the patient.

The hæmorrhage itself is sudden and profuse, the amount of blood coughed up being usually measured in ounces. It is rarely dangerous, and tends to stop spontaneously within half an hour or so, although residual blood may stain the sputum for a day or two.

Pulmonary apoplexy is attributed to rupture of a small intrapulmonary bronchial vein as a result of a rather sudden rise of left atrial pressure for which the pulmonary and bronchial venous systems are unprepared. In the early stage of mitral stenosis, as in normal individuals, these vessels are very thin walled; after being subjected to an increased pressure for several years, however, their walls thicken appreciably (Henry, 1952), and this may be one reason why attacks occur relatively early and after two or three years tend to cease spontaneously. Rupture of a dilated pleuro-hilar vein which is in anastomotic communication with the pulmonary venous system is another and perhaps more likely source of profuse hæmorrhage, for these small veins are forced to carry more than their fair share of blood and, though not subjected to high pressure, are often varicose (Gilroy *et al.*, 1952). The fall in pulmonary venous pressure likely to result from a brisk hæmorrhage may well discourage further bleeding.

As pointed out by Thompson and Stewart (1951), hæmoptysis of this kind is not a sign of pulmonary hypertension. On the contrary, it is exceedingly rare when the pulmonary vascular resistance is over 10 units, for the pulmonary venous system is then protected (Wood, 1954).

Congestive hæmoptysis is a convenient title for blood-stained sputum accompanying an attack of acute bronchitis, paroxysmal dyspnœa or pulmonary œdema. The mild hæmorrhage in these cases is never as important as the condition with which it is associated. The ruptured vessels are presumably very small, for hæmorrhage is never profuse: with bronchitis and paroxysmal dyspnœa a bronchial vessel is almost certainly at fault; with acute pulmonary œdema, however, the uniformly pink froth suggests capillary rupture into alveoli.

Hæmoptysis due to pulmonary infarction is a late complication of mitral stenosis, and is usually caused by an embolus secondary to phlebo-thrombosis in the legs in advanced cases with heart failure. This will be discussed later.

Winter bronchitis

Recurrent attacks of winter bronchitis occur in about a third of cases of well-developed mitral stenosis. Cough with blood-stained sputum, wheezing and breathlessness may be very distressing. The turgid or œdematous state of the bronchial mucosa caused by the high bronchial venous pressure is believed to be responsible for the severity of symptoms if not for the susceptibility to infection, although a convincing relationship between the frequency of bronchitis and the height of the left atrial pressure cannot be demonstrated statistically (Wood, 1954). Compression of the left bronchus by a greatly dilated left atrium, which has been known to cause collapse of the left lung (King, 1838), or splaying of either bronchus, plays little part in the syndrome.

It is unusual for recurrent bronchitis to have any permanent ill effect on lung function or the pulmonary circulation in cases of mitral stenosis and fears that bronchitis may be primary or that secondary bronchitis has already caused emphysema and cor pulmonale are rarely justified. On the contrary, one of the many remarkable results of technically successful valvotomy is the abolition of these tiresome attacks.

Systemic embolism

In any large series of living cases of mitral stenosis a history of systemic embolism is likely to be obtained in 9 to 14 per cent (Sellors, Bedford and Somerville, 1953; Wood, 1954). The embolism is cerebral in at least 60 per cent of instances, visceral in 10 per cent and peripheral in 30 per cent. In about 20 per cent of afflicted cases emboli are multiple, and in 60 per cent recurrent (Daley *et al.*, 1951; Wood, 1954).

Atrial fibrillation is a contributing factor in about three-quarters of all cases, and is particularly dangerous at its onset when the ventricular rate is uncontrolled.

Little correlation has been found between the size of the left atrium or of its appendage and the frequency of embolism, and giant left atria are rarely to blame. There is no correlation between the incidence of embolism and the pulmonary vascular resistance or the size of the mitral orifice. Embolism may be the first symptom of mitral stenosis, occurring at a time when there is no effort intolerance and when the rest of the data indicate a relatively mild stricture; this was so in 12.5 per cent of embolic cases studied by the author.

At operation a clot in the left atrium or its appendage is found in about 22 per cent of all cases, whether there has been a history of embolism or not. Left atrial thrombi are admittedly nearly twice as common in post-mortem material (Wallach *et al.*, 1953), but even then some 36 per cent of cases with a history of embolism have none (Daley *et al.*, 1951). Operative embolism, the frequency of which has dwindled from 10 to 5 per cent as more effective precautionary measures have been taken, is no more common in patients with a history of embolism than in those without.

All this suggests that only fresh clots are likely to be flung out into the systemic circulation, and that once a thrombus is organised there is no further spontaneous danger from that source; only the surgeon's finger is liable to dislodge a fragment of old thrombus.

The local effects of systemic embolism have been described briefly in chapter I. It may be added here that out of 20 cases of cerebral embolism occurring in patients already under observation in mitral valve disease, only two died, and that the 49 per cent mortality cited by Daley *et al.* 1951) may well be biased by selected and post-mortem material. When trying to prevent cerebral embolism during valvotomy, both carotids should be temporarily occluded at critical moments, because experimental and necropsy evidence proves that emboli may pass into either carotid impartially (Hall, Dencker and Biorck, 1952).

Angina pectoris

Cardiac pain indistinguishable in all respects from that encountered in occlusive coronary disease occurs in about 10 per cent of cases of mitral stenosis that are otherwise severe enough to warrant valvotomy; it does not occur in mild cases. The angina is not caused by coincidental coronary atherosclerosis because the sex ratio of affected cases is 5 : 1 in favour of women, their average age is 36, pain always disappears following technically successful valvotomy, and in a limited number that have come to necropsy the coronary arteries have been normal. Angina is twice as common in cases with a high pulmonary vascular resistance as in those without, and also twice as common in cases with extreme stenosis as in those with an average stricture. It is tentatively attributed to functional impairment of the coronary blood flow due to strict limitation of the cardiac output, and is believed to affect the left ventricle more than the right, as long as the pulmonary artery pressure on effort is lower than the aortic (Wood, 1954).

Left vocal cord paralysis (Ortner's syndrome)

Huskiness of the voice due to paralysis of the left recurrent laryngeal nerve occurs in about 0.5 per cent of cases of mitral stenosis. Ortner (1897) thought that the nerve was compressed by the dilated left atrium, and essentially this may be true, but the actual compression is usually mediated by enlarged trachea-bronchial lymph nodes (Dolowitz and Lewis, 1948), and dilatation of the pulmonary artery is often contributory (Fetterolf and Norris, 1911). The voice may improve post-operatively (Ari, Harvey and Hufnagel, 1955).

Atrial fibrillation

Rapid irregular palpitations in cases of mitral stenosis are commonly due to paroxysmal or uncontrolled atrial fibrillation. The abnormality of rhythm occurs in about 40 per cent of all cases, and is related chiefly to the age of the patient, not to the degree of stricture (de la Chapelle, Graefe and Rottino, 1934). My own findings in live cases agreed almost exactly with those of the authors cited; in addition, left atrial biopsies denied that rheumatic activity played any part in encouraging atrial fibrillation, even in the youngest adults, and more than average left and right atrial dilatation could be interpreted as a result rather more easily than as a cause of the rhythm change.

Uncontrolled atrial fibrillation may cause acute dyspnœa, because the rapid heart rate tends to increase the output of the right ventricle while depriving the left of sufficient diastolic time in which to fill: it should be understood that shortening diastole interferes little with ventricular filling when the atrioventricular valve is normal, but considerably when it is stenosed.

When the pulmonary vascular resistance is high, atrial fibrillation with a rapid ventricular rate usually causes congestive heart failure; the tendency for the left atrial pressure to rise secondary to the increased rate is offset by the diminished right ventricular output, so that fatigue, œdema and swelling of the abdomen overshadow breathlessness. The cardiac output may be very low in these cases, because the shortened left ventricular diastolic filling time is not compensated for by an adequate rise of left atrial pressure.

When the ventricular rate is controlled by means of digitalis, these physiological difficulties are removed and recovery is prompt. This is why digitalis has always been expecially renowned for the benefit it bestows on cases of *rheumatic heart disease* with atrial fibrillation.

The circulatory hold-up when the ventricular rate is very fast also explains the frequency of fresh thrombosis in the left atrium at this time and the immediate danger of embolism.

PHYSICAL SIGNS

Mitral facies and cold blue hands

Peripheral cyanosis in the face and hands is due to peripheral vaso-constriction secondary to a low cardiac output, and is therefore seen especially in cases with a high pulmonary vascular resistance; it is not a feature of uncomplicated mitral stenosis of average severity in which a fair output is maintained with the help of a high left atrial pressure. In advanced pulmonary hypertensive cases the hands may be warm and the palms bright red as a result of impaired hepatic function.

Loss of weight is usual in severe mitral stenosis, unless counterbalanced by œdema, and the lean features contribute to the mitral facies.

Peripheral pulse

The brachial pulse in all well-developed cases of mitral stenosis is small in volume, but well sustained in quality, except in advanced cases with pulmonary hypertension and chronic heart failure, when vasodilatation due to impaired hepatic function may modify it.

Jugular venous pressure and pulse

In simple mitral stenosis the systemic venous pressure and the jugular pulse are both normal. The venous pressure may rise, however, as a result of improperly controlled atrial fibrillation, severe pulmonary hypertension, or associated tricuspid stenosis. Heart failure due to myocarditis or cardiac fibrosis is rare.

With uncontrolled atrial fibrillation the *x* descent of the jugular pulse disappears: *v* begins earlier and is followed by *y*, so that there is only one crest and one trough per cardiac cycle; the higher the *v* wave the quicker the *y* descent and the more conspicuous the *y* trough.

Both pulmonary hypertension and tricuspid stenosis usually give rise to a giant *a* wave when there is normal rhythm; with atrial fibrillation, however, cases of pulmonary hypertension show a rapid *y* descent and deep *y* trough, whereas cases of tricuspid stenosis show a relatively slow *y* descent and absent *y* trough.

Cardiac impulse

The left ventricle is characteristically impalpable in cases of pure mitral stenosis, only the tap of the first heart sound being appreciated in the region of the mid-clavicular or anterior axillary line. The degree of right ventricular thrust in the left parasternal line is proportional to the pulmonary vascular resistance; passive pulmonary hypertension causes very little right ventricular enlargement, and a dilated left atrium posteriorly only pushes the heart forwards appreciably when it is aneurysmal. Pulsation over the pulmonary artery is rare, and when present means an extreme pulmonary vascular resistance.

Auscultation

There are four important auscultatory signs of mitral stenosis—a presystolic murmur, a loud first heart sound, an opening snap and a mitral diastolic murmur (fig. 10.08).

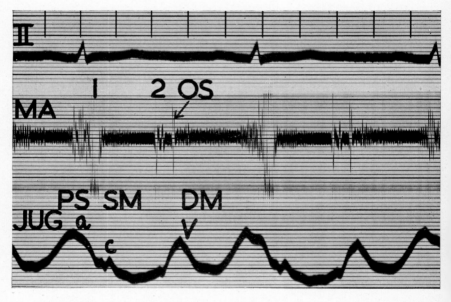

Fig. 10.08—Phonocardiogram from a case of mitral stenosis showing a crescendo presystolic murmur, loud first sound, opening snap, and mid-diastolic murmur timed against the electrocardiogram and phlebogram.

(*By courtesy of Drs. William Evans and Aubrey Leatham*

A *mitral presystolic* (Fauvel, 1843) *or left atrio-systolic* (Gairdner, 1861) *murmur* can be heard in practically all cases of physiological mitral stenosis with normal rhythm, even when the stricture is so mild as to be associated with a left atrial pressure of only 5 mm. Hg above the sternal angle. It is occasionally masked by gross enlargement of the right ventricle secondary to an extreme pulmonary vascular resistance, for the left ventricle may then be displaced so far posteriorly that mitral events cannot be heard at the apex beat, which is usurped by the right ventricle.

The *first heart sound is accentuated* in practically all cases of more or less pure mitral stenosis, provided the valve is not heavily calcified. In conjunction with the presystolic murmur a loud first sound can be heard in the mildest cases with left atrial pressures only a few mm. Hg above the sternal angle. The late diastolic or presystolic atrio-ventricular pressure gradient forces the mitral cusps to remain wide open to the very end of diastole, so that when the left ventricle contracts they slam together. Heavily calcified valves are usually so rigid that very little movement of the cusps is possible.

In cases with atrial fibrillation, the presystolic atrio-ventricular pressure gradient and therefore the intensity of the first sound, varies inversely with the length of the preceding diastole, as pointed out by Ravin and Bershof (1951). Exceptionally, however, the intensity of the first heart sound does

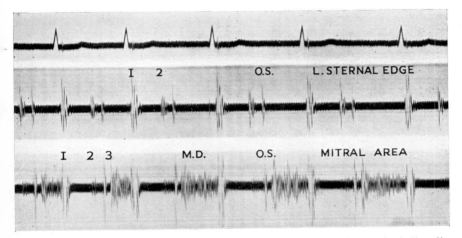

Fig. 10.09—Phonocardiogram showing an opening snap followed by a mitral diastolic murmur in a case of mitral stenosis with atrial fibrillation.

By courtesy of Dr. Aubrey Leatham)

not vary, or it may have a paradoxical relationship to the length of the preceding cycle. Such behaviour has not been satisfactorily explained, but it suggests relative fixation of the cusps so that they may not be able to billow into the ventricle beyond certain narrow limits whatever the atrioventricular pressure gradient; the intensity of the first sound then varies inversely with the pressure gradient, for the cusps close more sharply when the left ventricle is full and the left atrial pressure relatively low, than when the left ventricle is half empty and the left atrial pressure high.

The first heart sound is also slightly delayed in mitral stenosis because the first 0.01 second or so of systole is occupied with raising the left ventricular pressure to atrial level (Cossio and Berconsky, 1943). In cases with atrial fibrillation, the delay varies inversely with the length of the preceding cycle (Messer *et al.*, 1951).

The *opening snap* of Potain is a sharp, high-pitched sound made by the aortic cusp of the mitral valve when it is flung forwards into the cavity of the left ventricle as the atrio-ventricular pressure gradient is reversed at the end of the period of isometric relaxation, and therefore coincides temporally with the summit of the *v* wave of the left atrial pressure pulse (Margolies and Wolferth, 1932). It occurs 0.06 to 0.14 second (usually 0.08 to 0.10 second) after aortic valve closure (Braun-Menendez and Orias, 1935), and is best heard down the left sternal border over the root of the aorta or at the apex beat (fig. 10.09). The interval between the aortic second sound and the opening snap is inversely proportional to the height of the left atrial pressure and therefore directly proportional to the length of the preceding cardiac cycle (Messer *et al.*, 1951). Thus, if due allowance is made for cycle length (disregarding the cardiac output and the pulmonary vascular resistance), the more delayed the first heart sound and the earlier the opening snap, the tighter is the mitral stenosis (Wells, 1954).

The opening snap is heard in practically all cases of pure mitral stenosis of more than trivial degree, provided the valve is not heavily calcified and rigid. Exceptionally, an extreme pulmonary vascular resistance masks the snap, because a greatly enlarged right ventricle tends to prevent transmission of mitral sounds to the anterior chest wall. The opening snap may also be absent when there is associated aortic incompetence, probably because the regurgitant jet interferes with the forward movement of the aortic cusp of the mitral valve.

An *apical mid-diastolic murmur* is heard in all well-developed cases of mitral stenosis unless masked by a greatly enlarged right ventricle or a loud aortic diastolic murmur transmitted to the apex. It is usually low pitched and is heard best with the bell stethoscope when the patient lies on the left side. The murmur is not prevented by heavy calcification, nor altered by atrial fibrillation. It begins just after the opening snap, its onset coinciding with the period of rapid ventricular filling, i.e. with the steep part of the *y* descent (downstroke of *v*). It therefore gives rise to a form of triple rhythm, the cadence of which is very characteristic whether preceded by an opening snap or not.

Neither the intensity of the murmur nor the presence of a thrill matters much, but the length of the murmur is very important. In mild cases the murmur is relatively short, ending as soon as left atrial and ventricular diastolic pressures equalise; in more severe cases it extends right up to the next first heart sound, for left atrial and ventricular diastolic pressures do not equalise at all. The length of the murmur is easiest to gauge in cases with atrial fibrillation, for there is then no interference from atrial systole, and from time to time long pauses facilitate analysis.

THE ELECTROCARDIOGRAM

A well-defined P mitrale (fig. 10.10) is seen in practically all cases of moderate or severe mitral stenosis with normal rhythm, but is usually

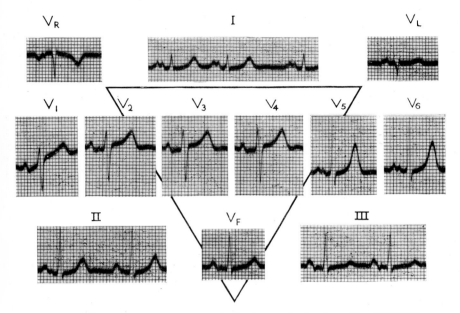

Fig. 10.10—Electrocardiogram in a case of mitral stenosis showing widened bifid P waves particularly in leads 1, 2, V_5 and V_6.

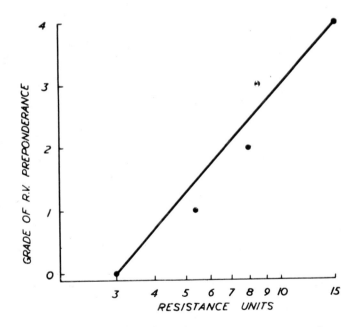

Fig. 10.11—Graph showing the relationship between the electrocardiographic grade of right ventricular preponderance and the pulmonary vascular resistance in cases of mitral stenosis (semi-logarithmic scale).

absent in mild cases. The P wave is bifid and widened to 0.12 second, the first peak representing right atrial activation, the second left atrial activation (Reynolds, 1953). The voltage is usually normal.

Tall peaked P waves in cases of mitral stenosis indicate a high pulmonary vascular resistance or associated tricuspid stenosis.

The ventricular complexes are strictly normal in uncomplicated cases, unless the S-T segments are depressed by digitalis therapy. Right ventricular preponderance means pulmonary hypertension secondary to a raised pulmonary vascular resistance, the degree of each correlating very closely with one another (fig. 10.11). Passive pulmonary hypertension does not cause right ventricular preponderance.

RADIOLOGICAL APPEARANCES

X-rays reveal characteristic changes in the size, shape and behaviour of the heart and great vessels and in the appearances of the lungs, which taken together are seen in no other condition.

The *aorta* is small unless the patient is over 45 years old, or unless the stenosis is sufficiently mild to allow a normal resting cardiac output.

The *left ventricle* is inconspicuous, hypodynamic, and fills relatively slowly. Apparent enlargement in otherwise uncomplicated cases of pure stenosis is usually an erroneous interpretation of a shadow that may represent pericardial effusion or a greatly enlarged right ventricle that is occupying the apex beat; occasionally it is genuine and may then be due to previous mitral incompetence or unusually severe carditis.

The left atrium is dilated in all but the mildest cases. In the anterior view it may be seen on both borders of the heart, forming a hump between the pulmonary arc and left ventricle on the left side, and lying above and overlapping the right atrium on the right side (fig. 10.12). In the lateral or oblique positions a dilated left atrium displaces the barium-filled œsophagus backwards (fig. 10.13). Rarely, the whole chamber is sharply outlined as a result of endocardial calcification.

The degree of left atrial enlargement is not related to the severity of the stenosis. The left atrium is apt to be relatively small in cases of pure stenosis in young adults with normal rhythm and a tendency to develop pulmonary œdema, and in cases with an extreme pulmonary vascular resistance; it is larger when there is atrial fibrillation, and especially when there is mitral incompetence as well.

Aneurysmal dilatation of the left atrium is more common with mitral incompetence, but it can occur with pure stenosis. The left atrial appendage may be enlarged disproportionately to the rest of the chamber; in such cases there is a conspicuous bulge on the left border of the heart just below the pulmonary arc, but little abnormal on the right border.

Heavy calcification of the mitral valve implies considerable destruction of the valve mechanism and is therefore uncommon in cases of pure

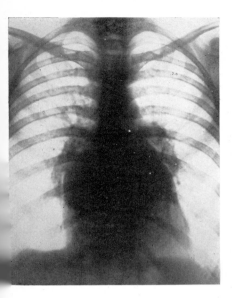

Fig. 10.12—Skiagram showing the characteristic appearances of dilatation of the left atrium in the anterior view in a case of mitral stenosis.

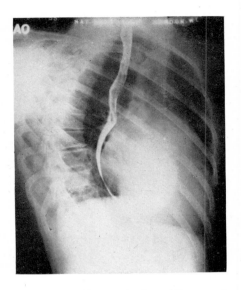

Fig. 10.13—Skiagram in first oblique position showing enlarged left atrium delineated by means of barium in the œsophagus in a case of mitral stenosis.

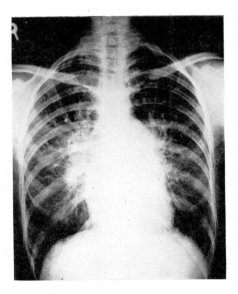

Fig. 10.14—Skiagram from a case of tight mitral stenosis showing intense "pulmonary venous congestion" (probably chronic interstitial œdema). Horizontal Kerley lines can be seen in the right lower zone. Dilatation of the pulmonary artery is due to passive pulmonary hypertension.

stenosis; on the other hand, it does not necessarily mean that incompetence is dominant.

Pulmonary venous congestion is supposed to be visible radiologically as fan-shaped mottling in the hilar regions (fig. 10.14). This traditional term has the advantage of familiarity, but the disadvantage of inaccuracy, for the pulmonary veins are not in fact congested—if congested means over-crowded—and the abnormal shadows are not venous. The pulmonary venous pressure is certainly raised considerably in all cases having this radiological sign, but the pulmonary veins themselves are constricted rather than dilated (Holling, 1951), and the pulmonary blood volume is normal at rest (Lagerlöf *et al.*, 1949). The precise nature of the hilar opacities awaits proof, but it is now believed that they are probably caused by a combination of chronic œdema and other changes in the interstitial connective tissue, engorged lymphatics, and dilated pleuro-hilar bronchial veins. These are the effects of pulmonary venous hypertension, caused by impedance to flow, the bottle-neck being situated at the mitral orifice. The radiological appearances themselves might well be called chronic interstitial œdema of the lungs.

Horizontal linear markings, best seen near the costophrenic angles, usually accompany the hilar opacities (Kerley, 1933, 1936). These are believed to represent œdematous inter-lobular septa (Grainger and Hearn, 1955).

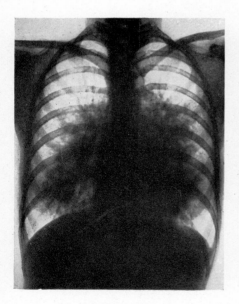
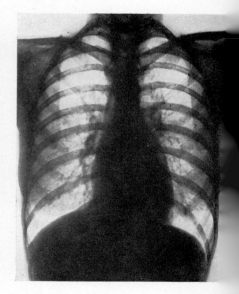

(a) 11th November 1942.   (b) Two days later after medical treatment

Fig. 10.15—Skiagram showing acute pulmonary œdema in a case of mitral stenosis.

Acknowledgments to Sir John Parkinson

In mitral stenosis (and left ventricular failure) the degree of chronic interstitial œdema, if this expression may be used, is directly proportional to the height of the left atrial pressure, and does not occur at all until the latter is over 10 mm. Hg above the sternal angle at rest. It is therefore proportional to the degree of stenosis and inversely proportional to the pulmonary vascular resistance.

Acute pulmonary œdema gives rise to a typical diffuse opacity spreading outwards from the hilum towards the periphery of the lung (fig. 10.15); it is always bilateral, but may be more conspicuous on one side than the other. The œdema is intra-alveolar and the shadows may develop and disappear within a matter of minutes or hours. Attacks are more likely to occur in patients with previously normal lungs than in those who already have chronic interstitial œdema, as explained earlier.

Pulmonary hæmosiderosis is seen in 10 per cent of moderate or severe cases of mitral stenosis. Fine or coarse miliary nodules are scattered throughout the lungs (fig. 10.16) and resemble those seen sometimes in certain hæmolytic anæmias of childhood (Gumpert, 1947). The lesions are closely linked with repeated hæmoptysis and develop relatively early in the course of mitral stenosis at a time when hæmorrhages are common (Laubry, Lenegre and Abbas, 1948) and the pulmonary vascular resistance

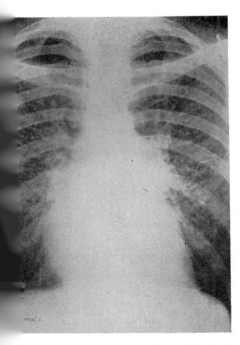

10.16—Skiagram of a case of mitral stenosis showing miliary nodules in the lungs due to hæmosiderosis.

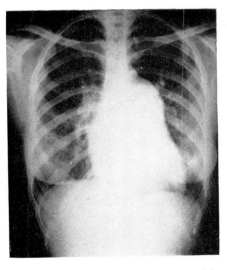

Fig. 10.17—Skiagram showing considerable dilatation of the pulmonary artery in a case of mitral stenosis with an extreme pulmonary vascular resistance; note the absence of chronic interstitial œdema of the lung.

low (Wood, 1954). The lesions represent focal accumulations of hæmo-siderin in groups of adjacent alveoli with resulting fibrosis (Lendrum, 1950), and are probably caused by hæmorrhages in the walls of the terminal bronchioles; secondary ossification occurs occasionally (Elkeles and Glynn, 1946). Since hæmorrhages resulting from a rising pulmonary and bronchial venous pressure tend to cease spontaneously, hæmosiderosis is never progressive beyond a certain point, and since the lesions represent a permanent change of structure, they never regress after successful valv-otomy. They have no greater significance than recurrent hæmoptysis, and point unmistakably to past miliary hæmorrhages even when there has been no history of hæmoptysis.

Dilatation of the pulmonary artery (fig. 10.17) is due to pulmonary hypertension and its degree is proportional to the pulmonary vascular resistance (fig. 10.18). Conspicuous dilatation of the pulmonary artery

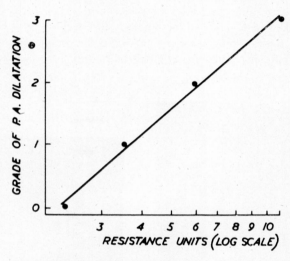

Fig. 10.18—Graph showing the correlation between the radiological grade of pulmonary artery dilatation and the pulmonary vascular resistance (semi-logarithmic scale).

therefore provides good evidence of at least critical stenosis, for a high resistance does not otherwise develop. Passive pulmonary hypertension alone is rarely severe enough to have much effect on the pulmonary artery.

Enlargement of the right ventricle is more easily recognised clinically and electrocardiographically than radiologically, but when the chamber respon-sible for cardiac enlargement has already been identified as the right ventricle by such means, its actual size is best determined radiologically. Like dilatation of the pulmonary artery, the degree of right ventricular enlargement is proportional to the pulmonary vascular resistance and to the duration of right ventricular failure when that has occurred. Right-sided enlargement is not a feature of simple mitral stenosis.

Dilatation of the right atrium usually accompanies enlargement of the right ventricle, and is difficult to distinguish from it by conventional radiological methods. The combination of an inconspicuous pulmonary artery and dilated right heart suggests isolated enlargement of the right atrium due to tricuspid stenosis; if the venous pulse and auscultatory signs deny such a diagnosis, pericardial effusion should be seriously considered; if that is excluded by means of cardiac catheterisation, primary impairment of myocardial function, due to fibrosis from old rheumatic carditis, may have to be invoked, although atrial fibrillation alone may be sufficient to explain some degree of dilatation.

General enlargement of the heart shadow is rare in cases of mitral stenosis, and when genuine is more likely to be caused by chronic pericardial effusion than rheumatic carditis or cardiac fibrosis. As a rule, however, the statement that the heart is enlarged or that the cardio-thoracic ratio is increased can be better expressed in terms of dilatation of the chamber or chambers responsible.

Angiocardiography is of little value as a diagnostic tool in cases of mitral stenosis. It helped, however, to prove that the hump on the left border of the heart between the pulmonary arc and left ventricle was the left atrium or left atrial appendage and not the conus of the right ventricle (Robb and Steinberg, 1939; Grishman *et al.*, 1944), and that in cases with a high pulmonary vascular resistance the branches of the pulmonary arteries changed calibre abruptly and considerably, instead of tapering off gradually (Davies *et al.*, 1953).

PHYSIOLOGICAL TESTS

Cardiac catheterisation is now chiefly employed to measure the degree of stenosis when it is doubted whether the stricture is tight enough to explain the symptoms, to determine whether mitral stenosis or incompetence is dominant in difficult borderline cases in which both are obviously present, to find out whether mitral stenosis is really responsible for a situation that is clinically indistinguishable from primary pulmonary hypertension, or to discover whether pericardial effusion, tricuspid stenosis or a myocardial fault is causing unexplained enlargement of the heart shadow.

The degree of stenosis can be estimated by measuring the left atrial pressure, the cardiac output, and the heart rate. A simple crude index of the size of the orifice is given by the ratio of the cardiac output (L./ min.) to the left atrial pressure (mm. Hg above the sternal angle) or C.O./L.A.P. Normally, this is 5/5 or 100 per cent. When mitral stenosis is trivial, the index is still close to 100 per cent; when the stricture is mild, the index is about 5/10 or 50 per cent; critical stenosis requiring valvotomy gives an average index of 4.5/22.5 or 20 per cent; while with extreme stenosis the index is about 3/25 or 12 per cent (Wood, 1954). For practical purposes this index works very well provided the heart rate does not exceed 90 beats per minute and there is no significant incompetence.

The size of the mitral orifice may be calculated more accurately by taking the heart rate into consideration, for forward flow through the valve can only take place in diastole. According to the Gorlins (1951)

$$\text{mitral valve area} = \frac{\text{mitral flow in c.c. per second}}{31\sqrt{\text{L.A.P.} - \text{diastolic L.V.P. (mm. Hg)}}}$$

where mitral flow (c.c. per sec.) is $\dfrac{\text{cardiac output (c.c. per min.)}}{\text{diastolic filling period (sec. per min.)}}$

For example, in an average case of critical stenosis with a cardiac output of 4.5 litres per minute, a heart rate of 70 beats per minute, and a left atrial pressure of 30 mm. Hg, the mitral flow in c.c. per second

would be $\dfrac{4.5 \times 1,000}{35 \text{ (approx)}} = 128$, so that the mitral valve area would be

$\dfrac{128}{31\ \sqrt{30-5}\text{ (assumed)}} = 0.83$ cm.^{2}.

Since the precise shape of the oval orifice is not known at operation, it is impossible to determine its exact cross section when its length and breadth are estimated by a surgeon, but it is likely to be about two-thirds of the quotient; e.g. an orifice measuring 1×0.5 cm. should have a cross section of about 0.33 cm.^{2}. A critical orifice measuring 0.83 cm.^{2} should have dimensions nearer 1.6×0.8 cm. Thus physiological calculations based on the Gorlin formula do not tally with Brock's estimates. This does not matter practically provided the order of the descrepancy is known.

Obstruction to forward flow may also be demonstrated by calculating the Ry/v ratio from the left atrial pressure pulse, as explained on page 513. With severe, critical and mild stenosis, the ratio averages 0.6, 1.0, and around 1.5 respectively. This test was introduced primarily to determine whether stenosis or incompetence was dominant in borderline cases in which both were known to be present: high ratios over 1.6 exclude obstruction to forward flow, so that under the clinical circumstances mitral incompetence can be diagnosed by inference.

The pulmonary vascular resistance in simple units is the pulmonary arterio-venous pressure gradient in mm. Hg, divided by the cardiac output in litres per minute, as explained elsewhere. In 80 per cent of cases of mitral stenosis it is normal or only slightly raised, but in 12.5 per cent it lies between 6 and 10 units, and in 7.5 per cent between 10 and 30 units. Patients with an extreme pulmonary vascular resistance may resemble cases of primary pulmonary hypertension, but cardiac catheterisation always reveals a left atrial pressure over 10 mm. Hg with reference to the sternal angle, a stenotic index of 10 to 25 per cent, and an Ry/v ratio under

1.3. The cardiac output is always low in these cases and the left atrial pressure strictly limited, even when stenosis is extreme.

The fourth reason for catheterising a case of mitral stenosis is to settle the question whether or not there is pericardial effusion, tricuspid stenosis, or a myocardial fault, when apparent cardiac enlargement is otherwise unexplained.

Pericardial effusion can at once be excluded if the tip of the catheter slides up and down the right border of the heart shadow when it is known to be in the right atrium. If part of the heart shadow extends beyond the catheter tip as it lies against the lateral border of the right atrium, however, a dilated left atrium is as likely to be causing the opacity as pericardial effusion. In either event, dilatation of the right side of the heart without physiological cause is excluded.

Tricuspid stenosis can be recognised at once if a continuous pressure tracing is recorded while the catheter is being withdrawn from the right ventricle to the right atrium, for if there is any obstruction at the valve the right atrial diastolic pressure is appreciably higher than the right ventricular diastolic pressure (vide infra).

It is not so easy to demonstrate a myocardial fault. Under routine conditions cases of primary myocardial failure associated with mitral stenosis should have a relatively low left atrial pressure, perhaps 5 to 10 mm. Hg above the sternal angle, a more or less normal pulmonary arterio-venous pressure gradient of 10 to 20 mm. Hg, raised right ventricular and right atrial diastolic pressures, and a low cardiac output. On exercise, or on tipping head-downwards, the right ventricular and right atrial diastolic pressures should rise and the cardiac output should fall or at least fail to increase. Cases that behave in this way are remarkably rare.

Technically, the left atrial pressure pulse, on which most of the above calculations depend, is recorded by wedging a catheter in a distal branch of the pulmonary artery, as described by Hellems et al. (1948), and Lagerlöf and Werkö (1949). If this cannot be accomplished, or if a satisfactory venous pulse is not so obtained, the left atrial pressure may be measured directly by means of a needle inserted through the left bronchus (Allison and Linden, 1953), or through the chest wall posteriorly (Björk et al., 1953). Excellent tracings of the left atrial and left ventricular pressure pulses can, of course, be obtained at operation (fig. 10.19).

Respiratory function tests may be required when the clinical features of a case suggest that cough and breathlessness may be due to chronic bronchitis and emphysema rather than to mitral stenosis. When breathlessness is due to mitral stenosis, the vital capacity and lung volume are reduced in proportion to the amount of chronic interstitial œdema present. The residual volume, mixing efficiency, and poorly ventilated space are normal. The maximum breathing capacity is diminished because of the mechanical difficulty in inflating and deflating the relatively rigid lungs, the intra-pleural pressure swings being greatly increased. As a rule the blood gases are normal, but in advanced cases with gross changes in the interstitial tissue there may be some difficulty in oxygen exchange, as with diffuse pulmonary fibrosis. The arterial oxygen saturation may then fall to 80 per cent, but rarely below this. Elimination of carbon dioxide, which diffuses more readily than oxygen in a fluid medium, is not hindered, so that hyperventilation due to anoxia may be associated with a low arterial pCO_2 and carbon dioxide content.

It will be appreciated that these findings at once distinguish the respiratory situation in mitral stenosis from that in emphysema (q.v.). In many respects, however, they resemble the findings in diffuse interstitial fibrosis.

The *pulmonary circulation time* is usually prolonged in well-developed cases of mitral stenosis, the delay being in the left atrium rather than in the pulmonary veins. The test is therefore of little value, because the dilated left atrium can be seen radiologically.

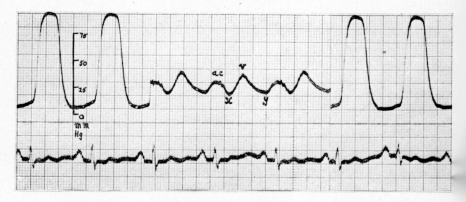

Fig. 10.19—Left ventricular and left atrial pressure pulses recorded in immediate succession from a case of mitral stenosis. Note presystolic and diastolic pressure gradients across the mitral valve, and the slow *y* descent following *v*.

COMPLICATIONS

Strictly speaking, acute pulmonary œdema, hæmoptysis, winter bronchitis, systemic embolism, laryngeal palsy, and atrial fibrillation may all be regarded as complications of mitral stenosis, but for convenience they have been treated as symptoms, and have already been discussed. There remain pulmonary hypertension, pulmonary incompetence, heart failure, tricuspid incompetence, pulmonary embolism, bacterial endocarditis, and massive thrombosis of the left atrium.

Pulmonary hypertension may be active or passive. The latter merely serves to keep the mean pulmonary artery pressure 10 mm. Hg or so above the left atrial pressure, and is clinically unimportant. Active pulmonary hypertension implies a high pulmonary vascular resistance and a pulmonary arterio-venous pressure gradient well above normal. Two grades of active pulmonary hypertension are recognised, moderate with a pulmonary vascular resistance of 6 to 10 units, and extreme with a pulmonary vascular resistance between 10 and 30 units.

In my own series 28 per cent of 275 critical cases of mitral stenosis developed a high resistance, moderate in 16 per cent and extreme in 12 per cent. The change begins early, just as the degree of stricture is becoming critical. High resistances are never encountered when stenosis is mild; on the other hand, extreme resistances may be encountered in young adults with only average stenosis (orifice 1 × 0.5 cm.). The available evidence favours the view that extreme resistances do not develop slowly over the years, but relatively suddenly, before pulmonary congestive symptoms have a chance to materialise. It has already been explained that a high resistance protects the pulmonary venous system from developing dangerously high pressures, and so prevents pulmonary œdema, paroxysmal cardiac dyspnœa, and orthopnœa. On injecting 1 mg. of acetylcholine into the pulmonary artery in these cases, the pulmonary vascular resistance and pulmonary blood pressure fall, the cardiac output rises, and the left atrial pressure rises (Wood and Besterman, 1956). In an ideal experiment the acetylcholine is totally inactivated before it reaches the systemic circulation, and so far there has been no fall in systemic blood pressure; on the contrary this has usually risen as a result of the increased output and there has been reflex cardiac slowing. These results provide conclusive proof of the protective effect of pulmonary vasoconstriction on the pulmonary venous system in mitral stenosis, and explain why high resistance cases do not suffer from pulmonary "congestive" symptoms. In a carefully analysed series of 300 cases of mitral valve disease of all types, 80 per cent of patients with an extreme pulmonary vascular resistance insisted that they had never had such symptoms. Again, if the high resistance were a late development it should be found more frequently in older patients; in fact, however, the average age of patients with a high resistance is exactly the same as the mean age for all cases of mitral stenosis. Finally, if a high resistance were due to sclerotic changes in the pulmonary arteries developing gradually over the years and secondary to passive pulmonary hypertension, it should not be influenced by mitral valvotomy; yet no case has so far been encountered in which the resistance did not fall appreciably after technically successful valvotomy.

Just what causes the pulmonary vasoconstriction is unknown. There is no experimental evidence that elevation of the pulmonary venous pressure per se has any such effect; on the contrary, the pulmonary artery pressure rises passively, as it does in 80 per cent of cases of mitral stenosis. Interstitial œdema can hardly excite the reflex, for as previously explained these patients do not have such œdema, and those that do usually have normal or only slightly raised resistances. A reduced alveolar oxygen tension is known to cause pulmonary vasoconstriction, but this does not occur.

Clinically, patients with an extreme pulmonary vascular resistance usually present with fatigue, œdema, angina pectoris or hæmoptysis from pulmonary infarction. In other words, the symptoms are those usually associated with a low cardiac output and not those associated with a high pulmonary venous pressure. There is either a florid mitral facies and other evidence of intense peripheral vasoconstriction, or, rarely, a palmar flush and signs of vasodilatation due to impairment of hepatic function. The arterial pulse is exceptionally small. The venous pressure is usually raised, and the jugular pulse may show a giant *a* wave in cases with normal rhythm or a conspicuous *v* wave and deep *y* trough in cases with atrial fibrillation with or without functional tricuspid incompetence. Occasionally, *y* may dominate the jugular pulse even when there is normal rhythm (fig. 10.20).

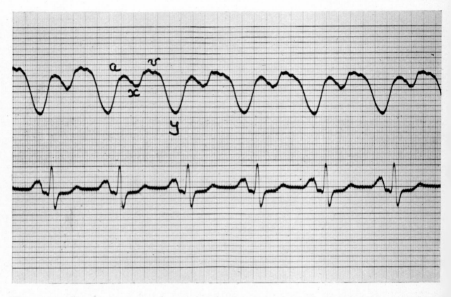

Fig. 10.20—Jugular venous pulse tracing from a case of mitral stenosis with an extreme pulmonary vascular resistance and heart failure, showing a rapid *y* descent and conspicuous *y* trough.

The left ventricle is always impalpable, but there is usually a substantial heave over the right ventricle, which may extend to the left as far as the anterior axillary line; occasionally there is a palpable impulse over the pulmonary artery. The auscultatory signs of mitral stenosis are often greatly damped, probably because the left ventricle, through which they are ordinarily heard, is unusually small, displaced posteriorly, and totally covered antero-laterally by the enlarged right ventricle. The mitral opening snap, however, may be detected at the aortic area. Right atrial gallop, a pulmonary ejection click, accentuation of the pulmonary component of the second heart sound, a pulmonary diastolic murmur due to functional pulmonary incompetence, and a tricuspid systolic murmur due to functional tricuspid incompetence, strongly confirms the diagnosis of severe pulmonary hypertension.

The electrocardiogram shows a combined P pulmonale and P mitrale, and considerable right ventricular preponderance. X-rays reveal conspicuous dilatation of the pulmonary artery and right side of the heart; the pulmonary interstitial and vascular markings are relatively light, and the left atrium may be only slightly dilated (fig. 10.17).

The physiological findings include a giant *a* wave in the right atrial pressure pulse when there is normal rhythm, or a conspicuous *v* wave followed by a sharp *y* descent and deep *y* trough in cases with atrial fibrillation; a left atrial pressure pulse characteristic of at least critical stenosis; a pulmonary artery pressure approaching, but rarely exceeding,

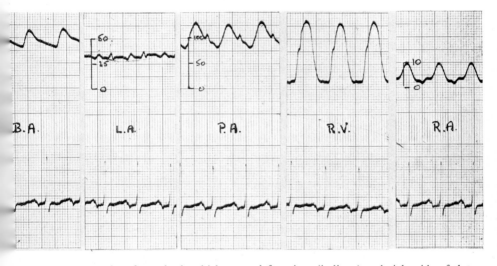

10.21—Pressure pulses from the brachial artery, left atrium (indirect) and right side of the in a case of mitral stenosis with an extreme pulmonary vascular resistance. The pulmonary y pressure is higher than that in the brachial artery and a giant *a* wave is seen in the right atrial tracing.

systemic level at rest (fig. 10.21); a pulmonary arterio-venous pressure gradient of some 30 to 70 mm. Hg; a high arterio-venous oxygen difference associated with a low cardiac output; and a pulmonary vascular resistance between 10 and 30 units (800 to 2,400 dynes sec./cm.^{5}).

These high resistance cases sooner or later develop right ventricular failure, and are especially prone to phlebothrombosis in the legs with secondary pulmonary embolism, which is often fatal.

Congestive heart failure

It has been stated more than once that uncomplicated cases of mitral stenosis with normal rhythm or controlled atrial fibrillation do not develop heart failure, although they may drown from pulmonary œdema. The complication above all others that causes failure is a high pulmonary vascular resistance. Thus in a consecutive series of 200 cases of mitral stenosis in which the resistance was measured, there was no single instance of heart failure when the resistance was less than 7 units, excluding cases with uncontrolled atrial fibrillation. When the resistance was 7 to 9.5 units, 50 per cent of the cases failed, and when it was 10 units or over 80 per cent failed (Wood, 1954). It was concluded from these unexpected findings that active carditis, residual myocardial fibrosis, or any other myocardial legacy from rheumatic fever could be dismissed as a practical cause for heart failure in cases of mitral stenosis. Since then, however, it must be admitted that rare exceptions to this general rule have been discovered.

The most dangerous precipitating cause of failure in these pulmonary hypertensive cases is pulmonary embolism secondary to phlebothrombosis in the legs.

The most common cause of reversible heart failure in cases of mitral stenosis is uncontrolled atrial fibrillation. The very rapid ventricular rate prevents adequate left ventricular filling; the cardiac output falls precipitously, the renal blood flow diminishes, sodium is retained and hydræmia causes œdema and raises the venous pressure; at the same time the left atrial pressure rises; passive pulmonary hypertension may be considerable, and if the resistance is moderately raised, the right ventricle may be easily overloaded; impairment of myocardial function secondary to an impoverished coronary blood flow adds to the difficulties. Congestive heart failure brought about in this way is far less serious than that accompanying severe pulmonary hypertension, and can be corrected rapidly by controlling the ventricular rate by means of digitalis.

An upper respiratory tract infection has been identified as the chief precipitating factor in 45 per cent of cases of heart failure from mitral stenosis (Werner, 1936). The effect may be due to tachycardia, paroxysmal atrial fibrillation, or a temporarily increased pulmonary vascular resistance.

Pulmonary embolism and infarction

Late hæmoptysis is usually caused by pulmonary infarction and is commonly associated with incipient or actual heart failure in high-resistance cases, the infarct resulting from pulmonary embolism secondary to phlebothrombosis in the legs. The low cardiac output, raised venous pressure, and immobilisation all encourage phlebothrombosis. Emboli are often recurrent, and by obstructing part of the pulmonary arterial tree increase the total pulmonary vascular resistance, so that heart failure increases, and a vicious circle is established. Pulmonary embolism is the commonest cause of death in this type of case. Pulmonary infarction may also result from pulmonary arterial thrombosis in cases of long-standing pulmonary hypertension, but this is believed to be relatively rare.

Pulmonary incompetence

Functional pulmonary incompetence in cases of mitral stenosis alway means a high pulmonary vascular resistance and considerable dilatation of the pulmonary artery. A basal diastolic murmur associated with a relatively normal pulmonary artery and normal resistance may be safely assumed to be aortic in origin, even when there is no other evidence of aortic incompetence.

Tricuspid incompetence

Functional tricuspid incompetence always means considerable dilatation of the right ventricle, and in cases of mitral stenosis implies a high pulmonary vascular resistance. The leak is usually reversible. The physical signs include a diminished *x* descent, high amplitude *v* wave, rapid *y* descent and deep *y* trough in the jugular pulse, systolic pulsation of the liver, and a pan-systolic murmur waxing on inspiration in the tricuspid area. In view of the great dilatation of the right ventricle in these cases, the tricuspid murmur may be very well heard at the apex beat, and may then be mistaken for the murmur of mitral incompetence.

If the pulmonary vascular resistance is not high, tricuspid incompetence should be regarded as organic, and careful re-examination is likely to disclose some evidence of stenosis, for organic tricuspid lesions are rarely purely incompetent.

Bacterial endocarditis

It is unusual for bacterial endocarditis to complicate established cases of mitral stenosis, and only one example has been seen by the writer while studying over 500 cases of mitral valve disease during the past seven years. When bacterial endocarditis involves the mitral valve, the latter is nearly always incompetent.

Massive thrombosis of the left atrium

Massive thrombosis occupying more than half of the left atrial cavity may be firmly adherent, pedunculated, or entirely free. It occurs in about 2 per cent of cases of mitral stenosis (Garvin, 1941), and is usually associated with atrial fibrillation. The left atrium shows no special features to account for the size of the clot. Free or pedunculated ball-valve thrombi may block the mitral orifice and virtually halt the circulation, causing sudden death; or partial obstruction may result in syncope, loss of peripheral pulses, and severe symmetrical ischæmia of the extremities, ears and tip of the nose, as emphasised by Fishberg (1940). More often, however, the symptoms of massive thrombosis do not differ qualitatively from those of uncomplicated mitral stenosis, but they may develop suddenly and tend to be severe. Angina pectoris was stressed by Evans and Benson (1948), and may be attributed to the unusually low output. It was hoped that angiocardiography might reveal an obvious filling defect of the left atrium in cases of massive thrombosis as it may experimentally in dogs (Read et al., 1955), but the clot has proved difficult to demonstrate by these or other pre-operative means.

ASSOCIATED CONDITIONS

Pregnancy. One of the most important events in the life history of a woman with mitral stenosis is pregnancy. The subject is discussed in detail elsewhere. It may be noted here, however, that one-third of all pregnancies in cases of mitral stenosis cause temporary (44 per cent) or permanent (56 per cent) deterioration. The chief symptoms are cough, dyspnœa, hæmoptysis, orthopnœa, paroxysmal dyspnœa and acute pulmonary œdema; atrial fibrillation, systemic embolism, and congestive failure are relatively rare. When symptoms develop they usually begin before the end of the first trimester. This tallies with physiological evidence that hydræmia and a moderate increase of cardiac output occur quite early in pregnancy, and can be demonstrated regularly during the third month (Burwell *et al.*, 1938; Palmer and Walker, 1949).

Anæmia, usually due to iron deficiency, may precipitate "congestive" symptoms in much the same way as pregnancy, the raised cardiac output being responsible. In practice the hæmoglobin is below 60 per cent, and usually below 50 per cent, before the output is sufficiently increased to raise the pulmonary venous pressure. Before advising valvotomy, therefore, it is wise to check the hæmoglobin, for symptoms may disappear after an iron deficiency anæmia is corrected.

Thyrotoxicosis aggravates the effects of mitral stenosis by causing tachycardia and a raised cardiac output, both of which are poorly tolerated as previously explained. The hyperthyroidism should be corrected medically before attempting to assess the severity of the mitral stenosis: if the latter requires valvotomy, there is a good case for treating the goitre first by means of radio-active iodine; if the stricture is relatively mild, the physician is at liberty to treat the thyrotoxicosis by any of the accepted methods that might seem most suitable on other grounds.

Active rheumatic carditis is present in at least one-third of relatively severe cases of mitral stenosis if Aschoff nodes in biopsy and post-mortem material may be so interpreted. The activity, however, is very low grade and rarely seems to influence the behaviour of the heart muscle; whether or not it has any bearing on the rate at which stenosis develops or increases however, is a moot point. Very occasionally, unexplained dilatation of the heart associated with a low cardiac output, left atrial pressure under 10 mm. Hg, and relatively normal pulmonary vascular resistance suggest serious myocarditis or myocardial fibrosis, but proof is lacking. In children with established mitral stenosis there is no doubt that a recurrence of active carditis may cause reversible heart failure, but fever, tachycardia and other hæmodynamic changes may be partly responsible. Considering the frequency of mitral stenosis it is quite likely that some cases of unexplained heart failure associated with a relatively mild stricture are due to non-rheumatic coincidental myocarditis of the type described by Gore and Sapphir (1947).

Rheumatoid arthritis may be associated with mitral stenosis and may b mistaken for a recurrence of rheumatic fever. The chief cardiac complication of rheumatoid is pericarditis, but a specific myocardial lesion occurs in about 2 per cent (Sokoloff, 1953). Mitral valve disease is never due to rheumatoid itself.

Chronic pulmonary tuberculosis occurs in about 2 per cent of cases, which is the same as in the general population. There is no evidence that the "congested" lung of mitral stenosis is antagonistic to tuberculosis.

Bronchitis and emphysema have already been discussed. Very rarely severe emphysema or *interstitial pulmonary fibrosis* may be incidentally associated with mitral stenosis and may be primarily responsible for breathlessness. Both should be carefully considered when dyspnœa seems disproportionate to the estimated degree of stenosis. It should be borne in mind that emphysema masks the auscultatory signs of mitral stenosis, that rhonci may well be due to œdematous bronchial mucosa secondary to mitral stenosis, that the radiological appearances of interstitial pulmonary fibrosis can be very similar to those of chronic interstitial pulmonary œdema, and that pulmonary physiology in these last two conditions can also be alike. If there is any doubt about what is causing the breathlessness, appropriate lung function tests should be carried out and the size of the mitral orifice calculated from data obtained at cardiac catheterisation, for mistakes are certainly being made both ways, patients with severe mitral stenosis being left to die in the belief that they are suffering from advanced emphysema, and patients with severe interstitial pulmonary fibrosis being operated on for relatively mild mitral stenosis under the false impression that the latter is causing the dyspnœa.

Essential hypertension (blood pressure 160/100 or above) occurred in only 3 per cent of the author's series, and the diastolic pressure was as high as 120 mm. Hg in only 1 per cent. Conversely, Bechgaard (1946) found that only 1 per cent of cases of essential hypertension had mitral stenosis. Following valvotomy any tendency towards hypertension may become more evident.

Congenital anomalies sometimes associated with congenital or acquired mitral stenosis include coarctation of the aorta, patent ductus arteriosus, and atrial septal defect. The effects of such combined lesions on the physiology of the circulation have already been described in chapter VIII. Since all are now repairable, double operations may be performed if necessary.

DIFFERENTIAL DIAGNOSIS

There is rarely much difficulty in recognising a case of mitral stenosis unless the characteristic physical signs are masked by a huge right ventricle or considerable emphysema; the diagnostic problem is more concerned with the degree of stricture, the amount of incompetence (if any), the height of the pulmonary vascular resistance, the state of the myocardium, the nature and degree of other valve lesions, the state of the lungs, and the presence or absence of the various complications or associated conditions enumerated and discussed above. No object would be achieved by commenting further on any of these things.

COURSE AND PROGNOSIS

The course of mitral stenosis may be summarised here with advantage. The initial rheumatic attack usually occurs between the ages of 8 and 12. The worst cases die within five years, the mortality in the active phase of the disease being 6.5 per cent. The vast majority of those that recover become temporarily free from symptoms, although some patients limit their activities on medical advice and others have a psychologically induced effort syndrome.

The symptom-free period lasts for an average of about 20 years. Approximately the first half of this period is occupied with the development of physiological stenosis, and is therefore a true latent interval; in the second half mitral stenosis can be readily detected, but the stricture is too mild to cause any symptoms. Around the age of 30 true effort dyspnœa develops and usually increases a grade every 2 to 3 years, so that total incapcity is reached in 7 to 8 years. The steps in this relentless deterioration often appear to be sudden, being precipitated by pregnancy, influenza, winter bronchitis, the onset of atrial fibrillation, a period of excessive worry or hard work, or some such factor. The course may also be punctuated by recurrent hæmoptysis, systemic embolism, acute pulmonary œdema, severe bronchitis, or paroxysmal atrial fibrillation.

A proportion of patients die prematurely from hemiplegia or acute pulmonary œdema. The development of structural changes in the interstitial tissue of the lungs helps to prolong life by allowing high left atrial pressures to be built up with relatively little danger of pulmonary œdema; and the development of a high pulmonary vascular resistance may prolong life by preventing the build-up of dangerously high left atrial pressures but at the expense of a low cardiac output and ultimate heart failure. Patients in the first group tend to die in an attack of acute bronchitis or bronchopneumonia, and those in the second group from heart failure, often aggravated or precipitated by phlebothrombosis and pulmonary embolism. The average duration of total incapacity is about three years, so that the total period of symptoms occupies about ten years, and the average age of death is about 40. There is, of course, a very wide variation in behaviour from case to case, some patients dying in adolescence, others reaching old age. The figures given indicate a better prognosis than in the series reported by De Graff and Lingg (1935), in which the average age of death was 2 for cases with normal rhythm and 38 for cases with atrial fibrillation, and a worse prognosis than in the follow-up series analysed by Olesen (1955) in which the average age of death was 47, and the interval between the onset of symptoms and total incapacity was 15 years.

TREATMENT

The management and treatment of cases of mitral stenosis is a joint concern, being partly medical and partly surgical. All agree theoretically that this should be so, but in practice there is a growing tendency for the physician's part to be dismissed as unnecessary and time wasting, so that more and more patients are being sent direct to surgical clinics. It is imperative that this tendency be halted abruptly and permanently, for the total physiological disturbance that results from mitral valve disease is very much a medical problem: it is often thoroughly complicated and proper selection of cases for surgical treatment demands a physician's knowledge, training and skill; moreover, there is a great deal more in the management of cases of mitral stenosis than surgical relief of the stricture, fundamental and epoch-making though the latter may be. The physician's therapeutic responsibilities include governing the patient's total activities, steering a woman through or away from pregnancy, recognising and treating important coincidental conditions such as psycho-neurosis, anæmia and thyrotoxicosis, managing recurrent hæmoptysis, preventing and treating paroxysmal cardiac dyspnœa and acute pulmonary œdema, respecting and treating attacks of winter bronchitis, controlling the rhythm, preventing systemic and pulmonary embolism as far as possible, appreciating the cause of heart failure and improving the circulation as much as possible, selecting cases that require valvotomy and preparing them for the operation, restoring normal rhythm post-operatively, accurately assessing the physiological situation three months later, and guiding the patient in the most advantageous way for the rest of his medically eventful life, for valvotomy does not cure rheumatic heart disease. The outstanding aims of medical research workers in this field must be to prevent rheumatic fever, to prevent or cure active endocarditis, or at least to prevent fusion of the cusps.

The patient's *work and other activities* should be regulated in accordance with the expected life-history of the lesion. If there is no detectable stenosis or no more than a trivial mitral leak 10 to 15 years after the initial rheumatic attack, the patient should be encouraged to lead an entirely normal life. If, on the other hand, stenosis can be detected at this time, even though trivial in degree, the patient should be advised to take up an occupation that will never involve him in more than light physical work, so that when symptoms develop he will not have to retire. During the symptom-free period, ordinary physical activities, including all but the most strenuous competetive sports such as rowing and long-distance running, should be allowed; on the other hand, such patients must be rejected for national service and are likely to be rejected or heavily loaded by life insurance companies. A woman wanting to have a family should take advantage of this latent period in which to complete it, for it may be her last safe opportunity to do so. At the average age of 30 or so, grade 1 effort intolerance develops and progresses to grade 2A over a variable time averaging about three years. During this period patients should be encouraged to continue all activities that do not cause dyspnœa, but to avoid those that do. If their occupations have been chosen wisely, they should have no difficulty in continuing with their work free from breathlessness. Any further deterioration usually means that dyspnœa is beginning to interfere seriously with the patient's happiness and comfort, and the time for valvotomy has arrived.

Pregnancy precipitates or aggravates symptoms in one-third of cases, the deterioration being permanent in half of them. If the valve lesion is obviously amenable to surgical treatment, a woman with grade 1 or 2A effort intolerance should not be advised against pregnancy if she is willing to have the operation should the necessity arise. If symptoms are not aggravated all is well. If she deteriorates seriously she usually begins to do so in the third month, and valvotomy can then be carried out if necessary, the pregnancy being allowed to continue to term. If the patient starts pregnancy with only grade 1 effort intolerance, any exaccerbation of symptoms can usually be controlled by medical means, and valvotomy is better deferred; patients starting pregnancy with grade 2A effort intolerance are more likely to cause anxiety and may well require valvotomy during the second trimester. Women with grade 2B effort intolerance should be advised against pregnancy unless valvotomy is carried out first; if they are already pregnant valvotomy should be advised without delay. If the nature of the valve lesion is such as to make surgical relief impracticable, women with more than slight effort intolerance should be advised against pregnancy and preferably sterilised. If she has already conceived, the pregnancy is best terminated during the first three or four months by therapeutic abortion or hysterectomy; if she is already five or six months pregnant and her life is not in imminent danger, she can usually be taken through to term and delivered naturally, symptoms being controlled by rest and appropriate medical measures. Urgent hysterotomy is rarely necessary or desirable.

Coincidental psycho-neurosis may be entirely responsible for any disability in cases of mitral stenosis, the symptoms being wholly psychosomatic, or it may encourage pulmonary congestive symptoms by raising the cardiac output and heart rate. This is an important diagnostic problem which must be solved correctly. Effective psychotherapy is as important as curing anæmia or controlling thyrotoxicosis, and should be undertaken before advising valvotomy.

Coincidental anæmia may be spontaneous or secondary to repeated hæmoptysis, usually the former. Iron deficiency is commonly responsible and replacement therapy rapidly effective. Transfusion is rarely required but packed cells may be given slowly if necessary. Intravenous infusion of any kind are highly dangerous in mitral stenosis.

Coincidental thyrotoxicosis is probably best treated by means of radioactive iodine. Mitral valvotomy can then be undertaken later, if necessary. Partial thyroidectomy is not without added risk in the presence of tight mitral stenosis, and antithyroid drugs are unlikely to be satisfactory in the long run. In view of the bad effect of a raised cardiac output on cases of mitral valve disease, it is imperative that the thyrotoxicosis should be properly and permanently controlled.

Suspected or proved rheumatic activity should be allowed to settle down before advising valvotomy when the latter is indicated, but the operation should not be deferred if it is urgent. There is no convincing evidence that cortisone improves the carditis or diminishes the operation risk.

Hæmoptysis from rupture of a broncho-pulmonary venous radicle usually ceases spontaneously within a few hours. If it is severe or repetitive it may be wise to lower the pulmonary venous pressure by means of rest, posture, mersalyl and a low sodium diet. The patient should be reassured that these hæmorrhages are not serious, occur relatively early in the course of mitral stenosis, are not in themselves an indication for valvotomy, and tend not to recur after certain natural adjustments to the circulation have taken place.

Acute pulmonary œdema is a medical emergency, but it is not a surgical emergency. The patient should be treated sitting bolt upright with the legs down. Venous tourniquets should be applied to the thighs as high up as possible. Morphine gr. ¼ or pethidine 100 mg. should be injected intramuscularly. The chief object of these measures is to lower the right ventricular output and so reduce the pulmonary venous pressure. Powerful sedatives may also have some indirect influence on the permeability of the pulmonary capillaries. Aminophylline, 0.24 G. intravenously, may help by relieving bronchospasm. Oxygen, administered through a simple light plastic mask, may help to correct the falling arterial oxygen tension, and counteract the adverse effect of anoxia on the pulmonary capillary permeability; whether or not anoxia helps to bring the attack to an end by causing pulmonary vasoconstriction is not yet known for certain, but a fall in alveolar oxygen tension is known to have this effect, and oxygen may yet prove to be a two-edged weapon.

If the patient does not improve, a suction catheter should be passed down the trachea via the nose or mouth in order to clear the air passages, or if facilities are available bronchoscopic suction may be employed. This may be life-saving when a patient is drowning in fluid which is filling the air passages. Finally, venesection should not be unduly delayed if the occasion seems to demand it; about a pint of blood should be removed.

Acute pulmonary œdema can usually be prevented when its imminence is recognised by limiting physical and emotional activities (sexual intercourse is a common precipitating agent), and prescribing a low sodium diet, mercurial diuretics and sedatives. Patients should sleep well propped up at night. Respiratory infections should be treated promptly in these dangerous cases, for they too may precipitate an attack. Paroxysmal atrial fibrillation, with a rapid ventricular rate, may also be responsible, and if this is suspected, digitalis should be given.

When the situation is under good medical control, but not before, valvotomy should be performed. It has been well said that the patient should not be allowed to leave hospital until the stricture has been relieved (Baker *et al.*, 1952).

Paroxysmal cardiac dyspnœa, in which the exudation from the capillaries does not extend beyond the interstitial tissues, calls for the same remedial and prophylactic treatment as acute pulmonary œdema, except that intra-tracheal suction is never indicated.

Acute bronchitis deserves considerable respect, for attacks are accompanied by much discomfort and dyspnœa, and blood spitting may add to the patient's alarm. Antibiotics should be supported by strong measures designed to lower the bronchial venous pressure, e.g. posture and mercurial diuretics, a low sodium diet, and strict control of the ventricular rate by means of digitalis in cases with atrial fibrillation. Aminophylline helps to relieve bronchospasm.

The onset of paroxysmal or permanent atrial fibrillation is usually accompanied by a very rapid ventricular rate, which in cases of mitral stenosis may have serious consequences, as previously explained. The chief dangers are acute pulmonary œdema, congestive heart failure, and cerebral embolism. The onset of atrial fibrillation in mitral stenosis should therefore be regarded as a medical emergency, and should be treated promptly with digitalis, heparin and dehydration until the ventricular rate is controlled. The object of the heparin is to prevent left atrial thrombosis, and 15,000 units should be given intravenously in the first instance, followed by similar doses two or three times daily intravenously or intramuscularly until digitalis is having the desired effect. Prophylactic dehydration by means of mercurial diuretics and a fruit and rice diet for 48 hours help to prevent pulmonary œdema and heart failure. If the patient happens to be in hospital at the time, and therefore under constant supervision, it may be best to give digoxin intravenously in an initial dose of 1 mg., followed by 0.5 mg. two-hourly until the ventricular rate is under 100 beats per minute, after which injections should be replaced by an oral maintenance dose. A single injection of heparin intravenously and 2 ml. of mersalyl intramuscularly should then suffice, for the ventricular rate should be controlled within six hours. If acute pulmonary œdema is present or threatened when the patient is first seen, the initial intravenous dose of digoxin may be 1.5 mg., but on no account more than this, and subsequent doses must never exceed 0.5 mg.

Permanent atrial fibrillation is best treated with a maintenance dose of digitalis, attempts to restore and maintain normal rhythm being rarely worth while prior to valvotomy. The matter is discussed more fully in chapter VI.

Systemic embolism is due to liberation of a fresh clot from the left atrium and though usually unpredictable, a limited number undoubtedly occur within a few days following the onset of atrial fibrillation with rapid ventricular rate, and these could probably be prevented by means of heparin if the danger were more widely recognised. Emboli are often recurrent, and in view of their serious consequences there is something to be said in favour of treating all embolic cases with dindevan until valvotomy is performed, or for life if for any reason valvotomy is contra-indicated. Embolism bears little relation to the degree of mitral stricture as previously pointed out, but its occurrence in otherwise uncomplicated mitral stenosis is usually sufficient reason for advising valvotomy, unless the mitral index is over 45 per cent. Treatment of the embolism is discussed in chapter I.

Pulmonary embolism is a late manifestation of a retarded circulation in cases with a high pulmonary vascular resistance and actual or incipient heart failure. In my own series this was the commonest cause of death in cases of mitral stenosis, partly because the danger was not at first recognised. Since treating all severe pulmonary hypertensive cases with dindevan until mitral valvotomy was carried out, there have been no further deaths from this source over a period of nearly three years. Prior to the adoption of this policy, seven out of eight medical deaths from mitral stenosis were due to pulmonary embolism, six of them in high resistance cases (Wood, 1954). During the same period there was only one death from acute pulmonary œdema and that was partly the result of bronchopneumonia.

If pulmonary embolism has already occurred, 15,000 units of heparin should be given at once intravenously, followed by adequate anticoagulant treatment, for the danger of further phlebothrombosis is imminent and any delay in preventing it may be lethal. There need be no fear that anti-coagulants may cause serious hæmorrhage from a pulmonary infarct, although hæmoptysis may be rather more prolonged. The risk with which we are concerned is not hæmorrhage from an infarct, but obstruction of the pulmonary circulation from recurrent embolism. If mitral valvotomy cannot be carried out in this type of case, because there is too much mitral incompetence, the patient is too old, or the operation is refused, then permanent anticoagulant therapy should probably be advised.

The immediate treatment of massive pulmonary embolism also includes nursing the patient flat, oxygen, respiratory stimulants such as amino-phylline or coramine, and digitalis, as described in chapter XVII.

Heart failure calls for complete rest, preferably in a cardiac bed, digitalis, mercurial diuretics and a low sodium diet, as detailed in chapter VII. In cases of mitral stenosis it is especially important to identify the cause of the failure, for it is far from being an inevitable consequence of the valve lesion. The only two common causes are uncontrolled atrial fibrillation and a high pulmonary vascular resistance. With the former rapid recovery follows adequate doses of digitalis alone, and the subsequent outlook may then be quite good; the latter is much more serious, and improvement can only be temporary unless mitral valvotomy is performed.

MITRAL VALVOTOMY

The treatment of mitral stenosis has been radically altered since the introduction of mitral valvotomy by Harken (1948) and Bailey (1949) in the United States, and independently by Brock (Baker, Brock an Campbell, 1950) in England. It is true that Souttar performed the first successful digital mitral valvotomy as early as 1925, but the operation did not gain favour at that time, perhaps because it was then believed that the myocardium was primarily at fault and the valve lesion relatively unim- portant; at that time, too, thoracic surgery was a formidable undertaking, anæsthesia was far less advanced, there were no antibiotics, and there was little to encourage cardiac surgery of any kind. In 1948, however, the situation was radically different, and mitral valvotomy was instantly acclaimed. Since then thousands of cases of mitral stenosis have been relieved of their stricture, and parallel physiological studies have placed the operation on a firm scientific footing. The easiest and best approach is through the left atrial appendage. In the simplest cases the fused com- missures are separated digitally, and the split is continued as far as the ring on both sides. More often dense cross fusion at the critical areas of tendinous insertion have to be cut with a special knife. Sometimes only one commissure can be split, and occasionally the architecture of the valve is so deranged that little can be done. Heavy calcification may also interfere with the operation, particularly on the medial side, but not necessarily. Clots in the left atrium can usually be recognised by the surgeon and may often be washed out by allowing a brief frank hæmorrhage to take place through the atrial appendix; a second precaution is to place tapes behind the common carotid arteries, so that these vessels may be occluded for a few vital seconds when there is any danger of embolism. For proper surgical details, however, the reader must consult appropriate surgical works.

Selection of cases for valvotomy

In general, any patient who is *suffering* from the effects of mitral *stenosis* requires valvotomy, and any patient who is able to continue his normal occupation without distress does not. There are several reasons for not operating prematurely: (1) the surgical mortality in relatively mild un- complicated cases is not negligible (1.7 per cent in my own series); (2) the risk of cerebral embolism at operation is not confined to advanced cases; (3) a technically good result is only achieved in 75 per cent of cases and is no more likely when the stricture is relatively mild than when it is extreme; (4) there is little doubt that post-operative re-stenosis is going to prove troublesome, for it is already occurring at the rate of about 2 per cent per annum, and second valvotomies are proving more difficult than the first. The chief dangers of waiting until effort intolerance is grade 2B are cerebral embolism and acute pulmonary œdema, both of which may occur unexpectedly in relatively mild cases.

Any patient, then, with simple mitral stenosis and grade 2B or greater effort intolerance should be advised to have the stricture relieved. The following remarks summarise briefly the various modifying factors that have been discussed in detail previously.

Age. Patients under 20 years old should be deferred as long as possible in view of the likelihood of activity and the presumed greater risk of re-stenosis; patients in the sixth decade, on the other hand, should not be deferred too long for they may soon be too old for the operation.

Rheumatic activity is obviously adverse, but is not a contra-indication if life is threatened by the stricture.

Recurrent bronchitis should encourage valvotomy, for it is usually the result of a high bronchial venous pressure. Secondary emphysema is rarely severe enough to prevent a successful outcome.

Systemic embolism is the one complication that demands valvotomy at a time that would be regarded as premature on other grounds.

Hæmoptysis, even when recurrent and profuse, rarely provides sufficient reason for surgical intervention.

Acute pulmonary œdema provides the strongest grounds for advising valvotomy as soon as intensive medical treatment has brought the situation under control.

A *high pulmonary vascular resistance* may mask the severity of mitral stenosis by inhibiting pulmonary venous "congestion". Since the resistance is never raised unless the stenosis is at least critical, valvotomy should be undertaken in all such cases. When the resistance is extreme the matter is urgent owing to the grave danger of heart failure and pulmonary embolism.

Atrial fibrillation has no direct bearing on the question of surgery; but if it has been associated with a rapid ventricular rate, breathlessness and œdema may give a false impression of the severity of the stenosis, and an operation may have been advised when only digitalis is needed.

Of the physical signs of uncomplicated mitral stenosis, only the brevity of the interval between the aortic second sound and the opening snap, and the length of the mitral diastolic murmur give any indication of the severity of the lesion. The louder and sharper the first sound and the opening snap the more mobile are the mitral cusps, and in such cases a good technical result may be expected from valvotomy (Sellors, Bedford and Somerville, 1953). Damping of the first sound and absence of the snap are usually due to heavy calcification, but this should not prevent a successful outcome although only one commissure may be split.

The *electrocardiogram* should show an obvious P mitrale in any case severe enough to warrant valvotomy, provided the rhythm is normal. Right ventricular preponderance, judged by the appearances in multiple chest leads, means a high pulmonary vascular resistance, and therefore indicates surgical treatment.

X-rays are particularly helpful in showing the amount of chronic interstitial œdema present, for this is closely related to the pulmonary venous pressure and therefore to the degree of stricture. Radiological evidence of pulmonary hypertension emphasises the need for valvotomy; it should be remembered that in these cases signs of pulmonary venous "congestion" may be absent.

Cardiac catheterisation should reveal a left atrial pressure well over 10 mm. Hg with reference to the sternal angle, a mitral stenotic index not exceeding 33 per cent, and an Ry/v ratio not exceeding 1.5; average figures for surgical cases are 22 mm. Hg, 15 to 20 per cent, and 0.8 to 1.0 respectively. A high pulmonary vascular resistance, which in case of mitral stenosis always indicates valvotomy, means that the pulmonary arteriovenous pressure gradient is at least 30 mm. Hg, and the gradient divided by the cardiac output in litres per minute is at least 6, and in extreme cases at least 10. If the Gorlin formula is used the critical mitral orifice is 1 cm.².

The chief difficulties in selecting cases for valvotomy, however, usually have less to do with the criteria and modifying factors just enumerated than with estimating the significance and degree of other valve lesions, especially mitral incompetence. To discuss the effect of other valve lesions on the varying physiology of mitral stenosis would entail too much repetition to be profitable, for the possible permutations and combinations are almost endless. Considerable experience is necessary to appreciate just what is going on in some of these complicated cases, and the decision to advise or withhold mitral valvotomy can be very difficult.

Pre-operative treatment

Medical measures designed to diminish the operative risk and postoperative complications include rest and sedatives, digitalis, dehydration, anticoagulants, and treatment of bronchitis.

Rest and sedatives are advisable for a few days beforehand while the total situation is being reviewed, but if unduly prolonged merely add to the patient's anxiety.

Digitalis should be given as a routine whether there is normal rhythm or otherwise, so that a rapid ventricular rate does not accompany postoperative atrial fibrillation should that occur. It is wise to start digitalis two or three weeks before valvotomy is planned, so that the right maintenance dose is arrived at in good time. This is not easily determined in cases with normal rhythm free from heart failure. It may be best to start with tabs. dig. folia gr. 2 t.d.s. for two days, followed by gr. 1 t.d.s. for two days, followed by gr. 1 twice daily thereafter. This should prove sufficient in most cases and rarely too much. If nausea develops, the maintenance dose should be reduced to gr. ½ t.d.s. or 0.1 mg. of digitoxin daily, which is its equivalent. When there is atrial fibrillation the ventricular rate must be properly controlled before valvotomy.

Quinidine is not advised. It has failed to prevent post-operative atrial fibrillation and unless full doses of digitalis are also given it then encourages a more rapid ventricular rate, slowing down the speed of the f waves so that the ventricles try to keep pace.

Dehydration by means of mercurial diuretics and a low sodium diet, supported or not with resins or diamox, should be strictly enforced in all cases liable to acute pulmonary œdema or paroxysmal dyspnœa, in all orthopnœa cases, when X-rays show considerable interstitial hilar mottling, and when there is heart failure secondary to a high pulmonary vascular resistance, but not otherwise.

Anticoagulants have already been discussed in relation to cases with an extreme pulmonary vascular resistance or recurrent systemic embolism. Dicoumarol, tromexan or dindevan is usually withheld four or five days before the operation.

Bronchitis should be improved as much as possible before valvotomy. This may mean a course of some suitable antibiotic—penicillin if the organism is believed to be the pneumococcus, streptomycin if H. influenzæ is responsible (May, 1953)—in addition to dehydration (to lower the bronchial venous pressure) and antispasmodics such as aminophylline.

Valvotomy should be deferred for several months following *hemiplegia* in view of the grave risk of post-operative pulmonary complications in these cases.

Post-operative course and management

Immediate post-operative management is a surgical responsibility and includes treatment of shock, peripheral embolism, hæmorrhage, collapse of the lungs, attending to pleural drainage and regulating fluid balance. The comments made here are confined to the more medical aspects of the case.

Hemiplegia occurs in about 5 per cent of cases, and is always due to cerebral embolism at the time of the operation, although it may not be discovered until the patient regains consciousness. Subsequent embolism is extremely rare. There is no effective treatment for embolic hemiplegia, but spontaneous improvement may be rapid and considerable.

Aortic saddle embolism or high femoral embolism is usually detected immediately if it occurs during the operation, because checking all peripheral pulses is part of the surgical routine. Embolectomy is always best carried out then and there.

Post-operative psychosis may be attributable to prolonged cardiac standstill or ventricular fibrillation during the valvotomy, or to hepatic failure in patients who have had prolonged heart failure. The first type is usually represented by a quietly confused, soporific or comatose state; the second by violently aggressive, abusive or paranoid behaviour. Both are serious in that they represent considerable functional damage to the cerebral cortex and liver respectively. As a rule, recovery is complete within a few weeks, but a minority lapse into coma and death. Little can be done to influence the issue.

Chest complications include hæmothorax, pleural effusion, collapse of the lung, and bronchitis or bronchopneumonia. They usually settle down satisfactorily with appropriate treatment.

Post-operative atrial fibrillation occurs in one-quarter of the cases with previously normal rhythm. This is not prevented by quinidine, but causes little disturbance if prophylactic digitalis has been given. It usually develops between the second and fifth day, and if left to nature stops spontaneously after an average of ten days in about half the cases, and becomes permanent in the other half. Attempts to restore normal rhythm at once usually fail; the natural course of events indicates that quinidine should be withheld until the end of the second post-operative week, and if given then proves successful in 95 per cent of cases in which the valvotomy has been technically successful (Wood, 1954).

Normal rhythm can also be restored in 50 per cent of patients with established pre-operative atrial fibrillation, but can only be maintained for long in three-fifths of these.

If the initial attempt to restore normal rhythm fails, a second attempt may be made a few weeks later, but usually without lasting success.

The chief contra-indications to quinidine therapy include technically unsuccessful valvotomy, too much mitral incompetence, extensive left atrial thrombosis, and grossly diseased left atrial muscle found at operation. The most important additional factor militating against prolonged maintenance of normal rhythm is advancing age.

Traumatic pericarditis is believed to be responsible for the recurrent attacks of left chest pain and fever that punctuate the post-operative course in 10 per cent of cases (Wood, 1954). The pain is pericardial in behaviour and distribution; there may be pericardial friction or radiological evidence of effusion; there are often electrocardiographic changes compatible with pericarditis. The fever lasts about a week and subsides without treatment. After an interval of two or three weeks a second attack may occur, and then perhaps a third or even a fourth. Sooner or later the attacks cease for good, and leave no sequelæ; they are not dangerous, but may interfere considerably with convalescence. Similar episodes occur when a bullet or piece of shrapnel is lying in or close to the pericardium, and have also been observed following direct cardiac surgery in cases of pulmonary stenosis.

"Heart failure" following mitral valvotomy may be due to post-operative sodium retention or chloride deficiency, to increased mitral incompetence, or to uncontrolled atrial fibrillation. An increase of pulmonary venous congestion is nearly always due to the unfortunate development of considerable mitral incompetence, which is one of the risks of surgical treatment. Convalescence should be very slow in these cases, to give the left ventricle time to adjust itself to the changed conditions. Should signs of "heart failure" develop with normal serum electrolytes, normal rhythm, controlled atrial fibrillation, and no mitral incompetence, pericardial effusion should be excluded before blaming the myocardium. A rare cause of post-operative heart failure is pulmonary embolism.

Patients are usually allowed to get up during the second week, as soon as their condition warrants it, and if there are no complications they may be discharged from hospital during the third week; but they should remain under close medical supervision for three months if possible, and should be warned of the possibility of recurrent pericarditis.

Results

In the first 260 patients operated on at the Brompton Hospital 6.9 per cent died. The results were excellent in 30 per cent, good in 40 per cent, fair in 15 per cent, and poor in 8 per cent. The best cases became symptom free or, if previously totally incapacitated, improved to the extent of having only slight effort intolerance. In other words, effort intolerance changed by three grades. The result was classed as good when effort intolerance changed by two grades, and fair when it changed by one grade. These results are more or less similar to those reported by other clinics (e.g. Janton, Glover and O'Neill, 1952; Sellors, Bedford and Somerville, 1953; Ellis and Harken, 1955).

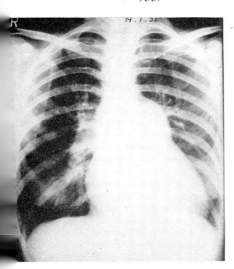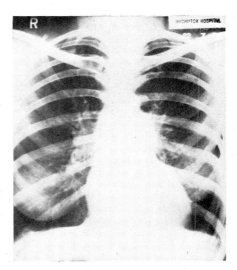

Fig. 10.22—Skiagrams (a) before, and (b) two years after mitral valvotomy in a case of mitral stenosis with an extreme pulmonary vascular resistance. In (b) there is considerable reduction in the size of the right ventricle, the pulmonary artery is less dilated and there is a gap on the left border of the heart which was previously occupied by the left atrial appendix.

When the results were analysed more fully it was found that the surgical mortality in uncomplicated cases of simple mitral stenosis was only 1.7 per cent, whereas it was 33 per cent in cases with an extreme pulmonary vascular resistance, 13 per cent when aortic valvotomy was carried out as well, and 6.2 per cent when mitral stenosis was complicated by significant incompetence.

Post-operative re-assessment

It has become customary to judge the results of valvotomy by the improvement in the patients' effort tolerance, and it has been stated repeatedly that the physical signs do not change much. It must be pointed out, however, that following a dramatic operation of this kind patients may become psychiatrically conditioned not to recognise cardiac symptoms and I have more than once found a patient in frank congestive failure who alleged that he was symptom free. Objective tests of effort tolerance and physiological studies of circulatory behaviour are more reliable. There is no doubt also that the physical signs may change materially; when a technically successful valvotomy has been performed, the presystolic murmur disappears, the first heart sound becomes far less accentuated, the opening snap is distinctly late, and the mitral diastolic murmur shortens considerably. Radiologically, "pulmonary venous congestion" diminishes, the left ventricle may fill out, and in pulmonary hypertensive cases the dilated right ventricle shrinks (fig. 10.22).

Post-operative cardiac catheterisation in successful cases reveals a considerable fall in left atrial and pulmonary artery pressures, a rise in cardiac output, a fall in pulmonary vascular resistance in cases with active pulmonary hypertension, and a gratifying increase of the Ry/v ratio, mitral stenotic index and calculated transverse section of the mitral orifice.

Subsequent course

In technically successful cases the marked improvement in effort tolerance has been well maintained in the majority of cases, but relapse due to re-stenosis has occurred at an approximate rate of 2 per cent per annum. In the absence of re-stenosis hæmoptysis, systemic embolism, winter bronchitis, angina pectoris, pulmonary œdema, paroxysmal cardiac dyspnœa and pulmonary embolism have not recurred, and in pulmonary hypertensive cases congestive failure has proved reversible in those that survived the operation.

Patients have been encouraged to return to work and resume active lives. Subsequent pregnancies have been encouraged and have caused no trouble apart from one instance in which toxæmia caused death from acute pulmonary œdema; the valve orifice at post-mortem was only slightly stenosed (2×1 cm.).

Poor or indifferent results have been due to technical failure to relieve the stricture sufficiently, the production or aggravation of mitral incompetence, or the presence or development of some other factor such as a myocardial fault, aortic valve disease (always more obvious after mitral valvotomy), independent bronchitis and emphysema, or psychoneurosis; occasionally, re-stenosis has occurred remarkably quickly, as in the case reported by Donzelot *et al.* (1953).

OTHER FORMS OF SURGICAL TREATMENT

Relief of pulmonary venous congestion has been achieved by *anastamosing the dorsal segment branch of the right inferior pulmonary vein to the azygos vein* (Bland and Sweet, 1949; D'Allaines *et al.*, 1949), and this type of operation may still have a place in cases that for one reason or another cannot have a mitral valvotomy, e.g. when there is too much mitral incompetence, or when valvotomy has proved technically too difficult.

Left atrial appendectomy was suggested as a means of preventing recurrent systemic embolism (Madden, 1949), and might still be considered in cases of combined stenosis and incompetence with an unusually large atrial appendage; but there is little guarantee that clots will not form in the body of the left atrium, and permanent anticoagulant therapy is probably the wiser course in these difficult cases.

Ligation of the inferior vena cava has been carried out with the dual object of relieving pulmonary venous congestion or heart failure and preventing pulmonary embolism secondary to phlebothrombosis in the legs (Cossio and Perianes, 1949). Although this operation has received a good deal of support in allegedly suitable cases, it is not physiological and there are better ways of achieving the objects stated.

AORTIC INCOMPETENCE

FREQUENCY

Rheumatic endocarditis accounts for 67 per cent of all cases of aortic regurgitation with or without stenosis, syphilis being responsible for 19 per cent, atherosclerosis for 7 per cent, and bacterial endocarditis for 2 per cent (Campbell, 1932). Congenital bicuspid or quadricuspid valve, congenital hypoplasia and dilatation of the ascending aorta, dissecting aneurysm, trauma, and simple severe hypertension without atherosclerosis of the valve account for the remaining 5 per cent. In cases of chronic rheumatic heart disease the aortic valve is involved in 44 per cent (Cabot, 1926). The present account deals primarily with the rheumatic type.

A good account of the history of aortic regurgitation was given by Rolleston (1940).

AGE AND SEX

About 90 per cent of cases of dominant rheumatic aortic incompetence are between 10 and 50 years of age, and have had the lesion since the original rheumatic attack. In Campbell's series the average age of the patients seen was 30. Males are affected twice as frequently as females.

CLASSIFICATION

There are five clinical types of rheumatic aortic valve disease:

1. Pure aortic incompetence.
2. Aortic incompetence with trivial stenosis.
3. Mixed aortic incompetence and stenosis.
4. Aortic stenosis with trivial incompetence.
5. Pure aortic stenosis.

While this appears to be obvious, it is stated for clarity, and is parallel to the five varieties of mitral valve disease. Types 1 and 2 are similar physiologically, as are types 4 and 5. In addition, any type may be complicated by any variety of mitral or tricuspid valve disease, by any degree of myocardial dysfunction, and by changes in the pulmonary vascular resistance. Cases may therefore be very complex. We are concerned here, however, with dominant aortic incompetence (type 1 or 2).

PATHOLOGY

Rheumatic inflammation of the aortic valve may cause immediate aortic incompetence. Healing usually results in thickening, retraction, and distortion of the cusps, with permanent regurgitation. In addition, the cusps often become adherent to one another at their bases (fusion of the commissures), so that some degree of aortic stenosis is usual. Secondary calcification is common when there is stenosis.

EFFECT ON FUNCTION

The stroke-volume of the left ventricle is increased by an amount which is at least equal to the quantity of blood that leaks back during diastole. The fibres of the left ventricle become considerably stretched in diastole: the force of the heart beat is therefore augmented according to Starling's law. The initial tension is increased, isometric contraction is abbreviated, maximum pressure is higher than normal and is attained earlier in systole, the ejection phase is shortened, and the pressure then falls away steeply in late systole. In other words, the shape of the pressure curve is altered so that early systole is loaded and late systole unloaded (Wiggers, 1935). The large quantity of blood pumped so quickly and powerfully into the relaxed arteries during early systole causes an abrupt percussion wave followed by late systolic collapse. The low diastolic pressure is due partly to the aortic reflux and partly to peripheral vasodilatation; the latter encourages forward flow. Both add to the collapsing quality of the pulse.

The cardiac output per minute remains about normal or may be even a little raised, as it is in patent ductus arteriosus and arterio-venous aneurysm, which have much in common with aortic incompetence. Effort tolerance is usually remarkably good until the disease is well advanced. Sooner or later, however, left ventricular failure develops, often suddenly and unexpectedly. The heart then becomes overloaded and the output falls below normal.

Zimmerman (1950) catheterised the left ventricle via the radial artery in 10 cases of aortic incompetence: when there was no clinical evidence of failure (three cases) the left ventricular diastolic pressure was normal, averaging 1.3 mm. Hg, whereas when there was congestive heart failure (seven cases) the left ventricular diastolic pressure ranged between 15 and 39 mm. Hg, and averaged 25 mm. Hg. It is hardly necessary to point out that in the absence of mitral stenosis the left ventricular diastolic pressure is the same as the left atrial diastolic pressure and can be measured accurately by more conventional methods.

Experimental aortic incompetence, brought about suddenly, markedly reduces the efficiency of the heart. After three or four months, however, left ventricular hypertrophy may be sufficient to compensate for the defect, and work capacity may be normal. If the valve lesion is then repaired the heart may be capable of performing more work than before. When two cusps are injured, however, full compensation is never achieved (Dieckhoff, 1936).

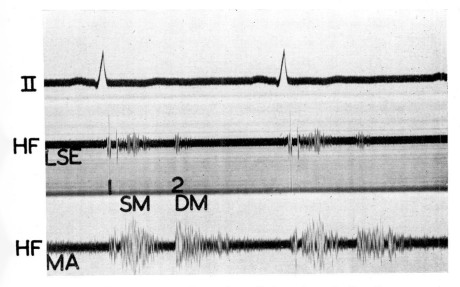

Fig. 10.23—Phonocardiogram illustrating a diminuendo aortic diastolic murmur.

CLINICAL FEATURES

Unlike mitral stenosis, aortic incompetence develops during the stage of active valvulitis, and may be at once permanent. Its early diagnosis depends entirely upon recognising an aortic diastolic murmur, heard best down the left border of the sternum, and closely resembling the sound of a whispered "R" (Hope, 1839). In contrast to the mitral diastolic murmur, there is little or no gap between it and the second heart sound, the one passing almost imperceptibly into the other. Thus the usual two-beat metre of the heart sounds is not altered (fig. 10.23). In distinguishing aortic from mitral diastolic murmurs, the greatest stress is laid on this difference in rhythm, for aortic murmurs may be heard best at the apex beat. It has already been explained that owing to the appreciable period that must elapse between the closure of the aortic and the opening of the mitral valves, mitral diastolic murmurs give rise to a three-beat dactylic cardiac metre. Only when aortic incompetence is trivial is there any clinically detectable delay in the onset of the bruit, for in these cases the murmur may only be audible when there is maximum turbulence, and this may not develop until the left ventricular diastolic pressure approaches zero. The appearance of the murmur phonocardiographically is then diamond-shaped (Wells, Rappaport and Sprague, 1949). As discussed under rheumatic carditis, aortic diastolic murmurs of this kind may be transient in about 20 per cent of active cases.

SYMPTOMS OF ESTABLISHED AORTIC INCOMPETENCE

Effort tolerance usually remains remarkably good until the left ventricle begins to fail, when breathlessness, orthopnœa and paroxysmal cardiac dyspnœa develop. Palpitations and throbbing, however, may cause discomfort earlier. Angina pectoris occurs in less than 5 per cent of cases and only when the leak is exceptionally free. Distressing attacks of pain accompanied by violent palpitations and tachycardia sometimes occur on the slightest provocation, even at rest at night. If the patient does not die from acute pulmonary œdema, congestive heart failure sets in sooner or later; sometimes it develops without clinical evidence of previous left ventricular failure, as in all left-sided lesions.

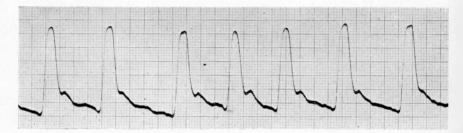

Fig. 10.24—Arteriogram illustrating the water-hammer pulse of aortic incompetence. The percussion wave is unusually abrupt; collapse precedes the pre-dicrotic notch, and is therefore a late systolic event.

PHYSICAL SIGNS

When incompetence is well developed, numerous changes in the heart and circulation may be recognised in addition to the characteristic aortic diastolic murmur. Owing to enlargement of the left ventricle, the apex beat is displaced downwards and to the left, and the cardiac impulse is heaving and hyperdynamic. At the mitral area a diastolic murmur may develop which has all the qualities of mitral origin: there is a gap between its commencement and the second heart sound; it is soft, low pitched, and rumbling; it may be accentuated in presystole. This is the Austin Flint murmur and may depend upon interference with mitral valve function by regurgitating blood. It is indistinguishable from the diastolic murmur of mitral stenosis, but is rarely accompanied by a thrill.

During systole the increased volume of blood flung into the circulation raises the systolic pressure and distends the aorta and large arteries. The upstroke of the pulse wave is abrupt and of high amplitude (fig. 10.24)

When an artery is palpated, this sudden shock feels like a water-hammer (a Victorian toy consisting of a small quantity of fluid in a glass vacuum tube—Watson, 1843), and on auscultation the sound heard may resemble a pistol shot. The pulse collapses in late "systole" almost as quickly as it is built up, and the diastolic blood pressure is low.

The abrupt distension and quick collapse of large arteries is well seen in the carotids, especially when the patient sits up. This characteristic visible behaviour of an artery above heart level is Corrigan's sign (Corrigan, 1832).

On auscultating the femoral or other large artery, a systolic murmur is heard when the vessel is compressed; when a critical pressure is applied to the artery just distal to the stethoscope, a diastolic murmur may also develop. The latter was first described by Durozier (1861), whose name is attached to the sign, and who attributed it to retrograde blood flow during diastole. Durozier's sign may occur, however, in any condition causing a large primary pulse wave, a steep predicrotic notch, and a conspicuous dicrotic wave. Such an obstacle halts the blood flow at the pre-dicrotic notch, but is overcome by the dicrotic wave. Above the obstacle the dicrotic wave is exaggerated; below it the dicrotic wave is flattened out. Hence the diastolic murmur is heard above but not below the constriction. The centrifugal direction of the passage of the wave which causes the murmur has been proved by means of simultaneous multiple phonoarteriograms (Luisada, 1943).

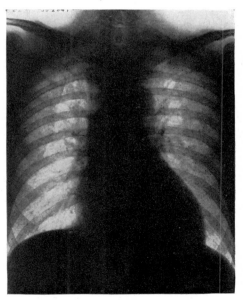

Vasodilatation exaggerates the collapsing quality of the pulse, further lowers the diastolic blood pressure, and causes capillary pulsation. The latter may be demonstrated by lightly compressing a finger nail, by transilluminating the tip of the finger, or by pressing a glass slide against the lips. Its presence depends upon direct transmission of the arterial pulse wave to the capillaries, and it occurs in any condition in which there is sufficient relaxation of the arterioles to allow this. Thus capillary pulsation may be seen in

Fig. 10.25—Skiagram showing prominence of the aortic arch and enlargement of the left ventricle in a case of aortic incompetence.

normal subjects after a hot bath, in thyrotoxicosis, arteriovenous aneurysm, fever, and in most hyperkinetic circulatory states. Pulsation of the retinal veins is another common finding.

Skiagrams show enlargement of the left ventricle and prominence of the aorta. The ascending aorta pushes the superior vena cava further to the right, the aortic knob is accentuated, and the descending limb appears further to the left (fig. 10.25). Unfolding of the arch is seen better in the left anterior oblique position. Fluoroscopy reveals exaggerated pulsation of the left ventricle and aorta. When there is left ventricular failure the usual fan-shaped hilar opacities of "pulmonary venous congestion" develop.

Electrocardiography may provide additional evidence of left ventricular enlargement (fig. 10.26).

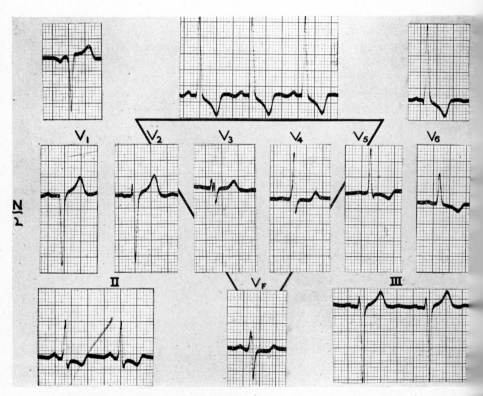

Fig. 10.26—Electrocardiogram in a case of aortic incompetence showing considerable left ventricular preponderance.

DIFFERENTIAL DIAGNOSIS

Most of the features described above are common to all forms of aortic incompetence.

A rheumatic etiology is favoured by a rheumatic history, relatively long duration, any age between 10 and 40 years, signs of associated aortic stenosis with or without calcification, the presence of other valve lesions absence of angina pectoris, and by a normal erythrocyte sedimentation rate

It is not always easy to be certain whether the mitral valve is stenosed when the chief lesion is obviously aortic incompetence, for then a mitral pre-systolic or diastolic murmur, backward displacement of the œsophagus, and widened bifid P waves may not have their usual significance. The practical point emerges that a case presenting as one of aortic incompetence, with doubtful signs of mitral stenosis, is better judged rheumatic on other grounds.

A *spirochætal etiology* is favoured by a history of syphilis, evidence of syphilis in some other system, short duration, age between 40 and 60, angina pectoris, absence of aortic stenosis and other valve lesions, calcification of the ascending aorta but not of the aortic valve, irregularities in calibre of the aortic arch or frank aneurysm, an accelerated erythrocyte sedimentation rate, and positive Wasserman and Kahn reactions.

Atherosclerosis is more likely in elderly men, although some of these cases are probably rheumatic primarily. Angina pectoris and some degree of calcific aortic stenosis are common in this group. Aortic calcification is confined to the knuckle and valve, the ascending aorta being spared. The erythrocyte sedimentation rate is normal, and the Wasserman reaction, of course, negative.

Severe hypertension presents no difficulty, because the aortic leak is usually trivial and does not alter the physiology of the circulation.

Bacterial endocarditis should be recognised by the rapid downhill course, changing murmurs and liability to perforation in addition to the fever, anæmia, petechiæ, clubbing, embolism, splenomegaly, hæmaturia, Osler's nodes, and positive blood culture.

Congenital aortic incompetence due to *anomalous cusps* alone may be suggested by the age of the patient, absence of rheumatic history and the presence of some other congenital lesion. *Congenital hypoplasia of the ascending aorta* with aortic ring dilatation may be part of Marfan's syndrome (arachnodactyly). The leak in these cases may be gross. Congenital aortic incompetence associated with *coarctation of the aorta or ventricular septal defect* should be obvious enough.

Dissecting aneurysm with survival may result in severe aortic incompetence; many of these cases have been mistaken for syphilis, in view of the age of the patient, short duration, free leak, absence of rheumatic history, absence of stenosis, and perhaps fusiform dilatation of the ascending aorta.

COURSE AND PROGNOSIS

The average life expectancy of rheumatic aortic incompetence is 20 to 30 years from its development. Prognosis should be based on the size of the left ventricle, and upon the degree of incompetence as judged by peripheral vascular behaviour. Effort tolerance often remains remarkably good until near the end. Failure is commonly with normal rhythm, and is usually left ventricular at first. Complications are practically limited to bacterial endocarditis.

TREATMENT

Medical care is a matter of guiding the patient in his choice of occupation, limiting physical activities wisely but not unnecessarily, steering a woman through or away from pregnancy, protecting the patient from bacterial endocarditis by the judicious use of prophylactic penicillin, and treating heart failure by means of all the usual remedies when it arises. Although trinitrin might be expected to aggravate rather than relieve angina pectoris, in fact it proves beneficial more often than not, presumably by having a relatively selective action on the coronary circulation.

Patients with aortic incompetence should be rejected for National Service and are usually rejected for insurance.

Surgical treatment has so far proved unsatisfactory, although Hufnagel (1954) has devised a polythene ball-valve which he inserts in the descending aorta below the left subclavian artery. This is said to prevent about 75 per cent of the regurgitant flow. Of the first 23 cases so treated there were 17 survivors, all said to be greatly improved. The valve makes a considerable noise, especially during the first few weeks, but patients usually become accustomed to it. Several cases have developed serious embolism in the legs following this operation, and a small number of post-operative physiological studies have revealed little if any improvement in left ventricular diastolic pressure or cardiac output. The attempt to relieve aortic incompetence by surgical means, however, must be encouraged, and better means of correcting this simple mechanical fault will no doubt be devised in due course.

AORTIC STENOSIS

FREQUENCY

Aortic stenosis may be congenital, rheumatic or possibly purely sclerotic. The frequency of rheumatic aortic stenosis partly depends on whether cases of calcific aortic stenosis in elderly subjects without a history of rheumatic fever are regarded as rheumatic or sclerotic. This point has been debated for at least half a century, ever since Mönckeberg (1904) recognised histologically both an inflammatory and a purely sclerotic form of stricture. Both macroscopic and microscopic differences between the two have been demonstrated since by many workers, e.g. Sohval and Gross (1936), but it is by no means easy to be sure of the initial etiology when confronted by a grossly distorted and heavily calcified valve, and the alleged differences are none too convincing. Two painstaking pathological studies, each of 200 cases of calcific aortic stenosis, were those by Clawson, Noble and Lufkin (1938) and Karsner and Koletsky (1947); both teams concluded that all cases were probably rheumatic. Assuming this to be so, rheumatic aortic stenosis is common, and must occur in at least one-quarter of all cases of chronic rheumatic heart disease.

PATHOLOGY

Fibrous scar tissue representing healed aortic valvulitis usually causes fusion of the cusps at their commissures. Slight narrowing at the aortic aperture is thus found in most cases'of rheumatic aortic valve disease. When fusion extends further up the margins of the cusps, true stenosis results. Valve leaflets become thick, rigid, distorted and often unrecognisable. Secondary valve calcification is common. The aorta and large arteries often remain remarkably free from atheroma (Clawson *et al.*, 1938), and both the frequency and severity of coronary atherosclerosis are inversely proportional to the degree of stenosis (Dry and Willius, 1939). The left ventricle hypertrophies and may finally become enormous; in a case reported by Lowe and Bate (1948), the heart weighed 2,340 G.

EFFECT ON FUNCTION

The aortic orifice must be reduced to about one-quarter of its natural size before changes in the circulation can be demonstrated (Wiggers, 1935). Left ventricular pressure curves then show a raised initial tension, steep isometric pressure gradient, and an elevated maximum pressure that is reached relatively early in systole, but there is no collapse as in aortic incompetence. Pressure curves obtained from the aorta show an initial relatively steep rise interrupted by an anacrotic notch and followed by a slower rise that reaches its maximum late in systole; the maximum pressure attained is less than normal (fig. 10.27). The more severe the stenosis, the earlier the anacrotic notch. The ejection phase is prolonged.

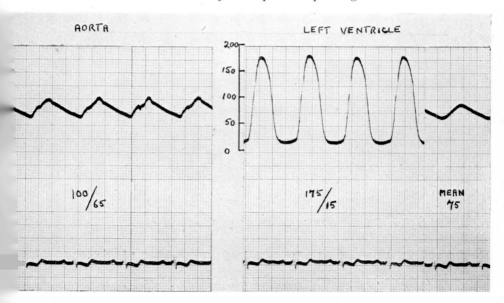

ɔ.27—Pressure pulses from the aorta and left ventricle in a case of aortic stenosis showing a systolic ɾe gradient of 75 mm. Hg. Note the anacrotic notch and the delayed summit in the aortic pulse.

The systolic pressure gradient between left ventricle and aorta may be anything between a few mm. Hg and over 150 mm. Hg according to the severity of the stricture and the integrity of the left ventricular myocardium. With a gradient of only 5 mm. Hg in mild cases, or in cases of mixed stenosis and incompetence, the aortic pulse may still show an anacrotic notch and slow secondary rise (fig. 10.28).

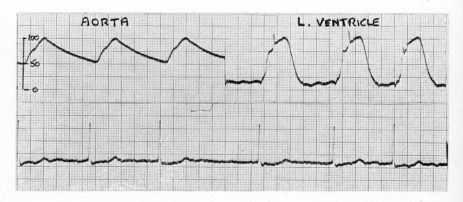

Fig. 10.28—Pressure pulses from the aorta and left ventricle in a case of aortic stenosis and incompetence. The pressure gradient is less than 5 mm. Hg, but the aortic pulse is stenotic in form.

To maintain the stroke volume and cardiac output great power must be developed by the left ventricle. The chamber is more hypertrophied and less dilated than in aortic incompetence. Its increased initial tension is partly due to more forceful left atrial systole; the left ventricle is deprived of this important help in cases of coincident mitral stenosis.

The cardiac output per minute is strictly limited, as in mitral, pulmonary and tricuspid stenosis, and in severe cases is reduced at rest. The low mean aortic pressure prevents the coronary blood flow from keeping pace with the increased demands of the left ventricle.

CLINICAL FEATURES

Sex and Age

Aortic stenosis is at least twice as common in men as in women. The lesion may be discovered at any time from adolescence to old age, usually in the sixth decade. Female patients tend to be younger than male.

Symptoms

Patients with aortic stenosis may complain of syncope (10–20 per cent), angina pectoris (20–36 per cent), or symptoms referabe to left ventricular or congestive heart failure (Contratto and Levine, 1937; Mitchell et al., 1954).

Syncope is of two kinds, cardiac and vasomotor. Cardiac syncope is abrupt and fleeting, and when it occurs on effort may be due to acute left ventricular failure or to a fixed low cardiac output, so that the blood pressure cannot be maintained when peripheral vasodilatation occurs. Cardiac syncope at rest may be due to paroxysmal ventricular fibrillation or possibly to locking of the valve (de Veer, 1938). Such attacks herald sudden death from a similar mechanism. The low blood pressure of aortic stenosis predisposes to vasomotor and orthostatic syncope.

Angina pectoris depends upon poor coronary filling due to the low mean blood pressure and low fixed cardiac output; on effort the heavy demands of the hypertrophied and overworking left ventricle have little chance of being adequately met. The pain is indistinguishable in site, quality, duration and behaviour to that associated with occlusive coronary athero-sclerosis, and may finally occur on the slightest effort, or even at rest, as in advanced coronary disease.

Breathlessness on effort is, of course, the commonest symptom, and sooner or later orthopnœa, paroxysmal cardiac dyspnœa or acute pulmonary œdema may occur as a result of left ventricular failure. Œdema, due to congestive heart failure, may occur later or may develop without previous evidence of left-sided failure, as in hypertensive heart disease.

The physical signs are as follows:

1. There is sometimes a delicate pale pink complexion – the Dresden china look.

2. The pulse is characteristic when relatively slow (fig. 10.29), being small and sustained (plateau or slow-rising pulse). It depends upon the longer duration of left ventricular systole, the low blood pressure, and upon the delayed development of maximum aortic pressure. These features tend

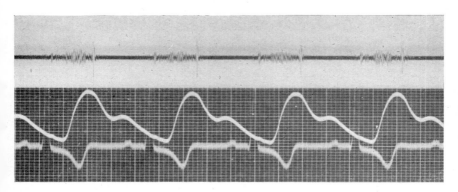

Fig. 10.29—Arteriogram in a case of aortic stenosis. The percussion wave is prolonged, and the maximum pressure is reached late in systole. The phonocardiogram above shows a typical mid-systolic murmur.

(*By courtesy of Drs. Frances Gardner and Max Zoob*)

to disappear as the heart rate quickens. The anacrotic notch of the aortic tracing may or may not be felt at the periphery, for it tends to be ironed out by the elasticity of the arteries (fig. 10.30). When aortic incompetence is present as well, the pulse assumes a "bisferiens" quality (fig. 10.31). To the palpating finger it feels double, and may even be mistaken for coupling

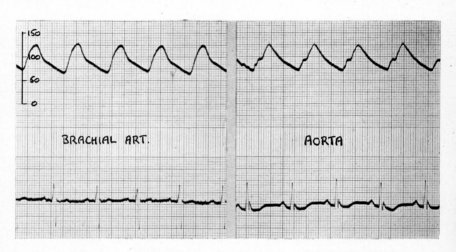

Fig. 10.30—Pressure pulses from the brachial artery and aorta in a case of aortic stenosis showing disappearance of the anacrotic notch in the more peripheral tracing.

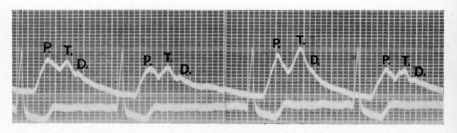

Fig. 10.31—Arteriogram illustrating pulsus bisferiens in a case of combined aortic stenosis and incompetence. P is the percussion wave, T the tidal wave; both are systolic events.
(*By courtesy of Drs. Frances Gardner and Max Zoob*)

due to premature ectopic beats. Both waves occur during the ejection phase. According to Bramwell (1937), the second impulse is tidal in nature, being due to overlapping and partial fusion between a forcible but prolonged percussion wave and its reflection from the periphery. Aortic incompetence increases the force of the percussion wave; aortic stenosis prolongs it. Neither alone will produce this pulse. Direct intra-arterial pressure tracings show a plateau rather than a dip following the percussion wave and preceding the tidal wave (fig. 10.32) The discrepancy may be due to the fact that both the palpating finger and any type of tambour used for

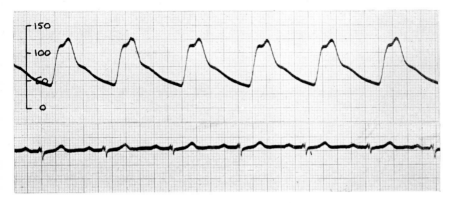

Fig. 10.32—Direct arteriogram from a case of aortic stenosis and incompetence showing a plateau instead of a dip between percussion and tidal waves. Clinically this was a classical pulsus bisferiens.

recording arterial pulsation from without must apply suitable pressure on the artery, usually approximating the diastolic pressure; both finger and tambour move through distances proportional to the pulse pressure, so that they record the sudden halting of the percussion wave as a negative pressure, for they have upward momentum at the time.

3. The blood pressure is variable. In severe cases it is low and the pulse pressure small, but in mild or moderate cases, or when there is recognisable aortic incompetence, it may be elevated and the pulse pressure may be increased. About 10 per cent are truly hypertensive—an incidence a good deal lower than in controls of the same age-group.

4. The apex beat is displaced downwards and to the left and the cardiac impulse is quietly heaving. The left ventricle is hypertrophied rather than dilated.

5. A basal systolic thrill is usually present. It is best appreciated when the patient leans forward and stops breathing in full expiration. It may be most intense either to the right or left of the sternum. A systolic thrill may also be felt over the carotid or subclavian arteries. Although such a thrill is not diagnostic of aortic stenosis, it is suggestive and encourages prolonged search at the base.

6. A rough, basal systolic murmur is almost invariable. It is conducted into the cervical arteries, and may be heard remarkably well at the apex beat over the left ventricle. The murmur is mid-systolic (fig. 10.29), starting when the aortic valve opens at the end of the period of isometric contraction, and finishing in physiological protodiastole, when the left ventricle begins to relax, appreciably before the aortic second sound (Leatham, 1951). When best heard at the apex beat, its timing at once distinguishes it from the pan-systolic murmur of mitral incompetence. When best heard at the base, an aortic systolic murmur may be distinguished from a pulmonary murmur not only by its shorter duration, but

also by its delayed return after the valsalva manœuvre (Zinsser and Kay, 1950).

7. An aortic systolic ejection click immediately precedes the murmur in many cases (Lian and Welti, 1937). When heard at the apex beat this click may be mistaken for the first heart sound, and the real first heart sound for presystolic left atrial gallop; the murmur is then erroneously believed to be early systolic, and a diagnosis of incipient left ventricular failure with functional mitral incompetence may be wrongly made.

8. The aortic component of the second heart sound is characteristically delayed in the majority of cases and absent in a minority: the delay is attributed to prolongation of left ventricular systole and to the time occupied by the relaxing left ventricle in abolishing the systolic pressure gradient across the valve; an absent aortic second sound is due to almost complete immobilisation of a heavily calcified rigid valve. These changes result in a single second heart sound, the aortic element being synchronous with the pulmonary or absent altogether, or in reversed splitting of the second heart sound, the aortic component falling after the pulmonary, so that the split widens during expiration instead of during inspiration (Leatham, 1952). When the second heart sound is single the two components are probably fused if the sound can be heard at the apex beat and over the right carotid artery; if the single second sound can be heard only at the pulmonary area, the aortic component is probably absent.

9. On fluoroscopy, the left ventricle looks dense and bulky. The aorta may be conspicuous, or relatively hypoplasic (fig. 10.33). Post-stenotic dilatation of the ascending aorta is usually more obvious at operation than in skiagrams, because the shadow of the aortic root tends to merge with that of the ventricles and right atrium. When the lower part of the ascending aorta is conspicuous, however, and the rest of it inconspicuous, the presence of aortic stenosis is strongly confirmed. Calcification of the aortic valve can be seen in most cases, particularly if the patient is over 50.

10. The electrocardiogram usually provides convincing

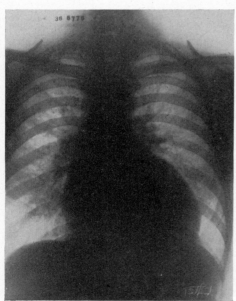

Fig. 10.33—Skiagram of a case of aortic stenosis showing great enlargement of the left ventricle, slight prominence of the ascending aorta, and hilar congestion.

evidence of left ventricular enlargement. Perhaps owing to the concentric type of hypertrophy and to the lack of dilatation, the heart is often electrically vertical. Standard leads then show the concordant pattern of left ventricular preponderance (fig. 10.34). Exceptionally high-voltage R waves are characteristic of aortic stenosis. T is frequently inverted in leads facing the surface of the left ventricle. Left bundle branch block, varying degrees of atrioventricular block, and atrial fibrillation each occur in about 10 per cent of cases (Mitchell *et al.*, 1954).

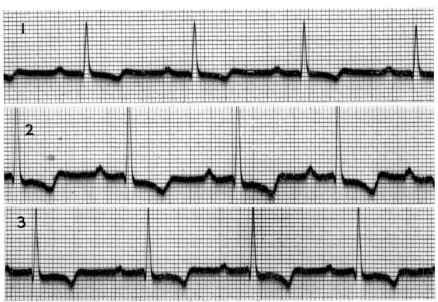

Fig. 10.34—Electrocardiogram in a case of aortic stenosis showing concordant left ventricular preponderance in standard leads, the heart being vertical.

SPECIAL TESTS

Indirect or direct arteriograms of the brachial pressure pulse confirm the anacrotic or bisferiens pulse that is felt. In doubtful cases these tracings may be helpful. A normal brachial pressure pulse occupies about 0.16 seconds from its onset to the beginning of the sharp downstroke, the initial upstroke or front of the percussion wave measuring 0.08 second, and the blunt peak also 0.08 second. In aortic stenosis the front of the percussion wave occupies 0.08 to 0.12 second to the anacrotic notch (fig. 10.32), or to the beginning of the blunt peak if the notch is ironed out (fig. 10.30), and the blunt peak itself occupies about 0.12 second, so that from its onset to the beginning of the sharp downstroke the pulse occupies at least 0.20 second, and usually 0.24 second.

In the pulsus bisferiens dominant aortic stenosis is favoured if the tidal wave is taller than the percussion wave, dominant aortic incompetence if it is the other way about (fig. 10.35).

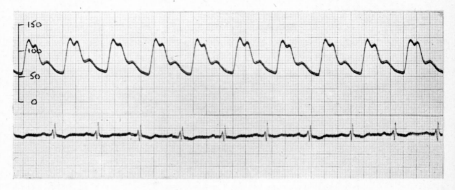

Fig. 10.35—Direct arterial tracing illustrating the pulsus bisferiens in a case of aortic stenosis and incompetence with a dominant leak; the percussion wave is taller than the tidal wave.

Cardiac catheterisation may be helpful in assessing the degree of co-incident mitral stenosis, measuring the force of left atrial systole, determining the left ventricular diastolic pressure, and estimating the cardiac output at rest and on effort.

Neither a powerful *a* wave in the indirect left atrial pressure pulse nor the level of the mean left atrial pressure provides any evidence of mitral valve disease in cases of severe aortic stenosis, for the former may be a manifestation of left ventricular stress and the latter the result of left ventricular failure (fig. 10.36). If the left atrial pressure is raised, only the Ry/v ratio indicates whether the mitral valve is obstructed or not. In figure 10.36 Ry/v measures at least 5, so that the high left atrial pressure is obviously due to left ventricular failure or gross mitral incompetence. In figure 10.37, on the other hand, Ry/v is 1.3, and the raised left atrial pressure is due to coincident mitral stenosis.

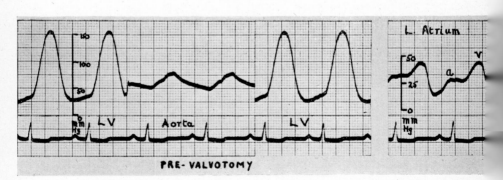

Fig. 10.36—Pressure pulses from the aorta, left ventricle and left atrium in a case of aortic ste with left ventricular failure. Note the very rapid *y* descent and conspicuous *y* trough in th atrial tracing. The Ry/v ratio is 5.

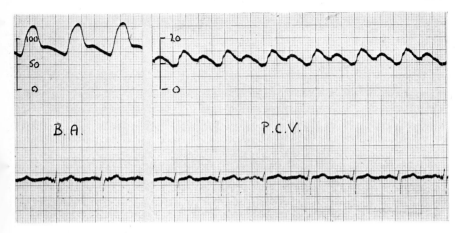

Fig. 10.37—Typical wedged pulmonary artery tracing (P.C.V.) from a case of combined aortic and mitral stenosis showing an Ry/v ratio of 1.3 in the indirect left atrial pressure pulse.

Giant a waves in the left atrial pressure pulse have been described by Gorlin (1955), and are believed to be the counterpart of giant *a* waves in the right atrium in cases of severe pulmonary stenosis. Extra care may be necessary at times, however, to make sure that what is taken for *a* at first sight is not in fact *c*, for accurate interpretation of wedged pulmonary artery tracings is not always easy.

The *left ventricular diastolic pressure* can only be measured from direct or indirect left atrial pressure tracings when mitral stenosis can be excluded, i.e. when the Ry/v ratio is over 1.6. A good example from a case with left ventricular failure is shown in figure 10.36, in which direct pressure tracings have been recorded from both left atrium and ventricle. The raised left ventricular diastolic pressure can, of course, be inferred from the patient's symptoms and from the radiological appearances of the lungs.

Estimation of the cardiac output at rest and on effort may be important when the severity of a case of aortic stenosis is in doubt. It also provides essential data for interpreting the significance of any given pressure gradient across the aortic valve. *Dye concentration curves* may be recorded with this object when the pressure gradient is being measured at operation. Good outputs at rest and on effort are maintained in cases of aortic stenosis until relatively late in their course (Goldberg, Bakst and Bailey, 1954).

The pressure gradient across the aortic valve may be measured by recording simultaneously or in immediate succession both left ventricular and brachial pressure pulses (fig. 10.36). The former may be achieved by threading a fine polythene catheter through a needle inserted directly into the left atrium from behind, and manipulating it until its tip passes through the mitral valve (Björk *et al.*, 1954, 1955). Alternatively, a needle may be passed directly into the left ventricle from the region of the apex beat. At Brompton the latter has proved safe and far less traumatic, but should be undertaken only by skilled surgeons who must be prepared to carry out an immediate aortic valvotomy should ventricular fibrillation occur. If the information is to be of any real value, forward flow should be measured at the same time, and if there is appreciable aortic incompetence this is impossible at the moment.

Phonocardiography is of real value when the nature of the systolic murmur is in doubt, when there is clinical difficulty in distinguishing left atrial gallop at the apex beat from an aortic ejection click, and when the timing of aortic valve closure cannot be ascertained clinically.

The *ballistocardiogram* in aortic stenosis has been studied by Van Lingen *et al* (1952). A characteristic angulated or outwardly bowed J-K segment was described in tracings obtained from a low frequency critically damped instrument.

Tomography is a good method of recording calcified aortic valves (Davies and Steiner, 1949).

COMPLICATIONS

If syncope, angina pectoris, changes of rhythm, left ventricular failure, congestive heart failure and heavy calcification are all regarded as manifestations of the disease itself, as they should be, then the only complication of rheumatic aortic stenosis is bacterial endocarditis, which sooner or later occurs in about 10 per cent of cases. In the large series reported by Mitchell *et al.* (1954) bacterial endocarditis accounted for 20 per cent of the deaths.

DIFFERENTIAL DIAGNOSIS

If as much attention were paid to the quality of the peripheral pulse as to cardiac murmurs, serious aortic stenosis would be both less frequently overlooked and less often diagnosed in error; nevertheless, the pulse is normal in mild cases. The chief sources of confusion include "functional" basal murmurs, mitral incompetence, ventricular septal defect, coarctation of the aorta, and a group of normotensive low-output cardiopathies that may involve mainly the left ventricle, such as acquired subendocardial fibrosis.

Innocent basal ejection murmurs are mid-systolic, especially when aortic. When associated with a high cardiac output, as in anæmia, they present little difficulty in diagnosis, but when occurring alone in young persons, or in association with atherosclerosis of the aorta in the elderly, slight aortic stenosis is difficult to exclude. A number of cases of advanced calcific aortic stenosis that have been seen in the last few years were diagnosed as having a functional systolic murmur during the first world war. A similar number of young people who have this murmur at the present time are therefore being watched with considerable interest, although strongly encouraged to lead normal lives.

Mitral incompetence should be distinguished by the sharper quality of the pulse, the hyperdynamic nature of left ventricular pulsation, the pan-systolic timing of the thrill and murmur, the small ascending aorta, and the enlarged left atrium. As previously stated, the murmur of aortic stenosis may be maximum at the apex beat over the surface of the left ventricle. When valve calcification is recognised, the position of the opacity should determine whether it is aortic or mitral.

Ventricular septal defect should also be distinguished by the hyperdynamic quality of ventricular pulsation and the pan-systolic timing of the bruit and thrill; in addition, characteristic changes in the electrocardiogram and skiagram help to prevent error. In doubtful cases cardiac catheterisation should demonstrate the shunt.

Certain cardiopathies, usually of unknown etiology, may present with clinical, electrocardiographic and radiological evidence of predominant left ventricular enlargement, a low or normal blood pressure, small rapid pulse, and a low cardiac output. If there is a murmur it is usually apical and pan-systolic, being caused by functional mitral incompetence. The absence of demonstrable valve calcification may be attributed to the size and density of the heart, so that the observer does not feel confident of his negative findings. Cases of this sort can be awkward, and diagnostic mistakes have been made in both directions. One of the sources of confusion is the belief that in about 10 per cent of cases of aortic stenosis no aortic systolic murmur can be heard at any time, as reported by Bergeron *et al.* (1952). A more convincing statement would be that no *mid-systolic murmur* could be heard at any time at base *or apex* by an experienced cardiologist; such a statement has yet to be made. In doubtful cases a phonocardiogram and intra-arterial pressure tracing should be recorded, and every effort made to reveal valve calcification. If the diagnosis is still uncertain the pressure gradient across the aortic valve should be measured, for aortic stenosis must not be missed.

In *combined aortic stenosis and incompetence* the difficulty is to decide which is dominant. This is essential when selecting cases for aortic valvotomy. Since the operation was introduced it has been discovered that physiologically in mixed cases there is often more incompetence and less stenosis than traditional evidence would lead one to suppose, rarely vice versa. For example, an obvious pulsus bisferiens seems to indicate dominant incompetence rather than stenosis; neither angina pectoris, a diastolic pressure of 80 mm. Hg, a coarse aortic systolic thrill, nor heavy valve calcification has proved reliable evidence of dominant stenosis. The mixed case, in fact, is causing great confusion, and even measuring the pressure gradient across the valve is useless without knowing the forward flow. At present, if a case has more than trivial aortic incompetence, so that a problem does in fact arise, the probability is that the leak is too great to warrant valvotomy, and until more is known this may be the best attitude to adopt. We have recorded pressure gradients up to 100 mm. Hg across the aortic valve in cases of dominant incompetence subsequently proved at operation.

Combined aortic valve disease and mitral stenosis usually presents less difficulty, because the degree of mitral stricture can be worked out with precision, and if this demands valvotomy then the pressure gradient across the aortic valve can be measured at operation easily enough. If the mitral stenosis is relatively unimportant, the problem reverts to that just discussed. It may be noted here, however, that well developed mitral valve disease damps all the signs of aortic valve disease, and these may become much more evident following mitral valvotomy.

Etiological diagnosis may also be difficult. Rheumatic aortic stenosis must be distinguished from congenital and calcific atherosclerotic varieties. Congenital stenosis may be clinically indistinguishable from the rheumatic variety; but the lesion is usually discovered in childhood, there is no rheumatic history, and incompetence is unusual.

It is uncertain whether calcific aortic stenosis in elderly or middle-aged subjects is atherosclerotic or rheumatic. Thus eleven of twenty-one cases reported by Christian (1931) gave a history of rheumatic fever. Dry and Willius (1939) obtained a rheumatic history in 22 per cent of 228 cases, and Clawson, Noble and Lufkin (1938) found a rheumatic history in 35 per cent of 200 cases. On the other hand, in the quoted series of Dry and Willius, there were 91 necropsied cases without disease of other valves; a rheumatic history was obtained in only four of these—the usual incidence in any series of normal controls. Again, in the quoted series of Clawson and his colleagues, 20.5 per cent of the patients were under 41 years of age, and 39 per cent were under 51; moreover, 89 had a mitral lesion as well. It is obvious that many of these cases were rheumatic; but this has little bearing upon the question of whether or not pure calcific aortic stenosis in elderly people is rheumatic. On the pathological side, Clawson (1931) particularly has drawn attention to the frequency of inflammatory stigmata of the rheumatic type, but others, notably Sohval and Gross (1936), have been unable to confirm such findings. The best evidence of a rheumatic or other inflammatory etiology is perhaps the remarkable absence of atherosclerosis in the aorta and coronary arteries in most cases. All observers have agreed on this point: that these vessels must have been long protected by the stenosis. However, Mönckeberg's original thesis that calcific aortic stenosis in elderly subjects may be degenerative (Mönckeberg, 1904) has not been altogether disproved.

Clinically, calcific aortic stenosis in elderly subjects behaves like rheumatic aortic stenosis.

COURSE AND PROGNOSIS

As already mentioned, the initial rheumatic attack in cases of more or less pure aortic stenosis is sub-clinical in about 80 per cent of cases. A mid-systolic murmur, however, is often heard when the patient is young and well; whether maximum at apex or base this murmur has usually been regarded erroneously as functional. Sooner or later, according to the severity of the lesion, attacks of syncope (15 per cent) or angina pectoris (33 per cent) may develop. Both are serious and limit future life expectancy to an average of 3.3 and 4.1 years respectively (Mitchell *et al.*, 1954). Abrupt death without immediate warning, presumably from ventricular fibrillation or cardiac standstill, occurs in 18 per cent of severe cases (Horan and Barnes, 1948; Mitchell *et al.*, 1954), and is by no means confined to those who have had syncope or angina pectoris. Subacute bacterial endocarditis may develop any time in 10 per cent of cases, and accounts for 20 per cent of the deaths (Contratto and Levine, 1937; Mitchell *et al.*, 1954). The majority of patients who survive these hazards succumb to left ventricular or congestive heart failure before reaching the age of 70. Heart failure accounted for 30 to 50 per cent of the deaths in the various series quoted above, and its onset usually limits further life expectancy to 2 years.

The total mortality from aortic stenosis increases in a linear manner from the third to the seventh decade (Dry and Willius, 1939), after which it falls again, but there are as many deaths in the eighth decade as in the sixth. No distinction is made here between rheumatic and calcific aortic stenosis. The average age at death is 55 to 65, women tending to be a decade younger than men.

In any given case the *prognosis* varies between excellent in those with no more than an aortic systolic murmur and a life expectancy of only 2, 3 or 4 years from the onset of heart failure, syncope or angina pectoris respectively. Between these two extremes the prognosis in symptom-free cases of unmistakable aortic stenosis may be assessed by recognising three grades of severity based on the physical signs, electrocardiogram and skiagram. Mild cases with only slight hypertrophy of the left ventricle, an aortic systolic thrill and murmur, aortic ejection click, and closely split or single second heart sound may be expected to remain symptom free for at least 20 to 30 years; cases of moderate severity with alteration of the peripheral pulse, hypertrophy of the left ventricle, moderately delayed aortic valve closure, grade 1 to 2 left ventricular preponderance electrocardiographically, and slight enlargement of the left ventricle radiologically may be expected to live 10 to 20 years; severe cases, as yet symptom free, having the fully developed physical signs, electrocardiogram, and fluoroscopic appearances described above—particularly an unmistakable anacrotic pulse, heaving left ventricle, reversed splitting of the second heart sound, inverted T waves in left ventricular surface leads on their equivalents, and obvious enlargement of the left ventricle radiologically—cannot be expected to survive more than 5 to 10 years.

TREATMENT

Medical management is similar to that of aortic incompetence. Little can be done to prevent syncope other than restricting physical effort. For

angina pectoris trinitrin is again of benefit more often than not, despite
its theoretical objections.

Aortic valvotomy (Bailey *et al.*, 1952) has proved more difficult and less
satisfactory than mitral valvotomy. The approach is through the anterior
wall of the left ventricle. Bailey uses a tri-fin expanding dilator on a swivel
head, which is said to adjust itself to the commissures (Larzelere and
Bailey, 1953), although cinematographic demonstration of aortic valve
function in cases of advanced aortic stenosis reveal so much fusion and
distortion of the cusps that three commissures can rarely be made out
(McMillan, 1955). Simple two-bladed expanding dilators may be just as
effective (or ineffective).

The present high mortality of 22 per cent from aortic valvotomy (Bailey
et al., 1954) is partly due to the very advanced type of case surgeons have
been invited to tackle, usually those with severe angina pectoris or heart
failure. The physician's difficult obligation is to advise the operation in
severe cases before these manifestations of impending disaster arise, i.e.
when the patient is still virtually symptom free, and that is no easy matter,
for the risk is still appreciable and the physiological result rarely excellent.

As previously stated, a common mistake is to under-estimate the degree
of aortic incompetence present; this should not be more than trivial clinically, if dominant stenosis is to be confirmed surgically. The error has
always been in the same direction, i.e. subsequent necropsies in cases
rejected for valvotomy on the grounds of too much aortic incompetence
have yet to show dominant stenosis. It is repeated here for emphasis that
neither angina pectoris, syncope, pulsus bisferiens, a diastolic blood
pressure of 80 to 85 mm. Hg, nor valve calcification can be accepted as
evidence of dominant stenosis in these mixed cases; even a systolic pressure
gradient of 50 to 100 mm. Hg across the aortic valve is inconclusive unless
the forward stroke flow is known. In classical cases of more or less pure
severe stenosis the gradient is usually 50 to 150 mm. Hg, but is greatly
influenced by the cardiac output at the time.

So far at Brompton, 50 cases have been operated on, mostly by Sir
Russell Brock, with a mortality of 22 per cent. All these cases were
advanced, many far too advanced. It is too early to assess the post-operative
results in the survivors with any precision, but it is fair to say that the
best tend to be good rather than excellent, and that the majority are fair
rather than good. In a technically successful case a ventricular-aortic
pressure gradient of 50 to 100 mm. Hg should be reduced to below
20 mm. Hg (fig. 10.38). Results of this kind are more likely to be achieved
if aortic valvotomy is carried out earlier.

Combined aortic and mitral valvotomy has proved very encouraging
(Likoff *et al.*, 1955). It is probable that in these cases symptoms due to
mitral stenosis have forced operative treatment at a time when the aortic
lesion itself might have caused no symptoms at all; in other words, some
of these cases are giving surgeons an opportunity to relieve aortic stenosis

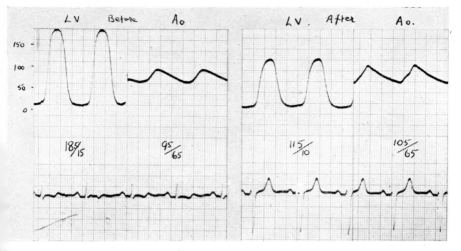

Fig. 10.38—Pressure pulses from the left ventricle and aorta in a case or aortic stenosis before and after aortic valvotomy; the pressure gradient across the aortic valve has been reduced from 90 to 10 mm. Hg.

when it is not too far advanced. Technically, most surgeons have so far preferred to undertake mitral valvotomy first, being the less hazardous of the two, for ventricular fibrillation or standstill occurring during aortic valvotomy might be very difficult to correct in the presence of unrelieved mitral stenosis.

TRICUSPID INCOMPETENCE

Tricuspid incompetence may be functional or organic, the former being secondary to right ventricular dilatation with expansion of the tricuspid ring, as may occur in cases of pulmonary hypertension, pulmonary stenosis with normal aortic root, atrial or ventricular septal defect, or right ventricular failure from any cause. When there is pulmonary hypertension secondary to mitral stenosis, clinical distinction between functional and organic tricuspid incompetence may be difficult in the first instance, but the course and response to digitalis and rest may clarify the issue: functional incompetence may be temporary; organic tricuspid disease is always permanent.

The majority of cases of chronic rheumatic tricuspid valve disease have some degree of stenosis, and the majority of cases of frank tricuspid incompetence are functional. Rheumatic tricuspid disease will therefore be discussed as a whole under tricuspid stenosis, and the following remarks apply chiefly to functional tricuspid incompetence.

FREQUENCY

At the present time it may be unwise to attempt to assess the frequency of functional tricuspid incompetence, because accurate criteria upon which its diagnosis may be based with confidence have yet to be set up. In my own cases considerable or gross tricuspid incompetence, with physical signs that would be generally accepted, occurred at one time or another in 22 out of 32 cases of mitral stenosis complicated by an extreme pulmonary vascular resistance (over 10 units), but in only one out of 14 cases of primary pulmonary hypertension, three out of 52 cases of severe pulmonary valve stenosis with normal aortic root (R.V. systolic pressure over 100 mm. Hg), and 10 out of 98 cases of severe atrial septal defect (pulmonary flow at least three times the systemic flow or high pulmonary vascular resistance). This curious discrepancy was found to be due to the presence or absence of atrial fibrillation. Thus in the mitral group atrial fibrillation occurred in 62 per cent; tricuspid incompetence was recognised in 91 per cent of these fibrillating cases and in only 10 per cent of those with normal rhythm. In the other three groups atrial fibrillation occurred in only 8.2 per cent; tricuspid incompetence was found in 87 per cent of these, but in only one out of 149 cases with normal rhythm. These rather startling figures make it only too clear that what is customarily taken for tricuspid incompetence is closely related to atrial fibrillation, whatever the explanation may be.

HÆMODYNAMICS

The effect of tricuspid incompetence on right ventricular output and filling, and on the right atrial and systemic venous pressure pulse, is similar in all respects to the effect of mitral incompetence on the left side of the heart and pulmonary venous circulation. Functional tricuspid incompetence occurs when the right ventricle and tricuspid ring dilate as a result of failure or a physiological situation close to failure. This results in initial diminution of forward flow by the amount of blood that regurgitates during systole. The larger volume of blood in the right atrium, however, increases the pressure of the v wave, so that when the right ventricle relaxes it is subjected to a higher filling pressure than before and dilates further to accommodate the extra blood. In this sense, augmented diastolic filling compensates for the leak. The increased right ventricular dilatation, however, may cause a greater degree of tricuspid incompetence, so that a vicious circle may become established; forces acting in the opposite direction are myocardial resistance to unlimited diastolic stretch and the restraining influence of the pericardium, so that the situation is quickly stabilised.

The right atrial pressure pulse is similar to the left atrial pressure pulse in cases of mitral incompetence, and is characterised by an unusually large v wave followed by a rapid y descent and deep y trough (fig. 10.39). The "overshoot" in the early part of the right ventricular diastolic pressure tracing slightly precedes the y descent, there being a strong potential pressure gradient from atrium to ventricle as the pressure within the latter falls rapidly to zero. These appearances are identical with those found in

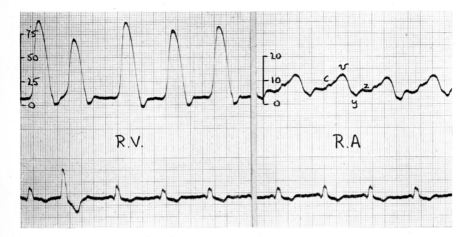

Fig. 10.39—R.V. and R.A. pressure pulses from a case of severe pulmonary valve stenosis with functional tricuspid incompetence. There is 2–1 atrial flutter (not well shown) and right B.B.B. Note the absence of the *x* descent, the steep *y* descent, and the conspicuous *y* trough in the R.A. tracing and the so-called "overshoot" in the R.V. tracing.

cases of Pick's disease, when the likelihood of tricuspid incompetence seems remote. In the illustration shown, there is 2–1 atrial flutter (not well seen in the electrocardiographic lead recorded) and right bundle branch block. The *x* descent is absent, as in most cases of atrial fibrillation (or flutter), just as it is in left atrial pressure tracings in cases of atrial fibrillation, even when it is known for certain that there is no mitral incompetence. Since nearly all cases of functional tricuspid incompetence that are recognised as such have atrial fibrillation, disappearance of the *x* descent does not provide convincing evidence of the diagnosis, despite traditional belief to the contrary. Certainly the magnitude of *v* can be so great in florid cases of tricuspid incompetence as to be hard to reconcile with any other diagnosis, but that is another matter. Certainly all cases of tricuspid incompetence with normal rhythm and with jugular pulses having two crests and two troughs (*a*, *x*, *v* and *y*) are being overlooked. For current expressions of the other view, based on careful physiological studies, the reader is referred to papers by Bloomfield *et al.* (1946), Müller and shillingford (1954), and Korner and Shillingford (1954).

CLINICAL FEATURES

Age and *sex* are related to the underlying disease, not to the tricuspid incompetence.

The only *symptoms* that are directly attributable to the leak are venous throbbing in the neck and abdomen, swelling of the abdomen from gross enlargement of the liver, and perhaps ascites and œdema, although these are partly due to the primary disease; tricuspid incompetence, however, diminishes the cardiac output further. In very advanced cases there may be impairment of hepatic function and hepatic psychosis.

The *physical signs* include an unusually large *v* wave in the jugular pulse, followed by a rapid *y* descent and conspicuous *y* trough (fig. 10.40),

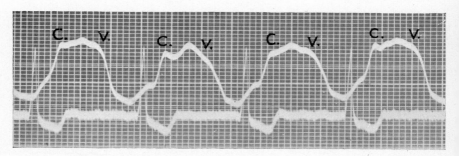

Fig. 10.40—Jugular phlebogram showing fusion of the *c* and *v* waves in a case of tricuspid incompetence; owing to atrial fibrillation the *a* wave is absent.
(*By courtesy of Dr. Max Zoob*)

systolic pulsation of the liver synchronous with the large *v* wave, occasionally systolic pulsation of peripheral veins also (when the venous valves have become incompetent), a hyperdynamic right ventricular thrust, a pansystolic murmur (with or without a thrill) that waxes during inspiration and which may be heard anywhere over the distended right ventricle from the left sternal edge to the apex beat (usually formed by the right ventricle in these cases), and sometimes a short functional tricuspid diastolic murmur as well.

The great majority of recognised cases are associated with atrial fibrillation, as previously pointed out, and either because of this or because

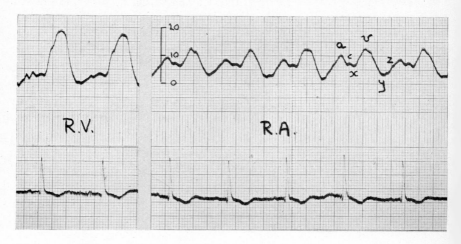

Fig. 10.41—Right ventricular and right atrial pressure pulses from a case of organic tricuspid incompetence with normal rhythm showing preservation of the *x* descent, and a conspicuous *y* trough.

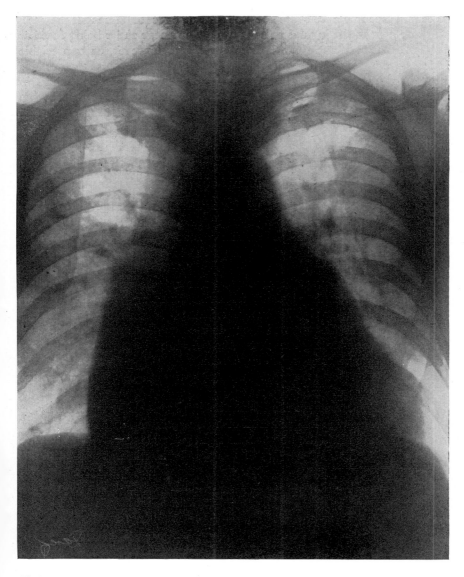

Fig. 10.42—Skiagram showing gross dilatation of the right atrium with a blunt right
cardio-phrenic angle in a case of tricuspid incompetence.

tricuspid incompetence overcomes the sucking effect of descent of the base, the x descent of the jugular pulse is usually absent, c and v being fused as in figure 10.40. When there is normal rhythm, however, an appreciable x descent may follow a powerful a wave, and the jugular pulse then retains its two crests (a and v) and two troughs (x and y). Good tracings of unquestionable tricuspid incompetence associated with normal rhythm are rare, but an example is shown in figure 10.41; the x descent in this case is admittedly small.

The *electrocardiogram* may show right ventricular preponderance in organic tricuspid incompetence without pulmonary hypertension; as a rule, however, the right ventricular preponderance is caused by the primary lesion.

X-rays show gross dilatation of the right atrium, the border of which may meet the diaphragm at a right angle, or even obtusely (fig. 10.42). In pericardial effusion this angle is usually acute. On fluoroscopy the right atrium rarely expands in systole; the right lobe of the diaphragm may reflect hepatic pulsation.

Catheter studies have demonstrated reversal of the central venous pressure gradient during systole, forward flow being limited to diastole (Bloomfield *et al.*, 1946). Venous valves take on the function of the tricuspid valve. The diagnosis of tricuspid incompetence may thus be confirmed by demonstrating a higher mean pressure in the right atrium and superior vena cava than in the subclavian vein (Sharpey-Schafer, 1947); moreover, as the catheter is withdrawn, pulsation ceases abruptly the moment the pressure falls (fig. 10.43).

Tricuspid incompetence should also be demonstrable by injecting Evans blue dye through the longer barrel of a double lumen catheter the tip of which is inserted into the body of the right ventricle, for some of the dye should then be recoverable from the right atrium via the shorter barrel. This technique was employed by Daley, McMillan and Gorlin (1953) to demonstrate functional mitral incompetence secondary to experimental atrial fibrillation in dogs.

By inserting the tip of a double lumen catheter into the right atrium so that the end of the shorter barrel lies in the superior vena cava, pressures from these two sites may be recorded simultaneously by means of two

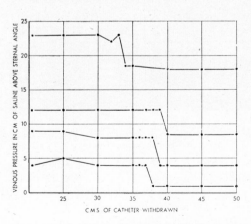

Fig. 10.43—Graph illustrating fall in mean central venous pressure as the catheter is withdrawn from right atrium and superior vena cava into the subclavian vein.

electromanometers and recording systems. If the electrical output from the two manometers is opposed, however, the resultant represents the differential pressure between right atrium and superior vena cava, and may be directly recorded as such (Lee, Matthews and Sharpey-Schafer, 1954). Using a specially constructed differential manometer, Müller and Shillingford (1954) found that in tricuspid incompetence there was a reversed pressure gradient between the superior vena cava and right atrium throughout ventricular systole, and that this was greater in early systole. They concluded that there must be a reversal of flow from right atrium to superior vena cava during this phase of the cardiac cycle.

DIFFERENTIAL DIAGNOSIS

The chief difficulty is to distinguish tricuspid incompetence from heart failure without tricuspid incompetence, and in view of the controversy concerning the correct interpretation of the venous pulse in cases with atrial fibrillation, it may be wise to rely more on the tricuspid pan-systolic murmur which waxes during inspiration. A point that needs settling, however, is whether an overloaded right ventricle does in fact leak more when its filling pressure is increased during inspiration; its forward output should fall under these circumstances, and its backward output could well fall also.

A second difficulty in cases of mitral valve disease is to distinguish a tricuspid systolic murmur from a mitral systolic murmur. Theoretically this is easy, but in practice they are not infrequently confused. This is because the tricuspid murmur may be very well heard at the apex beat, which in these cases is often formed by the right ventricle. Reliance should be placed not only on the way the bruit is influenced by respiration, but also on the clinical circumstances as a whole. For example, mitral incompetence is improbable in cases with an extreme pulmonary vascular resistance, functional tricuspid incompetence is rare in the absence of an extreme pulmonary vascular resistance, and organic tricuspid incompetence is rare without some evidence of tricuspid stenosis.

COURSE AND PROGNOSIS

Functional tricuspid incompetence is serious not so much in itself, but because of the severity of the underlying lesion that provokes it. The prognosis should be based on this lesion rather than the leak.

The two commonest causes are pulmonary hypertensive mitral stenosis and atrial septal defect, and in both of these conditions patients with tricuspid incompetence may continue to get about for years. Cases of pulmonary stenosis with tricuspid incompetence may also linger on. When tricuspid incompetence is caused by primary pulmonary hypertension or cor pulmonale, however, the outlook is bad, and life expectancy limited to a year or two at the most.

TREATMENT

Bed rest and full treatment for heart failure is advisable in the first instance to see whether the tricuspid incompetence is reversible. If not, the patient should be allowed up and about, although treatment for heart failure should be continued.

TRICUSPID STENOSIS

Although organic disease of the tricuspid valve is found at necropsy in 10 to 20 per cent of all cases of chronic rheumatic heart disease (Cooke and White, 1941; Smith and Levine, 1942), clinical tricuspid stenosis is infrequently recognised. It is nearly always accompanied by mitral stenosis (Pitt, 1909), often by aortic valve disease as well. In my own analysed series of some 500 cases of rheumatic heart disease tricuspid stenosis was found in 4 per cent; since the majority of these 500 cases were catheterised and the tracings inspected carefully for the tell-tale pressure gradient, the frequency given is believed to be accurate.

ETIOLOGY

Tricuspid stenosis is nearly always rheumatic. Both disseminated lupus and argentaffinoma, however, may cause it, and congenital cases have been reported.

PATHOLOGY

The development of chronic tricuspid valve disease following active endocarditis presumably resembles the march of events in mitral disease, but the end result is somewhat different in that fusion is said to result more often in a single valve curtain perforated by a central or eccentric roundish hole than in button-hole stenosis. Although some degree of incompetence would therefore be expected in the majority of cases, physiological studies suggest that stenosis is the commoner lesion. How this tallies with necropsy evidence to the contrary remains to be seen. Aceves and Carral (1947), for instance, found tricuspid valve disease in 33 per cent of 147 consecutive necropsies in cases of rheumatic heart disease; of these, 11 were stenosed, 28 incompetent and 11 mixed. It is possible, therefore, that cases of organic tricuspid incompetence are being overlooked clinically.

HÆMODYNAMICS

Tricuspid stenosis tends to prevent proper filling of the right ventricle and therefore both lowers the cardiac output and relieves pulmonary venous congestion caused by mitral stenosis, which is invariably present. The obstruction results in elevation of the right atrial pressure and in a presystolic (fig. 10.44) or diastolic pressure gradient (fig. 10.45) across the tricuspid valve, similar in all respects to the pressure gradient across the mitral valve in cases of mitral stenosis (fig. 10.46). The presystolic gradient

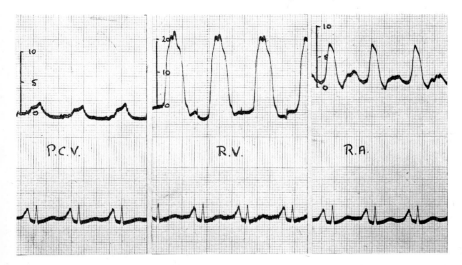

Fig. 10.44—Intracardiac pressure pulses from a case of tricuspid stenosis with normal rhythm showing giant *a* waves in the right atrial tracing, and a presystolic pressure gradient across the tricuspid valve.

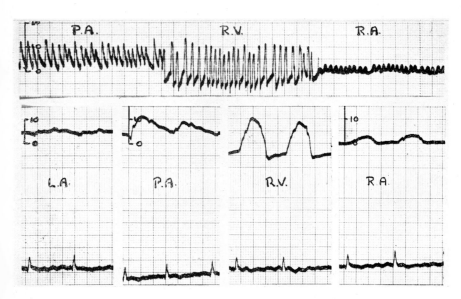

Fig. 10.45—Intracardiac pressure pulses in a case of tricuspid stenosis with atrial fibrillation showing a diastolic pressure gradient across the tricuspid valve, a rather slow *y* descent and absence of the *y* trough.

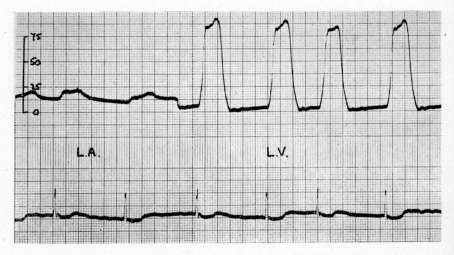

Fig. 10.46—Pressure pulses from the left atrium and left ventricle in a case of mitral stenosis with atrial fibrillation, showing a diastolic pressure gradient across the mitral valve, slow *y* descent and absent *y* trough.

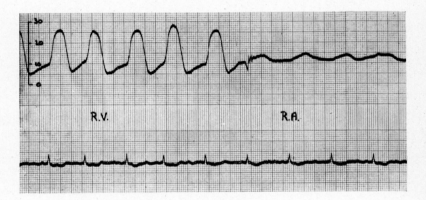

Tricuspid stenosis: pre-operative.

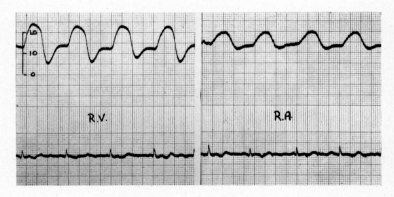

Post-operative tricuspid incompetence.

Fig. 10.47—Pressure pulses from the right ventricle and right atrium in a case of tricuspid stenosis before and after tricuspid valvotomy. The slow *y* descent and absent *y* trough have been abolished.

is seen with normal rhythm, the diastolic with atrial fibrillation. Filling of the right ventricle is retarded, so the rate of *y* descent following *v* in right atrial and jugular pressure pulses is relatively slow (fig. 10.47), and there is no appreciable *y* trough (Gibson and Wood, 1955). The change in the slope of *y* and the development of a *y* trough following surgical relief of the obstruction is well shown in the lower tracing of figure 10.47 (tricuspid incompetence was produced inadvertently in this case). The size of the orifice may be calculated from the cardiac output, pressure gradient and heart rate as described for mitral stenosis.

The right atrium becomes hypertrophied and distended, while the right ventricle remains quiet, underfilled, and small. The low cardiac output, high venous pressure and distended liver encourage œdema and ascites, as in Pick's disease, which in some respects it resembles (Thompson and Levine, 1937).

CLINICAL FEATURES

There were 16 women and 6 men in my small series of 22 cases. Their average age was 35, the range 21 to 48. Figures from the literature are not included because up till now the majority of mild and moderate cases have been overlooked clinically. Necropsy figures, however, show that the average age and sex ratio in tricuspid cases is much the same as for mitral stenosis (Aceves and Carral, 1947).

Symptoms

The first symptom may be fluttering discomfort in the neck caused by the development of a giant *a* wave in the jugular pulse. More often the pulse is seen in the mirror or noted by an interested relative. Hepatic pulsation is rarely mentioned by the patient.

Apart from this there are no complaints attributable to tricuspid stenosis until the cardiac output is sufficiently reduced to cause fatigue, or the liver sufficiently enlarged to cause obvious swelling of the abdomen; œdema and ascites follow. At the same time the patient is usually spared the distressing symptoms that would otherwise have developed on account of the associated mitral stenosis; thus hæmoptysis, acute pulmonary œdema, paroxysmal cardiac dyspnœa, orthopnœa and winter bronchitis are noticeably absent in the majority of cases.

Physical signs

There are so many characteristic and specific features of tricuspid stenosis that it is remarkable how frequently the clinical diagnosis is overlooked. In fact, a confident bedside diagnosis can be made in 80 per cent of cases if proper attention is paid to the following points:

1. If there is normal rhythm there is almost invariably a *giant a wave* in the jugular pulse (fig. 10.48), and *presystolic hepatic pulsation*, as noted by Mackenzie (1902).

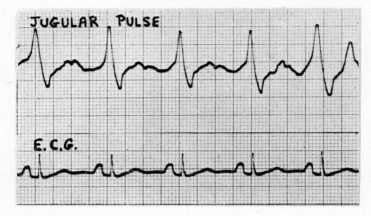

Fig. 10.48—Jugular phlebogram showing giant *a* waves in a case of tricuspid stenosis with normal rhythm.

2. If there is atrial fibrillation there is a prominent *v* wave in the jugular pulse, which characteristically subsides slowly; *there is no y dip* (fig. 10.47) as there is in all other conditions with venous pressures at this level (Owen and Wood, 1955; Gibson and Wood, 1955).

3. *The heart itself is quiet*, there being no appreciable lift over the right ventricle as there usually is in pulmonary hypertensive cases of mitral stenosis, which may also cause giant *a* waves in the jugular pulse. Pulmonary valve closure is also impalpable.

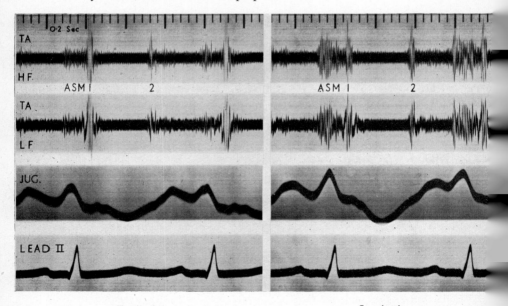

Expiration.   Inspiration.

Fig. 10.49—Phonocardiogram showing the effect of inspiration on the tricuspid atrio-systolic murmur. The prominent *a* wave in the jugular phlebogram also increases with inspiration

4. *Auscultation* at the left sternal edge in the fourth space reveals a tricuspid presystolic or diastolic murmur which is sharply accentuated during inspiration (fig. 10.49), when right ventricular filling is encouraged (Carvallo, 1950). A thrill may accompany the bruit. A tricuspid opening snap may also be heard (Kossman, 1955), but may be difficult to distinguish from the mitral opening snap which is usually present unless it is accentuated during inspiration. Accentuation of the tricuspid first sound, also increased by inspiration, is even less convincing. An associated tricuspid systolic murmur may be present, but is far from invariable. The pulmonary component of the second heart sound is not accentuated, as in pulmonary hypertensive cases of mitral stenosis, and there is never right atrial presystolic gallop which usually accompanies the giant *a* wave in other conditions.

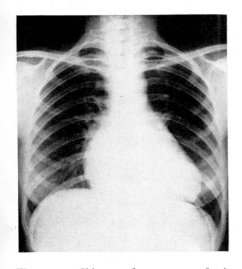

Fig. 10.50—Skiagram from a case of tricuspid stenosis showing conspicuous enlargement of the right atrium without dilatation of the pulmonary artery; note also the absence of "pulmonary venous congestion".

5. *Fluoroscopy* shows characteristic enlargement of the right atrium without conspicuous dilatation of the pulmonary artery, and the lung fields are relatively clear (fig. 10.50). Absence of enlargement of the right ventricle is difficult to demonstrate radiologically when the right atrium is dilated. Calcification of the tricuspid valve is very rare.

6. The *electrocardiogram* in cases with normal rhythm commonly shows the highly characteristic combination of an unusually tall widened P wave (combined P pulmonale and P mitrale) and absence of right ventricular preponderance (fig. 10.51).

DIFFERENTIAL DIAGNOSIS

The possibility of tricuspid stenosis should be borne in mind in any case of mitral valve disease in which the jugular venous pressure is unquestionably raised, the differential diagnosis then lying between this, uncontrolled atrial fibrillation, severe mitral incompetence, a high pulmonary vascular resistance and pericardial effusion, for in uncomplicated mitral stenosis the venous pressure is nearly always normal, a primary myocardial fault being rare (Wood, 1954).

Digitalis soon controls the ventricular rate, and allows the jugular pulse to be analysed more easily. Mitral incompetence should be recognised

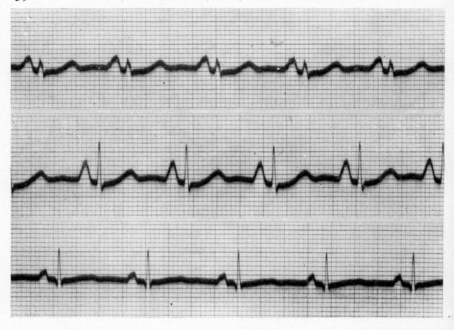

Fig. 10.51—Electrocardiogram showing exceptionally tall yet widened P waves in a case of mitral and tricuspid stenosis. Note also the absence of right axis deviation.

without difficulty, and if severe the likelihood of associated tricuspid stenosis is remote. If a high pulmonary vascular resistance is responsible for the giant *a* wave, it should be recognised by the heaving right ventricle, accentuated pulmonary second sound, conspicuously dilated pulmonary artery and strong right ventricular preponderance electrocardiographically. Pericardial effusion may have to be considered, but it does not cause a giant *a* wave, slow *y* descent, nor absent *y* trough; radiologically the appearances can be similar, but the P wave of the electrocardiogram is normal when there is sinus rhythm. Pathognomonic of tricuspid stenosis are the slow *y* descent and tricuspid bruits.

Ebstein's disease, certain cardiopathies usually of unknown or uncertain etiology, and chronic constrictive pericarditis may bear some superficial resemblance to rheumatic tricuspid stenosis, but their distinction is rarely difficult. They are more likely to be confused with isolated tricuspid stenosis from disseminated lupus.

SPECIAL TESTS

Cardiac catheterisation is the most convincing way of proving or disproving the existence of physiological tricuspid stenosis. By sliding the tip of a looped catheter up and down the lateral wall of the right atrium, pericardial effusion can be easily diagnosed or eliminated. After recording left atrial and pulmonary artery pressures and measuring the cardiac output in the usual way, the catheter is withdrawn slowly from the right ventricle to the right atrium, while intracardiac pressures are recorded continuously. In normal controls the diastolic and presystolic right atrial pressure is identical with the right ventricular diastolic and end-diastolic pressure respectively (fig. 10.52), whereas in tricuspid stenosis a presystolic or diastolic pressure gradient across the valve can be demonstrated routinely (fig. 10.53 and 10.47). If by ill fortune the right ventricle cannot be entered, the slow y descent in the right atrial tracing should still reveal the correct diagnosis. The Ry/v ratio has not yet been worked out for tricuspid valve disease.

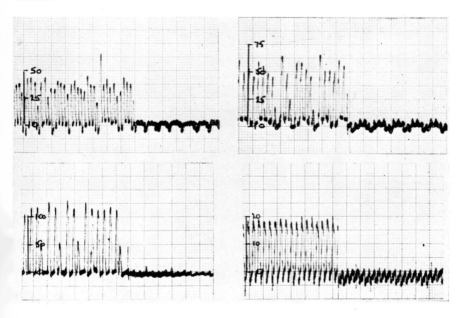

Fig. 10.52—Withdrawal tracings from right ventricle to right atrium showing identical
diastolic pressures in these two chambers in four controls.

Phonocardiography confirms the tricuspid origin of the murmurs and demonstrates their relationship to respiration (fig. 10.49).

PROGNOSIS

It has long been known that some patients with obvious tricuspid stenosis may carry on their occupations for a remarkably long time with relatively little disability. On the other hand, others linger on year after year in considerable distress from fatigue, chronic œdema, ascites and distended abdomen, whether they attempt to continue a sedentary occupation or not. A rigid low sodium diet, repeated injections of mersalyl, and occasional abdominal paracentesis may relieve these symptoms, but not without adding their own discomforts.

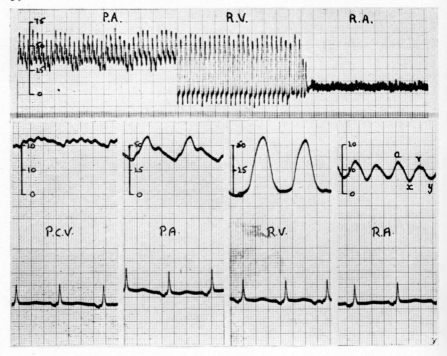

Fig. 10.53—Withdrawal tracings from the right ventricle to the right atrium in a case of tricuspid stenosis with normal rhythm showing a presystolic and diastolic pressure gradient across the tricuspid valve.

Aceves and Carral (1947) found that life expectancy averaged five years from the time the diagnosis was first made, but in the past the diagnosis has been made notoriously late. Thompson and Levine (1937) particularly have emphasised the relatively long life expectancy and surprising ability of patients to carry on despite the discomforts and gross physical signs alluded to above.

TREATMENT

Medical measures include all the usual means of combating chronic ascites and œdema; prior to their onset, however, the patient should not be unduly restricted, for there is little danger of acute pulmonary congestive symptoms despite coincident mitral stenosis.

Tricuspid valvotomy has only been undertaken in a few isolated cases so far (Trace *et al.*, 1954; Chesterman and Whittaker, 1954; O'Neill Janton and Glover, 1954; McCord, Swan and Blount, 1954). There may be considerable difficulty in locating the commissures and serious tricuspid incompetence may result from too bold an attack, as in the patient whose tracings are illustrated in figure 10.47. In the great majority of my own cases, the tricuspid stenosis was not severe enough to warrant interference although mitral valvotomy was carried out in several of them.

REFERENCES

Aceves, S., and Carral, R. (1947): "The diagnosis of tricuspid valve disease", *Amer. Heart J.*, **34**, 114.

Allison, P. R., and Linden, R. J. (1953): "The bronchoscopic measurement of left auricular pressure", *Circulation*, **7**, 669.

Ari, R., Harvey, W. P., and Hufnagel, C. A. (1955): "Etiology of hoarseness associated with mitral stenosis", *Amer. Heart J.*, **50**, 153.

Bailey, C. P. (1949): "The surgical treatment of mitral stenosis (mitral commissurotomy)", *Dis. Chest*, **15**, 377.

——, Bolton, H. E., Jamison, W. L., and Nichols, H. T. (1954): "Commissurotomy for rheumatic aortic stenosis. 1. Surgery", *Circulation*, **9**, 22.

——, Redundo-Ramirez, H. P., and Larzelere, H. B. (1952): "Surgical treatment of aortic stenosis", *J. Amer. med. Ass.*, **150**, 1647.

Baker, C., Brock, R. C., and Campbell M., (1950) "Valvulotomy for mitral stenosis". *B.M.J.*, *i*, **1283**.

——, ——, ——, and Wood, P. (1952): "Valvotomy for mitral stenosis", *Ibid.*, *i*, **1043**.

Bechgaard, P. (1946): "Arterial hypertension. A follow-up study of one thousand hypertonics", *Acta. med. Scand.*, Supp. 172.

Bergeron, J., Abelmann, W. H., Vazquez-Milan, H., and Ellis, L. B. (1954): "Aortic stenosis—clinical manifestations and course of the disease", *Arch. intern. Med.*, **94**, 911.

Björk, V. O., and Malström, G. (1955): "The diagnosis of aortic stenosis", *Amer. Heart J.*, **50**, 303.

——, ——, and Uggla, L. G. (1953): "Left auricular pressure measurements in man", *Ann. Surg.*, **138**, 718.

——, Blakemore, W. S., and Malmström, G. (1954): "Left ventricular pressure measurement in man", *Amer. Heart J.*, **48**, 197.

——, Kjellberg, S. R., Malmstrom, G., and Rudhe, U. (1955): "The diagnosis of mitral insufficiency", *Amer. Heart J.*, **49**, 719.

Bland, E. F., and Sweet, R. H. (1949): "A venous shunt for advanced mitral stenosis", *J. Amer. med. Ass.*, **140**, 1259.

Bloomfield, R. A., Lauson, H. D., Cournand, A., Breed, E. S., and Richards, D. W. (1946): "Recording of right heart pressures in normal subjects and in patients with chronic pulmonary disease and various types of cardiocirculatory disease", *J. clin. Invest.*, **25**, 639.

Boone, J. A., and Levine, S. A. (1938): "The prognosis in 'potential rheumatic heart disease' and 'rheumatic mitral insufficiency", *Amer. J. med. Sc.*, **195**, 764.

Bramwell, C. (1937): "Arterial pulse in health and disease", *Lancet, ii*, 239, 301, 366.

Braun-Menendez, E., and Orias, O. (1935): "Curacion de las fases del ciclo cardiaco en hipertensos", *Rev. Argent. Cardiol.*, **2**, 186.

Brigden, W., and Leatham, A. (1953): "Mitral incompetence", *Brit. Heart J.*, **15**, 55.

Brock R. C. (1950): See Baker.

—— (1952): "The surgical and pathological anatomy of the mitral valve", *Brit. Heart J.*, **14**, 489.

Burwell, C. S., Strayhorn, W. D., Flickinger, D., Corlette, M. B., Bowerman, E. P., and Kennedy, J. A. (1938): "Circulation during pregnancy", *Arch. intern. Med.*, **62**, 979.

Cabot, R. C. (1926): "Facts on the heart", Philadelphia.

Campbell, M. (1932): "Aortic valvular disease", *Brit. med. J.*, **1**, 328.

Carvallo, J. M. R. (1950): "El diagnóstico de la estenosis tricuspidea", *Arch. Inst. Cardiol. Mexico*, **20**, 1.

Chesterman, J. T., and Whitaker, W. (1954): "Mitral and tricuspid valvotomy for mitral and tricuspid stenosis", *Amer. Heart J.*, **48**, 631.

Christian, H. A. (1931): "Aortic stenosis with calcification", *J. Amer. med. Ass.*, **97**, 158.

Clawson, B. J. (1931): "Nonsyphilitic aortic valve deformity", *Arch. Path.*, **12**, 889.

——, Noble, J. F., and Lufkin, N. H. (1938): "The calcified nodular deformity of the aortic valve", *Amer. Heart J.*, **15**, 58.

Contratto, A. W., and Levine, S. A. (1937): "Aortic stenosis with special reference to angina pectoris and syncope", *Ann. intern. Med.*, **10**, 1636.

Cooke, W. T., and White, P. D. (1941): "Tricuspid stenosis", *Brit. Heart J.*, **3**, 147.

Coombs, C .F. (1924): "Rheumatic heart disease", Bristol.

Corrigan, D. J. (1832): "On permanent patency of the mouth of the aorta, or inadequacy of the aortic valves", *Edin. med. and surg. J.*, **37**, 225.

Cossio, P., and Berconsky, I. (1943): "El primer ruido cardiaco y el soplo presistolico en la estrechez mitral con fibrillación auricular", *Rev. Argent. Cardiol.*, **10**, 162.

——, and Perianes, I. (1949): "Surgical treatment of the 'Cardiac Lung'; ligation of the inferior vena cava and or tricuspid valvulotomy", *J. Amer. med. Ass.*, **140**, 772.

Cowan, J., and Ritchie, W. T. (1935): "Diseases of the heart", Edward Arnold & Co., London.

D'Allaines, F., Lenègre, J., Dubost, Ch., Mathivat, A., and Scébat, L. (1949): "Rétrécissement mitral. Anastomose veine pulmonaire-veine azygos. Premier cas opéré", *Mémoires de l' Académie de Chirurgie, Paris*, **75**, 318.

Daley, R., McMillan, I. K. R., and Gorlin, R. (1953): "Mitral incompetence in experimental auricular fibrillation", *Lancet*, **2**, 18.

——, Mattingly, T. W., Holt, L., Bland, E. F., and White, P. D. (1951): "Systemic arterial embolism in rheumatic heart disease", *Amer. Heart J.*, **42**, 566.

Davis, D., and Weiss, S. (1931): "Rheumatic heart disease. I. Incidence and rôle in the causation of death. A study of 5,215 consecutive necropsies", *Amer. Heart J.*, **7**, 146.

Davies, C. E., and Steiner, R. E. (1949): "Calcified aortic valve: clinical and radiological features", *Brit. Heart J.*, **11**, 126.

Davies, L. G., Goodwin, J. F., Steiner, R. E., and Van Leuven, B. D. (1953): "The clinical and radiological assessment of the pulmonary arterial pressure in mitral stenosis", *Ibid.*, **15**, 393.

Decker, J. P., *et al.* (1953): "Rheumatic activity as judged by the presence of Aschoff bodies in auricular appendages of patients with mitral stenosis. I. Anatomic aspects", *Circulation*, **8**, 161.

De Graff, A. C., and Lingg, C. (1935): "Course of rheumatic heart disease in adults", *Amer. Heart J.*, **10**, 459, 478, and 630.

de Veer, J. A. (1938): "Sudden death in aortic stenosis, explanation on a mechanical basis", *Ibid.*, **15**, 243.

de la Chapelle, C. E., Graef, I., and Rottino, A. (1934): "Studies in rheumatic heart disease; analysis of 119 hearts with special reference to relationship of auricular fibrillation, to mitral valvular deformity and certain rheumatic tissue changes", *Amer. Heart J.*, **10**, 62.

Dieckhoff, J. (1936): "Leistungs fahigkeit aortenklappeninsuffizienter Herzen ohne und mit Hypertrophie im Herz-Jungen-Praparat. (Nebst. Digitalisierungseffekten)", *Arch. f. Exper. Path. u. Pharmakol.*, **182**, 268.

Dolowitz, D. A., and Lewis, C. S. (1948): "Left vocal cord paralysis associated with cardiac disease", *Amer. J. Med.*, **4**, 856.

Donald, K. W., Bishop, J. M., Cumming, G., and Wade, O. L. (1953): "The effect of nursing positions on the cardiac output in man", *Clin. Sc.*, **12**, 199.

Donzelot, E., Dubost, Ch., Heim de Balzac, R., Metianu, C., and Gallemot, K. (1953): "Recurrence of mitral stenosis following commissurotomy", *Arch. mal. coeur*, **46**, 301.

Drinker, C. K. (1945): "Pulmonary edema and inflammation", Harvard University Press, Cambridge.

Dry, T. J., and Willius, F. A. (1939): "Calcareous disease of the aortic valve", *Amer. Heart J.*, **17**, 138.

Durozier, P. (1861): "Du double souffle intermittent crural, comme signe de l'insuffissance aortique", *Arch. gén. de Med.*, Paris, 107, 417, 588.

Elkeles, A., and Glynn, L. E. (1946): "Disseminated parenchymatous ossification in the lungs in association with mitral stenosis", *J. Path. Bact.*, 58, 517.

Ellis, L. B., and Harken, D. E. (1955): "Clinical progress: The clinical results in the first five hundred patients with mitral stenosis undergoing valvuloplasty", *Circulation*, 11, 637.

Evans, W. (1947): "Heart murmurs", *Brit. Heart J.*, 9, 1.

———, and Benson, R. (1948): "Massive thrombus of the left auricle", *Ibid.*, 10, 39.

Fauvel, S. A. (1843): "Memoire sur les signes stethoscopiques du rétrécisse-ment de l'orifice auriculo-ventriculaire gauche du coeur", *Arch. gén. de Med.*, Paris (ser. 4), 1, 1.

Fetterolf, G., and Norris, G. W. (1911): "The anatomical explanation of the paralysis of the left recurrent laryngeal nerve found in certain cases of mitral stenosis", *Amer. J. med. Sc.*, 141, 625.

Fishberg, A. M. (1940): "Heart failure", Lea and Febiger, Philadelphia, 2nd. ed., p. 521.

Flint, A. (1862): "On cardiac murmurs", *Amer. J. med. Sc.*, 44, 29.

Gairdner, W. T. (1861): "A short account of cardiac murmurs", *Edin. Med. J.*, 7, 445.

Garvin, C. F. (1941): "Mural thrombi in heart", *Amer. Heart J.*, 21, 713.

Gernandt, B., and Nylin, G. (1946): "The relation between circulation time and the amount of the residual blood of the heart", *Ibid.*, 32, 411.

Gibson, R. V., and Wood, P. (1955): "The diagnosis of tricuspid stenosis", *Brit. Heart J.*, 17, 552.

Gilroy, J. C., Marchand, P., and Wilson, V. H. (1952): "The rôle of the bronchial veins in mitral stenosis", *Lancet*, 2, 957.

Glover, R. P., O'Neill, T. J. E., and Bailey, C. P. (1950): "Commissurotomy for mitral stenosis", *Circulation*, 1, 329.

Goldberg, H., Bakst, A. A., and Bailey, C. P. (1954): "The dynamics of aortic valvular disease", *Amer. Heart J.*, 47, 527.

Gorlin, R., and Gorlin, S. G. (1951): "Hydraulic formula for calculation of the area of the stenotic mitral valve, other cardiac valves, and central circulatory shunts. 1.", *Ibid.*, 41, 1.

———, Lewis, B. M., Haynes, F. W., Spiegl, R. J., and Dexter, L. (1951): "Factors regulating pulmonary 'capillary' pressure in mitral stenosis. IV", *Ibid.*, 41, 834.

———, McMillan, I. K. R., Medd, W. E., Matthews, M. B., and Daley, R. (1955): "Dynamics of the circulation in aortic valvular disease", *Amer. J. Med.*, 18, 855.

Gouley, B. A. (1938): "The rôle of mitral stenosis and of post-rheumatic pulmonary fibrosis in the evolution of chronic rheumatic heart desease," *Amer. J. med. Sc.*, 196, 11.

Grainger, R. G., and Hearn, J. B. (1955): "Intrapulmonary septal lymphatic lines (B lines of Kerley). Their significance and their prognostic evaluation before valvotomy", *J. Fac. Radiol.*, 7, 661.

Gumpert, T. E. (1947): "Miliary appearances in the lungs in mitral stenosis", *Brit. med. J.*, ii, 488.

Hall, P., Dencker, S. J., and Björck, G. (1952): "Studies in mitral stenosis. III. Observations on the incidence and distribution of cerebral emboli with regard to the possibilities of their prevention during operative procedures", *Amer. Heart J.*, 44, 600.

Harken, D. E., Ellis, L. B., Ware, P. F., and Norman, L. R. (1948): "The surgical treatment of mitral stenosis. 1. Valvuloplasty", *New England J. Med.*, 239, 801.

Harrison, T. R. (1935): "Failure of the circulation", Baltimore.

Harvey, R. M., Ferrer, M. I., Samet, P., Bader, R. A., Bader, M. E., Cournand, A., and Richards, D. W. (1955): "Mechanical and myocardial factors in rheumatic heart disease with mitral stenosis", *Circulation*, 11, 531.

Hayward, G. W. (1955): "Pulmonary œdema", *Brit. med. J.*, 1, 1361.

Hellems, H. K., Haynes, F. W., Gowdy, J. F., and Dexter, L. (1948): "The pulmonary capillary pressure in man", *J. Clin. Invest.*, 27, 540.

Henry, E. W. (1952): "The small pulmonary vessels in mitral stenosis", *Brit. Heart J.*, 14, 406.

Holling, H. E. (1951): "The pulmonary circulation", *Guy's Hosp. Gaz.*, 65, 271.

Hope, J. (1839): "A treatise on the diseases of the heart and great vessels", 3rd ed., London.

Horan, M. J., Jr., and Barnes, A. R. (1948): "Calcareous aortic stenosis and coronary artery disease", *Amer. J. Med. Sc.*, 215, 451.

Hufnagel, C. A., Harvey, W. P., Rabil, P. J., and McDermott, T. F. (1954): "Surgical correction of aortic insufficiency", *Surgery*, 35, 673.

Janton, O. H., Glover, R. P., and O'Neill, T. J. E. (1952): "Indications for commissurotomy in mitral stenosis", *Amer. J. Med.*, 12, 621.

Karsner, H. T., and Koletsky, S. (1947): "Calcific disease of the aortic valve", J. B. Lippincott Company, Philadelphia and London.

Kerley, P. (1933): "Radiology in heart disease", *Brit. med. J.*, 2, 594.

King, T. W. (1838): "On morbid flattening or compression of the left bronchus produced by dilatation of the left auricle", *Guy's Hosp. Rep.*, 175.

Korner, P., and Shillingford, J. (1954): "The right atrial pulse in congestive heart failure", *Brit. Heart J.*, 16, 447.

Kossman, C. E. (1955): "The opening snap of the tricuspid valve; a physical sign of tricuspid stenosis", *Circulation*, 11, 378.

Kuttner, A. G., and Markowitz, M. (1948): "The diagnosis of mitral insufficiency in rheumatic children", *Amer. Heart J.*, 35, 718.

Lagerlöf, M., and Werkö, L. (1949): "The pulmonary capillary venous pressure pulse in man", *Scandinav. J. Clin. and Lab. Invest.*, 1, 147.

——, ——, Bucht, H., and Holmgren, A. (1949): "Separate determination of blood volume of right and left heart and lungs in man with aid of dye injection method", *Scand. J. Clin. and Lab. Invest.*, 1, 114.

Larzelere, H. B., and Bailey, C. P. (1953): "Aortic commissurotomy", *J. thorac. Surg.*, 26, 31.

Lasser, R. P., and Loewe, L. (1952): "Esophageal pressure pulse patterns (esophageal piezocardiogram). 1. Experimental observations", *Amer. Heart J.*, 44, 531.

——, —— (1954): "Cardiac and pulmonary artery pressure pulses in experimental mitral stenosis", *Ibid.*, 48, 801.

Leatham, A. (1951): "The phonocardiogram of aortic stenosis", *Brit. Heart J.*, 13, 153.

—— (1954): "Splitting of the first and second heart sounds", *Lancet*, ii, 607.

Lee, G. de J., Matthews, M. B., and Sharpey-Schafer, E. P. (1954): "The effect of the Valsalva manœuvre on the systemic and pulmonary arterial pressure in man", *Brit. Heart J.*, 16, 311.

Lendrum, A. C. (1950): "Pulmonary hæmosiderosis of cardiac origin", *J. Path. Bact.*, 62, 555.

——, Scott, L. D. W., and Park, S. D. S. (1950): "Pulmonary changes due to cardiac disease, with special reference to hæmosiderosis", *Quart. J. Med.*, 19, 249.

Lewis, B. M., Gorlin, R., Houssay, H. E., Haynes, F. W., and Dexter, L. (1952): "Clinical and physiological correlations in patients with mitral stenosis", *Amer. Heart J.*, 43, 2.

Lian, C., and Welti, J. J. (1937): "Le claquement artériel pulmonaire proto-systolique", *Arch. Mal. du Coeur*, 30, 946.

Likoff, W., Berkowitz, D., Denton, C., and Goldberg, H. (1955): "A clinical evaluation of the surgical management of combined mitral and aortic stenosis", *Amer. Heart J.*, 49, 394.

Liljestrand, G. (1948): "Regulation of pulmonary arterial blood pressure", *Arch. intern. Med.*, **81**, 162.

Logan, A., and Turner, R. (1952): "The diagnosis of mitral incompetence accompanying mitral stenosis. Review of eleven cases treated surgically", *Lancet*, **2**, 593.

Lowe, T. E., and Bate, E. W. (1948): "Hyperplasia of cardiac muscle fibres", *Med. J. Austral.*, **1**, 618.

Luisada, A. A. (1943): "On the pathogenesis of the signs of Traube and Durozier in aortic insufficiency. A graphic study", *Amer. Heart J.*, **26**, 721.

——, and Fleischner, F. G. (1948): "Dynamics of the left auricle in mitral valve lesions", *Amer. J. Med.*, **4**, 791.

McCord, M. C., Swan, H., and Blount, S. G. (1954): "Tricuspid stenosis: clinical and physiologic evaluation", *Amer. Heart J.*, **48**, 405.

MacKenzie, J. (1902): "The study of the pulse arterial, venous and hepatic, and of the movements of the heart", *Young J. Pentland*, London.

McKeown, F. (1953): "The left auricular appendage in mitral stenosis", *Brit. Heart J.*, **15**, 433.

McMillan, I. K. R. (1955): "Aortic stenosis. A post-mortem cinephotographic study of valve action", *Ibid.*, **17**, 56.

Madden, J. L. (1949): "Resection of the left auricular appendix: a prophylaxis for recurrent arterial emboli", *J. Amer. med. Ass.*, **140**, 769.

Magarey, F. R. (1951): "Pathogenesis of mitral stenosis", *Brit. med. J.*, **1**, 856.

Margolies, A., and Wolferth, C. C. (1932): "The opening snap (Claquement d'ouverture de la mitrale) in mitral stenosis, its characteristics, mechanism of production and diagnostic importance", *Amer. Heart J.*, **7**, 443.

Marchand, P., Gilroy, J. C., and Wilson, V. H. (1950): "Anatomical study of bronchial vascular system and its variations in disease", *Thorax*, **5**, 207.

Marshall, R., McIlroy, M. B., and Christie, R. V. (1954): "The work of breathing in mitral stenosis", *Clin. Sci.*, **13**, 137.

May, J. R. (1953): "The bacteriology of chronic bronchitis", *Lancet*, **2**, 534 and 899.

Messer, A. L., Counihan, T. B., Rappaport, M. B., and Sprague, H. B. (1951): "The effect of cycle length on the time of occurrence of the first heart sound and the opening snap in mitral stenosis", *Circulation*, **4**, 576.

Miller, W. S. (1947): "The Lung", 2nd ed., Blackwell Scientific Publications, Oxford.

Mitchell, A. M., Sackett, S. H., Hunzicker, W. J., and Levine, S. (1954): "The clinical features of aortic stenosis", *Amer. Heart J.*, **48**, 684.

Mönckeberg, J. G. (1904): "Der normale histologische Bau und die Sclerose der Aortenklappen", *Virchows Arch. f. path. Anat.*, **176**, 472.

Müller, O., and Shillingford, J. (1954): "Tricuspid incompetence", *Brit. Heart J.*, **16**, 195.

Olesen, K. H. (1955): "Mitral stenosis: a follow-up of 351 patients", Munksgaard, Copenhagen.

O'Neill, T. J. E., Janton, O. H., and Glover, R. P. (1954): "Surgical treatment of tricuspid stenosis", *Circulation*, **9**, 881.

Ortner, N. (1897): "Recurrenslahmung bei mitralstenose", *Wien. klin. Wschr.* **10**, 753.

Owen, S. G., and Wood, P. (1955): "A new method of determining the degree or absence of mitral obstruction", *Brit. Heart J.*, **17**, 41.

Palmer, A. J., and Walker, A. H. C. (1949): "The maternal circulation in normal pregnancy", *J. Obst. Gynæ. Brit. Emp.*, **56**, 537.

Parkinson, J. (1945): "Rheumatic fever and heart disease", *Lancet*, ii, 657.

——, and Hartley, R. (1946): "Early diagnosis of rheumatic valvular disease in recruits", *Brit. Heart J.*, **8**, 212.

Pitt, G. N. (1909): "The system of medicine", ed. Allbutt and Rolleston, London, **6**, 330, and **7**, 310.

Ravin, A., and Bershof, E. (1951): "The intensity of the first heart sound in auricular fibrillation with mitral stenosis", *Amer. Heart J.*, **41**, 539.

Read, J. L., Bosher, L. H., Ferraru, F., Richman, S., and Porter, R. R. (1955): "Angiocardiographic demonstration of occlusive auricular thrombi in dogs", *Circulation*, **12**, 247.

Reynolds, G. (1953): "The atrial electrogram in mitral stenosis", *Brit. Heart J.*, **15**, 250.

Rolleston, H. (1940): "History of aortic regurgitation", *Ann. Med. Hist.*, **2**, 271.

—— (1941): "The history of mitral stenosis", *Brit. Heart J.*, **3**, 1.

Sellors, T. H., Bedford, D. E., and Somerville, W. (1953): "Valvotomy in the treatment of mitral stenosis", *Brit. med. J.*, **2**, 1059.

Sharpey-Schafer, E. P. (1947): Unpublished observations.

Smith, J. A., and Levine, S. A. (1942): "The clinical features of tricuspid stenosis", *Amer. Heart J.*, **23**, 739.

Sohval, A. R., and Gross, L. (1936): "Calcific sclerosis of the aortic valve", *Arch. Path.*, **22**, 477.

Sokoloff, L. (1953): "The heart in rheumatoid arthritis", *Amer. Heart. J.*, **45**, 635.

Sprague, H. B., and White, P. D. (1926): "Comparative study of rheumatic mitral regurgitation and mitral stenosis", *Amer. Heart J.*, **1**, 629.

Steel, G. (1888): "The murmer of high pressure in the pulmonary artery", *Med. Chronicle, Manchester*, **9**, 182.

Thompson, A. C., and Stewart, W. C. (1951): "Hemoptysis in mitral stenosis", *J. Amer. med. Ass.*, **147**, 21.

Thompson, W. P., and Levine, S. A. (1937): "Note on duration of symptoms and age at death in chronic rheumatic valvular disease, especially in tricuspid stenosis", *Amer. J. med. Sc.*, **193**, 4.

Trace, H. D., Bailey, C. P., and Wendkos, M. H. (1954): "Tricuspid valve commissurotomy with a one-year follow-up", *Amer. Heart J.*, **47**, 613.

Van Lingen, B., Gear, J. H., Whidborne, J., and Lister, M. L. (1954): "The ballistocardiogram in aortic stenosis", *Amer. Heart J.*, **47**, 560.

Wallach, J. B., Lukash, L., and Angrist, A. A. (1953): "An interpretation of the incidence of mural thrombi in the left auricle and appendage with particular reference to mitral commissurotomy", *Ibid.*, **45**, 252.

Warren, M. F., and Drinker, C. K. (1942): "Flow of lymph from lungs of dogs", *Amer. J., Physiol.*, **136**, 207.

Watson, T. (1843): "Principles and practice of physic", London.

Wells, B. (1954): "The assessment of mitral stenosis by phonocardiography", *Brit. Heart J.*, **16**, 261.

——, Rappaport, M. B., and Sprague, H. B. (1949): "The graphic registration of basal diastolic murmurs", *Amer. Heart J.*, **37**, 586.

Werner, S. C. (1936): "Rheumatic cardiac disease. Association of active rheumatic fever with heart failure", *Arch. intern. Med.*, **57**, 94.

Wiggers, C. J. (1928): "Pressure pulses in the cardiovascular system", London.

—— (1935): "Physiology in health and disease", London.

Wood, P. (1954): "An appreciation of mitral stenosis", *Brit. med. J.*, **1**, 1051, 1113.

——, and Besterman, E. M. M. (1956): "Proof of the protective effect of a high pulmonary vascular resistance in the pulmonary venous system in mitral stenosis", to be published.

Wynn, A. (1953): "Gross calcification of the mitral valve", *Brit. Heart J.*, **15**, 214.

Zimmerman, H. A. (1950): "Left ventricular pressures in patients with aortic insufficiency studied by intracardiac catheterization", *J. clin. Invest.*, **29**, 1601.

Zinsser, H. F., and Kay, C. F. (1950): "The straining procedure as an aid in the anatomic localization of cardiovascular murmurs and sounds", *Circulation*, **1**, 523.

Zoob, M. (1954): "The œsophageal pulse in mitral valve disease", *Brit. Heart J.*, **16**, 39.

CHAPTER XI

NON-RHEUMATIC MYOCARDITIS AND MISCELLANEOUS CARDIOPATHIES

U NDER this heading are grouped together all those varieties of heart disease that have in common a primary or predominant myocardial fault. That only one chapter should be devoted to what might appear to be the very essence of cardiology emphasises the curious fact that the great majority of so-called diseases of the heart are simply those conditions that hinder filling mechanisms, increase cardiac work, or interfere with fuel supplies, i.e. mechanical disadvantages of one kind or another. What greater compliment could be paid to the general health and integrity of the myocardium itself than this?

Incidence

At present no definite figure can be given for the prevalence of non-rheumatic myocarditis and clinically similar cardiopathies, for there are wide discrepancies between clinical, instrumental and pathological data.

However, out of approximately 10,000 new patients with cardiovascular disease examined personally by the author only 30 were in this category, excluding cases of diphtheria, thyrotoxicosis, myxœdema, and digitalis or quinidine intoxication. This gives a relative clinical frequency of 0.3 per cent for cases presenting like isolated myocarditis.

Age and sex

The average age of the patients in this series was 44, the range 14 to 63; but a primary myocardial fault may occur at any age. In infants a congenital cause, such as fibroelastosis, von Gierke's disease, or anomalous origin of the left coronary artery from the pulmonary artery, is more likely.

The male/female sex ratio was 2 : 1.

Classification

The group comprises numerous infections and infestations, the collagen diseases and allied allergic states, disorders of metabolism or nutrition, certain endocrine disturbances, neuro-muscular dystrophies, primary or secondary tumours of the heart, and a number of drugs and poisons; included also are at least two important cardiopathies of unknown origin—isolated myocarditis and endomyocardial fibrosis. For convenience, a list of the more important members of each sub-group is given below.

ETIOLOGY

Bacterial infections
  1. Invasive
       Pyogenic organisms
       Syphilis
  2. Toxic
       Bacterial endocarditis
       Diphtheria
       Meningococcal septicæmia
       Pneumonia
       Streptococcal infections
       Tuberculosis
       Typhoid fever
       Typhus (especially scrub-
         typhus)

Fungus or yeast infections
  Actinomycosis
  Coccidioidomycosis
  Histoplasmosis

Parasitic or protozoal infections
  Bilharziasis
  South American trypanosomiasis
    (Chagas' disease)
  Toxoplasmosis
  Trichiniasis

Virus infections
  Common cold
  Infective mononucleosis
  Influenza
  Mumps
  Poliomyelitis

Isolated myocarditis
  Endomyocardial fibrosis
  Fiedler's type

Allergic or other tissue reactions
  Löffler's syndrome
  Sarcoidosis

Collagen diseases
  Dermatomyositis
  Disseminated lupus
  Periarteritis nodosa
  Rheumatoid arthritis
  Scleroderma

Congenital anomalies
  Anomalous left coronary artery
  Familial cardiomegaly
  Fibroelastosis
  Friedreich's disease
  Gargoylism
  Von Gierke's disease

Drugs
  Adrenalin   Emetine
  Calcium   Potassium
  Digitalis   Quinidine

Endocrine disorders
  Acromegaly and gigantism
  Myxœdema
  Thyrotoxicosis

Metabolic or nutritional disorders
  Alcoholism
  Amyloidosis
  Beri-beri
  Diabetes mellitus
  Hæmochromatosis
  Malnutrition

Neuromuscular dystrophies
  Progressive muscular dystrophy

Tumours
  Fibroma
  Leukæmia
  Myxoma
  Rhabdomyoma
  Sarcoma
  Secondary tumours
  Argentaffinoma

Hæmodynamics

   The chief physiological fault common to nearly all groups is inability on the part of the weakened myocardium to maintain an adequate cardiac output despite normal pressure and volume loads, normal coronary flow, and normal rhythm. Hypertrophy of relatively healthy muscle fibres, a high filling pressure in both venous systems giving increased diastolic stretch, and tachycardia may compensate for the defect for a while, but sooner or later prove inadequate, one or other or both ventricles becoming overloaded.

BACTERIAL INFECTIONS

The great majority of cases of myocarditis secondary to bacterial infection are toxic and the best example is diphtheritic myocarditis. Bacteria may actually invade the myocardium, however, in certain instances, e.g. in syphilitic myocarditis (q.v.) and suppurative myocarditis. Miliary or solitary abscesses of the myocardium may occur in staphyllococcal or pneumococcal septicæmia and may cause purulent pericardial effusion or cardiac rupture (Weiss and Wilkins, 1937). The outlook in these previously fatal cases has altered considerably since the advent of penicillin and other antibiotics.

THE HEART IN DIPHTHERIA

Diphtheria may cause peripheral circulatory collapse, or toxic myocarditis. Cutaneous diphtheria, so easily overlooked and so often untreated until too late, may be as lethal as the common faucial type. Early and adequate treatment with antitoxin has greatly reduced the incidence of toxic complications, but has by no means abolished them. Experimentally in dogs, diphtheria toxin causes peripheral vasodilatation, conduction defects, and weakness of myocardial contraction ending in failure (Witt, Lindner and Katz, 1937).

CIRCULATORY COLLAPSE

Towards the end of the first week or during the second week of the illness, the blood pressure may fall well below 100 mm. Hg; the patient becomes faint, sick, and restless; the skin pale, cold, and clammy; the pulse rapid and thready. Loss of vasomotor tone may be due to toxic depression of the vasomotor centre, perhaps to peripheral sympathetic paresis, or possibly to poisoning of the vessels themselves. Occasionally it is brought about by suprarenal failure due to necrosis or hæmorrhage. The earlier the onset of circulatory collapse, the worse the prognosis. Patients usually remain in a critical state for several days; in those who recover improvement may then occur, but the blood pressure usually remains low for two or three weeks.

The course of diphtheria may be complicated (as well as alleviated) by serum therapy; for this may induce not only immediate collapse from anaphylactic shock in a sensitised individual, but also later collapse from loss of plasma into the tissue spaces associated with serum sickness. Urticaria and œdema, usually on the ninth day, may be extreme, and result in a diminished blood volume and hæmoconcentration. Diphtheritic circulatory collapse and allergic "shock" may thus be expected at about the same time, and diagnostic difficulties may arise.

Treatment of serum sickness includes subcutaneous adrenalin 0.5 mg. two- to four-hourly, sodium salicylate gr. 15 to 20 (1 to 1.25 G.) three-hourly, and one of the anti-histamine drugs such as diphenhydramine (benadryl) 50 mg. six-hourly.

Treatment of diphtheritic circulatory collapse consists of raising the foot of the bed and maintaining the blood pressure by means of a slow drip infusion of some suitable pressor amine such as noradrenalin, at a rate of about 5 to 15 μg. per minute. In view of the uncertain state of the myo-cardium in these cases too much saline must not be given and the blood pressure should not be raised above 120 mm. Hg. It is best to use a strength of 1 mg. of noradrenalin to 100 ml. of normal saline; 15 drops (1 ml.) of such a solution per minute should contain 10 μg. of noradrenalin. Alterna-tively, mephentermine may be given intramuscularly in doses of 25 to 50 mg. (usually 30 to 35 mg.), and repeated when necessary; or mephenter-mine may be given by slow intravenous drip at a rate of 0.5 to 1 mg. per minute, until the blood pressure is satisfactory.

The *prognosis* is grave.

TOXIC MYOCARDITIS

Pathology. Diphtheritic carditis, being toxic in nature, may prove fatal without causing advanced changes in morbid histology. The characteristic finding is hyaline degeneration or necrosis of muscle, the fibres losing their striations and presenting a swollen granular appearance. Lesions are patchily distributed, and only short segments of individual muscle fibres may be affected. Monocytes cluster round the debris, and fibroblastic repair follows (Gore, 1948).

Clinical features. Disturbances of rhythm tend to occur first, usually during the second week of the disease. Partial or complete heart block, and bundle branch block are the best known, and in patients who recover from the illness are usually, but not invariably, transient (Perry, 1939). Both heart block and bundle branch block commonly denote severe carditis, most such cases proving fatal (Burkhardt, Eggleston, and Smith, 1938). Ectopic beats are common, and although often innocent and unrelated to carditis, should be viewed with suspicion in diphtheria. Auricular fibrilla-tion and paroxysmal tachycardia are rare. Ventricular fibrillation may be responsible for sudden death.

Other evidence of carditis tends to occur a little later, usually during the third week. Sinus tachycardia, gallop rhythm, enlargement of the heart and reduction of the pulse pressure are usual. The onset of heart failure may be suggested by pallor, breathlessness, præcordial oppression and vomiting. Congestion is systemic rather than pulmonary, the jugular venous pressure being raised and the liver distended; there is rarely orthopnœa, paroxysmal cardiac dyspnœa, or pulmonary œdema. Significant murmurs and peri-cardial friction are absent.

The *electrocardiogram* is especially helpful in the diagnosis of diphtheritic carditis, much more so than in rheumatic carditis. Depression of the RS-T segment or primary inversion of the T wave in most leads is characteristic, and is found during the second week in the majority of cases which develop clinical carditis, and in some that do not. A similar pattern may be produced in cats within 48 hours by injecting diphtheritic toxin (Nathanson, 1928). Of 600 cases of diphtheria studied by Altshuler *et al.* (1948), 108 or 18 per cent developed these changes, while only 11 showed heart block.

Radiological studies on diphtheritic carditis are rare, because patients are not allowed to stand or sit, and should not be moved to the X-ray department. Portable skiagrams give little information about the size of the heart. General dilatation, however, may be expected if the venous pressure is raised.

Prognosis. The outlook is grave, for sudden death is common, and presumably results from ventricular fibrillation or asystole. Some patients die from congestive heart failure. Not infrequently, associated circulatory failure complicates the picture. Those who survive usually develop polyneuritis later, and this is apt to be severe. The total mortality rate is difficult to assess, for mild cases may well be overlooked; but it is usually put at 50 per cent.

If the patient survives, the ultimate prognosis is excellent (White *et al.*, 1937), and complete recovery may be promised without reserve. It is important that the patient should be convinced of this from the start, in order to prevent anxiety neurosis and to maintain good morale.

Treatment. Antitoxic serum will already have been administered in most cases; if not, it is too late to give it by the time cardiovascular symptoms develop. The axiom that antitoxin cannot do any harm and might as well be given even at this stage is untrue; for serum reactions are common and may prove fatal when there is toxic circulatory collapse or carditis.

Prophylactic treatment, in addition to early and adequate doses of antitoxin, consists of complete rest in bed for a minimum period of one month in all cases of diphtheria. If by the end of this time there is no evidence of cardiovascular or neuro-intoxication, there is little further risk to life. Should any such intoxication have occurred, however, bed rest must be extended for another month; otherwise sudden death may occur during convalescence in the second month. Patients may be treated with far less respect subsequently, even when they have extensive polyneuritis.

The treatment of recognised carditis is unsatisfactory. Absolute rest is essential, for sudden slight effort, even sitting up in bed, may prove fatal during the critical period. Patients should be nursed flat, with one pillow, and should have everything done for them, including being fed and washed.

Diet should be light and fluids limited to two pints daily. If there is congestive failure the sodium intake should not exceed 0.5 G. daily.

Digitalis is dangerous and should only be used in rare cases when atrial fibrillation with a rapid ventricular rate is associated with severe congestive heart failure. Quinidine is also dangerous in view of its depressive effect on conduction.

THE HEART IN OTHER INFECTIONS

Up to the beginning of the twentieth century it was generally believed that toxic carditis was a common complication of certain fevers, such as influenza. It came to be recognised, however, that although "cloudy swelling" and "fatty degeneration" were often found at autopsy in cases dying from severe general infections, clinical evidence of cardiac involvement was rare. The change of view followed the establishment of stricter criteria for diagnosing organic heart disease: palpitations and irregularities of the heart were shown to be due to autonomic disturbance or to innocent ectopic beats; systolic murmurs lost their previous significance; effort syndrome following infections was proved attributable to anxiety; X-rays failed to confirm clinical cardiac enlargement (based on the position of the apex beat); standard lead electrocardiograms were rarely abnormal. The weight of negative evidence was considerable, and it became the custom to recognise no form of carditis other than that due to rheumatism or diphtheria. In recent years, however, the earlier view has gained some support particularly owing to the work of Gore and Saphir (1947), who found that diphtheria and rheumatism accounted for less than 25 per cent of fatal cases of myocarditis; they contended that carditis was common in a host of infectious diseases, including especially scrub typhus, bacterial endocarditis, and meningococcal septicæmia. It may be as well, therefore, t review the known facts critically, for there is grave danger that thi modern swing-back may go too far.

FAILURE OF THE PERIPHERAL CIRCULATION

Cardiovascular disturbances in acute infections are commonly of tw kinds, and neither is due to a cardiac fault. The first is peripheral circulato failure. This may be due to depression of the vasomotor centre, to tox paresis of the vessels themselves, to suprarenal failure, or to diminutic of the blood volume from dehydration or from loss of plasma into the tissu spaces through damaged vessels. The essential mechanism is critical di crepancy between the effective vascular capacity and the blood volum so that the central venous pressure falls, the cardiac output is reduced ar the blood pressure low, as in shock.

A good sign of vascular relaxation is a markedly dicrotic pulse, ar although not necessarily serious, should put the physician on guar Another significant feature is pallor and coldness of the extremities, due vasoconstriction in the skin; this appears to be a compensatory mechanis helping to maintain the venous pressure and blood pressure when da gerous vasodilatation occurs elsewhere, e.g. in muscle. Impending failu of compensatory vasoconstriction may be indicated by waxing and waning of the systolic blood pressure through a range of 10 to 20 mm. Hg. A fourth indication of circulatory failure is mental confusion or faintness in the sitting posture. Whilst tachycardia is the rule, and the half-hourly pulse chart of some value, it should be understood that deceleration sometimes accompanies a falling blood pressure, and that the character of the pulse is as important as its rate.

Circulatory failure should be treated by nursing the patient flat or with the foot of the bed raised, and by the intravenous administration of serum or plasma by the drip method, with or without noradrenalin in doses of about 10 μg. per minute.

The second common cardiovascular reaction to acute fevers is vasomotor neurosis during convalescence. This is discussed in Chapter XXII.

TOXIC MYOCARDITIS

True toxic myocarditis does occur, however, especially perhaps in pneumonia. Sections reveal focal hyaline necrosis, i.e. granular degeneration and loss of striation of the muscle fibres, patchily distributed. Cellular reaction with monocytes predominating, and fibroblastic repair, follow—as in diphtheritic carditis, which it resembles. This histological picture is common to most forms of carditis—hence the difficulty in making an etiological diagnosis from autopsy findings. For example, 35 cases of sudden death following tonsillitis or common cold were reported by Gore and Saphir (1947), and ascribed to toxic myocarditis. Thirty-one of them, however, could have been due to diphtheria or pneumonia; a negative throat swab does not exclude diphtheria.

Myocarditis and diffuse glomerulonephritis have long been known to complicate bacterial endocarditis; but when the death-rate of the septicæmic stage was 98 per cent, they received scant attention. Since the introduction of penicillin, however, heart failure from myocarditis has been said to be chiefly responsible for the present 25 per cent mortality; nevertheless, heart failure is rare in the absence of severe aortic or mitral incompetence, and the rapidly progressive mechanical fault could well be to blame.

Histological examination of the heart in cases dying from meningococcal infection may disclose evidence of carditis; but clinical signs of cardiac involvement are most unusual, and the total mortality rate in adults is less than 1 per cent (Daniels *et al.*, 1943).

Pneumococcal and *streptococcal* myocarditis, accompanying pneumonia and scarlet fever respectively, are perhaps the most convincing forms of non-diphtheritic bacterial toxic myocarditis, especially the former. Streptococcal myocarditis of this kind bears no resemblance to rheumatic carditis, which is a more likely complication of scarlet fever.

Tuberculous myocarditis, sometimes accompanied by erythema nodosum, has been reported in association with primary tuberculosis (Neidhart and Amrich, 1950), but is believed to be allergic in type. Six out of 30 cases of otherwise idiopathic myocardial fibrosis described by Perrin, Froment and Lenègre (1953) had pulmonary or mediastinal tuberculosis.

Collapse in *typhoid fever* is usually due to peripheral circulatory failure, evidence of true myocarditis being unconvincing (Porter and Bloom, 1935). Electrocardiographic changes during the course of typhoid have been reversed within 48 hours of giving 300–600 mg. of niacin (nicotinic acid) daily by mouth (Rachmilewitz and Braun, 1948), suggesting deficiency of at least one of the B group of vitamins.

Carditis accompanying scrub typhus (Tsutsugamushi fever) is clinically unconvincing. Although histology may reveal myocardial damage and cellular infiltration in fatal cases (Corbett, 1943), the clinical course of the disease seems to be little influenced by them (Williams *et al.*, 1944; Berry *et al.*, 1945). In a series of 184 cases seen within one to four weeks after the acute symptoms had subsided, and 10 cases seen during the stage of fever, the electrocardiogram was virtually normal (Howell, 1945). For further information the reader is referred to the issue of the *American Journal of Hygiene*, May 1945, which is devoted to studies on scrub typhus.

Certain *virus infections* are known to cause myocarditis occasionally: these certainly include infective mononucleosis, mumps and poliomyelitis; Saphir (1949) gives a much longer list and includes infective hepatitis and virus pneumonia. In the war, however, I encountered no clinical example of myocarditis associated with infective hepatitis or virus pneumonia despite having well over a thousand cases of the former and nearly 300 of the latter under my care. This discrepancy between clinical and patho logical data permeates the whole subject. In poliomyelitis, for example Ludden and Edwards (1949) found microscopic evidence of myocarditis in 14 out of 35 fatal cases, whereas Spain *et al.* (1950) reported only one instance of clinical myocarditis in 140 cases, although typical microscopic changes were found in 12 out of 14 that were fatal. I have, however, seen unquestionable examples of clinical myocarditis in adults associated with glandular fever and mumps.

The common cold, influenza, and other upper respiratory tract infection have been held responsible for many cases of alleged myocarditis, but the rarity of any such complication is much more impressive considering the frequency of these maladies; in a widespread epidemic of influenza in which clinical evidence of myocarditis was carefully sought, no single example could be found (Wood, 1941).

To assess the clinical value of the work of Gore and Saphir quoted above it is worth noting that 16 per cent of their 1,402 cases of myocarditis were due to scrub typhus, and there was no evidence that myocarditis was the cause of death. Their cases were highly selected, excluded children, and were based entirely on autopsy findings: there were 227 examples of scrub typhus, 208 of bacterial endocarditis, 144 of diphtheria, 130 of rheumatic carditis, and 105 of sulphonamide allergy. The reader will draw his own conclusions.

Clinically significant carditis accompanying acute infections in Great Britain (other than rheumatic fever, diphtheria, and bacterial endocarditis) is undoubtedly rare.

Clinical features of toxic myocarditis. In acute cases the signs and symptoms are similar to those of diphtheritic myocarditis, except that they may occur earlier, during the febrile stage of the infection. Symptoms attributable to cardiac involvement may be absent; on the other hand, there may be dyspnœa, unexpected vomiting, pallor and peripheral cyanosis due to congestive failure, substernal oppression or discomfort, or palpitations associated with changes of rhythm. It may be difficult to distinguish cardiac symptoms from those due to general toxæmia, particularly when there is peripheral circulatory failure. Sudden death is not infrequently the first tragic proof of myocarditis.

Physical signs include a small, rapid, thready pulse, low systolic blood pressure, small pulse pressure, gallop rhythm, dilatation of the heart,

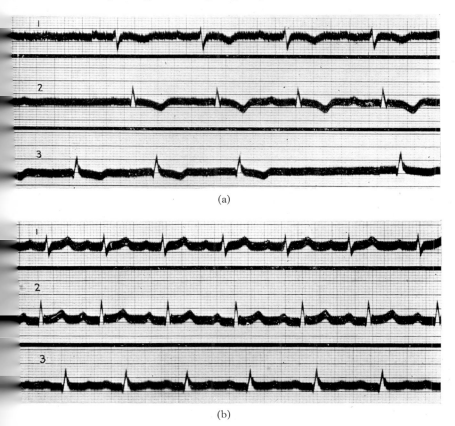

(a)

(b)

Fig. 11.01—Electrocardiogram in a case of toxic myocarditis due to pneumonia. Shows partial heart block with dropped beats and inversion of the T wave in all leads. (b) After recovery.

congestive heart failure, abnormalities of rhythm and electrocardiographic changes. The small rapid pulse and the low blood pressure may equally well be due to peripheral circulatory failure, and the gallop rhythm to fever (especially when there is anæmia). The size of the heart may be difficult to assess under the clinical circumstances, and the patient should not be moved to the X-ray department for more exact information. The importance of recognising early signs of congestive heart failure will thus be appreciated. Abnormalities of rhythm are also important, and include all grades of heart block, auricular flutter or fibrillation, and paroxysmal tachycardia. The electrocardiogram is especially helpful, not only in establishing the nature of a rhythm change, but also in revealing partial heart block and abnormalities of the T wave (fig. 11.01).

Sometimes the course of toxic myocarditis is subacute or chronic. The clinical features then closely resemble those of isolated myocarditis (q.v.)

Prognosis. If the diagnosis is beyond doubt, the outlook is grave, the mortality rate probably approaching 50 per cent. Whether central or peripheral in mechanism, the combination of hypotension and a small rapid pulse is always dangerous; and congestive heart failure often proves fatal. Abnormalities of rhythm and alterations of the T wave, without the manifestations just mentioned, are less serious.

Many cases of mild toxic myocarditis must pass unrecognised; but this is not a matter for concern, for recovery appears to be complete in all non fatal cases.

Treatment. Bed-rest and specific chemotherapy (when applicable) for a acute infections are axiomatic; bed-rest should be absolute if the cardio vascular system is involved. The patient should be nursed in the position of maximum comfort; but if the blood pressure is below 100 mm. Hg an there is no evidence of congestive failure, he should be kept horizontal; there is congestive failure he should be propped up at 30 to 45 degree against a back-rest. Digitalis should be avoided unless there is frank con gestive failure, for it increases the risk of sudden death from ventricula fibrillation, and may aggravate minor degrees of heart block. If the venou pressure is well raised and the liver distended, however, it should not be withheld; and it may be invaluable in cases of auricular flutter or fibrilla tion. Mersalyl and a low sodium diet may be given if there is fluid retentio Quinidine or procaine amide may have to be used in cases of paroxysm ventricular tachycardia, but its depressive effect on conduction can be ve dangerous if there is already partial heart block.

It must be admitted, however, that toxic myocarditis is little influenc by therapy, and is apt to be fatal or otherwise according to its severity.

MYOCARDITIS DUE TO PARASITES

A most convincing form of protozoal myocarditis may accompa *South American trypanosomiasis* or Chagas' disease (Chagas, 1909). Leis manial forms of T. *cruzi* multiply chiefly in the cells of the heart, brain and liver; the affected cells finally rupture and liberate the parasites into the blood stream. An intense local inflammatory reaction follows. The signs and symptoms of a typical acute or subacute myocarditis may dominate the clinical picture, and sudden death is common (Mosely and Miller, 1945). The clinical diagnosis may be suggested by associated encephalitis and may be proved by demonstrating the parasites in the blood stream.

Of the protean manifestations of *toxoplasmosis* myocarditis must be relatively rare, but three cases have been reported recently by Paulley *et al.* (1954), and others may come to light now that serological tests are likely to be performed in cases of myocarditis of uncertain etiology. The protozoal intracellular parasite known as toxoplasma seems to be far more widespread in man than originally suspected, but the majority of individuals with positive serological tests give no indication of disease. The best-known clinical reactions are cerebral and ophthalmic, whether congenital or acquired (Vail *et al.*, 1943; Ridley, 1949). If there is a myocardial reaction, however, a clinical picture resembling that of isolated myocarditis may arise, or myocarditis may complicate more familiar manifestations of the disease. The diagnosis is strongly supported by a specific complement-fixation test at titres of 1/16 or higher.

Trichiniasis is rarely complicated by myocarditis, and even minor electrocardiographic abnormalities are uncommon. Thus of 44 cases investigated by Beecher and Amidon (1938) only one had a slightly prolonged P-R interval, and one sino-auricular block. Solarz (1947) found transient flat or inverted T waves in 16 out of 114 cases (14 per cent), but no clinical evidence of myocarditis in any of them. Allergic reactions to trichiniasis occur, however, and rare instances of myocarditis may perhaps be of this kind.

Schistosomiasis is more likely to affect the heart by causing pulmonary hypertension from obliterative pulmonary endarteritis than myocarditis, although I have seen a pathological specimen of the latter in South Africa.

Cor pulmonale due to bilharzia is described in chapter XVIII.

There is little evidence that *malaria* causes myocarditis; collapse is usually due to peripheral circulatory failure.

A *hydatid cyst* may be found in the heart or pericardium as a result of a routine skiagram of the chest, but is rarely recognised clinically unless it ruptures. This is a space-filling lesion rather than a myocarditis. The electrocardiogram may show reduced R waves and inverted T waves in chest leads taken from points overlying the cyst. Rupture may be into the pericardial sac or into any of the cardiac chambers (Canabal *et al.*, 1955). The differential diagnosis is from other pericardial cysts, cardiac tumours, mediastinal cysts and neoplasms, and cardiac aneurysm. Echinococcal cysts elsewhere, the Casoni test and the complexion fixation test help to establish the diagnosis.

MYOCARDITIS DUE TO FUNGI AND YEASTS

Actinomycosis involves the heart in less than 2 per cent of cases (Kasper and Pinner, 1930). When it does so the fungus usually reaches the heart by direct extension from infected neighbouring structures, so that pericarditis occurs first, but initial myocarditis from hæmatogenous spread has also been reported (Cornell and Shookhoff, 1944). Clinically, the majority of cases have been recognised owing to the development of congestive heart failure; signs of pericarditis have been detected less frequently. Treatment includes heavy and prolonged doses of sulphonamides, penicillin, and surgery (Lyons *et al.*, 1943; Zoeckler, 1951).

Myocardial *coccidioido-mycosis* was found in 11 out of 48 cases included in the series reported by Gore and Saphir (1947). Clinically, however, myocardial involvement is rare. Thus in a large epidemic of 75 cases described by Goldstein and Louie (1943), all but one recovered without evidence of carditis. In this group the incubation period was 14 days. Symptoms and signs included fever, pleurisy, cough with brownish or blood-stained sputum, cervical adenitis, erythema nodosum or multiforme, and bilateral hilar opacities extending outwards into the central zone of the lungs. Leucocytosis, eosinophilia, and a high sedimentation rate were the rule. The diagnosis can be confirmed by a specific skin sensitivity test, a complement-fixation test, and by identifying the fungus in the sputum.

Histoplasmosis is sometimes mentioned as a cause of myocarditis by yeast-like organisms, but in a review of 71 cases Parsons and Zarafonetis (1945) found little evidence to support this statement. There were four instances of vegetative endocarditis, two of them involving the tricuspid valve, but no convincing examples of frank myocarditis.

ISOLATED MYOCARDITIS

Isolated myocarditis (Scott and Saphir, 1929) is a subacute or chronic "inflammation" of the heart of unknown etiology, characterised by patchy myocardial necrosis, cellular infiltration and fibroblastic repair, as in other forms of myocarditis. It was first properly described by Fiedler (1899). The disease may not be a specific entity and is difficult to distinguish pathologically from known forms of toxic or infective myocarditis of relatively long duration.

Incidence. Although still relatively rare, isolated myocarditis is being recognised with increasing frequency. The majority of cases have occurred in subjects between the ages of 20 and 50, but infants, children, and old people are not exempt. The disease has been reported sporadically in most countries and races, and accounts for about half of all cases that present clinically with heart failure of unknown etiology.

Pathology. Patchy necrosis of muscle is thought to be the primary lesion (fig. 11.02). Cellular reaction may be focal or more diffusely interstitial

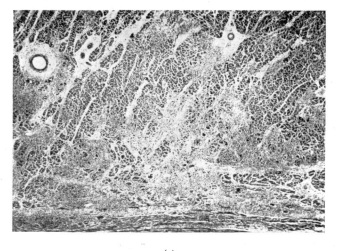

(a)

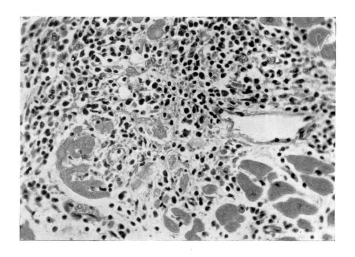

(b)

Fig. 11.02—Focal necrosis in a case of Fiedler's carditis.
(a) Low power.

(b) High power. The cells are macrophages, plasma cells,
lymphocytes and eosinophils.

(*By courtesy of Prof. C. V. Harrison*)

Monocytes predominate, but in the acute stage polymorphs may be more numerous. Hæmorrhage and exudate may occur. Giant cells, eosinophils, and arteritis suggest another etiology—allergy. Fibroblastic repair follows. As a rule, all stages of activity and healing are seen in the same specimen; occasionally, extensive interstitial fibrosis is found alone, and is believed to represents the end-result of the same process. As a rule these hearts weigh 500–600 G., and are usually very dilated.

The pericardium, endocardium and valves are not involved, but mural thrombi are common, and may give rise to emboli and infarcts in other organs (Scott and Saphir, 1929; Davies *et al.*, 1951).

Clinical features. The history is invariably short, rarely longer than a few months. The chief symptoms are increasing dyspnœa and fatigue; sometimes there is atypical angina pectoris or substernal discomfort (Hansmann and Schenken, 1938), or an attack of pain may be so severe and prolonged as to suggest cardiac infarction (Gillis and Walters, 1954); occasionally hemiplegia or hæmoptysis signals the onset (Josserand and Gallavardin, 1901; de la Chapelle and Graef, 1931).

The physical signs are usually those of congestive heart failure with a normal or low blood pressure, small pulse pressure, sinus tachycardia, peripheral cyanosis and pallor, cold extremities, general enlargement of the heart (fig. 11.03), gallop rhythm, and normal valves. Disturbances of rhythm, particularly paroxysmal tachycardia, atrial flutter and partial heart block, are not uncommon.

The *electrocardiogram* often shows left bundle branch block. Not infrequently rather low voltage and simple inversion of the T waves in most leads may suggest Pick's disease. Occasionally a relatively large zone of necrosis in the wall of the left ventricle may give rise to pathological Q waves and inverted T waves resembling the pattern of cardiac infarction. In one case Bayley (1946) recorded typical anoxic depression of the RS-T segment, and attributed it to the fact that the lesions were mainly close to the endocardium of both ventricles.

Radiographic appearances include moderate or considerable enlargement of the heart shadow, particularly the left ventricle, varying degrees of "pulmonary venous congestion", and dilatation of the right atrium and superior vena cava; the aorta, pulmonary artery and left atrium usually look normal.

There is no fever, no leucocytosis, no eosinophilia, and no rise of sedimentation rate. No special diagnostic tests are available.

Differential diagnosis. The case usually presents as one of heart failure of uncertain etiology. It is at once distinguished from the *hyperkinetic circulatory states* (e.g. anæmia, beri-beri, arteriovenous aneurysm, Paget's disease of bone, thyrotoxicosis, anoxic pulmonary heart disease, uræmia, and certain diseases of the liver) by the obviously low cardiac output and signs of peripheral vasoconstriction.

In middle-aged or elderly subjects *ischæmic heart disease* may be difficult

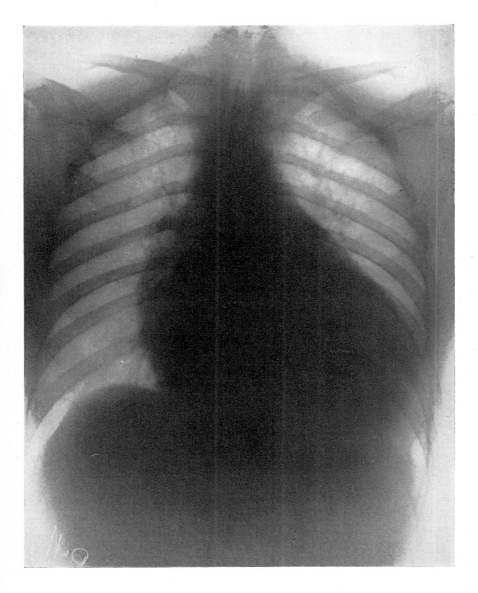

Fig. 11.03—Skiagram showing general enlargement of the heart in a case of Fiedler's myocarditis.

to exclude if there is a history of angina pectoris or electrocardiographic evidence suggesting active ischæmia or an actual infarct. In these unusual cases, however, there is apt to be some discrepancy between the clinical situation and the suggested diagnosis of coronary disease; for example, there may be advanced congestive failure with minimal "ischæmic" changes in the electrocardiogram; persistent heart failure may ante-date pain; the QT pattern suggesting infarction is rarely well developed, and the S-T segment is never conspicuously elevated. A normal blood cholesterol and normal lipo-proteins should add to the doubt.

Hypertensive heart disease in which the blood pressure has temporarily fallen is seen occasionally, but such a diagnosis should never be accepted readily without historical or subsequent proof (Kaplan, Clark and de la Chapelle, 1938).

Aortic stenosis with a minimal murmur heard best at the apex beat may be mistaken for isolated myocarditis with left ventricular failure and functional mitral incompetence. The quality of the peripheral pulse, an aortic ejection click, the timing of the aortic murmur, reversed splitting of the second heart sound (in the absence of left bundle branch block), and careful screening for calcium in the aortic valve should prevent error.

Pericardial effusion may be closely simulated. The apex beat, however, is usually more forceful in isolated myocarditis and much displaced to the left, pronounced gallop rhythm points to a myocardial fault, as does left bundle branch block. Diagnostic paracentesis or cardiac catheterisation settles any lingering doubts.

Chronic constrictive pericarditis without calcification can be clinically impossible to distinguish from isolated myocarditis, as emphasised by Davies *et al.* (1951). A paradoxical pulse, impalpable cardiac impulse and absence of gallop rhythm are all in favour of Pick's disease, whilst a strong cardiac impulse, functional tricuspid incompetence, and left bundle branch block are all in favour of myocarditis: but a small peripheral pulse, high venous pressure, steep y descent, conspicuous y trough, positive or negative Kussmaul sign, absence of murmurs, gallop rhythm, T wave inversion maximal in leads V_5 and V_6, and moderate general enlargement of the heart shadow all occur frequently in both conditions. *Routine cardiac catheterisation* does not distinguish them, for in both the cardiac output is low, left and right atrial pressures are high and more or less equal, steep y descents followed by conspicuous y troughs and ventricular overshoots are seen on both sides of the heart, and the pulmonary vascular resistance is normal (fig. 11.04). Special physiological tests for distinguishing the two are under trial, but have so far proved unreliable, for cases of Pick's disease sometimes behave physiologically like cases of heart failure; it is doubtful, however, if cases of heart failure ever behave like cases of uncomplicated Pick's disease. The tests include direct measurement of change in cardiac output brought about by alterations in right ventricular filling pressure, the

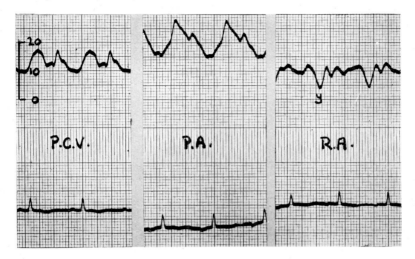

Fig. 11.04—Pressure pulses from a case of isolated myocarditis showing high atrial pressures and a conspicuous *y* trough in the right atrial tracing.

effect of Valsalva's manœuvre on the brachial arteriogram, and the effect of change of posture on the digital pulse (see pages 292 and 293).

A *primary change of rhythm*, particularly paroxysmal ventricular tachycardia in young persons, or paroxysmal atrial flutter or fibrillation in later life, may cause considerable diagnostic difficulty when attacks are prolonged, recurrent, and difficult to control, for severe heart failure may well occur under such circumstances, and if the patient is examined during a short period of normal rhythm there is likely to be a raised venous pressure, gallop rhythm, low blood pressure, small pulse, considerable cardiac enlargement and widespread inversion of the T waves in the electrocardiogram; it is easy then to assume that the rhythm change was secondary to myocarditis. The life and future good health of the patient may well depend on a more enlightened view, which is that every case of heart failure of uncertain etiology associated with an important change of rhythm should be regarded as secondary to that rhythm change until proved otherwise. Every effort must be made to restore normal rhythm, and to maintain it for at least six weeks; by the end of that time nutritional changes in the myocardium should have cleared up completely if the change of rhythm was primary.

Once it has been concluded that the case is one of isolated myocarditis or one of the many other cardiopathies described in this chapter, a serious attempt should be made to identify its nature. This may involve much time and labour, and the results are usually negative and disheartening, but any other attitude must halt progress in this baffling field.

Course and prognosis. All proven cases have naturally been fatal; even so, there have been no reports of probable cases that have survived. Death has usually occurred within a few weeks to a year or two of making the diagnosis or of admitting the patient to hospital.

Treatment. Absolute rest in bed, digitalis, mercurial diuretics, and a low sodium diet may help, but the general response is poor. Neither cortisone nor A.C.T.H. has proved of any value, even in large doses.

ENDOMYOCARDIAL FIBROSIS

In recent years considerable interest has been aroused by an obscure cardiopathy characterised by extensive endocardial and subendocardial fibrosis. When the endocardium is thick and white it resembles congenital fibroelastosis; when the fibrosis is chiefly subendocardial the pathology is more like the most chronic form of isolated myocarditis or the most fibrotic form of nutritional cardiopathy described later. It is therefore difficult to classify and until its etiology is understood it may be best to regard it as a special form of isolated myocarditis; this at least emphasises our ignorance concerning its nature.

The 40 cases in African troops serving in the Middle East described by Bedford and Konstam (1946) were having an adequate diet, "far better than they were accustomed to at home". There were 17 necropsies in this series and the fibrosis was mainly subendocardial; the authors thought the pathology resembled that of isolated myocarditis more closely than any other disease. Davies (1948) described a very similar disease in 36 East African natives (32 male); at autopsy the heart was dilated rather than hypertrophied, as in the series just quoted, but the fibrosis involved the endocardium as well as the subendocardial myocardium. The left ventricle was again chiefly involved, and there was the same frequency of mural thrombosis as has been noted in nearly all forms of heart failure of obscure origin, whether inflammatory, allergic or nutritional. A third series of 25 cases similar to Davies' was reported by O'Brien (1954) in the Sudan. The diet was normal in 23 of them, and alcoholism could be excluded. The patients were older than the others, averaging 54 years. Functional mitral and tricuspid incompetence was stressed, but it is doubted whether this had any special significance.

Becker, Chatgidakis and Van Lingen (1953) claimed that endomyocardial fibrosis was a diffuse collagen disease. There were 32 Bantu subjects amongst their 40 cases, but they did not blame the diet. They also stressed cardiac dilatation rather than hypertrophy and the frequency of mural thrombosis. The earliest lesion demonstrable was focal endocardial mucinous œdema; similar lesions occurred as "eccentric foci in the sub-intimal tissues of the small blood vessels of the myocardium". In addition, interstitial myocardial œdema, attributed to increased capillary permeability, caused muscle bundles to be widely separated. Fibrinous exudation was closely related to the areas of mucinous œdema and was the fore-runner of mural thrombosis. Foci of fibrinoid necrosis were seen in well-established areas of mucinous œdema. In subacute cases cellular infiltration and granulomatous tissue appeared in the affected zones. In chronic cases, "progressive fibrosis resulted in endocardial sclerosis, myocardial fibrosis, and eccentric subintimal connective tissue cushions". The authors' thesis was that the general design of the changes described was characteristic of all collagen diseases.

Clinically, cases of endomyocardial fibrosis usually present as examples of heart failure of uncertain etiology. Failure may be chiefly left sided or "congestive". Details are identical with those of isolated myocarditis.

COLLAGEN DISEASES AND ALLERGIC STATES

These include rheumatoid arthritis, periarteritis nodosa, disseminated lupus, scleroderma, dermatomyositis, and Löffler's syndrome. In all these conditions the clinical features of the cardiopathy closely resemble those of isolated myocarditis, and will not, therefore, be discussed in detail again; but each has specific features by which it may often be identified at the bedside or in the laboratory, and these must be briefly described.

Rheumatoid arthritis

Rheumatoid itself is too familiar to warrant detailed description here, but it should be borne in mind that joint manifestations superficially resembling rheumatoid may occur in any of the collagen diseases, particularly scleroderma.

The heart may be involved in cases of rheumatoid in three different ways: (1) chronic valve lesions indistinguishable from and probably identical with those following rheumatic fever are found in about 10 per cent; (2) clinical pericarditis is not uncommon, and necropsy evidence of healed pericarditis is found in 40 per cent of cases; (3) a specific focal granulomatous myocarditis has been described by many authors in 1 to 3 per cent of cases (Sokoloff, 1953). In addition, severe secondary anæmia may affect the cardiovascular system.

In differential diagnosis the following general rules may be found helpful in practice:

1. Acute or subacute endocarditis in children with Still's disease and chronic valve lesions in adults with frank rheumatoid arthritis should be attributed to coincident or past rheumatic carditis respectively.

2. Isolated pericarditis in children with Still's disease or in adults with rheumatoid may be attributed to the rheumatoid state with reasonable confidence, but not to the neglect of excluding tuberculosis.

3. A patient presenting with the combination of clinical rheumatoid arthritis and a cardiopathy resembling isolated myocarditis is more likely to have scleroderma or one of the other collagen diseases than true rheumatoid; even cor pulmonale with secondary osteo-arthropathy is more likely.

Periarteritis

Periarteritis nodosa or polyarteritis is a manifestation of hypersensitivity (Rich, 1942; Rich and Gregory, 1943), and may be provoked by a variety of antigens (Miller and Daley, 1946). It is characterised by disseminated or patchily distributed segmental arteritis, the initial lesion being fibrinoid necrosis of the media and internal elastic lamina, cellular infiltration and secondary thickening of the intima. Small aneurysms develop in about 16 per cent of cases (Harris, Lynch and O'Hara, 1939). Serious disturbances of function occur in the systems chiefly affected.

The disease may occur at any age, but particularly in young adults, and is three times as frequent in males as in females.

Cases tend to sort themselves into well-defined patterns, according to the system or combination of systems chiefly involved. These patterns include pyrexia of uncertain origin, peripheral neuritis (Kernohan and Woltman, 1938), nephritis (Davson, Bell and Platt, 1948), hypertension, bronchial asthma (Harkavy, 1941), obscure abdominal pain (Harris, Lynch and O'Hara, 1939), and myocarditis. It is only the last of these with which we are here concerned, but when an obscure cardiopathy is accompanied by any of the other manifestations mentioned, periarteritis should be seriously considered.

Confirmatory evidence includes almost any form of allergic rash, visible or palpable nodules along the course of a superficial artery such as the temporal, changes in the ocular fundus (including exudates, hæmorrhages, papillœdema, retinal detachment, vascular irregularities, and occlusion of the central artery of the retina (Sampson, 1945)), leucocytosis, eosinophilia, rapid blood sedimentation rate, positive C-reactive protein test, and, above all, a positive muscle or liver biopsy.

Löffler's syndrome

Löffler (1932, 1936) described a subacute condition of the lungs, characterised by transitory infiltrative lesions and eosinophilia. This seems to be similar to pulmonary periarteritis as described by Elkeles and Glynn (1944).

Allergic myocarditis

Eosinophilic myocarditis, as described by Reinhart (1946) and others, is also likely to be a variant of polyarteritis.

Sulphonamides have been accused of acting as antigens that may provoke allergic myocarditis (French and Weller, 1942; French, 1946), but a careful control study by Fawcett (1948) does not support this hypothesis.

Disseminated lupus

Disseminated lupus is regarded as a widespread necrosis of connective tissue, particularly fibrinoid degeneration of collagen fibres (Klemperer,

Pollack and Baehr, 1941), resulting from some crucial disturbance of antigen-antibody reaction.

Like periarteritis, it affects chiefly young adults, but unlike periarteritis it attacks women in 90 per cent of cases. A previous history of lupus erythematosis (butterfly rash) is obtained in at least one-third of all cases. The illness is apt to be precipitated by some infection, drug therapy or physical agent (such as sunburn).

The clinical features include fever, patchy erythematous rashes, painless erythematous macules (usually in the thenar or hypothenar emminences), tender nodules more deeply situated in the skin (like Osler's nodes), hyperæmia of the nail folds, petechiæ or purpura, small hæmorrhagic necrotic lesions in the fingers or mouth, polyarthritis not unlike that seen in rheumatic fever, generalised adenopathy, transient infiltrative lesions in the lungs which may cause hæmoptysis, vascular lesions in the ocular fundus, and cardiac manifestations consisting of pericarditis, myocarditis, and the verrucous endocarditis of Libman and Sachs (1924). Pericardial effusion may occur (Humphreys, 1948). The myocarditis itself behaves functionally like isolated myocarditis. Endocarditis, when present, is apt to affect the tricuspid as well as the mitral or aortic valve. The vegetations are larger than in rheumatic valvitis, but less damaging than in bacterial endocarditis. Histological details have been given by Gross (1940), and the subject has been well reviewed by Griffith and Vural (1951).

The diagnosis of disseminated lupus may be confirmed by leucopenia, thrombocytopenia, hypochromic anæmia, a raised sedimentation rate, absence of C-reactive protein, the presence of cold agglutinins, L.E. cells in the bone marrow and peripheral blood, hyperglobulinæmia, increased gamma-globulin, reversal of the albumin/globulin ratio, and increased heparin tolerance. These tests have been reviewed by Gold and Gowing (1953).

Scleroderma

Another collagen disease that may affect the heart is scleroderma. Here the connective tissue of the skin, œsophagus, joints and heart is chiefly and diffusely involved.

The sexes are about equally affected, and the average age is nearer 40 than 30.

In addition to the smooth, shiny, fixed skin of the affected areas, the majority of cases have Raynaud's syndrome (often the first symptom), polyarthritis (like rheumatoid), and pigmentation of the exposed surfaces of the skin (Weis et al., 1943). About half the cases have some difficulty in swallowing, and reduced peristalsis with delay in the passage of barium through the œsophagus may be demonstrated radiologically (Olsen et al., 1945). Occasionally the lungs are involved, and rarely the kidneys.

Many cases of scleroderma heart disease have been reported, the majority proving fatal within a year or two. There is an increase of cellular vascular connective tissue with secondary degeneration of muscle fibres followed by replacement fibrosis.

There are no specific laboratory tests for scleroderma except the microscopic appearances of biopsied skin. Patients are usually afebrile, but may have a raised sedimentation rate. The C-reactive protein test is negative, but the serum globulin may be increased. For diagnostic purposes clinical hall-marks are more helpful.

Dermatomyositis is similar to scleroderma in most of the above respects, but involves muscle as well as skin (Tager and Grossman, 1944).

Treatment of myocarditis due to collagen diseases

Few cases of myocarditis due to any of the collagen diseases or allergic states (except rheumatic carditis) survive more than two years whatever treatment is given. A.C.T.H., cortisone, hydrocortisone or preferably one of the newer compounds, such as decortisyl (delta-1-dehydrocortisone), that do not cause sodium retention may be tried. The usual dose of cortisone in these cases is 200–300 mg. daily for the first week, 100–150 mg. daily for the second, and 50–75 mg. daily for the third; it is then gradually reduced to the minimum that seems to control the disease. A strict low-sodium diet and mercurial diuretics help to combat sodium retention. The dose of decortisyl is one-quarter of the dose of cortisone. Withholding the drug all too frequently results in a violent exacerbation of activity, and few cases derive much benefit. Disseminated lupus responds best (Cohen and Cadman, 1953).

Sarcoidosis

The precise nature of sarcoidosis is still uncertain (Scadding, 1950). I may affect the cardiovascular system in two ways, both of which are rare extensive pulmonary involvement may cause cor pulmonale (q.v.), or ther may be an actual sarcoid myocarditis.

The clinical features of the cardiopathy resemble those of isolate myocarditis; cases may present with congestive failure (Yesner and Silve 1951) or with cardiac pain, suggesting ischæmic heart disease (Stepher 1954); sudden death may occur.

The diagnosis may be suggested by coincident pulmonary lesion mediastinal or generalised lymphadenopathy, splenomegaly, erythem nodosum, iridocyclitis and hyperglobulinæmia; it may be confirmed b biopsy of an enlarged gland, skin lesion or liver. In doubtful cases a salin emulsion of sarcoid tissue may be injected intradermally (Kveim test); th insidious development of a dusky red nodule at the site of injection havin the histological appearances of sarcoid is diagnostic (James and Thompso 1955).

METABOLIC AND NUTRITIONAL CARDIOPATHIES

These include primary amyloidosis, hæmochromatosis, diabetes mellitus, beri-beri, alcoholism and perhaps endomyocardial fibrosis; a congenital group comprising fibroelastosis, anomalous origin of the left coronary artery from the pulmonary artery, Von Gierke's disease, gargoylism, and possibly familial cardiomegaly, has already been described in Chapter VIII, and is therefore omitted here.

Primary amyloidosis

This is a rare metabolic disorder of unknown etiology affecting middle-aged or elderly persons of either sex. The heart is involved in 85 per cent of cases (Eisen, 1946), seriously so in at least 50 per cent (Lindsay, 1946). Amyloid material accumulates in the interstitial spaces between secondarily atrophic muscle fibres, and in the walls of the blood vessels (Larsen, 1930).

The majority of cases present clinically like isolated myocarditis, i.e. with congestive heart failure of obscure etiology. There are very few clues pointing to the true nature of the cardiopathy—only the age of the patient, which is usually over 50 (Jones and Frazier, 1950), macroglossia and profound asthenia (Eisen, 1946). There is, of course, no history of chronic suppuration or other infection in these primary cases, and the congo red test is negative. Virtually all laboratory tests selected in the hope of identifying the nature of an obscure cardiopathy are negative except biopsies of the tongue, or possibly skeletal muscle, which may reveal amyloid.

The two most important diagnostic errors are: (1) mistaking amyloid for Pick's disease, which may lead to a fruitless and dangerous thoracotomy (Couter and Reichert, 1950), and (2) misinterpreting abnormal Q or QS waves and inverted T waves in the electrocardiogram as evidence of cardiac infarction (Wessler and Freedberg, 1948; Holzmann, 1950). The differential diagnosis between both these conditions and isolated myocarditis has already been discussed.

Hæmochromatosis

The disorder of iron metabolism known as hæmochromatosis may affect the heart, as well as the pancreas, liver, testicles, adrenals, skin and other organs. Althausen and Kerr (1933) emphasised the serious consequences of cardiac involvement, and in his classic monograph Sheldon (1935) stated that heart failure was the cause of death in 15 per cent of 119 cases. Iron absorbed avidly from the intestinal tract, reaches a relatively high level in the blood, is poorly excreted and is deposited in the organs mentioned above. Diabetes mellitus, muddy pigmentation of the skin, loss of axillary and pubic hair, testicular atrophy and impotence, cirrhosis of the liver, and heart failure are the chief consequences. Deposition of iron in the muscle fibres of the heart is common in cases without disturbance of cardiac function (de Gennes *et al.*, 1936), but it has usually been more conspicuous in cases of heart failure, and secondary fibrosis more evident.

Of the 311 cases reviewed by Sheldon (1935) about 95 per cent were men. The usual age is between 45 and 60, but cardiac cases tend to be younger, all but three out of 25 such cases reviewed by Petit (1945) being under 45.

The chief cardiac manifestations are disturbances of rhythm (including heart block and ventricular fibrillation), and heart failure, which may be mainly left ventricular or "congestive"; but pain resembling that in ischæmic heart disease may occur (Horns, 1949), as in isolated myocarditis.

The diagnosis is usually obvious owing to the many characteristic features of the disease as a whole, but when the heart bears the brunt of the attack in a young adult it may be overlooked. Hæmochromatosis may be proved by biopsy of the skin or liver (King and Downie, 1948). Absorption, storage and excretion of iron may be studied by giving radioiron and following its course in the fæces, blood, and body organs (Bothwell *et al.*, 1952).

Diabetes mellitus

The relationship between diabetes, blood lipids, atherosclerosis, peripheral vascular disease and coronary disease is familiar if not fully understood. In addition, some confusion may be caused by the presence of depressed S-T segments or inverted T waves in the electrocardiogram in patients without other evidence of coronary disease: these appearances have been attributed to a low blood potassium following treatment for diabetic acidosis (Liebow and Hellerstein, 1949; Henderson, 1953); too much insulin therapy may also precipitate or aggravate latent angina pectoris for hypoglycæmia causes hyperadrenalism, and this too may alter the electrocardiogram. Finally, circulatory collapse in diabetic coma may temporarily impair the nutrition of the myocardium. Apart from these considerations diabetes mellitus does not injure the heart.

The heart in malnutrition and chronic alcoholism

The heart may be seriously affected by nutritional anæmia and beri beri; both conditions give rise to a hyperkinetic circulatory state and are discussed under that heading. The term *nutritional cardiopathy* is best reserved for that form of heart disease that may result from an unbalanced high carbohydrate, low protein diet, as described by Gillanders (1951). The disorder is common amongst the adult Bantu population of South Africa and something very similar may be seen in chronic alcoholics anywhere. At necropsy the heart is dilated and hypertrophied, and microscopy shows hypertrophy of the muscle fibres without loss of striation or hydropic degeneration; intracellular œdema may occur but is not specific, being found in many types of heart failure; patchy interstitial fibrosis is also described, but may be inconspicuous. There are no inflammatory foci and the endocardium is normal except where it underlies organised mural thrombi, which are common in both ventricles and atria. In other words the findings are simply those of chronic heart failure without demonstrable cause (Higginson, Gillanders and Murray, 1952). Varying degrees of cirrhosis of the liver, thought to be due to the same malnutrition, are found in nearly all cases; heavy deposits of hæmosiderin are common in the liver and other abdominal organs, but not in the heart itself.

The post-mortem findings in chronic alcoholics dying from heart failure are similar, although the intracellular œdema has been specially emphasised (Merle and Eelin, 1953). The hepatic hypoprotinæmic metabolic cardiopathy described by Oppenheim (1950) in cases of cirrhosis of the liver may be similar, but may also include hepatic hyperkinetic circulatory states.

Clinically cases present with the characteristic dietetic or alcoholic history and congestive heart failure with a low cardiac output. Atrial flutter is particularly common in alcoholic cases.

The *differential diagnosis* is from beri-beri, hæmochromatosis, and hepatic cardiopathy. Beri-beri is excluded by the low cardiac output, absence of response to aneurin, and negative biochemical and biological tests for aneurin deficiency. Cases may occur, however, in which B1 deficiency is also present, and therapeutically it is wise to cover the possibility. Hæmosiderosis may be found in hepatic biopsies and is believed to be another result of chronic malnutrition (Gillman and Gillman, 1951); hæmochromatosis involving the heart is unlikely in the absence of any other evidence of that disease. Associated cirrhosis of the liver may be advanced, especially in chronic alcoholics, and may lead to vasodilatation and an attempt to raise the cardiac output. The combination of nutritional and hepatic cardiopathies may be confusing and may result in an erroneous diagnosis of beri-beri; but the hepatic palms, spider nævi, small volume collapsing pulse, low blood pressure, and absence of response to thiamine should soon correct the mistake.

Treatment consists of a high protein, well-balanced diet, which if given in time may reverse the myocardial fault. Too often, however, it is already too late, or the diet is not maintained. The usual remedies for heart failure must also be prescribed.

ENDOCRINE CARDIOPATHIES

Thyrotoxicosis and *myxœdema* are by far the most important endocrine diseases that affect the cardiovascular system. They are discussed separately in Chapter XIX.

Acromegaly may cause considerable cardiac hypertrophy and hyperplasia of interstitial fibrous tissue. Enlargement of other viscera usually accompanies the cardiomegaly. Many hearts from acromegalics have weighed over 1,000 G. (Courville and Mason, 1938). Hypertension and coronary disease associated with diabetes complicate some of the cases, but heart failure may occur in their absence (Hejtmancik, Bradfield and Herrman, 1951). Failure is attributed to enlargement outstripping nutritional supplies.

NEUROMUSCULAR DYSTROPHIES

Friedreich's ataxia has been discussed in the congenital section.

Progressive muscular dystrophy involves the heart in about 50 per cent of cases (Rubin and Buchberg, 1952). There is muscular atrophy and fibrous tissue replacement (Weisenfeld and Messinger, 1952). There seems to be little relationship between the degree and severity of the skeletal myopathy and the cardiac lesion.

The great majority of cases are male, and the average age 25 (Zatuchni *et al.*, 1951).

Clinically the most common finding is some abnormality in the electrocardiogram, such as bundle branch block or T wave changes, without serious disturbance of cardiac function. Arrhythmias also occur, and in a minority congestive heart failure. Sudden death has been reported in several instances.

The diagnosis should be suggested by the prominent yet weak calf muscles, the awkward gait, and the habit of climbing up the legs when getting up; it may be proved by muscle biopsy.

TUMOURS OF THE HEART

Primary tumours are rare and include myxoma (35 per cent), sarcoma (21 per cent), fibroma (12 per cent), rhabdomyoma (19 per cent), and lipoma (12 per cent) (Yater, 1931). Secondary tumours are sixteen times more common (Reeves and Michael, 1936); they have been found a necropsy in 10 per cent of all cases of malignant disease, but have given rise to clinical manifestations in only 1 per cent (Goudie, 1955). The majority are secondary to carcinoma of the bronchus or breast, but almost any malignant tumour may metastasise to the heart (Raven, 1948; Young and Goldman, 1954). Leukæmia must also be considered in this section.

MYXOMA OF THE LEFT ATRIUM is the commonest primary tumour of the heart. It arises from the atrial septum to which it is attached by a pedicle close to the foramen ovale.

The majority of patients have been women between the ages of 30 and 60.

Symptoms may develop relatively suddenly and are attributable to acute, subacute, chronic or paroxysmal obstruction at the mitral orifice. Severe syncopal attacks, during which the pulse may be imperceptible, acute pulmonary œdema or paroxysmal nocturnal dyspnœa may occur. A chronic course ending in congestive heart failure has also been described. Arrhythmias are said to be infrequent, but paroxysmal atrial tachycardia and atrial fibrillation have both been recorded (Gilchrist and Miller, 1934; Fawcett and Ward, 1939).

The physical signs include a small peripheral pulse and remarkably variable mitral systolic and diastolic murmurs. In some cases, however, no murmurs are heard at all (Von Reis, 1949). The records in the literature rarely mention the first heart sound or the presence or absence of a mitral opening snap, but Burnett and Davidson (1945) stated that the first heart sound was accentuated in their case, as did Jones and Julian (1955), and all observers have likened the signs to those of variable mitral stenosis with or without pulmonary hypertension (Mahaim, 1947). The P wave of the electrocardiogram has usually been more or less normal, and as a rule X-rays have revealed little enlargement of the left atrium and pulmonary artery. Few illustrations of chronic pulmonary interstitial œdema have been published.

The physiological findings on cardiac catheterisation may prove as variable as the murmurs and this itself may suggest the correct diagnosis; myxoma should also be suspected if the left atrial pressure is found to be normal in a case of supposed mitral stenosis giving a history of paroxysmal cardiac dyspnœa. Angiocardiography may reveal a filling defect of the left atrium (Goldberg and Steinberg, 1955).

In the case reported by Jones and Julian (1955) the mean left atrial pressure was 44 mm. Hg and the mean pulmonary artery pressure 80 mm. Hg. Left atrial pressures as high as this at rest are very unusual in mitral stenosis, particularly in cases with so short a history. Even passive pulmonary hypertension of this degree could well cause right ventricular failure.

The downhill course is usually rapid, few patients surviving more than a year after the onset of symptoms. Death may terminate a syncopal attack or result from acute pulmonary œdema.

Treatment is surgical. In cases of acute pulmonary œdema or loss of consciousness it is worth changing the position of the patient in the hope that the tumour may slip away from the mitral orifice.

PRIMARY SARCOMA of the heart arises from the right atrium in at least half the cases (Weir and Jones, 1941), and as it grows tends to fill the cavities of both the right atrium and right ventricle. Hæmangioendothelio-sarcoma behaves similarly (Cheng and Sutton, 1955; Amsterdam *et al.*, 1949). These tumours may be highly vascular and are composed chiefly of nests of hæmangioblasts in a groundwork of endothelial cells.

The clinical features of sarcoma of the right atrium closely resemble those of rapidly progressive tricuspid stenosis, the obstruction of the circulation being more or less at the level of the tricuspid valve through which the tumour usually grows.

FIBROMA is most likely to involve the wall of the left ventricle. The only example I have seen was in a female child who presented with paroxysmal ventricular tachycardia, heart failure which finally proved fatal, an electro-cardiogram with a QT pattern suggesting cardiac infarction in anterolateral

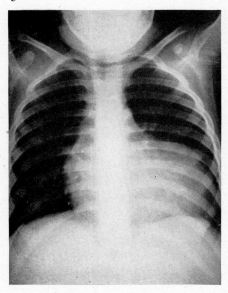

Fig. 11.05—Fibroma of the left ventricle.
(*Acknowledgment to Dr. Ursula James*).

left ventricular surface leads or their equivalents, and radiological appearances resembling a large left ventricular aneurysm (fig. 11.05).

RHABDOMYOMA is a congenital glycogen-containing "tumour" of heart muscle fibres ($\rho\alpha\beta\delta\sigma\varsigma$, a rod), and is more often multiple than solitary. The nodules are usually found in the wall of the left ventricle, and may be associated with tuberose sclerosis. Most cases die in infancy or childhood (Batchelor and Maun, 1945).

SECONDARY TUMOURS involve the heart or pericardium in about 10 per cent of all cases of cancer (Scott and Garvin, 1939). The majority are secondary to bronchial carcinoma, and invade the heart by direct extension, the pericardium being affected first. Thymic and other mediastinal neo-plasms may spread to the heart in the same way.

Clinically, such cases tend to present with hæmopericardium, often with cardiac tamponade; in others, paroxysmal atrial tachycardia or flutter is the first manifestation. Sometimes pericardial pain and inverted T waves in the electrocardiogram are mistaken for cardiac infarction, especially when followed by intractable heart failure.

Discrete blood-born secondary nodules from remote malignant growths are less frequent, and when present may be associated with more obvious secondaries in the lungs.

LEUKÆMIA may give rise to infiltrative myocardial or pericardial lesions but they are rarely of much clinical importance. Associated severe anæmia is more likely to embarrass the cardiovascular system. I have only seen five cases of leukæmia amongst my last 10,000 patients with cardiovascular disease: three of these presented with acute cardiac infarction from coronary thrombosis, one with acute coronary insufficiency after a long history of angina pectoris, and one with a hyperkinetic circulatory state due to severe anæmia. The patients with occlusive coronary disease were all elderly men, and the leukæmia was discovered as a result of a routine white count. Whether the two diseases were coincidental or related is unknown. The leukæmia was monocytic in three cases, and myeloid in the other two.

Argentaffinoma

In 1952, Biörck, Axen and Thorson described the unusual association of pulmonary valve stenosis, gross tricuspid incompetence, and carcinoid of the small intestine with metastases in the liver in a boy of 19; a remarkable feature of the case was intense, patchy and variable reddish blue cyanosis and attacks of flushing; there was also a nine-year history of asthma and diarrhoea. In 1954 Thorson, Biörck and Bjorkman reported seven definite cases of this interesting syndrome and concluded that the secretion of large quantities of serotonin (5-hydroxytryptamine) by the carcinoid and its metastases was responsible for the acquired pulmonary and tricuspid valve lesions as well as for flushing, patchy cyanosis, bronchospasm, and diarrhoea. The syndrome has excited considerable interest and a number of similar cases have been reported by others since (e.g. Bean *et al.*, 1955).

Biochemically, serotonin (5-hydroxytryptamine) has been demonstrated in high concentration in the serum and urine of patients with argentaffinoma of the small intestine (Pernow and Waldenström, 1954), as well as in the tumour itself and its metastases (Lembeck, 1953). Serotonin is inactivated by a lung enzyme—monoamine oxidase (Bradley *et al.*, 1950)—which breaks it down to 5-hydroxyindoleacetic acid (5-H.I.A.A.), and an enormous increase of this substance has been found in the urine of patients with argentaffinoma (Page *et al.*, 1955). In a case of my own there was good evidence that serotonin was inactivated in the lungs because its concentration in the serum and plasma fell from 56 and 62 μg. per cent respectively in samples from the pulmonary artery to 19 and 22 μg. per cent respectively in samples obtained from the brachial artery (Goble, Hay and Sandler, 1955). It is not yet clear how serotonin causes fusion of the pulmonary and tricuspid valve cusps, but its inactivation in the lung explains why the valve lesions are right sided.

Clinically the syndrome is easily recognised by anyone familiar with its manifestations. The combination of the peculiar mottled or patchy cyanosis, the attacks of flushing and bronchial asthma, the diarrhoea, large liver (from metastases), and signs of mild or moderate pulmonary and tricuspid stenosis are too characteristic to be mistaken for any other condition. In my own case (a 33-year-old woman) the pulmonary stenosis was of moderate degree (P.A.P. 9/4; R.V.P. 45/-5; C.O. 3.5 L/min. at rest), and the tricuspid stenosis mild (presystolic pressure gradient 4 mm. Hg). There was a two-year history of blotchy erythema, marked flushing and asthma, attacks being precipitated by meals, so that she became afraid to eat. The primary tumour was removed from the ileum, but there was little improvement owing to the extensive metastases in the liver, and she died within six months of her first admission to hospital. Necropsy confirmed the diagnosis. Full details of this case are being reported by Goble *et al.* (1956).

MYOCARDITIS DUE TO DRUGS

Certain therapeutic drugs have earned the reputation of being dangerous to the heart, either by causing transient toxic myocarditis or by inducing ventricular fibrillation or asystole. In the first group the best known are digitalis and emetine; in the second, choloroform, adrenaline, and potassium. Toxic myocarditis due to drug allergy is in a different category, and has already been discussed.

DIGITALIS

Digitalis is undoubtedly the best example of a therapeutic drug that may cause dangerous myocardial poisoning.

Pathology. Büchner (1934) first demonstrated that necrotic myocardial lesions could be produced in animals (cats) by means of digitalis. Dearing, Barnes, and Essex (1943), also working on cats, produced focal necrosis, cellular reaction, and fibroblastic repair. Similar necrotic lesions may be provoked by acetylcholine and by continuous direct vagal stimulation (Banting and Hall, 1936, 1937), and have been ascribed to coronary constriction. In the belief that the lesions due to digitalis were caused by the activity of acetylcholine, Kyser, Ginsberg and Gilbert (1946) succeeded in

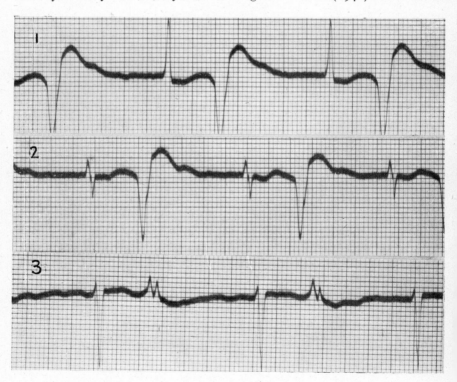

Fig. 11.06—Electrocardiogram showing coupling from ventricular ectopic beats due to digitalis.

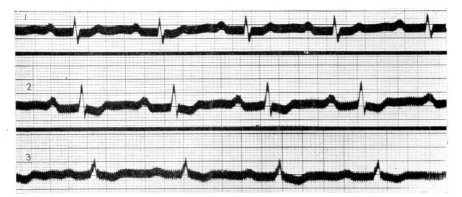

Fig. 11.07—Electrocardiogram showing partial heart block due to digitalis.

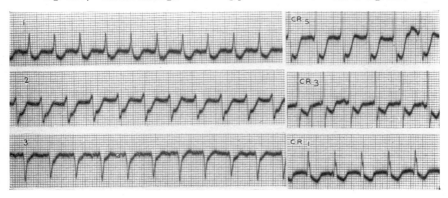

Fig. 11.08—Electrocardiogram showing paroxysmal tachycardia due to digitalis.

preventing them by the simultaneous administration of atropine or a coronary vasodilator, such as theophylline. Whether digitalis intoxication in man is characterised by similar patchy myocardial necrosis, and whether this is mediated by vagal stimulation, remain to be proved; but it is a reasonable hypothesis. Certainly, the effect of acetylcholine is augmented in the presence of strophanthin or digitalis (Danielopolu, 1946).

Clinical features. Anorexia, nausea or vomiting, and diarrhœa, usually give sufficient warning of digitalis overdosage, but there may be no such indication when carditis from other causes is already present. Disturbances of rhythm are common, and include coupling due to premature ectopic beats (fig. 11.06), nodal rhythm, partial or complete heart block (fig. 11.07), multiple ectopic beats, atrial fibrillation, paroxysmal tachycardia (fig. 11.08), and sudden death from ventricular fibrillation.

The electrocardiogram shows characteristic sagging depression of the RS-T segment (fig. 11.09), maximum in leads V_{4-6} when there is normal or increased left ventricular dominance, or in leads V_{1-2} when there is right ventricular preponderance. The depression is transmitted chiefly to lead V_L or V_F and thence to the appropriate standard lead according to the electrical position of the heart. At first, the peak of T remains upright, but later becomes absorbed in a sharply depressed RS-T segment, the Q-T interval being shortened (fig. 11.10). The electrocardiogram offers by far the most reliable evidence of digitalis saturation, even when the patient denies having taken the drug.

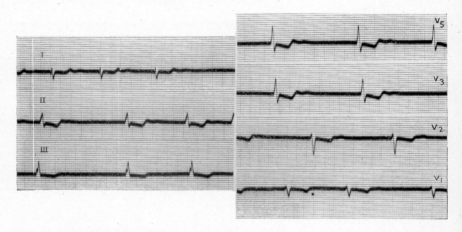

Fig. 11.09—Electrocardiogram showing depression of the RS-T segment due to digitalis.

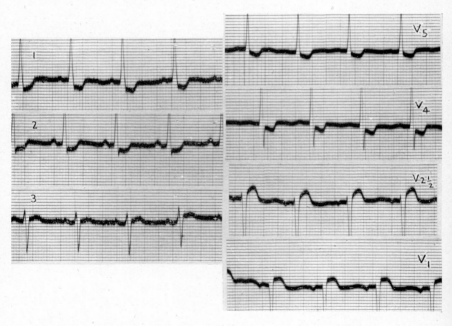

Fig. 11.10—Shortening of the Q-T interval due to digitalis. Q-T$_C$—0.3 sec.

Treatment. The best remedy, apart from stopping digitalis, is atropine, but it is rarely necessary. If the degree of intoxication appears dangerous, however, it may be given in doses of 0.5 mg. four-hourly for a day or two.

EMETINE

Emetine is another therapeutic drug with a reputation for causing toxic myocarditis, the chief danger being abnormalities of rhythm, particularly ventricular fibrillation. Emetine was used a great deal amongst British troops in the Mediterranean theatre during the second world war, but ill-effects on the heart were very rare if they occurred at all. Patients receiving emetine, however, were always confined to bed throughout the course.

Fatal cases of toxic myocarditis described in the literature received a total dose of 1.04 to 2.65 G. of emetine over a period of two to six weeks (Brown, 1935). Emetine is highly cumulative, being excreted very slowly, and the minimum lethal dose is said to be around 20 mg./kilo.

OTHER DRUGS

Potassium, when used in large single doses (8 to 16 G.) to stop paroxysmal tachycardia or multiple ectopic beats, or to differentiate between ischaemic and other causes of T wave inversion, is undoubtedly dangerous, and may cause sudden death from ventricular asystole, preceded by increasing heart block and bundle branch block. Spontaneous potassium poisoning may cause sudden death in uraemia (Marchand and Finch, 1944). The electrocardiogram in such cases shows widened QRS complexes and tall peaked T waves (fig. 11.11).

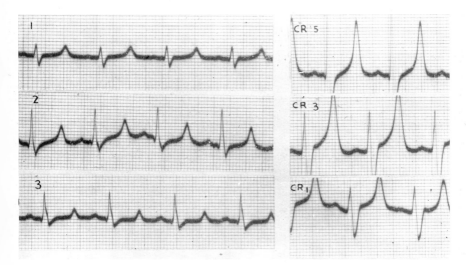

Fig. 11.11—Widening of the QRS complex and accentuation of the T wave due to a high blood potassium in a case of uraemia. The long Q-T is due to hypocalcaemia.

The normal serum potassium is 15 to 21 mg. per cent (4 to 5.5 m.eq. per litre). It may be reduced in a variety of conditions including familial periodic paralysis, diabetic acidosis, ulcerative colitis, idiopathic steator-rhœa, vomiting from interstinal obstruction, and as a result of prolonged treatment with resins. Electrocardiographic changes include flattening of the T wave, augmentation of the U wave, depression of the S-T segment, and prolongation of the P-R, Q-T and Q-U intervals (Perelson and Cosby, 1949; Bellet et al., 1950). The amplitude of T declines when the serum potassium is at 13 to 14 mg. per cent, U becomes prominent at 10 to 12 mg. per cent, and depression of the S-T segment at about 8 mg. per cent (Metzger and Blum, 1950). Ectopic beats and perhaps other arrhythmias may result from these low potassium levels, and McAllen (1955) found widespread myocardial fibrosis at necropsy in two cases.

Adrenaline in large doses may excite ectopic beats or almost any change of rhythm except heart block. Transient hypertension and inversion of the T wave in leads V_{4-6} are common. Violent palpitations and substernal discomfort may occur, and patients with ischæmic heart disease usually develop a severe attack of angina pectoris. Clinical examples may result from errors in the dose of adrenaline administered, or from spontaneous hyperadrenalism in cases of pheochromocytoma.

Chloroform is an example of a group of drugs, mostly anæsthetics, which may cause sudden death from ventricular fibrillation, especially in the presence of an excess of adrenaline.

Nocotine, as absorbed by heavy smokers, may provoke ectopic beats and cause slight coronary and peripheral vasoconstriction, and so aggravate angina pectoris, hypertension and peripheral vascular disease. *Barium chloride* causes ectopic beats.

Alcohol is a vasodilator, and in moderate amounts may benefit ischæmic heart disease; on the other hand, it may increase the work of the heart, especially if the blood volume is temporarily raised. Heavy drinkers may suffer from an inadequate supply of aneurin, and may develop heart failure in consequence, or their high carbohydrate low protein diet may lead to another form of nutritional cardiopathy as described on page 628. Finally, under the influence of alcohol, patients are apt to be careless of medical advice, and may exert themselves more than they should.

THE HEART IN ACUTE NEPHRITIS

Carditis accompanying acute nephritis (Whitehill et al., 1939) and toxæmia of pregnancy (Szekely and Snaith, 1947) is particularly interesting. The chief clinical features are elevation of the venous pressure, a tendency to develop acute pulmonary œdema, general enlargement of the heart, and inversion of the T wave in leads facing the surface of the left ventricle (Master, Jaffe, and Dack, 1937). The degree of hypertension is often insufficient to explain these findings. Nephritic œdema is usually present, the blood volume is raised, and the circulation time normal (Klein, 1947).

That there may be some form of cardiopathy is suggested in certain cases by the behaviour of the cardiac output, which may fail to rise as expected when the venous pressure is high; moreover, the Valsalva test yields a square wave response (Sharpey-Schafer, 1955). On the other hand,

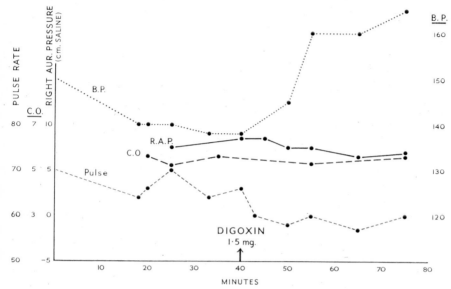

Fig. 11.12—Graph illustrating a high right atrial pressure that is not reduced by digitalis in a case of acute nephritis. There is a conspicuous rise of blood pressure and slight slowing of the pulse; the cardiac output is unchanged.

the lack of response to digitalis (fig. 11.12) shows that the heart is not overloaded. Histological examination of the heart muscle in fatal cases of acute nephritis presenting cardiac signs seldom reveals any structural abnormality; sometimes, however, the muscle fibres are dispersed by serous exudate, lymphocytes and endothelial cells—even then there is little, if any, necrosis (Gore and Saphir, 1948).

It is probable, therefore, that the raised venous pressure is mainly due to an increased blood volume from retention of sodium and water, and that, as a rule, the heart responds normally; but that in certain instances cardiac function is impaired, owing perhaps to biochemical rather than structural changes in the heart muscle; whether acute pulmonary œdema is a manifestation of left ventricular failure or whether it is due to a toxic or allergic effect on the pulmonary capillaries is not yet known.

REFERENCES

Althausen, T. L., and Kerr, W. J. (1933): "Hemochromatosis. Report of three cases with discussion of etiology", *Endocrinology*, **17**, 621.

Altshuler, S. S., Hoffman, K. M., and Fitzgerald, P. J. (1948): "Electrocardiographic changes in diphtheria", *Ann. Intern. Med.*, **29**, 294.

Amsterdam, H. J., Grayzel, D. M., and Louria, A. L. (1949): "Hemangioendothelioblastoma of the heart", *Amer. Heart J.*, **37**, 291.

Banting, F. G., and Hall, G. E. (1937): "Experimental production of myocardial and coronary artery lesions", *Tr. Ass. Amer. Phys.*, **52**, 204.

——, ——, and Ettinger, G. H. (1936): "Experimental production of coronary thrombosis and myocardial failure", *Canad. med. Ass. J.*, **34**, 9.

Batchelor, T. M., and Maun, M. E. (1945): "Congenital glycogenic tumors of heart", *Arch. Path.*, **39**, 67.

Bayley, R. H. (1946): "The electrocardiographic effects of injury at the endocardial surface of the left ventricle", *Amer. Heart J.*, **31**, 677.

Bean, W. B., Olch, D., and Weinberg, H. B. (1955): "The syndrome of carcinoid and acquired valve lesions of the right side of the heart", *Circulation*, **12**, 1.

Becker, B. J. P., Chatgidakis, C. B., and Van Lingen, B. (1953): "Cardiovascular collagenosis with parietal endocardial thrombosis. A clinico-pathologic study of forty cases", *Ibid.*, **7**, 345.

Bedford, D. E., and Konstam, G. L. S. (1946): "Heart failure of unknown aetiology in Africans", *Brit. Heart J.*, **8**, 236.

Beecher, C. H., and Amidon, E. L. (1938): "Electrocardiographic findings in 44 cases of trichinosis", *Amer. Heart J.*, **16**, 219.

Bellet, S., Steiger, W. A., Nadler, C. S., and Gazes, P. C. (1950): "Electrocardiographic patterns in hypopotassemia: observations on 79 patients", *Amer. J. med. Sci.*, **219**, 542.

Berry, M. G., Johnson, A. S., and Warshauer, S. E. (1945): "Tsutsugamushi fever. Clinical observations in one hundred and ninety-five cases", *War Med.*, **7**, 71.

Biörck, G., Axen, O., and Thorson, A. (1952): "Unusual cyanosis in a boy with congenital pulmonary stenosis and tricuspid insufficiency. Fatal outcome after angiocardiography", *Amer. Heart J.*, **44**, 143.

Bothwell, T. H., Van Lingen, B., Alper, T., and du Preez, M. L. (1952): "The cardiac complications of hemochromatosis", *Ibid.*, **43**, 333.

Bradley, T. R., Butterworth, R. F., Reid, G., and Trautner, E. M. (1950): "Nature of the lung enzyme which inactivates serum vasoconstrictor", *Nature*, **166**, 911.

Brown, P. W. (1935): "Results and dangers in treatment of amebiasis; summary of fifteen years' clinical experience at Mayo Clinic", *J. Amer. med. Ass.*, **105**, 1319.

Büchner, F. (1934): "Herzmuskelnekrosen durch hohe Dosen von Digitalisglykosiden", *Arch. Exp. path. Pharmakol.*, **176**, 59.

Burch, G., and Reaser, P. (1947): "A primer of cardiology", Philadelphia.

Burkhardt, E. A., Eggleston, C., and Smith, L. W. (1938): "Electrocardiographic changes and peripheral nerve palsies in toxic diphtheria", *Amer. J. med. Sc.*, **195**, 301.

Burnett, W., and Davidson, J. (1945): "A case of myxoma of the heart", *Brit. Heart J.*, **7**, 180.

Canabal, E. J., Aguirre, C. V., Dighiero, J., Purcallas, J., Baldomir, J. M., and Suzacq, C. V. (1955): "Echinococcus disease of the left ventricle. A clinical radiologic and electrocardiographic study", *Circulation*, **12**, 520.

Chagas, C. (1909): "Nova tripanozomiase humana. Estudos sobre a morfolojia e o ciclo evolutivo do Schizotrypanum cruzi n. gen., n. sp., agente etiolojio de nova entidade morbida do homenen", *Mem. de Inst. Oswaldo Cruz, Rio de Jan.*, **1**, 159.

Cheng, T. O., and Sutton, D. C. (1955): "Primary hemangioendotheliosarcoma of heart diagnosed by angiocardiography. Review of the literature and report of a case", *Circulation*, **11**, 456.

Cohen, Sir Henry, and Cadman, E. F. B. (1953): "The natural history of lupus erythematosus and its modification by cortisone and corticotrophin (A.C.T.H.)", *Lancet*, **ii**, 305.

Corbett, A. J. (1943): "Scrub typhus", *Bull. U.S. Army med. Dept.*, **70**, 34.

Cornell, A., and Shookhoff, H. (1944): "Actinomycosis of the heart stimulating rheumatic fever. Report of three cases of cardiac actinomycosis with a review of the literature", *Arch. intern. Med.*, **74**, 11.

Courville, C., and Mason, V. R. (1938): "The heart in acromegaly", *Arch. intern. Med.*, **61**, 704.

Couter, W. T., and Reichert, R. E. Jr. (1950): "Primary systemic amyloidosis mimicking chronic constrictive pericardial disease", *Circulation*, **2**, 441.

Danielopolu, D. (1946): *La Digitale et les Strophantines*, Pharmacodynamie-Thérapeutique, Paris, Masson et Cie.

Daniels, W. B., *et al.* (1943): "Meningococcic infection in soldiers", *J. Amer. med. Ass.*, **123**, 1.

Davies, J. N. P. (1948): "Endocardial fibrosis in Africans", *E. Afr. med. J.*, **25**, 10.

Davies, R. R., Marvel, R. J., and Genovese, P. D. (1951): "Heart disease of unknown etiology", *Amer. Heart J.*, **42**, 546.

Davson, J., Ball, J., and Platt, R. (1948): "The kidney in periarteritis nodosa", *Quart. J. Med.*, **17**, 175.

Dearing, W. H., Barnes, A. R., and Essex, H. E. (1943): "Experiments with calculated therapeutic and toxic doses of digitalis; effects on myocardial cellular structure", *Amer. Heart J.*, **25**, 648.

de Gennes, L., Delarue, J., and de Vericourt, R. (1936): "Le syndrome endocrino-hepato-cardiaque", *Pr. méd.*, **44**, 377.

de la Chapelle, C. E., and Graef, I. (1931): "Acute isolated myocarditis", *Arch. intern. Med.*, **47**, 942.

Elkeles, A., and Glynn, L. E. (1944): "Serial röntgenograms of chest in periarteritis nodosa as aid to diagnosis, with notes on pathology of pulmonary lesions", *Brit. J. Radiol.*, **17**, 368.

Eisen, H. N. (1946): "Primary systemic amyloidosis", *Amer. J. Med.*, **1**, 144.

Fawcett, R. M. (1948): "Myocardium after sulfonamide therapy", *Arch Path.*, **45**, 25.

Fawcett, R. E. M., and Ward, E. M. (1939): "Cardiac myxoma. A clinical and pathological study", *Brit. Heart J.*, **1**, 249.

Fiedler, A. (1889): "Ueber akute interstitielle Myokarditis. Festschrift zur Feier des 50 jahr. Bestehens des Stadtkrankenhauses zu Dresden-Friedrickstadt", Dresden, part **2**, 3.

French, A. J. (1946): "Hypersensitivity in the pathogenesis of the histopathological changes associated with sulfonamide chemotherapy", *Amer. J. Path.*, **22**, 679.

——, and Weller, C. V. (1942): "Interstitial myocarditis following the clinical experimental use of sulfonamide drugs", *Ibid.*, **18**, 109.

Gilchrist, A. R., and Miller, W. G. (1936): "Paroxysmal auricular tachycardia associated with primary cardiac tumour, with pathological report", *Edin. med. J.*, **43**, 243.

Gillanders, A. D. (1951): "Nutritional heart disease", *Brit. Heart J.*, **13**, 177.

Gillis, J. G., and Walters, M. B. (1954): "Acute isolated myocarditis simulating coronary occlusion", *Amer. Heart J.*, **47**, 117.

Goble, A. J., Hay, D. R., and Sandler, M. (1955): "5-hydroxytryptamine metabolism in acquired heart disease associated with argentaffin carcinoma", *Lancet*, ii, 1016.

——, ——, Hudson, R. J., and Sandler, M. (1956): "Acquired heart disease associated with argentaffin carcinoma", *Brit. Heart J.* (to be published).

Gold, S. C., and Gowing, N. F. C. (1953): "Systemic lupus erythematosus: a clinical and pathological study", *Quart. J. Med.*, **22**, 457.

Goldberg, H. P., and Steinberg, I. (1955): "Clinical progress. Primary tumors of the heart", *Circulation*, **11**, 963.

Goldstein, D. M., and Louie, S. (1943): "Primary pulmonary coccidioidomycosis. Report of an epidemic of 75 cases", *War Med.*, **4**, 299.

Gore, I. (1948): "Myocardial changes in fatal diphtheria. A summary of observations in 221 cases", *Amer. J. med. Sci.*, **215**, 257.

——, and Saphir, O. (1947): "Myocarditis associated with acute nasopharyngitis and acute tonsillitis", *Amer. Heart J.*, **34**, 831.

——, —— (1947): "Myocarditis. A classification of 1,402 cases", *Ibid.*, **34**, 827.

——, —— (1948): "Myocarditis associated with acute and subacute glomerulonephritis", *Ibid.*, **36**, 390.

Goudie, R. B. (1955): "Secondary tumours of the heart and pericardium", *Brit. Heart J.*, **17**, 183.

Griffith, G. C., and Vural, I. L. (1951): "Acute and subacute disseminated lupus erythematosus. A correlation of clinical and post-mortem findings in eighteen cases", *Circulation*, **3**, 492.

Gross, L. (1940): "Cardiac lesions in Libman-Sacks disease, with consideration of its relationship to acute diffuse lupus erythematosus", *Amer. J. Path.*, **16**, 375.

Hansmann, G. H., and Schenken, J. R. (1938): "Acute isolated myocarditis", *Amer. Heart J.*, **15**, 749.

Harkavy, J. (1941): "Vascular allergy; pathogenesis of bronchial asthma with recurrent pulmonary infiltrations and eosinophilic polyserositis", *Arch. intern. Med.*, **67**, 709.

Harris, A. W., Lynch, G. W., and O'Hare, J. P. (1939): "Periarteritis nodosa", *Ibid.*, **63**, 1163.

Hejtmancik, M. R., Bradfield, J. Y., and Herrman, G. R. (1951): "Acromegaly and the heart: a clinical and pathologic study", *Ann. intern. Med.*, **34**, 1445.

Henderson, C. B. (1953): "Potassium and the cardiographic changes in diabetic acidosis", *Brit. Heart J.*, **15**, 87.

Higginson, J., Gillanders, A. D., and Murray, J. F. (1952): "The heart in chronic malnutrition", *Ibid.*, **14**, 213.

Holzmann, M. (1950): "Amyloidosis of the heart. With special reference to the electrocardiogram", *Z. Kreisl. Forsch.*, **39**, 401.

Horns, H. L. (1949): "Hemochromatosis", *Amer. J. Med.*, **6**, 272.

Howell, W. L. (1945): "Absence of electrocardiographic changes in tsutsugamushi fever (scrub typhus)", *Arch. intern. Med.*, **76**, 217.

Humphreys, E. M. (1948): "The cardiac lesions of acute disseminated lupus erythematosus", *Ann. intern. Med.*, **28**, 12.

Jager, B. V., and Grossman, L. A. (1944): "Dermatomyositis", *Arch. intern. Med.*, **73**, 271.

James, D. G., and Thompson, A. D. (1955): "The Kveim test in sarcoidosis", *Quart. J., Med.*, **24**, 49.

Jones, G. P., and Julian, D. G. (1955): "Left atrial tumour simulating mitral stenosis", *Brit. med. J.*, **ii**, 361.

Jones, R. S., and Frazier, D. B. (1950): "Primary cardiovascular amyloidosis: its clinical manifestations, pathology and histogenesis", *Arch. Path.*, **50**, 366.

Josserand, E., and Gallavardin, L. (1901): "De l'asystolie progressive des jeunes subjets par myocarditis subaigue primitive", *Arch. gén. de méd.*, **78**, 513.

Kaplan, B. I., Clark, E., and de la Chapelle, C. E. (1938): "A study of myocardial hypertrophy of uncertain etiology, associated with congestive heart failure", *Amer. Heart J.*, **15**, 582.

Kasper, J. A., and Pinner, M. (1930): "Actinomycosis of the heart", *Arch. Path.*, **10**, 687.

Kernohan, J. W., and Woltman, H. W. (1938): "Periarteritis nodosa; clinico-pathologic study with special reference to nervous system", *Arch. Neurol Psychiat.*, Chicago, **39**, 655.

King, W. E., and Downie, E. (1948): "Hæmochromatosis. Observations on the incidence and on the value of liver biopsy in diagnosis", *Quart. J. Med.*, **17**, 247.

Klein, F. (1947): "Acute glomerulo-nephritis", *Acta med. Scand.*, **129**, 156.

Klemperer, P., Pollack, A. D., and Baehr, G. (1941): "Pathology of disseminated lupus erythematosus", *Arch. Path.*, **32**, 569.

Kyser, F. A., Ginsberg, H., and Gilbert, N. C. (1946): "The effect of certain drugs upon the cardiotoxic lesions of digitalis in the dog", *Amer. Heart J.*, **31**, 451.

Larsen, R. M. (1930): "A pathological study of primary myocardial amyloidosis", *Amer. J. Path.*, **6**, 147.

Lembeck, F. (1953): "5-hydroxytryptamine in a carcinoid tumour", *Nature*, **172**, 910.

Libman, E., and Sacks, B. (1924): "A hitherto undescribed form of valvular and mural endocarditis", *Arch. intern. Med.*, **33**, 701.

Liebow, I. M., and Hellerstein, H. K. (1949): "Cardiac complications of diabetes mellitus", *Amer. J., Med.*, **7**, 660.

Lindsay, S. (1946): "The heart in primary systemic amyloidosis", *Amer. Heart J.*, **32**, 419.

Löffler, W. (1936): "Die fluchtigen lungen-infiltrate mit eosinophilie", *Schweiz. med. Wschr.*, **66**, 1069.

Ludden, T. E., and Edwards, J. E. (1949): "Carditis in poliomyelitis. An anatomic study of thirty-five cases and review of the literature", *Amer. J. Path.*, **25**, 357.

Lyons, C., Owen, C. R., and Ayers, W. B. (1943): "Sulfonamide therapy in actinomycotic infections", *Surgery*, **14**, 99.

McAllen, P. M. (1955): "Myocardial changes occurring in potassium deficiency", *Brit. Heart J.*, **17**, 5.

Mahaim, I. (1947): "The problems evoked by polypus of the left auricle", *Acta cardiol. Brux.*, **2**, 136.

Marchand, J. F., and Finch, C. A. (1944): "Fatal spontaneous potassium intoxication in patients with uræmia", *Arch. intern. Med.*, **73**, 384.

Master, A. M., Jaffe, H. L., and Dack, S. (1937): "The heart in acute nephritis", *Arch. intern. Med.*, **60**, 1016.

Merle, E., and Belin, J. (1953): "Alcoholic enlargement of the heart (alcoholic myocarditis)", *Sem. Hôp. Paris*, **29**, 1454.

Metzger, H., and Blum, A. (1950): "Changes in the normal ECG in the course of two recent cases of hypopotassæmia. Definition of the types of ECG in accordance with the degree of hypopotassæmia", *Bull. Soc. méd. Hôp. Paris*, **66**, 1236.

Miller, H. G., and Daley, R. (1946): "Clinical aspects of polyarteritis", *Quart. J. Med.*, New Series, **15**, 255.

Moseley, V., and Miller, H. (1945): "South American trypanosomiasis (Chagas' disease)", *Arch. intern. Med.*, **76**, 219.

Nathanson, M. H. (1928): "Electrocardiogram in diphtheria", *Ibid.*, **42**, 23.

Neidhart, K., and Rumrich, R. (1950): "Myocarditis in tuberculosis", *Dtsch. med. Wschr.*, **75**, 667.

O'Brien, W. (1954): "Endocardial fibrosis in the Sudan", *Brit. med. J.*, ii, 899.

Olsen, A. M., O'Leary, P. A., and Kirklin, B. R. (1945): "Esophageal lesions associated with acrosclerosis and scleroderma", *Arch. intern. Med.*, **76**, 189.

Oppenheim, M. (1950): "Myocardosis in liver cirrhosis", *Schweiz. med. Wschr.*, **80**, 795.

Page, I. H., Corcoran, A. C., Undenfriend, S., Sjoerdsma, A., and Weissbach, H. (1955): "Argentaffinoma as endocrine tumour", *Lancet*, i, 198.

Parsons, R. J., and Zarefonetis, C. J. D. (1945): "Histoplasmosis in man. Report of seven cases and a review of seventy-one cases", *Arch. intern. Med.*, **75**, 1.

Paulley, J. W., Jones, R., Green, W. P. D., and Kane, E. P. (1954): "Myocardial toxoplasmosis", *Lancet*, ii, 624.

Perelson, H. N., and Cosby, R. S. (1949): "The electrocardiogram in familial periodic paralysis", *Amer. Heart J.*, **37**, 1126.

Pernow, B., and Waldenström, J. (1954): "Paroxysmal flushing and other symptoms caused by 5-hydroxytryptamine and histamine in patients with malignant tumours", *Lancet*, ii, 951.

Perrin, A., Froment, R., and Lenègre, J. (1953): "Insuffisance cardiaque des jeunes sujets par sclérose myocardique dense et diffuse d'origine tuberculeuse, incertaine ou inconnue", *Cardiologia*, Basel, **22**, 257.

Perry, C. B. (1939): "Persistent conduction defects following diphtheria", *Brit. Heart J.*, **1**, 111.

Petit, D. W. (1945): "Hæmochromatosis with complete heart block", *Amer. Heart J.*, **29**, 253.

Porter, W. B., and Bloom, N. (1935): "Heart in typhoid fever; clinical study of 50 patients", *Amer. Heart J.*, **10**, 793.

Rachmilewitz, M., and Braun, K. (1948): "Electrocardiographic changes in typhoid fever and their reversibility following niacin treatment", *Amer. Heart J.*, **36**, 284.

Raven, R. W. (1948): "Secondary malignant disease of the heart", *Brit. J. Cancer*, **2**, 1.

Reeves, J. M., and Michael, P. (1936): "Primary tumor of the heart", *Amer. Heart J.*, **11**, 233.

Rejnhart, W. (1946): "Isolated diffuse interstitial eosinophilic myocarditis", *Cardiologia*, **11**, 219.

Rich, A. R. (1942): "The role of hypersensitivity in periarteritis nodosa, as indicated by seven cases developing during serum sickness and sulfonamide therapy", *Bull. Johns Hopk. Hosp.*, **71**, 123.

——, and Gregory, J. E. (1943): "The experimental demonstration that periarteritis nodosa is a manifestation of hypersensitivity", *Ibid.*, **72**, 65.

Ridley, H. (1949): "Toxoplasmosis, summary of disease with report of case", *Brit. J. Ophthal.*, **33**, 397.

Rubin, I. L., and Buchberg, A. S. (1952): "The heart in progressive muscular dystrophy", *Amer. Heart J.*, **43**, 161.

Sampson, R. (1945): "Periarteritis nodosa affecting eye", *Brit. J. Ophthal.*, **29**, 282.

Saphir, O. (1949): "Virus myocarditis", *Mod. Conc. cardiovasc. Dis.*, **6**, 43.

Scadding, J. G. (1950): "Sarcoidosis, with special reference to lung changes", *Brit. med. J.*, **i**, 745.

Scott, R. W., and Saphir, O. (1929): "Acute isolated myocarditis". *Amer. Heart J.*, **5**, 129.

——, and Garvin, C. F. (1939): "Tumours of the heart and pericardium", *Amer. Heart J.*, **17**, 431.

Sharpey-Schafer, E. P. (1955): "The response of the heart in acute nephritis", *Lancet*, **ii**, 841.

Sheldon, J. H. (1935): "Hæmochromatosis", London, Oxford University Press.

Sokoloff, L. (1953): "The heart in rheumatoid arthritis", *Amer. Heart J.*, **45**, 635.

Solarz, S. D. (1947): "An electrocardiographic study of 114 consecutive cases of trichinosis", *Amer. Heart J.*, **34**, 230.

Spain, D. M., Bradess, V. A., and Parsonnet, V. (1950): "Myocarditis in poliomyelitis", *Amer. Heart J.*, **40**, 336.

Stephen, J. D. (1954): "Fatal myocardial sarcoidosis", *Circulation*, **9**, 886.

Szekely, P., and Snaith, L. (1947): "The heart in toxæmia of pregnancy", *Brit Heart J.*, **9**, 128.

Thorson, A., Biörck, G., Bjorkman, G., and Waldenström, J. (1954): "Malignant carcinoid of the small intestine with metastases to the liver, valvular disease of the right side of the heart (pulmonary stenosis and tricuspid regurgitation without septal defects), peripheral vasomotor symptoms, broncho-constriction, and an unusual type of cyanosis", *Amer. Heart J.*, **47**, 795.

Vail, D., Strong, J. C. Jr., and Stephenson, W. V. (1943): "Chorioretinitis associated with positive serologic tests for toxoplasma in older children and adults" *Amer. J. Ophthal.*, **26**, 133.

Von Reis, G. (1949): "Clinical aspects of endocardial myxoma situated in the left atrium", *Acta med. Scand.*, **133**, 213.

Weir, D. R., and Jones, B. C. (1941): "Primary sarcoma of the heart", *Amer Heart J.*, **22**, 556.

Weisenfeld, S., and Messinger, W. J. (1952): "Cardiac involvement in progressive muscular dystrophy", *Ibid.*, **43**, 170.

Weiss, S., Stead, E. A. Jr., Warren, J. V., and Bailey, O. T. (1943): "Scleroderma heart disease (with consideration of certain other visceral manifestations of scleroderma)", *Arch. intern. Med.*, **71**, 749.

——, and Wilkins, R. W. (1937): "Myocardial abscess with perforation of heart", *Amer. J. med. Sci.*, **194**, 199.

Wessler, S., and Freedberg, A. S. (1948): "Cardiac amyloidosis. Electrocardiographic and pathologic observations", *Arch. intern. Med.*, **82**, 63.

White, P., *et al.* (1937): "Heart 15–20 years after diphtheria", *Amer. Heart J.*, **13**, 534.

Whitehill, M. R., Longcope, W. T., and Williams, R. (1939): "The occurrence and significance of myocardial failure in acute hæmorrhagic nephritis", *Bull. Johns Hopk. Hosp.*, **64**, 83.

Williams, S. W., Sinclair, A. J. M., and Jackson, A. V. (1944): "Mite-borne (scrub) typhus in Papua and the Mandated Territory of New Guinea: Report of 626 cases", *Med. J. Australia*, **2**, 525.

Witt, D. B., Lindner, E., and Katz, L. N. (1937): "The dynamic effect of acute experimental poisoning of the heart with diphtheria toxin", *Amer. Heart J.*, **13**, 693.

Wood, P. H. (1941): "Differential diagnosis of Da Costa's syndrome", *Proc. Roy. Soc. Med.*, **34**, 543.

Yater, W. M. (1931): "Tumours of heart and pericardium; pathology, symptomology, and report of nine cases", *Arch. intern. Med.*, **48**, 627.

Yesner, R., and Silver, M. (1951): "Fatal myocardial sarcoidosis", *Amer. Heart J.*, **41**, 777.

Young, J. M., and Goldman, I. R. (1954): "Tumor metastasis to the heart", *Circulation*, **9**, 220.

Zatuchni, J., Aegerter, E. E., Molthan, L., and Shuman, C. R. (1951): "The heart in progressive muscular dystrophy", *Circulation*, **3**, 846.

Zoeckler, S. J. (1951): "Cardiac actinomycosis", *Ibid.*, **3**, 854.

CHAPTER XII

BACTERIAL ENDOCARDITIS

BACTERIAL or infective endocarditis means bacterial infection of any of the heart valves or of certain congenital anomalies of the heart or great vessels (bacterial endarteritis). It occurs in two main forms: acute (malignant), due to infection with any of the pyogenic bacteria; and subacute, due mainly to the *Streptococcus viridans*; but many other organisms have been isolated from both types. This broad classification is necessarily artificial, the course of the disease depending on the virulence of the organism and the resistance of the host. There is no clear division between the two types, and they are better considered as one disease.

There is usually some underlying fault, congenital (10 per cent) or acquired. The most susceptible congenital anomalies are pulmonary stenosis, bicuspid aortic valve, ventricular septal defect and patent ductus arteriosus; atrial septal defect is remarkably immune. Any acquired valve lesion may become infected, including syphilitic aortic incompetence (Martin and Adams, 1938) and calcific aortic stenosis (Brink and Smith 1937), but old rheumatic valvulitis is to blame in 80 per cent of cases (Clawson, 1948). In quite a number, active rheumatic infection is still present when bacterial endocarditis is superimposed. The most susceptible valve fault is mild mitral incompetence.

PATHOLOGY

The lesion is superficial and is not a valvulitis in the sense that rheumatic endocarditis is: bacteria invade the surface of a damaged or congenital deformed valve, and are encouraged by the formation of small superficial thrombi which provide an excellent culture medium. Both in the natural disease and experimentally in dogs, there appears to be a paucity of granulation tissue and of cellular reaction; the microbes are not destroyed and healing does not take place. Elsewhere in the body similar foci of bacteria are rapidly walled off by granulation tissue and the lesion is invaded by leucocytes: the microbes are destroyed and the inflammation soon subsides (Friedman, Katz, Howell et al., 1938).

The macroscopic appearances vary according to the infecting organism, tending to be finely granular with streptococcus viridans, ulcerative and haemorrhagic with the haemolytic streptococcus and pneumococcus, proliferative with the gonococcus. When associated with congenital defect the site of the vegetations depends upon the direction of blood flow through the defect: thus, in the maladie de Roger vegetations are found on the right side of the patent interventricular septum, and on the wall of the right ventricle opposite the defect; with patent ductus arteriosus they are found at the pulmonary artery end. Ulceration may lead to perforation of a valve cusp or sinus of Valsalva. In old rheumatic cases vegetations may spread on to the endocardium of the left atrium (Thayer, 1926).

The myocardium may show scattered focal lesions similar to those seen in isolated or toxic myocarditis, or small collections of lymphocytes, or lymphocytes and polymorphs, known as Bracht-Wachter bodies (Bracht and Wachter, 1909). The latter are believed to be embolic in origin and represent a local inflammatory reaction to bacterial nests (Perry, 1936). They are the non-suppurative counterpart of the miliary abscesses seen in staphylococcal cases. Saphir, Katz and Gore (1950) found myocardial lesions in all of 76 fatal cases; they included emboli, micro-infarcts, perivascular infiltration, micro-abscesses, interstitial infiltration, and myocardial necrosis.

OCCURRENCE

Bacterial endocarditis accounts for about 2 per cent of all cases of organic heart disease (White, 1937), and for 9 per cent of all deaths from heart disease (Clawson, 1948). It may occur at any age, but is most common in young adults of either sex. Auricular fibrillation occurs in only 2.5 per cent of cases (McDonald, 1946); presumably because it is not a feature of the congenital lesions mentioned, is uncommon in rheumatic aortic valve disease, and occurs late in the life-history of patients with mitral stenosis. There is no evidence that the two conditions are mutually antagonistic.

CLINICAL FEATURES

Patients may present themselves with cardiac symptoms, pyrexia of unknown origin, anæmia, a cerebral vascular lesion, subacute rheumatism, nephritis, broncho-pneumonia, or with other patterns which depend upon the nature of the invading organism, the underlying cardiac lesion, and the caprice of the disease process. At the onset, symptoms are often ascribed to influenza, but fail to clear up. A history of dental sepsis or recent tooth extraction is obtained in 48 per cent of cases (Gates and Christie, 1951). The diagnosis rests upon the combination of a variety of signs which will be considered individually.

Cardiac abnormalities. There should be evidence of one or other of the various underlying valve lesions or congenital defects already mentioned, especially mitral or aortic incompetence, and if there are no abnormal auscultatory signs of heart disease, the diagnosis is rarely tenable. The development of a new valve lesion, or of the whining diastolic murmur and thrill of a perforated aortic cusp may be highly suggestive.

Toxic myocarditis is not uncommon and may cause heart failure and death whether the infection yields to treatment or not. Its importance has been more widely recognised since the introduction of penicillin (Saphir,

Katz and Gore, 1950). Heart failure occurs most frequently towards the end of the course of antibiotic treatment or during convalescence and was detected in no less than 63 per cent of the 442 cases analysed by Cates and Christie (1951).

Pyrexia. Acute cases are always febrile; subacute cases are always febrile at some stage in the disease, but bouts of fever may alternate with afebrile periods. The fever is irregular in type, usually low grade or moderate in degree, and may continue for weeks, months or years.

Anæmia. Anæmia nearly always develops early, and is already present in about three-quarters of the patients when first seen. It is indeterminate in type, being normocytic and orthochromic, even when associated with hæmolytic infections. The red cells may be reduced to about three million and the hæmoglobin to about 60 per cent, giving a normal colour index. Stained films and bone marrow samples reveal no specific features. If microcytic hypochromic anæmia is found, the diagnosis should be doubted, for iron-deficiency anæmia itself may cause many of the signs and symptoms of bacterial endocarditis, e.g. functional systolic murmurs at the base or the apex of the heart, splenomegaly, petechiæ, red cells in the urine, and even low grade pyrexia.

The white count is variable. It may be normal; on the other hand there may be moderate leucocytosis or leucopenia. Leucocytosis is usually associated with acute septicæmic cases, normal or leucopenic counts with subacute infections.

Splenomegaly. The spleen is usually palpable. It may be soft as in typhoid when due to septicæmia; it may enlarge rather suddenly as a result of splenic infarction, when it is tender; it may be firm in subacute cases; or it may be so large as to cross the mid-line in chronic cases.

Petechiæ. Petechiæ are common and sometimes appear in successive crops. They may be seen under the nails, in the ocular fundi, in the conjunctivæ, or anywhere in the skin or mucous membranes. Under the nails they resemble small splinters (Horder, 1926); in the fundi they may have white centres of exudate; in the skin they must be distinguished from minute telangiectases—Campbell de Morgan's spots. Petechiæ, in successive crops or otherwise, are in no way diagnostic of bacterial endocarditis. They are due to capillary hæmorrhage and may occur in any condition in which the capillaries are suitably damaged, including most forms of septicæmia, acute rheumatic fever (especially when associated with acute glomerulonephritis), and severe anæmia. In bacterial endocarditis the capillary lesion may be due to toxins, to allergy or to anæmia.

Increased capillary fragility may be demonstrated by the capillary resistance test.

A cuff is placed on the upper arm, inflated to a pressure of 50 mm. of mercury and maintained for five minutes; alternatively a pressure of 80 mm. of mercury may be maintained for three minutes. The arm below the cuff is then inspected. Most normal subjects are unaffected, but some develop a few tiny petechiæ in the ante-cubital fossa. The result of the test may be expressed as slightly, moderately, considerably or grossly positive, or as negative, the four positive grades representing transitions from a few tiny hæmorrhages to gross purpura.

The test may be positive or negative in bacterial endocarditis when spontaneous petechiæ are present. When positive it is well to make sure that vitamin deficiency is not responsible, or to cover this possibility by giving adequate doses of ascorbic acid, rutin and crude vitamin P.

Small hæmorrhagic pustules in the skin may occur in the acute pyogenic forms of bacterial endocarditis, and are embolic in origin.

Clubbing of the fingers (and toes). Clubbing occurs in about half of the subacute cases, but as it takes at least 3 to 6 weeks to develop, it is rare in malignant endocarditis. Early clubbing may be recognised by noting congestion and thickening of the nail-fold, and loss of the normal angulation between the nail-fold and the base of the nail. Slight clubbing should be interpreted with caution, however, for it may occur in many conditions including active rheumatic carditis. Conspicuous clubbing, on the other hand, provides excellent supportive evidence of bacterial endocarditis, if cyanotic congenital heart disease, pulmonary abscess, bronchogenic carcinoma, and a congenital origin can be excluded.

Nodes. Osler's nodes are small, transient, erythematous lesions about the size of a pea, lasting a few days, and vivid pink in colour when fresh, bluish when fading, often with a darker centre; they are raised, palpable, and tender, and may be found particularly on the pads of the fingers and toes, on the sides of the fingers, or on the thenar or hypothenar eminences (Osler, 1909). They are due to infected cutaneous emboli, and the responsible organism may sometimes be cultured from them.

More important, perhaps, because more common, are larger deeper nodes which vary from the size of a pea to that of a grapefruit. They are red, painful, hot and tender, may occur anywhere in the limbs, and may be mistaken for osteomyelitis or periostitis. When a lesion involves the finger it closely resembles an ordinary infected pulp; it is non-suppurative, however, and disappears in about a week if left alone. Cultures from the inflamed tissue may yield *Streptococcus viridans*. Red, tender macules are equally characteristic and even more common, and may also yield positive cultures from biopsies.

Emboli. In addition to the minute emboli which cause white-centred petechiæ and the nodes just mentioned, larger emboli may block any artery —cerebral, visceral, or peripheral. They are more common in the radial, ulner, posterior tibial, and dorsal artery of the foot, than in the axillary or femoral artery, because their size is limited. For this reason peripheral emboli are often symptomless and are only discovered by those who look for them. In cases of suspected bacterial endocarditis the peripheral vessels should always be palpated, and their patency noted for future reference. In the series of 442 cases reported by Cates and Christie (1951), a major arterial embolism occurred in 35 per cent.

Mycotic aneurysm. Ulceration or degeneration of the wall of an artery due to local inflammation from an infected embolus lodging within the vessel or in its vasa vasorum may result in the formation of a small aneurysm. Severe hæmorrhage results from rupture of a mycotic aneurysm, and may prove fatal if cerebral or visceral.

Pulmonary emboli. When bacterial endocarditis involves the pulmonary or tricuspid valve, or when it is associated with a left to right cardiac shunt, as in patent interventricular septum, emboli may be flung into the pulmonary circulation. Numerous small pulmonary infarcts result, and may give rise to a clinical picture resembling recurrent or subacute hæmorrhagic bronchopneumonia.

Renal lesions. The various renal lesions that may occur in bacterial endocarditis represent almost every aspect of the disease.

(1) An embolus lodging in a small renal artery leads to simple infarction of the kidney, with hæmaturia, or without signs or symptoms.

(2) Minute bacterial emboli may cause embolic nephritis, which in greater or less degree is found in the majority of cases. Only some of the glomeruli are involved, rarely more than 60 per cent, and most of these have some of their capillary loops intact, so that the tuft is not entirely avascular, and the health of the tubules is not seriously threatened. Affected capillaries are converted into a hyaline mass and red cells may be found in the capsular space and in the urine. Embolic nephritis does not cause renal failure because a sufficient number of glomeruli are always spared (Baehr, 1921).

(3) In acute pyogenic forms of bacterial endocarditis, particularly when pneumococcal or staphylococcal in origin, miliary abscesses may be found in the substance of the kidney.

(4) Petechiæ due to simple capillary hæmorrhage may occur on the surface of the kidney in the absence of embolic nephritis. They are then similar to those found in the pericardium, pleura and skin.

(5) Acute diffuse glomerulo-nephritis may occur as with other streptococcal infections, and may progress to renal failure; but not more than 5 to 10 per cent of all cases take this course.

(6) Simple congestion of the kidney may result from heart failure and give rise to albuminuria and to a few red cells in the urine.

It will be appreciated that these six types of renal lesion represent thrombotic emboli, benign bacterial emboli, septic emboli, simple hæmorrhage, toxæmia or allergy, and heart failure respectively, and that nearly all the features of bacterial endocarditis may be understood in terms of these six factors.

Changes in the ocular fundus. Simple petechiæ, like those in the skin, are fairly common. Occasionally, they have white centres, and may be embolic in origin. It should be understood that these white centres represent exudate, and that identical lesions may be seen in other conditions, particularly leukæmia and malignant hypertension. The exudate may be surrounded by hæmorrhage or may be to one side of it. Embolism of the central artery of the retina or of one of its main branches may cause complete or partial loss of vision, but is fortunately rare. Finally, papillædema or papillitis, with or without widespread hæmorrhages and exudates, is not uncommon when there is diffuse glomerulo-nephritis, the appearances resembling those of malignant hypertension.

DIAGNOSIS

It is emphasised that pyrexia, anæmia, splenomegaly, petechiæ, and diffuse glomerulo-nephritis may occur wherever the site of the cardiac lesion; that systemic emboli, mycotic aneurysms, nodes, and embolic nephritis signify left-sided lesions, e.g. aortic or mitral valve disease; that multiple hæmorrhagic infarcts in the lungs are the prerogative of right-sided valve lesions and of left to right congenital shunts, such as patent ductus and maladie de Roger (Barker, 1949).

Clinically, bacterial endocarditis should be considered in all cases of unexplained fever with suspicious auscultatory signs in the heart. If an indeterminate anæmia is also present, a determined search should be made for other evidence; if splenomegaly, petechiæ, and red cells in the urine are added the diagnosis becomes probable, but is still uncertain. On the other hand, clubbing of the fingers, nodes, peripheral emboli, mycotic aneurysm, nephritis, and characteristic fundal changes may, each one of them, be diagnostic of bacterial endocarditis when associated with fever and an appropriate cardiac lesion.

The diagnosis is confirmed by a positive blood or bone-marrow culture. Six tubes are usually set up from each sample; and 4 to 6 samples should be obtained at different times, preferably when the temperature is high, before a negative result is accepted. It should be pointed out, however, that blood cultures from patients with pyorrhœa or with dental abscess may grow *Streptococcus viridans* when the specimen is obtained after chewing, so that the diagnosis of bacterial endocarditis should never rest on a positive blood culture alone.

NATURAL COURSE

Untreated patients with acute infection die in a matter of days or weeks, usually from septicæmia or from the effects of embolism; those with sub-acute infection usually live for months and occasionally for years, bouts of fever with exacerbation of signs and symptoms alternating with afebrile quiescent phases, described by Libman as bacteria-free periods. Death may result from heart failure, cerebral or other visceral embolism, hæmorrhage, uræmia, or other causes. According to Libman and Friedberg (1941), about 3 per cent of all patients recover spontaneously; but Lichtman (1943) found that only 1 per cent of 2,596 cases collected from the literature so recovered.

PROGNOSIS

Penicillin and streptomycin have radically altered the course of bacterial endocarditis, for the infection can now be controlled in 90 per cent of cases. However, about 25 per cent still die during or shortly after treatment, mostly from heart failure. This high mortality may be due to the frequency of serious toxic myocarditis and to the relatively rapid increase in severity of valve lesions, particularly aortic or mitral incompetence. Uræmia accounted for only 6 per cent of the 131 deaths in the combined hospitals series reported by Christie (1948); emboli for 11 per cent and hæmorrhage for 8 per cent. The most important factors influencing the mortality rate proved to be the presence and degree of heart failure, the duration of the infection, and the nutritional state of the patient.

Relapses are common in inadequately treated cases, but should not exceed 10 per cent in patients who have received at least 0.5 mega unit of penicillin daily for a minimum period of 28 days. Nearly all those who relapse do so within one month of ceasing treatment. The frequency of recurrence (as distinct from relapse) is not yet known.

TREATMENT

Prophylactic. Surgical repair of patent ductus arteriosus not only cures the defect, but protects the patient from infective endarteritis. Repair of coarctation of the aorta may be less successful in the second respect because infection may yet complicate an associated bicuspid aortic valve. It is not expected that surgical relief of pulmonary stenosis will reduce the frequency of bacterial endocarditis in that disease.

Dental hygiene is particularly important in all patients who have congenital heart disease or chronic valve disease. Tooth extractions, tonsillectomy, and other E.N.T. operations should be covered by 300,000 units of procaine-penicillin twice daily for five days, or perhaps 600,000 units daily. A single intramuscular injection of benzathene penicillin, 600,000 units, the day before tooth extraction, may also suffice, but awaits longer trial.

Chemotherapy. Sulphonamides have proved disappointing, and although they may temporarily sterilise the blood stream and lower the temperature, they rarely cure the disease. Of 489 cases treated with sulphonamides alone, only 4 per cent recovered (Lichtman, 1943).

The situation has greatly improved since the introduction of penicillin. Patients should be treated early, as soon as the diagnosis is clinically probable, without waiting for positive results of blood cultures. Every effort should be made to counter malnutrition, and a blood transfusion should be given if there is serious anæmia.

The minimum dose of penicillin is 0.5 mega unit daily, given in divided doses of 60,000 units three-hourly, 80,000 units four-hourly or 120,000 units six-hourly, and continued for twenty-eight days. Nothing less than this will suffice, and larger doses, averaging 2 mega daily, prolonged for six to eight weeks are preferred (Cates and Christie, 1951). One of my patients was not controlled until she received a million units three-hourly and a total of 250 million units. If the resistance of the organism is known, so much the better; but even then the optimum dose cannot be calculated exactly, because it depends partly on the physical properties of the lesion. Swift and maintained clinical response is the only reliable criterion by which to judge the correct dose. If, however, the resistance of the organism is known to be more than eight times that of the standard test strain of Oxford staphylococcus, the dose of penicillin should certainly be increased proportionately (Christie, 1948). If the coefficient of resistance is 10, not less than 100,000 units three-hourly will suffice; if 20, then at least 200,000 units three-hourly will be necessary—and so on (Baehr and Gerber, 1947). Peak (15 to 30 minutes after intramuscular injection) or constant (with the intravenous drip method) blood-serum levels of penicillin expressed in units per ml. may also be measured and checked against tables giving the expected level for the dose employed. Peak levels should range from 2 to 25 units per ml. with doses of 60,000 to 500,000 units intramuscularly; constant levels between 1 and 10 units per ml. with daily doses of 500,000 to 4 million units.

A practical method of arriving at the right dosage that has given good results for many years is to start with 100,000 units four-hourly, and to double the dose every second day until the fever abates; the dose to which the patient responds is thus known and is promptly doubled for maintenance purposes and continued for six weeks. This method has the advantage of testing the sensitivity of the organism to penicillin *in vivo*, and ensuring an adequate therapeutic maintenance dose. The theoretical objection that it might breed penicillin-resistant organisms has not been substantiated in practice.

To avoid the discomfort of frequent needling, there is an increasing tendency to give massive doses of penicillin (0.25 to 0.5 mega unit) three or four times daily. As these massive doses have a penetrating power denied to more modest quantities, there is something to be said for this method, but they should not be given too infrequently.

Another way of avoiding such frequent injections is to use one of the longer-acting penicillins, such as procaine-penicillin. As an aqueous suspension this may be injected intramuscularly in doses of 600,000 units twice daily. It should never be used at the start, however, and is only advised later in cases that have responded quickly and dramatically to the minimum daily dose of sodium penicillin G.

Finally, the blood level of penicillin may be increased up to fourfold by the oral administration of certain substances such as benzoic acid (Bronfenbrenner and Favour, 1945), sodium benzoate, or caronamide (4'-carboxyphenylmethane sulphonanilide) which interfere with penicillin excretion by the renal tubules. The dose of each of these substances is 2–3 G. four-hourly (Boger *et al.*, 1948). Caronamide may be combined with sodium benzoate with some advantage and is a valuable adjunct to treatment in highly resistant cases. Probenecid (Benemid) now seems to be replacing caronamide; the dose is o.5 G. six hourly.

Treatment of relapses or resistant cases. If the previous course of treatment was inadequate in dosage or duration, the standard course of 2 mega units daily for six weeks should be instituted; but if a relapse follows adequate treatment, every effort should be made to culture the organism and to determine its sensitivity to penicillin. If its resistance is not greater than eight times the standard, the dose of penicillin should be doubled, and treatment should be continued for six weeks. If the coefficient of resistance is greater than 8, the dose of penicillin should be increased proportionately. If the organism is highly resistant, or if it has not been isolated and the infection remains uncontrolled, streptomycin may be tried. The dose is 1 G. twice daily for two weeks, followed by 1 G. daily for four more weeks. Caronamide does not influence the blood level of streptomycin, for the latter is excreted by the glomeruli.

Combined penicillin and streptomycin treatment is advised for enterococcal infections (Hunter, 1947; Geraci and Martin, 1954). The dose of penicillin in these cases should be at least 10 million units daily (Hunter, 1953).

Innumerable reports of resistant cases of bacterial endocarditis caused by a wide variety of organisms have appeared in the literature in recent years, and the majority have responded in the end to one or other of the newer antibiotics when given in sufficient doses. To review all these reports would be profitless. The resistant case is a bacteriological problem. The organism should be identified and its sensitivity to all available antibiotics tested in the laboratory; treatment may then be instituted on a proper foundation.

Toxic reactions of penicillin. Apart from local pain from subcutaneous or superficial intramuscular injections, and phlebothrombosis from intravenous injections, the only toxic manifestations which can be attributed to penicillin are fever and urticaria. Fever was common when crude penicillin was used, but is rarely seen nowadays. Urticaria develops in about 5 per cent of cases and may be extreme; soft tissue œdema and hydrarthrosis are occasionally associated. This allergic reaction is alleviated by adrenaline and by the antihistamine group of drugs. Penicillin may be continued in mild cases, but may have to be stopped if the reaction is severe, or the dose may have to be reduced.

The chief toxic effect of streptomycin is on the vestibular nerve: loss of the sense of balance may be permanent if heavy doses are continued after giddiness has developed. A conservative dose of 1 G. daily, however, may be continued in the presence of minor vestibular symptoms if the latter are controlled by means of antihistamine drugs.

Other considerations. An infected ductus should be controlled by penicillin, then ligated as soon as the patient is fit enough.

Heart failure should be treated in the customary fashion; but the prognosis is grave in these cases.

Diffuse glomerulo-nephritis may be mistaken for a relapse of bacterial endocarditis. If the renal function is impaired, the blood level of penicillin may rise considerably and thus aid the primary treatment; unfortunately, however, the nephritis usually proves fatal. According to Spain and King (1952), diffuse glomerular nephritis rarely occurs if treatment is started within the first two months of the illness.

REFERENCES

Baehr, G. (1921): "The significance of the embolic glomerular lesions of subacute streptococcus endocarditis", *Arch. intern. Med.*, **27**, 262.

——, and Gerber, I. E. (1947): "Penicillin treatment of subacute bacterial endocarditis", *Advances intern. Med.*, **2**, 308.

Barker, P. S. (1949): "A clinical study of subacute bacterial infection confined to the right side of the heart or the pulmonary artery", *Amer. Heart J.*, **37**, 1054.

Boger, W. P., Miller, A. K., Tillson, E. K., and Shaner, G. A. (1948): "Caronamide: plasma concentrations, urinary recoveries, and dosage", *J. lab. and clin. Med.*, **33**, 297.

Bracht, E., and Wächter (1909): "Beitrag zur aetiologie und pathologischen anatomie der myokarditis rheumatica", *Deut. Arch. f. klin. Med.*, **96**, 493.

Brink, J. R., and Smith, M. L. (1937): "Subacute bacterial endocarditis; clinicopathological study of 37 cases", *Amer. Heart J.*, **14**, 362.

Bronfenbrenner, J., and Favour, C. B. (1945): "Increasing and prolonging blood penicillin concentrations following intramuscular administration", *Science*, **101**, 673.

Cates, J. E., and Christie, R. V. (1951): "Subacute bacterial endocarditis. A review of 442 patients treated in 14 centres appointed by the penicillin trials committee of the M.R.C.", *Quart. J. Med.*, **20**, 93.

Christie, R. V. (1948): "Penicillin in subacute bacterial endocarditis", *Brit. med. J.*, **1**, 1.

Clawson, B. J. (1948): "Rheumatic and bacterial endocarditis. 1,740 cases", *Minn. med.*, **31**, 1094.

Friedman, M., Katz., L. N., Howell, K. M., Lindner, E., and Mendlowitz, M. (1938): "Experimental endocarditis due to streptococcus viridans", *Arch. intern. Med.*, **61**, 95.

Geraci, J. E., and Martin, W. J. (1954): "Antibiotic therapy of bacterial endocarditis. VI. Subacute endocarditis: clinical, pathologic and therapeutic consideration of 33 cases", *Circulation*, **10**, 173.

Herrell, W. E., Nichols, D. R., and Heilman, F. R. (1947): "Procaine penicillin G (duracillin); a new salt of penicillin which prolongs the action of penicillin", *Proc. Mayo Clinic*, **22**, 567.

Horder, T. (1926): "Lumleian lectures on endocarditis", *Lancet*, i, 695, 745, 850.

Hunter, T. H. (1947): "Use of streptomycin in the treatment of bacterial endocarditis", *Amer. J. Med.*, **2**, 436.

—— (1953): "Bacterial endocarditis", *Mod. Conc. cardiovasc. Dis.*, **12**, 172.

Leach, C. E. (1941): "Chemo-therapy and heparin in subacute bacterial endocarditis; further experiences", *J. Amer. med. Ass.*, **117**, 1345.

Libman, E., and Friedberg, C. K. (1941): "Subacute bacterial endocarditis", New York.

Lichtman, S. S. (1943): "Treatment of subacute bacterial endocarditis; current results", *Ann. intern. Med.*, **19**, 787.

McDonald, R. K. (1946): "The coincidence of auricular fibrillation and bacterial endocarditis", *Amer. Heart J.*, **31**, 308.

Martin, H. E., and Adams, W. L., Jr. (1938): "Bacterial endocarditis superimposed on syphilitic aortitis and valvulitis", *Ibid.*, **16**, 714.

Osler, W. (1909): "Chronic infectious endocarditis", *Quart. J. Med.*, **2**, 219.

Perry, C. B. (1936): "Bacterial endocarditis", Bristol.

Saphir, O., Katz, L. N., and Gore, I. (1950): "The myocardium in subacute bacterial endocarditis", *Circulation*, **1**, 1155.

Spain, D. M., and King, D. W. (1952): "The effect of penicillin on the renal lesions of subacute bacterial endocarditis", *Ann. intern. Med.*, **36**, 1086.

Thayer, W. S. (1926): "Studies on bacterial (infectious) endocarditis", *Johns Hopk. Hosp. Rep.*, **12**, 1.

White, H. J., and Parker, J. M. (1938): "Bacterial effect of sulphanilamide upon beta hæmolytic streptococci in vitro", *J. Bact.*, **36**, 481.

White, P. D. (1937): "Heart disease", New York.

CHAPTER XIII

PERICARDITIS

THE features of pericarditis depend upon its etiology, the presence or absence of effusion, the nature and hydrostatic pressure of such effusion, and the development or otherwise of constriction in chronic or adhesive cases.

ETIOLOGY

Pericarditis may be benign, rheumatic, tuberculous, pyogenic, allergic, traumatic, uræmic or secondary to myocardial infarction; malignant growths may invade the pericardium; hæmopericardium may result from rupture of a syphilitic or dissecting aneurysm, from perforation of a myocardial infarct or ventricular aneurysm, or from stab or gun-shot wounds of the heart; hydropericardium may complicate congestive heart failure or myxœdema; sometimes the etiology is obscure. All these types have their own special characteristics which will be described subsequently; but they have also certain features in common.

DRY (FIBRINOUS) PERICARDITIS

All varieties of pericardial inflammation may present in this form. The diagnosis rests on three cardinal signs: pain, pericardial friction, and a specific electrocardiographic pattern. Disturbances of temperature, pulse rate, sedimentation rate, etc., of course, may occur, but are of little help in diagnosis.

Pain. Capps (1932) found that the pericardium was insensitive to stimuli calculated to produce pain, except in that part of it, roughly its lower third, which is supplied by the phrenic nerve. It follows that pericarditis should be painless unless the pain has phrenic distribution, or unless it is pleural in type from secondary involvement of that structure. In fact this is only partly true: in many cases there is no pain; in some, pain is referred to the neck or shoulder tip; in others it is precordial and pleural in type, catching the breath on inspiration or on coughing; but not infrequently the pain has none of these characteristics, being præcordial, constant, sharp in quality, and uninfluenced by respiration; pericardial pain of this type may be aggravated by rotating the trunk or by swallowing (McGuire, Kotte and Helm, 1954).

Pericardial friction. Friction sounds may be heard anywhere over the heart, according to the site and nature of the pathological process, but are most common at the left sternal border in the fourth intercostal space over the area of maximum cardiac dullness, where the pericardium lies in contact with the chest-wall. They are superficial, rough or smooth, loud or

657

soft; their timing is peculiar, being out of step with the heart sounds. Sometimes, they are confused with the to and fro murmur of aortic valve disease or with artificial stethoscopic sounds; sometimes they escape detection. Pleuro-pericardial friction can usually be distinguished by its relationship to respiration.

Electrocardiographic changes. A diagnostic electrocardiographic T_2 pattern, first described by Porte and Pardee (1929), may be found in the majority of cases of genuine pericarditis, whatever the etiology, and whether

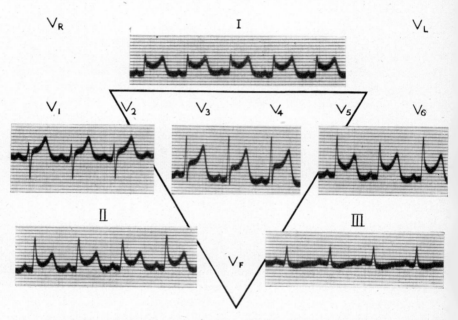

Fig. 13.01—Electrocardiogram showing the early phase of the pericardial T_2 pattern. This graph is atypical in that the R-T segment is not elevated in lead 3.

or not there is effusion (Wood, 1937). It develops in two stages, early and late, the changes usually appearing in all leads and therefore especially in lead 2. In the early phase (fig. 13.01) the RS-T segment is elevated, but retains its natural concavity. Within a few days it regains the iso-potential level or becomes depressed, and the T wave becomes flattened, diphasic, or inverted (fig. 13.02), QRS remaining unchanged throughout or losing voltage. When the inflammation subsides the graph returns to normal, except when a tuberculous pericarditis merges into the chronic constrictive form, when flat or inverted T waves and low-voltage QRS complexes become permanent. The T_2 pattern may only be appreciated in serial electrocardiograms, because changes may be confined to leads 1 and 2 in one record, and to leads 2 and 3 in another. Similar appearances are seen in all chest leads, and may be found when limb leads are normal (fig. 13.03).

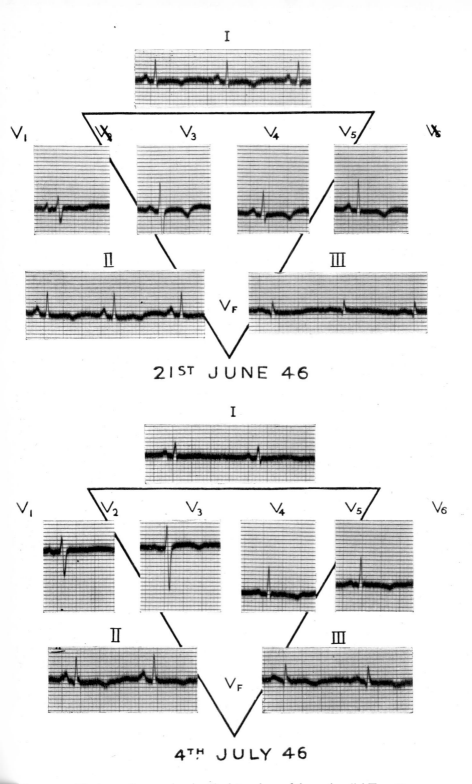

I

V₁   V₂   V₃   V₄   V₅   V₆

II   V_F   III

21ST JUNE 46

I

V₁   V₂   V₃   V₄   V₅   V₆

II   V_F   III

4TH JULY 46

Fig. 13.02—Electrocardiogram showing the later phase of the pericardial T₂ pattern: case of pyogenic pericarditis secondary to bronchopneumonia.

Both early and late stages appear to be due to alterations in the bio-physical properties of the sub-epicardial myocardium, whether or not there are recognisable structural changes (Kisch *et al.*, 1940). The early pattern of generalised pericarditis may be distinguished from that of myocardial infarction by the absence of a conspicuous Q wave, by the preservation of the upward concavity of the RS-T segment, and by the occurrence of maximum RS-T deviation in lead 2 (cf. T_1 and T_3 types in myocardial infarction). When pericarditis is localised, however, changes may be maximum in leads 1 or 3 (Burchell, Barnes and Mann, 1939). The later stage

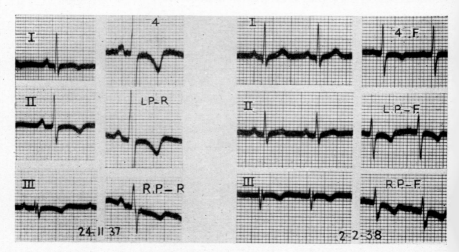

Fig. 13.03—Electrocardiogram showing late changes due to pericarditis; in the second record (2nd February 1938) they are limited to the chest leads.

may be confused with isolated myocarditis, myxœdema, carbon monoxide poisoning, severe anæmia, and most of the cardiopathies described in the previous chapter. On the other hand, the characteristic initial phase, the changing picture in serial graphs, and the clinical features of the case usually make the diagnosis easy.

PERICARDIAL EFFUSION

Fluid in the pericardial sac may be a simple transudate (hydropericardium), a straw-coloured sterile exudate, a purulent exudate, or blood (hæmopericardium). It may disturb the patient in one or more of four ways: (1) stretching of the pericardium may induce præcordial discomfort; (2) large effusions exerting pressure on surrounding structures, especially on the bronchi and lungs, may produce reflex cough and dyspnœa; (3) if the fluid is purulent, there may be constitutional effects similar to empyema; (4) as the pressure rises in the pericardial sac, cardiac filling is hampered, the pressure rises in both venous systems, the ventricular stroke-output diminishes, and the blood pressure tends to fall. The raised venous pressure is partly beneficial, for it aids cardiac filling; the diminished stroke-volume is countered by tachycardia; reflex vasoconstriction serves to maintain the blood pressure (Stewart, Crane and Deitrich, 1938). When these compensatory adjustments fail to meet the circulatory demands, the situation becomes critical (cardiac tamponade). There is reason to believe that cardiac tamponade seriously interferes with the coronary blood flow, not only because the cardiac output is reduced and the blood pressure low, but because the pressure gradient between the aorta and coronary circulation is significantly reduced. The myocardium appears to suffer accordingly and true heart failure may result. This may explain those cases that fail to recover after decompression, and suggests that tamponade should be regarded as a medical emergency.

Clinically, the *pulse* may be normal, small or paradoxical, according to the intra-pericardial pressure. During inspiration, descent of the diaphragm stretches the already tense parietal pericardium and increases the pressure within it; cardiac filling is then impaired and the stroke output and pulse pressure fall. As in constrictive pericarditis it is easier for the heart to increase its output by means of tachycardia than by raising the venous filling pressure.

The venous pressure varies directly with the intrapericardial pressure, and may rise appreciably during inspiration (Kussmaul's sign). The jugular pulse usually shows a rapid y descent and conspicuous y trough, as in Pick's disease.

Effusions in excess of 250 ml. may be detected by *percussion*. Dullness may be elicited in the second left space when the patient lies flat, to the left of the apex beat when the latter can be located, in the xiphisternal angle, and to the right of the sternum in the 4th and 5th intercostal spaces (Rotch's sign, 1878).

Auscultation reveals pericardial friction in the majority of instances, even with gross effusions. The first heart sound is soft because late diastolic ventricular filling is virtually at a standstill and the atrio-ventricular valves are therefore more or less closed before the ventricles contract; the second sound is soft because the blood pressure is low. The fluid layer between the heart and chest wall may also damp the sounds, but this is less certain. Theoretically, an accentuated third heart sound might be expected in view of the rapid ventricular filling in early diastole, but it is rarely heard.

Dullness to percussion and bronchial breathing at the left base, usually attributed to collapse of the lung (Ewart, 1896), are more likely to be due to associated pleural effusion, at least in rheumatic cases (Thomas, Besterman and Hollman, 1953).

Fluoroscopy reveals a large, relatively still, cardiac silhouette with the natural contours of individual chambers obliterated (fig. 13.04). It is doubted whether any of the special radiological points that have been said to favour effusion are really tenable, e.g. short vascular pedicle, divergent vascular shadows at the base, change of shape with alteration of posture,

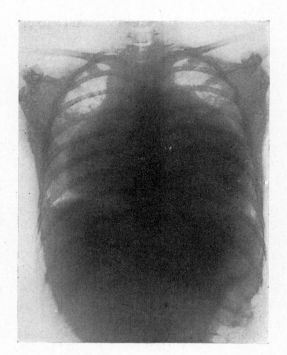

Fig. 13.04—Skiagram of a case of pericardial effusion.

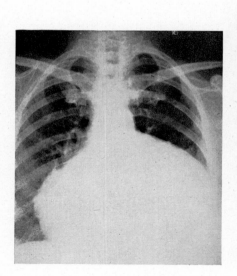

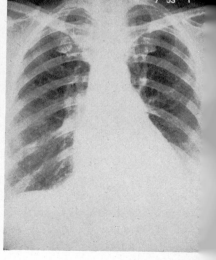

(a) Before treatment.   (b) Two weeks later.

Fig. 13.05—Gross pericardial effusion.

acute right cardio-phrenic angle, and convex posterior-inferior cardio-phrenic angle in the first oblique position (Besterman and Thomas, 1953). Rapid changes in the size of the cardiac shadow are more reliable (fig. 13.05), but even these may be seen in cases of acute dilatation of the heart with rapid recovery. Since more accurate methods of diagnosis have been adopted there have been many surprises; the more common error has been to mistake pericardial effusion for cardiac enlargement, but the reverse has also been true.

There are three good ways of determining the presence and degree of pericardial effusion—*cardiac catheterisation*, angiocardiography and paracentesis. If a cardiac catheter is looped in the right atrium, its tip may be

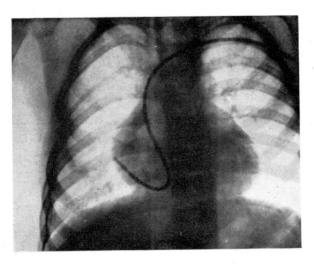

Fig. 13.06—Catheter looped in the right atrium proving the absence of pericardial effusion.

rotated laterally and guided up and down the lateral wall of the right atrium. When there is no effusion the tip of the catheter is then separated from the translucent lungs only by the thin wall of the right atrium (fig. 13.06). When there is pericardial effusion, however, the tip of the catheter is separated from the lungs by an opaque band of fluid (Wood, 1950, 1951). If 10 to 20 ml. of diaginol are injected rapidly through the catheter when its tip is directed upwards against the lateral wall of the right atrium and a film is exposed towards the end of the injection, the degree of effusion can be estimated accurately (fig. 13.07). Routine *angiocardiography* (Williams and Steinberg, 1949) reveals the degree of pericardial effusion with greater precision (fig. 13.08), but may be undesirable when the alternative diagnosis is severe heart failure. *Paracentesis* may prove the presence of effusion but only indicates its degree if all the fluid is removed or if sufficient air is introduced. The safest of these three methods is right atrial catheterisation. This does not, of course, distinguish pericardial effusion from gross dilatation of the left atrium.

The *differential diagnosis* of pericardial effusion includes any general cardiac enlargement of uncertain nature, heart failure from rheumatic carditis or any of the more obscure cardiopathies described in Chapter XI, and certain congenital anomalies such as Ebstein's disease. Under the clinical circumstances the best indication of pericardial effusion is a friction rub, and the best evidence of cardiac dilatation is loud diastolic gallop rhythm. A paradoxical pulse certainly favours effusion, but too much reliance should not be placed on Kussmaul's sign, the presence or absence of a palpable cardiac impulse, the intensity of the heart sounds, or inverted T waves in the electrocardiogram, for all these may occur in either condition.

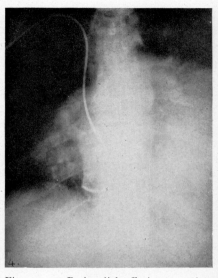

Fig. 13.07—Pericardial effusion seen beyond the right atrial border, which is delineated by the tip of a looped catheter through which a jet of diodone has been injected.

In addition to the three semi-radiological methods of diagnosis described above, certain physiological tests may prove useful, although they have not been tested sufficiently yet. These include Valsalva's manœuvre, and the effect of alterations of posture on the cardiac output and therefore on the blood pressure, pulse rate, forearm blood flow and digital pulse. In pericardial effusion the physiological response to the Valsalva manœuvre should be normal, i.e. the period of strain should be followed by a rise of blood pressure and slowing of the pulse, whereas in heart failure these changes do not occur. Tilting the patient foot down lowers the venous pressure: in pericardial effusion this should lower the cardiac output and so diminish the blood pressure and pulse pressure increase the heart rate, reduce the forearm blood flow and diminish

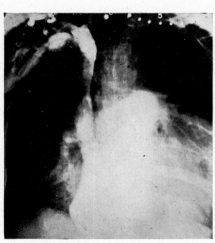

Fig. 13.08—Angiocardiogram demonstrating pericardial effusion.

the digital pulse; in heart failure, lowering the venous pressure increases the cardiac output and therefore has the opposite effect on the phenomena mentioned. The essential principle underlying all physiological tests for pericardial effusion is that the heart behaves normally (Isaacs, Berglund and Sarnoff, 1954), whereas cardiopathies with considerable cardiac dilatation are overloaded.

Cardiac catheterisation in both pericardial effusion and most of the obscure cardiopathies reveals that pulmonary venous and left atrial pressures are raised to just about the same level as the right atrial pressure; in Ebstein's disease, of course, this is not so.

Treatment. The object of treatment is to prevent death from cardiac tamponade, and is achieved by avoiding therapeutic agents that may lower the venous pressure, such as mersalyl, a low sodium diet and venesection, and by decompression if necessary. In practice it is rarely necessary to tap a pericardial effusion, for critical tamponade is rare in medical cases. The combination of a small pulse, venous pressure over 10 cm. of water at 90 degrees, and systolic blood pressure below 90 mm. Hg provides the necessary indication. Paracentesis may be carried out to the left of the apex beat, or at any point where there is reason to believe there is plenty of fluid. If the needle touches the heart, forcible pulsation can be felt, and it should be withdrawn a little, or inserted elsewhere; with due care the risk of causing hæmopericardium from puncturing a coronary vessel is small. Fluid may also be removed if purulent or if untoward symptoms are caused by pressure on surrounding structures. Traumatic hæmopericardium, which is responsible for many cases of tamponade, requires surgical evacuation and repair of the underlying injury.

CHRONIC CONSTRICTIVE PERICARDITIS

Although Richard Lower described the paradoxical pulse and calcified pericardium as early as 1669, he was not in a position to grasp their full significance, and it was Chevers who really drew attention to the disease, giving an excellent account of it, with considerable understanding of the circulatory dynamics involved, in 1842. The term "Pick's disease" is unfortunate, for Pick (1896) merely emphasised the accompanying "pseudo-cirrhosis of the liver", and because priority undoubtedly goes to Chevers. The issue is best avoided by adhering to the descriptive title—chronic constrictive pericarditis.

Morbid anatomy. The condition may be regarded as a complication of the healing process following tuberculous and perhaps certain other forms of pericarditis, the fibrous tissue laid down so extensively in the active phase contracting on maturation, and limiting diastolic expansion of the heart. Calcium is often deposited in large quantities, and the whole heart may become encased in "stone".

Etiology. Tuberculosis accounts for at least three-quarters of the cases, and may still be active when constriction first develops. The pyogenic bacteria appear to be responsible for a few, and the cause is uncertain or unknown in the remainder. None are rheumatic (White, 1935). Some regard tuberculosis as the sole cause of chronic constrictive pericarditis (Andrews, Pickering and Holmes Sellars, 1948).

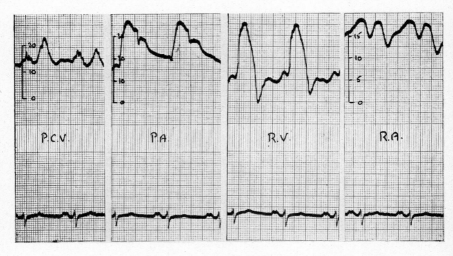

Fig. 13.09—Intracardiac pressure pulses from a case of Pick's disease.

Hæmodynamics

The essential physiological fault in Pick's disease is inadequate cardiac filling. It is uncertain to what extent ventricular contraction is also hampered, but that it is so in some measure can scarcely be doubted. The rigid limit imposed on diastolic filling is more or less the same for both ventricles so that the rise of pressure in the two venous systems is always similar, if not identical. This was true in all of eight consecutive cases that we have investigated, and in a series of six cases reported by Dexter's group (Sawyer et al., 1952). The elevated atrial and venous pressures usually measure between 10 and 20 mm. Hg above the sternal angle (fig. 13.09). As a rule the dominant wave is the y descent and trough (fig. 13.10). This represents the sudden fall in venous pressure that follows the opening of the tricuspid valve, when blood pours into the momentarily relaxed right ventricle. Owing to the unyielding pericardium the right ventricle is filled to its maximum

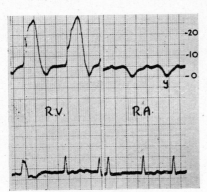

Fig. 13.10—Typical right atrial and right ventricular pressure pulses in a case of Pick's disease showing conspicuous y troughs.

capacity very quickly, and both right ventricular and right atrial diastolic pressures therefore rise again smartly. The right ventricular pressure pulse is characterised by a conspicuous dip in early diastole which is the counter-part of the *y* trough in the venous pulse. The same phenomenon may be recorded in left atrial and left ventricular pressure pulses (fig. 13.11). Typical tracings have been published and discussed by Bloomfield *et al.* (1946), Eliasch, Lagerlöf and Werkö (1950), Hansen *et al.* (1951), and McKusick (1952).

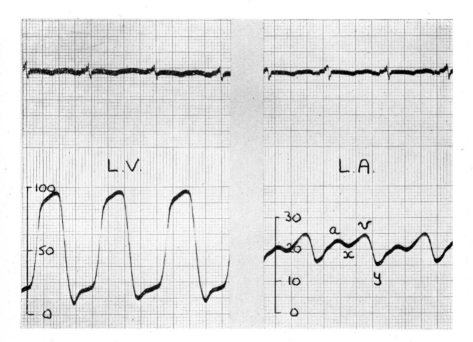

Fig. 13.11—Left atrial and left ventricular pressure pulses from a case of Pick's disease.

Since the stroke output is strictly limited and more or less fixed, alterations of cardiac output per minute depend chiefly on changes in heart rate (Stewart and Heuer, 1939). Raising or lowering the venous pressure makes relatively little difference. Since maximum filling is accomplished very quickly, doubling the heart rate may almost double the minute output.

The Valsalva manœuvre may give rise either to a normal or to a square wave response (fig. 13.12), and may therefore fail to distinguish constrictive pericarditis from heart failure. It is presumed that an intrathoracic pressure of 40 mm. Hg may fail to compress the calcified box that encloses the heart. The assumption that cases giving a square wave response are really in a state of myocardial failure is unwarranted; on the other hand, it is not denied that true heart failure may occur, and can sometimes be demonstrated post-operatively.

Other physiological phenomena such as Kussmaul's sign and pulsus paradoxus are discussed with the physical signs.

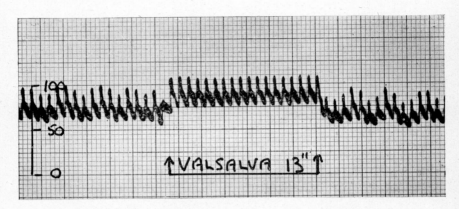

Fig. 13.12—Valsalva manœuvre in a case of Pick's disease showing a square wave response in the arterial pressure pulse.

Clinical features

The patient may be of either sex and almost any age, but is usually an adult between 20 and 50. A previous history of tuberculous pericarditis or peritonitis is unusual.

The onset of symptoms is insidious and signs may be well developed when the patient complains of little beyond fatigue, slight breathlessness on effort, fullness of the abdomen and perhaps a tendency to œdema. Obvious ascites and dropsy are late symptoms, although they may be the first that make the patient seek medical advice. Cases with active tuberculous pericarditis, of course, are in a different category.

On examination, the pulse is rather small and sometimes paradoxical, almost disappearing with inspiration. This is due to interference with cardiac filling when the pericardial tension is increased by descent of the diaphragm; although it is the forward counterpart of Kussmaul's sign (*vide infra*), it is far less common. The blood pressure is usually low. The venous pressure is high and may rise appreciably during inspiration (Kussmaul, 1873). A similar inspiratory rise of left atrial and pulmonary venous pressures may be recorded with the wedged catheter technique (fig. 13.13). The chief wave in the venous pulse (fig. 13.10) is usually the *y* trough (Friedreich's sign, 1864), but in relatively mild cases with normal rhythm the *x* descent may be equally conspicuous. Atrial fibrillation occurs in about one-third of all cases; its frequency is directly proportional to the age of the patient as in mitral stenosis and thyrotoxicosis.

On palpation the heart is usually quiet, the left ventricular impulse being barely perceptible and there being no lift over the right ventricle. There may be an appreciable diastolic shock, as if the heart, filling rapidly under the influence of a high venous pressure, suddenly met the unyielding resistance of a rigid pericardium, which, from a state of relaxation, was thrown abruptly into tension; on auscultation, this is represented by an

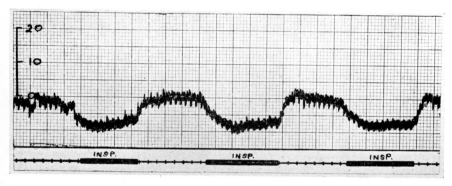

(a) Normal response, the pressure falling during inspiration and rising during expiration.

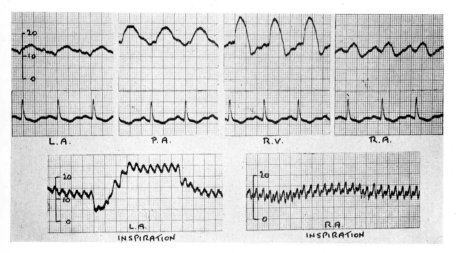

(b) Paradoxical response in a case of Pick's disease; an even greater rise of pressure is seen in the left atrial pressure tracing.

Fig. 13.13—Effect of respiration on the left and right atrial pressure.

accentuated and early third heart sound (Evans and Jackson, 1952). Friction is absent. Splitting of the second heart sound may fail to widen on inspiration, for increasing the filling pressure of the right ventricle may not augment the stroke volume, as previously explained. In a minority of cases, however, not excluding those with the heaviest calcification, not only does inspiration delay pulmonary valve closure as in normal individuals, but it

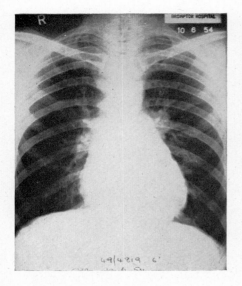

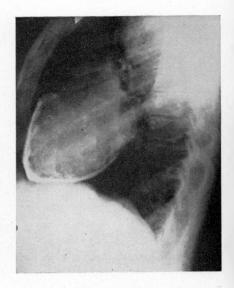

(a) Anterior view.

(b) Calcification seen in second oblique view.

Fig. 13.14—Skiagrams of a case of constrictive pericarditis.

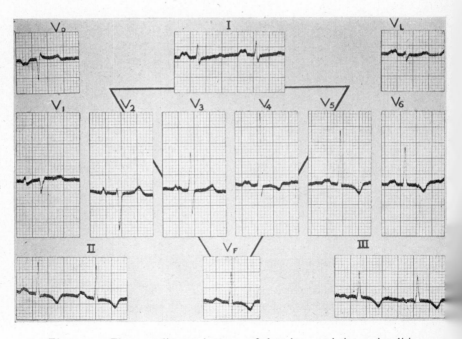

Fig. 13.15—Electrocardiogram in a case of chronic constrictive pericarditis.

may also increase the intensity of the first heart sound. In such cases the Valsalva manœuvre may be expected to give a normal response.

Considerable enlargement of the liver, ascites and œdema complete the clinical picture.

Fluoroscopy reveals little cardiac pulsation; the heart shadow is normal in size in 45 per cent, slightly enlarged in 17 per cent, moderately enlarged in 32 per cent, and greatly so in 6 per cent, and has an ill-defined outline (Paul, Castleman and White, 1948). Enlargement, when present, is due to the thickness of the pericardium which may measure as much as 26 mm. (Freedman, 1939). The shape of the heart shadow is also altered, being triangular in half the cases, with straight left and right borders and a small or absent aortic knuckle. Calcification occurs in about half the cases, and is best seen in the left anterior oblique position (fig. 13.14).

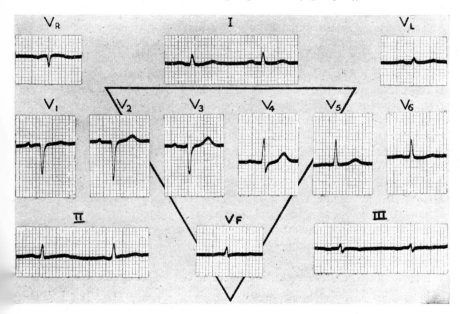

Fig. 13.16—Almost normal electrocardiogram from a woman of 67 with Pick's disease (proved at operation).

The electrocardiogram usually shows low-voltage QRS complexes, with flattening or inversion of T in most leads, representing the late stage of the pericardial T_2 pattern, which in these cases is permanent (fig. 13.15). A conspicuous or bifid P wave is not uncommon. Occasionally, the electrocardiogram is almost normal (fig. 13.16).

Differential diagnosis. It is insufficiently appreciated that the only pathognomonic sign of chronic constrictive pericarditis is a calcified pericardium, and even this can occur without constriction. Kussmaul's sign, Friedreich's sign, a loud and early third heart sound, and the characteristic electrocardiographic pattern can all occur in cases of isolated myocarditis or other cardiopathy of clinically obscure origin. A paradoxical pulse and the lack of much cardiac enlargement are highly suggestive of Pick's disease under the clinical circumstances, but are not pathognomonic and are not necessarily present. Poor ventricular pulsation on fluoroscopy is characteristic of most low output states.

Because of these difficulties special efforts have been made to find some reliable physiological test that would distinguish Pick's disease without calcification from cardiopathies of clinically obscure nature, but on the whole these efforts have failed, and many fruitless thoracotomies have been undertaken in consequence. This comment applies to intracardiac pressure pulses, measurement of the cardiac output in relation to changes of posture and heart rate, and the Valsalva manœuvre. Unfortunately, chronic constrictive pericarditis not infrequently behaves like heart failure, and the tests themselves may give indeterminate results.

Treatment. Treatment consists of cardiac decompression, achieved by surgical removal of the constricting tissue (Churchill, 1929, 1936). It has been assumed that the left side of the heart should be freed first to avoid the theoretical risk of acute pulmonary œdema, but evidence is accumulating which suggests that constricting forces tend to be distributed equally over both ventricles, and that division of constricting bands in any situation may result in generalised diminution of pericardial tension. Removal of calcium may be difficult and time-consuming, but is amply rewarded. The chief dangers during the operation are hæmorrhage and cardiac arrest or ventricular fibrillation. The post-operative course has been smoother since the advent of antibiotics, for pulmonary and pleural sepsis can now be avoided or treated effectively. The frequency of positive cultures obtained from pericardial tissue removed at operation has proved that activity is no direct bar to surgical treatment, but has encouraged the concomitant use of streptomycin. Even in subacute cases of tuberculous pericarditis of only six to twelve months' duration, pericardiectomy should not be withheld on the grounds of florid activity if mechanical interference with forward flow is endangering life (Andrews, Pickering and Sellors, 1948).

The results of surgical treatment were good in 62 per cent of 415 cases reviewed by Chambliss *et al.* (1951), and may be expected to be so in about three-quarters of clinically inactive cases. The surgical mortality over the last ten years has fallen from 33 per cent (Sellors, 1946) to about 15 per cen (Chambliss *et al.*, 1951; Evans and Jackson, 1952). The oldest patien operated on (successfully) in my own series was 67 years of age.

Follow-up studies in successfully treated cases reveal improved cardia filling and forward flow, reduction of left and right atrial pressures, an disappearance of fatigue, dyspnœa, ascites and œdema; but the physiolog of the circulation is still abnormal, venous pressures are higher than the should be, Kussmaul's sign may remain, the third heart sound may sti be heard, although it may be softer and appreciably later (Mounsey, 1955 normal rhythm is rarely restored, the electrocardiogram is usually ur changed, and the X-ray appearances are much the same, although the amplitude of cardiac pulsation may be greater. Re-constriction, presumably as a result of low-grade activity, has necessitated a second operation in roughly 5 to 10 per cent of surviving cases over a period of 10 to 15 years; precise figures on this point are not yet available.

ADHERENT PERICARDIUM

During the first quarter of this century adherent pericardium was still considered an important complication of pericarditis. Extensive adhesions anchoring the heart to adjacent resistant structures were believed to add a heavy burden to ventricular systole. The theory was coloured by the patho-logical observations of Cabot (1926), who recorded gross cardiac enlarge-ment associated with rheumatic adherent pericarditis. The clinical picture included Broadbent's sign (indrawing of the postero-lateral aspect of the ribs during ventricular systole, resulting from fixation of the visceral peri-cardium to the diaphragm), paradoxical pulse, diastolic shock or rebound of the ribs, fixation of the apex beat so that it failed to shift with change of posture, similar fixation of the electrical axis of the heart, and unexplained cardiac enlargement. To cure this unhappy condition, the operation of cardiolysis (Brauer, 1903) was devised to free the heart of its encumbrances by dividing adhesions between it and the surrounding tissues, and especially by extensive rib resection, so that the heart could pull against less resistant structures. In more recent years, however, the serious consequences of adherent pericardium have been denied, and its surgical treatment is no longer favoured.

Hosler and Williams (1936) failed to produce any cardiac enlargement or alteration of cardiac function by suturing the heart and pericardium to the diaphragm in 13 dogs: nor could they find a single instance of cardiac enlargement in 76 cases of adherent pericarditis in which there was not an adequate organic intracardiac cause, chiefly valvular disease. Similar clini-cal and autopsy evidence was obtained by Armstrong (1940) in 72 cases and by Evans (Parkinson, 1936) in 49 cases.

All Cabot's cases of gross cardiac enlargement with adherent pericardium were complicated by serious valve disease. Although Broadbent's sign (if not confused with indrawing of the left antero-lateral aspect of the thorax, which may occur whenever the heart is grossly enlarged) and diastolic rebound of the ribs are reliable signs of extrapericardial adhesions, para-doxical pulse favours constriction, and fixation of the apex beat or of the electrical axis is too variable to be of diagnostic value (France, 1938).

TYPES OF PERICARDITIS BASED ON ETIOLOGY

Rheumatic pericarditis. The dry form may give rise to nothing more serious than transient pericardial friction; but it has an important bearing on diagnosis, its advent during the course of rheumatic fever proving beyond question the presence of active carditis. More extensive pericarditis is usually associated with gross rheumatic infection, so that serious carditis may be assumed. These patients are often very ill, with high fever, considerable dyspnœa or hyperpnœa, and much pain. The development of cardiac dilatation and failure, under similar circumstances, is apt to be mistaken for pericardial effusion with cardiac compression, and indeed the differential diagnosis may not be easy. The position of the apex beat, the ease with which it can be felt, and the presence or absence of dullness in the second left intercostal space are good guides; but the electrocardiogram may be indeterminate and the interpretation of skiagrams difficult (see page 488). Occasionally, special diagnostic techniques may be necessary. The safest of these is right atrial catheterisation (page 663). Angiocardiography is equally conclusive, but less safe in these very sick children. The results of paracentesis should be interpreted with more caution: fluid may be obtained when there is a trivial amount present, and failure to obtain fluid may be due to technical fault.

Rheumatic pericardial effusion is a clear, straw-coloured, sterile exudate; it rarely compresses the heart, tends to be resorbed spontaneously without undue delay, appears to respond to salicylates and is usually best left alone.

Fortunately, there are no significant after-effects, for chronic constrictive pericarditis is never rheumatic, and adherent pericardium, though not uncommon, is of little importance. Pericardial calcification is seen occasionally, but is scanty and harmless.

Treatment is limited to relief of pain, when present, and to cardiac decompression in rare cases of high-pressure effusion. For the former antiphlogistine is comforting; but when the pain is severe morphine should be given. For the latter, paracentesis is required, and should be repeated when necessary. Salicylates may also help. Otherwise, treatment should be directed towards the rheumatic illness as a whole.

Tuberculous pericarditis. Tuberculous pericarditis is uncommon in Great Britain; it affects all age-groups, but favours coloured races and the male sex. The infection usually spreads from mediastinal lymph glands or pleura (Peel, 1948). Effusion is the rule, and if the patient survives constriction may follow. The onset is insidious, and in cases with effusion a large quantity of fluid may collect before symptoms are noticed. Dyspnœa and an irritable dry cough, due to pressure on the lungs and bronchi, are the usual complaints. The absence of constitutional disturbances is often remarkable, but continued fever, anorexia, loss of weight, night sweats and secondary anæmia may occur in the more active cases. Diagnosis depends upon the absence of rheumatic manifestations, the subacute or chronic course of the malady, the discovery of tuberculosis elsewhere, and the results of culture and guinea-pig inoculation of specimens of fluid obtained by paracentesis. The effusion is usually a clear straw-coloured exudate containing lymphocytes, but is sometimes blood-stained. Occasionally, the effusion is encapsulated and resembles a pericardial cyst radiologically (Freedman, 1937); a tuberculous pericardial abscess presents a similar appearance. The course is prolonged, usually ranging between three and eighteen months, and is often downhill, with progressive emaciation, toxæmia, and anæmia; cardiac compression may become dangerous, when frequent tapping adds to the patient's misery.

It is doubtful if more than 20 per cent of untreated cases with positive cultures survive, and of these the majority develop chronic constrictive pericarditis subsequently; not infrequently active and constrictive stages are telescoped. The prognosis is very different when tubercle bacilli cannot be recovered from the pericardial fluid, the mortality rate being then less than 10 per cent (Harvey and Whitehill, 1937); but of course the etiological diagnosis in many of these cases is open to question, and very few constrict later. Out of 71 untreated cases of tuberculous pericarditis reported by Carroll (1951), 53.5 per cent died within two years.

Treatment with streptomycin, 1 G. intramuscularly daily or 2 G. every third day, in conjunction with para-aminosalicylic acid (PAS) or its sodium salt, 5–10 G. twice daily by mouth, or with isoniazid, 100 mg. twice daily by mouth, for four to six months, has reduced the mortality from at least 70 per cent to 15 per cent in proved cases (Goyette, Overholt and Rapaport, 1954). The immediate results of such treatment are good in 70 per cent of cases, but it is too soon to assess the frequency of subsequent constriction. It is already evident, however, that constriction is the rule if treatment is delayed more than four months from the recognised onset of the disease.

Polyserositis. Whilst tuberculosis may affect the pleura and peritoneum as well as the pericardium, the term polyserositis (Concato's disease) is usually reserved for a somewhat similar inflammatory process of unknown origin. Large effusions collect in the serous sacs, the fluid being a clear or opalescent, straw-coloured, sterile exudate. The process is obliterative, and in the pleural cavity paracentesis must be performed ever higher, as the two layers of pleura become fused together in a thick dense white matting. Over the liver and spleen the greatly thickened peritoneum resembles a thick coating of sugar-ice. When the pericardium is involved, resorption of fluid is followed by total obliteration of the pericardial cavity, and constriction may ensue. The course and prognosis are similar to those of tuberculous pericardial effusion.

Benign (idiopathic) pericarditis. Idiopathic pericarditis has been recognised for at least a century (Christian, 1951). The newer title, *benign pericarditis* (Logan and Wendkos, 1948), has the advantage of emphasising its most important feature.

The M/F sex ratio is 3 : 1. The patient may be young, middle aged or elderly with almost equal frequency; the average age is 35 years. About two-thirds of reported cases have developed after an average latent period of twelve days following an upper respiratory tract infection (McGuire et al., 1954). The onset is usually acute, with fever, malaise, pericardial pain, friction, leucocytosis, and raised sedimentation rate. Effusion develops in about two-thirds of all cases, but is rarely extensive. The fluid is usually a straw-coloured, sterile exudate containing 3 to 4 G. of protein per cent and a variable number of lymphocytes. The electrocardiogram nearly always shows the typical changes of pericarditis.

The course averages about six weeks, with a range of two weeks to three months, but nearly 20 per cent relapse, occasionally several times, the intervals between attacks varying between two and eight weeks. This relapsing tendency is similar to that seen in traumatic and post-operative pericarditis.

Recovery is finally complete without calcification or constriction (Carmichael et al., 1951); subsequent Pick's disease suggests that the initial diagnosis was wrong.

In differential diagnosis benign pericarditis can usually be distinguished from cardiac infarction by the antecedent history of upper respiratory tract infection, malaise and fever preceding pain, the special characteristics of pericardial pain, an early extensive and persistent friction rub, the develop ment of pericardial effusion, and the absence of abnormal Q waves in the electrocardiogram.

No treatment has so far proved effective, although most of the newer antibiotics have been tried.

Malignant infiltration of the pericardium. When a male over 40 years of age complains of recent cough and breathlessness of insidious onset, and is found to have a large pericardial effusion, a malignant or tuberculous etiology is probable. If there is no fever and the fluid is blood-stained, the diagnostic scales tip sharply in favour of malignancy. When the pericardium is extensively invaded, hæmorrhagic effusion and cardiac tamponade are the rule; but when it is infiltrated by a single small nodule, the fluid usually clear and straw-coloured, and the sac being more distensible, tam ponade is less frequent. The condition is invariably fatal, and death never long delayed. Autopsy usually reveals a primary bronchial carcinoma.

Pyogenic pericarditis. Streptococcal, pneumococcal and staphylococcal infection may each give rise to pericarditis. Fever, leucocytosis and toxæmia are more conspicuous than in other forms. Effusion is common and usually purulent. It is generally believed that recovery may be followed by con striction, but this is certainly unusual if it occurs at all. Streptococcal pericarditis may complicate tonsillitis, erysipelas, broncho-pneumonia, any other streptococcal infection. It usually occurs during the acute stage of the illness, and is then readily distinguished from rheumatic pericarditis but when there is an appreciable latent interval, this distinction is not easy. Pneumococcal pericarditis is usually a complication of left basal pneumonia, organisms gaining access to the pericardium by direct spread from the pleura. Staphylococcal pericarditis may complicate myocardial abscess from staphylococcal septicæmia.

The course and prognosis of pyogenic pericarditis have been radically altered by chemotherapy. Penicillin is more effective than the sulphona mides, and should be given in divided doses of 1 mega unit daily, for seven to ten days. Surgical drainage is only necessary when there is frank suppuration. With such treatment, initial recovery is the rule, but the ultimate outcome is uncertain. The lower mortality rate may result in an increased incidence of chronic constrictive pericarditis; on the other hand, the prevention of frank suppuration may have the opposite effect. The few cases so far followed up by the author have not constricted.

Hæmopericardium and traumatic pericarditis. Hæmorrhage into the pericardial sac may be caused by stab or gun-shot wounds, by rupture of a syphilitic or dissecting aneurysm of the aorta, or by perforation of a myocardial infarct or ventricular aneurysm. Wounds of the heart are not necessarily fatal, and if the patient survives the initial insult, relief of cardiac tamponade and surgical repair may be life-saving. Rupture of the heart or aorta into the pericardium is always fatal, but not necessarily immediately. A patient with a perforated infarct, for example, may live as long as ten days.

Severe blows, crush-injuries, or blast, may cause myocardial bruising and pericardial ecchymoses. Transient pericardial friction and characteristic electrocardiographic changes usually provide evidence of the lesion. If there is no damage to the superficial coronary arteries, complete recovery is the rule.

An interesting form of traumatic pericarditis may be due to pericardial foreign body (usually a metallic fragment) or to a foreign body lying close to the pericardium. In these cases recurrent attacks of pericarditis with clear sterile effusion may occur at any time up to four months after the original injury. The interval between attacks is usually two to six weeks, during which the patient seems perfectly well. The attacks themselves, which last about a week, tend to be severe, with fever, rapid effusion, cardiac tamponade, and considerable pain and distress. Of seven cases that I reported in 1945, however, none died. If the foreign body is easily accessible it is best removed in a quiescent period; if not, it may be safer to leave it *in situ.*

Post-operative pericarditis may follow any direct operation on the heart, including mitral valvotomy, aortic valvotomy via the left ventricular route, pulmonary valvotomy and infundibular resection. Its frequency is about 5 per cent. Pericardial pain and fever, usually lasting about a week, are the chief manifestations; pericardial friction, common enough during the first week or two, may reappear, and a small effusion may develop. The first episode usually occurs during the third or fourth post-operative week, sometimes just after the patient has been discharged from hospital. Attacks are apt to be recurrent, with intervals of two to three weeks, over a period of two or three months.

The syndrome is sharply reminiscent of the recurrent pericarditis associated with pericardial foreign body described above, and may well be traumatic in nature (Wood, 1954).

Uræmic pericarditis. Pericardial friction is not uncommonly heard in patients dying with uræmia. Symptoms are rare, effusion absent, and electrocardiographic changes minimal. At autopsy, needle-like crystals of urea may be found massed in the pericardium.

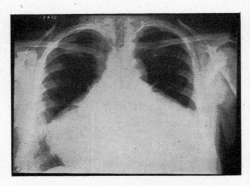

Fig. 13.17—Pericardial effusion of three years' duration in a case of extreme essential hypertension.

Pericarditis secondary to myocardial infarction. Acute myocardial infarction may give rise to a local (60 per cent) or general (15 per cent) pericardial reaction, and perforation may lead to hæmopericardium. Local pericarditis is limited to the surface area of the infarct, gives rise to no symptoms, and does not interfere with the electrocardiographic pattern of the underlying lesion. A fleeting friction rub may be heard if the infarct is anterior.

General pericarditis is less common but more important; it may cause additional pain, allows anterior friction to be associated with posterior infarction (Stewart and Turner, 1938), influences the electrocardiographic pattern, and may even give rise to effusion.

Chronic idiopathic pericardial effusion. Large pericardial effusions of unknown cause may remain virtually unchanged for years. It seems more than a coincidence that in my own series of six such cases, all had hypertension, two of them malignant. The effusion was usually gross (fig. 13.17) and had lasted for at least three or four years in four of them. There was no fever, pain, leucocytosis or raised sedimentation rate; indeed, the effusion was virtually silent in all of them, and in the two cases of malignant hypertension seemed to have prevented serious dyspnœa and orthopnœa by limiting the inflow to the right ventricle. In the case illustrated, for instance, the intrapericardial pressure was 9 cm. of saline and the venous pressure was raised proportionally; the patient was able to lie flat and could even be tilted head downwards without distress; after paracentesis orthopnœa and paroxysmal cardiac dyspnœa developed within three or four days and had to be controlled by dehydration until the pericardial effusion reaccumulated.

The fluid in these cases has always been clear and acellular, but has contained at least 4 G. of protein per cent.

In cases with severe hypertension it may be best not to disturb the physiological situation unless the blood pressure can be well controlled. In cases without serious hypertension, however, partial pericardiectomy should be advised if the effusion is gross and chronic. Mr. W. C. Cleland undertook this operation in one of my cases at the Brompton Hospital after repeated tapping and dehydration had failed to prevent rapid reaccumulation of fluid (fig. 13.05). The condition had been present for at least four years, and possibly for ten years. The pericardium itself looked normal enough, and there has been no trouble since.

Chronic effusive pericarditis may also occur in children; a good example in which the effusion was observed over a period of four years was reported by Contro *et al.* (1955) in a child of 7 to 11.

Hydropericardium. Hydropericardium associated with congestive failure is rarely conspicuous and is of little clinical significance. Pericardial effusion may also complicate myxœdema, when it frequently contains cholesterol (Creech *et al.*, 1955).

Pericardial cyst. A rounded opacity deforming the border of the heart shadow may represent a fibroma, lipoma, hydattid cyst, cardiac aneurysm, hæmatoma, loculated pericardial effusion, cold abscess or pericardial diverticulum or cyst.

Cardiac tumours usually alter the electrocardiogram and interfere with cardiac function, hydattid disease can be recognised by Casoni and complement fixation tests, cardiac aneurysm by paradoxical pulsation and characteristic electrocardiogram, hæmatoma by the history of stab or gunshot wound, and localised tuberculous abscess by subacute pericardial pain and local electrocardiographic changes. A pericardial cyst

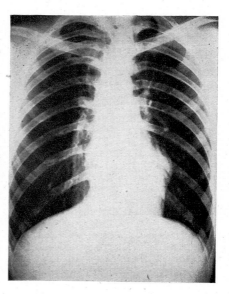

Fig. 13.18—Pericardial cyst or diverticulum on the left border of the heart.

or diverticulum, however, is silent, does not disturb the electrocardiogram, and is discovered only on routine radiography (fig. 13.18). It may be safely disregarded.

Mediastinal tumours are more likely to be confused with aortic aneurysm and are therefore considered in the next chapter.

REFERENCES

Andrews, G. W. S., Pickering, G. W., and Holmes Sellors, T. (1948): "The ætiology of constrictive pericarditis, with special reference to tuberculous pericarditis, together with a note on polyserositis", *Quart. J. Med.*, **17**, 291.

Armstrong, T. G. (1940): "Adherent pericardium constrictive and non-constrictive", *Lancet*, **ii**, 475.

Besterman, E. M. M., and Thomas, G. T. (1953): "Radiological diagnosis of rheumatic pericardial effusion", *Brit. Heart J.*, **15**, 113.

Bloomfield, R. A., *et al.* (1946): "Recording of right heart pressures in normal subjects and in patients with chronic pulmonary disease and various types of cardio-circulatory disease", *J. clin. Invest.*, **25**, 639.

Brauer, L. (1903–4): "Die kardiolysis und ihre indicationen", *Arch. f. Chir.*, **71**, 258.

Broadbent, W. H., and Broadbent, J. F. H. (1897): "Heart disease with special reference to prognosis and treatment", New York.

Burchell, H. B., Barnes, A. R., and Mann, F. C. (1939): "The electrocardiographic picture of experimental localised pericarditis", *Amer. Heart J.*, **18** 133.

Cabot, R. C. (1926): "Facts on the heart", Philadelphia.

Capps, J. A. (1932): "An experimental and clinical study of pain in the pleura, pericardium and peritoneum", New York.

Carmichael, D. B., Sprague, H. B., Wyman, S. M., and Bland, E. F. (1951): "Acute nonspecific pericarditis. Clinical, laboratory, and follow-up considerations", *Circulation*, **3**, 321.

Carroll, D. (1951): "Streptomycin in the treatment of tuberculous pericarditis", *Bull. Johns Hopk. Hosp.*, **8**, 425.

Chambliss, J. R., Jaruszewski, E. J., Brofman, B. L., Martin, J. F., and Feil, H. (1951): "Chronic cardiac compression (chronic constrictive pericarditis). A critical study of sixty-one operated cases with follow-up", *Circulation*, **4**, 816.

Chevers, N. (1842): "Observations on the disease of the orifice and valves of the aorta", *Guy's Hosp. Rep.*, **7**, 387.

Christian, H. A. (1951): "Nearly ten decades of interest in idiopathic pericarditis", *Amer. Heart J.*, **42**, 645.

Churchill, E. D. (1929): "Decortication of the heart (Delorme) for adhesive pericarditis", *Arch. Surg.*, **19**, 1457.

—— (1936): "Pericardial resection in chronic constrictive pericarditis", *Ann. Surg.*, **104**, 516.

Contro, S., DeGiuli, G., and Ragazzini, F. (1955): "Chronic effusive pericarditis", *Circulation*, **11**, 844.

Creech, O. Jr., Hicks, W. M. Jr., Snyder, H. B., and Erickson, E. E. (1955) "Cholesterol pericarditis. Successful treatment by pericardiectomy", *Circulation* **12**, 193.

Eliasch, H., Lagerlöf, H., and Werkö, L. (1950): "Diagnosis of adhesive pericarditis with special reference to heart catheterization", *Nord. Med.*, **44**, 112

Evans, W., and Jackson, F. (1952): "Constrictive pericarditis", *Brit. Heart J* **14**, 53.

Ewart, W. (1896): "Practical aids in the diagnosis of pericardial effusion, connection with the question as to surgical treatment", *Brit. med. J.*, **i**, 717.

France, R. (1938): "The use of the electrocardiogram in the diagnosis of adhesi pericardio-mediastinitis", *Bull. Johns Hopk. Hosp.*, **63**, 104.

Freedman, E. (1937): "Inflammatory diverticula of the pericardium", *Amer. Roentgenol. and Radium Therapy*, **37**, 733.

—— (1939): "Inflammatory diseases of pericardium", *Amer. J. Roentgenc* **42**, 38.

Friedreich, N. (1864): "Zur Diagnose der Hertzbeutelverwachsungen *Virchows Arch.*, **29**, 296.

Goyette, E. M., Overholt, E. L., and Rappaport, E. (1954): "The treatment of tuberculous pericarditis", *Circulation*, 9, 17.

Hansen, A. T., Eskildsen, P., and Gotzsche, H. (1951): "Pressure curves from the right auricle and the right ventricle in chronic constrictive pericarditis", *Circulation*, 3, 881.

Harvey, A. M., and Whitehill, M. R. (1937): "Tuberculous pericarditis", *Medicine*, 16, 45.

Hosler, R. M., and Williams, J. E. (1936): "Study of cardio-pericardial adhesions", *J. thorac. Surg.*, 5, 629.

Isaacs, J. P., Berglund, E., and Sarnoff, S. J. (1954): "Ventricular function. III. The pathologic physiology of acute cardiac tamponade studied by means of ventricular function curves", *Amer. Heart J.*, 48, 66.

Kisch, B., Nahum, L. H., and Huff, H. E. (1940): "The predominance of surface over deep cardiac injury in producing changes in the electrocardiogram", *Amer. Heart J.*, 20, 174.

Kussmaul, A. (1873): "Ueber schwielige Mediastino-Pericarditis und den paradoxen Puls.", *Berl. Klin. Wchnschr.*, 10, 433, 445, 461.

Logue, R. B., and Wendkos, M. H. (1948): "Acute pericarditis of benign type", *Amer. Heart J.*, 36, 587.

Lower, R. (1669): "Tractatus de Corde", Leyden ed., 1728. Quoted by Major, R. H. (1932): "Classic descriptions of disease", Springfield, Illinois.

McGuire, J., Kotte, J. H., and Helm, R. A. (1954): "Clinical progress. Acute pericarditis", *Circulation*, 9, 425.

McKusick, V. A. (1952): "Chronic constrictive pericarditis. I. Some clinical and laboratory observations", *Bull. Johns Hopk. Hosp.*, 90, 3.

Mounsey, P. (1955): "The early diastolic sound of constrictive pericarditis", *Brit. Heart J.*, 17, 143.

Parkinson, J. (1936): "Enlargement of the heart", *Lancet*, i, 1341.

Paul, O., Castleman, B., and White, P. D. (1948): "Chronic constrictive pericarditis", *Amer. J. med. Sc.*, 216, 361.

Peel, A. A. Fitzgerald (1948): "Tuberculous pericarditis", *Brit. Heart J.*, 10, 195.

Pick, F. (1896): "Uber chronische unter dem Bilde der Lebercirrhose verlaufende Perikarditis (perikarditische Pseudolebercirrhose) mebste Bemerkungen uber die Zuckergussleber (Curschmann)", *Ztrschr. F. klin. med.*, 29, 385.

Porte, D., and Pardee, H. E. B. (1929): "Occurrence of coronary T wave in rheumatic pericarditis", *Amer. Heart J.*, 4, 584.

Rotch, T. M. (1878): "Absence of resonance in the fifth right interspace diagnostic of pericardial effusion", *Boston med. & surg. J.*, 99, 389, 421.

Sawyer, C. G., et al. (1952): "Chronic constrictive pericarditis: further consideration of the pathologic physiology of the disease", *Amer. Heart J.*, 44, 207.

Sellors, T. H. (1946): "Constrictive pericarditis", *Brit. J. Surg.*, 33, 215.

Stewart, H. J., Crane, N. F., and Deitrick, J. E. (1938): "Studies of the circuation in pericardial effusion", *Amer. Heart J.*, 16, 189.

——, and Heuer, G. J. (1939): "Chronic constrictive pericarditis", *Arch. intern. Med.*, 63, 504.

——, and Turner, K. B. (1938): "A note on pericardial involvement in coronary thrombosis", *Amer. Heart J.*, 15, 232.

Thomas, G. T., Besterman, E. M. M., and Hollman, A. (1953): "Rheumatic pericarditis", *Brit. Heart J.*, 15, 29.

White, P. D. (1935): "Chronic constrictive pericarditis (Pick's disease) treated by pericardial resection", *Lancet*, ii, 597.

Williams, R. G., and Steinberg, I. (1949): "The value of angiocardiography in establishing the diagnosis of pericarditis with effusion", *Amer. J. Roentgenol.*, **61**, 41.

Wood, P. H. (1937): "Electrocardiographic changes of a T_2 pattern in pericardial lesions and in stab wounds of the heart", *Lancet, ii*, 796.

—— (1945): "War wounds of the heart", Proc. Conf. Army Phys., Rome, 23.

—— (1950): "The management of rheumatic fever and its early complications. Cardiac complications", *Proc. Royal Soc. Med.*, **43**, 195.

—— (1951): "Diagnosis of pericardial effusion by means of cardiac catheterization", *Brit. Heart J.*, **13**, 574.

—— (1954): "An appreciation of mitral stenosis", *Brit. med. J., i*, 1113.

CHAPTER XIV

SYPHILITIC AORTITIS

SYPHILITIC inflammation of the aorta is clinically unrecognisable unless it results in fusiform dilatation, saccular aneurysm, aortic incompetence, angina pectoris, or possibly heart block. It is true that many museums contain a specimen of syphilitic myocarditis, and even of syphilitic endocarditis, but these are oddities. The various manifestations of syphilitic aortitis commonly appear from ten to thirty years after primary infection, usually between the ages of 30 and 60, account for about 3 per cent of all cases of organic heart disease in Britain, and are approximately five times more common in men than in women. Aortic incompetence is about twice as common as aneurysm.

There can be little doubt that the disease is becoming less frequent and will become rare. This is the result of educating the public in venereology and the improved treatment of early syphilis. Thompson, Comeau and White (1939) found cardiovascular syphilis had developed clinically in 10 per cent of 241 patients known to have had syphilis fifteen to twenty-five years previously; all had been inadequately treated by 1939 standards. Uncomplicated aortitis, rarely recognised except at necropsy, is undoubtedly more frequent; but its exact clinical incidence is difficult to assess, published figures depending on the criteria upon which the diagnosis rests. According to Moore, only 16 per cent of 105 cases of uncomplicated syphilitic aortitis proved at necropsy were recognised clinically prior to 1932 (Moore et al., 1932), whereas 68 per cent of 79 proved cases were correctly diagnosed in life between 1932 and 1941 (Mattman and Moore, 1943). He ascribed this improved diagnosis to recognising the importance of a local substernal continual aching pain, a tympanitic aortic second sound, and slight dilatation of the ascending aorta in cases already known to have late syphilis. It is pointed out, however, that the interpretation of such signs in patients who are *not* known to have late syphilis is another matter, and their true value can only be judged properly under such circumstances.

Whilst the clinical features may be diagnostic of a syphilitic etiology, the latter may be confirmed by a history of syphilis, signs of syphilis in other systems (particularly neurosyphilis), a positive Wassermann or Kahn reaction in the blood in about 85 per cent of cases, a positive treponema pallidum immobilisation test (Nelson and Mayer, 1949; Friedman and Olansky, 1955), and a persistently raised erythrocyte sedimentation rate.

Congenital syphilis does not cause aortitis (McCulloch, 1930); although spirochætes may be present in the aorta, there is practically no tissue reaction.

Pathology. The initial lesion occurs in the adventitia, and consists of syphilitic endarteritis of the vasa vasorum and of focal granulomatous tissue. Although the inflammation spreads deeply into the media, atrophy and necrosis of muscular and elastic fibres are partly due to ischæmia. The damage is patchy and is repaired by fibrous tissue, the cross section of the aortic wall being correspondingly thinned at such points. These medial scars are indicated on the inner surface of the vessel by depressions of the intima, which presents a pock-marked appearance. Secondary athero-sclerosis and extensive calcification are common.

ANEURYSM

Sooner or later the diseased media may yield to the force of the blood pressure, either generally or at its weakest point, and a fusiform or saccular aneurysm results. A fusiform aneurysm is little more than an exaggeration of the inevitable dilatation of a syphilitic aorta, and has no greater consequences. It is usually associated with aortic incompetence, but may be seen radiologically when still uncomplicated (Rich and Webster, 1952); it then affords acceptable clinical evidence of relatively early syphilitic aortitis. The diagnosis should be confirmed by a history of syphilis or by positive serological tests, however, for fusiform aneurysm may result from congenital hypoplasia of the ascending aorta or from non-specific medial necrosis with or without dissection, and slight dilatation of the aorta may be due to atherosclerosis and hypertension. A ringing or amphoric second heart sound at the base of the heart may denote dilatation of the ascending aorta, but does not indicate its cause. Again, a suspicious aortic second sound must be disregarded if the ascending aorta is seen to be normal in size and shape. Irregularities in the calibre of the ascending aorta or aortic arch, which may be clearly demonstrated by means of angiocardiography, and calcification of the ascending aorta provide good evidence of syphilitic aortitis.

The syphilitic aneurysm proper is saccular (fig. 14.01), and may occur in any part of the thoracic aorta, particularly in the arch. Aneurysm of the abdominal aorta is relatively rare, and is less frequently due to syphilis. Thus Mills and Horton (1938) attributed only 8.8 per cent of 80 abdominal aneurysms to syphilis, and Estes (1950) only 5 per cent of 102 cases; on the other hand, Scott (1944) stated that syphilis was the cause of 58 per cent of his 96 cases. The selective influence of specialised clinics no doubt explains the discrepancy.

The M/F sex ratio in cases of saccular aneurysm is 10 : 1 (White, 1937), partly perhaps because the aorta tends to be subjected to greater physical stresses in men than in women. It is significant that saccular aneurysm rarely develops when there is aortic incompetence, occurring in little over 10 per cent of such cases (Welty, 1939), and that symptoms due to pressure

descending aorta. In the anterior skiagram they usually project either to the right of the ascending aorta or to the left in the region of the pulmonary artery or left atrial appendix (fig. 14.07). In the latter position they may compress the pulmonary artery and cause physiological stenosis with all

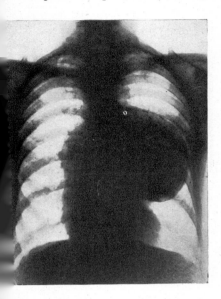

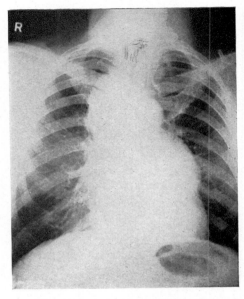

g. 14.06—Calcified dermoid cyst proved at post-mortem.
(*By courtesy of Sir John Parkinson*).

Fig. 14.07—Lymphatic cysts (proved by resection).

the characteristic physical signs and catheter findings. In the case illustrated in figure 14.08, for instance, in which there was a typical pulmonary systolic thrill and murmur, the right ventricular pressure was 70/3 mm. Hg and the pulmonary artery pressure beyond the point of compression 18/12 mm. Hg when the cardiac output was 8 L/min.

Thymic tumours or cysts are also anterior and often malignant. I have seen two calcified thymic cysts of many years' duration, both of which finally became malignant and invaded the pericardium and myocardium. In anterior skiagrams the cyst or tumour presented to the left of the mid-line just below the aortic knuckle (fig. 14.09a), and in lateral views was seen to be well anterior (fig. 14.09b). Pericardial pain, effusion, atrial flutter or fibrillation and characteristic electrocardiographic changes developed in both instances.

Retrosternal goitre is easily recognised if it moves upwards on swallowing, but may be mistaken for aneurysm if malignant and fixed.

Bronchial carcinoma with secondary invasion of mediastinal glands and partial obstruction of the superior vena cava may sometimes be mistaken for aneurysm.

Tuberculous cold abscess secondary to Pott's disease of the dorsal spine

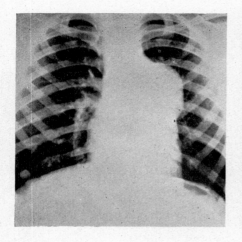

(a) Anterior view.

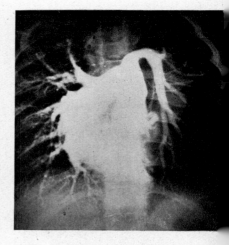

(b) Angiocardiogram of pulmonary artery

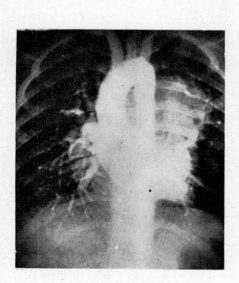

(c) Angiocardiogram of aorta.

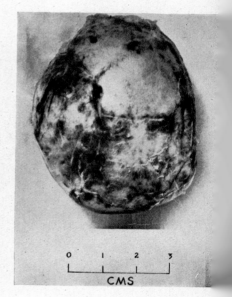

(d) The cyst after removal.

Fig. 14.08—Lymphatic cyst compressing the pulmonary artery.

may sometimes be identified by its irregular ramifications, especially when old and calcified. In its active stage, however, it may present as a fusiform swelling behind the heart and may be mistaken for a syphylitic or dissecting aneurysm of the descending aorta.

Tomography and *angiocardiography* have proved of great value in distinguishing aortic aneurysm from these and other mediastinal masses.

Retrograde aortography is rarely necessary and in cases of syphilitic aortitis is probably dangerous.

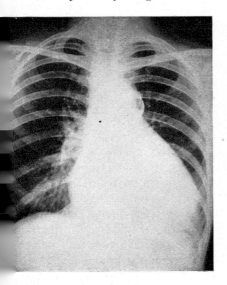
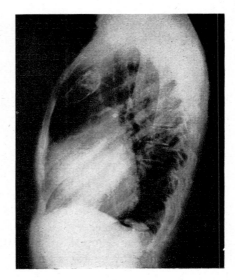

Anterior view: enlargement of the heart shadow is due to pericardial effusion.

(b) Second oblique view showing the anterior superior position of the tumour.

Fig. 14.09—Calcified cystic malignant tumour of the thymus invading the pericardium and myocardium.

The differential diagnosis between syphilitic and other forms of fusiform dilatation of the aorta is considered later in relation to aortic incompetence.

COURSE

Many aneurysms remain silent and are discovered accidentally by radiography; others cause much suffering. One of the worst features is the severe pain produced by pressure on bone, especially the root pain associated with vertebral erosion. This may last for months and be very resistant to treatment.

The prognosis varies greatly, but the average duration of life is little more than eighteen months from the onset of symptoms (Colt, 1926–27). Cases have been reported, however, which have survived for fifteen to thirty years (Kauntze, 1947). The chief dangers are infection of the lungs distal to bronchial compression, and rupture. Aortic aneurysm may rupture into the pericardium, the pulmonary artery, the trachea or bronchus, the œsophagus, or the pleura, giving rise to hæmopericardium with cardiac compression, acute right ventricular failure with signs and symptoms of an aorto-pulmonary shunt, dramatic hæmoptysis, hæmatemesis, or hæmothorax, respectively, usually with fatal results.

SPECIAL TREATMENT

The object of treatment apart from anti-syphilitic measures is to promote thrombosis and calcification in the aneurysmal sac, or to protect it by means of external fibrosis, in order to prevent rupture or further expansion.

Bed rest is necessary at first while routine anti-syphilitic treatment is given. During this period a course of calcium lactate, 10 grains (0.6 G.) t.d.s., with vitamin D may be added to promote calcification in the wall of the aneurysm.

If pain is not relieved by these measures, surgical interference may be considered. The old operation of inserting a wire into the sac in order to induce thrombosis is unsatisfactory: the risk is considerable and effective clotting cannot be guaranteed. Babcock's operation—the creation of an arterio-venous communication between the carotid and jugular vessels (Babcock, 1926, 1932)—reduces the mean aortic pressure and may relieve pain (Ranson, 1947). A more promising surgical method is to wrap the aneurysm in polythene cellophane: this causes an intense fibroblastic reaction which protects the sac from without, prevents further expansion and relieves pain (Poppe, 1948). Resection of the aneurysm and replacement by an aortic homograft may be feasible when the lesion is below the left subclavian artery (Debakey and Cooley, 1953; Rob, 1954).

AORTIC INCOMPETENCE

Pathology. Weakening of the mesaorta in the region of the aortic valve leads to dilatation of the aortic ring, and to separation of the cusps at their commissures, so that the valve becomes incompetent. Granulomatous tissue may also drive a wedge between the junctions of the cusps (fig. 14.10). The cusps themselves become rolled and thickened at their free margins and present a dwarfed stunted appearance. There is no stenosis, and calcification is absent unless there is much secondary atherosclerosis. Owing to the site of the lesion, which is necessarily at the root of the aorta the mouths of the coronary vessels are often partly occluded, either by active granulation tissue or fibrotic scarring. Ischæmic fibrosis of the myocardium results.

Incidence. Syphilis used to account for about one-third of all cases of aortic valve disease and for about one-half of those in subjects between the ages of 40 and 60 (Cowan and Ritchie, 1935). Of Campbell's series 300 cases of aortic valve disease syphilis was responsible for 19 per cent only half of his cases, however, had aortic incompetence alone, and of these syphilis was the cause in 38 per cent (Campbell, 1932). At the present tim syphilis is probably still the most common cause of pure aortic incompetence between the ages of 40 and 60, but its frequency is declining.

The sex ratio in syphilitic aortic incompetenc is about 3 : 1 in favour of men (Campbell, 1932), and is thus less remarkable than in aneurysm.

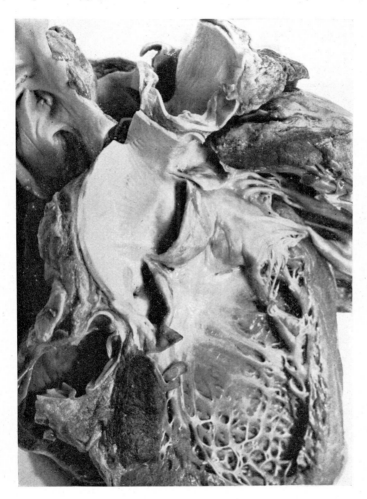

Fig. 14.10—Active syphilitic aortitis in a man of 26 showing granulomatous thickening around the coronary orifices and between the commissures of the thickened aortic cusps.

Clinical features. Syphilitic aortic incompetence has all the features of aortic incompetence in general (page 564) and some special characteristics of its own. Only the latter will be considered here.

1. The history of symptoms or of the discovery of the lesion is relatively recent, usually a matter of weeks or months and rarely more than a year or two.

2. Angina pectoris is common, occurring sooner or later in about half the cases.

3. The aortic incompetence is pure, there being no stenosis (unless there is secondary atherosclerosis).

4. The incompetence is usually very free so that peripheral vascular manifestations are marked.

5. The murmur is apt to be "to and fro", replacing the heart sounds at the base, and is often heard better at the aortic area than down the left border of the sternum, owing to dilatation of the ascending aorta.

6. A basal diastolic thrill is suggestive, being very rare in other types of aortic valve disease except when a cusp is perforated or ruptured.

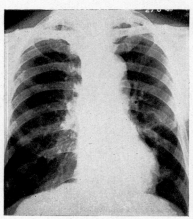

Fig. 14.11—Slightly dilated and irregular aorta in a case of syphilitic aortic incompetence.

7. Skiagrams may reveal differences in the diameter of the aorta at different points (fig. 14.11), or fusiform aneurysm; but a well-developed saccular aneurysm is uncommon. Irregularity of the lumen may be seen well in angiograms. In relatively young subjects, however, when the aortitis is in the active granulomatous stage, the aorta may look much the same as it does in rheumatic cases (fig. 14.12).

8. Calcification of the aortic valve is against syphilis, but may occur when there is secondary atherosclerosis calcification of the ascending aorta (fig 14.13) is much in favour of syphilis (Thorner et al., 1949).

9. The electrocardiogram more often shows bundle branch block, or various degrees of heart block, than it does in rheumatic aortic incompetence; but no more so than in calcific aortic stenosis. The changes are attributable to ischæmic fibrosis, rarely to gummatous lesions.

10. The diagnosis may be confirmed by obtaining other evidence of syphilis, as previously described. The E.S.R. is more often raised in syphilitic aortic incompetence than in any other variety of late syphilis including aneurysm, and is probably as good a guide to activity as the Wassermann reaction. In a consecutive series of 50 of my own cases averaged 45 mm. in one hour (Westergren) and ranged between 9 and 11 prior to treatment (excluding two cases in advanced congestive failure).

Differential diagnosis. In spite of all these highly characteristic features there may be clinical difficulty in distinguishing syphilitic from other forms of aortic incompetence.

Rheumatic aortic incompetence only resembles syphilitic aortitis when

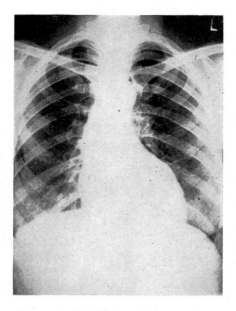

Fig. 14.12—Syphilitic aortic incompetence:
the appearances here differ little from other
forms of aortic valve disease.

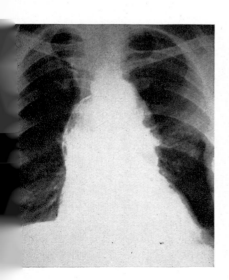

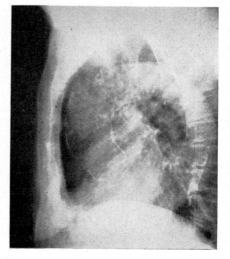

(a) Anterior view.   (b) Second oblique position.

Fig. 14.13—Calcification of the ascending aorta in a case of syphilitic aortitis.

(*By courtesy of Dr. J. S. McCann and Dr. D. C. Porter*).

there is no stenosis, no valve calcification, no mitral valve disease and no rheumatic history. Most syphilitic cases under the age of 30 are at first mistaken for rheumatic aortic incompetence, especially because in these active granulomatous cases there is little, if any, dilatation of the ascending aorta, or no more so than in any other type of free aortic incompetence. A rheumatic etiology is favoured if the lesion is known to have been present for many years, if there is no angina pectoris, and if the sedimentation rate is normal.

Old dissecting aneurysm of the ascending aorta involving the aortic valve and causing free incompetence is frequently mistaken for syphilitic aortitis; even a fresh dissection with rapidly developing aortic incompetence may be confused with syphilis, the new and severe valve lesion then being attributed to a ruptured cusp. The dilated appearance of the ascending aorta and the free regurgitation lend credence to the error. Occlusion of one or more of the great vessels arising from the arch of the aorta does not distinguish dissecting aneurysm from syphilitic aortitis—indeed, the latter is the commonest cause of what has been termed "reversed coarctation", meaning normal femoral pulses and diminished or absent pulses in the subclavians and carotids. This syndrome, also known as pulseless disease or Takayasu's disease, is sometimes caused by a primary arteritis of the aortic arch, especially when it occurs in young women (Ross and McKusick, 1953), but in such cases there is no aortic incompetence.

Old dissecting aneurysm (q.v.) should be suggested by the history, the presence of hypertension, the negative serology and the normal sedimentation rate.

Congenital hypoplasia of the ascending aorta (q.v.) may cause conspicuous dilatation of the aorta from the valve ring to the origin of the innominate artery, with free aortic incompetence. Associated arachnodactyly, some other congenital anomaly, or the long history may at once suggest the correct diagnosis.

Bacterial aortic endocarditis, active or old, is sometimes confused with syphilitic aortitis. Aneurysm of an aortic sinus, perforation of a cusp, free aortic incompetence, high sedimentation rate, and the development of severe heart failure towards the end of penicillin treatment, are common to both diseases. If the fever is low grade, blood culture negative and W.R. doubtful, the differential diagnosis may be very difficult in the absence of other pathognomic signs of bacterial endocarditis.

Atherosclerotic aortic incompetence is suggested by the age of the patient, some evidence of stenosis, calcium in the aortic knuckle but not in the ascending aorta, and valve calcification. Angina pectoris is common owing to the frequency of associated coronary disease, but the sedimentation rate is normal and serology negative.

Course. The prognosis is bad, the average duration of life being about two years (Campbell, 1932). Left ventricular failure develops sooner or later in many cases, and congestive heart failure follows. The downhill

Hunter (1796). Erosion or ulceration of atheromatous lesions forms an excellent nidus for secondary thrombosis. This is the common cause of acute coronary obstruction. Organisation of such thrombi leads to microscopical appearances similar to atherosclerotic lesions; indeed it has been

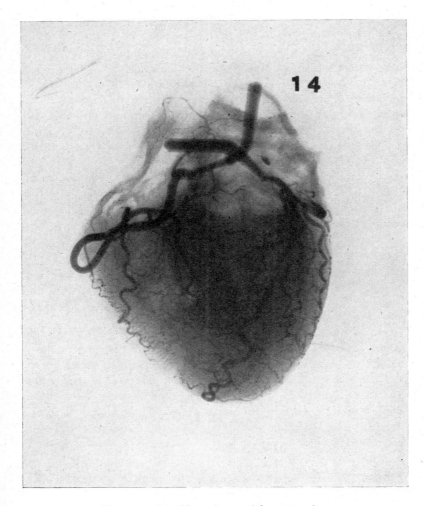

Fig. 15.01 (b)—Normal control for comparison.

suggested that atheroma may represent nothing more than intravascular clotting (Duguid, 1946, 1948).

Etiology of atherosclerosis

As a result of a vast amount of work on this important subject the sterile doctrine that atherosclerosis is an inevitable consequence of growing old has been largely abandoned; instead, it is now believed that atherosclerosis is closely related to disturbances of fat metabolism, usually acting over a long period of time (Katz and Stamler, 1953), and perhaps also to some alteration in the biophysical properties or biochemical structure of the intima itself (Page, 1954). The evidence upon which these conclusions are based can be summarised only very briefly here, but before doing so, it may be helpful to digress for a moment on the nature of the blood lipids.

The blood lipids

Fatty substances in normal blood include neutral fat, fatty acids, free cholesterol, cholesterol esters, and phospholipids.

Following a fatty meal the plasma may become opalescent; this is due to the transport of neutral fat and fatty acids combined with protein in the physical form of "chylomicrons", which are microscopically visible fatty bodies less than 1μ in diameter. Moreton's view that these bodies might play an etiological role in atherosclerosis (Moreton, 1948) has not been shared by subsequent workers (Gofman et al., 1950). Chylomicrons contain less than 5 per cent of cholesterol, have very high S_f values around 40,000 units (vide infra), and change their structure after an injection of heparin when they develop S_f values under 10 (Graham et al., 1951).

Cholesterol and phospholipids, also of course insoluble in water, are carried in combination with a and β globulins as a and β lipoproteins which are microscopically invisible macromolecules of various sizes and densities. The total serum cholesterol, which is normally around 150 to 300 mg. per cent, is certainly related to atherosclerosis, but has been found to be only a crude measure of blood lipid disturbance.

Gertler et al. (1950) emphasised the part played by the cholesterol ester and the phospholipids and suggested that the cholesterol/phospholipid ratio was more closely related to atherosclerosis than the total serum cholesterol. This ratio is normally about 0.85 to 1.0 (Barr, 1953), the amount of phospholipid tending to be proportional to the amount of free cholesterol present, rather than to the quantity of cholesterol esters. Ratios above unity mean that the cholesterol esters have risen more than the free cholesterol. High ratios are found in all diseases known to encourage atherosclerosis.

Such measurements, however, give no information about the biophysical properties of the macromolecules in which these substances are incorporated. The lipoproteins, however, may be fractionated biochemically (Cohn et al., 1946) or by means of electrophoresis (Pearsall and Chanutin, 1949) or the ultracentrifuge (Gofman et al., 1950). Russ, Eden and Barr (1951) found that practically all the serum cholesterol was incorporated in Cohn's fractions A and C, i.e. in the a_1 and β_1 lipoproteins, 30 per cent in the former and 70 per cent in the latter. They also found that the cholesterol/phospholipid ratio was about 0.5 for the a_1 lipoproteins and 1.35 for the β_1 lipoproteins. (If phospholipids are expressed in terms phosphorus, these ratios should be multiplied by 25). In atherosclerosis and diseases known to encourage it, there is a relative and usually absolute increase in the β_1 lipoproteins, even when the total blood cholesterol is normal, and the cholesterol/phospholipid ratio less than unity (Barr, Russ and Eden, 1951; Oliver and Boyd, 1955).

In the hands of Gofman and his associates (1950) the ultracentrifuge proved a useful tool for separating lipoproteins of different densities. The density of the macromolecules believed to be most closely related to atherosclerosis is close to 1 G./cc. If the density of the solution containing them is adjusted to 1.063 by means of sodium chloride, they will float with varying degrees of facility according to their densities. The α_1 lipoproteins, being denser than the solution, will not float and are therefore immediately separated out. In the Svedberg ultracentrifuge molecules that sediment at a rate of 5×10^{-13} cm. per second per unit field of force are said to have a value of 5 S (Svedberg) units. For flotation rates the same Svedberg unit s used with the suffix f. Thus molecules that float at rates of 20×10^{-13} cm. per second per unit field of force are said to have an S_f value of 20. It will be understood, therefore, that the higher the S_f value the lighter the molecule. Using this technique Gofman et al. (1950) have divided the lipoproteins into classes according to their flotation rates. Those not analysed, being denser than 1.063 (the arbitrary density of the solution), are the α_1 lipoproteins, which do not seem to be closely correlated with atherosclerosis. Of the large β_1 lipoprotein fraction the chief S_f classes are to 10, 12 to 20, 20 to 35, 35 to 100, and 100 to 40,000. The lipoproteins known to be closely related to atherogenesis are those with S_f values of 2 to 20 and 35 to 100 (Gofman et al., 1952).

Evidence that atherosclerosis is related to altered blood lipids

The chief evidence supporting the view that atherosclerosis and ischæmic eart disease are related to disturbances of blood lipid transport or metaolism may now be summarised.

1. In the animal kingdom man alone suffers commonly from atherolerotic disease; the total blood cholesterol, cholesterol esters, cholesterol/hospholipid ratio, β_1 lipoproteins and the concentration of lipoprotein acromolecules of the S_f 10–20 and 35–100 class, are all considerably igher in man than in any other mammal (Barr, 1953).

2. Only the new-born normal infant is immune from atherosclerosis; aildren, young adults and women during the child-bearing age are latively immune; the frequency of atherosclerosis in men increases with re, at least up to the end of the sixth decade. The blood concentration of e particular classes of lipoprotein mentioned above is relatively low in e more or less immune groups, but relatively high and increases with e in susceptible men (Gofman et al., 1950).

3. Œstrogens tend to restore the normal blood lipid pattern (Barr, 1953); drogens have the reverse effect (Russ et al., 1955). Atherosclerosis creases after bilateral oophorectomy in women (Wuest, Dry and

Edwards, 1953). By the age of 70 the M/F sex ratio in ischæmic heart disease is unity.

4. All diseases known to be associated with the altered blood lipid pattern described above are also associated with a high incidence of severe atherosclerosis: these diseases include diabetes mellitus, myxœdema, xanthomatosis, nephrosis, and familial hypercholesterolæmia (Gofman et al., 1951; Katz and Stamler, 1953). The same abnormal blood lipid pattern is the rule in spontaneous ischæmic heart disease.

5. Atherosclerosis has been produced experimentally in animals only by means of a high cholesterol intake; first in rabbits (Anitschkow, 1913; Leary, 1934), then in chicks (Dauber and Katz, 1942), dogs, with the aid of thiouracil (Steiner, Kendall and Bevans, 1949), hamsters (Goldman and Pollack, 1949), and guinea pigs (Altschul, 1950). Experimental atherosclerosis in omnivorous animals has the same distribution as in man.

6. The atheromatous lesions themselves contain a high proportion of cholesterol (Windaus, 1910), as has been known for a century (Cowdry, 1933).

7. Atherosclerosis is rare in people who live on a vegetarian diet low in fat (Steiner, 1946), and the incidence of clinical diseases due to atherosclerosis fell sharply in Northern Europe during the second world war parallel to the decline in the consumption of foods rich in cholesterol (Malmros, 1950). According to Wilens (1947) severe atherosclerosis is ten times as common in obese subjects as in the lean. Keys (1952) emphasised the importance of total fat intake rather than cholesterol intake per se. Gofman and Jones (1952) have shown that obese subjects tend to have a higher concentration of lipoprotein of the S_f 35–100 class than lean subjects; there was less relationship, however, between obesity and lipoproteins of the S_f 12–20 class. Gofman et al. (1950, 1951) have also shown that prolonged low fat diets gradually reduce the blood concentration of the abnormal lipids.

The part played by the intima

While it is now generally agreed that abnormal blood lipids are an important factor in the production of atherosclerosis, it is far from clear just how they operate.

Wilens (1951) showed that serum could filter through an artery from the lumen outwards. Experimentally, the filtrate was unchanged serum in respect of most inorganic substances, but contained very little cholesterol, relatively little protein, and a diminished amount of calcium, these substances becoming highly concentrated in the serum within the vessel. The rate of filtration was proportional to the filtration pressure, i.e. to the blood pressure. Some of the cholesterol penetrated the intima, but its further progress was barred by the internal elastic lamina.

The filtration theory of atherogenesis (Page, 1954) is based on observ tions of this kind, and implies that cholesterol deposits may accumulate gradually over the years in normal individuals, but that they may do so much more rapidly and in far greater degree in the presence of raised blood lipoproteins of the kind best adapted to penetrating the intima, especially if the filtration pressure is high (as in hypertension), and if there are changes in the ground substance of the intima increasing its permeability.

The presence of abnormal lipoproteins with particular biophysical properties has certainly been demonstrated in atherosclerosis, but whether these are best adapted to penetrate the intima and be prevented from passing through the internal elastic lamina is as yet unknown. Certainly, also, atherosclerosis is twice as frequent in hypertensive subjects as in those with normal blood pressures (Wilens, 1947). There is evidence that most atherosclerotic lesions are preceded by some change in the ground substance of the intima and by subendothelial fibroblastic proliferation (Moon and Rinehart, 1952). A certain degree of protection against cholesterol-induced atherosclerosis in rabbits and chicks is afforded by both potassium iodide and thyroid hormone, whether the blood lipids are favourably influenced by these substances or not (Katz and Stamler, 1953); it has been suggested that this favourable effect is due to the decreased permeability of the vascular endothelium which is known to follow the administration of these drugs.

ANGINA PECTORIS

Physiology. Angina pectoris and its close relative, the pain of intermittent claudication, are believed to be due to certain metabolites that are formed in ischæmic working muscle (Lewis, 1934). Whatever the precise explanation for the development of pain there can be no doubt that attacks depend upon relative myocardial ischæmia, an idea first enunciated by Parry (1799). The term angina pectoris is customarily applied to transient pain only, and refers to ischæmic attacks provoked by temporary stress, during which the metabolic demands of the myocardium are beyond the capacity of the coronary circulation.

Such a situation may arise during effort (1) if the coronary vessels are more or less occluded either at their mouths, as in syphilitic aortitis, or during their course, as in atherosclerosis, various forms of angiitis, and embolism; (2) if the coronary flow is diminished by other means, such as aortic stenosis, gross aortic incompetence, tight mitral stenosis, a high pulmonary vascular resistance, or severe pulmonary stenosis; (3) if the blood itself carries insufficient available oxygen as in anæmia or at high altitudes; or (4) if the regular work of the heart is increased by such conditions as hypertension, valve disease, or hyperkinetic circulatory states.

Although only angina pectoris resulting from coronary atherosclerosis concerns us here, the other factors mentioned often play a contributory role; thus anæmia may precipitate angina in a case of previously silent coronary disease, not only because of the limited oxygen transport, but also because the work of the heart is increased in order to maintain a high cardiac output. Hypertension is particularly important in so far as it increases the work of the heart and contributes to the development of atheroma: on the other hand, it tends to iron out the plaques and so may prevent coronary narrowing; in fact most cases of hypertensive heart disease have dilated coronary arteries (Harrison and Wood, 1949). Clinically, although more than half of all cases of ischæmic heart disease have blood pressures above 160/100 mm. Hg (Cassidy, 1946), systolic pressures over 200 mm. Hg are rare (Riseman and Brown, 1937).

CLINICAL FEATURES

Angina is a symptom, and must be distinguished from other pains in the upper half of the body by a careful analysis of its qualities and behaviour.

Site. The pain is central, mid-sternal, and tends to radiate bilaterally: across or round the chest; into the sides of the neck and jaws, or even into the face or nose; into the shoulders and down the inner or outer sides of the arms, sometimes as far as the little fingers or thumbs; occasionally through to the back between the shoulder-blades (fig. 15.02). This full distribution was experienced by John Hunter (1796). It is not situated in the left inframammary area, although it may be more left pectoral than sternal. Radiation may be unilateral, and it is true that the left side then suffers more often than the right; but it must not be thought that spread down the left arm is either especially typical or diagnostic, for bilateral spread is mor typical, and many other pains may radiate down the left arm, including le inframammary pain. Although centrifugal spread is the rule, radiation occasionally centripetal, the pain starting in the wrists, upper arms, or fac and spreading thence to the chest. Pain may even be confined to one of th points of radiation, e.g. to the face, back, or wrist, not being felt in th front of the chest at all.

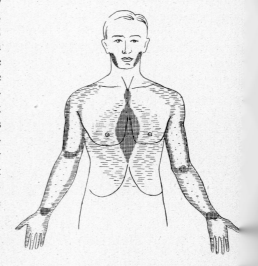

Fig. 15.02—Diagram illustrating radiation of pain in ischæmic heart disease.

Character. Angina pectoris is classically constricting, squeezing, pressin or crushing; it is sometimes stinging, numbing, or burning; sometimes cannot be described adequately by the patient. It is not sharp, shooting or stabbing, which are the usual adjectives applied to left inframammary pain. An important characteristic is its constancy, the pain being steady while it lasts, apart from initial waxing and final waning; no pain which repeats itself in a succession of jabs or knife-like thrusts is angina.

Duration. Attacks are measured in minutes; usually they last two or three minutes, occasionally five or ten; they are not momentary, nor do they continue for hours, and any pain that behaves in either of these ways is not angina pectoris (as defined above).

Provocation. Angina is characteristically produced by any effort that increases the metabolic demands of the myocardium beyond the capacity of the coronary circulation, and patients often know or learn the precise amount of effort necessary to provoke pain. When the critical point is reached the patient usually feels compelled to stop whatever he is doing, and to stand still until the pain passes off. Attacks are brought on especially by walking uphill, or against the wind, by hurrying after meals, by going out of a warm room into the cold, or by any unaccustomed exercise; less so by manual work to which the subject is trained. Pain may also be induced by excitement, anger, fear or apprehension. In advanced cases, pain is provoked by lying down (angina decubitus) or stooping, tending to occur when the patient first gets into bed at night, or waking him from sleep. It may then depend upon the rise in cardiac output that follows change of posture from vertical to horizontal, or upon anxiety dreams.

Pain that occurs after effort but not during it, or that is provoked by lying on the left side, or by the adoption of some particular posture (other than stooping or lying), is not angina; these features are characteristic of left inframammary pain.

The degree of angina pectoris (grade of effort intolerance) may be assessed according to the speed with which the patient is able to walk—not the distance. In grade I pain is only provoked by hurrying or walking up hills or several flights of stairs; in grade II walking on the level at an average speed causes pain, usually within the first 300 yards; in grade III pain occurs even when walking slowly; and in grade IV there is pain at rest and total incapacity.

As implied above, patients with moderate angina usually complain of pain soon after the beginning of effort or not at all (Kemball Price, 1951); if they do not have pain in the first quarter-mile then can very likely walk indefinitely at the same speed. Again, if the pain is not severe, patients can often walk it off. This behaviour is presumably related to the effect of exercise on vasomotor tone, i.e. to "second wind".

DIAGNOSIS OF ANGINA

If a pain conforms in site, quality, duration and relation to cardiac work, to the features mentioned above, it is angina pectoris, and the diagnosis must stand under any conditions except malingering. The diagnosis should stand likewise when pain conforms to the required features in three out of the four respects mentioned, provided it is not untenable in the fourth. For example, if a constricting pain, brought on only by exertion, and lasting but two or three minutes, is localised in the left inframammary area, it is probably not angina, for the site makes the diagnosis untenable, even though it conforms in the other three respects. On the other hand, if the same pain is situated in the left pectoral region between breast and clavicle, it is almost certainly angina, because this site, though atypical, is not contradictory. Again, a midsternal pressing pain, brought on only by effort but lasting fifteen minutes, is probably angina, for the long duration though unusual, is not altogether conflicting; but should it last two hours it is not angina as defined above.

It is sometimes said that certain associated symptoms, such as breathless ness, dizziness or faintness, flushing, sweating, weakness, and a feeling o impending death, help to confirm the diagnosis. It cannot be stressed to strongly that these symptoms carry little weight, for they are vasomotor i origin, and although they may be provoked by an attack of angina, they ar in no way characteristic of it, and are much commoner in the anxiet states.

The differential diagnosis includes anxiety states, functional disorder o organic disease involving the dorsal spinal ligaments, œsophageal or gastri spasm or distension, diaphragmatic hernia, and conditions causing respira tory distress.

Anxiety states with left inframammary pain present no diagnostic diff culty; but when pain is parasternal, or even central, it may be very cor fusing. The patients are usually women near the menopause, and they ma describe a central pain radiating to the throat, jaws and arms, during after effort, when reaching up to a high shelf, when washing or using the arms in other ways, and sometimes when emotionally upset. As noted t Cassidy (1946), the attacks are apt to be widely spaced, unrestricted effc causing no distress between them. Complete investigations may reve nothing significant in any system, and the nature of the attacks remai obscure. Angina can only be excluded, and then with some uncertainty, obtaining a normal electrocardiogram during spontaneous or induced pai

Referred pain from the dorsal spinal ligaments may be felt across the fro of the chest, as in the experimental work of Lewis and Kellgren (193 Attacks may be related to posture or reproduced by spinal movements pressure over the interspinous ligaments from D2 to D4.

Œsophageal spasm may cause central chest pain radiating down bo arms and tight or bursting in quality. There is no close relationship effort, and bouts may be periodic like any other gut colic. The diagno may be proved by demonstrating œsophageal spasm by means of fluor scopy and by obtaining a normal electrocardiogram during attacks (Wolfe and Edeiken, 1942).

Diaphragmatic hernia may cause pain on effort similar to angina pectoris, but attacks also occur without provocation, especially when the patient lies down, and at times even strenuous effort may be symptom free. Severe attacks may be mistaken for cardiac infarction. The diagnosis is made by means of a barium meal, fluoroscopy being carried out with the patient tilted head-down (Dwyer, 1937).

Relief of pain by belching in any disorder of the œsophagus or stomach is less helpful in distinguishing such conditions from angina pectoris than might be supposed, for ischæmic pain may be similarly relieved in about 10 per cent of cases (Riseman and Brown, 1937). Pain after meals is also common in cases of angina pectoris, although slight effort may be necessary to provoke it.

Bronchial asthma or extreme dyspnœa from any cause may be associated with a feeling of substernal tightness that should not be confused with angina pectoris; for breathlessness is not a feature of transient myocardial ischæmia.

PHYSICAL EXAMINATION

Having made the diagnosis on historical grounds, the patient should be examined with a view to ascertaining the cause of the ischæmia. Aortic valve disease and severe anæmia should be recognised by their characteristic features, the presence of obesity or of hypertension noted, the mental state of the patient assessed, and attention should be paid to any other factor that may have a bearing on the frequency or severity of attacks. In this respect, diabetes mellitus and polycythæmia must be borne in mind. In the majority of cases, however, there are no physical signs: the rhythm is normal, the heart is not enlarged, there are no murmurs, and there is no evidence of congestive failure; the peripheral and fundal arteries and the blood pressure may provide no evidence of general vascular disease; fluoroscopy shows a heart shadow normal in size, shape and pulsation; and the electrocardiogram may be normal at rest. It is repeated for emphasis that this apparent normality of the cardiovascular system is typical of pure angina pectoris due to coronary atherosclerosis, and that with few exceptions, physical signs, radiological changes, or electrocardiographic abnormalities, are due to complications or associated disease; even the demonstration of peripheral atherosclerosis proves little, for it is common enough without serious involvement of the coronary vessels, and is often missing with advanced coronary disease.

SPECIAL TESTS

Most of the special tests are of little help, for the circulation is usually normal at rest. Effort tolerance tests based on the behaviour of the pulse rate and venous pressure are of no value. Reproduction of pain by prescribed effort for purposes of accurate analysis is sometimes useful with a

bad witness, or pain may be induced to ascertain the prophylactic or curative effect of trinitrin. The only reliable test, however, is to obtain an
electrocardiogram immediately after effort (Scherf and Goldhammer,
1933), when characteristic depression of the RS-T segment, with or
without inversion of the U wave, clinches the diagnosis (fig. 15.03). The
depression should measure 1 mm. or more below the level of the atrial
T wave, and should remain flat or slope downwards for at least 0.08 second.
A depressed RS-T junction followed by an upwardly sloping RS-T
segment is normal. The best method is to make the patient exercise until
he is in pain; if he stops on account of fatigue or breathlessness without
developing pain, angina is unlikely. In the author's experience (Wood *et al.*,
1950) only 5 per cent of electrocardiograms remain normal during or
immediately after an attack of true angina or after sufficient effort to cause
breathlessness and fatigue (in ischæmic subjects).

This test is not entirely without danger and should only be carried out
when the diagnosis is really in doubt and the resting electrocardiogram
normal or equivocal.

The other method is to take serial electrocardiograms while the patient
breathes 10 per cent oxygen for twenty minutes, or for a shorter time if
pain is produced. As depression of the RS-T segment occurs in normal
subjects with this test, a positive result is only accepted if the depression
exceeds 2.5 mm. in any lead or if the T wave becomes inverted in left
ventricular surface leads or their counterparts (Larsen, 1938; Levy *et al.*,
1938, 1939, 1941). The test is positive in 3 to 5 per cent of normal controls
(Biorck, 1946; Weintraub and Bishop, 1947), in 15 to 20 per cent of cases
of doubtful angina, and in 50 to 55 per cent of cases of undisputed angina
(Levy *et al.*, 1941; Biorck, 1946). In the opinion of the writer this test is
less useful than the effort test, being more difficult to carry out, more
difficult to interpret, more dangerous, and far less frequently positive. The
subject is well reviewed by Stewart and Carr (1954).

COURSE

The onset of angina pectoris is more often sudden than gradual, and is
usually due to a small coronary thrombosis, insufficient to cause cardiac
infarction. The patient may say he was capable of climbing mountains a
week ago, yet now he can scarcely walk 100 yards. Less commonly, pain is
first experienced during unusually heavy exertion, and gradually becomes
more easily provoked. This represents the slow development of occlusive
atherosclerosis.

The subsequent course is apt to be punctuated by short periods of relatively sudden deterioration, followed by long periods of gradual improvement: these episodes signify thrombotic occlusion of a medium-sized
coronary artery, followed by the development of a collateral circulation
(Schlesinger, 1938), and perhaps by recanalisation.

Sooner or later in the majority of cases thrombosis occludes one of the

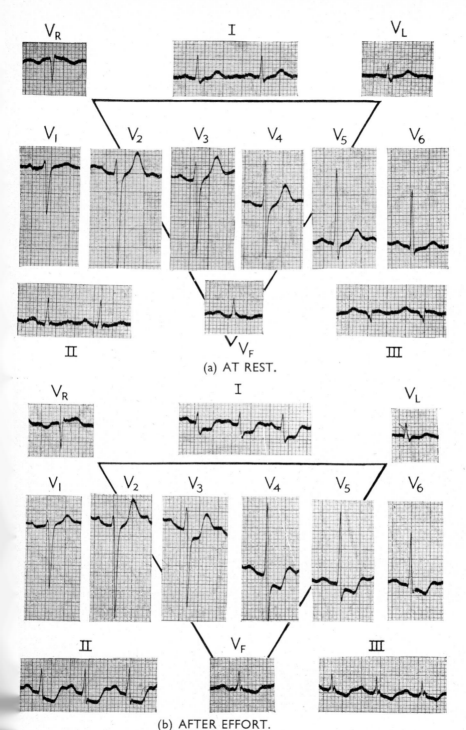

(a) AT REST.

(b) AFTER EFFORT.

Fig. 15.03—Electrocardiogram (a) before and (b) after exertion in a case of angina pectoris: the control record (a) is practically normal; the second record (b) shows significant depression of the ST segment.

main coronary arteries, and cardiac infarction results; but a major thrombosis may occur without infarction, infarction may occur without thrombosis, and ventricular fibrillation may terminate the illness in the absence of both (Appelbaum and Nicolson, 1935; Nathanson, 1936).

Angina may cause total incapacity in really severe cases, and may finally occur at rest (status anginosus or acute coronary insufficiency).

Some cases, severe or otherwise, improve after cardiac infarction; others lose their pain on developing congestive heart failure. It is not clear why this should be so, but the explanation may be related to the fact that ligation of the coronary vein appears to improve the coronary circulation (Beck and Mako, 1941).

PROGNOSIS

The average life expectancy from the onset of angina pectoris is nine to ten years (White, Bland and Miskall, 1943); about 10 per cent live well nigh twenty years, e.g. John Hunter, 1773–93; Sir James Mackenzie, 1907–25; Sir Thomas Lewis, 1927–45. Of 6,882 cases followed for 5 to 23 years at the Mayo Clinic, the mortality was 15 per cent in the first year, and 9 per cent per annum thereafter (Block *et al.*, 1952). Women have a better prognosis than men, and subjects over 40 years of age at the onset fare better than those under 40 (Parker *et al.*, 1946). Cardiac infarction, hypertension, enlargement of the heart, changes of rhythm, bundle branch block and other electrocardiographic abnormalities (at rest) all influence the prognosis adversely (Montgomery, Dry and Gage, 1947).

TREATMENT

Conservative. The majority of patients with uncomplicated angina of mild or moderate severity are able to carry out sedentary or light manual work. Any mental or physical activity that increases the frequency of attacks or that causes pain directly should be avoided, whilst adequate rest and relaxation should be assured. Diet should be light and its fat content low; although hypercholesterolæmia is difficult to influence by such means atherogenic macromolecular lipoproteins of the S_f 10–20 class tend to be inhibited (Gofman *et al.*, 1950). Alcohol in moderation is not harmful in fact, as a vasodilator it may be beneficial, although it does not prevent electrocardiographic S-T segment depression on effort (Russek *et al.*, 1950). Contributory factors such as hypertension, obesity, anæmia, diabetes mellitus, and anxiety, should be corrected as far as possible.

Cigarette smoking should be limited to 10 to 15 per day, or given up altogether if it is found to precipitate attacks. Intravenous nicotine bitartrate (2 mg.), equivalent to five inhalations from a cigarette in one minute, quickens the heart rate by about 15 beats per minute, raises the blood pressure by an average of 12/8 mm. Hg, increases the cardiac output 1 to 2 litres per minute, and frequently causes dizziness or slight

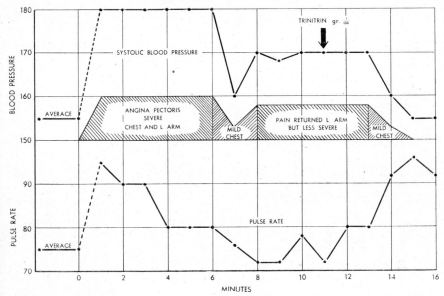

Fig. 15.04—Graph showing close correlation between the height of the blood pressure and the degree or extent of pain during an attack of angina pectoris treated with trinitrin.

faintness; in ischæmic cases angina pectoris is provoked in 8 per cent, and the electrocardiogram significantly altered in 12 per cent (Boyle *et al.*, 1947). Smoking cigarettes also inhibits diuresis, an effect that has been attributed to stimulation of the posterior pituitary (Walker, 1949); liberation of vasopressin (pitressin) may also explain the prolonged reduction of coronary blood flow that occurs in dogs (Bulbring, Burn and Walker, 1949). Since ischæmic heart disease is now alleged to be at least one and a half times more common in cigarette smokers than non-smokers it may be wise to abandon the habit altogether. As with lung cancer, cigars and pipe-smoking seem relatively innocuous.

Trinitrin, 1/100 to 1/120 of a grain (0.5 mg.), introduced by Murrell in 1879, may be slipped under the tongue as required, either to relieve an attack or before some unavoidable effort which might induce one. Trinitrin is absorbed quickly through the oral mucosa, and acts as a coronary vasodilator relieving pain without necessarily altering the blood pressure (Wayne and Laplace, 1933–34); but if the blood pressure is lowered as well, so much the better (fig. 15.04). Ischæmic S-T depression in the electrocardiogram is corrected quickly (fig. 15.05). Trinitrin tablets (B.P.) deteriorate with age, losing about 10 per cent of their potency per annum; preparations such as angised (B.W.) and nitrocine (M-C.) overcome this drawback.

Amyl nitrite, 5 minims (0.3 ml.) is also effective but less convenient (fig. 15.06): a capsule may be broken in a handkerchief and inhaled; the noise of the procedure, the pungent smell of the vapour, and the

ANGINA PECTORIS

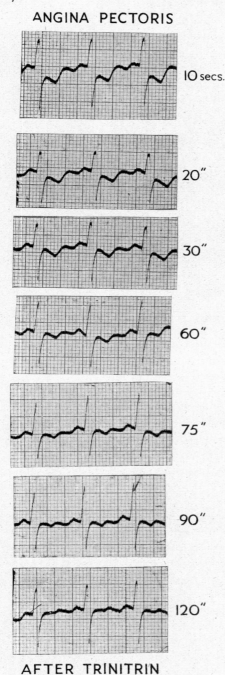

10 secs.

20"

30"

60"

75"

90"

120"

AFTER TRINITRIN

Fig. 15.05—Graph illustrating rapid correction of ischæmic depression of the S-T segment in lead V₃ in a patient with angina pectoris by means of trinitrin.

vivid facial flush that accompanies its use, are apt to embarrass the patient in public. Amyl nitrite is a powerful vasodilator and relief of pain is associated with considerable tachycardia and conspicuous elevation of the cardiac output. Much interest is also attached to the frequent paradoxical effect of amyl nitrite on the electrocardiogram, for the depression of the S-T segment that occurs during an attack of angina often becomes further depressed when the drug is inhaled and pain passes off (fig. 15.07).

Few of the drugs used as longer acting coronary vasodilators are of much value (Master, Jaffe and Dack, 1939). *Aminophylline* has the best reputation, and is employed widely in doses of 0.1 to 0.2 G t.d.s. It is difficult to demonstrate a physiological effect with such doses, but severe angina may be relieved by 0.3 G four-hourly, if the patient can tolerate it. Epigastric pain and nausea prohibit larger doses. Aminophylline, however, may be given in conjunction with aluminium hydroxide as *theodrox*, and in this form 0.2 G. is usually well tolerated. Theophylline may also be given as *etophylate:* this is the neutral salt of theophylline-ethanoic acid and the base diethylenediamine, and may be taken orally in doses of 0.25 to 0.5 G. t.d.s. without dyspepsia. *Choline theophyllinate*, in oral doses of 0.2 to 0.5 G. t.d.s., is also said to be well tolerated.

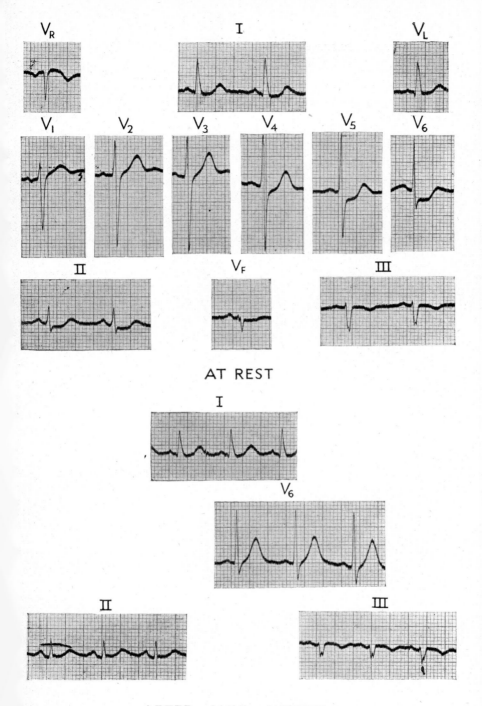

AT REST

AFTER AMYL NITRITE

Fig. 15.06—Electrocardiogram during an attack of myocardial ischæmia treated with amyl nitrite.
Expected response showing prompt correction of the depressed S-T segment.

Amongst the long-acting nitrites and nitrates there is *pentaerythritol-tetranitrate* (nitropent), which has a mild coronary vasodilator action lasting for about four hours. In Great Britain it is marketed as mycardol (Bayer) and peritrate (Warner); the former is made up in 30-mg. tablets, the latter in 10-mg. tablets. In oral doses of 10 to 30 mg. one hour before meals nitropent not only tends to relieve pain but also inhibits electrocardiographic S-T segment depression on exercise (Russek *et al.*, 1955). Larger doses of nitropent usually cause dyspepsia.

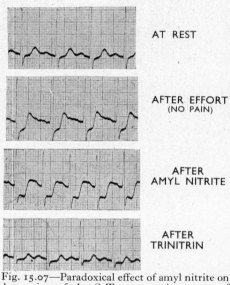

AT REST

AFTER EFFORT
(NO PAIN)

AFTER
AMYL NITRITE

AFTER
TRINITRIN

Fig. 15.07—Paradoxical effect of amyl nitrite on depression of the S-T segment in a case of angina pectoris.

Recent reports have claimed that khellin, an extract from the seeds of an Eastern Mediterranean wild plant, *ammi visnaga*, is an effective coronary vasodilator with a prolonged action. The dose is 100 mg. by mouth, three times daily. Angina pectoris is said to be relieved in 74 per cent of cases (Anrep *et al.*, 1946, 1947). Unfortunately, khellin is so badly tolerated by the majority of patients that in its present form it can hardly be considered a therapeutic agent.

Enthusiastic reports from Canada concerning the beneficial effect of vitamin E in doses of 200 to 600 mg. (Shute, 1945) have not been confirmed.

Since *œstrogens* not only inhibit experimental atherogenesis in cockerels, but also reduce the severity of atherosclerotic lesions already present (Katz and Stamler, 1953), they have naturally been tried therapeutically in man, and as previously stated they tend to restore the normal blood lipid pattern (Barr, 1953). Improvement of ischæmic heart disease, however, has not yet been demonstrated and the side effects, such as mammary development in the male, are undesirable. There may be a stronger case for the use of œstrogens in cases of angina pectoris in relatively young women who have undeveloped ovaries or who have had bilateral oophorectomy.

Testosterone propionate has no place in the treatment of angina pectoris for androgens are contra-indicated.

Other agents that may inhibit atherogenesis or actually help to clear lesions already present are under trial: they include inositol (Felch *et al* 1952), beta-sitosterol (Barber and Grant, 1955), and heparin (Engelberg 1952). No such drug can yet be recommended therapeutically.

Artificial myxœdema. Total ablation of the thyroid gland was introduced by Blumgart, Levine, and Berlin (1933) in the hope that an appreciable reduction on the circulatory demands would benefit cases of angina pectoris (and congestive heart failure). Fair results were obtained (Cutler and Schnitker, 1934), improvement being partly attributed to decreased sensitivity to adrenaline (Eppinger and Levine, 1934). The operation gained little favour in England. The high blood cholesterol that results does not favour the natural course of the disease, and the doubtful benefits obtained hardly justify the risks and complications of total thyroidectomy.

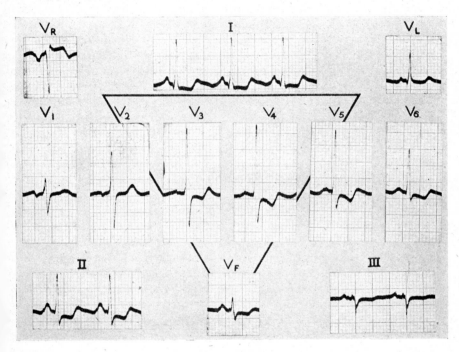

Fig. 15.08—Acute coronary insufficiency showing persistent inversion of the S-T segment in all indirect surface leads.

Thiouracil, however, offers a simple and more easily controlled means of achieving the same object, and can be abandoned at any time if the result is unsatisfactory (Raab, 1945; Ben-Asher, 1947). The dose recommended is 200 to 600 mg. of methyl or propyl thiouracil daily, beginning with the larger dose and gradually reducing it to the minimum that proves effective. If more heroic doses are required, equal quantities of propyl and methyl thiouracil may be given together in the hope of avoiding toxic reactions such as fever, rash and agranulocytosis, the principle being that drug combinations (e.g. sulphonamide mixtures) cause less sensitisation than the same total dose of a single member of the group, while retaining the same therapeutic effect (Lehr, 1948). Cases of severe angina pectoris do not tolerate thiouracil fever well. In the experience of the author, fever and

rash are less common with propyl than with methyl thiouracil. Mercazole, 20–30 mg. three times daily, finally reduced to about 10 mg. t.d.s.,
is equally effective and seems relatively free from complications.

The blood cholesterol should be watched, and if it rises above 300 mg.
per cent the question of reducing the dose of thiouracil or mercazole
should be considered. A low fat diet may help to keep the blood lipids
within bounds.

Radioactive iodine (I^{131}) performs the same service as thyroidectomy
and is equally permanent. It may be given in a single dose of 20 millicuries
or in three divided doses of 10 millicuries at weekly intervals. The B.M.R.
may then be maintained at minus 20–25 per cent by means of small doses
of thyroid. In view of the poor prognosis in these difficult cases the danger
of late malignancy may be disregarded. In their latest review of 720
resistant cases of angina pectoris treated by means of artificial myxœdema,
Blumgart et al. (1955) reported a good result in 75 per cent. I have never
myself been able to develop much enthusiasm for this form of treatment,
partly because of the rise in blood cholesterol that usually takes place, and
partly because it is very difficult to keep patients relatively free from pain
without provoking distressing features of myxœdema; but then I have only
embarked on antithyroid treatment in advanced cases that have been
almost totally incapacitated.

Surgical methods. Several surgical procedures designed to relieve angina
have been evolved in recent years. Few have gained much support, but
there is something to be said in favour of abolishing pain by sensory
denervation of the heart achieved by means of section of the upper four
dorsal spinal nerve roots, or by stellate and upper dorsal ganglionectomy
(White, Garrey and Atkins, 1933). Destruction of the ganglia by alcoholic
injection is less certain, and may cause intractable root pain in about
10 per cent of cases. Despite the theoretical argument that ganglionectomy may remove nature's warning signal, and so allow patients to
exercise themselves beyond the limits of safety, there is no doubt that
some cases do remarkably well (White and Bland, 1948; Lindgren, 1950).
Sensory denervation of the heart does not entirely abolish the subjective
recognition of an anginal attack, although the sensation experienced is not
painful. There is good reason to believe also that sympathectomy tends to
prevent ventricular fibrillation (Leriche et al., 1931; McEachern, 1940),
and seems to improve the coronary circulation either by preventing reflex
spasm (Levy and Moore, 1941), or by causing coronary vasodilatation
(Katz and Jochim, 1939).

A more drastic surgical procedure aims at improving the coronary circulation by supplying it with a new source of collateral vessels. The idea
was based on necropsy observations which showed that the heart might
function remarkably well despite almost complete coronary occlusion, if for
some reason an adequate collateral circulation had developed through the
pericardium. These natural results of accident and disease have been man

shalled and developed by Claud Beck (1935–36) in the U.S.A., and by O'Shaugnessy (1936–37) in England. Beck sutured a flap of pectoral muscle to the surface of the heart; O'Shaugnessy preferred cardio-omentopexy, the omentum being brought up through the diaphragm and stitched or glued on to the surface of the heart after scarification. Whilst experimental evidence affords convincing proof of the establishment of a collateral circulation by such means, the results obtained in clinical cases of ischæmic heart disease scarcely justify the risk entailed.

A simpler means of achieving the same object is to introduce bone dust into the pericardial sac; when the pericardial reaction subsides, vascular adhesions offer a collateral source of blood supply to the myocardium (King, 1941). Powdered magnesium silicate serves equally well (Thompson and Plachta, 1953).

ACUTE CORONARY INSUFFICIENCY

The term *acute coronary insufficiency* (Master *et al.*, 1947) is now widely used to describe those cases of ischæmic heart disease that cannot properly be called angina pectoris or cardiac infarction, but rather something between the two. Some cases are subacute or even chronic.

Physiologically the coronary circulation is insufficient to meet the full demands of the myocardium at rest, yet sufficient to prevent myocardial necrosis. Since the situation commonly develops relatively suddenly, it is usually attributed to coronary thrombosis or possibly to subintimal hæmorrhage.

Special forms of acute coronary insufficiency may be caused by any agent that temporarily interferes with the coronary blood flow, e.g. hæmorrhage (Master *et al.*, 1950), shock (Wiggers, 1947), vaso-vagal syncope, asphyxia, and carbon monoxide poisoning; especially if the work of the heart is increased simultaneously, as in paroxysmal tachycardia, atrial flutter (or fibrillation), massive pulmonary embolism, and ruptured aortic cusp; greatly increased cardiac work alone may also cause coronary insufficiency (especially when there is latent coronary disease), as in hypertensive or thyrotoxic crises.

Clinically, the onset is usually acute or subacute: from a state of normal or relatively good health, the patient suddenly finds himself unable to walk more than a few yards without pain, and may have prolonged attacks of angina at rest, particularly after food and when he lies flat; but the pain is still relieved by trinitrin, there is no fever, leucocytosis, elevation of the sedimentation rate or increased transaminase activity, the blood pressure does not fall, there is no pericardial friction or other clinical evidence of cardiac infarction, and the electrocardiogram shows nothing more than ischæmic depression of the RS-T segment in left ventricular surface leads or their equivalents (fig. 15.08). These electrocardiographic changes usually persist for several days or weeks and are not confined to attacks of pain.

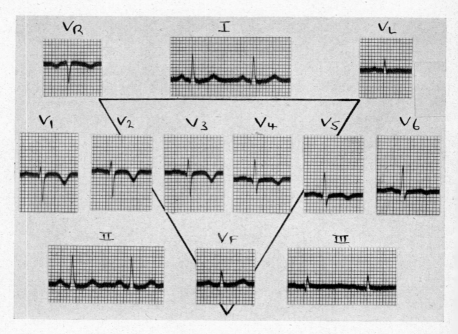

Fig. 15.09—Transient inversion of the T waves in all chest leads in a case of acute coronary insufficiency.

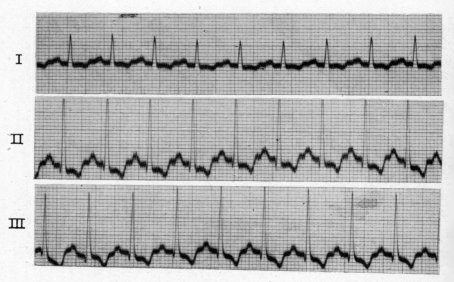

Fig. 15.10—Electrocardiogram showing transient inversion of the T waves following prolonged circulatory collapse with extreme tachycardia, without evidence of structural disease of the heart.

Transient inversion of the T waves proper, without abnormal Q waves and without elevation of the RS-T segment, may also occur in coronary insufficiency (fig. 15.09), but is more difficult to interpret, for it is also compatible with a small cardiac infarction. Simple transient inversion of the T waves is common in the special forms of coronary insufficiency mentioned above (fig. 15.10), especially following prolonged paroxysmal tachycardia, in paroxysmal hypertension from pheochromocytoma, and in carbon monoxide poisoning (fig. 15.11).

Treatment

Patients with acute coronary insufficiency should be put to bed for a minimum period of three weeks and treated with anticoagulants (page 746) in order to prevent extension of thrombosis; the fear that a subintimal hæmorrhage may be aggravated by such treatment is not substantiated in practice. Treatment should be continued for at least three weeks after attacks of pain have ceased, which may mean for two to three months in obstinate cases. These prolonged subacute cases may be very trying to all concerned, and it might seem better to abandon treatment in the hope that the ischæmic zone would then necrose and the pain cease. While it is agreed that this may happen and the patient be the better for it, it is unfortunately impossible to predict the consequences, which are just as likely to be disastrous. "Controlled cardiac infarction" is beyond our present therapeutic powers. It is far better, therefore, to continue anti-coagulant treatment, with or without the temporary help of an antithyroid drug, for sooner or later the situation is likely to ease as the result of an improved collateral circulation.

That anticoagulant therapy alters favourably the immediate outcome and future course of cases of acute coronary insufficiency has not yet been proved, but I have little doubt that it does. Cardiac infarction is preceded by symptoms of acute coronary insufficiency in at least one-quarter of all cases (Mounsey, 1951); of a personal series of 25 cases of acute coronary insufficiency not treated with anticoagulants no less than 12 developed acute cardiac infarction within three weeks, and five of these died; of 33 similar cases treated with anticoagulants only two developed cardiac infarction within the month, neither of which died, and a third steadily deteriorated and died suddenly a week after the onset of treatment. Both series are small because the criteria on which the diagnosis was based were strict (Wood, 1948).

Prognosis

Long-term follow-up studies of cases proved at the time to have acute coronary insufficiency rather than cardiac infarction await analysis. The immediate outcome depends largely on whether cardiac infarction develops or not, as explained above. Less than 5 per cent die abruptly from ventricular fibrillation without infarction.

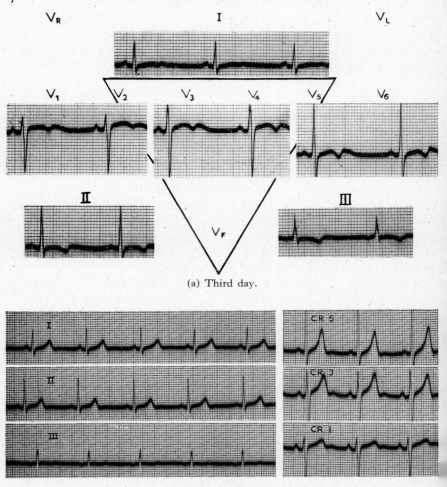

(a) Third day.

(b) Twelve days later.

Fig. 15.11—Transient inversion of the T waves due to carbon monoxide poisoning.

CARDIAC INFARCTION

Myocardial infarction occurs when a mass of heart muscle is sufficiently deprived of its blood supply for an adequate time. The common cause of such an event is coronary thrombosis; but coronary embolism, subintimal hæmorrhage in an atherosclerotic vessel, dissection, and critical lowering of the blood pressure, as from shock or hæmorrhage, in a patient with occlusive coronary atherosclerosis or syphilitic aortitis may each produce it. Again, coronary thrombosis does not cause myocardial infarction if the collateral circulation is sufficient to preserve the life of the threatened tissue. It follows that coronary thrombosis and myocardial infarction are not synonymous terms and should not be confused; the former means no more than its literal sense implies; the latter means death of a localised mass of heart muscle.

ANATOMY OF THE CORONARY CIRCULATION

The site and extent of the infarct depend upon the vessel or vessels occluded, upon the capacity and efficiency of collateral channels, and upon the anatomy of the coronary circulation.

There are two main coronary arteries, left and right. The left divides early into an anterior descending branch and into a left circumflex: the large anterior descending branch runs down the interventricular groove to the apex of the heart, and nourishes the anterior part of the right ventricle, the interventricular septum, and the anterior and apical part of the left ventricle; the smaller left circumflex branch curls round the back between the left atrium and ventricle, and supplies the upper lateral and posterior basal portion of the left ventricle. The right coronary artery does not divide, but runs round to the back between the right atrium and ventricle, sending branches to the region of the sinus node, to the anterior part of the right ventricle and to the posterior base of both ventricles. There is a considerable degree of anastomosis between the terminal branches of these vessels, an anastomosis that increases rapidly when the blood supply to any area is threatened (Prinzmetal *et al.*, 1947). The right ventricle, supplied as it is by the two biggest coronary arteries, and offering little resistance to systolic coronary blood flow, is rarely the seat of infarction. The upper and lateral part of the left ventricle is supplied by proximal branches from both anterior descending and left circumflex vessels, and is therefore relatively safe. The posterior basal region is less secure, for it is supplied only by terminal branches, some from the right coronary artery and some from the left circumflex. In having this double source of nourishment, however, it is still more fortunate than the anterior apex of the left ventricle, which is fed almost entirely by terminal rami from the anterior descending branch of the left coronary artery, although anastomotic channels can develop rapidly from the posterior descending branch of the right coronary artery. The interventricular septum is supplied anteriorly by perforating branches from the anterior descending coronary artery, and posteriorly by perforating branches from the right. Anastomoses are more conspicuous in the superficial layers of the myocardium than in the inner layers (Prinzmetal *et al.*, 1948); they are also at a physiological disadvantage when near the endocardium because they are subjected to a higher intramyocardial pressure (Johnson *et al.*, 1939).

SITE OF THROMBOSIS AND INFARCTION

Clinically, major coronary thrombosis involves the anterior descending branch of the left coronary artery in 66 to 75 per cent of cases, the right coronary artery in 25 to 40 per cent, and the left circumflex in 5 to 33 per cent (Barnes and Ball, 1932; Appelbaum and Nicolson, 1935; Munck,

1946); thrombosis of the left main trunk is relatively rare. These figures are conservative, for careful study of the whole coronary tree by means of radio-opaque injections reveals multiple thromboses in the majority of instances.

The relative incidence of the various sites of infarction harmonises with the anatomical and physiological data, and with the sites of thrombosis. In an analysis of 160 cases, Wartman and Hellerstein (1948) found chiefly anterior infarction in 72 per cent and chiefly posterior infarction in 28 per cent, but there were multiple infarcts in 41 per cent. Half the anterior infarcts and a quarter of the posterior infarcts also involved the inter-ventricular septum. Right ventricular infarction rarely occurs alone, but may complicate anteroseptal infarction of the left ventricle (Zaus and Kearns, 1952). Atrial infarction has also been described (Hellerstein, 1948).

Combining figures published by Appelbaum and Nicolson (1935), Nathanson (1936), Clawson (1939), and Munck (1946), it is found that coronary thrombosis occurs without cardiac infarction in 20 per cent of cases, and that cardiac infarction occurs without coronary thrombosis in 29 per cent; in the latter group atherosclerotic occlusion may be complete or incomplete.

PATHOLOGY

A cardiac infarct may be difficult to distinguish with the naked eye when less than twenty-four hours old; microscopically, however, acute necrosis of the muscle fibres may be recognised by their swollen appearance and by the loss of their nuclei and striations. When a few days old an infarct is discoloured and may be surrounded by a red zone of hæmorrhage or congestion. Microscopically the necrosed muscle is seen to be invaded by polymorphs. Older infarcts are yellowish white in colour and represent scar tissue.

When necrosis involves the inner layers of the myocardium, mural thrombi frequently form against the damaged endocardium; in fact they are found in 40 to 50 per cent of all cases (Hellerstein and Martin, 1947). Local pericarditis occurs over superficial necrosis and has been reported in 30 to 75 per cent of all cases (Wartman and Hellerstein, 1948; Stewart and Turner, 1938); diffuse pericarditis develops in about 10 per cent.

Myocardial softening (myomalacia cordis) may result in rupture of the heart (5 to 15 per cent) or in the formation of a cardiac aneurysm (10 to 30 per cent, according to published necropsy figures and according to the definition of an aneurysm).

Precipitating agents. If due allowance is made for the average time occupied by sleep, ordinary activities, and physical effort during each twenty-four hours, then coronary thrombosis (at least in men under 40) occurs six times more frequently during physical effort than during sleep, and twice as frequently during physical effort as during ordinary day-to-day activities (Yater *et al.*, 1948). Unaccustomed effort, particularly, may precipitate an attack.

The peak incidence of coronary thrombosis is in December (Brown and Pearson, 1948), but according to Teng and Heyer (1955) is more related to sudden changes of temperature than to the cold *per se*. Certainly, going out into the cold after leaving a warm room very commonly provokes an attack of angina pectoris in ischæmic subjects. Clearing the drive of snow includes both unaccustomed effort and the change from a warm to a cold temperature, and is a known precipitating cause of coronary thrombosis.

A heavy meal is often blamed, but statistical evidence on the point is not available. Sexual intercourse is in the same category. Both are notorious causes of an attack of angina pectoris. There is likewise as yet no proof that a prolonged period of excessive mental stress can be responsible, although experience favours the view that it can.

Other known precipitating agents include surgical "shock", the post-operative state, trauma, and a sudden fall of blood pressure.

SYMPTOMS

Although the onset of cardiac infarction is sudden, premonitory symptoms are common during the preceding week or so and take the form of typical or atypical angina pectoris. Then, or without warning of any kind, and often without any obvious precipitating cause, the major attack overwhelms the patient, and is commonly signalled by pain indistinguishable in site, radiation, and quality, from angina pectoris; but instead of passing off in a few minutes, it lasts for hours. Its intensity varies from a feeling of pressure to extreme agony, and gives no indication of the size of the infarct. There may be no other symptoms; on the other hand there may be collapse, weakness, faintness, sweating, restlessness, breathlessness, and vomiting. Whilst a classical attack is characterised by pain, others present with syncope, and yet others with suffocation. In the syncopal type, which represents a vaso-vagal reaction, loss of consciousness may prevent appreciation of pain; when paroxysmal cardiac dyspnœa or acute pulmonary œdema dominates the scene, the patient usually admits pain on close questioning. The lack of agreement in the literature concerning the frequency of painless infarction (0–61 per cent) may be explained by the heterogeneous manner in which historical data is collected and by lack of uniformity with regard to the definition of the word *painless*. In about one-third of all cases patients deny pain in its ordinary sense, preferring words like discomfort, pressure, tightness, oppression or heaviness—as in angina pectoris. Less than 5 per cent of cases of cardiac infarction have no ischæmic sensation at all; about half of these are entirely silent and discovered by routine electrocardiography.

PHYSICAL SIGNS

Unlike angina pectoris, myocardial infarction provides a wealth of physical signs and special findings. When first seen the patient is usually grey, cold, sweating, obviously ill and in pain; he may be breathless and cyanosed, or he may be pale and collapsed—perhaps unconscious; on the other hand, he may present none of these features. Within two or three days mild cases may look and feel well.

The jugular venous pressure is sometimes a little raised during the first day or two, and the pulse rate accelerated; but in cases with a vaso-vagal reaction there may be bradycardia. There may be orthopnœa, paroxysmal cardiac dyspnœa or frank pulmonary œdema in severe cases.

The *blood pressure* falls initially only in cases with a vaso-vagal reaction, and indeed may be elevated during the first twelve hours or so (Weiss, 1939); in animals it is similarly maintained for the first twenty-four hours (Gross *et al.*, 1938); but it drops later, commonly reaching its lowest level on the third or fourth day, when systolic pressures of 80 to 90 mm. of mercury are often found. Thereafter it remains low for several days, or even for weeks, and then in all who survive, climbs slowly back towards its previous level, which it may or may not reach (fig. 15.12). In 67 per cent of fatal cases Chambers (1947) observed no such recovery. In hypertensive subjects this drop in pressure may not be recognised unless the original level is known.

The *heart sounds* are often faint, particularly when the blood pressure is low, and there may be presystolic or diastolic gallop rhythm. Transient *pericardial friction* is heard in about 10 per cent of cases, especially when the infarct is anterior. *Disturbances of rhythm* are not uncommon and include ectopic beats, paroxysmal ventricular tachycardia, auricular flutter or fibrillation, and any grade of heart block.

Low-grade fever is the rule and may continue for several days, but rarely for more than a week. Transient polymorphonuclear *leucocytosis* also occurs during the first few days, and the C-reactive protein test is positive. The *sedimentation rate* begins to accelerate after a day or two, reaches maximum velocity towards the end of the first week, and then gradually returns to normal in an average period of six weeks from the onset (fig. 15.13) (Wood, 1936).

During the first 48 hours the *serum glutamic oxalacetic transaminase* (S.G.O.-T) activity is sharply increased from the normal of 10 to 40 units to any level up to 800 units, the height to which it rises being proportional to the mass of necrosed myocardium (La Due *et al.*, 1954, 1955). S.G.O.-T is an enzyme employed in the synthesis of glutamic and oxalacetic acids, and is widely distributed in the tissues, especially in heart muscle. It is not increased in infectious, neoplastic, metabolic, or degenerative diseases unless there is destruction of cardiac, hepatic or muscular tissue.

ELECTROCARDIOGRAPHIC APPEARANCES

These have already been described and explained in Chapter III. Leads facing the surface of the infarct show a prominent or monophasic Q wave, initial elevation of the RS-T segment, and subsequent inversion of the T wave. Anterior infarcts may be mapped out with precision by means of multiple unipolar chest leads, and may be chiefly anterolateral (fig. 15.14) or anteroseptal (fig. 15.15). The Q-T pattern is usually transmitted to lead V_L and hence mainly to standard lead I; but if the heart is electrically vertical a V_5 Q-T pattern may be transmitted to lead V_F, and hence to standard leads II and III. The Q-T pattern of posterior infarcts is seen in œsophageal leads over the posterior surface of the left ventricle, and is transmitted to lead V_F and hence to standard lead III (fig. 15.16), while chest leads usually show initial depression of the RS-T segment, followed by unusually tall T waves (fig. 15.17).

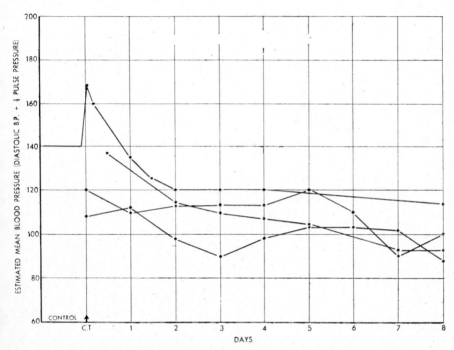

Fig. 15.12—Behaviour of the blood pressure in four cases of acute myocardial infarction.

The abnormal Q wave develops early and may persist indefinitely. Elevation of the R-T segment is usually transient; but a monophasic Q wave associated with persistent elevation of the Q-T segment is often seen with ventricular aneurysm (fig. 15.18). Primary inversion of the T wave appears in a few days, reaches a maximum within two or three weeks, and then gradually reverts towards normal; but slight inversion, with Pardee coving of the RS-T segment, may persist in one or more leads (fig. 15.19).

The diagnosis of acute cardiac infarction is practically untenable if serial electrocardiograms remain normal in all the recognised leads, but an initial electrocardiogram may be normal occasionally if taken within a few hours

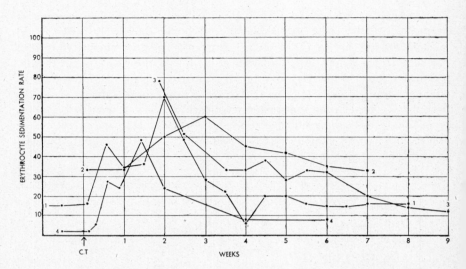

Fig. 15.13—Behaviour of the sedimentation rate in four cases of acute myocardial infarction.

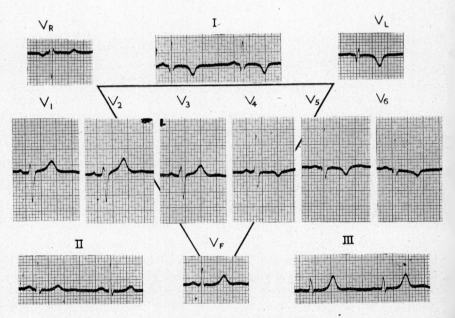

Fig. 15.14—Electrocardiogram showing anterolateral cardiac infarction. Maximum changes are seen in leads V_5, V_6, V_L and standard lead I.

of the onset. This statement may have to be tempered in the light of Prinzmetal's evidence that the inner third of the myocardium may be electrically silent (Prinzmetal *et al.*, 1953), at least in respect of the initial

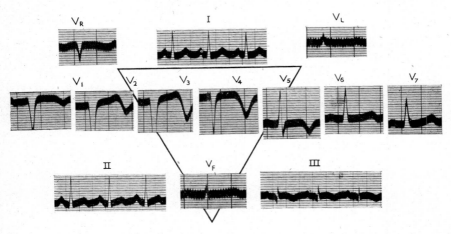

Fig. 15.15—Electrocardiogram showing anteroseptal cardiac infarction. Maximum changes are seen in leads V_3 and V_4.

ventricular complex. The belief that subendocardial infarcts cause depression of the RS-T segment in overlying surface leads (Levine and Ford, 1950) is not supported by Prinzmetal's experimental work (Rakita *et al.*, 1954).

In differential diagnosis great stress is laid on the abnormal Q wave, for this always means appreciable necrosis of heart muscle, however produced. It must, of course, be distinguished from a normal Q wave measuring 2 or 3 mm., and a monophasic downward deflection in standard lead III should not be accepted as a Q wave unless Q is also prominent in standard lead II and in lead V_F (fig. 15.20). Pathological Q waves, however, may be seen occasionally in cases of myocardial necrosis caused by non-ischæmic agents, e.g. isolated myocarditis, amyloidosis, tumour, hydattid, and other rare cardiopathies.

Elevation of the RS-T segment is also seen in pericarditis, and opposite large S waves in appropriate leads in left ventricular preponderance and left bundle branch block; but the contour of the S-T segment and the general pattern is different, as described elsewhere.

Primary inversion of the T wave alone is less conclusive evidence of infarction, for it may be seen in a variety of conditions including toxic myocarditis, pericarditis, carbon monoxide poisoning, myxœdema, certain biochemical states, most of the relatively obscure cardiopathies, and following paroxysmal tachycardia. However, the depth and sharpness of the inversion usually exceed that in all other types, and its association with upward coving of the RS-T segment is practically diagnostic. Changes in

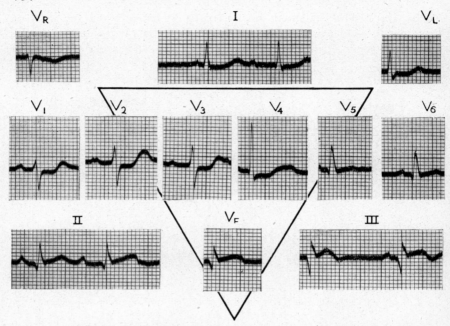

Fig. 15.16—Electrocardiogram showing posterior cardiac infarction. Characteristic changes are seen in leads V_F and hence in leads II and III. The ST segment is depressed in lead V_4.

serial graphs are less helpful, because many of the primary T wave changes mentioned above are also transient.

Bundle branch block, mostly left, occurred in 7.3 per cent of 700 cases of angina pectoris and in 8.9 per cent of 328 cases of cardiac infarction reported by Salcedo-Salgar and White (1935). Conversely they found that ischæmic heart disease accounted for approximately 50 per cent of 181 cases of intraventricular block of all types. Master, Dack and Jaffe (1938) found the

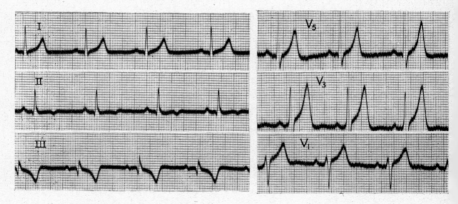

Fig. 15.17—The later stage of posterior infarction showing unusually tall T waves in chest leads.

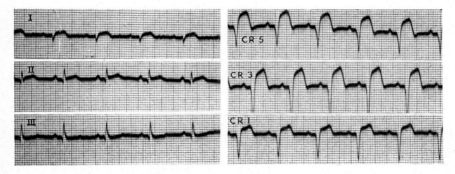

(a) 29th November 1941.

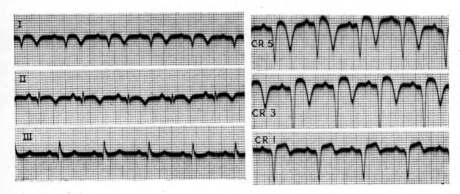

(b) 15th December 1941.

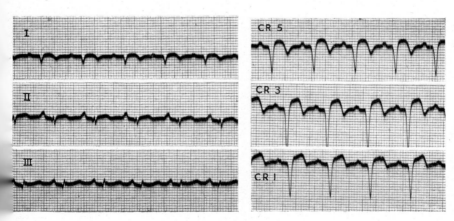

(c) 3rd March 1942.

Fig. 15.18—Electrocardiogram showing widespread monophasic Q waves and persistent elevation of the ST segment associated with ventricular aneurysm.

735

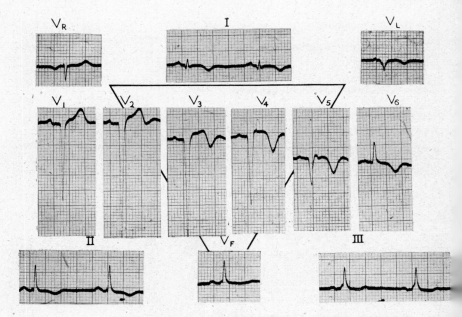

Fig. 15.19—Electrocardiogram of a case of old cardiac infarction showing persistent Q waves and Pardee coving of the ST segment in anterior left ventricular surface leads and their counterparts (leads V_L and standard lead I). The infarct occurred 14 months previously.

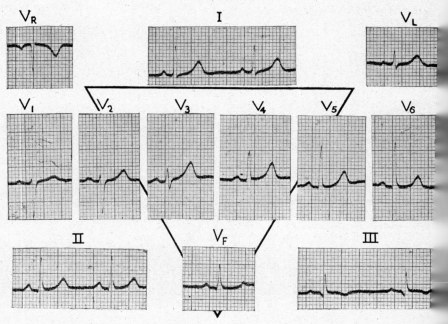

Fig. 15.20—Electrocardiogram in a case of pregnancy showing a prominent Q wave and inversion of the T wave in lead 3 due to cardiac rotation: note the absence of pathological Q wave in lead V_F and the presence of an S wave in standard lead I.

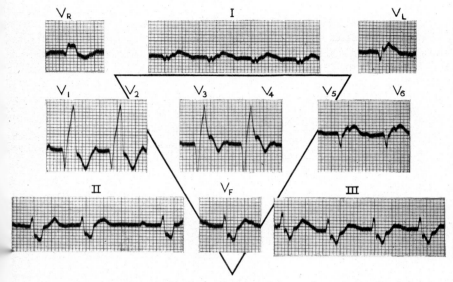

Fig. 15.21—Electrocardiogram showing typical appearances of anterior cardiac infarction in the presence of right bundle branch block.

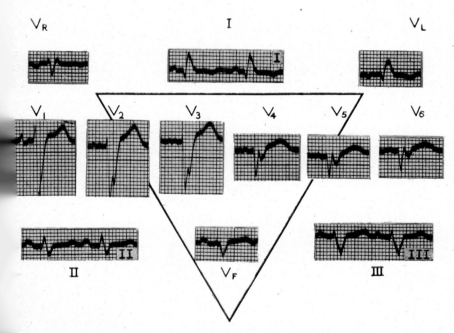

ig. 15.22—Electrocardiogram showing typical appearances of anterior cardiac infarction in the presence of left bundle branch block.

incidence of bundle branch block in acute coronary occlusion to be 12 per cent in 1,058 cases collected from the literature, and 15 per cent in 375 cases of their own. Intraventricular block does not necessarily imply septal infarction in these cases, and, of course, may precede the acute episode. Its importance lies in the fact that it may mask the electrocardiographic signs of cardiac infarction; for as explained on page 99 there can be no Q wave in leads facing the surface of the left ventricle in cases of left bundle branch block unless the septum is also necrosed, and the gross deformity of the R-T component may overshadow RS-T changes due to the infarct. Somerville and Wood (1949), however, found that the characteristic Q-T pattern of an infarct could be recognised in nearly all cases complicated by right bundle branch block (fig. 15.21), and in about half those with left bundle branch block (fig. 15.22).

Electrocardiography may be of great value in the diagnosis of myocardial infarction months or years after the event, an abnormal Q wave, local dwarfing of R, or primary inversion of the T wave in one or more left ventricular surface leads or their counterparts being particularly helpful. Complete restitution of the normal electrocardiographic pattern occurs in only 10 per cent of survivors from acute myocardial infarction (Mills et al., 1949).

RADIOLOGICAL FINDINGS

Fluoroscopy is impracticable during the acute stage of the illness, but may be useful later. An infarct on the left border of the heart near the apex may form a ledge (fig. 15.23). In normal hearts pulsation is seen around the whole surface of the left ventricle; in myocardial infarction there may be local absence of pulsation, or pulsation may be locally paradoxical, a portion of the ventricle expanding while the rest contracts this area of absent or paradoxical pulsation represents the infarct, and may be seen on the left border of the heart towards the apex, or on the disphragmatic surface of the left ventricle (with the aid of gas in the stomach for some reason posterior basal infarcts are less easily visualised. Interpretation of pulsation as seen on the fluoroscope is by no means easy, an requires considerable experience of normal variation. The kymograph, simple device for obtaining a permanent skiagraphic record of cardiac pulsation, has been used with some success as an aid in analysing the findings, and the electrokymograph is even better; but absence of pulsatic at the apex may also be seen occasionally in hypertensive and other form of heart failure.

Ventricular aneurysm is more easily recognised, particularly when situated towards the apex or left lateral border (fig. 4.34). It should not be confused with a dilated left atrium, an intrapericardial hæmatoma, pericardial cyst, or cardiac tumour. Rarely, a ventricular aneurysm may become calcified (fig. 4.35). Increased density and unfolding of the aorta, de to atheroma, with or without calcification, may be seen in many cases, but cannot be regarded as evidence of coronary atherosclerosis; calcified coronary arteries (Snellen and Nauta, 1937) offer more convincing proof, but even these do not necessarily signify ischæmic heart disease.

Apart from the changes mentioned, the size and shape of the heart are usually normal in cases of uncomplicated cardiac infarction (Miller and Weiss, 1928); enlargement is commonly due to heart failure or to coincident hypertensive heart disease.

With the aid of retrograde aortography via the right radial artery the entire coronary tree may be seen and the exact site of any obstruction identified (Coelho *et al.*, 1953); but the method is certainly not without risk and cannot be recommended as a safe diagnostic procedure.

COMPLICATIONS

(first 28 days)

	PERIOD (early, mid or late)	FREQUENCY (per cent)	MORTALITY (per cent of all cases)
Abrupt death (ventricular fibrillation or asystole) .	Onset	?25	?25
	Early or mid	10	10
Shock	Early	10 to 15	7 to 12
Conventional heart failure .	Mid and late	10 to 15	3 to 5
Rupture			
of heart	Early	1.5 to 3	1.5 to 3
of septum . . .	Early	Rare	Rare
of papillary muscle . .	Early	Rare	Rare
Cardiac aneurysm . .	Early (recognised late)	5 to 10	(See rupture; those recognised commonly survive)
Pericarditis . . .	Early	10	(See rupture; majority survive)
Thrombo-embolism			
Pulmonary . . .	Mid and late	15	2 to 3
Systemic (chiefly cerebral)	Mid	5 to 10	1 to 2
Changes of rhythm			
Atrial fibrillation . .	Early	10	Changes of rhythm increase the mortality from cardiogenic shock and heart failure.
Atrial flutter or tachycardia	Early	2	
Ventricular tachycardia .	Early	2	
Complete heart block .	Early	1	
TOTAL (excluding abrupt death at onset) . .	—	—	25 to 30

COURSE AND COMPLICATIONS

The acute stage lasts on the average for six weeks, during the earlier part of which many complications may arise (see table), the gravest danger being abrupt death from *ventricular fibrillation* (fig. 15.24). About 10 per cent of all cases that survive long enough to be admitted to hospital die in this way, and there must be many others that go to the coroner. Thus of 866 cases in relatively young men reported by Yater *et al.* (1948) 16 per cent died at once, and another 10 per cent within 15 minutes; none of these cases would have had time to be admitted to hospital. If coroners' cases are included, therefore, it is likely that at least one-third of all cases of acute cardiac infarction die from ventricular fibrillation or asystole.

Other disturbances of rhythm are also relatively common and include ventricular ectopic beats, paroxysmal ventricular tachycardia (2 per cent), paroxysmal auricular flutter (2 per cent) and fibrillation (10 per cent), nodal rhythm and heart block. They should be regarded seriously because they may herald ventricular fibrillation or precipitate heart failure. Complete heart block (1 per cent) is particularly lethal (Mintz and Katz, 1947).

Shock attending the first stage of acute cardiac infarction is characterised clinically by pallor, sweating, vomiting, coldness of the extremities and exposed surfaces, faintness or loss of consciousness, great weakness, restlessness, oliguria or anuria, small pulse, tachycardia or bradycardia, and low blood pressure; physiologically the cardiac output is much reduced, the peripheral resistance raised, the circulation time prolonged and the venous pressure raised (Freis *et al.*, 1952; Gilbert *et al.*, 1954). Fundamentally, therefore, there is a state of acute and severe heart failure although peripheral circulatory failure may complicate the picture, and sweating, vomiting and a slow pulse rate suggest powerful vagal activity "Cardiogenic shock" occurs in 10 to 15 per cent of cases and is fatal in two-thirds to three-quarters of them (Selzer, 1952).

Heart failure may present more conventionally either as left ventricular failure or congestive heart failure. Acute left ventricular failure with pulmonary œdema may occur at the onset, or a more insidious form with dyspnœa and orthopnœa may develop later, not infrequently during convalescence. Congestive failure, with a rise of venous pressure, distension of the liver and œdema may also be a relatively late complication, and increases the risk of phlebothrombosis and pulmonary embolism. Conventional heart failure, distinct from cardiogenic shock, usually responds to treatment in the first instance, but is a common cause of death during the ensuing twelve months. During the acute stage of cardiac infarction (first 28 days) it occurs as frequently as shock (10 to 15 per cent of cases) and proves fatal in approximately 3 to 5 per cent. It is very difficult to obtain precise figures from the literature, for cardiogenic shock and conventional heart failure are frequently grouped together.

Thrombo-embolic lesions in various situations are detected clinically in about 20 per cent of cases, and may be found at necropsy in about 45 p

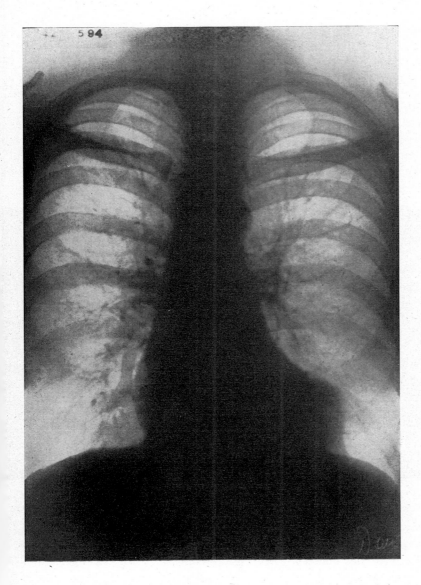

Fig. 15.23—Skiagram in a case of anterior cardiac infarction showing a ledge on the left border of the heart.

cent (Hellerstein and Martin, 1947). The dangerous period is from the fifth or sixth day to the end of the third week, when the clotting time is shortened (Ogura *et al.*, 1946). Phlebothrombosis in the legs resulting in pulmonary embolism is by far the most common clinical manifestation, and is responsible for death in 2 to 3 per cent of all cases of acute cardiac infarction. In a series of 200 fatal cases of coronary thrombosis reported by Eppinger and Kennedy (1938), pulmonary embolism was directly responsible for death in 6.5 per cent, was present in 24.5 per cent, and complicated 32.7 per cent of those with heart failure. The usual frequency of pulmonary embolism in all cases of cardiac infarction that survive long enough to be admitted to hospital is 15 per cent (Evans, 1954).

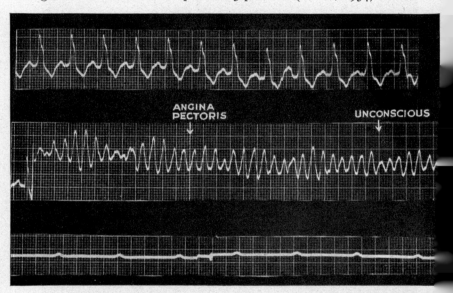

Fig. 15.24—Electrocardiogram showing the mode of death in a case of ischæmic heart disease: ventricular fibrillation developed while a routine graph was being taken.

Systemic embolism (or thrombosis) is detected *clinically* in 5 to 10 per cent of cases, the majority of them cerebral. Only 1 to 2 per cent of all cases of acute cardiac infarction die from cerebral or other systemic embolism. Hellerstein and Martin give the actual incidence of various thrombo-embolic lesions as follows:

	Per cent
Pulmonary	23.5
Renal	14.4
Splenic	8.8
Cerebral	7.7
Peripheral arteries	5.5
Mesenteric	1.9
Carotid or aortic	0.5

Mural thrombosis is found at necropsy in 44 per cent of all fatal cases of cardiac infarction, and is presumed to be the source of the peripheral vascular lesions; the fact that these lesions have been found in 46 per cent of cases with mural thrombosis (Wang, Bland and White, 1948), and in 39 per cent of cases without mural thrombosis does not invalidate this view, for fresh intraventricular clots may be dislodged and leave no evidence of their origin. On the other hand, pulmonary embolism is nearly always attributable to phlebothrombosis in the legs, not to right ventricular mural thrombosis, and cerebral vascular lesions may certainly result from coincidental local thrombosis (Bean, 1938).

Cardiac rupture occurs in 1.5 to 3 per cent, or in 5 to 10 per cent of fatal cases (Oblath, Levinson and Griffith, 1952), usually within the first four days of the illness, and chiefly in the older patients (Gans, 1951); it is not necessarily a dramatic event, for the perforation may be small, and the signs and symptoms often those of cardiac compression from hæmoperi-cardium rather than sudden catastrophe, such cases sometimes living a week or more. *Perforation of the interventricular septum* is seen occasionally, and gives rise to the sudden development of a coarse systolic thrill and murmur in the third and fourth intercostal spaces towards the sternum (Fowler and Failey, 1948). Heart failure has ensued rapidly in most of the cases reported (e.g. Leonard and Daniels, 1938). Although the perforation may look small at necropsy and the track tortuous, the shunt during life may be considerable, as has been proved (inadvisedly) by means of cardiac catheterisation. More than half the cases have died within the month.

Rupture of one of the papillary muscles is a rare complication of cardiac infarction and results in the sudden development of severe mitral in-competence with secondary acute and intractable left ventricular failure, usually ending in death (Craddock and Mahe, 1953).

Left ventricular aneurysm may be found at necropsy in as many as 22 per cent of fatal cases (Wartman and Hellerstein, 1948), but is recognised clinically in less than half of them. In the series referred to above, 25 were anterior and 10 posterior; five of them ruptured. The condition arises early and may be well developed by the time the patient is allowed up for fluoroscopy. The X-ray appearances have already been described (page 38). Clinically it is suggested by an unusual pulsation in the region of the apex beat when left ventricular enlargement is improbable on other grounds. Scherf and Brooks (1949) described an odd, high-pitched, rushing, soft diastolic murmur over the aneurysm in three of their cases, but this is unusual. The electrocardiogram usually shows a monophasic R wave and conspicuous and rather persistent elevation of the Q-T segment over the aneurysm, while the main QRS deflection is often upright in lead V_R (Goldberger and Schwartz, 1948) (fig. 15.25). If rupture does not occur during the first few weeks the prognosis is little, if at all, influenced by the aneurysm (Moyer and Hiller, 1951).

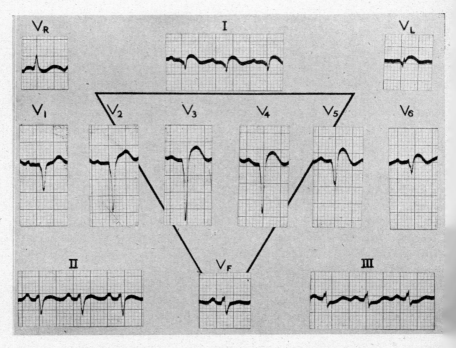

Fig. 15.25—Monophasic Q waves and persistent elevation of the S-T segment in all chest leads in a case of left ventricular aneurysm.

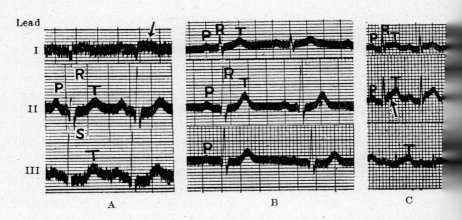

Fig. 15.26—Cardiac infarction complicated by perforation and hæmopericardium.

A. Original anterior cardiac infarction.

B. After recovery.

C. After perforation of infarct (hæmopericardium).

Pericarditis may be of three kinds: (1) a transient friction rub may be heard over an anterior apical infarct, and represents a local pericardial reaction; (2) there may be widespread pericarditis with friction heard at all areas or at a distance from the lesion, which may complicate either anterior or posterior infarcts; (3) there may be hæmopericardium resulting from ventricular perforation. Local pericarditis does not alter the electrocardiographic pattern of infarction; but widespread pericarditis may do so, and hæmopericardium invariably does (fig. 15.26). Pericardial friction of one kind or another is heard in about 10 per cent of cases.

After-effects. The subsequent course is determined by the effect of the occlusion on the total coronary circulation and the amount of healthy muscle left. Angina pectoris may develop, or if it was present before it may be worse; on the other hand, if previous pain was due to local ischæmia at the site of the recent infarct, angina may improve or temporarily disappear. Left ventricular or congestive heart failure may develop during convalescence or subsequently, and may cause the disappearance of angina. Later cardiac rupture is rare, and usually denotes fresh coronary occlusion. Less than 10 per cent of ruptured hearts are due to an old ventricular aneurysm (Munck, 1946).

DIFFERENTIAL DIAGNOSIS

In the differential diagnosis of myocardial infarction, many conditions must be borne in mind; the most confusing are massive pulmonary embolism, acute pericarditis, dissecting aneurysm of the aorta, diaphragmatic hernia, œsophageal or gastric dysfunction, and acute pancreatitis; but diaphragmatic pleurisy, especially when bilateral, disease of the gallbladder, perforated duodenal ulcer, epidemic myalgia, and pain referred from the spine may give rise to difficulty. In *pulmonary embolism* the most important clue is early engorgement of the cervical veins and immediate hypotension, whilst rhythm changes are very rare; otherwise, both symptoms and signs may be indistinguishable from those of coronary thrombosis, and even limb-lead electrocardiograms may resemble those of posterior cardiac infarction. Fortunately, however, chest-lead graphs are diagnostic (page 813). *Acute pericarditis* may simulate cardiac infarction closely, but may be distinguished by the electrocardiogram (page 658). *Dissecting aneurysm* is characterised by radiation of pain to the back and downwards, by hypertension, by the absence of electrocardiographic change, by the development of aortic incompetence, and perhaps by signs of involvement of carotid, subclavian, renal or femoral arteries (page 924). *Diaphragmatic hernia* should be considered when there are no changes in temperature, white count, E.S.R., and electrocardiogram, and may be diagnosed by means of a barium meal with the patient in the head-down position. *Œsophageal or gastric pain* may be felt in the centre of the chest and may resemble the pain of cardiac infarction; but physical examination is entirely negative, the electrocardiogram remains normal, and the subsequent course is benign. *Acute pancreatitis* may be recognised by the urinary diastase test.

TREATMENT

Patients should be *confined to bed* at once and should remain there for three to six weeks, or longer, according to the severity of the illness and to the behaviour of the sedimentation rate and electrocardiogram. If the blood pressure is low and the patient faint or dizzy, he may have to lie flat; otherwise, and particularly if there is any sign of failure, he should be propped up against a back-rest in order to reduce the work of the heart.

Semi-starvation for the first few days, followed by an 800-calorie diet during the dangerous period, practically halves the mortality rate (Master *et al.*, 1936). Fruit drinks and soft, stewed or fresh fruit with sugar and a little milk is all that should be allowed for the first forty-eight hours. The quality of the later light diet matters less than its bulk and calorific value, but should contain little sodium if there is any evidence of failure, and little fat.

The most beneficial drug in the acute phase is *morphine*, which should be given in adequate doses and as often as required to relieve pain and distress, and to induce rest and sleep. Excellent results are obtained when pain is severe by giving it intravenously in a dose not exceeding $\frac{1}{4}$ of a grain (15 mg.) dissolved in at least 2 ml. of sterile water or saline, and at a slow rate, three minutes being taken over the injection. *Pethidine*, 50 to 100 mg. by mouth, may be taken subsequently at four- to six-hourly intervals, if necessary.

Quinidine, 3 to 5 grains (0.25 G.) t.d.s., has been given in the hope of preventing ventricular fibrillation and other changes of rhythm, but with little success (Cutts and Rapoport, 1952), although it prevents ventricular fibrillation in dogs (Wegria and Nickerson, 1943).

Heparin and certain prothrombin inhibitors such as dicoumarol, tromexan (ethyl biscoumacetate), and dindevan (phenylindanedione) have been used widely in recent years to prevent extension of coronary thrombosis, mural thrombosis and phlebothrombosis.

Heparin, 15,000 units, should be given intravenously at once, followed by 15,000 units intramuscularly or subcutaneously eight-hourly during the first two days. Dindevan should also be given as soon as possible, starting with 150 mg. on the first day, 100 mg. on the second, and 50 mg. on the morning of the third, subsequent doses being regulated according to the prothrombin time, which should be maintained at two and a half times the prothrombin time in a normal control, i.e. at a ratio of 2.5. The treatment should be started at once in the patient's home, for laboratory control is unnecessary until the third day.

The results of such treatment in 432 cases were compared with those of conservative management in 368 controls by a special committee of the American Heart Association, and were reported by Wright, Marple and Beck (1948). The chief findings were as follows:

	Controls per cent	Cases treated with anticoagulants per cent
Mortality	24	15
Thrombo-embolic deaths . .	10	3
Thrombo-embolic complications .	25	11

Very similar figures for 301 cases treated with anticoagulants and 160 controls were published by Kerwin (1953): in the treated group the mortality was 17.9 per cent and the incidence of thrombo-embolic complications 7.6 per cent; in the control series the mortality was 29.4 per cent and the incidence of thrombo-embolic complications 20 per cent. In Great Britain the results of anticoagulant therapy have been much the same. Gilchrist and Tulloch (1954), for instance, treated 321 cases over a period of seven years and claimed to have halved the mortality rate.

Considering the uniformity of published results of anticoagulant therapy it is remarkable that many critical observers still feel uneasy about their reliability (e.g. Evans, 1954). The difficulty in accepting the figures arises from the disbelief that drugs like dicoumarol, tromexan and dindevan could diminish the mortality from ventricular fibrillation, shock, cardiac rupture and heart failure, which together should be responsible for the great majority of deaths. Prior to anticoagulant treatment deaths from pulmonary and systemic embolism were put no higher than 5 per cent, so that allowing for a five-fold decrease in thrombo-embolic mortality (Wright, Marple and Beck, 1954), it is still difficult to see why the total death rate should fall more than 4 per cent. It is possible, however, that extension of coronary thrombosis is a more important cause of disaster than at present believed, and that anticoagulants tend to prevent this. Of 95 deaths from cardiac infarction analysed by Selzer (1948), for instance, five were attributed to secondary coronary thrombosis. Both heparin and dicoumarol also appear to be coronary vasodilators (Gilbert and Nalefski, 1949) and may therefore improve the total coronary flow.

According to Schnur (1953) and Russek and Zohman (1954), the risk of serious hæmorrhage (1 per cent) does not justify the use of anticoagulants in mild cases, for in these the natural mortality is only 3 per cent, and the frequency of thrombo-embolism 0.8 per cent. By mild is meant a first attack, absence of shock, disappearance of severe pain within a few hours, normal rhythm, absence of heart failure, absence of gallop rhythm, no cardiac enlargement, and no diabetes. Against this attitude may be set the negligible risk of hæmorrhage when dindevan is used and when good laboratory facilities are available, and the disastrous consequences that may follow extension of the thrombosis.

Permanent anticoagulant treatment to prevent further attacks of coronary thrombosis is under trial (Nichol and Borg, 1950). An encouraging report comes from Suzman, Ruskin and Goldberg (1955), who treated 82 cases continuously over periods ranging between three months and six years. Comparing the results with those of 88 untreated controls observed over the same period, they found the mortality was reduced from 33 to 7.3 per cent, and the frequency of recurrences of coronary thrombosis from 24 to 7 per cent. When severe cases only were considered (67 cases) the mortality was still only 9 per cent in the treated group, compared with 46.7 per cent in 60 untreated controls, and the frequency of recurrences 7 per cent against 21 per cent in the controls. Owren (1954) treated 128 cases of uncomplicated angina pectoris with dicoumarol or dindevan for one to five years; coronary thrombosis occurred in ten instances during this period, and the mortality during the first year of treatment was 5 per cent; of 108 patients who had had one previous attack of cardiac infarction, seven developed a second coronary thrombosis during the same one- to five-year period of anticoagulent treatment. These results compare favourably with the natural course of ischæmic heart disease.

The *coronary vasodilators*, with the possible exception of aminophylline, do not relieve the pain of cardiac infarction, and do not influence its course; aminophylline may perhaps improve the collateral circulation and may help to prevent cardiac asthma.

Oxygen may be given in severe cases, but is not routine therapy in Great Britain. There may be some advantage in supersaturating the arterial blood, particularly when respiration is depressed spontaneously or as a result of morphine.

Cortisone has been said to halve the mortality from experimental cardiac infarction in animals (Johnson *et al.*, 1953); moreover, infarcts produced in the treated animals were found to be far smaller than in the controls. Healing, however, was delayed and fibroblastic proliferation much decreased. Opdyke (1953), on the other hand, found no diminution in the size of experimentally induced infarcts in cortisone-treated animals.

Treatment of complications

Shock has been treated actively in recent years and its mortality has been reduced from 80 to 50 per cent. Blood transfusion was tried (Epstein and Relman, 1949), but soon abandoned, and intra-arterial infusion proved no better (Berman *et al.*, 1952); but encouraging results have been obtained with vasopressor drugs such as mephentermine, noradrenaline, and aramine.

Mephentermine (wyamine) may be given intramuscularly in a dose of 30 to 40 mg., and repeated when necessary, or intravenously at the rate of 1 mg. per minute until the blood pressure is 120 mm. Hg, which is usually reached in 5 to 20 minutes (Hellerstein, Brofman and Caskey, 1952).

Noradrenaline, or L-noradrenaline (levophed) 10 mg. dissolved in a litre of 5 per cent glucose solution, may be given by intravenous drip infusion at the rate of 10 to 20 drops per minute; each ml. (15 drops) of the solution contains 10μg. of noradrenaline. The rate of infusion should be regulated to maintain the blood pressure at 120 mm. Hg, and continued as long as necessary (up to 72 hours). In England Shirley Smith and Guz (1953) reported encouraging results with this treatment. In the United States, Griffiths et al. (1954) reduced the mortality of shocked cases from 80 to 47.8 per cent: prior to the treatment 128 out of 161 shocked patients died in their series of 816 proved cases of acute coronary thrombosis; since starting treatment with pressor amines 64 out of 134 shocked cases died, and when treatment was begun within three hours of the onset, only 13 per cent died. These figures are impressive.

Aramine in doses of 0.01 to 0.1 mg. per kilo body weight improves cardiac function and coronary blood flow while maintaining the blood pressure in cardiogenic shock (Sarnoff et al., 1954). It may be given orally, intramuscularly or by drip infusion (0.1 to 0.5 mg. per minute).

Since appreciating that "shock" in acute cardiac infarction is a form of acute heart failure, it is rational to try digitalis. Gorlin and Robin (1955) reported good results with lanatoside C or Ouabain intravenously in four cases, although they used very small doses (0.4 mg. of lanatoside C and 0.05 to 0.2 mg. of Ouabain). This lead should be followed up.

Conventional heart failure usually responds well to routine treatment with posture, a low sodium diet, mercurial diuretics, and digitalis. The danger of the digitalis glycosides (Travell, Gold and Modell, 1938) should not be over-emphasised and they must not be withheld when the need for them arises.

Serious disturbances of rhythm call for their standard treatment. Ventricular tachycardia can usually be controlled with adequate doses of quinidine or procaine amide; atrial fibrillation, flutter, or tachycardia with digitalis; heart block with ephedrine. Under the appropriate circumstances these drugs may have to be used boldly without fear that they may cause cardiac standstill or ventricular fibrillation in the presence of cardiac infarction.

The "frozen shoulder" syndrome (left) that can prove troublesome for months after cardiac infarction may often be relieved by cortisone according to Russek et al. (1953). Hydrocortisone, 50 mg. in a 2 ml. suspension, with the addition of 1,000 units of hyaluronidase and 2 ml. of 2 per cent procaine, may be injected weekly into the subacromial bursa anteriorly, into the long head of the biceps antero-laterally, and into the joint capsule posteriorly, as described by Crisp and Kendall (1955).

Subsequent management

If the course is benign and the patient looks and feels well, he may be allowed up after three weeks, provided the sedimentation rate has returned to normal and the electrocardiogram does not show a large infarct. Most cases require a month in bed and a further fortnight resting at home on a couch; but those with complications should remain in bed for six weeks or longer.

Six weeks' to three months' convalescence is usually needed, while the patient regains his confidence and gradually resumes his ordinary activities. Radical change of employment is rarely practicable in this age-group, but lighter work and less responsibility may have to be advised. Relatively good recovery from the first attack is the rule; but severe angina or recurrent congestive failure may cause total incapacity after second or third attacks.

PROGNOSIS

With conservative treatment the mortality during the first month of acute cardiac infarction is 25 per cent. This figure is based on 3,948 cases collected from ten unselected series in the literature, mostly first attacks, and does not take into account all those cases that failed to survive long enough to receive skilled medical attention and hospital care. The mortality was also 25 per cent for 2,733 first attacks only; for second and third attacks it is said to be higher. Doscher and Poindexter (1950) found a combined mortality rate of 23.5 per cent in over 4,000 cases in the literature.

When assessing the influence of any new therapy on the mortality rate of acute cardiac infarction many factors must be taken into consideration:

1. First attacks are believed to have a lower mortality than subsequent attacks, assuming (possibly without justification) that abrupt death at the onset is not more frequent in first attacks.

2. Four-fifths of all deaths from acute cardiac infarction occur in the first twenty-four hours, 60 per cent in the first two hours, and 50 per cent within the first fifteen minutes, at least in men under 40 years of age having their first attack (Yater *et al.*, 1948).

3. The mortality in women averages 50 per cent higher than in men (Mintz and Katz, 1947; Doscher and Poindexter, 1950).

4. Mortality in men is proportional to age: in a group of 276 cases studied by Fitzgerald Peel (1955) it ranged from 5 per cent in men under 44 years old to 35 per cent in men over 65; in women it was 25 per cent at all ages.

5. The following complications adversely influence the mortality, which is given in brackets when known: complete heart block (80–90 per cent), shock (75–80 per cent), paroxysmal tachycardia of any type or atrial flutter (66 per cent), pneumonia (57 per cent), left ventricular or congestive heart failure (50 per cent), gallop rhythm, a pulse pressure under 20 mm. Hg,

a blood pressure under 90 mm. Hg, bundle branch block, unquestionable cardiac enlargement, intractable pain, diabetes mellitus, and marked obesity (Mintz and Katz, 1947; Russek and Zohman, 1952).

6. The following factors do not influence the mortality rate: previous angina pectoris, previous hypertension, absence of pain, the site of the infarct, ectopic beats and pericarditis (Mintz and Katz, 1947).

7. The mortality in favourable cases without any of the adverse features listed above is only 3 to 5 per cent, and the incidence of thrombo-embolism in this group is only 1 to 3 per cent (Russek and Zohman, 1952, 1954).

8. Particularly favourable are those cases with electrocardiograms that show simple inversion of the T wave only, without pathological Q waves and without initial elevation of the RS-T segment (East and Oram, 1948; Papp and Smith, 1951; Holzman, 1955), especially when there is no significant fever, leucocytosis or rise of sedimentation rate (Helander, 1950).

Mortality of specially treated cases

With prompt skilled medical and nursing attention, early intravenous heparin, proper use of vasopressor drugs within three hours of the onset of shock, a semi-starvation diet (800 calories approximately) containing not more than 0.5 G. of sodium for the first few days, prothrombin inhibitors for four to six weeks either in all cases or at least in those with one or more unfavourable features, early recognition and efficient treatment of left ventricular or congestive heart failure, immediate antibiotic therapy for complicating pneumonia, good control of diabetes mellitus, and the intelligent treatment of serious changes of rhythm, the natural mortality of 25 per cent in all cases that survive the first fifteen minutes of the attack should be reduced to about 10 per cent.

Ultimate prognosis

Of patients who survive the first acute attack of cardiac infarction about a third make a complete functional recovery, 50 per cent have angina pectoris or limited cardiac reserve, but are able to lead useful lives, and 20 per cent are seriously incapacitated with severe angina or heart failure (Mussafia and Masini, 1948; Master and Jaffe, 1951; Cole, Singian and Katz, 1954). If the ultimate prognosis of any particular case is to be based on statistical evidence, these three groups must be considered separately.

Patients with good functional recovery are not only free from angina pectoris but are also able to increase their cardiac output normally on effort (Chapman and Fraser, 1954). About 90 per cent of such patients survive five years, and 70 per cent ten years (Master and Jaffe, 1951; Cole et al., 1954).

Of the patients with mild or moderate angina pectoris about three-quarters survive five years and one-half survive ten years (Cole et al., 1954).

In the severe group, however, the majority die within five years.

The crude average life expectation following recovery from the first attack of cardiac infarction is about eight years. The chief causes of death include fresh cardiac infarction (66 per cent) and heart failure (20 per cent) (Katz *et al.*, 1949).

REFERENCES

Altschul, R. (1950): "Experimental cholesterol arteriosclerosis. II. Changes produced in golden hamsters and in guinea pigs", *Amer Heart J.*, **40**, 401.

Anitschkow, N. (1913): "Uber die Veränderungen der Kaninchenaorta bei experimenteller Cholesterinsteatose", *Beitr. path. Anat.*, **56**, 379.

Anrep, G. V., Barsoum, G. S., Kenawy, M. R., and Misrahy, G. (1946): "Ammi visnaga in the treatment of the anginal syndrome", *Brit. Heart J.*, **8**, 171.

——, ——, ——, —— (1947): "Therapeutic uses of Khellin. Method of standardisation", *Lancet*, *i*, 557.

Appelbaum, E., and Nicolson, G. H. B. (1935): "Occlusive diseases of coronary arteries; analysis of pathological anatomy of 168 cases with electrocardiographic correlation in 36 of these", *Amer. Heart J.*, **10**, 662.

Barber, J. M., and Grant, A. P. (1955): "The serum cholesterol and other lipids after administration of sitosterol", *Brit. Heart J.*, **17**, 296.

Barnes, A. R., and Ball, R. G. (1932): "The incidence and situation of myocardial infarction in one thousand consecutive post-mortem examinations", *Amer. J. med. Sc.*, **183**, 215.

Barr, D. P. (1953): "Some chemical factors in the pathogenesis of atherosclerosis", *Circulation*, **8**, 641.

——, Russ, E. M., and Eden, H. A. (1951): "Protein-lipid relationships in human plasma. II. In atherosclerosis and related conditions", *Amer. J. Med.*, **11**, 480.

Bean, W. B. (1938): "Infarction of the heart. 3. Clinical course and morphological findings", *Ann. intern. Med.*, **12**, 71.

Beck, C. S. (1935): "The development of a new blood supply to the heart by operation", *Ann. Surg.*, **102**, 901.

—— (1936): "Further data on the establishment of a new blood supply to the heart by operation", *J. thoracic Surg.*, **5**, 604.

——, and Mako, A. E. (1941): "Venous stasis in the coronary circulation", *Amer. Heart J.*, **21**, 767.

Ben-Asher, S. (1947): "Further observations on the treatment of the anginal syndrome with thiouracil", *Ibid.*, **33**, 490.

Berman, E. F., *et al.* (1952): "Intra-arterial infusion in the treatment of shock resulting from coronary occlusion", *Ibid.*, **43**, 264.

Biorck, G. (1946): "Anoxæmia and exercise tests in the diagnosis of coronary disease", *Ibid.*, **32**, 689.

—— (1946): "Hypoxæmia tests in coronary disease", *Brit. Heart J.*, **8**, 17.

Block, W. J., Crumpacker, E. L., Dry, T. J., and Gage, R. P. (1952): "Prognosis of angina pectoris. Observations in 6,882 cases", *J. Amer. med. Ass.*, **150**, 259.

Blumgart, H. L., Levine, S. A., and Berlin, D. D. (1933): "Congestive heart failure and angina pectoris: the therapeutic effect of thyroidectomy on patients without clinical or pathological evidence of thyroid toxicity", *Arch. intern. Med.*, **51**, 866.

——, Freedberg, A. S., and Kurland, G. S. (1955): "Treatment of incapacitated euthyroid cardiac patients with radioactive iodine", *J. Amer. med. Ass.*, **157**, 1.

Boyle, M. N., Wégria, R., Cathcart, R. T., Nickerson, J. L., and Levy, R. L. (1947): "Effects of intravenous injection of nicotine on the circulation", *Amer. Heart J.*, **34**, 65.

Brown, H. R., and Pearson, R. (1948): "Seasonal variations in heart and coronary disease as related to various environmental factors", *Ibid.*, **35**, 763.

Bulbring, E., Burn, J. H., and Walker, J. M. (1949): "Reduction in coronary flow by pituitary (posterior lobe) extract in relation to the action of nicotine and to smoking", *Quart. J. Med.*, **18**, 73.

Cassidy, M. (1946): "Coronary disease", *Lancet*, ii, 587.

Chambers, W. N. (1947): "Blood pressure studies in 100 cases of coronary occlusion with myocardial infarction", *Amer. J. med. Sc.*, **213**, 40.

Chapman, C. B., and Fraser, R. S. (1954): "Studies on the effect of exercise on cardiovascular function. III. Cardiovascular response to exercise in patients with healed myocardial infarction", *Circulation*, **9**, 347.

Clawson, B. J. (1939): "Coronary sclerosis. An analysis of nine hundred and twenty-eight cases", *Amer. Heart J.*, **17**, 387.

Coelho, E., Fonseca, J. M., Nunes, A., and Rocha Pinto (1953): "Arteriography of the coronary circulation in man", *Cardiologia*, **22**, 45.

Cohn, E. J., *et al.* (1946): "Preparation and properties of serum and plasma proteins. IV. A system for the separation into fractions of the protein and lipo-protein components of biological tissues and fluids", *J. Amer. chem. Soc.*, **68**, 459.

Cole, D. R., Singian, E. B., and Katz, L. N. (1954): "The long-term prognosis following myocardial infarction, and some factors which affect it", *Circulation*, **9**, 321.

Cowdry, E. V. (1933): "Arteriosclerosis. A survey of the problem", New York.

Craddock, W. L., and Mahe, G. A. (1953): "Rupture of papillary muscle of heart following myocardial infarction", *J. Amer. med. Ass.*, **151**, 884.

Crisp, E. J., and Kendall, P. H. (1955): "Treatment of periarthritis of the shoulder with hydrocortisone", *Brit. med. J.*, **1**, 1500.

Cutler, E. C., and Schnitker, M. T. (1934): "Total thyroidectomy for angina pectoris", *Ann. Surg.*, **100**, 578.

Cutts, F. B., and Rapoport, B. (1952): "The routine use of quinidine in acute myocardial infarction", *New Engl. J. Med.*, **247**, 81.

Dauber, D. V., and Katz, L. N. (1942): "Experimental cholesterol atheromatosis in an omnivorous animal, the chick", *Arch. Path.*, **34**, 937.

Doll, R., and Hill, A. B. (1954): "The mortality of doctors in relation to their smoking habits", *Brit. med. J.*, i, 1451.

Doscher, N., and Poindexter, C. A. (1950): "Myocardial infarction without anticoagulant therapy", *Amer. J. Med.*, **8**, 623.

Duguid, J. B. (1946): "Thrombosis as a factor in the pathogenesis of coronary atherosclerosis", *J. Path. Bact.*, **58**, 207.

—— (1948): "Thrombosis as a factor in pathogenesis of aortic atherosclerosis", *Ibid.*, **60**, 57.

——, and Robertson, W. B. (1955): "Effects of atherosclerosis on the coronary circulation", *Lancet*, i, 525.

Dwyer, M. F. (1937): "Hernia of cardiac end of stomach through diaphragm", *Radiology*, **28**, 315.

East, T., and Oram, S. (1948): "Cardiac pain with recovery of the T wave", *Brit. Heart J.*, **10**, 263.

Engelberg, H. (1952): "Heparin therapy of severe coronary atherosclerosis, with observations of its effect on angina pectoris, the two-step electrocardiogram and the ballistocardiogram", *Amer. J. med. Sc.*, **224**, 487.

Eppinger, E. C., and Kennedy, J. A. (1938): "The cause of death in coronary thrombosis with special reference to pulmonary embolism", *Amer. J. med. Sc.*, **95**, 104.

——, Levine, S. A. (1934) "The effect of total thyroidectomy on the response to adrenaline", *Proc. Soc. exper. Biol. and Med.*, **31**, 485.

Epstein, F. H., and Relman, A. S. (1949): "Transfusion treatment of shock due to myocardial infarction", *New Engl. J., Med.*, **241**, 889.

Evans, W. (1954): "Anticoagulant therapy in coronary occlusion", *Proc. Roy. Soc. Med.*, **47**, 318.

Felch, W. C., *et al.* (1952): "The depressing effect of inositol on serum cholesterol and lipid phosphorus in hypercholesteremic myocardial infarct survivors", *Amer. Heart J.*, **44**, 390.

Fitzgerald Peel, A. A. (1955): "Age and sex factors in coronary artery disease", *Brit. Heart J.*, **17**, 319.

Fowler, N. O., Jr., and Failey, R. B., Jr. (1948): "Perforation of the infarcted interventricular septum; report of two cases, one diagnosed ante-mortem", *Amer J., med. Sc.*, **215**, 534.

Freis, E. D., Schnaper, H. W., Johnson, R. L., and Schreiner, G. E. (1952): "Hemodynamic alterations in acute myocardial infarction. 1. Cardiac output, mean arterial pressure, total peripheral resistance, 'central' and total blood volumes, venous pressure and average circulation times", *J. clin. Invest.*, **31**, 131.

Gans, R. H. (1951): "Acute myocardial infarction with rupture of the ventricle", *Amer. Heart J.*, **41**, 332.

Gertler, M. M., Garn, S. M., and Lerman, J. (1950): "The interrelations of serum cholesterol, cholesterol esters and phospholipids in health and in coronary artery disease", *Circulation*, **2**, 205.

Gibson, A. G. (1925): "The clinical aspects of ischæmic necrosis of the heart muscle", *Lancet*, **2**, 1270.

Gilbert, N. C., and Nalefski, L. A. (1949): "The effect of heparin and dicumarol in increasing the coronary flow volume", *J. Lab. and Clin. Med.*, **34**, 797.

Gilbert, R. P., Goldberg, M., and Griffin, J. (1954): "Circulatory changes in acute myocardial infarction", *Circulation*, **9**, 847.

Gilchrist, A. R., and Tulloch, J. A. (1954): "Anticoagulants in coronary disease", *Brit. med. J.*, ii, 720.

Gofman, J. W., and Jones, H. B. (1952): "Obesity, fat metabolism and cardiovascular disease", *Circulation*, **5**, 514.

——, Jones, H. B., Lindgren, F. T., Lyon, T. P., Elliott, H. A., and Strisower, B. (1950): "Blood lipids and human atherosclerosis", *Ibid.*, **2**, 161.

——, Lindgren, F., Elliott, H., Mantz, W., Hewitt, J., Strisower, B., Herring, V., and Lyon, T. P. (1950): "The role of lipids and lipoproteins in atherosclerosis", *Science*, **111**, 166.

——, ——, Jones, H. B., Lyon, T. P., and Strisower, B. (1951): "Lipoproteins and atherosclerosis", *J. Gerontol.*, **6**, 105.

——, *et al.* (1952): "Blood lipids and human atherosclerosis", *Circulation*, **5**, 119.

Goldberger, E., and Schwartz, S. P. (1948): "Electrocardiographic patterns of ventricular aneurysm", *Amer. J. med.*, **4**, 243.

Goldman, J., and Pollak, O. J. (1949): "The hamster as experimental animal for the study of atheromatosis", *Amer. Heart J.*, **38**, 474.

Gordon, K. (1947): "Mechanism of lipophage deposition in atherosclerosis", *Arch. Path.*, **44**, 247.

Gordon, W. H., Bland, E. F., and White, P. D. (1939): "Coronary artery disease analysed post mortem", *Amer. Heart J.*, **17**, 10.

Gorlin, R., and Robin, E. D. (1955): "Cardiac glycosides in the treatment of cardiogenic shock", *Brit. med. J.*, **1**, 937.

Graham, D. M., *et al.* (1951): "The influence of heparin in lipoprotein metabolism and atherosclerosis", *Circulation*, **4**, 465.

Griffiths, G. C., *et al.* (1954): "The treatment of shock associated with myocardial infarction", *Circulation*, **9**, 527.

Gross, L., Schauer, G., and Mendlowitz, M. (1938): "Hemodynamic studies in experimental coronary occlusion", *Amer. Heart J.*, **16**, 278.

Hammond, E. C., and Horn, D. (1954): "The relationship between human smoking habits and death rates", *J. Amer. med. Ass.*, **155**, 1316.

Harrison, C. V., and Wood, P. H. (1949): "Hypertensive and ischæmic heart disease; a comparative clinical and pathological study", *Brit. Heart J.*, 11, 205.

Heberden, W. (1802): "Commentaries on the history and cure of diseases", London.

Hedley, O. F. (1939): "Analysis of 5,116 deaths reported as due to acute coronary occlusion in Philadelphia, 1933–7", *Public Health Rep.*, Washington, p. 972.

Helander, S. (1950): "The prognosis of myocardial infarction and the comparability of different degrees of infarction", *Cardiologia*, 15, 347.

Hellerstein, H. K. (1948): "Atrial infarction with diagnostic electrocardiographic findings", *Amer. Heart J.*, 36, 422.

——, and Martin, J. W. (1947): "Incidence of thromboembolic lesions accompanying myocardial infarction", *Ibid.*, 33, 443.

——, Brofman, B. L., and Caskey, W. H. (1952): "Shock accompanying myocardial infarction: treatment with pressor amines", *Ibid.*, 44, 407.

Herrick, J. B. (1912): "Clinical features of sudden obstruction of the coronary arteries", *J. Amer. med. Ass.*, 59, 2015.

Holzman, M. (1955): "Experiences with the rudimentary anterior wall infarction", *Amer. Heart J.*, 50, 407.

Hunter, J. (1796): "A treatise on the blood, inflammation, and gunshot wounds", Philadelphia.

Johnson, A. S., *et al.* (1953): "Effect of cortisone on the size of experimentally produced myocardial infarcts", *Circulation*, 7, 224.

Johnson, J. R., and Di Palma, J. A. (1939): "Intra-myocardial pressure and its relations to aortic blood pressure", *Amer. J. Physiol.*, 125, 234.

Katz, L. N., and Jochim, K. (1939): "Observations on innervation of coronary vessels of dog", *Ibid.*, 126, 395.

——, and Mintz, S. S. (1947): "An analysis of immediate mortality in 572 cases of recent myocardial infarction", *J. lab. clin. Med.*, 32, 325.

——, Mills, G. Y., and Cisneros, F. (1949): "Survival after recent myocardial infarction", *Arch. int. Med.*, 84, 305.

——, and Stamler, J. (1953): "Experimental atherosclerosis", Charles C. Thomas, Springfield, Illinois.

Kemball Price, R. (1951): "First effort angina. Second wind in angina pectoris", *Brit. Heart. J.*, 13, 197.

Kerwin, A. J. (1953): "Anticoagulants in the treatment of cardiac infarction", *Amer. Heart J.*, 46, 865.

Keys, A. (1952): "Human atherosclerosis and the diet", *Circulation*, 5, 115.

King, E. S. J. (1941): "Surgery of the heart", Baltimore.

La Due, J. S., and Wróblewski, F. (1955): "The significance of the serum glutamic oxalacetic transaminase activity following acute myocardial infarction", *Circulation*, 11, 871.

——, ——, and Karmen, A. (1954): "Serum glutamic oxalacetic transaminase activity in human acute transmural myocardial infarction", *Science*, 120, 497.

Larsen, K. H. (1938): "Om forandringer 1 Elecktrokardiogrammet hos sunde ; Syge under experimental iltmangel", Copenhagen, Ejnar Munksgaards, Forlag.

Leary, T. (1934): "Experimental atherosclerosis in the rabbit compared with iman (coronary) atherosclerosis", *Arch. Path.*, 17, 453.

——, (1938): "Vascularisation of atherosclerotic lesions", *Amer. Heart J.*, 16, 9.

Lehr, D. (1948): "Lowered incidence of sensitisation through the use of sulphomide combinations", *Brit. med. J.*, ii, 4576.

Leonard, B. W., and Daniels, W. B. (1938): "Perforation of the interventricular ptum caused by coronary occlusion", *Amer. Heart J.*, 16, 751.

Leriche, R., Hermann, L., and Fontane, R. (1931): "Ligature de la coronaire uche et fonction cardiaque chez l'animal intact", *C.R. Soc. Biol.*, 107, 545.

Levine, H. D., and Ford, R. V. (1950): "Subendocardial infarction: report of cases and critical survey of the literature", *Circulation*, 1, 246.

Levy, R. L., Barach, A. L., and Bruenn, H. G. (1938): "Effects of induced oxygen want in patients with cardiac pain", *Amer. Heart J.*, 15, 187.

——, Bruenn, H. G., and Russell, N. G. (1939): "The use of the electrocardiographic changes caused by induced anoxæmia as a test for coronary insufficiency", *Amer. J. med. Sc.*, 197, 241.

——, and Moore, R. L. (1941): "Paravertebral sympathetic block with alcohol for relief of cardiac pain; report of 45 cases", *J. Amer. med. Ass.*, 116, 2563.

——, Williams, N. E., Bruenn, H. G., and Carr, H. A. (1941): "The anoxemia test in the diagnosis of coronary insufficiency", *Amer. Heart J.*, 21, 634.

Lewis, T. (1934): "Clinical science", London. ——, Kellgren, J. H. (1939): "Observations relating to referred pain, viscero-motor reflexes and other associated phenomena", *Clin. Sc.*, 4, 47.

Leyden, E. (1883–4): "Ueber die scleroseder coroner-arterien und davon abhaugigen Krankheitszustande", *Ztschr. f. Klin. Med.*, 7, 459 and 539.

Lindgren, I. (1950): "Angina pectoris: A clinical study with special reference to neurosurgical treatment", *Acta. med. Scand.*, 138, suppl. 243, 1.

McEachern, C. G., Manning, G. W., and Hall, G. E. (1940): "Sudden occlusion of coronary arteries following removal of cardio-sensory pathways, an experimental study", *Arch. intern. Med.*, 65, 661.

McNee, J. W. (1925): "Clinical syndrome of thrombosis of coronary arteries", *Quart. J. Med.*, 19, 44.

Malmros, H. (1950): "Relation of nutrition to health; statistical study of effect of war-time on arteriosclerosis, cardiosclerosis, tuberculosis and diabetes", *Acta. md. Scand.*, suppl. 246, 137.

Master, A. M. (1936): "Treatment and immediate prognosis of coronary artery thrombosis; 267 attacks", *Amer. Heart J.*, 12, 549.

—— (1947): "Incidence of acute coronary artery occlusion", *Ibid.*, 33, 135.

——, Dack, S., and Jaffe, H. L. (1938): "Bundle branch and intraventricular block in acute coronary artery occlusion", *Ibid.*, 16, 283.

——, ——, Horn, H., Freedman, B. I., and Field, L. E. (1950): "Acute coronary insufficiency due to acute hæmorrhage: an analysis of 103 cases", *Circulation*, 1, 1302.

——, Grisham, A., Field, L. E., and Horn, H. (1947): "Acute coronary insufficiency: an entity", *J. Mount Sinai Hosp.*, 14, 8.

——, and Jaffe, H. L. (1951): "Complete functional recovery after coronary occlusion and insufficiency", *J. Amer. med. Ass.*, 147, 1721.

——, Jaffe, H. L., and Dack, S. (1939): "The drug treatment of angina pectoris due to coronary artery disease", *Amer. J. med. Sc.*, 197, 774.

Miller, H. R., and Weiss, M. M. (1928): "Disease of coronary arteries; it occurrence without gross cardiac hypertrophy", *Arch. intern. Med.*, 42, 74.

Mills, G. Y., Simon, A. J., Cisneros, F., and Katz, L. N. (1949): "Myocardia infarction. Observations on 100 patients who survived up to six years", *Ibid.* 84, 632.

Mintz, S. S., and Katz, L. N. (1947): "Recent myocardial infarction", *Ibid.* 80, 205.

Montgomery, G. E., Dry, Th. J., and Gage, R. P. (1947): "Further observation on the prognosis in angina pectoris due to coronary sclerosis", *Minnesota Med* 30, 162.

Moon, H. D., and Rinehart, J. F. (1952): "Histogenesis of coronary athero sclerosis", *Circulation*, 6, 481.

Moreton, J. R. (1948): "Physical state of lipids and foreign substances producin atherosclerosis", *Science*, 107, 371.

Morris, J. N., *et al.* (1953): "Coronary heart-disease and physical activity work", *Lancet*, ii, 1053 and 1111.

——, Heady, J. A., and Barley, R. G. (1952): "Coronary heart disease in medic practitioners", *Brit. med. J.*, i, 503.

Mounsey, P. (1951): "Prodromal symptoms in myocardial infarction", *Bri Heart J.*, 13, 215.

Moyer, J. B., and Hiller, G. I. (1951): "Cardiac aneurysm: clinical and electro-cardiographic analysis", *Amer. Heart J.*, **41**, 340.

Munck, W. (1946): "Pathological anatomy of sudden heart death", *Acta. Path. et Micro. Scand.*, **23**, 107.

Murrell, W. (1879): "Nitro-glycerine as a remedy for angina pectoris", *Lancet*, i, 80.

Mussafia, A., and Masini, V. (1948): "The prognosis in myocardial infarction. 1. The prognosis after the acute stage. Study of 100 cases", *Cuore e Circol.*, **32**, 193.

Nathanson, M. H. (1936): "Pathology and pharmacology of cardiac syncope and sudden death", *Arch. intern. Med.*, **58**, 685.

Newman, M. (1946): "Coronary occlusion in young adults. A review of fifty cases in the Services", *Lancet*, ii, 409.

Nichol, E. S., and Borg, J. F. (1950): "Long-term dicumarol therapy to prevent recurrent coronary artery thrombosis", *Circulation*, **1**, 1097.

Oblath, R. W., Levinson, D. C., and Griffith, G. C. (1952): "Factors influencing rupture of the heart after myocardial infarction", *J. Amer. med. Ass.*, **149**, 1276.

Ogura, J. H., Fetter, N. R., Blankenhorn, M. A., and Glueck, H. I. (1946): "Changes in blood coagulation following coronary thrombosis measured by the heparin retarded clotting test (Waugh and Ruddick Test)", *J. clin. Invest.*, **25**, 586.

Oliver, M. F., and Boyd, G. S. (1955): "Serum lipoprotein patterns in coronary sclerosis and associated conditions", *Brit. Heart J.*, **17**, 299.

Opdyke, D. F. (1953): "Failure to reduce the size of experimentally produced myocardial infarcts by cortisone treatment", *Circulation*, **8**, 544.

O'Shaugnessy, L. (1936): "An experimental method of providing a collateral circulation to the heart", *Brit. J. Surg.*, **23**, 665.

—— (1937(: "Surgical treatment of cardiac ischæmia", *Lancet*, i, 185.

——, Slome, D.: "Surgical revascularisation of the heart", *Ibid*, i, 617.

Owren, P. A. (1954): "Long-term anticoagulent therapy in coronary artery disease", *Schweiz. med. Wschr.*, **84**, 822.

Page, I. H. (1954): "Atherosclerosis. An introduction", *Circulation*, **10**, 1.

Papp, C., and Shirley Smith, K. (1951): "Prognosis and treatment of cardiac infarction. A survey of 200 patients", *Brit. med. J.*, **1**, 1471.

Parker, R. L., Dry, T. J., Willius, F. A., and Gage, R. P. (1946): "Life expectancy in angina pectoris", *J. Amer. med. Ass.*, **131**, 95.

Parry, C. H. (1799): "An inquiry into the symptoms and causes of the syncope anginosa, commonly called angina pectoris; illustrated by dissections", London.

Paterson, J. C. (1936): "Vascularisation and hæmorrhage of intima of arterio-sclerotic coronary arteries", *Arch. Path.*, **22**, 313.

—— (1939): "Capillary rupture with intimal hæmorrhage as cause of pulmonary thrombosis", *Amer. Heart J.*, **18**, 451.

—— (1941): "Some factors in causation of intimal hæmorrhages and in precipitation of coronary thrombi", *Canad. med. Ass. J.*, **44**, 114.

Pearsall, H. R., and Chanutin, A. (1949): "Electrophoretic nitrogen and lipid analyses of plasma fractions of healthy young men", *Amer. J. Med.*, **7**, 297.

Poe, W. D. (1947): "Fatal coronary artery disease in young men", *Amer. Heart J.*, **33**, 76.

Prinzmetal, M., Bergman, H. C., Kruger, H. E., Schwartz, L. L., Simkin, B., and Sobin, S. S. (1948): "Studies on the coronary circulation. III. Collateral circulation of beating human and dog hearts with coronary occlusion", *Ibid.*, **35**, 9.

——, Simkin, B., Bergman, H. C., and Kruger, H. E. (1947): "Studies on the coronary circulation. II. The collateral circulation of the normal human heart by coronary perfusion with radioactive erthyrocytes and glass spheres", *Ibid.*, **33**, 420.

——, *et al.* (1953): "Intramural depolarisation potentials in myocardial infarction. A preliminary report", *Circulation*, **7**, 1.

Raab, W. (1945): "Thiouracil treatment of angina pectoris", *J. Amer. med. Ass.*, **128**, 249.

Ratika, L., Borduas, J. L., Rothman, S., and Prinzmetal, J. (1954): "Studies on the mechanism of ventricular activity. XII. Early changes in the RS-T segment and QRS complex following acute coronary artery occlusion; experimental study and clinical applications", *Amer. Heart J.*, **48**, 351.

Registrar General's statistical review of England and Wales for the year 1953, London, Her Majesty's Stationery Office (1954).

Riseman, J. E. F., and Brown, M. G. (1937): "Analysis of diagnostic criteria of angina pectoris; critical study of 100 proved cases", *Amer. Heart J.*, **14**, 331.

Russ, E. M., Eden, H. A., and Barr, D. P. (1951): "Protein-lipid relationships in human plasma. I. In normal individuals", *Amer. J. Med.*, **11**, 468.

———, ———, ——— (1955): "Gonadal hormones on protein-lipid relationships in human plasma", *Amer. J. Med.*, **19**, 4.

Russek, H. I., Naegele, C. F., and Regan, F. D. (1950): "Alcohol in the treatment of angina pectoris", *J. Amer. med. Ass.*, **143**, 355.

———, Russek, A. S., Doerner, A. A., and Zohman, B. L. (1953): "Cortisone in treatment of shoulder-hand syndrome following acute myocardial infarction", *Arch. intern. Med.*, **91**, 487.

———, and Zohman, B. L. (1952): "Prognosis in the 'uncomplicated' first attack of acute myocardial infarction", *Amer. J. med Sc.*, **224**, 496.

———, ——— (1954): "The place of anticoagulants in coronary thrombosis", *Lancet*, ii, 910.

———, ———, Drumm, A. E., Weingarten, W., and Dorset, V. J. (1955): "Long-acting coronary vasodilator drugs: metamine, paveril, nitroglyn and peritrate", *Circulation*, **12**, 169.

Ryle, J. A., and Russell, W. T. (1949): "The natural history of coronary disease. A clinical and epidemiological study", *Brit. Heart J.*, **11**, 370.

Salcedo-Salgar, J., and White, P. D. (1935): "Relationship of heart block, auriculo-ventricular and intraventricular to clinical manifestations of coronary disease angina pectoris, and coronary thrombosis", *Amer. Heart J.*, **10**, 1067.

Sarnoff, S. J., Case, R. B., Berglund, E., and Sarnoff, L. C. (1954): "Ventricular function. V. The circulatory effects of aramine; mechanism of action of 'vaso pressor' drugs in cardiogenic shock', *Circulation*, **10**, 84.

Scherf, D., and Brooks, A. M. (1949): "The murmurs of cardiac aneurysm" *Amer. J. med. Sci.*, **218**, 389.

———, and Goldhammer, S. (1933): "Zur Fruehdiagnose der Angina Pectoris" *Wien. med. Wschr.*, **83**, 836.

Schlesinger, M. J. (1938): "An injection plus dissection study of coronary arter occlusions and anastomoses", *Amer. Heart J.*, **15**, 528.

Schnur, S. (1953): "Mortality and other studies questioning the evidence fo and value of routine anticoagulant therapy in acute myocardial infarction" *Circulation*, **7**, 855.

Selzer, A. (1948): "The immediate sequelæ of myocardial infarction. The relation to the prognosis", *Amer. J. med. Sc.*, **216**, 172.

——— (1952): "The hypotensive state following acute myocardial infarctior I. Clinical observations", *Amer. Heart J.*, **44**, 1.

Sharpey-Schafer, E P. (1944): "Circulatory dynamics of hæmorrhage", *Bri med. Bull.*, **2**, 171.

Shirley Smith, K., and Guz, A. (1953): "L-noradrenaline in treatment of shoc in cardiac infarction", *Brit. med. J.*, ii, 1341.

Shute, E. V. (1945): "Effect of vitamin E upon impaired kidney functic (preliminary note)", *Canad. med. Ass. J.*, **52**.

Snellen, H. A., and Nauta, J. H. (1937): "Roentgen diagnosis of corona calcification", *Fortschr. a. d. Geb. d. Röentgenstrahlen*, **56**, 277.

Somerville, W., and Wood, P. H. (1949): "The electrocardiogram of cardi infarction associated with bundle-branch-block", *Brit. Heart J.*, **11**, 305.

Steiner, A., Kendall, F. E., and Bevans, M. (1949): "Production of arteri sclerosis in dogs by cholesterol and thiouracil feeding", *Amer. Heart J.*, **38**, 34.

Stewart, C. F., and Turner, K. B. (1938): "A note on pericardial involvement in coronary thrombosis," *Amer. Heart J.*, 15, 232.

Stewart, H. J., and Carr, H. A. (1954): "The anoxemic test", *Ibid.*, 48, 293.

Suzman, M. M., Ruskin, H. D., and Goldberg, B. (1955): "An evaluation of the effect of continuous long-term anticoagulant therapy on the prognosis of myocardial infarction: a report of 82 cases", *Circulation*, 12, 338.

Teng, H. C., and Heyer, H. E. (1955): "The relationship between sudden changes in weather and the occurrence of acute myocardial infarction", *Amer. Heart J.*, 49, 9.

Thompson, S. A., and Plachta, A. (1953): "Experiences with cardiopericardiopexy in the treatment of coronary disease", *J. Amer. med. Ass.*, 152, 678.

Travell, J., Gold, H., and Modell, W. (1938): "Effect of experimental cardiac infarction on response to digitalis", *Arch. intern. Med.*, 61, 184.

Van der Veer, J. B., Marshall, D. S., and Kuo, P. T. (1948): "Experiences with the use of heparin and dicoumarol in the treatment of coronary thrombosis and thrombo-embolic disease". *Trans. Coll. Phys. Philadelphia*, 16, 67.

Walker, J. M. (1949): "The effect of smoking on water diuresis in man", *Quart. J. Med.*, 18, 51.

Wang, C. H., Bland, E. F., and White, P. D. (1948): "A note on coronary occlusion and myocardial infarction found post morten at the Massachusetts General Hospital during the twenty-year period from 1926 to 1945 inclusive", *Ann. intern. Med.*, 29, 601.

Wartman, W. B. (1938): "Occlusion of the coronary arteries by hæmorrhage into their walls", *Amer. Heart J.*, 15, 459.

——, Hellerstein, H. K. (1948): "The incidence of heart disease in 2,000 consecutive autopsies", *Ann. intern. Med.*, 28, 41.

Wayne, E. J., and Laplace, L. B. (1933-4): "Observations on angina of effort", *Clin. Sc.*, 1, 103.

Wegria, R., and Nickerson, N. D. (1943): "The benzol-adrenaline test as a reliable method of estimating changes in the sensitivity of the dog's ventricles to fibrillation. Application of the method to the study of quinidine sulfate", *Amer. Heart J.*, 25, 58.

Weintraub, H. J., and Bishop, L. F. (1947): "The anoxæmia test for coronary insufficiency", *Ann. intern. Med.*, 26, 741.

Weiss, M. M. (1939): "The early rise of blood pressure in coronary thrombosis", *Amer. Heart J.*, 17, 103.

White, J. C., and Bland, E. F. (1948): "The surgical relief of severe angina pectoris. Methods employed and end results in 83 patients", *Medicine*, 27, 1.

——, Garrey, W. E., and Atkins, J. A. (1933): "Cardiac innervation: experimental and clinical studies", *Arch. Surg.*, 26, 765.

White, P. D., Bland, E. F., and Miskall, E. W. (1943): "The prognosis of angina pectoris: a long-time follow-up of 497 cases, including a note on 75 additional cases of angina pectoris decubitus", *J. Amer. med. Ass.*, 123, 801.

Wiggers, C. J. (1947): "Myocardial depression in shock", *Amer. Heart J.*, 33, 33.

Wilens, S. L. (1947): "The relationship of chronic alcoholism to atherosclerosis", *Amer. med. Ass.*, 135, 1136.

——, (1947): "Resorption of arterial atheromatous deposits in wasting disease", *Amer. J. Path.*, 23, 793.

—— (1947): "Bearing of general nutritional state on atherosclerosis", *Arch. intern. Med.*, 79, 129.

—— (1951): "The experimental production of lipid deposition in excised arteries", *Science*, 114, 389.

Windaus, A. (1910): "Über den Gehalt normaler und Atheromatöser Aorten an Cholesterin und Cholesterinestern", *Ztschr. f. physiol. Chem.*, 67, 174.

Wolferth, C. C., and Edeiken, J. (1942): "The differential diagnosis of angina pectoris with special reference to œsophageal spasm and coronary occlusion", *Pennsylvania med. J.*, 45, 579.

Wood, P. (1936): "The erythrocyte sedimentation rate in diseases of the heart", *Quart. J. Med.*, **5**, 1.

—— (1948): "Therapeutic application of anticoagulants", *Trans. med. Soc. Lond.*, **66**, 80.

——, McGregor, M., Magidson, O., and Whittaker, W. (1950): "The effort test in angina pectoris", *Brit. Heart J.*, **12**, 363.

Wright, I. S., Marple, C. D., and Beck, D. F. (1948): "Report of the committee for the evaluation of anticoagulants in the treatment of coronary thrombosis with myocardial infarction", *Amer. Heart J.*, **36**, 801.

——, ——, —— (1954): "Myocardial infarction: its clinical manifestations and treatment with anticoagulants", Grune and Stratton, New York.

Wuest, J. H., Dry, T. J., and Edwards, J. E. (1953): "The degree of coronary atherosclerosis in bilaterally oophorectomised women", *Circulation*, **7**, 801.

Yater, W. M., Traum, A. H., Brown, W. G., Fitzgerald, R. P., Geisler, M. A., and Wilcox, B. B. (1948): "Coronary artery disease in men 18 to 39 years of age", *Amer. Heart J.*, **36**, 334, 481 and 683.

Zaus, E. A., and Kearns, W. M. (1952): "Massive infarction of the right ventricle and atrium. Report of a case", *Circulation*, **6**, 593.

CHAPTER XVI

HYPERTENSIVE HEART DISEASE

HYPERTENSIVE heart disease is but one facet of the whole problem of systemic hypertension. It is necessary to consider this problem first.

DEFINITION

Hypertension implies elevation of the basal blood pressure above the arbitrary normal limits of 145/90 mm. Hg. Physiological vasoconstriction or a transient increase of cardiac output due to emotion, cold, or other trivial cause, is common, and modifies the significance of casual high readings of the order of 160/90 mm. Hg. The basal pressure is that obtained when the subject is lying down, and when successive readings at five-minute intervals have dropped to a steady level. If there were an easy bedside method of measuring the cardiac output, hypertension would be expressed in terms of total peripheral resistance. In healthy young adults,

$$R \text{ (resistance)} = \frac{80 \text{ to } 100 \text{ mm. Hg (mean arterial pressure)}}{5 \text{ to } 8 \text{ L/min. (cardiac output)}}$$
$$= 10 \text{ to } 20 \text{ units}$$
$$= 800 \text{ to } 1{,}600 \text{ dynes sec./cm.}^5 \text{ (page 177)}.$$

Unquestionable hypertension means a peripheral resistance above 25 units (2,000 dynes sec./cm.^{5}). It is insufficiently realised that with an average peripheral resistance of 15 units, a cardiac output of 10 litres per minute, which is common in mildly excited young adults, would raise the blood pressure to around 210/110 mm. Hg (mean 150 mm. Hg). With a relatively high normal resistance of 18 units, and a cardiac output of 12 litres per minute, resulting from more marked excitement (also common enough), the physiology of the circulation could still be "normal" with a blood pressure of 300/150 mm. Hg (mean 210). That such hyperkinetic levels are not commonly encountered in healthy but apprehensive young adults is due to the fact that when the cardiac output rises in response to adrenergic stimuli the peripheral resistance falls. The figures given, however, should serve to emphasise the fact that measurement of the blood pressure without reference to the cardiac output provides no evidence of the state of vasomotor tone, and is therefore a poor method of detecting essential hypertension or of estimating its degree. Once this is understood many of the anomalies that surround the height of the blood pressure in "normal" and "hypertensive" subjects fall into line. *Hyperkinetic elevation of the blood pressure is not essential hypertension.*

When elevation of the blood pressure shows disproportion between systolic and diastolic levels, systolic bias favours rigidity of the aorta and large vessels as in atherosclerosis, or increased force of cardiac contraction as in thyrotoxicosis; whereas diastolic bias favours vasoconstriction, as in true hypertension.

VARIETIES OF HYPERTENSION

Hypertension may be paroxysmal, as in phæochromocytoma of the adrenal medulla; transient, as in acute nephritis and toxæmia of pregnancy; or persistent, as in chronic nephritis, chronic pyelonephritis, surgical kidney, coarctation of the aorta, Cushing's syndrome, and essential and malignant hypertension. High blood pressure accompanying thyrotoxicosis and the climacteric is coincidental: statistical analysis shows no significant correlation, and the pressure does not fall when these disorders are corrected (Bechgaard, 1946). The blood pressure in obese subjects may appear to be higher than it really is, owing to the unreliability of the cuff method of measurement when applied to a fat limb; lower pressures may be recorded by direct arterial puncture. Under certain conditions, e.g. during a rigor when there is intense vasoconstriction, or when the main artery to the limb is partly occluded, the blood pressure reading may be much lower when measured by the cuff method than when measured by direct arterial puncture; indeed it may be immeasurable by ordinary means when direct puncture proves it to be in the region of 100 mm. Hg. Such fallacies must be constantly borne in mind. Hypertension associated with mitral stenosis is almost certainly a matter of chance, apart from the transient rise of pressure that may result from heart failure.

INCIDENCE

In 1928 hypertension accounted for 14.8 per cent (Bell and Clawson) to 20 per cent (Fahr) of all deaths in the U.S.A. in people over 50 years of age. In England and Wales the Registrar General's Statistical Review for 1953 reveals that 4 per cent of all deaths (8 per cent of cardiovascular deaths) were due to hypertension, and another 13.5 per cent of all deaths (27 per cent of cardiovascular deaths) to stroke, chiefly cerebral hæmorrhage or thrombosis.

If a blood pressure of 150/100 mm. Hg or above means hypertension, then the prevalence of this disease is 5 per cent in young adults, 10 to 20 per cent in the fifth decade, 20 to 30 per cent in the sixth decade, and 35 to 40 per cent in those between the ages of 60 and 65 (Master et al., 1952). As pointed out by Hamilton et al. (1954) there is no sharp dividing line between what is normal and what is abnormal. If 180/105 mm. Hg is accepted as the lower limit of genuine hypertensive disease, then its prevalence is 0.7 per cent in young adults under 40 years of age, 3 per cent in the fourth decade, 6 per cent in the fifth decade, and 10 per cent between the ages of 60 and 65 (Master et al., 1952). Males are more prone to hypertension than females up to the age of 40, but thereafter it is the other way about.

At least 80 per cent of hypertensive subjects are between 40 and 70 years of age, the peak period being 50 to 59 (Janeway, 1913; Bechgaard, 1946). According to Platt (1948), severe persistent hypertension in persons under 40 years of age is commonly renal: less than a third of his series were essential, and he encountered no primary malignant cases under the age of 34.

The sex incidence is about equal, men being rather more frequently affected in the upper classes (Janeway, 1913; Ehrstrom, 1918), women in the lower (Blackford et al., 1930; Bechgaard, 1946). Malignant hypertension, however, affects three men to one woman.

About 80 to 85 per cent of cases of persistent hypertension are essential, about 2 per cent are primary malignant, and most of the remainder are renal. Brod (1955) found a particularly high incidence of malignant hypertension amongst his cases of chronic pyelonephritis (20 per cent).

High blood pressure appears to be linked with civilisation: it is said to be rare or uncommon in China, amongst orientals generally (Harris, 1927), and in negroes (Donnison, 1929); but it is as common or more common in civilised negroes in the U.S.A. as in the white population (Fishberg, 1939). The evidence has been reviewed by Smirk (1949).

PATHOGENESIS

Paroxysmal hypertension is due to an excess of circulating adrenaline released by a phæochromocytoma of the adrenal medulla (Beer, King and Prinzmetal, 1937); it is now known that there is also an excess of nor-adrenaline, sometimes one and sometimes the other predominating (Pitcairn and Youmans, 1950).

Transient hypertension in acute nephritis appears to depend upon a nervous rather than a humoral agent (Pickering, 1943), and may be due to extra-renal factors (Kylin, 1926). There is reason to believe that acute nephritis is an allergic vascular reaction to the products of remote bacterial infection (Cavelti and Cavelti, 1945) usually but not exclusively streptococcal, the brunt of the attack falling on the glomerular tufts, but the capillaries elsewhere not escaping entirely. General vasospasm may cause the hypertension. Wilson (1953), on the other hand, accepts the obvious, and assumes that the hypertension of acute nephritis is renal and humoral in origin.

Hypertension in *toxæmia of pregnancy* may be transient and behave like that in acute nephritis or it may be persistent and resemble essential or malignant hypertension (Golden, Dexter and Weiss, 1943). Since the blood volume and cardiac output are raised, the hypertension may be partly hyperkinetic. More measurements of the peripheral resistance in toxæmia of pregnancy are needed.

High blood pressure in *coarctation of the aorta* (page 332) probably

results from diminution of the renal blood flow. It does not occur experimentally if the aorta is constricted below the origin of the renal arteries
(Rytand, 1938).

Hypertension resulting from *chronic nephritis, chronic pyelonephritis*
(Schoen, 1930; Longcope and Winkenwerder, 1933), and certain *surgical
kidneys* (Braasch, Walters, and Hammer, 1940) is almost certainly attributable to a humoral agent liberated by the diseased kidney (Pickering,
1943), at least in the first instance.

Malignant hypertension may develop in any form of hypertension provided the diastolic blood pressure rises sufficiently, particularly when it
does so rapidly (Pickering, 1952).

ETIOLOGY OF ESSENTIAL HYPERTENSION

Certain predisposing factors must be considered first.

Heredity. According to Platt (1947), essential hypertension could be a
hereditary disease conveyed as a Mendelian dominant with a rate of expression of more than 90 per cent. This may be an extreme view, but the
importance of the hereditary factor cannot be denied. Thus Ayman (1934),
studying 277 families, found hypertension in the children in 3.1 per cent
of the families when both parents were normal, in 28.3 per cent when one
parent was hypertensive, and in 45.5 per cent when both parents were
hypertensive. Again, in an investigation based upon 256 members of 30
families, Hines (1940) found that the children were hyper-reactors to the
cold pressor test in 43.4 per cent when one parent was either hypertensive or a hyper-reactor, and in 95 per cent when both parents were
affected. In Bechgaard's series of over 1,000 cases of persistent hypertension, which included 20.7 per cent possible renal cases (in which there
is no hereditary factor), one or both parents were seriously hypertensive
in 75 per cent.

Hyper-reaction to pressor agents. The excessive reaction of hypertensive
subjects to the cold pressor test of Hines (1940) is the best example. The
test is carried out as follows: the basal blood pressure is first recorded in the
usual way; the subject's free hand is then plunged into ice-cold water
(3° to 5°C.) to just above the level of the wrist, and immersed for one
minute, while the blood pressure is recorded at half-minute intervals. In
8.5 per cent of normal persons the blood pressure rises an average of
12.4/10.1 mm. Hg, and returns to its previous level within two minutes.
If the immersed limb is anæsthetic there is no response, whether the
anæsthetic is organic or hysterical (Wolff, 1951). A rise of more than
20/15 mm. Hg is regarded as a hyper-reaction. Patients with established
essential hypertension show an average rise of 46.6/30.9 mm. Hg, 95 per
cent being hyper-reactors. Follow-up studies indicate that apparently normal individuals who are hyper-sensitive to the cold pressor test are likely
to develop persistent hypertension. Hines also claims that high casual
readings due to emotion have the same significance, and Harris *et al.* (1953)

agree; but this is not substantiated by the subsequent histories of patients with Da Costa's syndrome (Grant, 1925; Wood, 1941).

Holding the breath for 20 seconds may also be used as a pressor agent in much the same way, and compares favourably with the cold pressor test (Ayman and Goldshine, 1939).

Other factors. The influence of civilisation, and of sex in malignant hypertension, have already been mentioned.

Structural changes in the vessels. Certain structural vascular changes often found associated with hypertension have been proved to play no part in its production. Atherosclerosis is innocent in this respect unless a plaque constricts the renal artery; increased rigidity of the aorta and great vessels may raise the systolic pressure, increase the pulse volume, and accelerate the speed of the pulse wave, but it has little influence upon the mean blood pressure. Calcification of the media of medium-sized arteries has a similar effect. The characteristic vascular lesion which is the signature of malignant hypertension, necrosing afferent glomerular arteriolitis, is a result, not a cause, of extreme hypertension. Multiplication of the internal elastic lamina, and hypertrophy of the media of small arteries and arterioles, are also effects, not causes, of sustained hypertension. Hyaline thickening of the intima, especially of the afferent glomerular arterioles, found in 98 per cent of cases of essential hypertension, is the only vascular lesion possibly to blame which has not yet been proved to be a result of high blood pressure (Pickering, 1943).

Experimental studies. The classical experiments of Goldblatt (1934 *et seq.*) proved that persistent hypertension could be induced in dogs by constricting both renal arteries; unilateral constriction failed unless the other kidney was removed. Hypertensive retinopathy and widespread arteriolar necrosis similar to malignant hypertension in man were reproduced by more severe constriction; but the renal vessels distal to the clamp were spared. Similar results were obtained in rabbits by Wilson and Pickering (1937). In 1939, Wilson and Byrom succeeded in causing persistent hypertension, benign or malignant, in rats by constricting only one renal artery. The vessels in the other kidney then showed changes comparable in all respects to those seen in benign or malignant hypertension in man.

The conclusion that the difference between essential and malignant hypertension is merely one of degree is supported by the occasional development of malignant changes in practically all varieties of hypertension, including paroxysmal, transient and renal hypertension; moreover, in the early malignant stage, renal biopsy usually reveals no evidence of arteriolar necrosis, indicating that this is not an essential part of the picture, but merely a late consequence (Castleman and Smithwick, 1943).

Biochemical hypothesis concerning the cause of hypertension. Experimental hypertension of the kind just described is believed to depend upon the liberation of an excess of renin by the ischæmic kidney. Renin combines with an enzyme, hypertensinogen, which is a normal constituent of the plasma globulins, to form a pressor substance, hypertensin or angio-tonin (Braun-Menendez *et al.*, 1939). Hypertensin is said to be destroyed by another enzyme, hypertensinase (Pickering, 1943).

There is, as yet, no direct proof that essential hypertension in man is caused by this mechanism, although it seems to explain renal hypertension. It may also explain rare cases of hypertension associated with atherosclerotic obstruction of one or both renal arteries (Yuile, 1944). It should be noted that unilateral renal disease is capable of causing hypertension in man; in other words, man behaves like the rat in this respect, not like the dog or rabbit.

Physiology of the circulation in essential hypertension. In essential hypertension vasoconstriction affects chiefly the efferent glomerular arterioles of the kidney, the intraglomerular pressure being raised and the cortical blood flow diminished; obviously, if the latter were due to vasoconstriction proximal to the glomeruli, the intraglomerular pressure would be lowered. Blood appears to be diverted from the renal cortex into other channels. The classical studies of Trueta and his colleagues (1947) make it highly probable that the juxta-medullary by-pass provides the principal diversion. The vessels of the skin and brain are constricted more or less sufficiently to prevent an increased blood flow through these territories; on the other hand, the arterioles in skeletal muscle, and probably in the heart, are little if at all constricted, so that they may passively yield to the raised pressure, and take some of the shunt. The behaviour of the splanchnic vessels remains to be investigated, but in normal subjects their reactions tend to be opposite to those in the skin (Grayson, 1950). The cardiac output, blood volume, and blood viscosity are normal. Vasoconstriction appears to be humoral rather than nervous in mechanism (Pickering, 1943). Hypertensin causes a similar type of vasoconstriction: the chief effect is on the efferent glomerular arterioles; the skin is involved only to the extent of preventing secondary increase of blood flow; the skeletal muscles take some of the shunt. That hypertensin is the humoral cause of essential hypertension is therefore an attractive hypothesis. Pickering remarks that the brain and heart, being two of the most important organs in the body,  are provided with special pressor mechanisms, the carotid sinus and aortic arch, which respond to falling intravascular pressure by causing vasoconstriction; as the nature of these organs demands that appropriate adjustments are immediately executed, it is natural that the mechanism of this vasoconstriction is nervous. But the kidneys are just as vital, and it would therefore harmonise with general principles if they too were provided with a pressor mechanism to ensure adequate intraglomerular pressure without which filtration would cease; but there is no necessity for *sudden* adjustments, but rather for prolonged ones. A humoral mechanism would meet the requirements nicely.

Nevertheless, as previously stated, proof that essential hypertension in man is due to excessive liberation of renin is lacking. Transfusion experiments have failed to demonstrate a pressor agent in the venous blood of hypertensive subjects; and Light and I (1939) failed to demonstrate a pressor agent in a pint of blood taken from the renal vein of a patient with malignant hypertension, and transfused into a boy of nine. Even if the humoral mechanism were proved to be the renin-hypertensin system, we should still be ignorant of the cause of its hyperactivity.

A promising line of investigation seems to be that opened up by Trueta and his colleagues at Oxford. They have shown that blood reaching the kidney has two alternative routes: (1) through the glomeruli of the cortex, (2) through a juxta-medullary by-pass. Blood may be diverted from the cortex in varying degree as a result of emotion, shock, crushing injuries, hæmorrhages, certain drugs, certain bacterial toxins, and probably by innumerable other agents. In cases of Bright's disease they have noticed degenerative changes in the juxta-medullary glomeruli consistent with constant operation of the shunt. The significance of these findings will not be overlooked, particularly their suggestion that the juxta-medullary by-pass may act as a functional Goldblatt clamp.

It is possible that the cause of essential hypertension is simply physiological hypertension repeated too often or sustained for too long a period, as suggested by Smirk (1949). Whether repetitive physiological hypertension is chiefly hyperkinetic, neurogenic (vasoconstrictive) or humoral (vasoconstrictive) is immaterial to this hypothesis, which holds that a raised blood pressure, however produced, may initiate secondary reactions which themselves increase the total peripheral resistance and so perpetuate the hypertension. Agents capable of causing sufficiently repetitive or prolonged hypertension to excite these secondary changes include a particular type of personality that over-reacts to stress (hereditary factor), prolonged emotional strain (psychological factor), acute nephritis, toxæmia of pregnancy, paroxysmal hypertension from phæochromocytoma, and certain hyperkinetic circulatory states such as thyrotoxicosis. Secondary changes that may perpetuate the hypertension are renal ischæmia and arteriosclerosis in its broadest sense; but a more important unknown factor is postulated. A similar hypothesis has been put forward to explain pulmonary hypertension, for sustained pulmonary vasoconstriction also seems to result from pulmonary hypertension, *however caused* (page 839).

CLINICAL FEATURES

PAROXYSMAL HYPERTENSION

Paroxysmal hypertension, first described by Frankel (1886), is rare, being responsible for only 0.5 per cent of cases of severe persistent hypertension (Graham, 1951). It usually occurs in youthful or early middle-aged subjects of either sex, and is characterised by recurrent attacks of palpitation, headache, and vomiting; angina pectoris or even acute pulmonary œdema (Howard and Barker, 1937) may be associated. Abdominal compression, as occurs on stooping, may provoke an attack; but usually there is no previous precipitating cause. During the crisis, which may last for minutes or hours, the blood pressure (systolic and diastolic) is extremely high; most of the skin is cold, pale and mottled, but the forehead, face and neck may be flushed. Sweating and trembling may follow. Between attacks the patient is usually well, but persistent hypertension, occasionally malignant, develops sooner or later in the majority (Green, 1946).

The quality of the symptoms depends upon whether the tumour liberates chiefly adrenaline or noradrenaline, although both are usually present in excess. Adrenaline is the body's emergency hormone and is normally released by the suprarenal medulla in amounts proportional to physiological estimates (Cannon, 1940). It increases the heart rate, venous pressure (Iglauer and Altschule, 1940), and strength of cardiac contraction (Marsh et al., 1948), so that the cardiac output is increased by means of all three reserve mechanisms (McMichael and Sharpey-Schafer, 1944; Goldenberg et al., 1948), while the coronary blood flow is augmented (Anrep and Stacey, 1927), and the total peripheral resistance diminished (von Euler and Liljestrand, 1927). Although the blood flow through the skin (Barcroft and Swan, 1953) and through the kidneys (Barclay, Cooke and Kenney, 1947) is reduced, the blood flow through skeletal muscle (Allen, Barcroft and Edholm, 1946) and liver (Bearn, Billing and Sherlock, 1952) is greatly increased. Adrenaline also stimulates all impulse-forming foci in the heart, whether normal or abnormal. The chief clinical effects of an excess of circulating adrenaline are therefore pallor of the skin, tachycardia, abnormalities of rhythm, a bounding pulse, marked elevation of the systolic but less of the diastolic blood pressure (hyperkinetic hypertension), and a hyperdynamic heart action; the chief symptoms are palpitations and a sense of alarm.

Noradrenaline is liberated physiologically at sympathetic nerve endings, where it activates effector cells (von Euler, 1946, 1948), but it is also found in the adrenal medulla, where it forms up to 25 per cent of the total secretion (Swan, 1952). Noradrenaline is a powerful vasoconstrictor of all but the coronary vessels, and causes a sharp rise of systolic and diastolic blood pressures, and of total peripheral resistance. The pulse rate slows reflexly, owing to stimulation of carotid and aortic baroreceptors, and though the stroke volume and power of ventricular contraction may be enhanced, the minute output does not rise (Goldenberg et al., 1948). Noradrenaline does not stimulate impulse-forming foci in the heart and does not encourage changes of rhythm (Nathanson and Miller, 1952). The chief clinical effects of an excess of circulating noradrenaline are therefore pallor, systolic and diastolic hypertension, and bradycardia.

Mixtures of adrenaline and noradrenaline (arterenol), infused at the rate of 10 µg per minute, behave like adrenaline when there is less than 25 per cent of noradrenaline in the mixture (as in normal medullary secretion); with adrenaline/noradrenaline ratios of 3/1 to 1/3, the adrenaline effects still predominate, but with ratios of 1/8 or less the noradrenaline effects predominate; balanced effects are observed with ratios between 1/3 and 1/8 (De Largy *et al.*, 1950).

A mass about the size of an orange may be felt in the abdomen in one-third of the cases, or may be demonstrated by simple skiagrams, pyelograms, or other radiological methods. The adrenal medullary tumour is commonly unilateral and benign. There is usually a considerable excess of circulating adrenaline or nor-adrenaline all the time, and in attacks there may be a thousand times the normal quantity (Mackeith, 1944). The electrocardiogram may show the usual pattern associated with persistent hypertension, or it may show evidence of acute left ventricular stress during attacks—inversion of the T wave in leads facing the surface of the left ventricle.

Death may result from cerebral hæmorrhage, acute pulmonary œdema, or ventricular fibrillation.

Following the demonstration by Clerc and Sterne (1937) that a synthetic benzodioxan (diethyl-aminoethyl-benzodioxan) in oral doses of 0.05 G., six-hourly, relieved all symptoms immediately and prevented further attacks, the administration of this substance has been used as a diagnostic test for the condition (Goldenberg *et al.*, 1947; Cahill, 1948). The usual dose is 0.25 mg. per kilogram body weight intravenously. In cases of phæochromocytoma the systolic and diastolic blood pressures drop sharply for 10 to 15 minutes, whereas in other forms of hypertension they tend to rise a little, sometimes alarmingly so.

Of the newer adrenolytic drugs, such as dibenamine (3 to 5 mg./Kg intravenously), dibenyline or dibenzyline (0.25 to 0.5 mg./Kg intravenously or 20 to 50 mg. three or four times daily orally), rogitine (*vide infra*), and ilidar (25 to 50 mg. three or four times daily by mouth), rogitine is probably the most satisfactory for detecting or excluding phæochromocytoma. Rogitine (phentolamine) is related to priscoline, both being derivatives of amidazoline. For diagnostic purposes a dose of 5 mg. is given intravenously: in cases of phæochromocytoma the blood pressure falls more than 35/25 mm. Hg within two or three minutes and then gradually returns to the basal level over the next 10 to 15 minutes (Gifford, Roth and Kvale, 1952). Dangerous pressor reactions in essential or malignant hypertension, such as may occur with benzodioxane (Rosenheim, 1954), do not seem to occur with phentolamine. The drug may also be given orally in doses of 20 mg. three or four times daily.

A marked fall of blood pressure after intravenous dibenamine, dibenzyline, or ilidar is not specific for phæochromocytoma, for these drugs are all sympatholytic as well as adrenolytic in the doses used, whereas phentolamine is not.

The intravenous injection of 0.025 mg. of histamine (Roth and Kvale, 1945) or of 300 mg. of tetraethylammonium bromide is also helpful in diagnosis, for in cases of phæochromocytoma both *raise* the blood pressure

(La Due *et al.*, 1948). Mecholyl may have the same effect, but is unreliable (Anderson *et al.*, 1952). Hexamethonium (and presumably ansolysen) appears to excite similar responses to those of tetraethylammonium (Freis *et al.*, 1951).

The most reliable test for phæochromocytoma, however, is to estimate the plasma adrenaline and noradrenaline or the output of these catechol amines in the urine. In normal controls and in patients with essential hypertension they should not exceed 2.5 μg per litre in the plasma (mean 1.6), mostly noradrenaline, whereas in cases of phæochromocytoma with sustained hypertension and in paroxysmal cases after a test dose of histamine, they usually exceed 12 μg per litre, adrenaline alone exceeding 4 μg (Manger *et al.*, 1954). In normal subjects at rest in bed only infinitesimal amounts of adrenaline and noradrenaline are excreted, and in subjects leading quiet lives only about 5 μg of adrenaline and 20 to 40 μg of noradrenaline are excreted within 24 hours. In cases of phæochromocytoma, however, up to 100 times this quantity is excreted within 24 hours (Engel and von Euler, 1950).

Treatment is surgical and may be entirely successful; but the operative mortality is about 30 per cent (Mackeith, 1944). The chief dangers are extreme hyper-adrenalism during manipulation of the tumour, and a profound drop in blood pressure following its removal. Dibenyline, 20 mg. three or four times daily (Allen *et al.*, 1951) or phentolamine, 20 to 40 mg. t.d.s., may be given orally to control the pre-operative situation, and noradrenaline may be infused post-operatively, at a rate of approximately 10 μg per minute, to control the transient circulatory collapse that may follow removal of the tumour.

TRANSIENT HYPERTENSION

The clinical features of acute nephritis and toxæmia of pregnancy are beyond the scope of this work, and their effect upon the heart is discussed elsewhere (page 638).

PERSISTENT HYPERTENSION

It is doubtful whether any symptoms can be ascribed to high blood pressure itself. Certainly the majority of cases are discovered accidentally, or by reason of complications. Headaches, fatigue, dizziness, difficulty in concentration, and palpitations, are commonly due to anxiety, whether the blood pressure is raised or not. Redistribution of blood due to selective vasoconstriction may, however, determine the behaviour of two variables. It was stated previously that vasoconstriction in skin and brain was more or less sufficient to prevent an increase of blood flow through these territories as a result of raised pressure: the words "more or less" may now be amplified. Thus more cutaneous vasoconstriction may be responsible for the pale hypertensive, less for the red; more cerebral vasoconstriction may be responsible for dizziness, failing memory, and for general mental deterioration, less for headache. The more important symptoms associated with hypertension are due to cardiac, renal or cerebral complications, and will be discussed later.

The blood pressure is necessarily raised; a diagnosis of previous persistent hypertension, when the blood pressure is found to be normal, is nearly always wrong, unless there is severe hæmorrhage, shock, massive pulmonary embolism, or myocardial infarction. It is customary to recognise four grades of hypertension according to the level of the diastolic pressure: between 95 and 110 mm. Hg is considered mild; 110 to 125 moderate; 125 to 140 severe; above 140 gross. The systolic pressure may be at any level between 150 and 300 mm. Hg, and may modify the grade accordingly. With mild hypertension it is usually between 150 and 200; with moderate hypertension between 180 and 230; with severe, between 210 and 260; with gross, between 240 and 300. Essential and nephritic hypertension may be of any grade; malignant hypertension is always severe or gross. The frequent discrepancy between the grade of hypertension itself and the severity of the disease as a whole is explained by the fact that the blood pressure without reference to the cardiac output is only a rough guide to the total peripheral resistance.

The pulse is firm and varies considerably in amplitude from case to case. In the more severe grades it is apt to be small; in those with marked atherosclerosis, large. If the pulse is full and bounding the raised pressure is more likely to be due to a hyperkinetic circulatory state (high cardiac output). Hard, tortuous or calcified peripheral arteries indicate atherosclerosis or Monckeberg's sclerosis, not hypertension—although they may be associated. In the latter event, one or other carotid, usually the right, may be kinked, and then mistaken for an aneurysm; or carotid pulsation may be so increased in amplitude as to suggest aortic incompetence. A diminished and delayed femoral pulse associated with absent dorsalis pedis and posterior tibial pulses indicates coarctation of the aorta. Pulsus alternans may occur in severe cases, and is usually associated with heart failure, or with ectopic beats.

Retinoscopy may reveal arterial thickening, hæmorrhages, exudates or papillœdema (Liebrecht, 1859), and should never be omitted. There are five signs of arterial thickening: (1) increased tortuosity; (2) notching, pinching, or S-shaped bending of veins at arterio-venous crossings; (3) uniform or irregular narrowing of the arterial blood streams, owing to reduction in the diameter of the vascular lumina; (4) white arterial fringes or thin white lines bordering the red arterial streams, representing the thickened white walls of the arteries themselves—they are rarely seen in more than one or two places and then only for a short distance, usually on a bend; (5) the single white streak, representing a thrombosed artery with an obliterated lumen. Occasionally, the distal part of such an artery may be patent, due to the development of a collateral circulation.

By far the most important of these signs is narrowing of the arterial lumen. Normally, the apparent width of a retinal artery compared with its accompanying vein is as 5 : 5 or 4 : 5. When the artery is thickened this ratio is decreased, and may be about 3 : 5 or less. There is no better way of expressing the average calibre of the retinal arteries than by giving the approximate arterio-venous ratio.

In benign hypertension it is rare to find more than notching of veins and narrowing of the arterial lumina; white arterial fringes and obliteration of the lumen usually mean nephritic or malignant hypertension.

It should perhaps be added that the appearance of the fundal vessels gives little indication of the state of the cerebral vessels; the risk of stroke cannot be assessed from retinoscopy.

Retinal hæmorrhage may be superficial, when it is linear or fan-shaped in appearance; or deep, when it resembles a rounded smudge. Both kinds may be seen in hypertensive retinopathy, but the former is more common. Hæmorrhages are unusual in essential hypertension, and when present are usually minute. They are not uncommon in nephritic hypertension, and almost invariable, sooner or later, in the malignant type. Just what causes these small hæmorrhages is not clear, for the capillary blood pressure is normal in hypertension (Ellis and Weiss, 1929–30), and in any case healthy capillaries can withstand astonishingly high pressures. Hæmorrhage secondary to a venous thrombosis at an arterio-venous crossing is more easily understood.

Thrombosis of a retinal artery or vein usually causes a defect in the visual field of the affected eye, and thrombosis of the central artery or vein causes blindness. Unfortunately retinal thrombosis is apt to be recurrent.

Retinal exudates are of four distinct types: (1) large hæmorrhages sometimes reveal eccentric soft white cores which may persist after absorption of the blood; (2) soft fleecy patches scattered indiscriminately over the retina are characteristic of malignant hypertension; (3) complete or incomplete star patterns, composed of hard whitish particles or dots, radiating from the macula, may be seen in chronic nephritic or in malignant hypertension; (4) in diabetes mellitus, the exudate is waxy, sharply cut, and scattered, resembling pale yellow confetti. Small areas of retinal degeneration in old people should not be confused with exudates.

When *papillœdema* is added to the signs of hypertensive retinopathy already described, malignant hypertension should be diagnosed. Conversely, malignant hypertension should not be diagnosed in the absence of papillœdema (Ellis, 1938). Although chronic nephritis may be responsible little is lost by making the other diagnosis, for if there is papillœdema the course of the disease will certainly be malignant, if acute nephritis and toxæmia of pregnancy can be excluded. The appearances may be distinguished from those of cerebral tumour by the arterial changes, by the macular star figure, or by exudates independent of hæmorrhages.

Papillœdema is usually associated with a high cerebro-spinal fluid pressure, but not invariably; moreover, higher C.S.F. pressures are found without papillœdema in cases of superior vena cava obstruction. Evidence from experimental hypertension in rats suggests that papillœdema is due to cerebral œdema caused by intense vascular spasm and secondary increased capillary permeability (Byrom, 1954). Occasionally, progressive blindness occurs.

Examination of the heart usually reveals some degree of left ventricular hypertrophy. The apex beat becomes displaced slightly to the left and downwards; the cardiac impulse becomes heaving in quality, and unusually easy to feel. It is quite different from the short sharp thrust of the over-acting heart, for it is a quiet unhurried action, giving the impression of great strength. The hyperdynamic quality of the former may be compared with the first few strokes of a racing crew, galvanised into urgent action by the sound of the starting signal; the heaving impulse of left ventricular hypertrophy to the powerful steady drive maintained by the crew when it has settled down to a long hard struggle. If, with due care, the apex beat cannot be located, left ventricular hypertrophy is unlikely, even in obese subjects, unless masked by emphysema.

Presystolic gallop rhythm is common with severe hypertension, and means that the left ventricle is receiving atrial help to increase its diastolic stretch so that it may contract more powerfully. The second sound at the base is accentuated and high pitched. Functional aortic incompetence is not uncommon and may be associated with diastolic pressures of 130 to 170 mm. Hg; in other words, it may not affect the circulatory dynamics. It is due to dilatation of the aortic ring and may be compared with functional pulmonary incompetence in cases of pulmonary hypertension. Pulsus alternans may sometimes be heard, especially if there is a mitral systolic murmur (Levine, 1948).

Auricular fibrillation is found in about 7.5 per cent of unselected hypertensive patients (Rothstadt, 1938), and may precipitate congestive heart failure. At first, and particularly if untreated, it may be paroxysmal; but as a rule it soon becomes persistent, especially in elderly subjects. Permanent auricular fibrillation under digitalis control is less troublesome than paroxysmal fibrillation, and tends to protect the individual from paroxysmal cardiac dyspnœa and acute pulmonary œdema. Other rhythm changes are relatively rare, but include auricular flutter, paroxysmal tachycardia and all degrees of heart block.

Limitation of cardiac reserve is indicated by undue breathlessness on exertion and by poor responses to effort tolerance tests. Left ventricular failure develops sooner or later in the majority of those who survive the other hazards of hypertension, and may be recognised by a history of orthopnœa, paroxysmal cardiac dyspnœa or pulmonary œdema, and by finding a diminished vital capacity, maximum breathing capacity and lung volume, exaggeration of respiratory intrathoracic pressure swings, prolongation of the crude pulmonary circulation time, an increased pulmonary blood volume, and radiological evidence of chronic interstitial œdema ("pulmonary venous congestion"), as described on pages 273 to 279.

Congestive heart failure with elevation of the venous pressure, hepatic distension, and dependent œdema, follows left ventricular failure in practically all cases that survive other risks. Not infrequently, patients with hypertensive heart disease develop congestive heart failure without previous orthopnœa and paroxysmal cardiac dyspnœa. There are two chief explanations for this behaviour. (1) Left ventricular failure may result in a diminished cardiac output, which reduces the renal blood flow and leads to retention of sodium and water; the increased blood volume then raises the venous pressure, so that the clinical features resemble those of failure of both ventricles, although the right ventricle itself may not be overloaded. (2) As in mitral stenosis, passive pulmonary hypertension resulting from an elevated left atrial pressure may lead to active pulmonary vasoconstriction; when the pulmonary vascular resistance exceeds 10 units, right ventricular failure may be expected. It should be explained, perhaps, that the pulmonary artery pressure is not ordinarily raised in systemic hypertension of any type or severity, provided there is no left ventricular failure (Lenegre and Maurice, 1947).

The suggestion that the right ventricle is partly obstructed by displacement of the interventricular septum (Bernheim, 1910) lacks proof, but the grounds on which the existence of Bernheim's syndrome is now being rejected are premature and equally unconvincing. It may clarify matters to restate the present position. The syndrome implies a severe left-sided cardiopathy (such as hypertensive heart disease, aortic valve disease, mitral incompetence, or cardiac infarction) with a form of left ventricular failure that presents clinically with a high venous pressure, enlargement of the liver, œdema, and relatively little breathlessness, but without orthopnœa, paroxysmal cardiac dyspnœa, pulmonary œdema, or radiological evidence of "pulmonary venous congestion". Bernheim's suggestion, that a filling defect of the right ventricle caused by undue bulging of the interventricular septum might be responsible for the so-called right ventricular failure, was welcomed as a reasonable hypothesis to explain the physiological situation, and after holding sway for forty years should not be abandoned without adequate proof to the contrary.

Just as Eisenmenger's complex has had to be brought up to date by adding its most essential feature (a pulmonary vascular resistance at or above systemic level), so Bernheim's syndrome must be brought up to date by adding *absence of a high pulmonary vascular resistance*, a *small right ventricle*, and *considerable dilatation of the right atrium*. As explained above the development of a high pulmonary vascular resistance (10 to 20 units in cases of left ventricular failure can certainly prevent pulmonary congestive manifestations, just as it can in mitral stenosis, but in such instance the right ventricle is enlarged, and the electrocardiogram may provide evidence of this in life. This situation must be excluded before a diagnosis of Bernheim's syndrome is tenable. The high resistance can be proved b means of cardiac catheterisation in non-ischæmic cases, but the procedure is dangerous in patients with angina pectoris or previous cardiac infarction. But if the pulmonary vascular resistance is not unduly high, as in the case described by Selzer *et al.* (1955), in which it was only 5.7 units, what is protecting the lungs? Right ventricular failure should not occur from passive pulmonary hypertension (Wood, 1954).

In some individuals with high left atrial pressures, pulmonary congestive symptoms are curiously lacking despite the radiological demonstration of chronic interstitial œdema of the lungs, but we are not concerned with these in the present discussion, because one of the criteria upon which the modern diagnosis of Bernheim's syndrome rests is absence of this radiological sign.

Selzer *et al.*, in their argument against the validity of the Bernheim concept, compare the expected physiological situation with that in "right-sided constrictive pericarditis". This is unsound, partly because there is virtually no such thing as right-sided constrictive pericarditis, and partly because Bernheim's syndrome could not exist without left ventricular failure and a rise of left ventricular diastolic pressure. A filling defect of the right ventricle implies impairment of a *diastolic* physiological function, and the septum would not bulge unduly into the cavity of the right ventricle during diastole if the diastolic pressure relationship between the two ventricles was reversed. Pick's disease, however, considered conventionally, serves very well to illustrate the Bernheim concept. In this disease the left atrial pressure is usually of the order of 20 mm. Hg, which in uncomplicated mitral stenosis would certainly be sufficient to cause pulmonary congestive symptoms. Why then are these symptoms usually absent? The answer, of course, is because the cardiac output cannot rise sufficiently to raise the left atrial pressure well above the osmotic pressure of the plasma. This is just what might be expected if left ventricular failure were complicated by a filling defect of the right ventricle.

One way of proving whether the right ventricle is overloaded or suffering from a filling defect would be to raise or lower the right atrial pressure by tipping or other means: if the right ventricle is overloaded, raising its filling pressure should reduce its output and therefore lower the pulmonary systolic pressure and the mean left atrial pressure; if the right ventricle is suffering from a filling defect, then raising the right atrial pressure should increase its output and therefore raise the pulmonary systolic pressure and mean left atrial pressure. Or one might study the effect of inspiration and expiration upon the pulmonary component of the second heart sound: with an overloaded right ventricle P_2 should not be delayed by inspiration, whereas with a filling defect of the right ventricle it should be so delayed.

The cardiac output is low in hypertensive congestive heart failure, but may be near normal at rest in isolated left ventricular failure; moreover, paroxysmal cardiac dyspnœa may occur as the output rises (page 274).

The size of the heart in hypertension bears a close relationship to the duration of heart failure; it is largest in essential hypertension when failure has been protracted; least enlarged in chronic nephritic hypertension when death is due to renal failure, or in those who die from apoplexy or from other non-cardiac causes (Harrison and Wood, 1949). Again, serial skiagrams may show little alteration in the manifest size of the heart for long periods in essential hypertension, yet gross enlargement may develop rapidly when failure occurs. This is not only a matter of cardiac dilatation, because heart weights show similar correlation. Slight to moderate left ventricular hypertrophy probably results from hypertension alone, according to its degree and duration; but gross enlargement, which usually involves the right ventricle as well as the left, is always due to protracted failure.

Moderate hypertrophy should be regarded as a compensatory change of structure which is beneficial: it helps the heart to perform more work (Dieckhoff, 1936).

Electrocardiography provides the most accurate means by which the degree of left ventricular enlargement and stress may be assessed. Leads facing the surface of the left ventricle, such as V_5 and V_6, show high voltage and slightly widened R waves, with depressed R-T segments and inverted T waves (fig. 16.01). This fundamental pattern is reflected in right

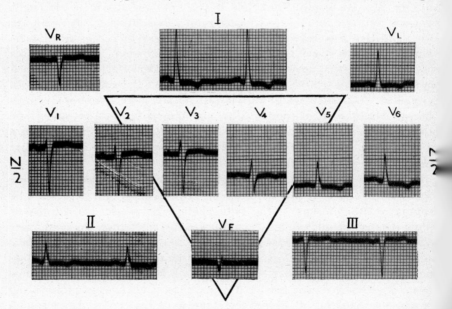

Fig. 16.01—Electrocardiogram in a case of hypertensive heart disease (see text). The heart is electrically horizontal.

ventricular surface leads, such as V_2, as small R waves followed by deep S waves, the S-T segment being elevated, and the T wave invariably upright. The heart is usually electrically horizontal, left ventricular surface potentials being transmitted to the left arm, right ventricular surface poter tials to the left leg. Lead V_L then resembles V_5 and V_6; lead V_F resembles V_1. Standard limb leads therefore show left axis deviation, lead I looking like V_L and lead III like V_F.

When the heart is rotated clockwise on its longitudinal axis (viewed from below), the anterior part of the inter-ventricular septum is displaced to the left, and the transition zone shifts to the left of V_4 (fig. 16.02); when the heart is rotated anti-clockwise, the transition zone moves to the right, and QR complexes or dominant R waves with inverted T waves may be found as far across as V_3.

When the heart is electrically vertical, left ventricular surface potentials are transmitted to the left leg, right ventricular surface potentials to the left

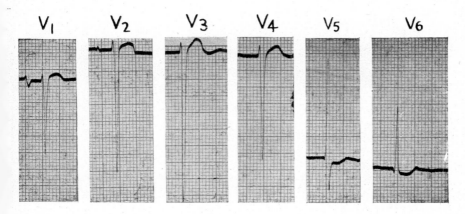

Fig. 16.02—Electrocardiogram in a case of hypertensive heart disease with clockwise rotation about the longitudinal axis: the transition zone is shifted to the left.

arm. Lead V_F then shows the tall R wave and inverted T, whilst lead V_L has a prominent S wave. Standard leads may then show right axis deviation with inversion of the T wave in leads 2 and 3.

Concordant left ventricular preponderance in standard leads (fig. 16.03) is due to a semi-vertical electrical position of the heart. Left ventricular surface potentials are transmitted to the left leg, and standard leads show high-voltage R waves and inversion of the T wave in all leads.

The higher and wider the R wave in lead V_5–V_6, and the deeper the S wave in lead V_1, the bigger the left ventricle. The pattern may be distinguished from left bundle branch block by the presence of Q in lead V_6. The cause of the R-T segment depression and the T wave inversion is less well understood: these changes may be associated with acute left ventricular stress without hypertrophy of the muscle, although they usually result from both; coronary disease is not responsible. They are not altered by exercise or by transient reduction of the blood pressure to normal levels by means of hexamethonium or tetraethylammonium (Hayward, 1948).

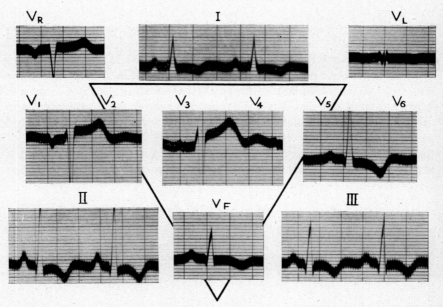

Fig. 16.03—Electrocardiogram showing concordant left ventricular preponderance due
to a semi-vertical position of the heart.

X-rays reveal left ventricular enlargement fairly well, but accurate
measurement is difficult in obese subjects. The left border of the heart is
not only displaced to the left, but is denser and more rounded than usual,
and may sink deeply into the shadow of the diaphragm (fig. 16.04a), whilst
the point of opposing movement is displaced upwards. In the second
oblique position the patient often has to be turned further to his right
than usual before the left ventricle clears the spine; the increased bulk of
the left ventricle is usually obvious (fig. 16.04b).

Hypertension also leads to unfolding of the aortic arch. The ascending
limb curves more forward and to the right, the descending more backward
and to the left. In the anterior view the aorta may thus appear widened,
but only because the two limbs throw adjacent instead of superimposed
shadows (fig. 16.05a). Unfolding is best seen in the left anterior oblique
position, especially with barium in the œsophagus, which is deflected back
with it (fig. 16.05b); the abrupt angulation so caused occasionally produces
dysphagia.

The combination of left ventricular enlargement and unfolding of the
aorta presents the characteristic appearance of two ovals set at right angles;
another descriptive term is "boot-shaped" (this should not be confused
with the "cœur en sabot", which compares the turned-up toe of the heart
in Fallot's tetralogy with that of the wooden shoe commonly worn by
Dutch peasants).

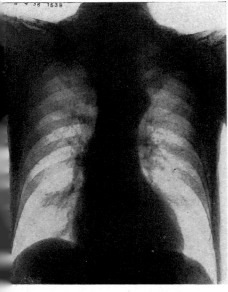

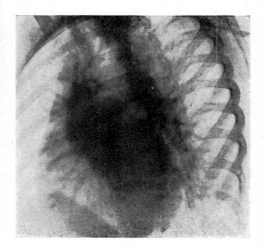

Anterior view: the apex of the left ventricle is buried in the diaphragm.

(b) Angiocardiogram in the second oblique position.

Fig. 16.04—Hypertensive heart disease showing left ventricular enlargement.

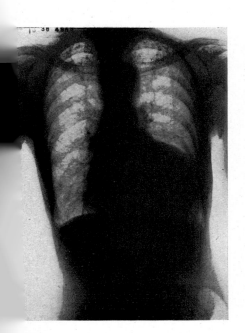

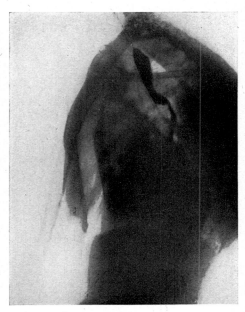

(a) Anterior view.

(b) Left anterior oblique position with barium in the œsophagus.

16.05—Skiagram of a case of hypertensive heart disease showing unfolding of the aortic arch.

779

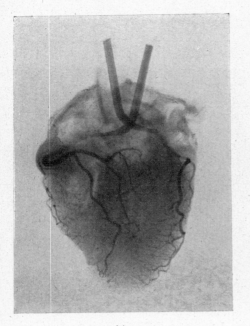

(a)

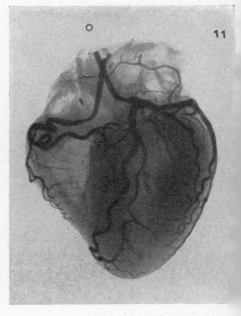

(b)

Fig. 16.06—Comparison of the coronary systems in a normal (a) and a hypertensive heart (b)
The coronary vessels have been injected with a radio-opaque gel (see text).

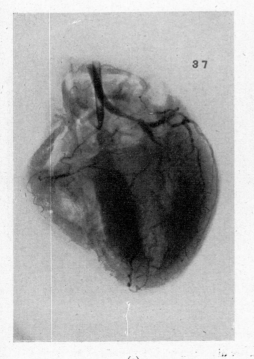

(a)

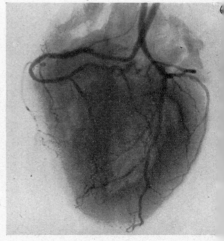

(b)

Fig. 16.07—Coronary systems of two case
hypertensive heart disease with angina pecto

(a) Showing occlusive coronary atheroscler
(mixed case).

(b) Showing failure of the coronary vessel
enlarge with the heart.

Angina pectoris occurs in 5 to 10 per cent of cases, and may be due to associated coronary atherosclerosis or to relative coronary insufficiency. Conversely, essential hypertension (past or present) has been found in 27 per cent of men and 71 per cent of women who present with coronary occlusion (Master, 1953). Angina may be typical, or it may tend to last longer than usual, even up to an hour or so, depending particularly upon transient rises of blood pressure such as occur, for example, in paroxysmal hypertension; strong emotion, e.g. fear or anger, and exposure to cold, may provoke such an attack.

It will be remembered that the coronary blood flow depends upon the mean blood pressure, and upon the state of the coronary arteries. During systole, the large extra-mural coronary vessels dilate, forming a tense elastic reservoir, the outflow being sealed by the intramural pressure. The higher the systolic pressure, the greater this elastic reservoir. As the ventricles relax, blood flows through the intra-mural branches, influenced not only by the aortic diastolic pressure, but also by the elastic recoil of the superficial coronary arteries.

Autopsy studies indicate that the coronary blood flow in essential hypertension is considerably increased. In figs. 16.06 the coronary systems of a normal and of a hypertensive heart are compared. The vessels have been injected with a radio-opaque substance at the calculated mean pressure, and skiagrams have been taken at a fixed distance, so that comparative measurements are valid. The large and luxuriant coronary tree of the hypertensive case is typical of the series studied (Harrison and Wood, 1949). It is probable that the coronary flow behaves like the blood flow through skeletal muscle, and is usually increased in all forms of hypertension. In cases of angina, however, skiagrams of the injected coronary vessels show either occlusive atherosclerosis (fig. 16.07a) or a meagre coronary system which has failed to enlarge with the heart (fig. 16.07b).

Renal behaviour varies greatly according to the type of hypertension. In the essential variety renal failure is rare, and when it does occur it is late, usually in patients over 70 years of age. Minor degrees of renal involvement, however, are common. Traces of albumin, and hyaline casts, are often found in the urine, due to glomerular fault, and diminished filtration may be revealed by inulin, creatinine, or urea clearance tests. Tubular re-absorption may be impaired, resulting in polyuria and in diminished power of urinary concentration. Nocturia may also be a feature.

In malignant hypertension there is always a fast race between renal failure, cardiac failure, and cerebral catastrophe. The end is sometimes a combination of all three. Nevertheless, despite the early occurrence of renal failure, it is rare for pronounced changes in renal function, or for conspicuous urinary findings, to precede the characteristic retinopathy (Wagener and Keith, 1924). The converse is true of nephritic hypertension. Nephrosclerosis in malignant hypertension differs from that found in essential hypertension only in the presence of afferent glomerular arteriolar necrosis.

In chronic nephritis there is usually considerable evidence of renal damage at a time when the heart is but little enlarged, and when the fundi are relatively normal. Albumin, hyaline and granular casts, and occasionally red cells, are found in the urine; inulin, creatinine, and urea clearance are greatly diminished; the blood urea may be raised; and there is commonly polyuria, nocturia, and failure of urinary concentration.

Cerebral manifestations occur sooner or later in about one-quarter of hypertensive cases. *Cerebral hæmorrhage* is an ever-present danger, and may at any time cut short the life of the patient. *Subarachnoid hæmorrhage* is by no means rare, congenital deficiencies in the media or elastica of certain arteries, particularly those forming the circle of Willis, with or without berry aneurysm, giving way to the high pressure. *Cerebral thrombosis* may also occur, but depends more upon associated cerebral atherosclerosis.

Hypertensive encephalopathy is characterised by attacks of severe headache, vomiting, coma or convulsions, lasting for hours, with or without transient localising signs, and is an important complication of malignant hypertension. It is probably due to local or general cerebral ischæmia and œdema, secondary to intense cerebral vascular spasm and increased capillary permeability (Scheinker, 1948; Byrom, 1954). It should be understood that the normal cerebral blood flow in uncomplicated malignant hypertension implies intense cerebral vasoconstriction, for if the cerebral vascular resistance remained normal the cerebral blood flow would be torrential with blood pressures in the region of 260/150. The rapid recovery that follows appropriate treatment (*vide infra*) and the ease with which appropriate prophylactic treatment prevents attacks deny both cerebral hæmorrhage and cerebral thrombosis, although both may have to be excluded in the first instance.

Deterioration of higher cerebral function has already been mentioned; when severe it is usually due to associated atherosclerosis and ischæmia. Occasionally, however, multiple pin-point hæmorrhages, scattered widely throughout the frontal lobes, are found at autopsy, and provide adequate explanation for dementia.

Hæmorrhages elsewhere are not uncommon and include epistaxis, hæmoptysis, and hæmatemesis. Whilst some local predisposing factor would seem probable, nothing significant is usually found. Clinical diagnosis in such cases may be obscure at first, for hypertension may not be recognised owing to the fall of blood pressure which accompanies the hæmorrhage. Moreover, when hæmodilution is slow, so that the hæmoglobin or hæmatocrit level is but little reduced, the apparently normal blood pressure may lead to gross error of judgment concerning the size of the hæmorrhage. Routine examination of the ocular fundi tends to prevent such mistakes.

DIFFERENTIAL DIAGNOSIS

If the blood pressure is found to be raised relative to standards already discussed, a diagnosis of hypertension can be made, and differential diagnosis is concerned only with its cause.

Acute nephritis should be obvious enough. The distinction between *toxæmia of pregnancy* and essential hypertension in a pregnant woman is not always easy unless the previous or subsequent history is known. Essential hypertension tends to be relieved during the second trimester, for the peripheral resistance is lowered during a normal pregnancy. Albuminuria, sodium and water retention, œdema, elevation of the venous pressure, breathlessness, and a demonstrably rising blood pressure all indicate toxæmia of pregnancy. It should be borne in mind, however, that the incidence of toxæmia in women with chronic essential hypertension is about seven times that in previously normal women (Browne, 1947), so both may well be present. *Coarctation of the aorta* is easily recognised if the femoral arteries are palpated as a routine. *Cushing's syndrome* is suggested by obesity, purple striæ, high coloured moon facies, hirsutism, and amenorrhœa; further studies are needed to elucidate the cause of the pituitary basophilism. Functional overactivity of the adrenal cortex may lead to a rather similar syndrome (Shrœder *et al.*, 1949). A *hyperkinetic circulatory state* with high systolic pressure and less conspicuously raised diastolic pressure should be recognised by the tachycardia, throbbing digital vessels, bounding pulse and overacting heart. Its cause may not be at all obvious and it should certainly not be attributed to an anxiety state or functional hyperadrenalism by a process of exclusion, but only on positive grounds. Hyperthyroidism, arteriovenous fistula, and Paget's disease of bone may be responsible for a hyperkinetic rise of blood pressure, especially when there is coincidental atherosclerosis, which increases the more proximal vascular resistance. The degree of vasodilatation in hepatic failure and beri-beri, the reduced blood volume in severe chronic anæmia, and the relatively slight increase of cardiac output in hypoxic cor pulmonale do not encourage hyperkinetic systemic hypertension. *Phæochromocytoma* with a predominant outpouring of adrenaline rather than noradrenaline can cause a hyperkinetic circulatory state with chiefly systolic hypertension; a test dose of rogitine is therefore advised in these difficult cases. *Functional hyperadrenalism* should respond to rogitine equally well. Personal experience suggests that there is also a non-psychiatric form of hyperkinetic hypertension of as yet undetermined cause.

Paroxysmal hypertension due to phæochromocytoma may be suggested by the history and confirmed by the rogitine or histamine type of test and by finding an excess of catechol amines in the plasm or urine (page 770).

The differential etiological diagnosis of persistent hypertension due to a high peripheral vascular resistance (after excluding phæochromocytoma and Cushing's syndrome) lies between chronic pyelonephritis, other "surgical kidneys", chronic nephritis, and essential hypertension.

Chronic pyelonephritis may be suggested by the history, the absence of hypertension in the parents, pus cells and micro-organisms in the urine, early limitation of tubular concentrating power and the development of the malignant course in a relatively young subject (Brod, 1955). Whether routine pyelography is justified, when there is nothing to suggest chronic unilateral pyelonephritis, is at least debatable. Out of 2,055 routine pyelograms in subjects with persistent hypertension reported by Ratcliff *et al.* (1947), less than 0.8 per cent were found to have an unsuspected unilateral renal lesion of a kind that led to nephrectomy, and of this small number only about a third were so relieved of hypertension. Since pyelography is not entirely without risk it is difficult to believe that its routine use is either wise or economically defensible for the sake of one patient out of 300 investigated. Perhaps it should be restricted to those cases that might reasonably be suspected of having chronic pyelonephritis on the grounds given above.

Chronic nephritis (chronic pyelonephritis and other "surgical kidneys" having been excluded) is a more likely etiological diagnosis than essential hypertension if impairment of renal function is far in advance of cardiac or cerebral disturbance, or if renal failure occurs without heart failure in subjects under 60 years of age. The differential etiological diagnosis between chronic nephritis and essential hypertension is no longer academic when hypertension is in the malignant phase.

Malignant hypertension itself is diagnosed whenever there is papilloedema. Etiologically almost any form of hypertension may take this course, including acute nephritis, visceral angiitis, toxaemia of pregnancy, phaeochromocytoma, Cushing's syndrome, pyelonephritis, chronic nephritis and essential hypertension; only coarctation of the aorta is exempt.

COURSE AND PROGNOSIS

The hypertension of *acute nephritis* is nearly always transient in those that recover. After a latent interval, which varies from a few weeks to very many years, the blood pressure rises again in those that develop chronic nephritis. The prognosis is then grave, the mortality rate in men being six times that which would be expected in unaffected men of the same age group (Frant and Groen, 1950).

Follow-up studies on cases with *toxaemia of pregnancy* reveal that 30 per cent develop permanent essential hypertension (Light, 1948). It is not clear, however, whether pre-eclampsia is responsible for the subsequent hypertension, or whether pregnancy merely precipitates the onset of essential hypertension. The prognosis, once persistent hypertension has developed, appears to be the same as for essential hypertension.

Perhaps the best follow-up studies of persistent hypertension in the literature are those by Janeway (1913), Blackford, Bowers and Baker (1930), and Bechgaard (1946). Janeway found that one-half of 458 patients were dead within five years, and three-quarters within ten years of the onset of symptoms. Blackford, Bowers and Baker reported a 50 per cent mortality (70 per cent of the men; 9 per cent of the women) amongst 222 cases within five to eleven years. Of Bechgaard's 1,000 patients, 41 per cent of the men and 22.4 per cent of the women were dead within five to ten years. The better outlook in women was emphasised in all three articles. Bechgaard found the mortality rate of hypertensive men was 2.9 times, and women 1.4 times, that of the general population, and was similar in all age groups (excluding renal cases).

Apart from sex the chief factors affecting prognosis include the type of hypertension, the degree of retinopathy, the height of the diastolic blood pressure, and the state of the heart. The natural outlook in malignant hypertension is uniformly bad, few cases surviving more than one or two years, and the average only 8.4 months after the diagnosis is first made (Schottstaedt and Sokolow, 1953). Chronic nephritic hypertension also has a grave prognosis, the mortality rate being about three times that of essential hypertension (Frant and Groen, 1950). This is partly because renal hypertension is often a late manifestation of chronic kidney disease— hence the frequency of a normal-sized heart in this group.

Wagener and Keith (1939) correlated life expectancy with changes in the ocular fundi; they followed the course of 209 patients for five to nine years. The survival rate according to whether retinal changes were mild, moderate, severe or gross was 80 per cent, 35 per cent, 9 per cent, and nil, respectively. When retinopathy was gross and included papillœdema, 80 per cent died within one year.

Although the height of the systolic blood pressure is often said to matter little, Sarre and Lindner (1948) found that in a series of 166 cases observed over a period of seven years, 48 per cent of those with systolic pressures under 200 mm. Hg survived, compared with only 11 per cent of those with systolic pressures over 200 mm. Hg. It is generally agreed that high diastolic pressures are sinister: in the series just quoted, for example, only 6 per cent of those with diastolic pressures above 140 mm. Hg when first seen survived seven years.

Cardiac behaviour in hypertension is determined by the amount of extra work involved, and by the ability of the heart to cope with it; it is chiefly influenced by the rapidity of hypertensive development, by the size and strength of the left ventricle, and by the efficiency of the coronary blood flow. The best defence is put up by a placid patient of voluntary or enforced sedentary habits and occupation, who has a naturally strong left ventricle with a good coronary blood flow, when hypertension is neither too severe nor too sudden. Under such circumstances the heart enlarges but little over the years, failure is indefinitely deferred, and the patient remains free from cardiac symptoms. The worst defence, leading to rapid failure, and perhaps to early death, occurs in an excitable individual of active physical habits and strenuous occupation, who tries to cope with a rapidly developing and extreme hypertension with an unprepared left ventricle indifferently nourished by a mean coronary system.

Evidence of any cardiac abnormality, e.g. diminished cardiac reserve, angina pectoris, enlargement, or electrocardiographic changes, at once doubles or trebles the mortality rate (Bechgaard, 1946). Inversion of the T wave in left ventricular surface leads or their equivalent is particularly grave, at least 60 per cent of such cases being dead in an average of eight months from the time of its discovery (Rykert and Hepburn, 1935). Auricular fibrillation means death within two years in 80 per cent of cases (Rothstadt, 1938).

Hypertensive heart failure is characteristically left ventricular at first and limits natural life-expectancy to about eighteen months. Systemic congestion follows sooner or later. Several congestive attacks usually occur, each responding less satisfactorily to treatment than its predecessor. The patient finally sinks into a stuporose condition with chronic venous congestion, hepatic engorgement and dependent dropsy; the blood pressure falls, Cheyne-Stokes breathing develops, and death comes slowly. Heart disease is responsible for death in 33 per cent (Janeway, 1913) to 55 per cent (Bell and Clawson, 1928) of hypertensive cases; stroke in 7.2 per cent (Paullin et al., 1927) to 16 per cent (Bechgaard, 1946); uræmia in 10 per cent (Bechgaard, 1946).

The average life expectancy in uncomplicated benign hypertension of slight or moderate grade is about fifteen years (Fahr, 1928). Obese subjects do as well or better than those with normal weight, probably because their blood pressures are not as high as they seem when measured by means of standard cuffs. Spontaneous recovery occurred in 5.4 per cent of Bechgaard's series (2 per cent of the women; 13 per cent of the men), but in none of those seen by Blackford, Bowers and Baker. After five to ten years 58 per cent of Bechgaard's cases were free from symptoms or only slightly inconvenienced.

Only about 0.2 per cent of cases of essential hypertension later become malignant, but 8 per cent of cases of chronic pyelonephritic hypertension do so.

TREATMENT

It must be said at once that as yet there is no satisfactory treatment for essential or malignant hypertension. When nephritic hypertension is due to a unilateral lesion such as chronic pyelonephritis, nephrectomy has proved curative in 19 per cent of 242 cases (Smith, 1948), but otherwise it can be but little influenced. Moreover, a causal relationship between a unilateral renal lesion and hypertension cannot be taken for granted, and before advising nephrectomy it is as well to make sure that neither parent was hypertensive (Platt, 1947). Normal renal function is also a necessary condition for successful nephrectomy; for severe hypertension may have so damaged the vessels of the originally healthy kidney as to have made it ischæmic and so to have established a vicious circle (Wilson and Byrom, 1941). Good results from nephrectomy may be expected in 25 to 50 per cent of cases when the renal lesion is chronic uncomplicated unilateral pyelonephritis (Ratcliff *et al.*, 1947; Pickering and Heptinstall, 1953).

The hypertension of Cushing's syndrome and that of phæochromocytoma both respond to removal of the offending tumour; and that due to coarctation of the aorta to surgical repair.

For essential hypertension there are six main lines of treatment: (1) conservative, (2) the low sodium or rice diet, (3) a miscellaneous group of drugs acting on the central nervous system, including rauwolfia, veratrum, hydrazinophthalazine and thiocyanate; (4) adrenergic blocking agents, such as hydergine; (5) lumbo-dorsal sympathectomy; (6) ganglionic blocking agents such as hexamethonium and pentolinium.

Conservative. When the grade of hypertension is mild or moderate, and when the prognosis is judged to be good on criteria previously outlined, radical medical or surgical treatment is hardly justified; but this does not mean that nothing else need be done. Conservative treatment seeks to correct adverse factors and to prevent complications or deterioration.

If circumstances permit, it is a good plan to begin treatment by putting the patient to bed, and to keep him there until the blood pressure has reached a static level. Symptoms usually disappear quickly, and the patient gains confidence. During this time, renal function may be fully and conveniently investigated; also, the reaction of the blood pressure to bed rest gives useful diagnostic and prognostic information, innocent labile types falling quickly to normal, nephritic and malignant hypertension responding least.

Patients should then be advised to live at a lower tempo: they should learn to refuse extra commitments and to relinquish the least important or most irksome of those they already have; they should keep Saturday and Sunday free for relaxation, should have at least nine hours rest in bed every night, and should insist on proper holidays each year, preferably six weeks. Long working hours, heavy mental or physical stress, and the general rush, hurry and struggle of modern life must be avoided or reduced. Occupation may require modification, but it is rarely practicable to change it radically. Sudden effort, especially in the cold or after a heavy meal, should be avoided; straining at stool should be prevented by regular habits, and if necessary by the use of liquid paraffin. Alcohol in moderation is permitted; smoking should be strictly limited.

Mental relaxation may be impossible without sedatives or psychiatric help. Phenobarbitone, $\frac{1}{2}$ to 1 grain (32 to 64 mg.) t.d.s. may be prescribed at times of unavoidable anxiety, alternated with potassium bromide, 5 to 10 grains (0.32 to 0.65 G.) t.d.s. Psychiatric help is invaluable, not necessarily from a psychiatrist, but by any experienced physician with the requisite knowledge. Many of the symptoms ascribed to hypertension are more often due to anxiety; moreover, hypertensive subjects usually have hyper-reactions to anxiety in the sense that their blood pressures rise unduly (Hines, 1940).

Symptoms attributed to hypertension at the menopause may respond to oral stilbœstrol 0.5 mg., ethinylœstradiol 0.02 mg., dienœstrol 1 mg., or mepilin tab. 1, daily, although the blood pressure does not fall; an associated anxiety state is also common at this time.

Obese patients tend to do well on a weight-reducing diet. One day's bed rest with semi-starvation per week, diet then being limited to fresh fruit, fruit juice and water only, may be most helpful; or such a régime may be instituted at less frequent intervals when the patient feels the need of it.

With this simple régime 60 per cent of patients with essential hypertension remain free from symptoms until cerebral, cardiac or renal complications arise.

Venesection has been advocated in the past and is still practised from time to time. It is only justified in phlethoric cases associated with polycythæmia. In essential hypertension its effect is fleeting, the blood pressure often regaining its previous level within twenty-four hours. In malignant hypertension and in chronic nephritis venesection is contra-indicated, for some degree of anæmia is usually present in both conditions.

Encephalopathy may be treated conservatively by means of rest and vigorous dehydration. Vestibular disturbances are relieved by dramamine or avomine, 25 mg. three times daily (Goldman et al., 1951). Heart failure responds to rest, digitalis, mercurial diuretics, aminophylline, and a low sodium diet. Renal failure resists all therapy.

Low sodium diet. Although Allen and Sherrill in 1922 showed that a low salt diet was a potent means of lowering the blood pressure, efficient dietetic treatment was not generally practised until re-introduced by Kempner in 1944. Kempner's fruit-rice diet consists essentially of fruit in any form, fruit juices, rice, sugar and a little milk; it contains approximately 2,000 calories, 20 G. of protein, 5 G. of fat, 200 mg. of chloride and 150 mg. of sodium (Kempner, 1946). Lean meat, fish and non-leguminous vegetables without salt and fat may be added when the blood pressure has been satisfactorily controlled (Kempner, 1948). Of 777 cases so treated, the majority severe, 70 per cent were unquestionably improved in an average time of three to four months (Kempner, 1949): objective evidence included a fall in the sum of the systolic and diastolic blood pressure of at least 40 mm. Hg, disappearance of papillœdema and of retinal hæmorrhages and exudates, restoration of an upright T wave in standard lead I (achieved in 50 per cent of cases in which it was previously inverted), and an appreciable reduction in the transverse diameter of the heart (51 per cent of 286 cases radiographed showed a reduction of about 6 per cent 37 per cent a reduction averaging 14 per cent, and 6.6 per cent a reduction averaging 24 per cent).

The efficacy of a diet very low in sodium was confirmed in rats with experimental hypertension by Grollman and Harrison (1945), and in human essential hypertension by Grollman (1945). It is now generally believed that its effect depends chiefly on its low sodium content (Pickering, 1952).

Treatment of this kind is invaluable to relieve hypertensive crises, including encephalopathy, and severe retinopathy with impairment of vision; it is also the best means of rapidly controlling left ventricular failure and congestive heart failure; but its monotony precludes its routine use in uncomplicated essential hypertension, for life expectancy may be ten years or more; nor can it be used when there is gross impairment of renal function, for it may then precipitate uræmia. For long-term treatment, however, a modified low sodium diet containing between 0.5 and 1 G. of sodium per day is advised. With the help of lemon and herbs of all kinds, such a diet (page 303) is well tolerated by the majority of patients whose personal experience has demonstrated its value, and after six to twelve months some of them develop an active dislike towards salt. A modified diet of this kind is insufficient by itself to control severe hypertension, but it is a helpful adjunct to other forms of treatment, and is imperative in cases with heart failure.

Rauwolfia serpentina

Although a preparation of the root of rauwolfia serpentina has been used in India as a sedative since ancient times, its value as a hypotensive agent has only recently been demonstrated (Vakil, 1940, 1949, 1955; Bhatia, 1942). The isolation of reserpine, one of the most active of the rauwolfia alkaloids, by Müller, Schlittler and Bein (1952), was a notable advance.

Reserpine, 0.25 mg., is as active as 50 mg. of the dried extract, and more or less equivalent to 1 or 2 mg. of preparations such as rauwiloid and hypertane, which contain several of the other alkaloids of rauwolfia. The initial dose of reserpine (serpasil) is 0.25 mg. t.d.s., but it may be increased up to 0.5 mg. t.d.s., or reduced to as low as 0.1 mg. daily, according to the response. There can be no doubt that reserpine is a moderately potent hypotensive agent (Vakil, 1953). It appears to act on the vasomotor centre itself in the hypothalamus. A spate of literature has confirmed Vakil's results (e.g. Wilkins and Judson, 1953).

Side effects include sinus bradycardia, nasal congestion, looseness of the bowels, gain in weight, coarse tremor or shakiness of the limbs, vivid dreams, drowsiness and mental depression.

Bradycardia is beneficial in cases that present initially with hyperkinetic features and is never a disadvantage. *Nasal congestion* may be very uncomfortable and should be treated with a suitable vasoconstrictor spray (such as privine). The *tendency to diarrhœa* helps to correct constipation in patients who are also treated with hexamethonium or pentolinium, and is otherwise innocuous. *Gain in weight* is due partly to the development of a hearty appetite and partly to retention of salt and water. Both are serious disadvantages, the former particularly in cases with coincident coronary disease, the latter when there is hypertensive heart failure (McGregor and Segal, 1955). Dexamphetamine, 5 mg. one hour before breakfast and lunch may correct the increase of appetite, and combat serpasil depression, but theoretically it would seem undesirable and is not advised until trials have established its safety in these cases. A low sodium diet, given in conjunction with reserpine therapy, prevents serious water retention. *Shakiness of the limbs* is rare with doses not exceeding 0.25 mg. t.d.s., and usually disappears if the dose is reduced. Coarse tremor seems to be Parkinsonian in type. *Drowsiness* is beneficial at night, but may interfere with efficiency by day; the midday dose may then have to be withheld. *Mental depression* may be intense and calls for immediate withdrawal of the drug, for reducing the dose will not suffice. This is fortunately unusual, but must never be disregarded. It has been suggested that depression is more common with reserpine than with preparations containing some of the other rauwolfia alkaloids, but this has not yet been fully substantiated.

Reserpine is not anti-thyroid and does not increase the blood lipids *per se*. As a rule, coincident angina pectoris is not influenced by the treatment; aggravation, when it occurs, may be attributed to gain in weight. There is no evidence that the renal blood flow is reduced by rauwolfia alkaloids.

Veratrum

Veratrum viride, in the form of its powdered dry rhizome and roots, was re-introduced as a hypotensive agent fot the clinical treatment of essential hypertension by Hite (1946) and Freis and Stanton (1948). A stable mixture of alkaloids, biologically standardised, was called veriloid (Stutzman *et al.*, 1949), and was found to be more easily managed clinically (Wilkins *et al.*, 1949). With initial doses of 2 mg. t.d.s. after meals, increased gradually to 12 or 16 mg. a day, the blood pressure can be lowered in about two-thirds of hypertensive cases (Kauntze and Trounce, 1951). But side effects are the rule and include nausea and vomiting, weakness and malaise, and occasional collapse. In the author's experience the patient's lack of well-being while on veriloid precludes its long-term use, especially since it does not rank highly as a permanent hypotensive agent.

Veratrum album has proved more valuable, perhaps, in that it has given us an active pure alkaloid, protoveratrine (Krayer *et al.*, 1944, 1946), which when given intravenously in doses of 0.1 to 0.15 mg. may produce a profound fall of blood pressure in hypertensive patients (Meilman and Krayer, 1950): thus it may be used intravenously with advantage in hypertensive crises. For maintenance treatment protoveratrine is usually given by mouth in doses of 0.4 to 2.0 mg. three times daily after meals, starting with the smallest dose and gradually increasing it until the desired therapeutic effect is achieved or until the limit of tolerance is reached. Toxic symptoms, similar to those of veriloid, are all too common, and the number of cases that can be successfully treated is less than 25 per cent (Doyle and Smirk, 1953; Currens, Myers and White, 1953).

Veratrum, like rauwolfia, appears to act directly on the central nervous system (Stutzman, Simon and Maison, 1951).

I-Hydrazinophthalazine is another hypotensive agent which may act centrally. It has been given by mouth in doses of 50 to 150 mg. four- to six-hourly, but an appreciable fall in blood pressure is obtained in relatively few cases, and side effects may be formidable—chiefly severe headache, tachycardia, and anxiety or depression (Shroeder, 1952); moreover, good results are transient (Johnson *et al.*, 1952). A short experience of this drug was sufficient for the author to abandon it permanently.

Thiocyanates. Thiocyanate was originally introduced as a hypotensive agent by Treupel and Edinger (1900), but gained no immediate favour in view of the difficulty experienced in avoiding serious toxic symptoms. Considerable interest was taken in the drug, however, when Barker (1936) showed that the dose could be properly controlled if the thiocyanate blood level was estimated weekly. The normal serum thiocyanate ranges between 0 and 2.77 mg. per cent and is not altered in hypertension (Connell, Wharton and Robinson, 1946). Levels above 15 mg. per cent are dangerous, and those between 12 and 15 mg. per cent are risky. Toxic symptoms include weakness, anorexia, indigestion, nausea, vomiting, limb pains, impotence, purpura, dermatitis, goitre, thrombophlebitis, mental lethargy and confusion. In fatal cases dysarthria, verbal aphasia, convulsions, hallucinations, delirium and mania have usually preceded death by three to nineteen days (Del Solar *et al.*, 1945). Progressive anæmia and emaciation have been attributed to chronic poisoning after five to ten years' continuous therapy (Wald, Lindberg and Barker, 1939).

The potassium salt was given by mouth in initial doses of 2 to 3 grains (0.13 to 0.2 G.) three times daily after meals. The serum thiocyanate was measured on the seventh day and then at weekly intervals, subsequent dosage being regulated as follows:

Thiocyanate level	*Dosage recommended*
Under 5 mg. per cent .	. 2 to 3 grains (0.13 to 0.2 G.) t.d.s.
5 to 7 ,, ,, .	. 1.5 grains (0.1 G.) t.d.s.
7 to 10 ,, ,, .	. 1 grain (64 mg.) t.d.s.
Over 10 ,, ,, .	. Stop drug for one week

The lowest blood level compatible with a satisfactory hypotensive effect was maintained for three to six months. Further courses were given as desired.

The drug was said to be unsafe in patients over 60 years old, who had had cerebral or other thrombosis, or who had poor renal function; but Watkinson and Evans (1947) observed no ill-effect in fifteen patients over 60, nor in sixteen cases of malignant or chronic nephritic hypertension.

Thiocyanates were particularly recommended for labile hypertensives who complained of headache and giddiness (Hines, 1946); but they were also used for severe or gross cases unsuitable for lumbo-dorsal sympathectomy, and as an adjunct to surgical treatment. Clinical benefit associated with a significant fall of blood pressure was claimed in about 60 per cent of cases (Watkinson and Evans, 1947). This figure is not impressive when it is recollected that Bechgaard found that 58 per cent of 1,000 persistent hypertensives did well without treatment. Carefully controlled observations such as those by Rusken and McKinley (1947) are more convincing, and throw considerable doubt on the efficacy of thiocyanates. It is well to remember that Pauli (1903), who is usually credited with introducing thiocyanate for the treatment of hypertension, actually used the drug in the hope that it would prove superior to bromide in allaying anxiety symptoms, and reported singular success in this respect. Whether thiocyanate acts in this way or whether it has a more specific central hypotensive effect is still unknown, but it is now considered too toxic for routine therapy and has been largely abandoned.

Adrenergic blocking agents

Some confusion is attached to words like sympatholytic and adrenolytic, and it may help to define these terms. A drug that blocks the response of effector cells to peripheral sympathetic nerve stimulation is said to be sympatholytic, and since noradrenaline is the normal chemical mediator between the sympathetic nerve ending and the effector cell, a sympatholytic substance is necessarily an adrenergic blocking agent. A substance that blocks excitatory responses to *circulating* adrenaline and noradrenaline is said to be adrenolytic rather than sympatholytic, but of course is also an adrenergic blocking agent. The difference in actions between the two groups of drugs (although they always overlap to greater or less degree) is well exemplified in some of the diagnostic tests for phæochromocytoma. For this purpose the best drugs are adrenolytic rather than sympatholytic, and include benzodioxane and phentolamine (rogitine); dibenamine, dibenzyline and ilidar have too powerful a sympatholytic effect to be reliable, for this may lower the blood pressure in any kind of hypertension. As therapeutic agents in essential hypertension it is the sympatholytic rather than the adrenolytic action that is needed, and to this end hydergine is perhaps the best of the adrenergic blocking agents.

Hydergine (1 ml.) contains 0.1 mg. of each of the three dihydrogenated alkaloids of ergotoxine (dihydroergocornine, dihydroergocrystine, and dihydroergokryptine). Dihydroergocornine or hydergine may be given in doses of 0.05 to 0.1 mg. intramuscularly, or 0.1 to 0.5 mg. orally, three times daily (Freis *et al.*, 1949; Gibbs, 1952), but seems to lose its effect after a few weeks (Moister, Stanton and Freis, 1949).

Dibenamine, priscoline and rogitine are of little value (Nickerson, 1951).

Lumbo-dorsal sympathectomy. In recent years numerous attempts have been made to lower the blood pressure by surgical means. The only operation that has proved eminently successful is nephrectomy in those relatively rare cases in which hypertension is due to unilateral renal disease, such as chronic pyelonephritis. Of other surgical measures the best known is lumbo-dorsal sympathectomy as elaborated by Smithwick (1940). This consists of bilateral resection of the whole sympathetic chain from D8 to L2, including preganglionic fibres, ganglia, and splanchnic nerves. The object is to release as much vasoconstrictor tone as possible, to prevent renal cortical vasoconstriction, to produce postural hypotension, and, of course, to lower the basal blood pressure if possible. With these aims there has been an increasing tendency to extend Smithwick's operation, and a number of surgeons, e.g. Grimson (1947) and Boyd (1948), favour either total or subtotal paravertebral sympathectomy, splanchnicectomy and cœliac ganglionectomy.

The results of these various procedures have been fair. The operative mortality has averaged 3.9 per cent, but about 25 per cent have died during the period of post-operative observation (usually three to five years). There is no doubt that headache, dizziness and other symptoms may be alleviated, the blood pressure lowered, the electrocardiogram improved, the heart size reduced, and retinopathy diminished by such means (Peet *et al.*, 1940); objective improvement of one kind or another has been demonstrable in about 66 per cent of cases (Smithwick, 1944, 1949).

In a series of 400 cases operated on for hypertension at the Massachusetts General Hospital (F : M sex ratio 1.8 : 1) follow-up studies showed that after one year postural hypotension had virtually disappeared, after two years 38 per cent were improved, and after five years 8 of 100 cases had normal blood pressures, 13 had significantly reduced blood pressures, 52 were much the same, and 27 were dead (Evelyn *et al.*, 1949).

Of 143 cases of malignant hypertension treated by splanchnic resection by Peat and Isberg (1948), 21.6 per cent were still alive and free from papillœdema five years later; the operative mortality was 10 per cent, and no patient with moderate or marked impairment of renal function or with considerable cardiac enlargement did well.

Although the long-term results of surgical treatment were indifferent, their historical value should not be underestimated, for sympathectomy first proved that the blood pressure in essential hypertension could be permanently lowered, occasionally even to normal, and that lowering the blood pressure abolished the malignant reaction, improved the patient's health and prolonged life, thereby disproving the ill-founded theoretical objection that to lower the blood pressure in essential hypertension without dealing with the disease itself (whatever that was supposed to mean) was unphysiological.

Surgical sympathectomy thus opened the way to medical sympathectomy and encouraged pharmacological research into blood pressure lowering drugs of all kinds.

Ganglionic blocking agents

The demonstration by Burn and Dale in 1915 that tetraethylammonium ions inhibited transmission of all sympathetic and parasympathetic nerve impulses at the autonomic ganglia, and the realisation how this action might be exploited (Acheson and Moe, 1945) opened the way to medical sympathectomy. Normally all autonomic impulses are chemically transmitted by means of acetylcholine, which is liberated by the preganglionic nerve terminal and which then excites the ganglionic cells. Ganglion blocking drugs prevent acetylcholine from acting on the ganglion cells (Paton, 1951). In doses of 3 to 5 mg. per kilo intravenously or about 10 mg. per kilo intramuscularly, tetraethylammonium releases vasoconstrictor tone: both the blood pressure and venous pressure fall, especially in the upright position, the peripheral blood flow increases, the skin temperature rises, and the heart rate quickens. These effects may be reversed immediately by peripherally acting adrenergic drugs such as noradrenaline. Simultaneous parasympathetic block results in temporary paralysis of the gut and bladder, dry mouth, dry skin, dilatation of the pupils and loss of accommodation (Berry *et al.*, 1946; Lyons *et al.*, 1947). Peripherally acting cholinergic drugs, such as acetylcholine, mecholyl, etc., reverse these effects.

Pentamethonium iodide (C_5) and *hexamethonium iodide* (C_6) or bromide, introduced by Paton and Zaimis (1949) were found to be more powerful and more prolonged ganglionic blocking agents than T.E.A., and were soon tried clinically for the relief of hypertension (Arnold and Rosenheim, 1949; Burt and Graham, 1950; Turner, 1950). None of these early reports was enthusiastic: fears that merely lowering the blood pressure was unphysiological still lingered, postural hypotension and fainting turns were regarded as serious drawbacks, and the side-effects from parasympathetic blockade were troublesome and occasionally dangerous. In New Zealand, however, Smirk (1949) had perhaps a more enlightened view, believing that the chief danger of hypertension was the high blood pressure itself, however produced, and that the object of treatment was to lower the blood pressure efficiently and keep it lowered; postural hypotension, properly harnessed, became an asset rather than a liability, and in conjunction with a low sodium diet methonium halides soon became the treatment of choice for the majority of cases of severe hypertension (Restall and Smirk, 1950; Smirk, 1950; Smirk and Alstad, 1951).

Hexamethonium bromide (vegolysen) may be given by subcutaneous injection in initial doses of 15 to 20 mg. approximately three times daily; the patient is preferably propped up in bed, or may have the head of the bed raised on blocks, so that orthostatic hypotension may be quickly recognised and corrected, if too severe, by lying the patient flat. The blood pressure should be recorded hourly, both lying and standing. Day by day the dose is increased by 10 to 20 mg. according to the reaction and the rate at which tolerance develops; the final dose may be 100 to 200 mg. three times daily, but may have to be limited owing to side effects (*vide infra*). The objective is to maintain the blood pressure around the upper limit of normal when the patient stands up, and to maintain it at this level for as long as possible during waking hours, without causing serious side effects.

Oral treatment requires doses of 250 to 750 mg. thrice daily, half to one hour before meals. Unfortunately hexamethonium is very irregularly absorbed from the gut, so that the correct dose is more difficult to arrive at, and serious side-effects may occur occasionally without warning.

After a suitable single subcutaneous or intramuscular injection the clinical effect begins in 10 to 15 minutes and persists for several hours. Within 24 hours 90 per cent of the drug is recoverable from the urine (Harrington, 1953). Glomerular excretion is necessarily retarded in the presence of impaired renal function, and if the blood urea is raised doses should be correspondingly small and infrequent if the drug is used at all.

Undesirable side-effects include constipation, rarely intestinal paralysis, retention of urine (particularly in patients with enlarged prostates), dry mouth, and disturbance of vision due to difficulty in accommodation. The most dangerous of these is paralytic ileus, which should be treated immediately with prostigmine, 1.5 to 2 mg. intravenously or intramuscularly, and repeated two-hourly if necessary, no further doses of hexamethonium being given for at least 48 hours. Laxatives are usually required as a routine to combat the tendency to constipation, and patients should be advised to open their bowels before the morning dose of hexamethonium. When serpasil is also used to help lower the blood pressure, constipation is less troublesome. Special reading glasses should be provided to compensate for the loss of accommodation.

Weakness, dizziness and pallor, when standing still, is due to orthostatic hypotension, and can be counteracted by walking about or lying down; if dizziness is severe, or if there is actual syncope, the dose of hexamethonium should be reduced.

Since bromine constitutes about 44 per cent by weight of hexamethonium bromide, doses of 2 or more Grams per day orally are likely to result in symptoms of bromism sooner or later, especially when patients are also on the low sodium diet. These occur when the blood bromide exceeds 150 mg. per cent, and sometimes when it is only 75 to 100 mg. per cent (Goodman and Gilman, 1941). Hexamethonium iodide has a similar drawback in respect of iodism, and the chloride is hygroscopic; but the bitartrate, 300 mg. of which is equivalent to 250 mg. of the bromide, has none of these defects and is usually well tolerated. Nevertheless, with doses under 2 G. daily, hexamethonium bromide is preferred, for its sedative action is an advantage.

Pentolinium tartrate (M & B 2050 A or ansolysen) is about five times more potent and lasts one and a half times longer than hexamethonium (Wien and Mason, 1953); moreover, it is better absorbed from the gut, more consistent results follow oral therapy (Maxwell and Campbell, 1953), and hypertensive symptoms and complications (such as retinopathy) are controlled more swiftly than with hexamethonium (Smirk, 1953).

If given by injection the initial dose should not exceed 4 mg., and increments should be small (2 mg.). The initial oral dose is 20 to 40 mg. three or four times daily, half an hour before meals, and this should not be increased by more than 20 mg. per dose per day. Management is otherwise the same as when using hexamethonium.

Combined methods of treatment

The best all-round results in the treatment of hypertension are undoubtedly obtained by combining rest, the low sodium diet, rauwolfia alkaloids and pentolinium by mouth (Smirk *et al.*, 1954). The treatment should be pressed home at the start until the blood pressure is normal or not above 160/90 in the standing position two hours after the last dose of pentolinium.

The amount of each of the four therapeutic agents should then be adjusted to suit the patient, until undesirable side-effects are minimal and the regime tolerable and compatible with a reasonably active and enjoyable life. This is usually possible while maintaining a good measure of control of the blood pressure.

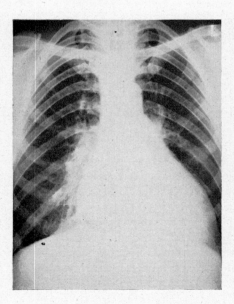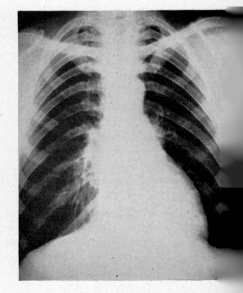

Fig. 16.08—Skiagrams (a) before and (b) after treatment of hypertensive heart failure by means of bed rest and a low sodium diet.

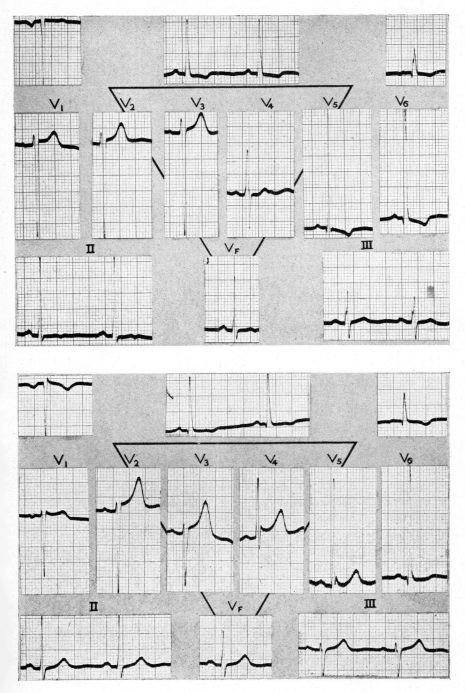

Fig. 16.09—Electrocardiogram in a case of hypertensive heart disease (a) before and (b) after treatment with hexamethonium bromide and a low sodium diet. Note the T wave changes in V_5 and V_6.

Of the various manifestations of hypertension virtually all are relieved by combined therapy except nephrosclerosis. Headaches, encephalopathy and retinopathy disappear rapidly in most instances. Cerebral thrombosis is discouraged rather than encouraged by the fall in blood pressure. The cerebral blood flow itself is not altered appreciably (Dewar *et al.*, 1953), the cerebral vascular resistance falling more or less in proportion to the drop in blood pressure. Left ventricular failure and congestive heart failure improve quickly, and even some reserve can be built up in the more favourable cases (fig. 16.08). Hypertensive T wave changes can be partly or wholly reversed (fig. 16.09) in about half the cases (Doyle, 1953). Angina pectoris is usually relieved, but may be aggravated occasionally when the blood pressure falls steeply in cases with advanced coronary disease; coronary thrombosis is no more common in treated than untreated cases (Doyle and Kilpatrick, 1954). On effort, the increased rise of blood pressure that ordinarily occurs in hypertensive subjects is suppressed (Fowler and Guz, 1954).

Long-term results of effectual medical treatment await the passage of the years, but already it is obvious that the prognosis of malignant hypertension and hypertensive heart failure is at least twice as good as formerly. Death from cerebral thrombosis, coronary thrombosis or renal failure rather than from heart failure is now the rule instead of the exception, and patients live longer and in a better state of health in consequence.

If treatment was undertaken much earlier, at a time when it is often said to be worse than the disease, the prospects might be brighter. The most promising regime for early treatment is probably a combination of emotional relaxation and the rauwolfia alkaloids.

While the treatment of transient hypertension cannot be considered here in detail, it may be noted that toxæmia of pregnancy responds very well to the low sodium diet, veratrum (Assali *et al.*, 1950), progesterone, 10 to 50 mg. daily (Dalton, 1954), and sympathectomy (Peat and Isberg, 1949): it seems likely, therefore, that it should also respond to the combined treatment outlined above for essential hypertension.

REFERENCES

Acheson, G. H., and Moe, G. K. (1945): "Some effects of tetra-ethyl ammonium on mammalian heart", *J. Pharmacol.*, **84**, 189.

Allen, E. V., *et al.* (1951): "A new sympatholytic and adrenolytic drug. Clinical studies in pheochromocytoma and essential hypertension", *Trans. Ass. Amer. Phys.*, **64**, 109.

Allen, F. M., and Sherrill, J. W. (1922): "Treatment of arterial hypertension", *J. metab. Res.*, **2**, 429.

Allen, W. J., Barcroft, H., and Edholm, O. G. (1946): "On action of adrenaline on blood vessels in human skeletal muscle", *J. Physiol.*, Lond., **105**, 255.

Anderson, W. H., *et al.* (1952): "The use of pharmacological tests in the diagnosis of pheochromocytoma", *Amer. Heart J.*, **43**, 252.

Anrep, G. V., and Stacey, R. S. (1927): "Comparative effect of various drugs upon the coronary circulation", *J. Physiol.*, Lond., **64**, 187.

Arnold, P., and Rosenheim, M. L. (1949): "Effect of pentamethonium iodide on normal and hypertensive persons", *Lancet*, ii, 321.

Assali, N. S., Brust, A. A., Garber, S. T., and Ferris, E. B. (1950): "Comparative study of the effects of tetra-ethyl-ammonium chloride and veratrum viride on blood pressure in normal and toxæmic pregnancy", *J. clin. Invest.*, 29, 290.

Ayman, A., and Goldshine, A. D. (1939): "The breath-holding test: a simple standard stimulus of blood pressure", *Arch. intern. Med.*, 63, 899.

Ayman, D. (1934): "Heredity in arteriolar (essential) hypertension: a clinical study of the blood pressure of 1,524 members of 277 families", *Ibid.*, 53, 792.

Barclay, J. A., Cooke, W. T., and Kenney, R. A. (1947): "Observations on effects of adrenaline on renal function and circulation in man", *Amer. J. Physiol.*, 151, 621.

Barcroft, H., and Swan, H. J. C. (1953): "Sympathetic control of human blood vessels", *Monographs of the Physiol. Soc.*, No. 1.

Barker, M. H. (1936): "Blood cyanates in treatment of hypertension", *J. Amer. med. Ass.*, 106, 762.

Bechgaard, P. (1946): "Arterial hypertension. A follow-up study of one thousand hypertonics", *Acta. med. Scand., Supp.* 172.

Beer, E., King, F. H., and Prinzmetal, M. (1937): "Pheochromocytoma with demonstration of pressor (adrenaline) substance in the blood, pre-operative, during hypertensive crises", *Ann. Surg.*, 106, 85.

Bell, E. T., and Clawson, B. J. (1928): "Primary (essential) hypertension", *Arch. Path.*, 5, 939.

Bernheim (1910): "De l'asystolic veineuse dans l'hypertrophie du coeur gauche par stenose concomitante du ventricule droit", *Rev. de Méd.*, 30, 785.

Berry, R. L., Campbell, K. N., Lyons, R. H., Moe, J. K., and Sutler, M. R. (1946): "The use of tetraethylammonium in peripheral vascular disease and causalgic states", *Surgery*, 20, 525.

Bhatia, B. B. (1942): "On use of rauwolfia serpentina in high blood pressure", *J. Ind. med. Ass.*, 11, 262.

Blackford, J. M., Bowers, J. M., and Baker, J. W. (1930): "Follow-up study of hypertension", *J. Amer. med. Ass.*, 94, 328

Boyd, A. M. (1948): "Discussion of the surgical treatment of hypertension", *Proc. Roy. Soc. Med.*, 41, 370.

Braasch, W. F., Waters, W., and Hammer, H. J. (1940): "Hypertension and the surgical kidney", *J. Amer. med. Ass.*, 115, 1837.

Braun-Menendez, E. (1939): "The blood pressure raising substance in the blood of ischæmic kidneys", *Rev. Soc. Argent. de Biol.*, 15, 420.

Brod, J. (1955): "Chronic pyelonephritis", Praha.

—— (1955): "The syndrome of malignant hypertension in chronic pyelonephritis", *Cas. Lék. ces.*, 94, 614.

Browne, F. J. (1947): "Chronic hypertension in pregnancy", *Brit. med. J.*, i, 283.

Burn, J. H., and Dale, H. H. (1915): "The action of certain quaternary ammonium bases", *J. Pharmacol.*, 6, 417.

Burt, C. C., and Graham, A. J. P. (1950): "Pentamethonium and hexamethonium iodide in investigation of peripheral vascular disease and hypertension", *Brit. med. J.*, ii, 455.

Byrom, F. B. (1954): "The pathogenesis of hypertensive encephalopathy and its relation to the malignant phase of hypertension. Experimental evidence from the hypertensive rat", *Lancet*, ii, 201.

Cahill, G. F. (1948): "Pheochromocytomas", *J. Amer. med. Ass.*, 138, 180.

Cannon, W. B. (1940): "Adrenal medulla", *Bull. N.Y. Acad. Med.*, 16, 3.

Castleman, B., and Smithwick, R. H. (1943): "The relation of vascular disease to the hypertensive state. Based on a study of renal biopsies from one hundred hypertensive patients", *J. Amer. med. Ass.*, 121, 1256.

Cavelti, P. A., and Cavelti, E. S. (1945): "Studies on the pathogenesis of glomerulonephritis: I. Production of auto-antibodies to kidney in experimental animals", *Arch. Path.*, 39, 148.

Clerc, A., and Sterne, J. (1937): "A case of repeated anginal crises with parox-ysmal hypertension and vasomotor disturbances: a record of medical treatment, two surgical interventions, and of the efficiency of a synthetic sympathicolytic drug", *Bull. et Mém. Soc. méd. d. hôp. d. Paris*, 53, 562.

Connell, W. F., Wharton, G. K., and Robinson, C. E. (1946): "The relationship of blood pressure and serum thiocyanate", *Amer. J. med. Sc.*, 211, 74.

Currens, J. G., Myers, S., and White, P. D. (1953): "The use of protoveratrine in the treatment of hypertensive vascular disease", *Amer. Heart J.*, 46, 576.

Dalton, K. (1954): "Similarity of symptomatology of premenstrual syndrome and toxæmia of pregnancy and their response to progesterone", *Brit. med. J.*, ii, 1071.

De Largy, C., Greenfield, A. D. M., McCorry, R. L., and Whelan, R. F. (1950): "The effects of intravenous infusion of mixtures of L-adrenaline and L-noradrenaline on the human subject", *Clin. Sci.*, 9, 71.

Del Solar, A. V., Dussaillant, G. G., Brodsky, M. B., and Rodrignez, G. C. (1945): "Fatal poisoning from potassium thiocyanate used in treatment of hyper-tension. Report of a case and review of the literature", *Arch. intern. Med.*, 75, 241.

Dewar, H. A., Owen, S. G., and Jenkins, A. R. (1953): "Effect of hexamethonium bromide on the cerebral circulation in hypertension", *Brit. med. J.*, ii, 1017.

Dieckhoff, J. (1936): "Leistungsfahigkeit aortenklappeninsuffizienter Herzen ohne und mit Hypertrophie im Herz-Lungen-Praparat. (Nebst Digitalisierungsef-fekten)", *Arch. f. Exper. Path. u. Pharmacol.*, 182, 268.

Donnison, C. P. (1929): "Blood pressure in African natives: its bearing upon ætiology of hyperpiesia and arteriosclerosis", *Lancet*, i, 6.

Doyle, A. E. (1953): "Electrocardiographic changes in hypertension treated by methonium compounds", *Amer. Heart J.*, 45, 363.

——, and Kilpatrick, J. A. (1954): "Methonium compounds in the angina of hypertension", *Lancet*, 1, 905.

——, and Smirk, F. H. (1953): "The use of pure veratrum alkaloids neo-germitrine and protoveratrine in hypertension", *Brit. Heart J.*, 15, 439.

East, T., and Bain, C. (1949): "Right ventricular stenosis (Bernheim's syn-drome)", *Brit. Heart J.*, 11, 145.

Ehrstrom, R. (1918): "Nefrosklerosen", *Finstra Läk.-säll sk., handl., Helsingfors*, 60, 365.

Ellis, A. (1938): "Malignant hypertension", *Lancet*, 1, 977.

Ellis, L. B., and Weiss, S. (1929-30): "Measurement of capillary pressure under natural conditions and after arteriolar dilatation in normal subjects and in patients with arterial hypertension and with arteriosclerosis", *J. clin. Invest.*, 8, 47.

Engel, A., and von Euler, U. S. (1950): "Diagnostic value of increased urinary output of noradrenaline in phæochromocytoma", *Lancet*, ii, 387.

Evelyn, K. A., Alexander, F., and Cooper, S. R. (1949): "Effect of sympathec-tomy on blood pressure in hypertension. A review of thirteen years' experience at the Massachusetts General Hospital", *J. Amer. med. Ass.*, 140, 592.

Fahr, G. (1928): "Hypertension heart", *Amer. J. med. Sc.*, 175, 453.

Fishberg, A. M. (1939): "Hypertension and nephritis", London, 4th ed.

Fowler, P. B. S., and Guz, A. (1954): "Blood pressure during exercise and the effect of hexamethonium", *Brit. Heart J.*, 16, 1.

Frankel, F. (1886): "Ein Fall von doppelsertigem, vollig latent verlaufenen Nebennierentumor und gleichzeitiger naphritis mit Veranderungen am circula-tions-apparat und Retinitis", *Virchows Arch*, 103, 244.

Frant, R., and Groen, J. (1950): "Prognosis of vascular hypertension. A nine-year follow-up study of four hundred and eighteen cases", *Arch. intern. Med.*, 85, 727.

Freis, E. D., et al. (1949): "The hemodynamic effects of hypotensive drugs in man: 11. Dihydroergocornine", *J. clin. Invest.*, 28, 1387.

——, MacKay, J. C., and Oliver, W. F. (1951): "The effect of 'sympatholytic' drugs on the cardiovascular responses to epinephrine and norepinephrine in man", *Circulation*, 3, 254.

——, and Stanton, J. R. (1948): "A clinical evaluation of veratrum viride in the treatment of essential hypertension", *Amer. Heart J.*, **36**, 723.

Gibbs, D. (1952): "Dihydrogenated alkaloids of ergot in the investigation and treatment of diastolic hypertension", *Brit. Heart J.*, **14**, 77.

Gifford, R. W., Roth, G. M., and Kvale, W. F. (1952): "Evaluation of new adrenolytic drug (Regitine) as test for pheochromocytoma", *J. Amer. med. Ass.*, **149**, 1628.

Goldblatt, H. (1937): "Studies in experimental hypertension. V. The pathogenesis of experimental hypertension due to renal ischæmia", *Ann. intern. Med.*, **11**, 69.

—— (1938): "Studies on experimental hypertension. VII. The production of the malignant phase of hypertension", *J. exper. Med.*, **67**, 809.

—— (1948): "The renal origin of hypertension", Springfield, Illinois.

——, Lynch, J. R. F., Hazal, F., and Summerville, W. W. (1934): "Studies on experimental hypertension. I. The production of persistent elevation of systolic blood pressure by means of renal ischæmia", *J. exper. Med.*, **59**, 347.

Golden, A., Dexter, L., and Weiss, S. (1943): "Vascular disease following toxæmia of pregnancy", *Arch. intern. Med.*, **72**, 301.

Goldenberg, M., Pines, K. L., Baldwin, E. de F., Greene, D. G., and Roh, C. E. (1948): "Hemodynamic response of man to nor-epinephrine and epinephrine and its relation to problem of hypertension", *Amer. J. Med.*, **5**, 792.

——, Snyder, C. H., and Aranow, H. Jr. (1947): "New test for hypertension due to circulating epinephrine", *J. Amer. med. Ass.*, **135**, 971.

Goldman, I. R., Stern, N. S., and Stern, T. N. (1951): "The use of dramamine in vestibular disturbances complicating hypertensive and arteriosclerotic heart disease", *Amer. Heart J.*, **42**, 302.

Goodman, L., and Gilman, A. (1941): "Pharmacological basis of therapeutics", New York, p. 161.

Graham, J. B. (1951): "Pheochromocytoma and hypertension; analysis of 207 cases", *Int. abstr. Surg.*, **92**, 105.

Grant, R. T. (1925): "Observations on the after-histories of men suffering from the effort syndrome", *Heart*, **12**, 121.

Grayson, J. (1950): "Observations on blood flow in human intestine", *Brit. med. J.*, ii, 1465.

Green, D. M. (1946): "Pheochromocytoma and chronic hypertension", *J. Amer. med. Ass.*, **131**, 1260.

Grimson, K. S. (1947): "The surgical treatment of hypertension", *Advances intern. Med.*, **2**, 173.

Grollman, A. (1945): "Sodium restriction in diet for hypertension", *J. Amer. med. Ass.*, **129**, 533.

——, and Harrison, T. R. (1945): "Effect of rigid sodium restriction on blood pressure and survival of hypertensive rats", *Proc. Soc. exper. Biol. and Med.*, **60**, 52.

Hamilton, M., Pickering, G. W., Fraser Roberts, J. A., and Sowry, G. S. C. (1954): "The ætiology of essential hypertension. 1. The arterial pressure in the general population", *Clin. Sci.*, **13**, 11.

Harrington, M. (1953): "The absorption and excretion of hexamethonium salts", *Ibid.*, **12**, 185.

Harris, H. A. (1927): "Vascular diseases and sympathetic system", *Brit. med. J.*, i, 789.

Harris, R. E., Sokolow, M., Carpenter, L. G., Freedman, M., and Hunt, S. P. (1953): "Response to psychologic stress in persons who are potentially hypertensive", *Circulation*, **7**, 874.

Harrison, C. V., and Wood, P. H. (1949): "Hypertensive and ischæmic heart disease", *Brit. Heart J.*, **11**, 205.

Hayward, G. W. (1948): "Tetraethylammonium bromide in hypertension and hypertensive heart failure", *Lancet*, i, 18.

Hines, E. A. (1940): "The significance of vascular hyper-reaction as measured by the cold pressor test", *Amer. Heart J.*, **19**, 408.

—— (1940): "The hereditary factor and subsequent development of hypertension", *Proc. Mayo Clin.*, **15**, 145.

Hines, E. A., Jr. (1946): "Thiocyanates in treatment of hypertensive disease", *M. Clin. N. Amer.*, **30**, 869.

Hite, W. K. (1946): "Hypertension and veratrum viride, a preliminary study", *Illinois med. J.*, **90**, 336.

Howard, J. E., and Barker, W. H. (1937): "Paroxysmal hypertension and other clinical manifestations associated with benign chromaffin cell tumors (phæochromocytomata)", *Bull. Johns Hopk. Hosp.*, **61**, 371.

Iglauer, A., and Altschule, M. D. (1940): "Effect of paredrine on venous system", *J. clin. Invest.*, **19**, 503.

Janeway, T. C. (1913): "A clinical study of hypertensive vascular disease", *Arch. intern. Med.*, **12**, 755.

Johnson, R. L., et al. (1952): "Clinical evaluation of L-hydrazinophthalazine (C-5968) in hypertension, with special reference to alternating treatment with hexamethonium", *Circulation*, **5**, 833.

Kaunzte, R., and Trounce, J. (1951): "Treatment of arterial hypertension with veriloid (veratrum viride)", *Lancet*, **ii**, 1002.

Kempner, W. (1944): "Treatment of kidney disease and hypertensive vascular disease with rice diet", *North Carolina med. J.*, **5**, 125.

—— (1946): "Some effects of rice diet treatment of kidney disease and hypertension", *Bull. N.Y. Acad. Med.*, **22**, 358.

—— (1948): "Treatment of hypertensive vascular disease with rice diet", *Amer. J. Med.*, **4**, 545.

—— (1949): "Treatment of heart and kidney disease and of hypertensive and arteriosclerotic vascular disease with the rice diet", *Ann. intern. Med.*, **31**, 821.

Krayer, O., and Acheson, G. H. (1946): "Pharmacology of veratrum alkaloids", *Physiol. Rev.*, **26**, 383.

Kylin, E. (1926): "Die Hypertoniekrankheiten", Berlin, pp. 32, 62.

La Due, J. S., Murison, P. J., and Pack, G. T. (1948): "The use of tetraethylammonium bromide as a diagnostic test for pheochromocytoma", *Ann. intern. Med.*, **29**, 914.

Lenegre, J., and Maurice, P. (1947): "The right ventricular pressure in arterial hypertension", *Arch. Mal. Coeur*, **40**, 173.

Levine, S. A. (1948): "Auscultation of the heart", *Brit. Heart J.*, **10**, 213.

Liebrecht, R. (1859): "Ophthalmoskopischer Befund bei Morbus Brightii", *Arch. Ophth.*, **5**, 265.

Light, A. L., and Wood, P. H. (1939): Protocol at Post-graduate Medical School of London.

Light, F. P. (1948): "A nine-year follow-up in cases of toxæmia of pregnancy", *Amer. J. Obstet. Gynec.*, **55**, 321.

Longcope, W. T., and Winkenwerder, W. L. (1933): "Clinical features of the contracted kidney due to pyelonephritis", *Johns Hopk. Hosp. Bull.*, **53**, 255.

Lyons, R. H., Moe, G. K., Neligh, R. B., Hoobler, S. W., Campbell, K. N., Berry, R. L., and Rennick, B. R. (1947): "The effects of blockade of the autonomic ganglia in man with tetraethylammonium. Preliminary observations on its clinical application", *Amer. J. med. Sci.*, **213**, 314.

McGregor, M., and Segel, N. (1955): "The rauwolfia alkaloids in the treatment of hypertension", *Brit. Heart J.*, **17**, 391.

MacKeith, R. (1944): "Adrenal-sympathetic syndrome. Chromaffin tissue tumour with paroxysmal hypertension", *Brit. Heart J.*, **6**, 1.

McMichael, J., and Sharpey-Schafer, E. P. (1944): "Cardiac output in man by direct Fick method: effects of posture, venous pressure change, atropine, and adrenaline", *Ibid.*, **6**, 33.

Manger, W. M., Flock, E. V., Berkson, J., Dollman, J. L., Roth, G. M., Baldes, E. J., and Jacobs, M. (1954): "Chemical quantitation of epinephrine and nor epinephrine in thirteen patients with pheochromocytoma", *Circulation*, **10**, 641.

Marsh, D. F., Pelletier, M. H., and Ross, C. A. (1948): "Comparative pharmacology of N-alkylarterenols", *J. Pharmacol.*, **92**, 108.

Master, A. M. (1953): "Hypertension and coronary occlusion", *Circulation*, **8**, 170.

——, Marks, H. H., and Dack, S. (1943): "Hypertension in people over 40", *J. Amer. med. Ass.*, **121**, 1251.

——, Garfield, C. I., and Walters, M. B. (1952): "Normal blood pressure and hypertension", Henry Kimpton, London.

Maxwell, R. D. H., and Campbell, A. J. M. (1953): "New sympathicolytic agents", *Lancet*, **1**, 455.

Meilman, E., and Krayer, O. (1950): "Clinical studies on veratrum alkaloids. I. The action of protoveratrine and veratridine in hypertension", *Circulation*, **1**, 204.

Moister, F. C., Stanton, J. R., and Freis, E. D. (1949): "Observations on the development of tolerance during prolonged oral administration of dihydroergocornine", *J. Pharmacol.*, **96**, 21.

Müller, J. M., Schlittler, E., and Beim, H. J. (1952): "Reserpin, der Sedative Wirkstoff aus Rauwolfia serpentina Benth", *Experientia*, Basel, **8**, 338.

Nathanson, M. H., and Miller, H. (1952): "The action of norephinephrine, epinephrine and isopropyl norepinephrine on the rhythmic function of the heart", *Circulation*, **6**, 238.

Nickerson, M. (1951): "Sympathetic blockade in therapy of hypertension", in "Hypertension, a symposium", ed. by E. T. Bell, p. 410, Univ. of Minnesota Press.

Paton, W. D. M. (1951): "The paralysis of autonomic ganglia, with special reference to the therapeutic effects of ganglion-blocking drugs", *Brit. med. J.*, **1**, 773.

——, and Zaimis, E. J. (1949): "The pharmacological action of cholinemethylene bistrimethylammonium salts", *Brit. J. Pharmacol.*, **4**, 381.

Pauli, W. (1903): "Ueber lonenwirkungen und ihre therapeutische Verwendung", *Munch. Med. Wchnschr.*, **50**, 153.

Paullin, J. E., Bowcock, H. M., and Wood, R. H. (1927): "Complications of hypertension", *Amer. Heart J.*, **2**, 613.

Peet, M. M., and Isberg, E. M. (1948): "The problem of malignant hypertension and its treatment by splanchnic resection", *Ann. intern. Med.*, **28**, 755.

——, —— (1949): "Some aspects of hypertensive disease of pregnancy treated by splanchnicectomy", *Amer. J. med. Sci.*, **217**, 530.

——, Woods, W. W., and Braden, S. (1940): "The surgical treatment of hypertension", *J. Amer. med. Ass.*, **115**, 1875.

Pickering, G. W. (1939): "The problem of high blood pressure in man", *Brit. med. J.*, **i**, 1.

—— (1943): "Circulation in arterial hypertension", *Ibid.*, **ii**, 1, 31.

—— (1952): "Blood pressure—treatment of hypertension", *Surgical Progress*, p. 155, Butterworth and Co., London.

—— (1952): "The pathogenesis of malignant hypertension", *Circulation*, **6**, 599.

——, and Heptinstall, R. H. (1953): "Nephrectomy and other treatment for hypertension in pyelonephritis", *Quart. J. Med.*, **22**, 1.

Pitcairn, D. M., and Youmans, W. B. (1950): "The nature of pressor substances in pheochromocytomas", *Circulation*, **2**, 505.

Platt, R. (1947): "Hypertension and unilateral kidney disease", *Quart. J. Med.*, **6**, 143.

—— (1947): "Heredity in hypertension", *Ibid.*, **16**, 111.

—— (1948): "Severe hypertension in young persons. A study of 50 cases", *Ibid.*, **17**, 83.

Ratliff, R. K., Nesbit, R. M., Plumb, R. T., and Bohne, W. (1947): "Nephrectomy for hypertension with unilateral renal disease. Report of 49 cases", *J. Amer. med. Ass.*, **133**, 296.

Restall, P. A., and Smirk, F. H. (1950): "Treatment of high blood pressure with hexamethonium iodide", *N.Z. med. J.*, **49**, 206.

Rosenheim, M. L. (1954): "The treatment of severe hypertension", *Brit. med. J.*, *ii*, 1181.

Roth, G. M., and Kvale, W. F. (1945): "Tentative test for pheochromocytoma", *Amer. J. med. Sci.*, **210**, 653.

Rothstadt, L. E. (1938): "The effect of auricular fibrillation on the course of hypertension", *Med. J. Australia*, **1**, 813.

Rusken, A., and McKinley, W. F. (1947): "Comparative study of potassium thiocyanate and other drugs in the treatment of essential hypertension", *Amer. Heart J.*, **34**, 691.

Rykert, H. E., and Hepburn, J. (1935): "Electrocardiographic abnormalities characteristic of certain cases of arterial hypertension", *Ibid.*, **10**, 942.

Rytand, D. A. (1938): "The renal factor in arterial hypertension with coarctation of the aorta", *J. clin. Invest.*, **17**, 391.

Sarre, H., and Lindner, E. (1948): "Retinal changes and blood pressure in relation to prognosis in arterial hypertension. (On the basis of 166 cases observed over seven years)", *Klin. Wschr.*, Berlin, **26**, 102.

Scheinker, I. M. (1948): "Hypertensive cerebral swelling, a characteristic clinico-pathologic syndrome", *Ann. intern. Med.*, **28**, 630.

Schoen, R. (1930): "Uber die Dobbeltseitige chronische pyelogene Nephritis", *Deutsches Arch. f. klin. Med.*, **169**, 337.

Schottstaedt, M. F., and Sokolow, M. (1953): "The natural history and course of hypertension with papilloedema (malignant hypertension)", *Amer. Heart J.*, **45**, 331.

Schroeder, H. A. (1952): "The effect of 1-hydrazinophthalazine in hypertension", *Circulation*, **5**, 28.

——, Davies, D. F., and Clark, H. E. (1949): "A syndrome of hypertension, obesity, menstrual irregularities and evidence of adrenal cortical hyper-function", *Proc. Central Soc. Clin. Research*, **22**, 73.

Selzer, A., Bradley, H. W., and Willett, F. M. (1955): "A critical appraisal of the concept of Bernheim's syndrome", *Amer. J. Med.*, **18**, 567.

Smirk, F. H. (1949): "Pathogenesis of essential hypertension", *Brit. med. J.*, *i*, 791.

—— (1950): "Methonium compounds in hypertension", *Lancet*, *ii*, 477.

—— (1953): "Action of a new methonium compound in arterial hypertension. Pentamethylene 1 : 5-Bis-N-(N-Methyl-Pyrrolidinium) Bitartrate (M. and B. 2050 A)", *Lancet*, *i*, 457.

——, and Alstad, K. S. (1951): "Treatment of arterial hypertension by penta- and hexa-methonium salts", *Brit. med. J.*, *i*, 1217.

——, Doyle, A. E., and McQueen, E. G. (1954): "Control of blood-pressure by combined action of reserpine and pentapyrrolidinium", *Lancet*, *ii*, 159.

Smith, H. W. (1948): "Hypertension and urologic disease", *Amer. J. Med.*, **4**, 724.

Smithwick R. H. (1940): "Technique for splanchnic resection for hypertension. Preliminary report", *Surgery*, **7**, 1.

—— (1944): "Surgical treatment of hypertension; the effect of radical (lumbo-dorsal) splanchnicectomy on the hypertensive state of one hundred and fifty-six patients, followed one to five years", *Arch. Surgery*, **49**, 180.

——, (1949): "An evaluation of the surgical treatment of hypertension", *Bull N.Y. Acad. Med.*, **25**, 698.

Stutzman, J. W., Maison, G. L., and Kusserow, G. W. (1949): "Veriloid, a new hypotensive extract of veratrum viride", *Proc. Soc. exper. Biol. and Med.*, **71**, 725

——, Simon, H., and Maison, G. L. (1951): "Role of vagus nerves in depresso action of veratrum derivatives", *J. Pharmacol.*, **101**, 310.

Swan, H. J. C. (1952): "Noradrenaline, adrenaline, and the human circulation" *Brit. med. J.*, *i*, 1003.

Treupel, G., and Edinger, A. (1900): "Untersuchungen übe Rhodan-verbin dungen", *Munch. Med. Wschr.*, **47**, 717.

Trueta, J., Barclay, A. E., Daniel, P. M., Franklin, K. J., and Prichard, M. M. L (1947): "Studies of the renal circulation", Oxford.

Turner, R. (1950): " 'Medical sympathectomy' in hypertension. A clinical study of methonium compounds", *Lancet*, ii, 353.

Vakil, R. J. (1940): "Hypertension", *Med. Bull.*, 8, 15.
—— (1949): "A clinical trial of rauwolfia serpentina in essential hypertension", *Brit. Heart J.*, 11, 350.
—— (1953): "Hypotensive action of another rauwolfia serpentina alkaloid: a clinical report", *J. Ind. med. Ass.*, 23, 97.
—— (1955): "Rauwolfia serpentina in the treatment of high blood pressure. A review of the literature", *Circulation*, 12, 220.
von Euler, U. S. (1946): "A specific sympathomimetic ergone in adrenergic nerve fibres (sympathin) and its relations to adrenaline and nor-adrenaline", *Acta. physiol. Scand.*, 12, 73.
—— (1948): "Identification of sympathomimetic ergone in adrenergic nerves of cattle (sympathin N) with lævo-noradrenaline", *Ibid.*, 16, 63.
——, and Liljestrand, G. (1927): "Die Wirkung des Adrenalins auf das Minutenvolumen des Herzens beim Menschen", *Skand. Arch. Physiol.*, 52, 243.

Wagener, H. P., and Keith, N. M. (1939): "Diffuse arteriolar disease with hypertension and the associated retinal lesions", *Medicine*, 18, 317.
——, —— (1924): "Cases of marked hypertension, adequate renal function and neuroretinitis", *Arch. intern. Med.*, 34, 374.
Wald, M. H., Lindberg, H. A., and Barker, M. H. (1939): "Toxic manifestations of thiocyanates", *J. Amer. med. Ass.*, 112, 1120.
Watkinson, G., and Evans, G. (1947): "Potassium thiocyanate in the treatment of hypertension", *Brit. med. J.*, i, 595.
Wien, R., and Mason, D. F. J. (1953): "Pharmacology of M. and B. 2050", *Lancet*, i, 454.
Wilkins, R. W., and Judson, W. E. (1953): "The use of rauwolfia serpentina in hypertensive patients", *New Engl. J. Med.*, 248, 48.
——, Stanton, J. R., and Freis, E. D. (1949): "Essential hypertension, therapeutic trial of veriloid, a new extract of veratrum viride", *Proc. Soc. exp. Biol.*, New York, 72, 302.
Wilson, C. (1953): "Renal factors in the production of hypertension", *Lancet*, ii, 579, 632.
——, and Byrom, F. B. (1939): "Renal changes in malignant hypertension. Experimental evidence", *Lancet*, i, 136.
——, —— (1941): "The vicious circle in chronic Bright's disease. Experimental evidence from the hypertensive rat", *Quart. J. Med.*, 10, 65.
——, Pickering, G. W. (1937–8): "Acute arterial lesions in rabbits with experimental renal hypertension", *Clin. Sc.*, 3, 343.
Wolff, H. H. (1951): "The mechanism and significance of the cold pressor response", *Quart. J. Med.*, 20, 261.
Wood, P. H. (1941): "Da Costa's syndrome", *Brit. med. J.*, i, 767, 805, 845.

Yuile, C. L. (1944): "Obstructive lesions of the main renal artery in relation to hypertension", *Amer. J. med. Sc.*, 207, 394.

CHAPTER XVII

PULMONARY EMBOLISM

PULMONARY embolism may cause sudden death from reflex ventricular fibrillation or cardiac standstill, acute or subacute obstructive
pulmonary hypertension, pulmonary infarction, or no ill-effects.
Emboli may be single or multiple, infected or sterile. They are usually
attributable to mobile venous thrombi originating in the legs, but are
occasionally due to fat, air, foreign body, or to fragments of some remote
malignant tumour.

THROMBO-EMBOLISM

General incidence. Massive pulmonary embolism is directly or chiefly
responsible for about 3 per cent of all hospital deaths, published figures
ranging from 2 to 6.5 per cent as shown below:

Author	Number of necropsies	Incidence of fatal pulmonary embolism, per cent
Belt (1934)	567	6.5
Collins (1936)	10,940	2.07
Pilcher (1939)	2,861	4.5
Hampton and Castleman (1940)	3,500	3.5
McCartney (1945)	25,771	2.62
Crutcher (1948)	2,580	2.14

The actual incidence of clinical thrombo-embolism among all hospital
patients is difficult to assess, but appears to be about 1 per cent in post-
operative cases (Nygaard *et al.*, 1940–41), and is believed to be equally
frequent in medical, obstetrical and gynæcological wards (Belt, 1939).

ETIOLOGY

Thrombo-embolism results from the breaking away of a blood clot
formed either in the right side of the heart or in the systemic venous
system, commonly the latter.

Intracardiac thrombosis. Clots may form in the right side of the heart in
cases of auricular fibrillation, congestive failure, myocardial infarction,
bacterial endocarditis, and isolated myocarditis or endomyocardial fibrosis.
Damaged endocardium, slowing of the blood flow, and backwater eddies
in dilated chambers are important contributory factors. Myocardial infarction practically always affects the left ventricle, and as mural thrombi

are limited to the area of devitalised tissue, emboli from the heart are usually systemic; exceptions are associated with septal infarction. Bacterial endocarditis is only a source of pulmonary embolism when it affects the pulmonary or tricuspid valve, a ventricular septal defect, or a patent ductus arteriosus; infarcts so produced are apt to be small and frequent, the clinical course resembling subacute or chronic hæmorrhagic broncho-pneumonia. In isolated myocarditis and endomyocardial fibrosis mural thrombi are commonly found in the left ventricle and emboli are therefore mostly systemic; but the right ventricle may also be involved.

Venous thrombosis. Intracardiac thrombosis, however, accounts for only about 10 per cent of pulmonary emboli (Belt, 1939), the remainder, including the majority of those associated with mitral stenosis, auricular fibrillation, myocardial infarction and congestive heart failure being due to venous thrombosis, particularly in the legs. Such emboli are common. Belt (1939) found them in 6 per cent of 1,990 consecutive necropsies, and as often in medical as in surgical cases. They were directly responsible for death in 22 instances (1.1 per cent) and a contributory factor in approximately 70 (3.5 per cent). Thrombosis begins in the calf and extends upwards.

The chief causes of venous thrombosis may be listed under three main headings:

1. *Local venous injury.*
   (a) Inflammatory—as in thrombophlebitis.
   (b) Chemical—from the injection of irritant solutions.
   (c) Traumatic—as in fractures.
   (d) Infiltrative—as in cancer.

2. *Slowing of the venous blood flow.*
   (a) By local obstruction—as by tight bandaging, immobilisation in an unfavourable posture, or space-filling lesions (including obesity and pregnancy).
   (b) As a whole—as in heart failure.

3. *Increased clotting tendency of the blood.*
   (a) Post-operative, post-traumatic and puerperal states.
   (b) Polycythæmia and hæmoconcentration.
   (c) Associated with tissue breakdown, e.g. carcinoma of the stomach, myocardial infarction.
   (d) Certain fevers, e.g. typhoid.

The mechanism of intravascular clotting is a complicated process and is not yet fully understood. Its discussion is beyond the scope of this work, and the reader is referred to the excellent monograph by Nygaard (1941), and to more recent articles by Quick (1950) and Wright (1952).

Thrombophlebitis is often said to be less dangerous than simple phlebo-thrombosis; but this is doubtful, for the former is less frequent but more easily diagnosed, whilst the latter is common but apt to be overlooked, so that the percentage incidence of embolism is likely to appear higher in phlebothrombosis. Fatal pulmonary embolism follows the injection treatment of varicose veins in 0.05 per cent of cases (Westerborn, 1937), and the operative treatment in 0.4 per cent (Westerborn, 1937; McPheeters and Rice, 1928).

Fractures, particularly of the legs or pelvis, may cause thrombo-embolism on account of injury to veins, immobilisation, and post-traumatic acceleration of the clotting time; they may also give rise to fat embolism. Malignant neoplasms, especially carcinoma of the stomach, may be responsible for thrombo-embolism as a result of venous infiltration, mechanical venous obstruction, and shortening of the clotting time (owing to tissue necrosis). They may also give rise to malignant cellular emboli.

The most common cause of phlebothrombosis is immobilisation in bed, especially in obese subjects over 40 years of age. Of 229 cases of fatal post-operative pulmonary embolism, Prettin (1936) found the average weight in women was 11 kg. above normal, and in men 4.2 kg. In a series at the Mayo clinic, 93 per cent of fatal post-operative pulmonary emboli occurred in patients over 40 years of age (Barnes, 1937).

Congestive heart failure encourages phlebothrombosis because the circulation is slowed. When the cardiac output remains elevated or is less reduced than usual, as in failure from the hyperkinetic circulatory states, thrombosis is rare. Congestive failure due to mitral stenosis or to myocardial infarction is particularly dangerous. Eppinger and Kennedy (1938) found that pulmonary embolism was the direct cause of death in 6.5 per cent of 200 fatal cases of coronary thrombosis, and a contributory cause in 32.7 per cent of those with congestive failure. The clotting time appears to shorten after myocardial infarction, perhaps owing to the products of tissue necrosis. The clotting time also appears to be shortened by digitalis (Massie et al., 1944) and by the organic mercurial diuretics (Macht, 1946). Clinically pulmonary embolism is recognised in about 10 per cent of cases with heart failure; it is more frequent (20 per cent) in those with valvular disease than in those without (6 per cent) (Rissanen, 1947).

Almost any major surgical procedure may result in thrombo-embolism; but abdominal and pelvic operations carry the highest embolic risk. Responsible factors include post-operative reduction of the clotting time (maximum at the tenth day), and immobilisation. Child-birth incurs a similar risk for similar reasons. McCartney (1945) found that pulmonary embolism was directly responsible for 5.28 per cent of obstetrical fatalities, and for 5.1 per cent of post-operative deaths.

HÆMODYNAMICS

Experiments in which the pulmonary arteries have been occluded in varying degree by ligature, or by artificial emboli, have shown that it is necessary to obstruct about 60 to 85 per cent of their total cross-section before the systemic blood pressure falls or before signs of right ventricular failure can be detected, and between 85 and 100 per cent before death ensues (Haggart and Walker, 1923; Gibbon, Hopkinson and Churchill, 1932). It is thus possible to undertake unilateral pneumonectomy without embarrassing the circulation (Barnes, 1941). In accord with these facts the majority of pulmonary emboli cause no cardiac disturbance; but when a large embolus lodges at the bifurcation of the main pulmonary artery, or when multiple emboli block more than two-thirds of the more distal trunks, the circulation is impeded and the left ventricular output falls. This is the condition known as massive pulmonary embolism, and implies acute obstructive pulmonary hypertension. Compensatory adjustments include vasoconstriction which combats the falling blood pressure, elevation of the right ventricular pressure which helps to squeeze blood past the obstruction, and elevation of the venous pressure which serves to encourage the right ventricle. It is as yet uncertain whether that chamber usually becomes overloaded or not. In cases which recover, the embolus is gradually packed to the side of the vessel, where it becomes organised, and finally shrinks to a mere thread. Infarction of the lung does not necessarily occur, because sufficient blood may pass through to nourish the tissues.

Subacute cases may occur in which repeated small emboli gradually block the pulmonary circulation over a period of weeks or months (Belt, 1939). There is reason to believe that secondary pulmonary vasoconstriction may develop in some cases as a reaction to this subacute obstructive pulmonary hypertension, and turn a potentially reversible situation into an irreversible state that closely resembles primary pulmonary hypertension (see page 833).

Pulmonary infarction. When an embolus lodges distally in a relatively small arterial trunk, there is no rise of pressure in the pulmonary artery, blood is not squeezed past the obstruction, and the block is complete; infarction of that part of the lung supplied by the occluded vessel follows (unless the collateral circulation is sufficient to nourish the ischæmic area). Of course, such an event is likely to complicate massive pulmonary embolism, and does so in 62 per cent of cases (Belt, 1934), but it is a complication, and not an essential part of the picture. Admittedly, experimental pulmonary embolism does not cause infarction in animals unless the circulation is otherwise impaired (Karsner and Ash, 1912), but no such condition appears to be necessary in clinical medicine. Infarcts of the lung are hæmorrhagic because blood from the bronchial arteries exudes into the devitalised area. If this second source of nutrition is adequate for the needs of the tissue, infarction does not occur. When the hæmorrhagic zone reaches the surface of the lung, a sero-fibrinous pleural reaction develops: pain may be severe as in any other pleurisy; effusion is common and is usually blood-stained.

Pulmonary infarcts are nearly always embolic in origin (Virchow, 1856); very few are due to primary pulmonary thrombosis, and they rarely complicate idiopathic pulmonary hypertension or Fallot's tetralogy, two diseases in which primary thrombosis is relatively common.

CLINICAL FEATURES

Massive pulmonary embolism. In a typical dramatic attack the patient feels as if he had been struck in the centre of the chest, and rapidly becomes faint, grey, cold, clammy and breathless. Central sternal pain may be indistinguishable from that of acute myocardial infarction. Consciousness may be lost. Peripheral cyanosis is evident in the ears, lips and nail-beds, but

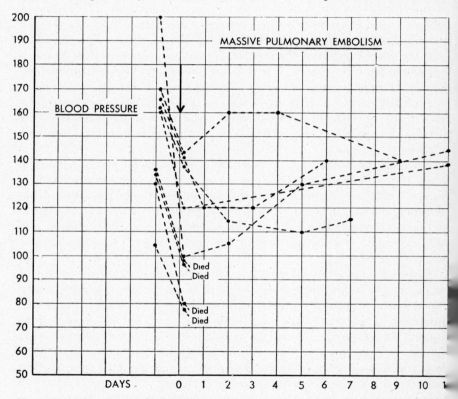

Fig. 17.01—Behaviour of the blood pressure in 9 cases of massive pulmonary embolism. There is invariably a profound initial drop. In the group shown, those with relatively high blood pressures previously recovered; whereas those with relatively low pressures previously died.

elsewhere pallor is usually more noticeable. Sweating is commonly profuse. The pulse is thready and rapid, or may be imperceptible; the blood pressure is low or immeasurable (fig. 17.01). The jugular venous pressure is invariably raised (fig. 17.02) and the liver may be palpable; cardiac œdema is not seen in acute cases, but may occur later in the subacute form. Examination of the lungs may reveal nothing abnormal. The heart sounds are usually soft, although the second sound at the base may be relatively accentuated or widely split (if there is right bundle branch block). Clinical and direct visual evidence of dilatation of the pulmonary artery proximal to the embolus have been described by McGinn and White (1935), and by Churchill (1934), respectively. The Graham Steele murmur of functional pulmonary incompetence has been heard (White and Brenner, 1933). Occasionally a pericardial friction rub develops over the base of the distended pulmonary artery (White, 1937).

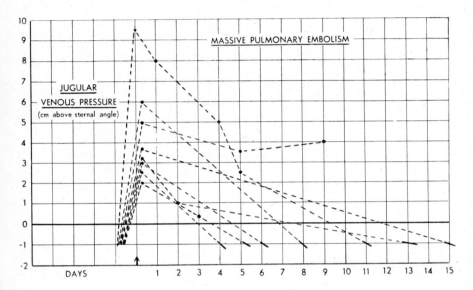

Fig. 17.02—Behaviour of the venous pressure in 8 cases of massive pulmonary embolism. There is initial elevation in all, but it is rarely maintained for more than a few days.

Rarely, patients die abruptly at the onset, presumably from reflex cardiac inhibition or ventricular fibrillation, such deaths being preventable by atropine in animals and being independent of the size of the embolus (Scherf and Schönbrunner, 1937). The great majority, however, survive the initial insult; but about one-third die subsequently from circulatory obstruction, approximately 10 per cent within 10 minutes, 30 per cent within an hour, and 60 per cent in a matter of hours or days (de Takats and Fowler, 1945). On the other hand, about two-thirds recover—within hours, days or weeks. Throughout this anxious period there is a 25 per cent risk of another, and perhaps fatal, embolus.

Massive pulmonary embolism, however, is not always dramatic, and mild cases are easily overlooked. Passing tightness of the chest, fleeting unexplained breathlessness, transient faintness, or a symptomless rise of systemic venous pressure may be the sole manifestation of an event that brought death very close.

Subacute cases may pass gradually into congestive heart failure without a single incident suggesting embolism: the clinical features of these rare cases resemble those of primary pulmonary hypertension.

It should be noted that "calling for the bed-pan and falling back dead" is not specially correlated with pulmonary embolism. The phenomenon appears to be associated with impending death from ventricular fibrillation

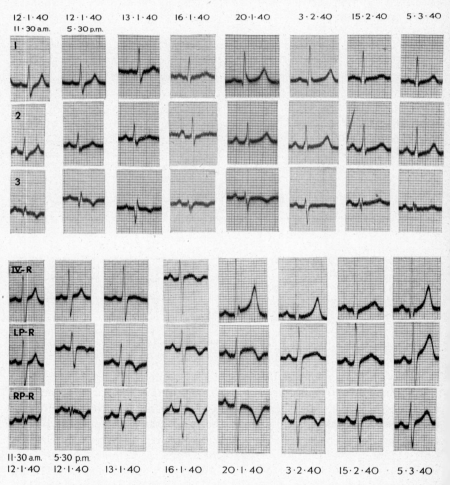

Fig. 17.03—Electrocardiogram showing the characteristic appearances associated with massive pulmonary embolism (lead IV-R=CR4; LP-R=CR2-3; RP-R=CR1).

or asystole, and may occur as a tragic climax to many forms of heart disease, including aortic stenosis and myocardial infarction. The colonic disturbance may be a vagal manifestation. Abrupt death from pulmonary embolism, preceded or not by a call to stool, is rare as already mentioned.

The diagnosis of acute right ventricular stress may be proved electrocardiographically (fig. 17.03). Limb leads show sinus tachycardia, a constant S wave in lead 1, a frequent Q wave in lead 3, inversion of T_3, flattening or slight inversion of T_2, and rather low voltage (Barnes, 1937). Occasionally P_2 becomes tall and sharp (Wood, 1948). These appearances are not unlike those of posterior myocardial infarction, although an absent S_1, conspicuous Q_2, and elevation of the R-T segment in lead 3 should be sufficient to distinguish the latter in standard leads. Again, Q_3 in cases of massive pulmonary embolism is caused by cardiac rotation, and is not seen

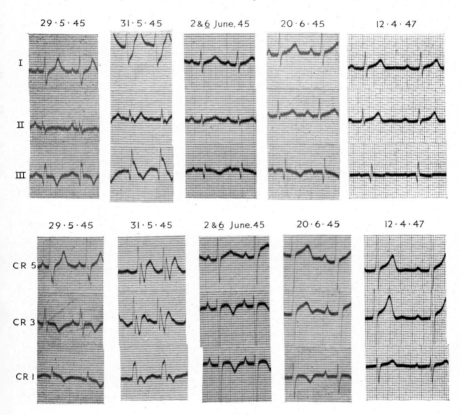

Fig. 17.04—Electrocardiogram showing transient right bundle branch block in a case of massive pulmonary embolism.

in lead V_F. In multiple chest leads appearances are equally characteristic (Wood, 1941): the T wave is nearly always inverted in leads V_{1-3} over the right ventricle, sometimes in V_4 and occasionally even in V_5 (fig. 17.03); and clockwise rotation or displacement of the interventricular septum to the left brings the RS pattern round as far as V_5 or even V_6. There are no pathological Q waves and the RS-T segment is not deviated from the baseline; but in about 15 per cent of cases there is transient right bundle branch block (fig. 17.04). These changes are not immediate, but develop within a few hours, and are usually maximum within one to three days. Recovery is relatively slow, three to six weeks elapsing before the T wave is finally upright again in leads V_1 or V_2.

The electrocardiographic pattern has been variously attributed to reflex coronary spasm (Scherf and Boyd, 1939), to interference with the coronary blood flow through the right ventricle owing to the combined effect of a low aortic and high right ventricular pressure (Durant, Long and Oppenheimer, 1947), and to right ventricular stress (Wood, 1941). There is no proof of coronary spasm, and, although usually ascribed to a vagal reflex, the electrocardiographic pattern is unaltered by vagal section in dogs (Malinow, Katz and Kondo, 1946). In experimental air embolism in dogs, Durant, Long and Oppenheimer (1947) directly observed the development of right ventricular ischæmia. Their thesis is supported by the 60 per cent frequency of constricting substernal pain in clinical cases (Wood, 1947). On the other hand, remarkably similar changes are found in any condition giving rise to right ventricular stress.

Pulmonary infarction. When an embolus lodges in a small or moderate sized pulmonary artery there are no immediate symptoms or signs. Within a variable time, however, impossible to determine clinically, a sudden pleural pain may signal the accident. Hæmoptysis may precede or follow the pain, may not occur at all, or may occur without pain. Coincident with these events, and especially if there is pleurisy, the respiratory rate rises and fever develops. Examination of the chest reveals little at first, except perhaps pleural friction, but within a day or two the percussion note may become impaired, the breath sounds diminished, and râles may be heard; sometimes there are frank signs of consolidation or of fluid. When the diagnosis is in doubt, a specimen of this fluid should be obtained, for it is hæmorrhagic in most cases of infarction. A skiagram is also helpful, the cone-shaped infarct casting a triangular, egg-shaped, or rounded shadow, according to its lateral, oblique, or antero-posterior lie (fig. 17.05). Unfortunately, the characteristic appearance is often obscured by the obliterating shadow of fluid. When embolism occurs without infarction, skiagrams occasionally show a segmental area of increased translucency owing to the absence of vascular shadows in the ischæmic area (Shapiro and Rigler, 1948); this is denied by Lenégre and Nèel (1950).

Pain, hæmoptysis, fever and tachypnœa may last a week or two, but the patient does not look or feel seriously ill unless the primary disease makes him so. Moderate leucocytosis and a rapid erythrocyte sedimentation rate are the rule, the former lasting a few days, the latter several weeks, as with cardiac infarction.

Whilst the above description applies to most cases, it should be added that infarcts may be clinically silent, and are often only discovered at necropsy. In other cases, secondary infection complicates the picture, or the embolus may be infected from the start; pulmonary abscess or empyema may then develop.

Venous thrombosis. In all cases of suspected pulmonary embolism a search

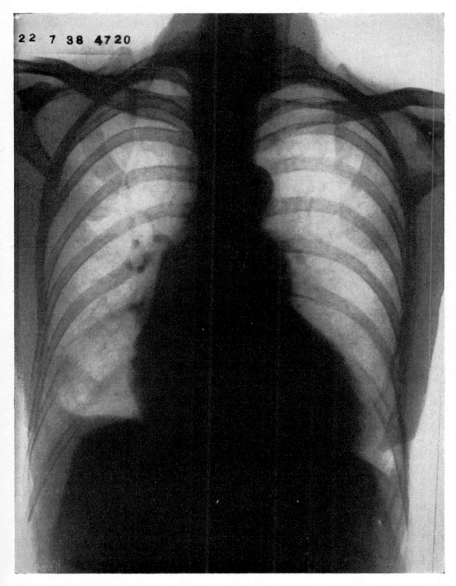

Fig. 17.05—Skiagram showing a small pulmonary infarct at the right base with a little hæmorrhagic effusion.

should be made for the source. As previously stated, this is commonly phlebothrombosis in the legs. It usually begins in the calf, where there may be deep muscle tenderness, or pain on dorsiflexing the foot (Homans' sign). If a pressure cuff is wrapped round the thigh and inflated to 40 mm. Hg, a characteristic pain develops in the calf when there is phlebothrombosis (Ortiz-Ramirez and Serna-Ramirez, 1955). Superficial thrombosis in the long saphenous vein may be felt as a solid cord, and is usually tender. With thrombophlebitis the overlying skin is hot, red, indurated and painful. Extension to the femoral vein causes a conspicuous rise of skin temperature in the affected limb, a most useful sign of serious phlebothrombosis; œdema also occurs in many cases, but is less constant.

PROGNOSIS

It is not easy to assess the true mortality rate in thrombo-embolism, for many mild cases are overlooked; but in a consecutive series of twenty clinically recognised cases of massive pulmonary embolism seen by the author, six died. In necropsy material, about two-thirds of all pulmonary emboli are major, involving more than 50 per cent of the cross-section of the pulmonary arteries (Belt, 1939); but it is naturally the more severe ones that are seen at necropsy. From evidence of this kind it is estimated that nearly two-thirds of all cases of massive pulmonary embolism recover, and that less than a third of clinical thrombo-emboli are massive; this gives a total mortality rate of about 10 per cent. In those that recover there are ordinarily no sequelæ; but there is an important though small group of cases in which subacute obstructive pulmonary hypertension leads to permanent and finally fatal chronic pulmonary hypertension.

TREATMENT

Prophylaxis is most important, and should be directed towards accelerating the venous circulation in the legs and preventing the clotting process in bed-ridden patients.

Breathing exercises, frequent changes of position, active movements of the legs for specified times every day, prevention of dehydration, and limitation of morphine, are simple, logical, and effective measures. Heart failure should be treated quickly and adequately. Rest in bed should never be prolonged unnecessarily.

Heparin is the quickest and safest anticoagulant; but it is too expensive for routine prophylactic use. It should certainly be employed, however, as soon as phlebothrombosis or thrombo-embolism is recognised, for 23 per cent are multiple (Nygaard *et al.*, 1940–41) and not more than a quarter of cases of massive pulmonary embolism are fatal at the first insult (de Takats and Fowler, 1945). Heparin may be given intravenously in doses of 50 mg. (5,000 units) four- to six-hourly, by continuous intravenous drip in doses of 150 to 300 mg. daily (50 to 100 mg. to a pint of normal saline), or intramuscularly or subcutaneously combined with 2 ml. of 2 per cent procaine in doses of 150 mg. twice daily. The last route is simple and effective. Procaine prevents pain and local bruising is rarely serious. The dose of heparin should be regulated so that the clotting time is maintained at about two to three times the normal (Murray and Best, 1938). Pitkin's menstruum (gelatin 18 per cent, dextrose 8 per cent, glacial acetic acid 0.5 per cent, distilled water to 100 per cent) as a vehicle for heparin to retard its absorption (Loewe et al., 1946), is usually too painful for routine use.

In the event of hæmorrhage the anticoagulant effects of 5,000 units (50 mg.) of heparin may be neutralised immediately by injecting 50 mg. of protamine sulphate intravenously (Parkin and Kvale, 1949).

Heparin is the sulphuric ester of a complex polysaccharide (Jorpes and Bergström, 1937), and in view of the difficulty in preparing it from liver, and therefore its expense, strenuous efforts were made to find a sulphuric ester of some other polysaccharide that could be used as a substitute. This search was rewarded by the discovery that several such esters had powerful anticoagulant properties, including paritol (Sorenson and Wright, 1950), treburon (Field et al., 1953), and dextran sulphate (Ricketts et al., 1953). The most promising and least toxic of these appears to be dextran sulphate. Weight for weight, paritol is one-seventh as potent as heparin, but its anticoagulant effect lasts two to three times longer; treburon is one-third as potent as heparin, but lasts one and a half times longer; dextran sulphate is put up in units that are equivalent to heparin, but its effects last two to three times longer. Paritol may cause swelling of the hands and feet, and serious vasomotor collapse; treburon has been reported to produce severe diarrhœa and late alopecia in some cases, but has the advantage of being painless when injected intramuscularly; dextran sulphate appears to be non-toxic. The heparin-like action of dextran sulphate includes its ability to clear the turbidity of lipid-laden plasma (Brown, 1952). Its chief disadvantage is that it can only be given intravenously.

Dicoumarol (3 : 3'-Methylene-bis-4-hydroxycoumarin), the cause of hæmorrhagic sweet-clover disease of cattle (Link, 1943), is a cheap and effective anticoagulant, but its action is delayed for forty-eight to seventy-two hours and is cumulative, so that it is difficult to control. It acts indirectly by preventing the liver from manufacturing prothrombin. Dicoumarol is given by mouth in single doses each day, beginning with 300 mg. the first day, 200 mg. the second, and 100 mg. the third, subsequent doses (usually 50 to 100 mg.) being adjusted according to the prothrombin time, which should be kept as close as possible to two and a half times the prothrombin time in a normal control, i.e. at a patient/control prothrombin ratio of 2.5, usually achieved with a maintenance dose of 50 to 100 mg. daily. In the past this ratio has been expressed reciprocally as an index, i.e. $\dfrac{\text{control time}}{\text{patient's time}} \times 100$, or 40 per cent for a ratio of 2.5. This means that with a control time of 12 seconds, the patient's prothrombin time should be kept at 30 seconds. The prothrombin time is inversely proportional to the prothrombin content of the plasma. If the former is measured with increasing dilutions of plasma a graph may be constructed by plotting the prothrombin times against the respective plasma dilutions (or their reciprocals if the graph is to be a straight line instead of an impracticable rectangular hyperbola). If the patient's prothrombin time is read off on such a graph (constructed for normal plasma) it may be expressed in terms of prothrombin activity or content. No practical advantage is gained by this manœuvre, which has been the source of much confusion where there is no room for any misunderstanding whatsoever. In fact, a prothrombin ratio of 2.5 or index of 40 per cent is usually equivalent to an activity or content of 15 to 20 per cent. It is solely to avoid any possibility of error that experienced physicians often prefer to chart the prothrombin time itself in seconds, and to record the control time separately below.

At first the prothrombin time should be measured daily, but as soon as the graph stabilises it may be estimated less frequently, e.g. every second day, then twice weekly, and finally once a week. Frequent adjustments of the daily dose of dicoumarol are usually necessary at first, but after a while it is easier to judge the right maintenance dose. About 10 per cent of individuals are unduly sensitive to dicoumarol and an equal number unduly resistant: the degree of sensitivity or resistance seems to be determined by heredity and changes little over the years.

If the prothrombin ratio exceeds 3, microscopic hæmaturia may occur, and if it exceeds 3.5 to 4, hæmorrhage may be serious or even fatal. Hæmaturia, malena and purpura occur in that order of frequency, but a fatal hæmorrhage may be cerebral, pericardial or retro-peritoneal. With proper laboratory control, however, clinical hæmorrhage is rare (1 per cent), and a safe level of prothrombin activity can be restored immediately by blood transfusion or within a few hours by injecting 200 mg. of vitamin K_1 intravenously (Douglas and Brown, 1952). It has since been shown that 25 to 50 mg. of vitamin K_1 orally is usually quite sufficient to restore normal prothrombin times, and 15 to 25 mg. to restore a satisfactory blood therapeutic level of prothrombin when it is desired to continue dicoumarol therapy (Toohey, 1954). In the event of serious hæmorrhage it is hardly necessary to add that dicoumarol must be withheld at once, whatever the prothrombin time, for bleeds have been reported occasionally when the prothrombin activity has been well within the desired therapeutic range.

When all goes well, treatment should be continued for at least three weeks and preferably for six weeks in all cases of thrombo-embolism, and there should be no hesitation in continuing for three to six months in cases giving a history of recurrent thrombo-embolic episodes.

In view of the delayed effect of dicoumarol, heparin is usually given as well during the first forty-eight to seventy-two hours. With this treatment the post-operative mortality rate from massive pulmonary embolism in cases specially selected as thrombo-embolic risks has been reduced from perhaps 5 per cent to 0.1 to 1.0 per cent (Barker *et al.*, 1945; Wright, 1946).

Many other coumarin derivatives have been shown to act like dicoumarol and have been used clinically as anticoagulants. Some of them, such as marcoumar [3-(1'-phenyl-propyl)-4-hydroxycoumarin], are even longer lasting and more cumulative than dicoumarol, and therefore have little to recommend them, for this property is a disadvantage. Cyclocumarol (cumopyran) is in the same category. Marcoumar, for example, inhibits the manufacture of prothrombin for five days after a single dose. Weight for weight it is very powerful, the loading dose being 21, 9, and 3 mg. at daily intervals, and the maintenance dose around 3 mg. daily (Bourgain *et al.*, 1954).

Ethyl biscoumacetate [bis-3,3'-(4-oxycoumarinyl)-ethyl acetate], introduced as "tromexan" and "pelentan", is in a different class, for its maximum effect occurs between eight and twenty-four hours after a single dose, and the prothrombin time returns to normal within the next eight to twenty-four hours, according to the size of the dose (Burt, Wright and Kubik, 1949). Being three to four times less active than dicoumarol the initial loading dose is high, usually 900, 600 and 300 mg. at daily intervals, whilst the maintenance dose is commonly 300 to 600 mg. daily; it is also best given in divided doses two or three times daily (a tablet contains 300 mg.). Ethyl biscoumacetate, however, is expensive, and has been largely replaced by "dindevan".

Sinthrone, which is 3-[α-(4'-nitrophenyl)β-acetyl-ethyl]-4-oxycoumarin, is probably the best of the coumarin derivatives for clinical purposes in that a therapeutic level of reduced prothrombin activity can be achieved easily in twenty-four to forty-eight hours and maintained steadily on a small daily maintenance dose, whilst there is little cumulative effect. The loading dose is 24 mg. the first day, 16 mg. the second and 4 to 8 mg. thereafter according to the prothrombin ratio (Moeschlin and Schorno, 1955). Sinthrome is put up in 4 mg. tablets.

Phenylindanedione (2-phenylindane-1 : 3-dione) or "dindevan" appears to approach the ideal therapeutic drug of its class, and is the most active prothrombopenic agent of the indanedione derivatives (Soulier and Gueguen, 1947, 1948); moreover, it is much cheaper than tromexan. Its effect on the prothrombin time is maximum between twenty-four and thirty-six hours after a single dose, and it has virtually no effect after forty-eight hours (Toohey, 1953). Given in divided doses twice daily it therefore keeps the prothrombin level steadier than tromexan; on the other hand, its relatively short period of activity, and the absence of a cumulative effect, make it much safer and easier to manage than dicoumarol. Phenindione, as it is now being called, is non-toxic, but dermatitis, apparently due to the development of hypersensitivity to the drug, developed in two of my own cases. The loading dose is 150 to 200 mg. on the first day, 100 mg. on the second, and 50 mg. on the morning of the third; for maintenance 50 to 150 mg. daily is usual. Tablets contain 50 mg., but are scored so that 25 mg. doses may be given.

Hæmorrhages are rare with the shorter-acting prothrombin depressors and relatively small doses of vitamin K_1 (10 to 15 mg. orally or 5 mg. intravenously) are usually sufficient to restore safe prothrombin levels within twenty-four hours if an overdose has been given (Toohey, 1954; Dawson, 1955). Nevertheless, it must never be forgotten that all anticoagulants are potentially dangerous, and should not be given lightly or without proper laboratory facilities; nor should they be given to any patient with an active peptic ulcer or with a recent history of spontaneous hæmorrhage from any source. They should be withheld temporarily in the event of any surgical operation, dental extraction or infective hepatitis.

Bilateral ligation of the femoral or common iliac veins or ligation of the inferior vena cava has been received with less enthusiasm, but it may be a life-saving procedure when anti-coagulants are contraindicated. Subsequent œdema, when present, usually passes off within three months, and little detrimental clinical or physiological effects can be detected as a rule (Burch and Ray, 1947). Recurrent superficial thrombophlebitis, however, may prove troublesome.

Treatment of acute obstructive pulmonary hypertension

Relatively mild cases recover spontaneously and require no special treatment. The majority of those clinically recognised, however, are seriously ill, and require urgent attention. The objective is very simple: it is to keep the patient alive long enough for the clot to retract and so relieve the obstruction; at the same time further emboli must be prevented at all costs. To this end the following procedures should be carried out immediately:

1. The patient should be nursed flat in order to encourage the cerebral circulation. Warmth should not be applied to the body and vasodilating agents should not be given with the idea of dilating the pulmonary artery, for these merely serve to lower the blood pressure, which is already critically reduced, and can have no influence on the large pulmonary vessels.

2. Oxygen should be given through a light plastic mask, or the patient may be nursed in an oxygen tent, so that the litre or two of blood that is passing through the lungs may be supersaturated with oxygen.

3. The basal vasomotor and respiratory centres must be supported, for their collapse means instant death. For this purpose nikethamide (coramine) has no equal, and it should be given in doses of at least 0.5 to 1 G. (2 to 4 ml. of the standard 25 per cent solution) intravenously, as often as required (even every five minutes in desperate situations); and if there is no response to 1 G. the dose should be doubled. Nikethamide is rapidly inactivated in the blood stream, and there is therefore no danger of a cumulative effect. An overdose, however, may give rise to convulsions.

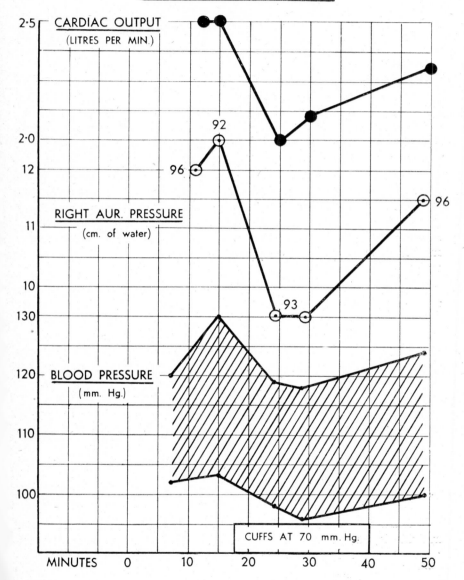

Fig. 17.06—Effect of a venous pressure lowering agent (cuffs on the thighs) on the blood pressure and cardiac output of a case of massive pulmonary embolism.

Morphine is contra-indicated in view of its depressing effect on respiration, and pethidine is also better withheld in view of its vasodilating action, at least until the situation is under control.

4. The blood pressure must be maintained by means of noradrenaline, aramine, or mephentermine (wyamine), as described on page 749.

5. Heparin, 10,000 to 15,000 units, should be given intravenously at once, and repeated in doses of 5,000 to 10,000 units four-to six-hourly during the first forty-eight hours. As soon as the patient is able to swallow, 200 mg. of phenylindanedione should be given, followed by 100 mg. the following day, subsequent doses being regulated according to the pro-thrombin ratio. Anticoagulant treatment must be maintained at a high therapeutic level (ratio nearer 3 than 2) for at least three weeks, or until the danger of recurrent embolism is passed.

6. Ouabain or digoxin, 1 mg. may be given intravenously if the venous pressure is more than 5 cm. above the sternal angle at 30 degrees, on the chance that the right ventricle is overloaded, and 0.5-mg. doses may be repeated twice at six-hourly intervals. In a typical case of the author's, however, lowering the venous pressure resulted in a fall of cardiac output and blood pressure (fig. 17.06), suggesting that the right ventricle was not overloaded.

The Trendelenburg operation (Trendelenburg, 1908)—exposure of the pulmonary artery and removal of the clot—is only possible if a well trained and thoroughly prepared surgical team is available, and is only practised when the situation is desperate: the operative mortality is over 90 per cent (Nygaard, 1938), and spontaneous recovery is the rule rather than the exception. The first successful embolectomy in Great Britain was reported by Ivor Lewis in 1939.

Treatment of pulmonary infarction. No specific treatment is required for pulmonary infarction itself; but secondary infection or septic embolism calls for penicillin or other suitable antibiotic; morphine may be necessary if there is severe pleural pain; and hæmorrhagic pleural effusion may need aspirating if extensive. Infarction does not contraindicate anticoagulants.

PARADOXICAL EMBOLISM

Valvular patency of the foramen ovale is present in about a third of all individuals, but the opening remains closed because the pressure in the left atrium is higher than that in the right. When the right ventricle fails, however, the atrial pressures may be reversed; the valve then opens and blood is shunted from right to left. This event is improbable in heart failure secondary to mitral stenosis, for the left atrial pressure remains too high. Ideal conditions are presented by acute right ventricular failure due to massive pulmonary embolism, for not only is the right atrial pressure then raised, but the left is lowered as in pulmonary stenosis, and emboli are

already forthcoming. Having passed through the foramen ovale, the embolus is carried into the systemic circulation, and may lodge in any cerebral, visceral, or peripheral artery.

AIR EMBOLISM

Small quantities of air may be injected into the systemic venous system of healthy subjects with little risk; indeed about 15 ml. per kg. body weight are required to kill a dog, even when injected rapidly (Wolffe and Robertson, 1935). Fatalities have occurred, however, when air has been accidentally introduced into a vein during an operation, intravenous infusion, therapeutic or diagnostic procedure. The clinical features are those of massive pulmonary embolism; but in addition a loud churning sound or millwheel murmur may be heard over the right ventricle and pulmonary artery. Death appears to result from circulatory obstruction due to air-lock in the outflow tract of the right ventricle. Treatment consists of turning the patient into the left lateral position in the hope of displacing the air into the right atrium (Oppenheimer, Durant and Lynch, 1953). A similar manœuvre has proved life-saving in dogs, but has not yet been tried in man.

FAT EMBOLISM

Globules of fat may penetrate the systemic venous circulation following fractures, usually of the femur, and accidents have occasionally occurred during therapeutic or diagnostic procedures involving the use of oil. Fat embolism has several characteristics which help to distinguish it from other forms. First, it happens within a few hours of the accident, perhaps while manipulating the injured limb under anæsthesia, or when moving the patient to the X-ray department. Second, signs of multiple systemic embolism usually complicate the picture owing to the passage of fat globules through the pulmonary capillaries. Thus, there may be severe headache, drowsiness or loss of consciousness, usually without localising signs; multiple petechial spots may appear in the skin; red cells, albumin, and droplets of oil may be found in the urine. Third, breathlessness and cyanosis are associated with the development of fine crepitations over all areas of the lungs, and skiagrams show an abundance of cotton-wool shadows in all zones. The mortality rate is similar to that of other forms of massive pulmonary embolism; but those who survive recover remarkably quickly – often within forty-eight hours.

EMBOLISM DUE TO FOREIGN BODY

Metallic fragments from gun-shot wounds, and even bullets, may enter the circulation in rare instances. Such an event should be considered if a skiagram shows an intra-thoracic foreign body when there is no wound of the chest or adjacent structures. An intravascular metallic foreign body may remain mobile for several days, and may move against the bloodstream if so directed by the force of gravity. Surgical attempts to remove the missile may be foiled by such behaviour. An excellent example was described by Bauer (1943).

MALIGNANT EMBOLI

Cancer cells may infiltrate the systemic venous system and be swept into the lungs in the form of cellular emboli. Subacute pulmonary hyper-

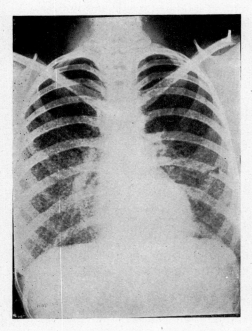

Fig. 17.07—Skiagram showing miliary embolic carcinomatosis of the lungs.

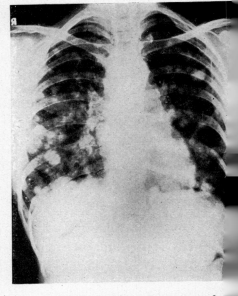

Fig. 17.08—Radiological appearances of lungs showing embolic secondaries due to chorionepithelioma.

(By courtesy of Dr. Phillip Ellman)

tension develops if more than two-thirds of the vessels are blocked, the clinical features resembling those of massive pulmonary embolism but with an insidious onset and progressive course. The diagnosis may be suggested by the skiagram which may show minute miliary lesions (fig. 17.07). Cases so far reported have been due either to carcinoma of the stomach (Brill and Robertson, 1937) or breast (Mason, 1940), or to chorionepithelioma (fig. 17.08).

Subacute pulmonary hypertension may also be due to multiple pulmonary thromboses secondary to perivascular lymphatic carcinomatous infiltration (Brill and Robertson, 1937). As a rule, however, these cases present with subacute hypoxic cor pulmonale (q.v.).

REFERENCES

Barker, N. W., Cromer, H. E., Hurn, M., and Waugh, J. M. (1945): "The use of dicoumarol in the prevention of post-operative thrombosis and embolism with special reference to dosage and safe administration", *Surg.*, **17**, 207.

Barnes, A. R. (1937): "Pulmonary embolism", *J. Amer. med. Ass.*, **109**, 1347.

Barnes, C. G. (1941): "Electrocardiogram after pneumonectomy", *Proc. Roy. Soc. Med.*, **34**, 606.

Bauer, K. H. (1943): "Penetrating gunshot wound of the heart – triple embolism by a bullet", *Der chirurg.*, **15**, 697.

Belt, T. H. (1934): "Thrombosis and pulmonary embolism", *Amer. J. Path.*, **10**, 129.

—— (1939): "Late sequelæ of pulmonary embolism", *Lancet, ii*, 730.

—— (1939): "The ætiology of lung infarction", *Brit. Heart J.*, **1**, 283.

—— (1939): "Autopsy incidence of pulmonary embolism", *Lancet, i*, 1259.

Bourgain, R., Todd, M., Herzig, L., and Wright, I. S. (1954): "Marcumar [3-(1′-phenyl-propyl)-4-hydroxycoumarin]. A new anticoagulant", *Circulation*, **10**, 680.

Brill, I. C., and Robertson, T. D. (1937): "Subacute cor pulmonale", *Arch. intern. Med.*, **60**, 1043.

Brown, W. D. (1952): "Reversible effects of anticoagulants and protamine on alimentary lipæmia", *Quart. J. exp. Physiol.*, **37**, 75, 119, 257.

Burt, C. C., Wright, H. P., and Kubik, M. (1949): "Clinical tests of a new coumarin substance", *Brit. med. J.*, **ii**, 1250.

Churchill, E. D. (1934): "The mechanism of death in massive pulmonary embolism", *Surg. Gynec. and Obstetr.*, **59**, 513.

Collins, D. C. (1936): "Pulmonary embolism based upon study of 271 instances", *Amer. J. Surg.*, **33**, 210.

Crutcher, R. R. (1948): "Venous thrombosis and pulmonary embolism", *Kentucky Med. J.*, **46**, 427.

Dawson, P. (1955): "Effects of intravenous vitamin K_1 on the action of phenindione", *Brit. med. J.*, **ii**, 1427.

de Takats, G., and Fowler, E. F. (1945): "The problem of thrombo-embolism", *Surg.*, **17**, 153.

Douglas, A. S., and Brown, A. (1952): "Effect of vitamin K preparations on hypoprothrombinæmia induced by dicoumarol and tromexan", *Brit. med. J.*, **i**, 412.

Dunn, J. S. (1920): "Effects of multiple embolism of pulmonary arterioles", *Quart. J. Med.*, **13**, 129.

Durant, T. M., Long, J., and Oppenheimer, M. J. (1947): "Pulmonary (venous) air embolism", *Amer. Heart J.*, **33**, 269.

Eppinger, E. C., and Kennedy, J. A. (1938): "The cause of death in coronary thrombosis, with special reference to pulmonary embolism", *Amer. J. med. Sc.*, **195**, 104.

Field, J. B., Ramsay, G. D., Attyah, A. M., and Starr, P. (1953): "The effect in man of a new heparinoid, Treburon", *J. lab. and clin. Med.*, **41**, 208.

Gibbon, J. H., Hopkinson, M., and Churchill, E. D. (1932): "Changes in circulation produced by gradual occlusion of pulmonary artery", *J. clin. Invest.*, **11**, 543.

Haggart, G. E., and Walker, A. M. (1923): "The physiology of pulmonary embolism as disclosed by quantitative occlusion of the pulmonary artery", *Arch. Surg.*, **6**, 764.

Hampton, A. O., and Castleman, B. (1940): "Post-mortem chest teleroentgenograms with autopsy findings", *Amer. J. Roentgenol.*, **43**, 305.

Homans, J. (1947): "Venous thrombosis and pulmonary embolism", *New Engl. J. Med.*, **236**, 196.

Jorpes, E., and Bergström, S. (1937): "Heparin: a mucoitin polysulpuric acid", *J. biol. Chem.*, **118**, 447.

Karsner, H. T., and Ash, J. E. (1912–3): "Studies in infarction. II. Experimental bland infarction of the lung", *J. med. Res.*, 27, 205.

Lenégre, J., and Nèel, J. (1950): "Embolies pulmonaire sans infarctus", *Arch. Mal. Coeur.*, 43, 385.

Lewis, I. (1939): "Trendelenburg's operation for pulmonary embolism", *Lancet*, i, 1037.

Link, K. P. (1943–4): "The anticoagulant from spoiled sweet clover hay", Harvey Lectures, p. 162, Pennsylvania.

——, (1943–4): "The anticoagulant dicumarol", Harvey Lectures, 39, 162.

Loewe, L., Rosenblatt, P., and Hirsch, E. (1946): "Venous thrombo-embolic disease", *J. Amer. med. Ass.*, 130, 386.

McCartney, J. S. (1945): "Post-operative pulmonary embolism", *Surgery*, 17, 191.

McGinn, S., and White, P. D. (1935): "Acute cor pulmonale resulting from pulmonary embolism: its clinical recognition", *J. Amer. med. Ass.*, 104, 1473.

McPheeters, H. O., and Rice, C. O. (1928): "Varicose veins; complications, direct and associated, following injection treatment. Review of the literature", *Ibid.*, 91, 1090.

Macht, D. I. (1946): "Thromboplastic properties of some mercurial diuretics", *Amer. Heart J.*, 31, 460.

Malinow, M. R., Katz, L. N., and Kondo, B. (1946): "Is there a vagal pulmono-coronary reflex in pulmonary embolism?", *Ibid.*, 31, 702.

Mason, D. G. (1940): "Subacute cor pulmonale", *Arch. intern. Med.*, 66, 1221.

Massie, E., Stillerman, H. S., Wright, C., and Minnich, V. (1944): "Effect of administration of digitalis on coagulability of human blood", *Ibid.*, 74, 172.

Moeschlin, S., and Schorno, H. (1955): "Clinical experience with a new 4-oxycoumarin derivative Sintrom (Geigy 23350)", *Schw. med. Wschr.*, 85, 590.

Murray, G. D. W., and Best, C. H. (1938): "Use of heparin in thrombosis", *Ann. Surg.*, 108, 163.

Nygaard, K. K. (1938): "Consideration of clinical diagnosis and possibilities for the Trendelenburg operation", *Proc. Mayo Clin.*, 13, 586.

—— (1941): "Hæmorrhagic diseases: photoelectric study of blood coagulability", London.

——, Barker, N. W., Walters, W., and Priestly, J. T. (1940): "A statistical study of post-operative venous thrombosis and pulmonary embolism. I. Incidence in various types of operation", *Proc. Mayo Clin.*, 15, 769.

——, ——, ——, —— (1941): "A statistical study of post-operative venous thrombosis and pulmonary embolism. II. Predisposing factors", *Ibid.*, 16, 1.

——, ——, ——, —— (1941): "A statistical study of post-operative venous thrombosis and pulmonary embolism. III. Time of occurrence during post-operative period", *Ibid.*, 16, 17.

Oppenheimer, M. J., Durant, T. M., and Lynch, P. (1953): "Body position in relation to venous air embolism and the associated cardiovascular-respiratory changes", *Amer. J. med. Sc.*, 225, 362.

Ortiz-Ramirez, T., and Serna-Ramirez, R. (1955): "New early diagnostic sign of phlebitis of the lower extremeties", *Amer. Heart J.*, 50, 366.

Parkin, T. W., and Kvale, W. F. (1949): "Neutralisation of the anticoagulant effects of heparin with protamine (salmine)", *Amer. Heart J.*, 37, 333.

Pilcher, R. (1939): "The rôle of obstruction in fatal pulmonary embolism", *Lancet, i*, 1257.

Prettin, F. (1936): "Thrombose und tödliche Lungen-embolie", *Virchows Arch. f. Path. Anat.*, 297, 535.

Quick, A. J. (1950): "A new concept of venous thrombosis", *Surg. Gynec. and Obst.*, 91, 296.

Ray, C. T., and Burch, G. (1947): "Vascular responses in man to ligation of the inferior vena cava", *Arch. intern. Med.*, **80**, 587.

Ricketts, C. R., *et al.* (1953): "Therapeutic trial of the synthetic heparin analogue dextran sulphate", *Lancet*, **ii**, 1004.

Rissanen, E. (1947): "Statistical study of the incidence of pulmonary embolism in connection with cardiac insufficiency", *Duodecim*, Helsinki, **63**, 126.

Scherf, D., and Boyd, L. J. (1939): "Cardiovascular diseases", London.

——, and Schönbrunner, E. (1937): "The pulmonary reflex in lung emboli", *Klin. Wchnschr.*, **16**, 340.

Shapiro, R., and Rigler, L. (1948): "Pulmonary embolism without infarction", *Amer. J. Roentgenol.*, **60**, 460.

Sorenson, C. W., and Wright, I. S. (1950): "A synthetic anticoagulant: a poly-sulfuric acid ester of polyanhydromannuronic acid (paritol)", *Circulation*, **2**, 658.

Soulier, J. P., Gueguen, J. (1947): "Action hypoprothrombinemiante (anti-K) de la phényl-indane-dione étudiée experimentalement chez le Lapin", *C.R. Soc. Biol.* (Paris), **141**, 1007.

——, —— (1948): "Action de la phényl-indane-dione sur le taux de la pro-thrombine; étude experimentale sur le Lapin", *Rev. Hematol.*, **3**, 180.

Toohey, M. (1953): "Clinical trial of phenylindanedione as an anticoagulant", *Brit. med. J.*, **i**, 650.

—— (1954): "Vitamin K_1 in anticoagulant therapy", *Ibid.*, **i**, 1020.

Trendelenburg, F. (1908): "Operation der Emboli der Lungenarterie", *Deutsch. med. Wchnschr.*, **34**, 1172.

Virchow, R. (1856): "Ueber die verstopfung de Lungenarterie", *Gesammelt als handlungen*, Frankfurt a.m., 224.

—— (1856): "Thrombose und Embolie, Gefässentzündung und Septische Infek-tion. (i) Ueber die Verstopfung der Lungenarterie", *Gesammelt. Abhandl. zur Wissenschaft. med.* (Chap. 4, p. 221), Frankfurt, A.M.

Westerborn, A. (1937): "Uber die Emboliegefahr bei Injektions behandlung von varizen nebst einen Bericht uber die in Schweden vorgekommenen Embolie-falle", *Acta. chir. Scand.*, 321.

White, P. D. (1937): "Heart disease", New York.

——, and Brenner, O. (1933): "Pathological and clinical aspects of the pulmonary circulation", *New Engl. J. Med.*, **209**, 1261.

Wolffe, J. B., and Robertson, H. F. (1935): "Experimental air embolism", *Ann. intern. Med.*, **9**, 162.

Wood, P. H. (1941): "Pulmonary embolism: diagnosis by chest lead electro-cardiography", *Brit. Heart J.*, **3**, 21.

—— (1947): "Discussion on pulmonary embolism", *Ibid.*, **9**, 308.

—— (1948): "Electrocardiographic appearances in acute and chronic pulmonary heart disease", *Ibid.*, **10**, 87.

Wright, I. S. (1946): "Practical considerations in the conservative treatment of thrombophlebitis", *N.Y. J. Med.*, **46**, 1819.

—— (1952): "The pathogenesis and treatment of thrombosis", *Circulation* **5**, 161.

CHAPTER XVIII

PULMONARY HYPERTENSION

Normal pulmonary blood pressure

The average normal pulmonary blood pressure is 16/7 mm. Hg (mean 11 mm. Hg) with reference to the sternal angle. This figure is based on fifty normal controls investigated by the author for one reason or another over the past eight years. The cardiac output at the time ranged between 5.8 and 12.8 litres per minute (average 8.6). As repeatedly pointed out, conditions are not basal during cardiac catheterisation. The normal mean left atrial pressure averages 2 to 3 mm. Hg above the sternal angle, so that the normal pulmonary artery–left atrial pressure gradient is 8 to 9 mm. Hg, and the pulmonary vascular resistance (page 177 is therefore $\frac{8 \text{ to } 9}{8.6}$ or around unity (80 dynes sec./cm.^{5}). Conventional figures are 10 mm. Hg for the gradient, 5 litres per minute for the cardiac output, and 2 units for the resistance.

Definition and classification of pulmonary hypertension

Pulmonary hypertension literally implies a pulmonary blood pressure above 30/15 mm. Hg, which is the upper limit of the normal range. Physiologically there are four entirely different mechanisms that may produce pulmonary hypertension, namely, appreciable elevation of the left atrial pressure, obstruction or obliteration of more than two-thirds of the total cross section of the pulmonary vascular bed at any level, a sufficiently increased pulmonary blood flow, and active pulmonary vaso-constriction: each of these mechanisms causes its own particular variety of pulmonary hypertension, which may be labelled respectively—passive, obstructive or obliterative, hyperkinetic and vasoconstrictive. There is no doubt that any form of pulmonary hypertension, if sufficiently severe and prolonged, finally produces sclerotic changes in the pulmonary arteries, with or without local thromboses, which may add an obliterative or obstructive element to the picture; and there is good reason to suspect that any form of pronounced pulmonary hypertension may also excite a vasoconstrictive reaction and so turn passive, obstructive or hyperkinetic pulmonary hypertension into the more serious vasoconstrictive type. Such a reaction would close a vicious circle and so transform a relatively innocent pulmonary hypertension into a more or less malignant form. The parallel between this hypothesis and current theory in respect of systemic hypertension will not pass unnoticed.

PASSIVE PULMONARY HYPERTENSION

Mean left atrial pressures of 20 to 30 mm. Hg at rest, and 40 to 50 mm. Hg on effort are common in mitral stenosis. In such cases the mean pulmonary artery pressure must be at least 10 mm. Hg higher if the normal pressure gradient is to be preserved. A similar situation arises in mitral incompetence and left ventricular failure. This may be called passive pulmonary hypertension because it represents no more than transmitted pulmonary venous hypertension. Left atrial pressures of 15 to 20 mm. Hg and therefore mean pulmonary artery pressures of 25 to 30 mm. Hg are usual in chronic constrictive pericarditis and in cases of congestive heart failure due to any generalised cardiopathy such as isolated myocarditis, but they do not rise on effort because the right ventricle is incapable of increasing its stroke output. Passive pulmonary hypertension in these cases is therefore trivial.

Reactive pulmonary vasoconstriction raised the pulmonary vascular resistance to between 6 and 10 units in 16 per cent of 275 critical cases of mitral stenosis studied by the author, and to over 10 units (average 17) in 12 per cent. By critical is meant sufficient stenosis (orifice around 1 × 0.5 cm.) to raise the left atrial pressure 20 mm. Hg or more when the cardiac output is 4 to 5 litres per minute and the heart rate normal, i.e. sufficient to cause a mean pulmonary artery pressure over 30 mm. Hg at rest. Reactive pulmonary vasoconstriction does not seem to occur in response to less passive pulmonary hypertension than this. Whether it is persistent pulmonary hypertension of the order of 50/25 mm. Hg, or repetitive pulmonary hypertension of a much higher degree that is responsible for the vasoconstrictive reaction is unknown; indeed, there is no direct proof that it is the pulmonary hypertension that is causing the vasoconstrictive reaction at all. Certainly, the historical and objective lack of chronic interstitial œdema of the lungs in cases with an extreme resistance exonerate that factor as a possible etiological agent.

The incidence of active pulmonary vasoconstriction in mitral incompetence appears to be lower. Of 58 cases severe enough to have warranted mitral valve repair, had such an operation been available, only 14 per cent had an appreciably increased pulmonary vascular resistance (9 per cent between 6 and 10 units and 5 per cent in the extreme range over 10 units). The lower *mean* left atrial pressure and lower mean level of passive pulmonary hypertension may explain this lower incidence of the vasoconstrictive response. Alternatively, the factor that seems to limit right ventricular filling in severe mitral incompetence (Bernheim effect or increased pericardial tension?) may prevent surges of right ventricular output and undue rises of pressure on effort. Certainly, an increased pulmonary venous or arterial pulse pressure, which is characteristic of mitral incompetence, cannot be responsible for reactive vasoconstriction, or the latter would be more common in mitral incompetence than stenosis.

No figures are available for the frequency of active pulmonary hypertension secondary to the passive pulmonary hypertension of left ventricular failure. It was observed on page 774, however, that many cases that present clinically with the Bernheim syndrome prove to be examples of right ventricular failure secondary to reactive pulmonary vasoconstriction.

No instance of extreme pulmonary vasoconstriction has yet been recorded secondary to the relatively mild passive pulmonary hypertension of Pick's disease and generalised cardiopathies. This again suggests that a critical level of pulmonary hypertension must be reached before significant reactive vasoconstriction occurs.

The clinical details of passive pulmonary hypertension and its vasoconstrictive response (Wood, 1954) have already been discussed in relation to mitral valve disease on page 540 and to left ventricular failure on page 774.

HYPERKINETIC PULMONARY HYPERTENSION

As the blood flow through the lungs increases, the vessels dilate to accommodate the extra volume, and temporarily closed vessels probably open up, so that the resistance falls; there is thus little or no rise of pressure at first (Hickam and Cargill, 1947; Riley *et al.*, 1948), but as the flow approaches three times the normal (15 litres per minute in an adult of average height and weight) a state of maximum vasodilatation is reached and no further drop in resistance is possible; thereafter the pulmonary blood pressure rises in proportion to the flow (Cournand, 1950). In other cases the pulmonary vascular resistance does not alter much with effort, the pulmonary blood pressure tending to rise with quite small changes of output (Dexter *et al.*, 1951; Donald *et al.*, 1955). In disease both types of response are seen. For example, pulmonary blood flows of 10 to 15 litres per minute, reduced resistance and no appreciable rise of pulmonary blood pressure are characteristic of many cases of atrial septal defect; in the majority of cases of patent ductus or ventricular septal defect, on the other hand, flows of this order are usually associated with some rise of pressure, the resistance being normal (or even slightly raised) rather than unduly low. With flows of 20 to 30 litres per minute the pulmonary blood pressure may approach and even reach systemic level. Hyperkinetic pulmonary hypertension, then, may be defined as a raised pulmonary blood pressure associated with an increased flow and normal resistance.

In the generalised hyperkinetic circulatory states, such as thyrotoxicosis, beri-beri, Paget's disease of bone, anæmia, cor pulmonale, hepatic failure, pregnancy, and phæochromocytoma of the adrenaline (rather than noradrenaline) type, the frequency of hyperkinetic pulmonary hypertension is not yet known, but there can be little doubt that it may occur, especially perhaps in beri-beri. The increased pulmonary blood flow in cor pulmonale is particularly important, because it may be associated with some degree of obliterative pulmonary hypertension, and the combination may be responsible for very high pulmonary blood pressures.

Of the congenital shunts there are at least five acyanotic and five cyanotic forms that may result in hyperkinetic pulmonary hypertension:

Acyanotic	*Cyanotic*
Partial anomalous pulmonary venous drainage	Total anomalous pulmonary venous drainage
Atrial septal defect	Single atrium
Ventricular septal defect	Single ventricle
Patent ductus arteriosus	Persistent truncus
Aorto-pulmonary septal defect	Transposition of the great vessels

These have all been discussed in detail in the chapter on congenital heart disease.

Appreciable reactive pulmonary vasoconstriction occurred in one-quarter of a consecutive series of 100 critical cases of atrial septal defect, and two-thirds of 100 critical cases of patent ductus or ventricular septal defect studied by the author. By critical is meant a defect of sufficient size to cause a pulmonary blood flow of at least three times the systemic flow in the presence of a normal pulmonary vascular resistance. Clinically this means that the case would be regarded as severe or gross rather than mild or moderate in degree. In the 93 cases that had developed the vasoconstrictive response, the pulmonary vascular resistance lay between 6 and 10 units in 29 and between 10 and 30 units (average 17) in 64. This suggests that if the reaction occurs at all it is likely to become extreme. The presence or absence of the vasoconstrictive response was obviously determined at birth in the great majority if not in all cases, and the idea that pulmonary hypertension due to a high pulmonary vascular resistance develops slowly over the years is totally unsupported by all available data. Obstructive pulmonary hypertension due to embolism or thrombosis may occur suddenly in the later stages of these diseases, but that is another matter altogether. The evidence suggests that in one group of individuals hyperkinetic pulmonary hypertension at once causes persistent pulmonary vasoconstriction, whereas in another group of individuals it does not. The secret of this difference in behaviour has not yet been discovered, nor is it yet understood why cases of atrial septal defect are less likely to develop the reaction than cases of patent ductus and ventricular septal defect of comparable severity.

The clinical features of hyperkinetic pulmonary hypertension and the effect of the vasoconstrictive reaction on the physiology of the circulation in all these congenital anomalies have already been described in Chapter VIII and cannot be further considered here.

OBSTRUCTIVE OR OBLITERATIVE PULMONARY HYPERTENSION

The word obstructive is best applied to massive pulmonary embolism or thrombosis, and to subacute miliary thrombo-embolism or widespread peripheral pulmonary thromboses; pneumonectomy also provides an example of artificial obstruction of half the total cross-section of the pulmonary vascular tree. Carcinomatous embolism and diffuse infiltrative lymphatic carcinomatosis behave rather differently and will be described as a form of subacute cor pulmonale in Chapter XIX, although secondary widespread thromboses may also cause obstructive pulmonary hypertension. The term obliterative more accurately describes the situation in respect of the capillaries in emphysema and the small arteries and arterioles when they are partially or wholly blocked by gross endocardial thickening as an anatomical reaction to severe and prolonged pulmonary hypertension of any kind, secondary to subacute thrombo-embolism, or as a result of certain forms of arteritis, including periarteritis nodosa, disseminated lupus, and schistosomiasis. Secondary thrombosis is common in these partially occluded vessels, so that obstructive and obliterative types may overlap.

Massive pulmonary embolism was considered fully in the last chapter.

Massive pulmonary thrombosis is relatively rare, but may complicate any form of long-standing pulmonary hypertension that has developed extensive pulmonary atherosclerosis. Its pathogenesis is comparable to thrombosis at the distal end of the descending aorta in elderly men with gross aortic atherosclerosis.

The degree of obstructive pulmonary hypertension produced obviously depends on the size and number of vessels thrombosed. As a rule only one major vessel is involved, and even if this is the main right or left pulmonary artery not more than half the total cross-section of the pulmonary arterial tree is cut off, and therefore pulmonary hypertension would not arise if the rest of the circulation were normal. But the pulmonary circulation is never normal in these cases, for otherwise neither the atherosclerosis nor the secondary thrombosis would occur. The complication, therefore, nearly always has serious consequences. In the congenital group with hyperkinetic pulmonary hypertension, massive thrombosis may greatly elevate the pulmonary blood pressure, overload the right ventricle and reverse the shunt. In obliterative or vasoconstrictive pulmonary hypertension, the relatively sudden increase of total pulmonary vascular resistance usually causes immediate right ventricular failure.

Clinically, massive thrombosis should be suspected in any advanced case of pulmonary hypertension of any type, if there is relatively sudden deterioration in effort tolerance, unexpected shunt reversal, or unexpected heart failure. Pulmonary thrombosis is never a dramatic event like massive pulmonary embolism, and deterioration may be quite insidious in some cases. As a rule, the breakdown associated with thrombosis is subacute rather than acute or chronic, and the majority of cases are fatal (Magidson and Jacobson, 1955).

The diagnosis may be confirmed by the skiagram, which may show an exceptionally dense, bulky, pulseless, comma-shaped shadow in the position of one or other main pulmonary artery (fig. 18.01), and an unduly translucent ischæmic lung distal to the block on one or other side (Keating *et al.*, 1953). Proof of the obstruction may be obtained by means of angio-cardiography, but this is rarely necessary.

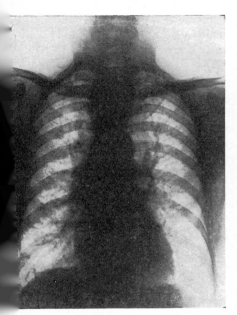 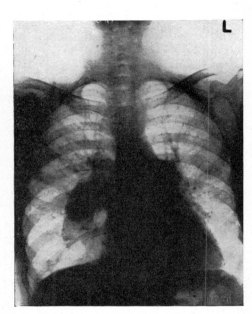

(a) 22nd March 1944.   (b) 5th December 1946.

Fig. 18.01—Development of thrombosis of the right pulmonary artery in a case of anoxic cor pulmonale.

Subacute thrombo-embolic pulmonary hypertension

This is one of the most important forms of severe pulmonary hyper-tension for several reasons: (1) socially and economically because it most commonly affects otherwise healthy young married women after childbirth; (2) therapeutically because it can be cured by swift diagnosis and adequate treatment, but is otherwise fatal; (3) experimentally because it can be wholly reproduced and investigated in animals; (4) academically because it is a most important and thoroughly understood link between simple obstructive pulmonary hypertension, secondary obliterative pulmonary hypertension, and so-called primary pulmonary hypertension (*vide infra*). The disease therefore repays close scrutiny.

Experimentally the condition has been reproduced in rabbits by the repeated intravenous injection of finely fragmented fibrin clot. With relatively large doses the rabbits died from heart failure secondary to obstructive pulmonary hypertension. When the dose was nicely judged for the purpose, however, the rabbits lived longer, the emboli became organised, the lumens of the obstructed small arteries were reconstituted, and the vessels were left with marked fibro-elastic intimal thickening which was indistinguishable from that seen in "primary" pulmonary hypertension (Harrison, 1948). This important work was confirmed by Barnard (1954), who produced similar lesions of the small arteries and arterioles of mice and rabbits by injecting thromboplastin into the systemic venous system so that fibrin emboli were formed *in vivo*.

Physiologically pulmonary hypertension is initially obstructive, then obliterative, and finally may well be vasoconstrictive in response to the hypertension itself.

Clinically, cases present in a subacute manner with right ventricular failure secondary to severe pulmonary hypertension. The majority are young married women and symptoms develop soon after childbirth; occasionally the condition arises during pregnancy, or is associated with some other cause of recurrent intravascular clotting of the appropriate kind. Thus one of my five cases occurred in a young man following a sprained ankle, small emboli being liberated from repeated phlebo-thrombosis in the vicinity. Death occurred within six months from right ventricular failure secondary to severe pulmonary hypertension. Repeated small hæmoptyses were a feature of this case. Of the other four, two (a woman aged 40 and a man aged 36) followed simple recurrent thrombo-phlebitis in the legs; one of them died after a typical course lasting 18 months, and the other is still alive on permanent anticoagulant treatment. The other two, aged 27 and 25, were both associated with phlebo-thrombosis following pregnancy. One of them, who appeared to be dying with advanced heart failure after inadequate treatment for two to three months, was cured by prolonged anticoagulant therapy, strict bed rest, and intensive treatment for heart failure over a period of three months. Final catheterisation in her case revealed complete restoration of the pulmonary vascular resistance to normal. The other was progressing favourably with similar treatment for six weeks when she discharged herself from hospital because her husband did not appear to believe that she was seriously ill and needed her services at home. At this time her pulmonary vascular resistance had fallen to 5.3 units (P.A.P. 50/13 mm. Hg; C.O. 5.1 L/min.), and she had improved considerably in all other respects. She has continued anticoagulant treatment as an out-patient since, and for a year has held her own, but the clinical signs indicate that she still has moderate pulmonary hypertension.

The case described by Castleman and Bland (1946) occurred in a woman of 35 following her third pregnancy; she survived nine years of increasing obstruction and obliteration of the tertiary branches of the pulmonary artery, the distal vessels remaining normal.

The physical signs, X-ray and electrocardiographic appearances, physiological findings, course, prognosis and detailed treatment of subacute thrombo-embolic pulmonary hypertension are the same as for "primary" pulmonary hypertension (page 839), and will not be further considered here except to re-emphasise the importance of prolonged rest and anticoagulant therapy, the goal being a normal pulmonary vascular resistance. It is not enough to prevent further embolism; it may well be essential to keep the pulmonary blood pressure as low as possible for several months so that secondary proliferative changes and reactive pulmonary vasoconstriction are discouraged. Only when the resistance has fallen to normal should ordinary activities be resumed and pulmonary blood pressure lowering agents abandoned.

Subacute obliterative pulmonary hypertension

The best examples of this condition are caused by periarteritis, disseminated lupus and pulmonary schistosomiasis. The first two have already been discussed to some extent in the section on cardiopathies of obscure origin, and it is only necessary to add that both may cause obliterative pulmonary hypertension as a result of widespread arteritis involving the small vessels (Eskelund, 1943). The clinical picture in this respect does not differ from any other kind of subacute pulmonary hypertension.

Schistosomiasis has been recognised as a cause of pulmonary hypertensive heart failure in Egypt for over twenty years (Azmy, 1932). Either intestinal bilharziasis due to S. Mansoni or urinary bilharziasis due to S. hæmatobium may be responsible (Shaw and Ghareeb, 1938). Ova from S. Mansoni only reach the lungs when sufficient cirrhosis has developed to have resulted in anastomotic channels between the portal and systemic venous systems, so that hepatosplenomegaly is invariably present in these cases; ova from S. hæmatobium can pass directly to the lungs. The ova lodge in the arterioles, where they set up an acute obliterative necrotising arteriolitis, which is the cause of the pulmonary hypertension. A specific angiomatoid lesion often develops in relation to capillary recanalisation of the occluded vessels (Shaw and Ghareeb, 1938). Ova that escape through the wall of the arteriole cause the characteristic parenchymatous giant-celled bilharzia tubercle (Sorour, 1928), but these play no part in the syndrome under discussion. Proximal to the sites of oval impaction the small arteries hypertrophy and develop marked intimal thickening—the usual reaction to pulmonary hypertension, however caused.

Clinically males are affected more often than females and the majority of patients are between 12 and 35 years of age. Once pulmonary hypertension has developed the clinical course and findings are like those of "primary" pulmonary hypertension (Bedford et al., 1946) and death from congestive failure is likely within two years.

A bedside diagnosis is usually possible, as demonstrated by Kenawy (1950). It is based on (1) clinical features resembling those of primary pulmonary hypertension in a young man who has lived in Bilharzia territory; (2) a history of urinary or intestinal schistosomiasis, or the demonstration of ova in urine or fæces; (3) hepatosplenomegaly independent of heart failure when S. Mansoni is responsible; (4) radiological evidence of scattered infiltrative parenchymatous lesions in the lungs.

No specific treatment is advised, for the damage is already done, and the cardiotoxic properties of antimony may adversely influence the course of the disease (Kenawy, 1950).

Chronic obliterative pulmonary hypertension

Although any of the subacute types of obstructive or obliterative pulmonary hypertension described above may take a relatively chronic course, the title is reserved for those cases of advanced emphysema that have two-thirds or more of their pulmonary capillaries obliterated (Cournand, 1950). This is unusual, but is one of the many factors that have to be taken into account in the complex pathogenesis of cor pulmonale (q.v.).

VASOCONSTRICTIVE PULMONARY HYPERTENSION

As implied by the title, the fundamental mechanism causing pulmonary hypertension in this group is pulmonary vasoconstriction at small arterial or arteriolar level. It is as yet uncertain whether reactive pulmonary hypertension (*vide infra*) and "primary" pulmonary hypertension (page 839) should be included under this heading or not, but to avoid controversy they have been considered separately.

Anatomical considerations

There has always been much uncertainty concerning the physiological behaviour of the small pulmonary arteries and arterioles and whether or not they play an active or passive role in the regulation of the circulation. It was at first argued that their delicate structure favoured passive behaviour: thus there is no muscle in a pulmonary arteriole, merely a layer or two of elastic tissue around the endothelium; in the small arteries (0.1 to 1.0 mm. in external diameter) the muscular media averages only 14 per cent of the external diameter of the vessel, compared with 36 per cent in a systemic artery of the same size (Brenner, 1935). The question therefore arises whether these vessels are capable of sufficient vasoconstriction to embarrass the right ventricle. To this may be said that it is unsound to argue about physiological events in terms of anatomical structure. Thus capillaries can constrict against astonishing pressures, a function retained by pulmonary capillaries although they have no Rouget cells (Wearn, 1934), and there is no valid reason for supposing that small pulmonary arteries and arterioles are not possessed of considerable contractile power. The belief that systemic veins were incapable of active vasoconstriction in view of their structure has long been abandoned.

Nervous and chemical control

The presence and degree of autonomic nervous control of the pulmonary blood vessels has also been a controversial subject. It is known that they are supplied with vasoconstrictor fibres through the sympathetic (Bradford and Dean, 1894), the cell stations being in the stellate and middle cervical ganglia, and that the post-ganglionic vasoconstrictor neurones are adrenergic (Daly *et al.*, 1954); it is also believed that the pulmonary vessels are supplied with vasodilator fibres (Daly and Euler, 1932). Normally, the pulmonary vascular resistance varies inversely with the inflow pressure and pulmonary blood flow (Williams, 1954), but whether the mechanism is active or passive is unknown.

There is little doubt that pressor drugs such as noradrenaline and phenylephrine cause pulmonary vasoconstriction and that systemic vaso-dilators such as acetylcholine, aminophylline and priscol cause pulmonary vasodilatation. When these drugs are injected into the pulmonary artery the effect is immediate and independent of both the left atrial pressure and cardiac output. There are certain important exceptions, however, to the general rule that systemic vasoconstrictors and vasodilators have a similar action on the pulmonary circulation. In the first place, the systemic vascular resistance is normally eight times the pulmonary, so that systemic vessels may be regarded as having greater normal tone than the pulmonary, and this may influence the effect of nitrites, for example, which only appear to lower the pulmonary vascular resistance when it is initially high (Halmagyi *et al.*, 1953). Then, of the vasoconstrictors, pitressin is selective and does not act on the pulmonary circulation (Nelson *et al.*, 1955), whilst noradrenaline sometimes raises the pulmonary blood pressure only passively by raising the pulmonary venous pressure (Fowler *et al.*, 1951; Nelson *et al.*, 1955). Again, histamine is a systemic vasodilator, yet it is believed to constrict the pulmonary vessels (Dixon and Hoyle, 1930), and although several of the dihydrogenated alkaloids of ergot are adrenolytic and sympatholytic and therefore lower the systemic peripheral resistance, dihydroergotamine (1 mg.) is a pulmonary vasoconstrictor by direct action on the vessels (Halmagyi, 1953). Finally, ganglionic blocking agents, such as hexamethonium bromide, appear to lower the pulmonary vascular resistance by releasing normal sympathetic vasomotor tone (Gilmore *et al.*, 1952).

A word of warning is necessary here. Much of the confusion surrounding the results of experiments on the physiological behaviour of the pulmonary circulation in health and disease is due to inadequate control of the many factors involved; to test the effect of any agent on the pulmonary vascular resistance in man it is necessary to measure simultaneously and con-inuously the left atrial or pulmonary venous pressure, the pulmonary artery pressure, and the pulmonary blood flow; and preferably the systemic blood pressure and flow, and the intrathoracic pressure as well; even then he behaviour of the bronchial circulation may influence the findings Daly, 1936).

Hypoxic pulmonary hypertension

Pulmonary vasoconstriction, which is not abolished by vagotomy or stellate ganglionectomy, undoubtedly occurs in response to reduced alveolar oxygen tension both in animals (von Euler and Liljestrand, 1946) and man (Motley *et al.*, 1947). This response to oxygen lack is opposite to what occurs in the systemic circulation, and has the advantage of deflecting the pulmonary blood flow from poorly ventilated zones (Liljestrand, 1948).

At first it seemed likely that this mechanism might be responsible for the pulmonary hypertension of anoxic cor pulmonale, but it was soon discovered that the vasoconstrictive response seemed to occur only in acute experiments or clinical situations and was not maintained in the presence of chronic anoxia from advanced emphysema (Mounsey *et al.*, 1952). Nevertheless, the reaction is clinically very important and explains why pulmonary hypertensive heart failure may be precipitated so easily by an attack of acute bronchitis in cases of chronic cor pulmonale, and why oxygen therapy in such cases is so much more important than digitalis and elimination of sodium.

REACTIVE PULMONARY HYPERTENSION

This group characteristically includes all those cases with a high or extreme pulmonary vascular resistance that has developed in response to passive or hyperkinetic pulmonary hypertension (Wood, 1952), e.g. pulmonary hypertensive mitral stenosis (page 540), "false Bernheim's syndrome" (page 774), and the whole of the Eisenmenger group (page 392); but it may also include many cases in which pulmonary hypertension was caused initially by obstructive, thrombo-embolic, or obliterative vascular lesions and has been perpetuated by a similar reaction. Whether or not hypoxic pulmonary hypertension is ever maintained long enough to be perpetuated in this way is uncertain, but it is a possibility that should be borne in mind when attempting to synthesise the variable manifestations of cor pulmonale.

The mechanism is not yet known for certain. The belief that structural changes, such as fibroelastic thickening of the intima of the small arteries and arterioles, develop in response to passive or hyperkinetic pulmonary hypertension, and gradually obliterate the pulmonary vascular bed and so cause secondary obliterative pulmonary hypertension, is in the author's view untenable in the light of the known clinical and physiological data. Evans (1951) went so far as to postulate a congenital deficiency of the media of the small pulmonary arteries in these cases, and believed that fibroelastic thickening was a protective reaction which finally obstructed the pulmonary circulation and caused obliterative pulmonary hypertension.

But it has been repeatedly pointed out that reactive pulmonary hypertension is *not* a late manifestation of mitral stenosis, left ventricular failure, patent ductus, ventricular septal defect or atrial septal defect, but if i occurs at all it develops early, pari passu with the critical passive or potentially hyperkinetic pulmonary hypertension caused by the lesions mentioned (Wood, 1952, 1954). This behaviour categorically denies that a secondary obliterative process is responsible for the initial reaction, although it no doubt increases the already raised resistance as the years go by.

Again, it is nearly always possible to lower the pulmonary vascular resistance in cases of reactive pulmonary hypertension by injecting acetyl-choline, aminophylline or priscoline into the pulmonary artery, and this would not be expected in obliterative pulmonary hypertension.

Finally, whenever passive or hyperkinetic pulmonary hypertension is relieved by surgical correction of the responsible lesion, the pulmonary vascular resistance falls, which does not harmonise with the mechanistic hypothesis.

For these reasons it is believed that reactive pulmonary hypertension is due to active vasoconstriction, and that anatomical changes in the small pulmonary blood vessels are secondary, but such a mechanism awaits proof. There is good evidence that neither an elevated pulmonary venous pressure, chronic interstitial œdema, an increased pulmonary pulse pressure, dilatation of the pulmonary artery, or alteration of the alveolar or blood gas tensions is responsible for the reaction. The tentative hypo-thesis that in certain individuals pulmonary vasoconstriction develops in response to pulmonary hypertension itself (Wood, 1952) fits the known facts best, and harmonises with the current theory that chronic essential hypertension in the systemic circulation may be initiated by any other form of systemic hypertension, and once developed may be self-per-petuating (Smirk, 1949). If the hypothesis is correct, reactive pulmonary hypertension should develop also in a proportion of cases of obstructive or obliterative hypertension, which should then be perpetuated in the same way long after the initial cause has subsided. The behaviour of certain thrombo-embolic cases does not deny this possibility.

Clinically, reactive pulmonary hypertension in cases of mitral valve disease, left ventricular failure, and the Eisenmenger group has already been discussed in detail, and will not be further considered here.

PRIMARY PULMONARY HYPERTENSION

There remains for discussion the enigma known as primary, idiopathic or essential pulmonary hypertension.

Incidence

In a consecutive clinical series of approximately 10,000 cases of cardio-vascular disease of all types personally examined by the author since the second world war there were 17 instances of primary pulmonary hyper-tension (0.17 per cent). These were all diagnosed clinically in the first instance, all but two were confirmed by cardiac catheterisation, and the ten that died (which include the two not catheterised) were confirmed at necropsy. So far, no case in which the final clinical diagnosis was primary pulmonary hypertension has been disproved by subsequent necropsy. This should be enough to emphasise the highly distinctive nature of the syndrome and to re-affirm that it is a disease entity in its own right, whatever the cause.

In my series there were 14 females and 3 males. In Brenner's exhaustive analysis of the literature up to 1935 he could only find 16 convincing cases of primary pulmonary vascular sclerosis, as it was then called, but he did not give their ages or sex. From my own files of the literature, however, I have records of another 20 acceptable cases, making 27 in all, although many more have been reported. These include the cases of Brenner (1935) 1, Seely (1938) 1, de Navasquez et al. (1940) 2 of their 3, East (1940) 3, Barrett and Cole (1946) 1, Gold (1946) 1, Gilmour and Evans (1946) 1, Rosenbaum (1947) 2, Dresdale et al. (1951) 3, and Soulie et al. (1955) 5. Of the total there were 28 females and 9 males. This female preponderance may well prove important.

The ages of these thirty-seven patients ranged between 4 and 68, the average being 31. Four were children or adolescents, twenty-two were young adults between the ages of 20 and 40, eight were between 40 and 50, and three were over 50. Primary pulmonary hypertension in infants has also been described (Wolman, 1950).

Pathology

Since Brenner's careful description the majority of authors have confirmed the great variability of the lesions. Considerable dilatation of the pulmonary artery is almost invariable. Atherosclerosis is common in the major arteries, particularly in the older patients, and is regarded as a secondary change; secondary thrombosis may occur. It is in the small arteries and arterioles that the most significant lesions are found: these include fibroelastic thickening of the intima (Barrett and Cole, 1946), and hypertrophy of the media (Brenner, 1935), but normal vessels are nearly always seen as well, and in several cases all the small vessels have looked normal (de Navesquez et al., 1940; East, 1940). McKeown (1952), moreover, demonstrated that all the peripheral vascular lesions that have been reported as characteristic of pulmonary hypertension may be found in controls in the same age groups, which makes accurate interpretation very difficult.

There are two other findings which must not be passed by. Gilmour and Evans (1946) described hypoplasia of the media of many small vessels, which they believed was congenital in origin, and found that endarteritis fibrosa was closely related and presumably secondary to the defect. In Gold's case (1946) there was also hypoplasia of the media and widespread secondary thromboses. When old and new clots are a feature of the case, thrombo-embolic obstructive hypertension with secondary obliterative changes is the more likely diagnosis.

In my own cases the degree and extent of proliferative changes in the small arteries and arterioles was usually quite outside the range of what may be seen in controls, but they could well have been secondary to the hypertension rather than its cause.

Physiology

The high pulmonary vascular resistance imposes a heavy burden on the right ventricle, which hypertrophies accordingly; the right atrium gives maximum support and increases right ventricular diastolic stretch. Despite these compensatory devices the cardiac output is low and on effort the right ventricle is readily overloaded (Howarth and Lowe, 1953), so that the output may fall and result in syncope, whilst the reduced coronary flow may cause angina pectoris. The arterial oxygen saturation remains normal until near the end, and cyanosis is peripheral unless there happens to be a patent foramen ovale, through which there may be a small reversed interatrial shunt.

Physiological measurements were completed in 12 of my cases and were very similar to those reported by Dresdale *et al.* (1951). *The pulmonary vascular resistance* averaged 15 units and ranged between 10 and 26. As Dresdale said, this is about eight times the normal; it is the same as is commonly found in fully developed reactive pulmonary hypertension in mitral stenosis and the Eisenmenger group.

The pulmonary systolic blood pressure was well over 100 mm. Hg (145 mm. Hg) in only one instance; in two cases it hovered round the 100 mark, and in the rest it was only 65 to 90 mm. Hg. The diastolic pressure averaged 40 per cent of the systolic. These unexpectedly low figures were attributed to right ventricular failure, although at the time of catheterisation after treatment for congestive failure the right ventricular diastolic pressure was rarely much elevated. Two of Dresdale's three cases also had pulmonary systolic pressures under 100 mm. Hg.

The cardiac output averaged 3.8 litres per minute in 11 adults, and ranged between 2.6 and 4.5 at rest. *The arterio-venous oxygen difference* averaged 64 ml. per litre, the range being 56 to 80. Dresdale's figures were similar.

The arterial oxygen saturation ranged between 88 and 95.5 per cent, and averaged 92 per cent. Each of Dresdale's cases was fully saturated.

Clinical features

Symptoms include increasing effort intolerance due to fatigue, breathlessness, angina pectoris or syncope. Fatigue and breathlessness are the prerunners of congestive heart failure. Angina pectoris occurred in two of my cases and in two of 18 collected from the literature; this gives an incidence of 11.5 per cent. Effort syncope occurred in four of my cases and in four of 18 collected from the literature, i.e. in 23 per cent. All my cases developed congestive failure, including those that are still alive.

On examination the *physical signs* are highly characteristic and since they constitute the prototype of all kinds of pulmonary hypertension they are given here in full.

1. Cyanosis, when present, is peripheral, not central, unless there is a reversed shunt through a patent foramen ovale, which has been mentioned in necropsy reports in several instances. The face may be highly coloured and bloated, as in severe pulmonary valve stenosis, but this is exceptional. The hands are cold and blue as a rule, unless hepatic failure causes vasodilatation and a palmar flush.

2. The peripheral pulse is small.

3. The rhythm is normal at first, but towards the end paroxysmal or permanent atrial flutter or fibrillation is not uncommon in the more chronic cases.

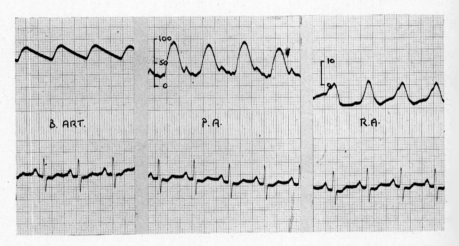

Fig. 18.02—Pressure pulse from the brachial artery, pulmonary artery and right atrium in a case of primary pulmonary hypertension showing giant *a* waves in the right atrial tracing.

4. The jugular venous pressure pulse reveals a giant *a* wave measuring 5 to 10 cm. above *v* in three-quarters of the cases (fig. 18.02). When there is advanced right ventricular failure the right atrium may also fail, and the giant *a* may then disappear, *v* becoming proportionately larger. Functional tricuspid incompetence may also have this effect.

5. Right atrial gallop rhythm and presystolic hepatic pulsation usually accompany the giant *a* wave.

6. The left ventricle is impalpable, but there is usually a powerful heave over the right ventricle between the left sternal border and mid-clavicula

line. Sometimes the right ventricle occupies the position of the apex beat. Pulmonary artery pulsation was palpable in 60 per cent of my cases.

7. There are five auscultatory signs: right atrial gallop, a tricuspid pan-systolic murmur sometimes accompanied by a thrill when there is functional tricuspid incompetence (often heard well to the left since the dilated right ventricle occupies the apex beat), a sharp high-pitched pulmonary ejection click over the dilated pulmonary artery, a closely split second heart sound with sharp accentuation of the second or pulmonary element, and a Graham Steell pulmonary incompetent diastolic murmur occasionally accompanied by a thrill in 40 per cent of cases. An appreciable pulmonary ejection murmur is rare.

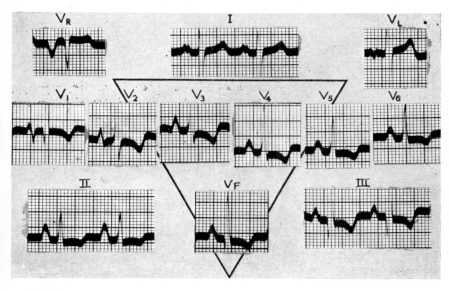

Fig. 18.03—Electrocardiogram from a case of primary pulmonary hypertension showing a conspicuous P pulmonale and gross right ventricular preponderance.

8. Signs of congestive heart failure are inevitable sooner or later.

The *electrocardiogram* classically shows a conspicuous P pulmonale and gross right ventricular preponderance (fig. 18.03).

X-rays reveal a small aorta, considerable dilatation of the pulmonary artery, a variable degree of enlargement of the right ventricle and atrium, an inconspicuous left ventricle and atrium, and light peripheral vascular markings (fig. 18.04).

Cardiac catheterisation reveals the physiological situation previously described. If acetylcholine 1 mg. is injected quickly into the pulmonary artery, the pulmonary vascular resistance falls, the pulmonary systolic and diastolic pressures fall, the cardiac output rises (by 20 per cent in the case illustrated), the systemic blood pressure rises, and the heart rate slows

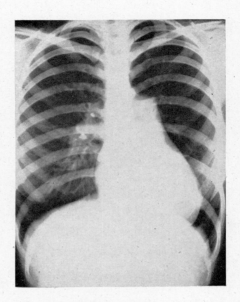

Fig. 18.04—Primary pulmonary hypertension showing a small aorta, conspicuous dilatation of the pulmonary arc, moderate enlargement of the right ventricle (which is occupying the apex beat), and light peripheral vascular markings.

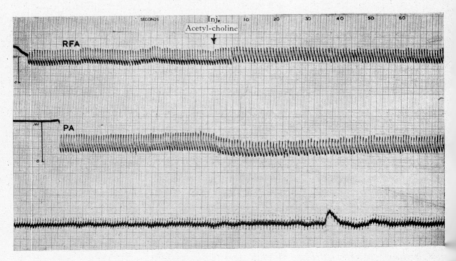

Fig. 18.05—Pressure pulses from the femoral and pulmonary arteries showing the effect of 1 mg. of acetylcholine injected into the pulmonary artery (paper speed 2.5 mm. per second).

reflexly (fig. 18.05). The advantage of using acetylcholine in these studies is that in the dose used it is virtually inactivated by the time it reaches the systemic circulation and therefore has a selective action on the pulmonary vessels. The effect is immediate, begins with the first heart beat following the injection, and proves conclusively that some degree of vasoconstriction, whether physiological or pathological, is present in these cases: if anatomical obstruction of more than two-thirds of the total cross-section of the pulmonary vascular bed is in fact present, then the relatively healthy vessels are maintaining disadvantageous vasoconstrictor tone; alternatively, the high resistance is due, at least in part, to abnormal functional vaso-constriction.

Differential diagnosis

Clinically the diagnosis of severe pulmonary hypertension secondary to a high pulmonary vascular resistance is usually obvious, the only question at issue being whether it is primary, obstructive, obliterative, or reactive, and at the bedside this may not be answered at all easily. If the onset of symptoms follows pregnancy, phlebothrombosis, a surgical or dental operation, or an accident, thrombo-embolic obstructive or secondarily obliterative pulmonary hypertension is more probable, if indeed this is not the cause of all cases. Disseminated lupus, periarteritis, and schistosomiasis should be considered, and tell-tale clues searched for. In primary pul-monary hypertension all laboratory tests are negative.

Reactive pulmonary hypertension due to mitral stenosis is probable if there is a history of rheumatic fever or chorea, if the mitral first sound is sharp, if a faint opening snap can be heard or recorded phonocardio-graphically, if slight dilatation of the left atrium can be demonstrated radiologically, or if the electrocardiogram shows a P mitrale. No difficulty, of course, arises if the classical signs of mitral stenosis are not masked by the large right ventricle. In one of the author's cases the only clinical evidence of mitral stenosis was slight calcification of the mitral valve, but this was considered conclusive and successful mitral valvotomy was carried out.

Reactive pulmonary hypertension associated with patent ductus, ven-tricular septal defect or atrial septal defect is at once suggested if there is any direct or indirect evidence of central cyanosis or reduced arterial oxygen saturation at rest or on effort, whether generalised as in atrial septal defect and ventricular septal defect, or chiefly confined to the lower half of the body as in patent ductus. In adults the history alone usually proves the congenital nature of the disease, but in acyanotic children the differential diagnosis may not be easy at the bedside. Giant a waves, however, deny an alternative route for blood ejected from the right ventricle and therefore exclude patent ductus and ventricular septal defect. A loud pulmonary ejection murmur is much in favour of one of the Eisenmenger group, in which the pulmonary blood flow averages twice that in primary pulmonary hypertension. A pure single second heart sound favours Eisenmenger's complex proper (with ventricular septal defect), and a relatively widely split second sound favours pulmonary hypertension with atrial septal defect. Any clinical, electrocardiographic or radiological evidence proclaiming a state of balanced ventricular work at once denies primary pulmonary hypertension and is strongly in favour of patent ductus or ventricular septal defect with reactive pulmonary hypertension.

When in doubt the correct diagnosis may be established in most cases by means of cardiac catheterisation with or without the help of Evans blue or other dye. Angiocardiography may also prove the presence and site of a reversed shunt. The simplest out-patient test, however, is to see whether or not the arterial oxygen saturation falls on effort: this may be detected by means of an ear oximeter in cases of Eisenmenger's complex and pulmonary hypertension with reversed interatrial shunt, and by means of femoral artery samples in cases of pulmonary hypertension with reversed aorto-pulmonary shunt through a patent ductus.

Course

The average duration of life from the onset of symptoms in 20 fatal cases was 3.2 years, the range one month to 10 years. It is not without significance that so far no early case has yet been diagnosed. It was at one time suspected that mass radiography might reveal an occasional early case, but this has not proved to be so: of 10 patients discovered to have unexplained dilatation of the pulmonary arc, for example, but who were symptom free and without abnormal physical signs, cardiac catheterisation revealed normal physiology. This persistent failure strongly suggests that the disease is subacute rather than chronic, and so it would be if it were initially thrombo-embolic in origin.

Treatment

No effective treatment has yet been devised for primary pulmonary hypertension. Dresdale (1951) suggested priscoline, but it has proved valueless in my cases, although when injected directly into the pulmonary artery in a dose of 10 mg. it undoubtedly lowers the pulmonary vascular resistance, as does acetylcholine and aminophylline. I have tried oral priscol 25 to 50 mg. t.d.s., aminophylline 0.2 G. t.d.s., etophylate 0.5 G. t.d.s., and hexamethonium bromide 500 to 750 mg. t.d.s. before meals, all without the slightest effect. I have also tried permanent anticoagulant therapy with dindevan on the chance that recurrent thrombo-embolism was responsible, but without avail. Cortisone merely aggravated heart failure as a result of sodium retention, and prednisone proved little less harmful in one case in which it was tried for several months. In desperation, on one occasion, Blalock's operation of subclavian-pulmonary artery anastomosis was attempted, in the hope of providing a safety valve for the pulmonary circulation, but the patient died of ventricular fibrillation on the operating table.

At the present time and in the light of what is known or suspected, there is a chance that a combination of strict bed-rest or total inactivity, priscol, theophylline and ansolysen, and permanent anticoagulant therapy may favourably influence a small number of cases which fulfil the clinical criteria for a diagnosis of primary pulmonary hypertension. When heart failure is present it should be treated in the usual way.

REFERENCES

Azmy, S. (1932): Pulmonary arteriosclerosis of Bilharzial nature", *J. Egyptian med. Ass.*, **15**, 87.

Barnard, P. J. (1954): "Thrombo-embolic primary pulmonary arteriosclerosis", *Brit. Heart J.*, **16**, 93.

Bedford, D. E., Aidaros, S. M., and Girgis, B. (1946): "Bilharzial heart disease in Egypt. Cor pulmonale due to Bilharzial pulmonary endarteritis", *Brit. Heart J.*, **8**, 87.

Castleman, B., and Bland, E. F. (1946): "Organized emboli of the tertiary pulmonary arteries. An unusual cause of cor pulmonale", *Arch. Path.*, **42**, 581.

Cournand, A. (1950): "Some aspects of the pulmonary circulation in normal man and in chronic cardiopulmonary diseases", *Circulation*, **2**, 641.

Daly, I. de Burgh (1936): "The physiology of the bronchial vascular system", Harvey Lectures, **31**, 235.

——, Linzell, J. L., Mount, L. E., and Waites, G. M. M. (1954): "Pulmonary vasomotor responses and acid-base balance in perfused eviscerated dog preparations", *Quart. J. exp. Physiol.*, **39**, 177.

de Navasquez, S., Forbes, J. R., and Holling, H. E. (1940): "Right ventricular hypertrophy of unknown origin: so-called pulmonary hypertension", *Brit. Heart J.*, **2**, 177.

Dexter, L., *et al.* (1951): "Effects of exercise on circulatory dynamics of normal individuals", *J. appl. Physiol.*, **3**, 439.

Dixon, W. E., and Hoyle, J. C. (1930): "Studies in pulmonary circulation; action of histamine", *J. Physiol.*, **70**, 1.

Donald, K. W., Bishop, J. M., Cumming, G., and Wade, O. L. (1955): "The effect of exercise on the cardiac output and circulatory dynamics of normal subjects", *Clin. Sci.*, **14**, 37.

Dresdale, D. T., Schultz, M., and Michtom, R. J. (1951): "Primary pulmonary hypertension. 1. Clinical and hemodynamic study", *Amer. J. Med.*, **11**, 686.

Evans, W. (1951): "Congenital pulmonary hypertension", *Proc. Roy. Soc. Med.*, **44**, 600.

Fowler, N. O., Westcott, R. N., Scott, R. C., and McGuire, J. (1951): "The effect of l-norepinephrine upon pulmonary arteriolar resistance in man", *J. clin. Invest.*, **30**, 517.

Gilmore, H. R., Kopelman, H., McMichael, J., and Milne, I. G. (1952): "The effect of hexamethonium bromide on the cardiac output and pulmonary hypertension", *Lancet*, *ii*, 898.

Gold, M. M. A. (1946): "Congenital dilatation of the pulmonary arterial tree", *Arch. intern. Med.*, **78**, 197.

Halmágyi, D., *et al.* (1953): "The role of the nervous system in the maintenance of pulmonary arterial hypertension in heart failure", *Brit. Heart J.*, **15**, 15.

Harrison, C. V. (1948): "Experimental pulmonary arteriosclerosis", *J. Path. Bac.*, **60**, 289.

Hickam, J. B., and Cargill, W. H. (1948): "Effects of exercise on cardiac output and pulmonary arterial pressure in normal persons and in patients with cardiovascular disease and pulmonary emphysema", *J. clin. Invest.*, **27**, 10.

Howarth, S., and Lowe, J. B. (1953): "The mechanism of effort syncope in primary pulmonary hypertension and cyanotic congenital heart disease", *Brit. Heart J.*, **15**, 47.

Keating, D. R., Burkey, J. N., Hellerstein, H. K., and Feil, H. (1953): "Chronic massive thrombosis of pulmonary arteries. A report of seven cases with clinical and necropsy studies", *Amer. J. Roentgenol.*, **69**, 208.

Kenawy, M. R. (1950): "The syndrome of cardiopulmonary schistosomiasis (cor pulmonale)", *Amer. Heart J.*, **39**, 678.

Liljestrand, G. (1948): "Regulation of pulmonary arterial blood pressure", *Arch. intern. Med.*, **81**, 162.

McKeown, F. (1952): "The pathology of pulmonary heart disease", *Brit. Heart J.*, **14**, 25.

Magidson, O., and Jacobson, G. (1955): "Thrombosis of the main pulmonary arteries", *Brit. Heart J.*, **17**, 207.

Motley, H. L., Cournand, A., Werko, L., Himmelstein, A., and Dresdale, D. (1947): "The influence of short periods of induced acute anoxia upon pulmonary artery pressures in man", *Amer. J. Physiol.*, **150**, 315.

Mounsey, J. P. D., Ritzman, L. W., Selverstone, N. J., Briscoe, W. A., and McLemore, G. A. (1952): "Circulatory changes in severe pulmonary emphysema", *Brit. Heart J.*, **14**, 153.

Nelson, R. A., May, L. G., Bennett, A., Kobayashi, M., and Gregory, R. (1955): "Comparison of the effects of pressor and depressor agents and influences on pulmonary and systemic pressures of normotensive and hypertensive subjects", *Amer. Heart J.*, **50**, 172.

Riley, R. L., Himmelstein, A., Motley, H. L., Weiner, H. M., and Cournand, A. (1948): "Studies of the pulmonary circulation at rest and during exercise in normal individuals and in patients with chronic pulmonary disease", *Amer. J. Physiol.*, **152**, 372.

Rosenbaum, F. F. (1947): "Right ventricular and auricular hypertrophy of obscure origin", *Ann. intern. Med.*, **26**, 76.

Seely, H. (1938): "Primary obliterative pulmonary arteriolar sclerosis", *J. Amer. med. Ass.*, **110**, 792.

Shaw, A. F. D., and Ghareeb, A. A. (1938): "Pathogenesis of pulmonary schistosomiasis in Egypt with special reference to Ayerza's disease", *J. Path. and Bact.*, **46**, 401.

Sorour, M. F. (1928): "Pathology of schistosomiasis", *C.R. Congrés. Internat. Méd. Trop. et d'Hygiene*, Cairo, **4**, 321.

Soulié, P., Tricot, R., di Matteo, J., Baillet, J., and Silvestre, J. (1953): "L'hypertension artérielle pulmonaire primitive", *Bull. Mém. Soc. med. Hôp. Paris*, **19** and **20**, 629.

von Euler, U. S., and Liljestrand, G. (1946): "Observations on the pulmonary arterial blood pressure in cat", *Acta Physiol. Scand.*, **12**, 301.

Williams, M. H. (1954): "Relationship between pulmonary artery pressure and blood flow in the dog lung", *Amer. J. Physiol.*, **179**, 243.

Wolman, M. (1950): "Hypertrophy of the branches of the pulmonary artery, and its possible relationship with the so-called primary pulmonary arteriosclerosis in 2 infants with hypertrophy of the right heart", *Amer. J. med. Sc.*, **220**, 133.

Wood, P. (1952): "Pulmonary hypertension", *Brit. med. Bull.*, **8**, 348.

—— (1954): "An appreciation of mitral stenosis", *Brit. med. J.*, i, 1051.

CHAPTER XIX

COR PULMONALE

Definition

The term cor pulmonale is best reserved to identify a specific cardio-vascular disorder secondary to disease of the lung parenchyma; although classically chronic, it may be subacute or even acute.

Incidence

It is difficult to estimate the prevalence of cor pulmonale for several reasons: (1) the disease is rarely so labelled until there is congestive heart failure; (2) its distribution is patchy, apparently being more common in large industrial cities than elsewhere; (3) in view of the frequency with which its clinical manifestations are precipitated by acute bronchitis or bronchopneumonia most cases are admitted to general hospitals rather than cardiovascular clinics, and the recognition of cor pulmonale often depends a great deal on the interest of the physician concerned. In the Registrar General's review for 1953 the disease is not listed at all as such, but there were 30,392 deaths from bronchitis (6 per cent of the total mortality for England and Wales for that year) and 15,661 deaths from bronchopneumonia. During the same year there were 61,751 deaths from ischæmic heart disease (12 per cent), 20,423 from hypertensive heart disease (4 per cent), and 8,837 from chronic rheumatic heart disease (1.8 per cent). Now in a general hospital in Sheffield, according to Flint (1954), cor pulmonale accounted for 25 per cent of 300 cases of *congestive heart failure*, ischæmic heart disease for 22 per cent, hypertensive heart disease for 21 per cent, and rheumatic heart disease for 23 per cent. At the other extreme there is my own small series of only 45 proved cases of cor pulmonale amongst a consecutive series of about 10,000 clinical cases of cardiovascular disease of all types seen at specialised clinics and in private practice. Realistic figures are therefore impossible to compile at the present time. A reasonable conservative guess for the frequency of chronic cor pulmonale might be 5 to 10 per cent of all cases of organic heart disease.

Cor pulmonale is at least five times more common in men than in women, and about 75 per cent of the patients are over 50 years old (Spain and Handler, 1946).

Pathogenesis

There are only two fundamental factors concerned with the develop-ment of cor pulmonale, hypoxia and obliterative changes in the pulmonary circulation. The degree to which each contributes determines the clinical features and course of the disease. Carbon dioxide retention may modify the symptoms, but not the essential cardiovascular hæmodynamics.

Hypoxia is commonly due to emphysema, and is much aggravated by attacks of bronchitis, bronchopneumonia and bronchial asthma, which themselves are usually responsible for the emphysema. The chief difficulty is ventilatory; an insufficient number of alveoli are filled with fresh air at each breath. Blood that perfuses unventilated alveoli cannot absorb oxygen or eliminate carbon dioxide. The arterial oxygen tension therefore falls and the carbon dioxide tension rises; in turn this results in reduced arterial oxygen saturation (McMichael and Sharpey-Schafer, 1944) and increased arterial carbon dioxide content (Taquini *et al.*, 1947).

Hypoxia, however, may also occur as a result of difficulty in oxygen perfusion across the alveolar-capillary interface, when the boundary zone is thickened in any way. Carbon dioxide, being twenty-five times more soluble in water than oxygen and therefore equally more diffusable, rarely experiences this difficulty, so that in these cases hypoxia is not associated with carbon dioxide retention (Baldwin, Cournand and Richards, 1949). Arnott (1955) gives the chief causes of difficulty in oxygen diffusion as diffuse interstitial pulmonary fibrosis, sarcoidosis, silicosis, inhalation of beryllium, scleroderma, radiation fibrosis, and diffuse carcinomatosis.

Hypoxia, however produced, results in central cyanosis, vasodilatation, an increased cardiac output (McMichael and Sharpey-Schafer, 1944) and polycythæmia. It is the hypoxia that is responsible for the hyperkinetic character of the circulation in cor pulmonale. During acute episodes of bronchitis, bronchopneumonia, or bronchial asthma, the alveolar oxygen tension falls as a result of the increased ventilatory difficulty. This causes transient pulmonary vasoconstriction (Motley *et al.*, 1947), further reduction in arterial oxygen saturation and a secondary rise of cardiac output: in a group of cases described by Donald (1953) the mean pulmonary artery pressure rose from an average of 25 mm. Hg to 50 mm. Hg during such episodes. This puts a heavy burden on the right ventricle, which is asked to increase its stroke volume against an increased resistance, and congestive failure is common.

Obliteration of a sufficient cross-section of the pulmonary vascular bed to raise the pulmonary blood pressure at rest is unusual in both emphysema and interstitial pulmonary fibrosis; but there is frequently sufficient obstruction to cause obliterative pulmonary hypertension when the cardiac output is raised in response to effort or hypoxia (Bloomfield *et al.*, 1946; Harvey *et al.*, 1951). In my own series of 45 cases of well-established cor pulmonale the pulmonary vascular resistance was between 6 and 10 units in 20 per cent, and over 10 units (extreme) in a further 20 per cent, but the arterial oxygen saturation in these two groups was no lower than in the 60 per cent of cases that had normal or only slightly raised resistances, averaging 85 per cent at rest when free from infection and bronchospasm irrespective of the resistance. This lack of correlation is not surprising, for the lower the arterial oxygen saturation the more the perfusion of un-ventilated alveoli, and this means non-obliterated capillaries in the non-functioning zones, which would not encourage pulmonary hypertension. Admittedly the pulmonary blood pressure may be higher in the more anoxic patients, but this may be explained by the higher cardiac output.

Whether or not the 20 per cent of cases with pulmonary vascular resistances in the extreme range have reactive vasoconstriction or merely advanced obliterative pulmonary hypertension remains to be seen. Such a group would be expected if there is anything in the hypothesis propounded in the last chapter. There is no doubt that secondary atherosclerosis, thrombosis, medial hypertrophy and fibroelastic intimal thickening may develop as a result of the long-standing pulmonary hypertension and add their own obstructive or obliterative burden.

Clinical features

The patient is usually a middle-aged or elderly man. He commonly gives a history of bronchial asthma or of recurrent winter bronchitis for many years, with increasing breathlessness over the last year or two, and may have sought advice because of recent swelling of the legs. Cross-examination yields little further information: he may have had attacks of tightness in the chest associated with breathlessness, but not paroxysmal cardiac dyspnœa; he may have had substernal discomfort, but not true angina; he may prefer to be propped up a little at night, but usually raises no objection to lying flat. Headache, attributed to a raised C.S.F. pressure, was noted in 55 per cent of Flint's series. Dyspnœa is attributed to oxygen lack, carbon dioxide retention (until the respiratory centre becomes insensitive), decreased pH, and mechanically to the extra effort required to inflate and deflate the lungs (Christie, 1944).

In a minority of cases there may be historical clues pointing to the nature of the underlying lung disease, e.g. symptoms of bronchiectasis, established pulmonary tuberculosis, pneumonectomy or thoracoplasty, Pott's disease of the spine, or bronchopneumonia in the last London fog. Cases with oxygen diffusion difficulty may give a history of severe and increasing breathlessness on effort for which they have received scant sympathy, or they may mention occupational hazards of silicosis, asbestosis, or beryllium poisoning, cutaneous or other lesions suggesting sarcoid or scleroderma, deep X-ray therapy for carcinoma of the lung, or just a single attack of virus pneumonia. Occasionally the onset of congestive heart failure is heralded by no previous symptoms whatsoever.

Physical signs

Emphysema is usually obvious: the chest is distended and moves little with respiration; cardiac dullness is absent and the percussion note is generally tympanitic; the breath sounds are faint. Wheezing and rhonchi denote bronchospasm or active bronchitis, and the latter may also cause widespread coarse râles and mucopurulent sputum. Central cyanosis may be gross or scarcely detectable. It may be recognised in warm situations, as in the conjunctivæ and inner sides of the lips, where it is unlikely to be confused with peripheral cyanosis. The hands are warm and the forearm veins distended; capillary pulsation, digital throbbing, a modified water-hammer pulse and increased pulse pressure may often be demonstrated (fig. 19.01). Clubbing may occur, but is unusual, and pulmonary osteo-

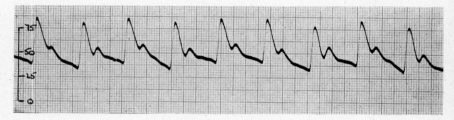

Fig. 19.01—Brachial arteriogram showing a typical waterhammer pulse in a case of anoxic cor pulmonale.

arthropathy is more so. Slight elevation of the jugular venous pressure and tachycardia may confirm the impression that the cardiac output is raised. Papillœdema sometimes occurs and may be attributed to a raised C.S.F. pressure associated with a greatly increased cerebral blood flow secondary to carbon dioxide retention (Simpson, 1948).

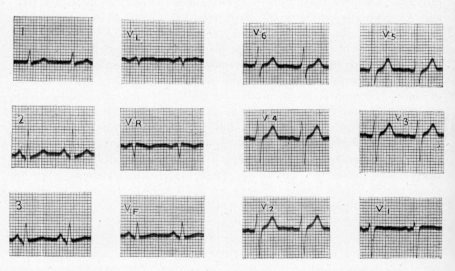

Fig. 19.02—Electrocardiogram in a case of emphysema showing a vertical electrical position and clockwise rotation (viewed from below).

The heart itself is apt to be camouflaged by over-expanded lung: the apex-beat is impalpable, the left cardiac border impossible to locate by percussion, the heart sounds difficult to hear, and the second sound at the base often inaudible; there are no murmurs, but right-sided summation gallop may be heard or felt just to the left of the sternum in the fourth intercostal space, or in the epigastrium.

When there is congestive heart failure the venous pressure is higher, the liver distended and tender, and œdema usually considerable; the signs of a hyperkinetic circulatory state may remain or disappear, gallop rhythm becomes diastolic in time, and there may be functional tricuspid incompetence. When the pulmonary vascular resistance is high in cor pulmonale the clinical findings are quite different; central cyanosis is still present, but there may be peripheral cyanosis as well; the hands are cold and blue, the forearm veins constricted, and there is no evidence of a hyperkinetic circulation; there may be a giant *a* wave in the jugular pulse and gallop rhythm is presystolic.

In severe cases vasomotor collapse is apt to occur when some superimposed broncho-pulmonary infection lowers the arterial oxygen saturation relatively suddenly: the blood pressure drops, the pulse becomes small and thready, the cardiac output low and the skin cold and clammy; the outlook is then very grave.

The electrocardiogram. Emphysema alone does not materially affect the electrocardiogram, although it may cause clockwise rotation about the antero-posterior and longitudinal axes (viewed from the front and below). Thus there may be right axis deviation in standard leads, an RS pattern in lead V_L, a QR pattern in lead V_F, and an RS pattern from V_1 as far as V_5 or even V_6 (fig. 19.02). When the heart is exceptionally vertical, V_R and V_L may be indistinguishable, or backward tilting of the apex may cause V_L to resemble an œsophageal lead from the back of the heart.

In 100 cases of chronic cor pulmonale analysed by the author (Wood, 1947), the following electrocardiographic appearances were found in *standard leads* (fig. 19.03a to e):

Pulmonary P wave 85
Right axis deviation—
    with T3 (and often T2) inverted (a) . . 20
    with T upright in all leads (b) . . . 30
Prominent S wave in all leads (c) . . . 9
Tendency to right axis deviation (d) . . . 11
Normal axis of QRS (e) 26
Right bundle branch block 4
Low voltage 40

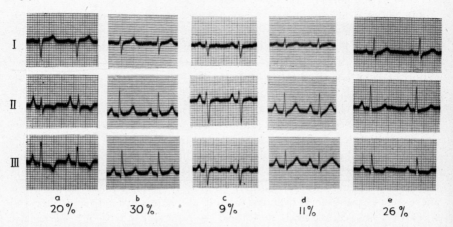

Fig. 19.03—Standard lead electrocardiographic findings in 100 cases of cor pulmonale.
(a) Right axis deviation with inversion of T3 (and often T2).
(b) Right axis deviation with upright T waves.
(c) Dominant S wave in all standard leads.
(d) Tendency to right axis deviation.
(e) Normal QRS axis.
The pulmonary P wave is seen in all.

Multiple chest leads revealed the following (fig. 19.04a to e):
Normal QRS deflections in the majority (a and b)
Inversion of T from V_1–V_3 (c) 13
Dominant R wave in V_1 with conspicuous S in
V_5 (d)   .   .   .   .   .   .   : 16
Dominant S wave from V_1–V_5 (e)   .   .   . 16

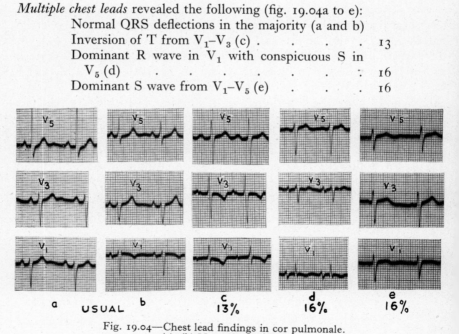

Fig. 19.04—Chest lead findings in cor pulmonale.
(a), (b) Normal chest leads.
(c) Inversion of T from V_1 to V_3.
(d) Dominant R wave in V_1 with conspicuous S in V_5.
(e) Dominant S wave from V_1 to V_5.

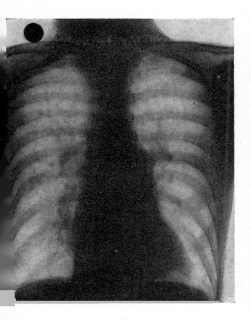
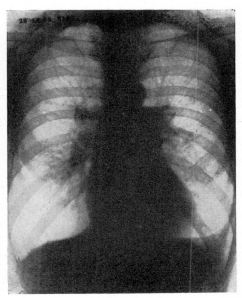

(a)   (b)

Fig. 19.05 (a), (b)—Skiagrams of two advanced cases of cor pulmonale showing dilatation of the pulmonary artery and of the left and right branches.

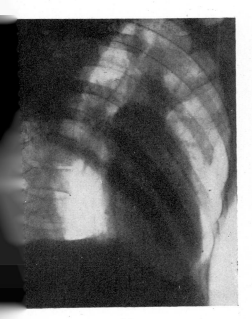
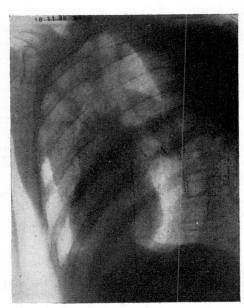

(a)   (b)

Fig. 19.06 (a)—Right anterior oblique position showing the increased density and diameter of the pulmonary artery at its bifurcation.
(b) Left anterior oblique position showing the left pulmonary artery forming an arc almost as dense and as large as the aortic arch.

855

Unipolar limb leads nearly always showed a vertical electrical position. The pulmonary P wave is probably the earliest sign of cardiovascular disturbance resulting from emphysema, or at least competes in this respect with elevation of the right ventricular pressure and slight reduction of the arterial oxygen saturation; it may develop several years before the onset of heart failure.

As would be expected, the degree of right ventricular preponderance is proportional to the pulmonary artery pressure and pulmonary vascular resistance (Johnson *et al.*, 1950).

Fluoroscopy. Prominence of the main branches of the pulmonary artery at the hila, with or without dilatation of the main pulmonary arc, is seen in over 50 per cent of cases of severe emphysema (Parkinson and Hoyle, 1937), but the changes are rarely conspicuous until cor pulmonale is well advanced (fig. 19.05 and 19.06). Associated hypertrophy of the right ventricle is less easily demonstrated.

Pulsation of the pulmonary artery and its main branches may be seen sometimes, but does not compare with that in atrial septal defect, and as a rule is absent. Peripheral vascular markings are relatively unimpressive. Enlargement of the right atrium is rare in the absence of failure. The left atrium is flat, and a prominence on the left border of the heart between the pulmonary and left ventricular arcs is never seen. Owing to the raised cardiac output and the average age of these patients, the aortic knuckle is usually well seen, and may be unduly prominent.

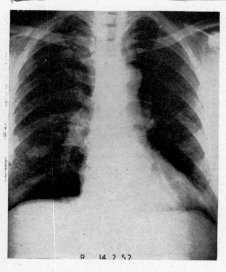

Fig. 19.07—Skiagram of a case of advanced anoxic cor pulmonale due to emphysema with a normal pulmonary vascular resistance showing a cardiovascular contour having no resemblance to the traditional descriptions.

The changes described are not as frequent as originally supposed and are much more typical of the 40 per cent of cases that have a high pulmonary vascular resistance than of the 60 per cent that have not (fig. 19.07). It is this unfamiliarity with the nondescript appearance of the cardiac shadow in many cases of advanced cor pulmonale with a raised cardiac output and normal resistance that has so often led to the diagnosis being overlooked. Indeed, when there is moderate coincident essential hypertension or ischæmic heart disease cases may actually present with left ventricular failure, as in any other hyperkinetic circulatory state when the left ventricle carries the heavier load or is weakened by intrinsic disease; such cases are erroneously diagnosed as hypertensive or ischæmic heart failure.

Then there may be evidence of emphysema: widening of the rib spaces, elevation of the ribs and clavicle, depression of the diaphragm, and increased translucency of the lung parenchyma. However, it is notoriously difficult to diagnose the degree of emphysema from the radiological appearances, and in any case emphysema is not cor pulmonale.

Finally, X-rays may reveal the nature of any underlying disease of the lungs that may be causing or behaving like emphysema, such as bronchiectasis, or honeycomb lung (fig. 19.11), any of the diseases listed earlier that may cause interstitial fibrosis (fig. 19.09), diffuse carcinomatosis (fig. 19.10), or perhaps a surprise such as a massive bulla, aneurysm or thrombosis of a main pulmonary artery (fig. 18.01). As Flint (1954) pointed out, pleural effusion is very uncommon in cor pulmonale, owing to the frequency of obliterative pleurisy.

Special investigations

The diagnosis of emphysema and its degree may be established by demonstrating static changes in the subdivisions of the lung volume: namely, a reduced vital capacity, greatly increased residual volume or dead space, diminished inspiratory capacity, and a normal or increased total lung volume. Typical findings were published by Whitfield *et al.* (1951) as follows (for men):

	Normal controls (litres)	Moderate emphysema (litres)	Severe emphysema (litres)
Vital capacity .	4.00	3.31	2.22
Residual volume	1.75	2.86	3.51
Expiratory reserve	1.27	1.05	0.70
Inspiratory capacity	2.73	2.26	1.52
Total lung volume .	5.74	6.17	5.74

All workers in the field of emphysema, however, have found poor correlation between the degree of these changes and the grade of effort intolerance. They are anatomical measurements and give little direct information about pulmonary function (Baldwin *et al.*, 1949).

The *maximum breathing capacity* is much reduced in emphysema, and of course even more so when there is bronchospasm. Over a 15-second test period of maximum respiratory effort only 20 to 30 litres per minute may be ventilated instead of the normal 75 to 100 litres per minute. These low figures are due to mechanical difficulty in inflating and deflating inelastic emphysematous lungs and the reduced number of functioning alveoli. It should be remembered that the maximum breathing capacity is an artificial test over a very short period of time, and that normal subjects become pyspnœic when ventilating more than half their test figure.

The *resting ventilation* (normally around 6 to 7 litres per minute) varies considerably according to the state of the blood gases, the arterial pH and the sensitivity of the respiratory centre. When the arterial pCO_2 and carbon dioxide content are high the respiratory centre is usually insensitive and respiration may be depressed in the presence of considerable anoxia. Resting ventilation is more likely to be increased in emphysema when CO_2 retention is minimal and anoxia slight. Much of the air inhaled is wasted in the increased dead space and unperfused alveoli, or by over-ventilation of relatively normal alveoli. It follows that for each 100 ml. of oxygen consumed more than the normal 2.5 litres of air must be breathed. Thus the *ventilation equivalent for oxygen*, as this relationship is called, is increased.

Ventilation on effort is limited by mechanical respiratory difficulty. It is usually expressed as a percentage of the maximum breathing capacity (Cournand and Richards, 1941). Patients with emphysema tend to develop very high ratios, and complain less when the figure is over 50 per cent than patients with other respiratory diseases (Baldwin *et al.*, 1949).

Mixing efficiency is impaired in emphysema (Meneely and Kaltreider, 1941). If an inert gas like helium is inhaled it should reach all parts of the lung quickly and uniformly, and the curve of its dilution should be rapid and uniform until mixing is complete. In emphysema complete mixing is delayed, for it takes longer for helium to reach the unventilated alveoli.

The volume of the *poorly ventilated space* in emphysema can also be measured by the helium method and increases with the degree of emphysema.

Analysis of the blood gases is the most important single measurement of the degree of emphysema. Baldwin *et al.* (1949) recognised four grades of severity: in mild cases the arterial oxygen saturation was over 92 per cent at rest and did not fall on effort; in moderate cases it was over 92 per cent at rest, but fell on effort; in grade 3 there was carbon dioxide retention in addition to a reduced arterial oxygen saturation at rest; and in grade 4 there was heart failure in addition.

Cor pulmonale only occurs in the two severe grades of emphysema and the average *arterial oxygen saturation* in my own cases was 85 per cent at rest. This explains why central cyanosis is so often borderline. The *arterial carbon dioxide content*, normally 44 to 53 ml. per cent, ranged between 62 and 71 vols. per cent in a group of cases with heart failure studied by Platts and Whitaker (1954). More sensitive than measurement of the arterial oxygen content is that of the partial pressure of oxygen in arterial blood, for this determines the quantity of oxygen that must combine with hæmoglobin. The normal *arterial pO_2* is about 100 mm. Hg. This may fall to as low as 62 while the arterial oxygen has only dropped to 90 per cent, as the familiar oxyhæmoglobin dissociation curve shows (fig. 19.08). Something is gained also by measuring the *arterial pCO_2*, for although a 5 per cent increase of CO_2 tension results in approximately a 5 per cent rise of carbon dioxide content, pCO_2 is normally fixed close to 40 mm. Hg, so that quite small alterations are significant, whereas the normal range of carbon dioxide content varies through 10 vols. per cent from 44 to 53.

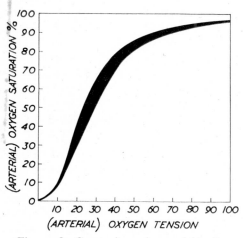

Fig. 19.08—Composite oxyhaemoglobin dissociation curve (after Barcroft).

Again, the CO_2 content of arterial blood is more helpful than the *CO_2 content of venous blood*, the normal range for the latter varying between 53 and as much as 75 vols. per cent.

The plasma pH, normally 7.41, is usually lowered in severe emphysema with cor pulmonale, and ranged between 7.29 and 7.39 in the group of cases studied by Taquini *et al.* (1947).

Finally, estimation of the *alveolar-capillary or alveolar-arterial oxygen tension gradient* may give valuable information concerning oxygen diffusion across ventilated alveolar-capillary membranes or the degree of perfusion of unventilated alveoli (venous admixture). High alveolar-capillary oxygen tension gradients are characteristic of diffuse interstitial fibrosis (Donald *et al.*, 1952).

The pulmonary blood pressure and cardiac output may be measured by means of cardiac catheterisation. Circulatory changes are unlikely to be present, however, unless the arterial oxygen saturation is below 92 per cent at rest and the arterial carbon dioxide content above 53 vols. per cent. When the pulmonary vascular resistance is normal or under 5 units, the cardiac output is then raised, but rarely above 10 litres per minute (McMichael and Sharpey-Schafer, 1944). When the resistance is high, however, the output is usually normal or even low. Thus when both types are analysed together, the net result is usually a high normal output around 6 litres per minute at rest.

When pressures are normal at rest they may yet rise smartly on effort (Riley *et al.*, 1948).

Diagnosis

The usual clinical problem is to decide whether the cardiovascular system is involved in a known case of emphysema: this is not at all difficult, for it is simply a matter of deciding whether the arterial oxygen tension and saturation are reduced and whether or not the pulmonary blood pressure is raised. If central cyanosis cannot be recognised, the arterial oxygen saturation is not likely to be below 85 per cent. If the oxygen tension is down there should be good evidence of peripheral vasodilatation and a hyperkinetic circulatory state. The ocular fundi may suggest carbon dioxide retention. Signs of pulmonary hypertension should not escape notice. If there is heart failure or simply œdema, a diagnosis of cor pulmonale can usually be made with confidence under the clinical circumstances. If there is any doubt blood gas analysis should resolve it.

Difficulty may arise in distinguishing cor pulmonale from other cardiopathies, and especially in unravelling a mixed etiology. Other hyperkinetic circulatory states may have to be excluded, particularly cirrhosis of the liver in emphysematous alcoholics, but also thyrotoxicosis, secondary carcinomatosis of the liver, and Paget's disease of bone in emphysematous subjects. The commonest mixed etiology is the association of emphysema and hypertension. Although the differences between hypertensive heart failure and cor pulmonale are many, it should be remembered that both may occur at the same time.

In the stage of low blood pressure and reduced cardiac output, clinical diagnosis may be more difficult. Toxic vasomotor collapse from bronchopneumonia may cause confusion; mitral stenosis, Pick's disease, mediastinal tumour, the Eisenmenger group, other forms of severe pulmonary hypertension, and many other conditions may have to be considered. The correct diagnosis can usually be made after full investigation, but the first clinical impression can be misleading.

Complications

Pulmonary hypertension, a raised cardiac output, the effects of a high C.S.F. pressure, polycythæmia, pulmonary osteoarthropathy, insensitivity of the respiratory centre, carbon dioxide narcosis, and a number of other features that might be considered as complications, have all been treated as part of the disease itself. Similarly, the absence of angina pectoris, rhythm changes, pleural effusion, phlebothrombosis, have also been referred to. *Congestive heart failure*, however, requires further comment.

It has already been explained that heart failure may result from overwork (pulmonary hypertension and raised cardiac output) under hypoxic conditions. According to Boniface and Brown (1953) a high carbon dioxide tension also depresses myocardial function. There is, however, another important aspect of these cases that has been a source of much confusion— the effect on the circulation of a diminished renal plasma flow and diminished glomerular filtation. This renal factor may come into play when the cardiac output is raised or well within the normal range (Lewis et al., 1952), and causes sodium retention, an increased blood volume (which masks polycythæmia), a rise of venous pressure, and œdema, when the heart is not overloaded. On several occasions patients in this physiological state, referred to the clinic because of "heart failure", have responded to physiological tests, such as tipping and the Valsalva manœuvre, like normal controls. What constitutes heart failure proper and what does not is largely a matter of definition, but from the prognostic point of view the outlook is better in these cases than when the heart is overloaded.

Prognosis

The diagnosis of chronic anoxic cor pulmonale usually carries with it a grave prognosis, few cases surviving two years; but such diagnoses are rarely made before the onset of failure. With the newer methods of investigation, circulatory involvement should be recognised much earlier, perhaps by five years, and appropriate treatment might then prolong life.

Treatment

Vigorous preventive and symptomatic treatment of bronchitis and asthma may delay the development of serious emphysema indefinitely. Half-hearted measures must be condemned when the ultimate fate of these patients is realised.

By the time the cardiovascular system is involved, emphysema is usually far advanced. A partly reversible state may be encountered however, when acute bronchitis, bronchopneumonia, or an asthmatic bout is superimposed on chronic changes of only moderate degree. In such cases, infection should be treated promptly with penicillin or other forms of chemotherapy, and bronchial spasm relieved by a dust-free atmosphere and antispasmodics.

Although details of such treatment cannot be considered in a work of this kind, one or two observations are necessary. Morphine is frequently lethal owing to its depressing effect on respiration; pethidine may quieten a restless patient just as well, is a good antispasmodic, and does not depress respiration. Subcutaneous adrenaline is still the most effective way of relieving bronchial spasm; in an emergency newer remedies, such as the antihistamine drugs, may be given in addition but not as a substitute. Isopropyl-*nor*-adrenaline, which may be administered in sublingual tablets in doses of 20 to 40 mg., is a useful preparation. Antispasmodics that improve the cardiac output or coronary circulation, such as aminophylline, may be chosen in preference to those that do not. An oral dose of 0.1 to 0.2 G., t.d.s., is usually insufficient, and since repeated intravenous injections are impracticable and the intramuscular route too painful, the only efficient way of giving aminophylline is by suppository, 0.4 to 0.5 G. twice daily. Etophylate, 0.5 G. t.d.s., or choline theophyllinate, 0.5 G. t.d.s., however, may be given by mouth as a substitute, and etophylate is painless intramuscularly.

Whether the case is complicated by infection and bronchial spasm or not, it is vitally important that the patient should be nursed in an oxygen tent. The effect of improving the arterial oxygen saturation is often dramatic: it prevents fatal vasomotor collapse, reduces the cardiac output, and may lower the pulmonary blood pressure. The fear of carbon dioxide narcosis is no excuse for withholding the one remedy these patients need above all others. It is true that some 10 per cent of patients with cor pulmonale have developed such insensitive respiratory centres that they no longer respond to carbon dioxide, but only to oxygen lack. When oxygen is provided, the increased arterial oxygen tension deprives the respiratory centre of its stimulus and respiration becomes depressed. The arterial carbon dioxide tension may then rise very high indeed and the patient may become drowsy and finally lapse into coma (Davies and MacKinnon, 1949), presumably with a high C.S.F. pressure and cerebral œdema. It is also true that oxygen is still given intermittently, but the fact remains that it is not given with sufficient enthusiasm nowadays, and patients are not recovering as quickly as they should in consequence. As implied above, 90 per cent of cases do not develop carbon dioxide narcosis when treated in an oxygen tent without any special precautions. Moreover, it has now been shown that the insensitivity of the respiratory centre is partly due to oxygen lack itself and may recover when oxygen is supplied (Westlake, Simpson and Kaye, 1955). Respiratory stimulants may also be given if drowsiness develops or an artificial respirator may be used. Aminophylline may help and nikethamide may be given repeatedly in emergency. Since aspirin may cause hyperventilation with secondary alkalosis by its direct action on the respiratory centre, it has been tried recently in the cases under discussion (Wégria, 1955), but since it also increases oxygen consumption by about 20 per cent (Tenney and Miller, 1955) it is far from ideal.

Mersalyl and a low sodium diet should be used with caution. Howarth, McMichael and Sharpey-Schafer (1947) have shown that in most cases with raised cardiac outputs the venous pressure is already at an optimum level, and that lowering it by any means may reduce the output and harm the patient. In a minority, however, the heart is overloaded and then responds to such treatment in the usual way. Although clinically it may not always be easy to judge the physiological state of the circulation, warm extremities and a full bounding pulse theoretically contraindicate all venous pressure-lowering agents, whereas cold extremities, a small pulse and low blood pressure demand them (when the venous pressure is raised). When œdema is considerable and the jugular venous pressure over 7 cm. above the sternal angle, mersalyl and a low sodium diet should be tried. Practical experience has proved their value and no harmful effects have been observed; part of their usefulness is in removing what is virtually renal œdema.

Venesection should certainly be avoided, not only because its venous pressure-lowering effect is too drastic and may be dangerous if ill judged, but because correcting physiological polycythæmia results in a further increase of cardiac output, a rise in pulmonary artery pressure, and a fall in arterial oxygen saturation (Lewis et al., 1952).

Digitalis or strophanthin may be used without fear if the heart is thought to be overloaded; if in fact the output is raised and at its physiological maximum no harm will result from therapeutic doses.

If, after relief of bronchial spasm and infection, the arterial oxygen saturation is still below 80 per cent when the patient is out of the tent, antithyroid drugs should be seriously considered as a means of reducing the oxygen requirement (page 312).

SPECIAL FORMS OF COR PULMONALE

Diffuse interstitial pulmonary fibrosis

In 1944 Hamman and Rich described a hitherto unknown type of parenchymatous disease of the lungs of uncertain etiology characterised by alveoli lined with cuboidal cells and separated from one another by marked proliferation of the interstitial connective tissue. In this condition the physical barrier between alveolar air and capillary blood is considerable and efficient oxygen diffusion difficult. Carbon dioxide, being 25 times more soluble in water than oxygen, has little difficulty in crossing the barrier. This results in reduced arterial oxygen tension and saturation without carbon dioxide retention; indeed, hyperventilation due to anoxia may result in reduction of the arterial pCO_2 and carbon dioxide content. The respiratory centre remains highly sensitive in this condition and responds vigorously to any rise in CO_2 tension.

The subdivisions of the lung volume, maximum breathing capacity, mixing efficiency and poorly ventilated space may be altered very little, although the increased rigidity of the fibrotic lungs may add to the work of respiration, the inspiratory reserve capacity may be reduced, and the intra-pleural pressure swings greater than normal.

Clinically these patients complain of severe dyspnœa at a time when little abnormal may be detected, and on this account may receive scant sympathy, an erroneous diagnosis of respiratory neurosis being made, for in the early stages the X-ray appearances of the lungs may be normal. But the reduced arterial oxygen tension leads to early peripheral vasodilatation and the warm hands, throbbing digital vessels, and distended forearm veins should not escape notice. On effort, the arterial oxygen saturation, which may be over 90 per cent at rest, drops sharply and central cyanosis may then be detected clinically.

The diffusion difficulty may be demonstrated by measuring the alveolar-arterial oxygen tension gradient, which is much increased above the normal of 5 to 10 mm. Hg; serious venous admixture is excluded by relatively normal ventilatory function tests.

As the disease advances the circulation becomes more hyperkinetic and cor pulmonale with heart failure develops sooner or later, as in the case described by Sloper and Williams (1955). Pulmonary hypertension has not been a feature of my own three cases, but is said to develop sooner or later in most (Arnott, 1955). Radiological evidence of the diffuse fibrotic change also becomes apparent as a fine reticular or ground glass appearance.

The prognosis and treatment are similar to emphysematous cor pulmonale except that antispasmodics are not required and there is no danger of carbon dioxide narcosis.

Other types of interstitial fibrosis

A very similar physiological situation may arise from any other disease that thickens the barrier between the alveoli and the capillaries of the lung. Donald (1953) lists the following causes of serious diffuse interstitial fibrosis: beryllium granuloma, asbestosis, scleroderma, sarcoidosis, reticuloses, and "interstitial pneumonitis", and Arnott (1955) adds radiation fibrosis, silicosis, and diffuse carcinomatosis.

Although the nature of the etiological agent is obviously important and every effort should be made to identify it, the development and course of cor pulmonale in each type follows the same familiar lines. How often a serious diffusion difficulty accompanies chronic interstitial œdema in mitral stenosis and left ventricular failure is at present uncertain. In figure 19.09 the radiological appearances in a case of interstitial fibrosis are illustrated. This woman, who was very breathless on exertion, also had signs of mild mitral stenosis, but cardiac catheterisation revealed a left atrial pressure under 5 mm. Hg, a mean pulmonary artery pressure of only 13 mm. Hg, a cardiac output of 4.1 litres per minute, and an arterial oxygen saturation of 86.5 per cent. The radiological appearances are not unlike those of chronic interstitial œdema, but in view of the findings independent interstitial fibrosis seemed inescapable.

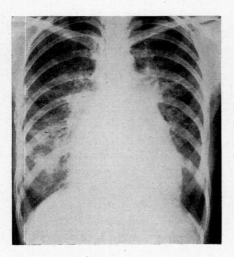

Fig. 19.09—Diffuse interstitial pulmonary fibrosis in a case of mild mitral stenosis.

Cor pulmonale from pneumoconiosis

Although many papers have described the frequency and course of cor pulmonale in pneumoconiosis (e.g. Coggin et al., 1938; Thomas, 1948), it is not yet clear whether emphysema, interstitial fibrosis or obliterative pulmonary hypertension is chiefly responsible, or whether a variable combination of all three factors are to blame. Further detailed physiological studies are awaited with interest.

Diffuse carcinomatosis

In previous classifications diffuse carcinomatosis has usually been regarded as a special form of subacute obstructive "cor pulmonale", when the term cor pulmonale included all forms of pulmonary hypertension.

Two chief types were recognised: (1) multiple embolic carcinomatosis behaving like subacute thrombo-embolic pulmonary hypertension, as in the case described by Mason (1940), which was secondary to carcinoma of the breast; (2) diffuse lymphatic carcinomatosis with secondary thrombosis of the small pulmonary arteries and arterioles, as in the case described by Brill and Robertson (1937), in which carcinoma of the stomach was responsible.

Of four cases of my own, however, none presented like subacute pulmonary hypertension, but all had the features of subacute cor pulmonale with doubtful or absent central cyanosis at rest, marked breathlessness and central cyanosis on effort, and a remarkably hyperkinetic circulation ending in congestive heart failure. Only the last of these four was investigated physiologically, and at the time clinical heart failure was present. Both right and left atrial pressures were raised, the right being 8/-1 with reference to the sternal angle, with *a* and *v* about equal in amplitude, and the left being 15/5 with *v* dominant. The pulmonary artery pressure was 45/20,

the right ventricular pressure 45/0/8, the cardiac output 7.3 litres per minute, the pulmonary vascular resistance only 2 units, and the arterial oxygen saturation 83 per cent. A low hæmoglobin (59 per cent) prevented central cyanosis at rest, as it may often do in this group. These findings excluded obstructive pulmonary hypertension. At the time these four cases were seen it was not at all clear what was causing the central cyanosis, for there was no evidence of emphysema. There seems little doubt in retrospect that they were suffering from a diffusion difficulty, and that physiologically they resembled cases with diffuse interstitial fibrosis. The case investigated showed diffuse lymphatic

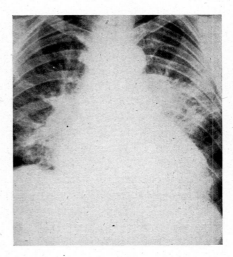

Fig. 19.10—Subacute anoxic cor pulmonale with heart failure and a normal pulmonary vascular resistance due to diffuse lymphatic carcinomatosis secondary to bronchial carcinoma.

spread from a bronchial carcinoma of the right middle lobe bronchus (fig. 19.10). Of the other three cases the primary growth was in the stomach in one, in the breast in one, and was not established in the third.

Of four cases described by Storstein (1951) two were secondary to carcinoma of the stomach, and two to carcinoma of the breast. Physiological investigations in two of the cases revealed pulmonary artery pressures of 36/17 and 26/7, cardiac outputs of 5 and 4 litres per minute, pulmonary vascular resistances of about 4 and 3 units, and arterial oxygen saturations at rest of 78 and 61 per cent respectively.

Reporting 24 new cases of this condition and reviewing 154 from the literature, Harold (1952) gives its frequency as 1.5 per cent of 836 consecutive necropsies at St. Bartholomew's Hospital, or 7.5 per cent of all cases of malignant disease. The essential pathological findings were distension of the peribronchial and perivascular lymphatics by tumour cells, with secondary interstitial fibrosis; intravascular tumour emboli, secondary thrombosis and obliterative endarteritis were seen occasionally. Of the total of 178 cases, the primary tumour was gastric in 53.5 per cent, bronchial in 13 per cent, mammary in 9.5 per cent, pancreatic in 6 per cent, and prostatic in 4 per cent. Although only one of Harold's 24 cases collected from the records at Brompton and St. Bartholomew's Hospitals was recognised as having terminal subacute cor pulmonale, his statement that the outstanding symptom was severe increasing breathlessness until the patient became distressed on the least exertion leaves little room for doubt as to what was happening physiologically. It seems unlikely, however, that pulmonary hypertension was a feature of any of these cases.

The clinical diagnosis is based on the combination of subacute hypoxic cor pulmonale, usually without marked pulmonary hypertension, the characteristic radiological changes of diffuse lymphatic carcinomatosis, evidence of the primary neoplasm, secondary anæmia instead of polycythæmia, relatively good ventilatory function, absence of carbon dioxide retention, and the demonstration of impeded oxygen diffusion.

The prognosis is hopeless, and treatment can only be symptomatic.

Honeycomb lung

The occurrence of small, thin-walled, air-containing cysts, measuring up to a maximum of 1 cm. in diameter and widely distributed throughout both lungs may be associated with interstitial fibrosis, however caused (Oswald and Parkinson, 1949). Known forms of interstitial disease that may develop these cysts include xanthomatosis (Rowland, 1928), reticuloses in infants (Mallory, 1942), tuberous sclerosis (Berg and Vejlens, 1939), and probably diffuse interstitial fibrosis itself (Oswald and Parkinson, 1949). A few may be congenital. Bronchograms reveal no filling of the cysts with lipiodol, but the frequency of pneumothorax, which is often recurrent and bilateral, suggests some communication between some of the cysts and the bronchial tree. The cysts are sometimes lined with flattened epithelium, sometimes not. Adjacent cysts are separated by thick-walled septa which may contain connective tissue and blood vessels. The bronchial tree itself appears to be normal.

Physiological studies in this group are scanty. There were only two examples in my series of 45 cases of chronic cor pulmonale. The first was a cyanosed woman of 26 with an obviously hyperkinetic circulatory state who finally developed congestive heart failure, opened up a valve paten foramen ovale, and died from paradoxical cerebral embolism. Her vital capacity was 2 litres, her arterial oxygen saturation 72 per cent in an oxygen tent, and from the modest (grade 2) electrocardiographic changes her pulmonary vascular resistance was probably between 6 and 9 units.

The second case was a man of 28 admitted with congestive heart failure and typical radiological evidence of honeycomb lung (fig. 19.11). The arterial oxygen saturation was 69 per cent, cardiac output 4.4 litres per minute, mean pulmonary artery pressure 43 mm. Hg, pulmonary vascular resistance 10 units, and hæmoglobin 115 per cent. The arterial carbon dioxide content was not estimated.

Necropsy confirmed the diagnosis in both these cases, but whether the physiological behaviour was like emphysema or interstitial fibrosis cannot be determined from the inadequate investigations carried out at the time.

Clinically, the majority of patients with honeycomb lung who survive the pneumothorax hazard develop cor pulmonale sooner or later. Anoxia and a

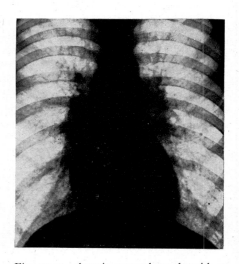

Fig. 19.11—Anoxic cor pulmonale with a high pulmonary vascular resistance due to honeycomb lungs.

hyperkinetic circulation are probably usual, but the pulmonary vascular resistance may also be high. Interstitial fibrosis is likely to impede oxygen diffusion across the alveolar-capillary interface and perfusion of unventilated air-containing cysts is likely to cause a high degree of venous admixture in the arterial blood.

Ayerza's disease

Much confusion has arisen from the use of this term: it has been applied to cases of intense cyanosis and polycythæmia associated with syphilitic or other disease of the pulmonary arteries (Boyd, 1931). The facts are that Ayerza, of Buenos Aires, in an unpublished clinical lecture (1901) described a single case of heart failure in which the patient was so cyanosed as to be almost black—a cardiac negro. Autopsy revealed much enlargement of the right side of the heart, dilatation of the bronchi, and peribronchitis. Neither syphilis nor the state of the pulmonary vessels was mentioned. Arrillaga (1913, 1924) was, perhaps, chiefly responsible for stressing the syphilitic origin of such cases, although other authors from the Argentine believed the arterial lesions to be atherosclerotic. Brenner (1935), after reviewing the evidence, concluded that there was no good reason for retaining the term Ayerza's disease, on the grounds that published cases described nothing but chronic cor pulmonale.

Cor pulmonale associated with deformities of the chest

Gross kyphoscoliosis accounts for perhaps 1.5 per cent of cases of chronic cor pulmonale. The condition is associated with extensive collapse-atrophy of part of the lung and severe emphysema of the remainder. Cardiovascular involvement is similar in type to that associated with other forms of emphysema; kinking of the aorta (Corvisart) plays no part in its development.

A curious form of syncope has been described in a number (Chapman, Dill and Graybiel, 1939), possibly due to sudden lowering of the right atrial pressure consequent upon compression of the inferior vena cava in certain postures (page 13). Otherwise the symptoms are similar to those of cor pulmonale from ordinary emphysema. There is also the same tendency to chest infection.

On the average death occurs five months after the onset of heart failure and at an average age of 30 years. An injection of morphine is particularly lethal (Fischer and Dolehide, 1954).

Aneurysm of the pulmonary artery

Aneurysm of the pulmonary artery is rare, being found in less than .01 per cent of all autopsies, and accounting for less than 0.5 per cent of all aneurysms (Deterling and Clagett, 1947). The sexes are represented equally, and about one-third of the patients are under 30 years of age (Boyd and McGarack, 1939). The etiology is believed to be a congenital defect in the wall of the pulmonary artery in about 40 per cent, syphilis in 30 per cent and chronic cor pulmonale with atherosclerotic pulmonary arteries in 30 per cent. The diagnosis may be obvious on fluoroscopy if gross pulsation is seen; if not, it may be proved by means of angiocardiography (Robb and Steinberg, 1940).

In pulmonary heart disease aneurysmal dilatation may develop remarkably quickly; underlying congenital weakness of the arterial wall is difficult to exclude. Thrombosis may occur in the sac, or the whole vessel may be occluded; but apart from such a complication the aneurysm is unlikely to influence the course of the primary disease. Rupture is very rare.

REFERENCES

Arnott, W. M. (1955): "Order and disorder in pulmonary function", *Brit. med. J.*, ii, 279.
Arrillaga, F. C. (1913): "Sclerose de l'artère pulmonaire secondaire à certains etats pulmonaires chroniques (cardiaques noirs)", *Arch. d. mal. du Coeur*, 6, 518.
—— (1924): "Sclerose de l'artere pulmonaire (cardiaques noirs)", *Bull. et mém. Soc. med. d. hôp. de Paris*, 1, 292.

Baldwin, E. de F., Cournand, A., and Richards, D. W. (1949): "Pulmonary insufficiency; study of 39 cases of pulmonary fibrosis", *Medicine*, **28**, 1.

——, "Pulmonary insufficiency; study of 122 cases of chronic pulmonary emphysema", *Medicine*, **28**, 201.

Barcroft, J., and Nagahashi, M. (1921): "Direct measurement of partial pressure of oxygen in blood", *J. Physiol.*, Lond., **55**, 339.

Berg, G., and Vejlens, G. (1939): "Maladie kystique du poumon et sclérose tubéreuse du cerveau", *Acta paediatr.*, Stockh., **26**, 16.

Boniface, K. J., and Brown, J. M. (1953): "Effect of carbon dioxide excess on contractile force of heart, *in situ*", *Amer. J. Physiol.*, **172**, 752.

Bloomfield, R. A., Lauson, H. D., Cournand, A., Breed, E. S., and Richards, D. W. (1946): "Recording of right heart pressures in normal subjects and in patients with chronic pulmonary disease and various types of cardio-circulatory disease", *J. clin. Invest.*, **25**, 639.

Boyd, L. J., and McGavack, T. H. (1939): "Aneurysm of the pulmonary artery: a review of the literature and a report of two cases", *Amer. Heart J.*, **18**, 562.

Boyd, W. (1931): "The pathology of internal diseases", Philadelphia.

Brenner, O. (1935): "Pathology of the vessels of the pulmonary circulation", *Arch. intern. Med.*, **56**, 211, 457, 724, 976, 1189.

Brill, I. C., and Robertson, T. D. (1937): "Subacute cor pulmonale", *Arch. intern, Med.*, **60**, 1043.

Chapman, E. M., Dill, D. B., and Graybiel, A. (1939): "The decrease in functional capacity of the lungs and heart resulting from deformities of the chest: pulmonocardiac failure", *Medicine*, **18**, 167.

Christie, R. V. (1944): "Emphysema of the lungs", *Brit. med. J.*, i, 143.

Coggin, C. B., Griggs, D. E., and Stilson, W. L. (1938): "The heart in pneumoconiosis", *Amer. Heart J.*, **16**, 411.

Cournand, A., and Richards, D. W. (1941): "Pulmonary insufficiency; discussion of physiological classification and presentation of clinical tests", *Amer. Rev. Tuberc.*, **44**, 26, 123, 272.

Davies, C. E., and Mackinnon, J. (1949): "Neurological effects of oxygen in chronic cor pulmonale", *Lancet*, ii, 883.

Deterling, R. A., and Clagett, O. T. (1947): "Aneurysm of the pulmonary artery: review of the literature and report of a case", *Amer. Heart J.*, **34**, 471.

Donald, K. W. (1953): "The definition and assessment of respiratory function", *Brit. med. J.*, i, 1068.

——, Renzetti, A., Riley, R. L., and Cournand, A. (1952): "Analysis of factors affecting concentrations of oxygen and carbon dioxide in gas and blood of lungs: results", *J. appl. Physiol.*, **4**, 497.

Fischer, J. W., and Dolehide, R. A. (1954): "Fatal cardiac failure in persons with thoracic deformities", *Arch. intern. Med.*, **93**, 687.

Flint, F. J. (1954): "Cor pulmonale. Incidence and ætiology in an industrial city", *Lancet*, ii, 51.

Griggs, D. E., Coggin, C. B., and Evans, N. (1939): "Right ventricular hypertrophy and congestive failure in chronic pulmonary disease", *Amer. Heart J.*, **17**, 681.

Hamman, L., and Rich, A. R. (1944): "Acute diffuse interstitial fibrosis of lungs", *Bull. Johns Hopk. Hosp.*, **74**, 177.

Harold, J. T. (1952): "Lymphangitis carcinomatosa of the lungs", *Quart. J. Med.*, **21**, 353.

Harvey, R. M., Ferrer, M. I., Richards, D. W., and Cournand, A. (1951): "Influence of chronic pulmonary disease on heart and circulation", *Amer. J. Med.*, **10**, 719.

Howarth, S., McMichael, J., and Sharpey-Schafer, E. P. (1947): "Effects of oxygen, venesection and digitalis in chronic heart failure from disease of the lungs", *Clin. Sc.*, **6**, 187.

Johnson, J. B., Ferrer, M. I., West, J. R., and Cournand, A. (1950): "The relation between electrocardiographic evidence of right ventricular hypertrophy and pulmonary arterial pressure in patients with chronic pulmonary disease", *Circulation*, 1, 536.

Lewis, C. S., Samuels, A. J., Daines, M. C., and Hecht, H. H. (1952): "Chronic lung disease, polycythæmia and congestive heart failure. Cardiorespiratory, vascular and renal adjustments in cor pulmonale", *Circulation*, 6, 874.

McMichael, J., and Sharpey-Schafer, E. P. (1944): "The action of intravenous digoxin in man", *Quart. J. Med.*, 13, 123.

Mallory, T. B. (1942): "Medical progress; pathology, diseases of bone", *New Engl. J. Med.*, 227, 955.

Mason, D. G. (1940): "Subacute cor pulmonale", *Arch. intern. Med.*, 66, 1221.

Meneely, G. R., and Kaltreider, N. L. (1941): "Use of helium for determination of pulmonary capacity", *Proc. Soc. exp. Biol.*, N.Y., 46, 266.

Motley, H. L., Cournand, A., Werko, L., Himmelstein, A., and Dresdale, D. (1947): "The influence of short periods of induced acute anoxia upon pulmonary artery pressure in man", *Amer. J. Physiol.*, 150, 315.

Oswald, N., and Parkinson, T. (1949): "Honeycomb lungs", *Quart. J. Med.*, 18, 1.

✔ Parkinson, J., and Hoyle, C. (1937): "The heart in emphysema", *Quart. J. Med.*, 6, 59.

Platts, M., and Whitaker, W. (1954): "The diagnostic importance of the blood carbon dioxide content of patients with central cyanosis", *Amer. Heart J.*, 48, 77.

Riley, R. L., Himmelstein, A., Motley, H. L., Weiner, H. M., and Cournand, A. (1948): "Studies of the pulmonary circulation at rest and during exercise in normal individuals and in patients with chronic pulmonary disease", *Amer. J. Physiol.*, 152, 372.

Robb, G. P., and Steinberg, I. (1940): "Visualisation of the chambers of the heart; the pulmonary circulation and the great blood vessels in man: summary of method and results", *J. Amer. med. Ass.*, 114, 474.

Rowland, R. S. (1928): "Xanthomatosis and reticulo-endothelial system; correlation of unidentified group of cases described as defects in membranous bones, exophthalmos and diabetes insipidus (Christian's syndrome)", *Arch. intern. Med.*, 42, 611.

Simpson, T. (1948): "Papilloedema in emphysema", *Brit. med. J.*, ii, 639.

Sloper, J. C., and Williams, E. (1955): "Diffuse interstitial pulmonary fibrosis. The Hamman-Rich syndrome", *Lancet*, ii, 533.

Spain, D. M., and Handler, B. J. (1946): "Chronic cor pulmonale—sixty cases studied at necropsy", *Arch. intern. Med.*, 77, 37.

Storsten, O. (1951): "Circulatory failure in metastatic carcinoma of the lung. A physiologic and pathologic study of its pathogenesis", *Circulation*, 4, 913.

Taquini, A. C., Fasciolo, J. C., Suarez, J. R. E., and Chiodi, H. (1947): "Circulatory adaptations in Ayerza's syndrome—black cardiacs", *Amer. Heart J.*, 34, 50.

Tenney, S. M., and Miller, R. M. (1955): "The respiratory and circulatory actions of salicylate", *Amer. J. Med.*, 19, 498.

Thomas, A. J. (1948): "The heart in the pneumoconiosis of coalminers", *Brit. Heart J.*, 10, 282.

Wégria, R., et al. (1955): "Effect of salicylate on the acid-base equilibrium of patients with chronic CO_2 retention due to pulmonary emphysema", *Amer. J. Med.*, 19, 509.

Westlake, E. K., Simpson, T., Kaye, M. (1955): "Carbon dioxide narcosis in emphysema", *Quart. J. Med.*, 24, 155.

Whitfield, A. G. W., Smith, O. E., Richards, D. G. B., Waterhouse, J. A. H., and Arnott, W. M. (1951): "The correlation between the radiological appearances and the clinical and spirometric state in emphysema", *Quart. J. Med.*, 20, 247.

Wood, P. H. (1947): "Electrocardiographic appearances in acute and chronic pulmonary heart disease", *Brit. Heart J.*, 10, 87.

CHAPTER XX

THYROTOXICOSIS AND THE HEART IN MYXŒDEMA

THYROTOXIC HEART DISEASE

THE cardiovascular system is clearly involved from the onset of thyrotoxicosis, although the term thyrotoxic heart disease is usually reserved for the late stage when auricular fibrillation or congestive heart failure dominates the scene. Such a distinction is artificial and simply means that a young and healthy heart can maintain a high output for years without distress, but that an aged heart cannot.

Historical note. Thyrotoxic heart disease was first adequately described by Caleb Hillier Parry (1815, 1825) of Bath, who witnessed his first case in 1786. Flajani's publication of the details of one case (1802) appeared first, but cannot be compared with Parry's account. Graves' description (1835) is also inferior. Carl von Basedow (1840), a general practitioner at Merseburg, Germany, called special attention to exophthalmos and drew a vivid picture of most of the features of primary exophthalmic goitre as we see it today, omitting only tremor, which was later recognised and added to the Merseburg triad (exophthalmos, goitre and palpitations) by Pierre Marie (1883). For further historical details the reader is referred to the classical monographs of Cecil Joll (1932) and of Means and Richardson (1938).

NATURE OF THYROID HORMONE

The exact composition of thyroid hormone is not yet known. In 1895, Baumann obtained from thyroid tissue a protein-free, physiologically active substance containing 10 per cent of iodine, which he called iodothyrin. In 1899, Oswald showed that the active principle stored in the gland was attached to a protein in the form of thyroglobulin: this is the chief constituent of colloid. Kendall isolated thyroxine in 1915, showed that it contained 65 per cent of iodine, and demonstrated its potency. These researches culminated in the synthesis of thyroxine by Harington and Barger in 1927.

Thyroxine, however, accounts for only 40 to 50 per cent of the total iodine in the thyroid gland, is relatively insoluble, and is not believed to be identical with thyroid hormone. The rest of the thyroid iodine is found in the practically inert substance, di-iodotyrosine, a likely precursor of thyroxine. According to Harington (1933), thyroxine and di-iodotyrosine are probably linked with amino-acids as constituents of thyroglobulin in colloid; and the natural thyroid hormone is perhaps a thyroxine-containing peptide.

871

PATHOLOGY OF GOITRE

The normal thyroid gland consists essentially of numerous acini lined with epithelium and containing colloid material rich in iodine, from which thyroid hormone appears to be liberated according to the demand. When the gland is stimulated, the epithelium assumes an active columnar form, and colloid tends to disappear. When there is little or none left, the walls of the acini may become crenated, like any other vesicle whose contents have been removed. In this phase the gland as a whole is soft and vascular, and is not enlarged. When the stimulus ceases, involution takes place: the epithelum flattens, colloid reappears, and the acini become distended. This is the resting phase, and is characterised by a firmer, less vascular gland of somewhat larger size. If the stimulus to activity is excessive the morphological changes described above are supplemented by true hyperplasia of the acinar epithelium, and subsequent involution may be incomplete, leading to permanent enlargement of the gland.

Simple goitre is due to benign hyperplasia, and develops when iodine supplies are short or diverted, especially when thyroid demands are heavy (Marine, 1927). This response to iodine lack is believed by some to be mediated by the production of excessive amounts of thyrotropic hormone from the anterior pituitary. Endemic goitre due to lack of iodine in the soil occurs in New Zealand, parts of Italy and North America, and in many other mountainous districts or places remote from the sea. Iodine diversion may be due to polluted water (Marine and Lenhart, 1910; McCarrison, 1927). Increased demands for thyroid hormone occur at puberty and during pregnancy.

Colloid goitre represents the resting involuted phase of previous benign hyperplasia (Marine, 1930). When the stimulus subsides, colloid reaccumulates in the acini, intervening walls between distended crowded vesicles break down to form cysts, and the whole gland becomes tense and big. This process is innocent and causes no symptoms except possible discomfort in the neck.

In primary Graves' disease persistent uncontrolled stimulation of the thyroid gland of unknown cause leads to marked hyperplasia and to wild manufacture and liberation of excessive amounts of thyroid hormone. The acinar epithelium is columnar and proliferated, the walls of the acini markedly crenated, and the colloid practically all gone. The gland as a whole is soft, vascular and enlarged.

Nodular goitre is usually regarded as the end-result of repeated cycles of hyperplasia and incomplete involution. The process probably begins with failure of complete involution of a previously stimulated and hyperplastic gland. Subsequent stimulation leads to local hyperplasia of these hypo-involuted nests, and subsequent involution to local nodules of colloid goitre. Such a process may be repeated indefinitely. Thyrotoxicosis from nodular goitre depends chiefly upon the activity of the hyperplastic nests the nodules themselves being mostly inert. The term adenomatous goitr is therefore incorrect when applied to this type of lesion, and should be reserved to describe those cases in which thyroid nodules (usually single) are composed of solid masses of cells of fœtal type. Compared with primary Graves' disease, nodular goitre usually runs a longer and less dramatic course, which by its very nature is necessarily phasic, periods of activity alternating with periods of relative quiescence. Why production of thyroid hormone should exceed the demand is no more understood than it is in primary Graves' disease. The implication of the anterior pituitary thyrotropic hormone may explain part of the mechanism, but in no way solves the problem.

Physiology of the circulation under the influence of thyroxin. The administration of thyroxin to man and mammals is followed, after a time-lag of several days, by an appreciable rise in the basal metabolic rate. The increased oxygen requirement is met by elevation of the cardiac output, not by greater utilisation of available oxygen (as occurs when the B.M.R. is raised by dinitrocresol), nor by polycythæmia. The high minute-output is maintained more by tachycardia than by a raised venous pressure, the stroke-volume being but little increased (Friedberg and Sohval, 1937). The strength of cardiac contraction is probably enhanced. These effects are usually attributed to the direct action of thyroxine on the heart.

At the same time the peripheral blood flow is greatly increased, there is obvious vasodilatation in the skin, and adrenergic responses are magnified.

Morbid anatomy of the thyrotoxic heart. There are no macroscopic changes in the thyrotoxic heart prior to the onset of auricular fibrillation and failure; until then the heart-weight remains normal. Cases exhibiting cardiac embarrassment during life may still show little at necropsy except some increase in heart-weight and evidence of congestive failure (Kepler and Barnes, 1932). In a few, however, there are scattered foci of fibrosis (Rake and McEachearn, 1932).

CLINICAL FEATURES

The hyperkinetic circulation of primary Graves' disease is usually well tolerated because the subjects are young; but in middle-aged or elderly people with toxic nodular goitre cardiac embarrassment is the rule. The sex-ratio favours women in the proportion of about 6 : 1 (Fraser and Dunhill, 1934). A family history of goitre is found in 45 per cent of cases (Bruun, 1945). Contributory factors include pregnancy, the climacteric, infection (such as tonsillitis) and perhaps emotional shock, although the scarcity of thyrotoxicosis amongst active service casualties in the first two world wars was noteworthy. The rôle of iodine has already been discussed.

Of the symptoms, loss of weight, heat intolerance, agitation or restlessness, palpitations and fatigue are the most important. Loss of weight associated with a voracious appetite is particularly suggestive. Palpitations may be due to vigorous and rapid action of the heart or to paroxysmal auricular fibrillation; the latter is especially significant.

Whilst the symptoms themselves are important, the manner in which they are told and the general behaviour and appearance of the patient are often more so. The subject is usually a woman; she is commonly thin and talks quickly, often gesticulating to lend emphasis to her remarks. She may wear a scarf to hide an unsightly swelling in her neck, but her clothing is otherwise light. One of Parry's patients liked to sit in a draught, stripped to the waist, in order to keep cool (Parry, 1815). A good moment to look for the goitre is towards the beginning of the interview, when the patient may lean forward in her chair, and swallow once or twice in nervousness. The eyes are characteristic, not so much because of exophthalmos, which is usually absent, but because of their typical stare. The trend of the patient's conversation is often illuminating, and in sharp contrast to that of the anxiety neurotic. The latter complains of symptom after symptom in a challenging fashion, exaggerating their severity, and stressing his inability to cope with them. The thyrotoxic patient tries to explain away her symptoms: she feels the heat, but of course it has been very warm recently; she is losing weight, but she supposes she was too fat before; she gets tired and irritable, but she knows she tries to do too much; and so on.

Physical examination may reveal a wealth of signs which are all directly or indirectly attributable to excess of thyroid hormone, except exophthalmos and goitre. They may be suitably described under four main headings.

1. *The eyes.* Exophthalmos may be present (fig. 20.01), but is uncommon in toxic nodular goitre. It is occasionally unilateral (fig. 20.02). Artificial glass eyes may also become proptosed. Its mechanism is still a subject of controversy (Zondek and Ticho, 1945), but exophthalmos is certainly not due to sympathetic stimulation, for it is not relieved by sympathectomy (Shaw, 1929); nor is it due to excess of thyroid hormone, which never reproduces it. Moreover, exophthalmos occasionally becomes more marked after thyroidectomy or treatment with thiouracil. In severe cases of exophthalmic ophthalmoplegia and malignant exophthalmos, thyrotoxicosis may be minimal, and the protrusion of the eye-ball appears to be secondary to intense œdema of the orbital contents (Brain and Turnbull, 1938). Of great interest is the exophthalmos that can be produced in guinea-pigs (also in rabbits and fish, but not so far in man) by injecting thyrotropic hormone, especially if the thyroid gland is first removed (Marine and Rosen, 1933). All these facts point to the likelihood of the pituitary being directly responsible, and provide further evidence that thyrotoxicosis may depend upon a primary pituitary disorder.

Retraction of the upper lid (fig. 20.03), revealing the white sclerotic above the iris (Dalrymple's sign), which may be unilateral, is also uncommon in toxic nodular goitre. It should be distinguished from exophthalmos, which reveals the white sclerotic below the iris by mechanically displacing the lower lid (Pochin, 1937–8).

If the patient looks up, and then lowers the eyes to watch a descending object, the upper lid lags behind the movement of the eye-ball, revealing

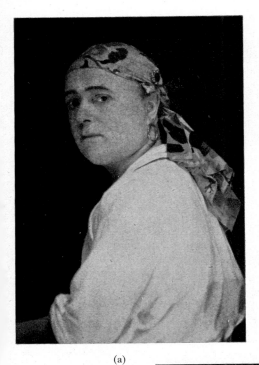

(a)

Fig. 20.01—Exophthalmic goitre. The first photograph (a) (in gipsy dress) was taken in 1933; the second (b) in 1936. The white sclerotics are seen below the iris due to mechanical displacement of the lower lid.

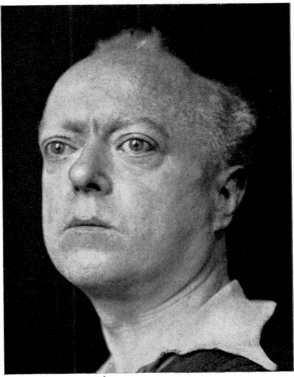

(b)

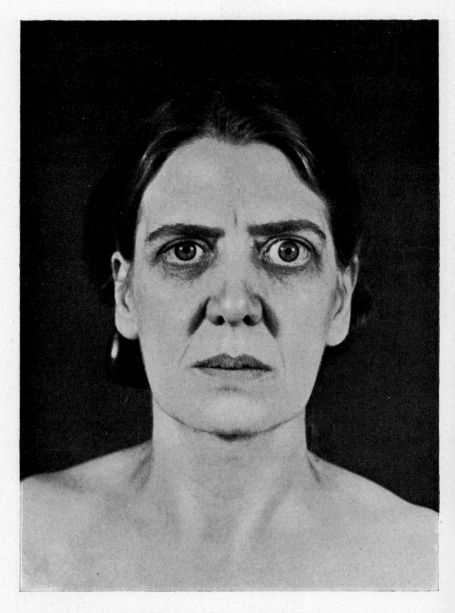

Fig. 20.02—Unilateral lid retraction and exophthalmos.

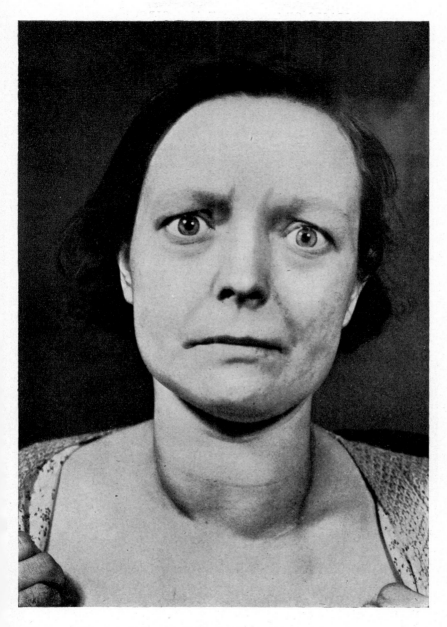

Fig. 20.03—Lid retraction and characteristic thyrotoxic stare.

the white sclerotic above the iris (von Graefe, 1864). Lid-lag and lid-retraction were for a long time attributed to stimulation of the sympathetic reinforcement of the levator palpabræ superioris (von Graefe, 1864), but if sympathetic stimulation were responsible, the lower lid would also be retracted, which it is not (Pochin, 1937–8, 1939). Moreover, both exophthalmos and lid-retraction may occur when the ocular sympathetic is paralysed (Brain, 1939). In the light of these findings von Graefe's hypothesis is untenable.

The characteristic stare has already been mentioned. It is more than lid retraction and infrequent blinking (Stellwag's sign); it is a look which may occur independently and which can be recognised with experience. The other eye-signs of the textbooks are less important: failure to wrinkle the forehead when the eyes are cast up (Joffroy's sign) may depend upon lid-retraction and exophthalmos; divergent strabismus as the eyes focus on an approaching object (Moebius' sign) may be due to weakness of the oculomotor muscles as a result of stretching.

2. *The hands*. The hands are warm, pink, and slightly moist on both surfaces; they are restless and expressive, and may show a fine, even, constant tremor. In contrast, the hands of a psychoneurotic are cold and clammy, being wet on the palms but not at the back; they tend to be inert and expressionless; tremor is coarse, irregular and inconstant.

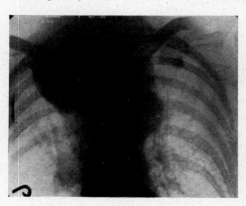

Fig. 20.04—Substernal goitre revealed by X-rays.

3. *The goitre*. If a goitre is not seen, it may be discovered by palpation. It is best to stand behind the patient, and to place the thumbs behind the sternomastoids, and the fingers in front. On asking the patient to swallow, a nodular swelling may be felt moving upwards. Posterior enlargement may be detected readily with this technique. Practically all cases of thyrotoxicosis have a goitre, although it is sometimes difficult to demonstrate (so-called masked hyperthyroidism). In such instances, it may become more convincing after a course of Lugol's iodine. Occasionally it is substernal and may be revealed by fluoroscopy (fig. 20.04).

The goitre of thyrotoxic heart disease is commonly nodular, irregular and asymmetrical. It may displace the trachea to one side, and the common carotid artery to the other, and on rare occasions it may compress the trachea, causing cough, dyspnœa, and stridor. Sudden enlargement is usually due to hæmorrhage within a nodule or cyst. Degenerated nodules may become calcified.

Primary exophthalmic goitres are uniformly enlarged, smooth, and fleshy

They are similar to simple hyperplastic goitres, but more vascular. Sometimes an arteriovenous continuous thrill and murmur may be detected over the gland. Colloid goitres are also smooth and symmetrical; but they are harder and, as a rule, larger. After a course of iodine, primary exophthalmic goitre may feel like colloid goitre. Nodular goitre should be distinguished from other causes of thyroid enlargement and from other swellings in the neck.

Fœtal adenoma (Wolfler, 1883), whether regarded as a true neoplasm arising in nests of embryonic epithelial cells, or as an ordinary hyperplastic nodule in which the vesicles are unusually small and devoid of colloid (Joll, 1932), presents clinically as a firm smooth single tumour within the substance of the thyroid gland. It is usually innocent.

What were believed to have been *malignant changes* were found by Wilson (1921) and by Speese and Brown (1921) in about 5 per cent of all goitres that were surgically removed, but their histological criteria have been disputed and the true incidence of malignancy is probably lower. In non-toxic goitres it may be between 1 and 4 per cent (Lerman, 1944), but in toxic nodular goitre it is extremely rare. Thus Means (1937) said he had not seen a single case, and Crile (1936) met no instance of toxicity amongst 249 malignant cases. Malignancy should be suspected when a goitre grows rapidly, becomes unduly hard, causes dysphagia, involves the recurrent laryngeal nerve, surrounds and buries the common carotid artery, obstructs the internal jugular vein, causes pain by involving adjacent sensory nerves, or when fixation can be demonstrated. Enlargement of neighbouring cervical lymph glands is particularly suggestive. Metastases are found especially in the lungs and bone.

Riedel's disease (Riedel, 1896) may be readily confused with malignant disease clinically. It is characterised by a brawny induration of part or all of the thyroid gland, sometimes involving surrounding tissues. It is a slow fibrotic process of unknown etiology, affecting individuals of either sex and of any age. Pain, dyspnœa, dysphagia, huskiness of the voice and obstruction of neighbouring vessels occur, and the gland is soon fixed; but lymph nodes are not enlarged and thyrotoxic symptoms are unusual.

Lymphadenoid goitre (Hashimoto's disease) is seen particularly in women over the age of 45. The whole gland is involved from the start, surrounding structures are not affected, and myxœdema usually develops (Joll, 1932). Microscopically, acinar remnants are scattered among masses of lymphoid tissue.

Acute thyroiditis may complicate a variety of infections, but is rare. It may be suppurative or non-suppurative according to the nature of the invading organism and to the severity of the attack. Clinically it is characterised by a painful, tender, uniform swelling of the gland accompanied by fever. Cellulitis with or without suppuration may invade surrounding tissues. Thyrotoxic symptoms may be associated, but usually subside with the inflammation.

Thyroglossal cyst is essentially a mid-line structure, developing from remnants of the thyroglossal duct, and moves upwards when the tongue is protruded. It is of cosmetic rather than medical significance.

4. *Cardiovascular signs*. Vasodilatation in the skin and muscle is nearly always present, and may be recognised by hot extremities, distended forearm veins, throbbing digital vessels, capillary pulsation, modified water-hammer pulse, and raised pulse pressure. Tachycardia is the rule, and persists during sleep (Boas, 1932). The action of the heart is vigorous, the cardiac impulse being forceful and displaced a little to the left, and the heart sounds slapping. A systolic murmur may be heard at apex or base, and a thrill may be felt on compressing the carotid or subclavian artery. Rarely, a functional mitral diastolic murmur may be heard.

Auricular fibrillation may be initiated by overdosage of thyroxine in patients with normal hearts. It occurs in 10 per cent of all cases of thyrotoxicosis, and in 84 to 96 per cent of those with cardiac failure, and may be paroxysmal or persistent. It is rare in young subjects, but becomes progressively frequent with advancing years. During attacks the ventricular rate is apt to be very fast, and the patient may complain of violent palpitations.

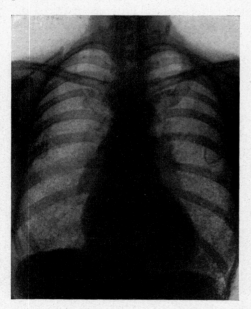

Fig. 20.05—Skiagram showing slight prominence of the aortic knuckle and of the left pulmonary arc in a case of thyrotoxicosis.

Cardiac enlargement and failure are also relatively late developments, and are unusual with normal rhythm, but often follow the onset of auricular fibrillation. An appreciable proportion of such cases (over 50 per cent according to Magee and Smith, 1935) are complicated by hypertension or other forms of heart disease.

X-rays may show slight prominence of both the aortic knuckle and left pulmonary arc (Parkinson and Cookson, 1931), and general fullness of all chambers, probably due to the high cardiac output (fig. 20.05). The electrocardiogram may be within normal limits, unless it shows auricular fibrillation, or the voltage of P and QRS may be augmented (fig. 20.06).

5. *Other and less constant features*. Neurological signs are rare; they include exophthalmic ophthalmoplegia and myasthenia—sometimes resembling myasthenia gravis, but not responding to prostigmine. Curious

patches of local myxœdema occasionally occur on the legs, koilonychia has been described, and the skin may be unduly pigmented.

Decalcification of bone is not uncommon; a negative calcium and nitrogen balance may be demonstrated; the blood cholesterol may be rather low; sugar tolerance may be reduced; and impairment of hepatic function has been reported.

THIOURACIL TREATMENT

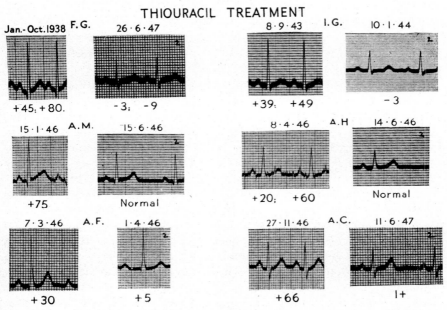

Fig. 20.06—Electrocardiograms (all lead 2) showing relatively high voltage P and QRS waves in 6 cases of thyrotoxicosis. After treatment with thiouracil the voltage falls considerably. The B.M.R. is recorded under each record.

SPECIAL INVESTIGATIONS

1. *The basal metabolic rate* (B.M.R.), introduced by Magnus-Levy in 1895, has proved a useful guide to the degree of hyperthyroidism, and is a measurement of the amount of oxygen consumed by the patient per minute when at complete rest, i.e. fourteen hours after the last meal, and after lying down undisturbed for at least half an hour. The patient breathes in and out of a closed system containing equal proportions of air and oxygen for ten minutes, carbon dioxide being removed by means of soda-lime; the amount of gas disappearing from the system represents the total amount of oxygen consumed. This is then recorded in terms of oxygen consumption per square metre of body surface per minute, and expressed as a percentage of what a normal person of the same age and sex would require. In thyrotoxicosis, the B.M.R. commonly ranges between plus 10 and plus 80 per cent. Read's formula for estimating the B.M.R. by the pulse rate and pulse pressure is unreliable, and worth no more than the knowledge that the com-

bination of tachycardia and a bounding pulse suggests a raised cardiac out-put. (Read's formula is: B.M.R. equals $\frac{3}{4}$ [pulse rate plus $\frac{3}{4}$ pulse pressure] minus 72.)

It should be understood that a single B.M.R. of plus 20 per cent does not necessarily mean that the disease is milder than one with a B.M.R. of plus 40 per cent, for the course of thyrotoxicosis is variable. Serial readings may give a truer picture of the degree of activity. Another important point is that auricular fibrillation and heart failure are more often associated with low grade activity acting over a long period of time, than with acute thyro-toxicosis, so that the level of the B.M.R. is no guide to the degree of cardiac disability.

The B.M.R. is more difficult to interpret when measured for diagnostic purposes, but if it is below plus 10 per cent thyrotoxicosis is improbable. High readings, however, may be due to faulty basal conditions or to other causes, such as leukæmia, and relatively high readings may be obtained in congestive heart failure of any etiology. According to Foote *et al.* (1952) 23 per cent of thyrotoxic patients have basal metabolic rates within the normal range.

2. *The administration of* 10 *minims* (0.6 *ml.*) *of Lugol's iodine* three times daily for a week or ten days, may be used as a test for hyperthyroidism in two ways: (1) to see whether it unmasks a goitre, for a hyperplastic gland enlarges and hardens under its influence; (2) to determine its effect on the sleeping pulse, body weight, and B.M.R., for these are beneficially in-fluenced in thyrotoxic cases, but not when the B.M.R. is raised from other causes.

3. *Measurements of the cardiac output, peripheral blood flow, and circula-tion time* provide valuable data. Outputs of 8 to 12 litres per minute are usual, and are correlated more with the heart rate than with the venous filling pressure. When the heart fails, the output drops, usually to sub-normal levels. The fore-arm blood flow is invariably increased, and usually remains so when the cardiac output falls as a result of failure; moreover, the augmented flow does not subside for several weeks after the B.M.R. has been restored to normal by means of thyroidectomy or thiouracil ther-apy (Howarth, 1948). Circulation times under 10 seconds are characteristic (Goldberg, 1938) and may remain well within normal limits when there is systemic congestion.

The demonstration of a high cardiac output at rest places a case in the hyperkinetic group: the differential diagnosis then includes severe anæmia anoxic cor pulmonale, arterio-venous aneurysm, Paget's disease of bone secondary carcinoma involving the liver or other serious hepatic disorders and beri-beri. The majority of these can be recognised or excluded at once on clinical grounds.

4. *Urinary creatine test.* Up to 200 mg. of creatine may be excreted dail in the urine by normal women and children in an irregular manner, bu very little, if any, by normal men. Excessive creatinuria occurs durin

pregnancy, and increased amounts may appear in the urine of either sex in fevers, wasting diseases and certain muscular dystrophies.

Most thyrotoxic subjects excrete an excess of creatine (Sohval, King and Reiner, 1938), and its detection may be used as a diagnostic test if the above considerations are borne in mind. Thyroid responsibility may be proved by the disappearance of creatinuria within ten days of first giving iodine or thiouracil treatment (fig. 20.07) (Schrire, 1938). On the other

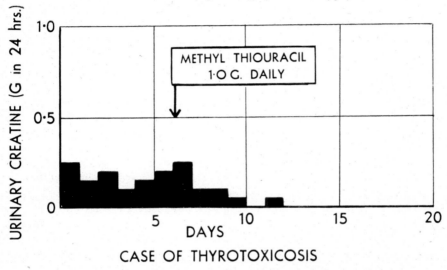

CASE OF THYROTOXICOSIS

Fig. 20.07—Effect of thiouracil on the excretion of creatine in the urine.

hand, absence of creatinuria does not exclude thyrotoxic heart disease, for such cases are apt to be associated with low grade toxicity acting over a long period of time rather than with a high degree of hyperthyroidism, and creatine excretion may be well within normal limits.

5. *Electrocardiography* may reveal abnormally high voltage of P and QRS (fig. 20.06) as previously stated. It may also be of value in proving the nature of an irregularity of rhythm, or in excluding certain other causes of a hyperkinetic circulation (e.g. pulmonary heart disease and anæmia).

6. *Radioactive iodine* (I^{131}), which has a half-life of eight days, may be given orally or intravenously in single test doses of 10 to 30 microcuries to see how the thyroid gland deals with it (Keating *et al.*, 1945). The body does not distinguish between radio-iodine and ordinary iodine. The concentration of I^{131} in liquids such as the plasma and urine can be estimated by means of liquid counters that detect the beta ray emanation; the concentration of I^{131} in any tissue zone can be estimated by means of surface Geiger-Muller counters that detect gamma rays, which unlike the soft beta rays penetrate the skin. Normally, the concentration of I^{131} in the thyroid gland reaches a maximum of about 33 per cent of the test dose in two or three days, and then slowly declines (Myant and Pochin, 1949).

Simultaneously, about 60 per cent of the test dose is excreted in the urine within two days, the actual quantities extracted by the thyroid or excreted in the urine depending on the concentration of I^{131} in the plasma. The plasma concentration necessarily falls to a very low level by the end of the second day, for 93 per cent of the test dose is by then in the thyroid gland or excreted in the urine. Subsequently, however, I^{131} again appears in the plasma, as protein-bound radiothyroxine. The more active the thyroid gland the greater the quantities of iodine extracted and radiothyroxine manufactured, the quicker the turn-over, and the less iodine excreted in the urine (Myant and Pochin, 1949); the more inactive the gland the more does the reverse hold true.

All radioactive iodine tests of thyroid function are based on these four fundamental principles:

(i) *The concentration of I^{131} in the thyroid gland* at the end of four hours in normal subjects averages 20 to 25 per cent of a 10 microcurie test dose (range 10 to 40 per cent); in thyrotoxicosis it is usually 40 to 90 per cent (Wayne, 1954). This type of test is sometimes expressed as a neck/thigh ratio, the concentration of I^{131} in the thigh serving as a control, so that the amount of iodine in the thyroid gland can be distinguished from the amount in the soft tissues of the neck (Pochin, 1950).

(ii) Thyroxine, as manufactured and released by the thyroid gland, is closely bound to protein, and when circulating in the plasma may therefore be precipitated with the plasma proteins. Radiothyroxine, of course, is similarly protein-bound. As stated above, the amount of protein-bound radiothyroxine circulating in the plasma 24 to 48 hours after a 25 microcurie test dose of I^{131} is negligible in normal subjects, being less than 0.4 per cent of the test dose per litre of plasma at the end of 48 hours; and usually less than 0.1 per cent (Goodwin et al., 1951); in thyrotoxicosis, however, it ranges between 0.04 and 3.5 per cent per litre (Wayne, 1954).

(iii) The *thyroid clearance* test is the best measure of the speed at which the thyroid gland extracts iodine from the plasma. After an intravenous test dose of 30 microcuries of I^{131} the thyroid gland normally extracts about 6 per cent of the test dose per hour when the plasma concentration is around 4 per cent of the test dose per litre; this means that 1.5 litres of plasma are cleared of radio-iodine per hour, or that the thyroid clearance is 25 ml. per minute. In normal subjects the thyroid clearance ranges between 7 and 42 ml. per minute. In thyrotoxicosis, however, iodine extraction is speeded up, and the thyroid clearance averages 240 ml. per minute, ranging between 80 and 500 (Pochin, 1950).

(iv) *The quantity of I^{131} excreted in the urine* is proportional to its concentration in the plasma, provided renal function is unimpaired. Normally, over 40 per cent of a 10 microcurie test dose is excreted in 24 hours, whereas in cases of thyrotoxicosis less than 25 per cent is usually excreted in this time (Pochin, 1950). This test is an indirect measure of the amount of I^{131} extracted by the thyroid gland during the 24 hours, for the more extracted the lower the plasma concentration and therefore the less excreted in the urine. Mason (1949) and Fraser *et al.* (1953) have shown that the urinary excretion test is more helpful if the amount of I^{131} excreted during the first six or eight hours is considered separately, for excretion is only diminished when the plasma concentration has fallen owing to increased thyroid extraction. In practice the amount of I^{131} excreted from the sixth or eighth to the twenty-fourth hour after the test dose seems to be the most sensitive index of thyroid activity. In normal subjects Mason (1949) found that 10 to 25 per cent of the test dose was excreted during the critical 6- to 24-hour period, whereas in cases of thyrotoxicosis less than 4.5 per cent was excreted during this time.

According to Wayne (1954) the most reliable of these tests is the estimation of protein-bound radiothyroxine in the plasma at 48 hours, thyroid clearance coming second, and the amount of I^{131} taken up by the thyroid gland in four hours, third.

TREATMENT

The most satisfactory method of treating thyrotoxic heart disease is subtotal thyroidectomy as developed by Dunhill (1908, 1929, 1937). The best results are obtained when physician and surgeon work in the closest harmony, success depending as much upon the skill and judgment of the physician as upon the experience and dexterity of the surgeon (Fraser and Dunhill, 1934), adequate premedication being all-important.

The patient should be put to bed, and fed on a liberal and nourishing diet. The addition of 5 to 10 mg. of aneurin daily may be helpful on the grounds that an abundant supply of this vitamin is needed for the increased carbohydrate metabolism. Fatigue and weakness may respond to 50 mg. of pyridoxine daily (Soskin and Levine, 1944). Phenobarbitone, $\frac{1}{2}$ a grain (32 mg.) t.d.s., or potassium bromide, 10 grains (0.64 G.) t.d.s., may also be prescribed with benefit, and a nocturnal sedative is usually necessary.

During this preliminary stage of treatment, which usually induces some remission of symptoms, the degree of thyrotoxicosis may be assessed clinically and by means of the special tests detailed above. Prior to the introduction of thiouracil and the newer antithyroid drugs, iodine was then given by mouth in doses of 10 minims (0.06 ml.) of Lugol's solution three times daily, preferably in milk. Within ten days there was usually marked improvement: the pulse rate fell, the B.M.R. was lowered and the patient felt better (Waller, 1914; Plummer, 1923). The moment for operation was usually ten to fourteen days after beginning iodine. Nowadays, however, preliminary treatment with antithyroid drugs is preferred (*vide infra*).

The introduction of thiouracil by Astwood (1943) following the discovery by the Mackenzies (1941) that the administration of sulphaguanidine to rats caused thyroid hyperplasia and reduction of colloid, has proved an important therapeutic advance. Thyroid hyperplasia was attributed to increased production of thyrotropic hormone by the anterior pituitary in an endeavour to compensate for deficiency of thyroid hormone brought about by sulphaguanidine. Astwood found that many substances had a similar effect, including all the sulphonamides, p-aminobenzoic acid, thiourea, and its compounds; and that of these, thiouracil offered the best prospects, being potent and relatively non-toxic. It is held that thiouracil and the other substances mentioned act by interfering with the union of iodine and tyrosine and so prevent the formation of di-iodotyrosine, a known precursor of thyroxine (Riker and Wescoe, 1945). The histological appearance of the thyroid gland under their influence resembles the hyperplastic gland of iodine deficiency.

Since then several other more potent and less toxic antithyroid drugs have been developed, and several of them have superseded thiouracil. These include methylthiouracil, propylthiouracil, and neomercazole. The initial dose of thiouracil and its derivatives is 50 to 100 mg. three times daily for two weeks, followed by 25 to 50 mg. two or three times daily thereafter (Astwood, 1949). Neomercazole (Lawson et al., 1951) is in a different category, the equivalent dose being only 10 mg. two or three times daily initially and 5 mg. once or twice daily for maintenance.

Extensive trials have established what may be expected from treatment with antithyroid drugs (Astwood, 1944; Williams, 1944, 1946; Himsworth, 1948; Goodwin et al., 1954). Amelioration of all symptoms, except exophthalmos and those due to the size of the goitre, and objective evidence of reduced thyroxine output can be demonstrated in 90 per cent of cases, but when the drug is withheld after a year or so, there is a 2 : 1 chance in favour of relapse within forty-eight months (Goodwin et al., 1954). Moreover, toxic symptoms such as fever, dermatitis, purpura, adenopathy, and agranulocytosis, which develop in 13 per cent of cases having thiouracil (Van Winkle, 1946), prevent long-term treatment even with the less toxic propylthiouracil or neomercazole in about 5 per cent of cases. The mortality from agranulocytosis due to thiouracil is 0.5 per cent (Moore, 1946). Increasing exophthalmos and the development of a highly vascular expanding goitre are attributed to over-activity of the pituitary thyrotropic hormone in response to subnormal thyroxine output and may be prevented by the simultaneous administration of a maintenance dose of thyroid (Williams and Bissell, 1943) or thyroxine (Fraser and Wilkinson, 1953).

Despite the high relapse rate, antithyroid drugs may be the treatment of choice in acute cases of primary Grave's disease in young people. It is usually unsatisfactory in the long run in well established cases of toxic nodular goitre, relapse in this group being more or less inevitable when the drug is withheld.

The antithyroid drugs, however, have proved invaluable for preparing patients for partial thyroidectomy, and if L-thyroxine sodium 0.1 to 0.3 mg. daily or thyroid gr. 1 to 3 daily is given in addition, increased vascularity of the gland can be avoided. Lugol's iodine may be used instead of thyroid for the same purpose (Means, 1946), but is probably less efficient. The great advantage of the antithyroid drugs over Lugol's iodie-in preparing patients for operation is the abolition of the sense of urgency, for patients do not relapse while taking antithyroid drugs.

Cardiac complications do not contraindicate partial thyroidectomy (Dunhill, 1937). More careful preparation, however, is needed; auricular fibriln lation must be controlled and heart failure relieved before it is safe to operate, but normal rhythm should not be deliberately restored at this stage.

The commonest post-operative complication used to be paroxysmal auricular fibrillation with rapid ventricular rate, but this is less frequent if the patient is prepared with an antithyroid substance. It should not occasion undue alarm, for the rhythm usually reverts to normal spontaneously within 48 hours. If auricular fibrillation persists, however, whether previously well established or of recent onset, every effort should be made to restore normal rhythm by means of quinidine before the patient leaves hospital. The risk of embolism is slight, perhaps because the hyperkinetic circulation lessens the chance of venous thrombosis.

Treatment with radioactive iodine

Deep X-ray therapy was curative in about a third of cases, resulted in some improvement in a third, and was without benefit in the remainder (Means and Holmes, 1923). In the treatment of thyrotoxicosis it has now been wholly superseded by radioactive iodine.

Radioactive iodine, introduced as a potent therapeutic agent by Hertz and Roberts (1942, 1946), has fulfilled its early promise (Chapman, 1948; Prinzmetal *et al.*, 1949; Moe *et al.*, 1950). Until a sufficient number of patients have lived 20 years after the irradiation the risk of subsequent carcinoma cannot be accurately assessed. In the meantime all workers are disinclined to advocate it in patients under 45 years of age with a life expectancy of at least 20 years. In older patients, in subjects with other diseases that have a relatively poor prognosis, such as V.D.H. or ischæmic heart disease, when thyroidectomy is refused or considered too dangerous, or when thyrotoxicosis has recurred post-operatively, radioactive iodine is the treatment of choice. An absolute contra-indication, however, is pregnancy, for the fœtal thyroid may concentrate I^{131} and be destroyed or seriously damaged.

The therapeutic dose of I^{131} is approximately 100 to 200 microcuries per gram of estimated thyroid mass, the exact dose depending upon the degree to which the gland concentrates radioactive iodine and the duration of its activity in the gland (Blomfield *et al.*, 1951).

The results of so treating 140 patients were reviewed after one year by Blomfield *et al.* (1955). Symptoms usually abated within three to six months, and finally 84 per cent became euthyroid, myxœdema developed in 12 per cent and 4 per cent remained thyrotoxic. There were no deaths.

The thyroid gland usually became smaller in size and exophthalmos did not increase in the series reviewed (but may do so occasionally). The only side effect was rheumatism, which occurred four to eight weeks after treatment in about 10 per cent of cases, half of them non-articular and recovering spontaneously.

These results are impressive and certainly suggest that radioactive iodine would be the treatment of choice in all cases of thyrotoxicosis if the risk of subsequent carcinoma proves to be less than 2 per cent.

Thyrotoxic crises. Owing to the impossibility of neutralising thyroid hormone that has already been manufactured, both iodine and thiouracil do not benefit the patient for several days (graphs illustrating the effect of partial thyroidectomy, iodine and thiouracil on the basal metabolic rate are remarkably similar). The treatment of thyrotoxic crises by massive doses of iodine (by mouth or intravenously) as advocated by Boland and Kepler (1938), for example, is therefore questionable. Absolute rest, heavy sedation, and replacement of salt and water lost in sweating and vomiting, are probably more important. Aneurin, 100 mg. intravenously, may also help.

If toxic goitre is recognised and treated promptly, however, crises should not occur.

Thyrotoxicosis and tonsillitis. Cases are encountered in which an attack or repeated attacks of tonsillitis are associated with thyrotoxicosis. The problem then arises whether to perform partial thyroidectomy or tonsillectomy first. Before the introduction of thiouracil most authorities agreed that it was safer to remove the thyroid gland before the tonsils, for tonsillectomy in thyrotoxic patients sometimes precipitated a crisis. Thiouracil has simplified the problem, however, and allows tonsillectomy to be undertaken first without risk.

Thyrotoxicosis and rheumatic heart disease. Thyrotoxicosis may be associated with acute rheumatic carditis or with established rheumatic valve lesions Both Parry's and Basedow's first cases were so related. The association, if more than a coincidence, is indirect, and may depend upon their joint relationship to streptococcal tonsillitis. Rheumatic heart dis-

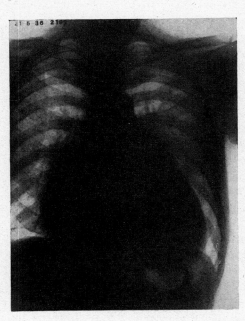

Fig. 20.08—Skiagram showing gross cardiac enlargement in a case of thyrotoxicosis plus mitral stenosis.

ease with fixed valve lesions may result in enormous enlargement of the heart owing to the excessive work induced by thyrotoxicosis (fig. 20.08), and the sooner the latter is treated the better. Radioactive iodine is ideal for these cases.

Thyrotoxicosis and hypertension. There is a group of cases, sometimes designated thyrotoxic hypertension, in which thyrotoxicosis is associated with high blood pressure, both systolic and diastolic levels being raised. There is little evidence of any direct relationship between the two diseases, and the blood pressure does not fall following thyroidectomy (Bisgard, 1939).

Thyrotoxicosis and angina pectoris. Ischæmic heart pain occurs when the blood supply to the myocardium is insufficient to meet the demand. By increasing the demand, thyrotoxicosis may induce angina in a patient with

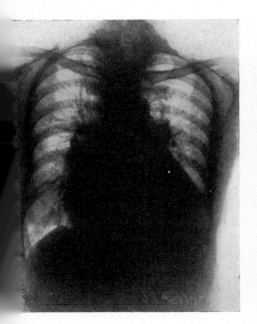 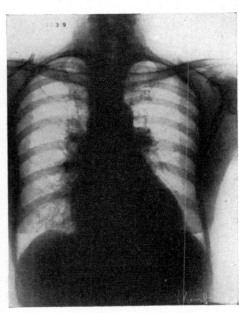

Fig. 20.09 (a)—Thyrotoxic heart failure.   (b)—After subtotal thyroidectomy.

a relatively minor degree of coronary atherosclerosis, behaving in this respect like anæmia. Thyroid hormone also sensitises the organism to adrenalin. When ischæmic and thyrotoxic heart disease are associated, angina may be completely relieved, at least temporarily, by successful treatment of the thyrotoxicosis, preferably by means of radioactive iodine.

Thyrotoxicosis and pregnancy. Thyrotoxicosis developing during pregnancy may be due to primary exophthalmic or nodular goitre. With the aid of thiouracil, in combination with small doses of iodine or thyroid, patients should be taken safely to term. If the condition does not then subside, subtotal thyroidectomy may be carried out. The danger of goitre developing in the fœtus is minimised by the iodine (or thyroid); but it is well to keep the dose of antithyroid drug as small as possible.

PROGNOSIS

There are few forms of heart disease that respond better to adequate treatment than thyrotoxic heart disease. Cases with gross congestive failure and well established auricular fibrillation may be cured, and the largest hearts may resume their normal size (fig. 20.09). On the other hand, heart failure and death are inevitable if the disease remains unchecked. In the hands of the best surgeons the mortality rate of subtotal thyroidectomy in cases of toxic nodular goitre has been 1.6 per cent (Cole, 1944) to 2.6 per cent (Dunhill, 1937); but it may be less with thiouracil preparation. No reliable figures are available upon which to assess the total relapse rate. Post-operative tetany and paralysis of the vocal cord each occurs in approximately 1 per cent (Means, 1946).

Myxœdema, which may follow otherwise successful treatment of thyrotoxicosis however accomplished, is easily controlled by a maintenance dose of thyroid gr. 3 or L-thyroxine sodium 0.3 mg. daily.

THE HEART IN MYXŒDEMA

Artificial myxœdema, produced by total ablation of the thyroid gland or by antithyroid drugs, benefits the heart by lessening the circulatory demands, and so relieves angina pectoris and congestive heart failure. Yet well developed myxœdema from natural causes gives rise to cardiac enlargement, pericardial effusion, and ultimately to congestive heart failure; moreover, angina pectoris may be associated. Enlargement cannot be due to overwork; it must depend upon some intrinsic change in the heart muscle. Histological examination, however, is usually disappointing. The fault is probably biochemical, and is unlikely to be properly understood until studies in tissue chemistry are more advanced.

The diagnosis of myxœdema is suggested by the placid sleepy character (unless there is manic psychosis), poor memory, sensitivity to cold (Raynaud's phenomenon is common), dry coarse skin, thickened lips and tongue, low thick voice, baggy eyes, scanty dry hair, podgy hands, supraclavicular pads of fat, and general pallor. It is confirmed by an impalpable thyroid gland, by a B.M.R. of minus 30 to 40 per cent, by prolongation of the arm-to-tongue circulation time to 19 to 25 seconds, by a high blood cholesterol of 300 to 400 mg. per cent, by relative insensitivity to atropine and adrenaline, by a characteristic form of anæmia, and by a pathognomonic electrocardiogram. If further proof is needed it may be obtained by demonstrating failure of the thyroid gland to extract radioactive iodine after a test dose, so that the neck : thigh ratio remains unaltered (Foote et al., 1952), a thyroid clearance of only 1 to 4 ml. per minute (Pochin, 1950), or an abnormally high urinary excretion of radio-iodine (Mason, 1949; Fraser et al., 1953). Estimation of the protein-bound radiothyroxine 48 hours after a test dose of I[131] does not distinguish myxœdema from normal controls (Wayne, 1954).

The type of anæmia that responds to thyroxine alone is normocytic and orthochromic, and may be regarded as a compensatory adjustment to diminished oxygen requirement (Bomford, 1938). The electrocardiogram shows sinus bradycardia, low voltage atrial and ventricular complexes, and flat or inverted T waves in all leads (fig. 20.10). The cause of these changes is not yet understood: they do not depend upon the presence of pericardial effusion, nor upon the state of the subcutaneous tissues. The response to thyroxine is quick and complete, and accompanies beneficial changes in the B.M.R. The electrocardiogram in cretinism behaves similarly (fig. 20.11) (Schlesinger and Landtman, 1949).

Whilst a well developed case of myxœdema is difficult to overlook (fig. 20.12), cases of short duration, especially in younger women (the sex incidence is 8 : 1 in favour of women), may easily escape notice. The diagnosis should be considered in any case of congestive heart failure or of peri-

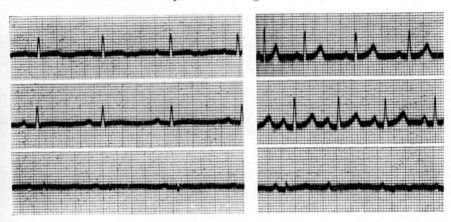

Fig. 20.10 (a) —Electrocardiogram showing sinus bradycardia, low voltage atrial and ventricular complexes and flat T waves in all leads in a case of myxœdema.
(b) Normal electrocardiogram after treatment.

cardial effusion of unknown etiology. Congestion, when it occurs, is systemic, and is associated with a low cardiac output. Pericardial effusion is due to simple transudation. Cardiac enlargement is general and pulsation of all chambers poor. Angina pectoris has been said to occur in only 1 to 2 per cent of cases (Smyth, 1938), but is surely much more frequent (Hueper, 1944, 1945). Coronary atherosclerosis may result from the high blood cholesterol. Myocardial infarction without coronary thrombosis has been described in such cases when treated too vigorously with thyroxine. The blood pressure is little influenced by myxœdema, and is as often elevated as low. When congestive failure is present, measurements of the B.M.R. give unduly high readings; more reliance should then be placed on other tests, especially on the electrocardiogram.

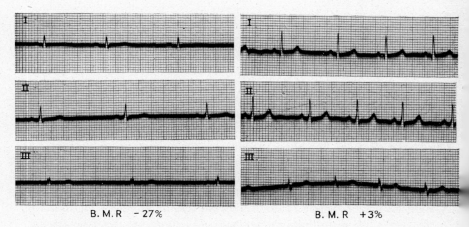

B. M. R − 27%   B. M. R +3%

Fig. 20.11—Electrocardiogram before and after treatment in a case of cretinism.

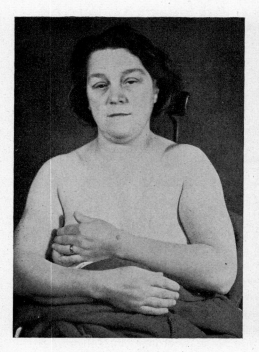
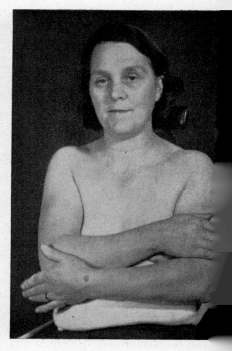

Fig. 20.12 (a)—Myxœdema.   (b) After seven weeks' treatment.

Treatment. If there is no evidence of coronary disease, thyroxine may be given intravenously in a single dose of 10 mg., or thyroid may be given by mouth in doses of 3 grains (0.2 G.) daily. The response is delayed but dramatic. Within five to ten days the B.M.R. rises, the blood cholesterol falls, the T wave begins to change, and clinical improvement is obvious. Signs of failure or of pericardial effusion soon disappear, and the heart gradually resumes its normal size (Lerman, Clark and Means, 1933).

Initial treatment is easier than maintenance. With the aid of the B.M.R. it is not difficult to regulate dosage for a patient at rest in bed; but when she leaves hospital and varies her activities, it is not so easy, and supervision is required for life. The average maintenance dose of thyroid is 3 grains (0.2 G.) daily by mouth, or 0.3 mg. of L-thyroxine sodium.

If there is any suspicion of associated coronary disease, initial treatment should be cautious, and the oral route advised. Not more than 1 grain (65 mg.) of thyroid should be given daily, and in cases with angina pectoris not more than ½ a grain (32 mg.). The dose may be increased slowly, week by week, if well tolerated, or reduced and maintained at a minimum if not tolerated.

The chief complication arising during treatment is the development of angina pectoris: should this occur the dose of thyroid may have to be less than ideal, but enough to keep the blood cholesterol below 300 mg. per cent.

REFERENCES

Astwood, E. B. (1943): "Treatment of hyperthyroidism with thiourea and thiouracil", *J. Amer. med. Ass.*, **122**, 78.
—— (1944–5): "Chemotherapy of hyperthyroidism", The Harvey Lectures, series **40**, 195.
—— (1949): "Treatment of hyperthyroidism with antithyroid compounds", *Advances in internal medicine*, **3**, 237.
——, and VanderLaan, W. P. (1945): "Thiouracil derivation of greater activity for treatment of hyperthyroidism", *J. clin. Endocrinol.*, **5**, 424.

Baumann, E. (1895): "Ueber das normale Vorkommen von Jod im Thierkorper", *Z. f. physiol. Chem.*, **21**, 319.
Bisgard, J. D. (1939): "Relation of hyperthyroidism to hypertension", *Arch. intern. Med.*, **63**, 497.
Blomfield, G. W., Jones, J. C., MacGregor, A. G., Miller, H., and Wayne, E. J. (1951): "Treatment of thyrotoxicosis with radioactive iodine", *Brit. med. J.*, ii, 373.
——, ——, ——, ——, ——; and Weetch, R. S. (1955): "Treatment of thyrotoxicosis with radioactive iodine. Review of 140 cases", *Brit. med. J.*, ii, 1223.
Boas, E. P. (1932): "Heart rate during sleep in Graves' disease and in neurogenic sinus tachycardia", *Amer. Heart J.*, **8**, 24.
Boland, E. W., and Kepler, E. J. (1938): "Crisis of exophthalmic goitre. Report case", *Proc. Mayo Clin.*, **13**, 817.
Bomford, R. R. (1938): "Anæmia in myxœdema: and rôle of thyroid gland in erythropoiesis", *Quart. J. Med.*, **7**, 495.
Brain, W. R. (1939): "Exophthalmos in Graves' disease despite sympathetic paralysis", *Lancet*, ii, 1217.

Brain, W. R., and Turnbull, N. M. (1938): "Exophthalmic ophthalmoplegia, with pathological report on ocular muscles and thyroid glands", *Quart. J. Med.*, **7**, 293.

Bruun, E. (1945): "Exophthalmic goitre developing after treatment with thyroid preparation", *Acta. med. Scand.*, **122**, 13.

Chapman, E. M. (1948): "Treatment of Graves' disease with radioactive iodine", *West. J. Surg., Obst. and Gynæ.*, **56**, 47.

Cole, W. H. (1944): "Factors influencing operability and mortality rate in goitre", *Surg.*, **16**, 688.

Crile, G., Jr. (1936): "Hyperthyroidism associated with malignant tumours of the thyroid gland", *Surg. Gynec. and Obstet.*, **62**, 995.

Dunhill, T. (1908): "The surgical treatment of exophthalmic goitre", *Intercolon. med. J. Australia*, **13**, 293.

—— (1929): "Toxic goitre", *Brit. J. Surg.*, **17**, 424.

—— (1937): "Surgery of the thyroid gland", The Lettsomian Lectures, London.

Flajani, G. (1802): "Sopra un tumor freddo nell' anterior parte del collo detto broncocele", **3**, 270, Rome.

Foote, J. B., MacKenzie, D. H., and Maclagan, N. F. (1952): "A comparison of radioactive and metabolic methods of investigating thyroid function", *Lancet, i*, 486.

Fraser, F. R., and Dunhill, T. P. (1934): "Lectures on toxic goitre", London.

Fraser, R., *et al.* (1953): "The urinary excretion of radioiodine as a clinical test of thyroid function", *Quart. J. Med.*, **22**, 99.

——, and Wilkinson, M. (1953): "Simplified method of drug treatment for thyrotoxicosis using a uniform dosage of methylthiouracil and added thyroxine", *Brit. med. J., i*, 481.

Friedberg, C. K., and Sohval, A. R. (1937): "Occurrence and pathogenesis of cardiac hypertrophy in Graves' disease", *Amer. Heart J.*, **13**, 599.

Goldberg, S. J. (1938): "Circulation time as diagnostic aid in hyperthyroidism", *Ann. intern. Med.*, **11**, 1818.

Goodwin, J. F., Macgregor, A. G., Miller, H., and Wayne, E. J. (1951): "The use of radioactive iodine in the assessment of thyroid function", *Quart. J. Med.*, **20**, 353.

——, Steinberg, H., and Wilson, A. (1954): "Long-term therapy of thyrotoxicosis with thiouracil compounds", *Brit. med. J., i*, 422.

Graves, R. J. (1835): "Newly observed affection of the thyroid gland in females", *London med. and surg. J.*, **7**, 516.

Harington, C. R. (1933): "The thyroid gland", London.

——, and Barger, G. (1927): "Chemistry of thyroxine. II. Constitution and synthesis of thyroxine", *Biochem. J.*, **21**, 169.

Hertz, S., and Roberts, A. (1942): "Application of radioactive iodine in therapy of Graves' disease", *J. clin. Invest.*, **21**, 624.

——, —— (1946): "The use of radioactive iodine therapy in hyperthyroidism" *J. Amer. med. Ass.*, **131**, 81.

——, ——, and Evans, R. D. (1938): "Radioactive iodine as indicator in the study of thyroid physiology", *Proc. Soc. exper. Biol. and Med.*, **38**, 510.

Himsworth, H. P. (1948): "Thiouracil and its derivatives in the routine treatment of thyrotoxicosis", *Brit. med. J. ii*, 61.

Howarth, S. (1948): Personal communication.

Hueper, W. C. (1944): "Arteriosclerosis", *Arch. Path.*, **38**, 162, 245, 350.

—— (1945): *Ibid.*, **39**, 117, 187.

Joll, C. A. (1932): "Diseases of the thyroid gland", London.

Keating, F. R., Rawson, R. W., Peacock, W., and Evans, R. D. (1945): "Collection and loss of radio-active iodine compared with anatomic changes induced in thyroid of chick by injection of thyrotropic hormone", *Endocrinol.*, **36**, 13'

Kendall, E. C. (1915): "The isolation in crystalline form of the compound containing iodine which occurs in the thyroid; its chemical nature and physiolog activity", *J. Amer. med. Ass.*, **64**, 2042.

Kepler, E. J., and Barnes, A. R. (1932): "Congestive heart failure and hyperthrophy in hyperthyroidism. Clinical and pathological study of 178 fatal cases", *Amer. Heart J.*, **8**, 102.

Lawson, A., Rimington, C., and Searle, C. E. (1951): "Antithyroid activity of 2- carbethoxythio-1-methylglyoxaline", *Lancet, ii*, 619.
Lerman, J. (1944): "The endocrine activity of thyroid tumours and the influence of the thyroid hormone on tumours in general", *Surg.*, **16**, 266.
——, Clark, R. J., and Means, J. H. (1933): "Heart in myxœdema: electrocardiograms and roentgen-ray measurements before and after therapy", *Ann. intern. Med.*, **6**, 1251.

McCarrison, R. (1927): "Experiment in goitre prevention", *Brit. med. J.*, *i*, 94.
Mackenzie, J. B., Mackenzie, C. G., and McCollum, E. V. (1941): *Science*, **94**, 518.
Magee, H. R., and Smith, H. L. (1935): "Auricular fibrillation in hyperthyroidism; influence of age", *Amer. J. med. Sc.*, **189**, 683.
Magnus-Levy, A. (1895): "Ueber den respiratorischen Gaswechsel unter dem Einfluss der Thyreoidee sowie unter verschiedened pathologischen Zuslanden", *Berl. klin. Woch.*, **32**, 650.
Marie, P. (1883): "Sur la nature et sur quelques-uns des symptomes de la maladie de Basedow", *Arch. de Neurol.*, **6**, 79.
Marine, D. (1927): "Iodine in the treatment of diseases of the thyroid gland", *Medicine*, **6**, 127.
—— (1930): "The essential thyroid changes in goitre", *Amer. J. Path.*, **6**, 607.
——, and Lenhart, C. H. (1910): "Observations and experiments on the so-called thyroid carcinoma of brook trout (salvelinus fontinalis) and its relation to ordinary goitre", *J. exper. Med.*, **12**, 311.
——, and Rosen, S. H. (1933): "Exophthalmos in thyroidectomised guinea pigs by thyrotropic substance of anterior pituitary, and the mechanism involved", *Proc. Soc. exper. Biol. and Med.*, **30**, 901.
Mason, A. S. (1949): "Urinary excretion of radioactive iodine as a measure of thyroid activity", *Proc. Roy. Soc. Med.*, **42**, 961; and *Lancet, ii*, 456.
Means, J. H. (1937): "The thyroid and its diseases", Philadelphia.
—— (1946): "Evaluation of the several methods for treating Graves' disease available to-day", *Ann. intern. Med.*, **25**, 403.
——, and Holmes, G. W. (1923): "Further observations on the Roentgen-ray treatment of toxic goitres", *Arch. intern. Med.*, **31**, 303.
——, and Richardson, E. P. (1938): "The diagnosis and treatment of diseases of the thyroid", New York.
Moe, R. H., Adams, E. E., Rule, J. H., Moore, M. C., Kearns, J. E., Jr., and Clark, D. E. (1950): "An evaluation of radioactive iodine in the treatment of hyperthyroidism", *J. clin. Endocrinol.*, **10**, 1022.
Moebius, P. J. (1886): "Ueber Insufficienz der Konvergenz bei morbus Basedowii, *Centralbl. f. nerventik. u. Psychiat.*, **9**, 356.
Moore, F. D. (1946): "Toxic manifestations of thiouracil therapy: a co-operative study", *J. Amer. med. Ass.*, **130**, 315.
Myant, N. B. (1952): "Radioiodine tests of thyroid function in man", *Brit. med. Bull.*, **8**, 141.
——, and Pochin, E. E. (1949): "The thyroid clearance rate of plasma iodine as a measure of thyroid activity", *Proc. Roy. Soc. Med.*, **42**, 959.
——, Honour, A. J., and Pochin, E. E. (1949): "Estimation of radioiodine in thyroid gland of living subjects", *Clin. Sci.*, **8**, 135.

Oswald, A. (1899): "Die Eiweisskorper der Schilddrüse", *Z. f. physiol. chem.*, **27**, 14.

Parkinson, J., and Cookson, H. (1931): "Size and shape of heart in goitre", *Quart. J. Med.*, **24**, 499.
Parry, C. H. (1825): "Collected works", **1**, 478, London. (Extracted by Major, R. H., in "Classic descriptions of disease", Springfield, Illinois, 1932.)

Plummer, H. S. (1923): "Results of administering iodine to patients having exophthalmic goitre", *J. Amer. med. Ass.*, 80, 1955.

Pochin, E. E. (1937–8): "Unilateral retraction of upper lid in Graves' disease", *Clin. Sc.*, 3, 197.

—— (1939): "Ocular effects of sympathetic stimulation in man", *Ibid.*, 4, 79.

—— (1939): "Mechanism of lid-retraction in Graves' disease", *Ibid.*, 4, 91.

—— (1950): "The investigation of thyroid function and disease with radioactive iodine", *Lancet*, ii, 41, 84.

Prinzmetal, M., Agress, C. M., Bergman, H. C., and Simkin, B. (1949): "The use of radioactive iodine in the treatment of Graves' disease", *California Medicine, San Francisco*, 70, 235.

Rake, G., and McEachern, D. (1932): "Study of heart in hyperthyroidism", *Amer. Heart J.*, 8, 19.

Riedel (1896): "Die chronische, zur Bildun eisenharter Tumoren fuhrende Enzundung der Schilddrüse", *Verhandl. d. deut. Ges. f. Chir.*, 25, 101.

Riker, W. F., and Wescoe, W. C. (1945): "The pharmacology and therapeutic application of anti-thyroid compounds", *Amer. J. med. Sc.*, 210, 665.

Schlesinger, B., and Landtman, B. (1949): "Electrocardiographic studies in cretins", *Brit. Heart J.*, 11, 237.

Schrire, I. (1948): "The effect of 2-thiouracil on the creatinuria of thyrotoxicosis and its use in the diagnosis of thyrotoxicosis", *Clin. Sc.*, 7, 49.

Shaw, R. C. (1929): "Cervical sympathetic and its relation to thyroid gland in exophthalmic goitre", *Brit. med. J.*, i, 495.

Smyth, C. J. (1938): "Angina pectoris and myocardial infarction as complications of myxœdema", *Amer. Heart J.*, 15, 652.

Sohval, A. R., King, F. H., and Rainer, M. (1938): "The creatine tolerance test in the diagnosis of Graves' disease and allied conditions", *Amer. J. med. Sc.*, 195, 608.

Soskin, S., and Levine, R. (1944): "Recent advances in physiology of the thyroid and their clinical application", *Arch. intern. Med.*, 74, 375.

Speese, J., and Brown, H. P., Jr. (1921): "Malignant degeneration in benign tumours of the thyroid gland", *Ann. Surg.*, 74, 684.

Van Winkle, W. (1946): "Clinical toxicity of thiouracil; survey of 5,745 cases", *J. Amer. med. Ass.*, 130, 343.

von Basedow, C. A. (1840): "Exophthalmos durch Hypertrophie das Zellgewebes in der Augenhohle", *Wochenschrift fur die gesammte Heilkunde*, Berlin, 28th March.

von Graefe, A. (1864): "Concerning Basedow's disease", *Deutsch. Klinik.*, 16, 158.

Waller, H. E. (1914): "On the value of iodine, taken internally, in Graves' disease", *Prescriber*, 8, 153.

Wayne, E. J. (1954): "The diagnosis of thyrotoxicosis", *Brit. med. J.*, i, 411.

acil", *Arch. intern. Med.*, 74, 479.

Williams, R. H. (1944): "Antithyroid drugs with particular reference to thiouracil", *Arch. intern. Med.*, 74, 479.

—— (1946): "Thiouracil treatment of thyrotoxicosis. I. Results of prolonged treatment", *J. clin. Endocrinol.*, 6, 1.

Williams, R., and Bissell, J. (1943): "Treatment of hyperthyroidism with thiouracil", *New Engl. J. Med.*, 229, 97.

Wilson, L. B. (1921): "Malignant tumours of the thyroid", *Ann. Surg.*, 74, 129.

Wolfler, A. (1883): "Uber die Entwickelung und den Bau des Kropfes", *Arch. f. klin. Chir.*, 29, 1, 754.

Zondek, H., and Ticho, A. (1945): "Observations on so-called thyrotropic exophthalmos", *Brit. med. J.*, i, 836.

CHAPTER XXI

HYPERKINETIC CIRCULATORY STATES

(ANÆMIA, PREGNANCY, ARTERIO-VENOUS FISTULA, BERI-BERI, PAGET'S DISEASE OF BONE, HEPATIC FAILURE)

IN addition to the diseases enumerated above, hyperkinetic circulatory states (Harrison, 1935) include thyrotoxicosis, anoxic cor pulmonale, fever and exercise. The first two have been considered fully elsewhere, and the last two have a purely physiological basis.

All these conditions are characterised by a raised cardiac output maintained by means of tachycardia, a raised venous filling pressure, or both; moreover the heart may beat more strongly. Conspicuous evidence of vasodilatation in skin and muscle is found in all of them: the skin is warm and flushed, the forearm veins are distended, the pulse is bounding, the digital vessels throb, and there may be capillary pulsation. The forearm and calf blood flows are increased. Whilst young and healthy hearts may cope with the situation without distress, older or unhealthy hearts may fail to meet the requirements. The chief symptoms are palpitations and breathlessness.

It may be difficult clinically to recognise congestive failure in these cases, for the usual signs may have other interpretations. Thus, a raised venous pressure may be part of the physiological mechanism maintaining a high cardiac output (McMichael, 1947), enlargement of the liver may be due to secondary carcinoma or to hepatitis, and œdema is commonplace in severe anæmia and beri-beri for other reasons. Indeed, it is by no means easy to be sure what is meant by failure in this group; for example, McMichael uses the term "high output failure" to describe a state in which a raised venous pressure and œdema are associated with a high cardiac output, whether or not the latter is capable of being raised further. Yet failure ordinarily denotes an overloaded heart or ventricle, one incapable of raising its output further. But this question has already been discussed (page 264).

THE HEART IN ANÆMIA

Physiology. Severe chronic or post-hæmorrhagic anæmia may affect the heart in three ways: (i) it may cause a hyperkinetic circulatory state as described above; (ii) it may cause or precipitate angina pectoris or acute coronary insufficiency; (iii) it may result in nutritional degenerative changes in the cardiac muscle, which may reduce its reserve.

With an oxygen consumption of 240 ml. per minute, an anæmic subject with a hæmoglobin of 20 per cent could not have a cardiac output less than

6 litres per minute if all the available oxygen were utilised (20 per cent Hb.=3 G. Hb. per cent=3×1.34 ml. oxygen per cent=4 ml. oxygen per cent or 40 ml. per litre. Thus cardiac output $= \dfrac{240}{40} = 6$ litres per minute). If half the available oxygen were utilised the cardiac output would be 12 litres per minute.

In anæmic subjects investigations have shown that the resting cardiac output may reach 13 litres per minute and utilisation of available oxygen may be increased from the normal 33 per cent to as much as 90 per cent (Liljestrand and Stenstrom, 1925–6; Nielson, 1934; Sharpey-Schafer, 1944). These changes do not occur at rest with hæmoglobin values above 50 per cent, but become increasingly apparent at lower levels (Bouchut and Froment, 1934). The high cardiac output is maintained both by tachycardia and a raised venous pressure. The latter must be due to widespread capillary or peripheral venoconstriction, for the blood volume is reduced (McMichael et al., 1943), and the small arteries and arterioles are dilated (McMichael, 1947).

Clinical features. The chief symptoms of severe anæmia are breathlessness, fatigue and palpitations. Angina pectoris occurs in about 30 per cent (Coombs, 1926; Pickering and Wayne, 1934), occasionally even when there is no underlying coronary disease. Thus the author has treated a boy of 17 with pernicious anæmia and angina pectoris, and also a young man of 21 who presented himself with classical ischæmic heart pain due to iron deficiency anæmia resulting from bleeding hæmorrhoids. Œdema may be due to congestive heart failure, but is more often nutritional. It is especially prone to develop during the first three weeks of blood regeneration in response to treatment of the anæmia.

Paroxysmal cardiac dyspnœa or acute pulmonary œdema is rare as a spontaneous event, but may arise during blood transfusion or saline infusion. These procedures should not be lightly undertaken in cases of severe chronic or post-hæmorrhagic anæmia: precautionary measures include the use of concentrated red cells instead of whole blood, and venous pressure lowering agents, such as cuffs applied to the thighs. Transfusion should be temporarily abandoned if the venous pressure is seen to rise appreciably.

Physical signs. A hyperkinetic circulation and peripheral vasodilatation may be recognised by the features detailed previously.

A functional systolic murmur (so-called hæmic murmur) at apex or base is common, and is due to the increased blood flow through the aortic and pulmonary valves. Functional mitral or aortic diastolic murmurs may also be heard occasionally, earlier observations such as those by Von Noorden (1891), Sahli (1895) and Kraus (1905), having been amply and repeatedly confirmed (Goldstein and Boas, 1927). Mitral presystolic or d¹astolic murmurs are probably due directly or indirectly to the increased velocity of blood flow, the mechanism being the same as that responsible for mitral diastolic murmurs in patent ductus arteriosus, ventricular septal defect and thyrotoxicosis. Basal diastolic murmurs are attributed to dilatation of the aortic or pulmonary ring.

The electrocardiogram. Despite several publications emphasising the normality of the electrocardiogram in anæmia (e.g. Smith, 1933; Pickering and Wayne, 1934), there can be no doubt that significant changes occur in at least a third of cases with hæmoglobin values under 40 per cent (Block, 1937). In a consecutive series of twenty such cases analysed by the author,

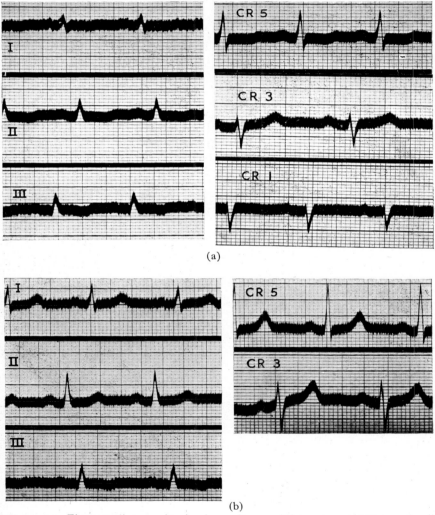

(a)

(b)

Fig. 21.01—Electrocardiogram showing low voltage and flat or inverted T wave in all leads in a case of pernicious anæmia.

(a) Before treatment.
(b) After correction.

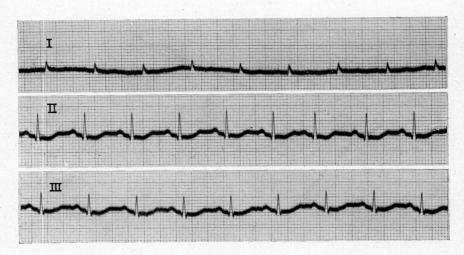

Fig. 21.02—Electrocardiogram showing depression of the ST segment due to acute coronary insufficiency resulting from post-hæmorrhagic anæmia.

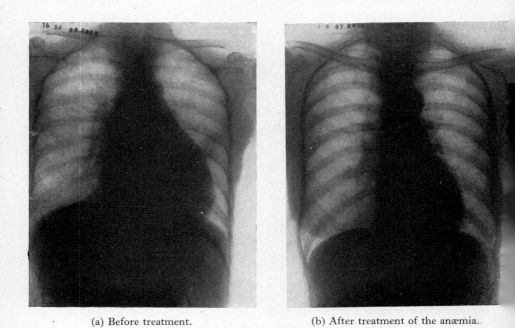

(a) Before treatment.   (b) After treatment of the anæmia.

Fig. 21.03—Skiagram showing general cardiac enlargement in a case of severe pernicious anæmia.

eight showed low voltage, depressed S-T segments, or flat or inverted T waves in left ventricular surface leads or their equivalents. As the anæmia improved under treatment these faults were corrected (fig. 21.01). Several instances of bundle branch block have also been observed, but these have always persisted when the anæmia was cured. Depression of the S-T segment is common following gross hæmorrhage, and is believed to represent temporary coronary insufficiency (fig. 21.02).

Fluoroscopy. X-rays often reveal slight enlargement of all chambers of the heart and prominence of both the aorta and pulmonary artery in cases with hæmoglobin levels below 40 per cent (fig. 21.03).

Necropsy studies have revealed slight increase of heart weight (350 to 450 G.) in the majority of cases of severe anæmia, and considerable increase occasionally (Cabot and Richardson, 1919). Experimental anæmia in rats has resulted in slight cardiac hypertrophy at hæmoglobin levels of 10 G. per cent, and considerable hypertrophy (weight at least twice normal) at levels of 2 to 3 G. per cent (Forman and Daniels, 1930–1). According to Grunberg (1930), hypertrophy is invariable in man when the hæmoglobin is 15 per cent or less, and does not occur at all when the hæmoglobin is 66 per cent or more.

These findings harmonise with the behaviour of the cardiac output in relation to hæmoglobin levels, and there can be little doubt that enlargement depends on increased work.

Clinical diagnosis. Knowledge of cardiovascular behaviour is of little value in making a diagnosis of anæmia, and is of no value at all in determining the nature of the anæmia. It is helpful, however, in differential diagnosis, especially between anæmia, the anxiety states, and bacterial endocarditis. Thus, an anxiety state may present with the same group of symptoms, including pallor, and there may be cardiac over-action and functional systolic murmurs. The pallor, however, is due to peripheral vasoconstriction, and does not affect the conjunctivæ or the mucous membranes, and it is less obvious in the palms of the hands; the nail beds too are more likely to be cyanosed than pale. In anæmia, pallor is often waxy, chalky, or lemon tinted according to its severity and type. The cardiovascular dynamics are quite different. Over-action of the heart and tachycardia in the anxiety states are associated with little or no rise in cardiac output; there is peripheral vasoconstriction rather than vasodilatation, and the diastolic blood pressure tends to be raised in casual readings; the stroke-volume tends to be reduced, and the pulse may be small; the circulation time and venous pressure are normal. There are, however, exceptions to this general pattern, about 10 per cent of patients with an anxiety state having a hyperkinetic circulation probably caused by an excess of circulating adrenaline.

A type of case that may cause confusion is one that presents with pallor, low-grade fever, petechiæ, splenomegaly, over-action of the heart, and a loud systolic murmur at apex or base. Bacterial endocarditis may be suspected, especially when there is a diastolic basal murmur as well, and the pulse is collapsing; yet all these features may be due to anæmia alone.

Treatment. All cardiovascular changes due to anæmia are reversible, if the anæmia is treated successfully. Cardiac remedies are rarely required, apart from urgent measures in the event of acute pulmonary œdema. The danger of ill-judged or too rapid intravenous infusion has already been mentioned.

THE HEART IN PREGNANCY

PHYSIOLOGY

There is now sufficient evidence to state with confidence that the hyperkinetic circulation of pregnancy begins to develop during the second month, is well established by the end of the third month, increases slightly and gradually to the thirty-second week, and thereafter declines. Much of this evidence has been summarised by Morgan Jones (1951).

Clinically the palms flush, the extremities are hot, the digital vessels throb, capillary pulsation may be demonstrated, the pulse is full and bounding, the heart rate quickens, the venous pressure rises, the soft tissues become more tense, and there may be slight œdema. The heart itself is hyperdynamic: the cardiac impulse is forcible and displaced slightly to the left, aortic and pulmonary systolic murmurs heard at apex and base advertise the increased blood flow, a loud third sound confirms rapid ventricular filling, and X-rays may reveal slight diastolic enlargement. Ectopic beats are common. The electrocardiogram often shows a prominent S wave in lead I and a conspicuous Q wave and inverted T wave in lead III (fig. 21.04), due to rotation of the heart.

Special tests reveal the following:

(1) Oxygen consumption is increased by 15 to 20 per cent (Burwell, 1937, 1938).

(2) The cardiac output increases by 50 per cent (Palmer and Walker, 1949; Hamilton, 1949).

(3) Retention of sodium and water results in considerable hæmodilution, the increase of plasma volume reaching a maximum of 45 per cent above normal by the thirty-second week (Cohen and Thomson, 1936; Thomson *et al.*, 1938), after which diuresis sets in (Chesley, 1943).

(4) The general venous pressure rises as a result of the increased blood volume, sometimes considerably; the venous pressure in the legs is particularly high owing to the local obstructing effect of the enlarged uterus (Burwell *et al.*, 1938). Compression of the inferior vena cava is common in the supine position, and the fall in right atrial pressure and cardiac output that may result from pooling of blood in the legs may cause faintness and seriously interfere with physiological studies.

The circulatory effects of pregnancy are attributed chiefly to the increased blood volume, whilst the rise in oxygen consumption and a uterine arterio-venous shunt (Burwell, 1938) are contributory.

Whilst the normal heart tolerates the added load easily enough, diseased hearts may not. When trouble occurs it usually *begins* early, often by the end of the third month. The *onset* of heart failure proper occurs with increasing frequency up to the end of the thirty-second week, after which it steadily declines (Hamilton and Thomson, 1942).

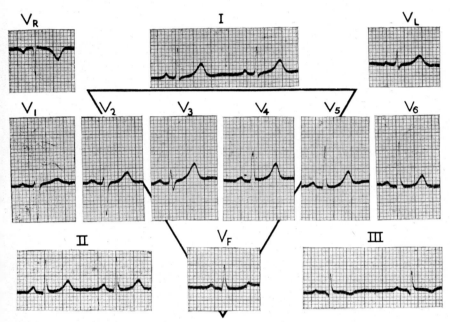

Fig. 21.04—Electrocardiogram showing characteristic appearances associated with pregnancy.

Frequency and types of heart disease associated with pregnancy

Heart disease was recognised in 1.3 per cent of 80,422 pregnant women analysed by Haig and Gilchrist (1949). Of their 1,100 heart cases 94 per cent were rheumatic, 3.6 per cent congenital, 1.8 per cent hypertensive and 0.6 per cent miscellaneous. Similar figures (see table) have been published by Hamilton (1935), Morgan Jones (1951) and many others.

Hypertension associated with toxæmia of pregnancy is obviously excluded from these statistics, since this occurs in 5 per cent of all pregnancies. Toxæmia is particularly dangerous in cases of heart disease, not because of the hypertension (except in relatively rare cases of hypertensive heart disease), but because of the sodium and water retention.

The mortality from heart disease in pregnancy averages 4.5 per cent (Jensen, 1938; Jones, 1951), but naturally varies greatly according to the

NO. OF PREGNANT WOMEN WITH HEART DISEASE	NATURE OF HEART DISEASE (frequency per cent)				AUTHORS
	RHEUMATIC	CONGENITAL	HYPER-TENSIVE	MISC.	
1,335	93	5.2	—	1.8	Hamilton (1935)
1,100	94	3.6	1.8	0.6	Haig and Gilchrist (1949)
485	90	6.8	2.1	1.1	Morgan Jones (1951)

severity of the lesion. If patients are classified according to their grade of previous effort intolerance as defined on page 521, then the mortality from heart disease increases from about 0.4 per cent in grades 0 to 2A, 5.3 per cent in grade 2B, and 22.6 per cent in grades 3 and 4 (Jensen, 1938). These figures were based on 1,428 cases collected from the literature, over 90 per cent of them rheumatic. Hamilton (1947) reported somewhat similar figures in a series of 1,335 cases of heart disease in pregnancy (93 per cent rheumatic): the mortality in grades 0 to 2A was 2 per cent, as it was in non-pregnant controls with heart disease of similar degree, whereas in grades 2B to 4 the mortality was 18 per cent, compared with 6.7 per cent in non-pregnant controls. When there was atrial fibrillation the maternal mortality was 32 per cent (8 per cent in non-pregnant controls).

Infant mortality should also be considered. In Hamilton's series this was 8.6 per cent in the favourable group, 31 per cent in the unfavourable group, and 50 per cent when there was atrial fibrillation.

Figure 21.05, which has been constructed from data published by Jensen (1938), shows that mortality increases steadily throughout pregnancy and reaches its climax during labour itself and the ensuing 24 hours,

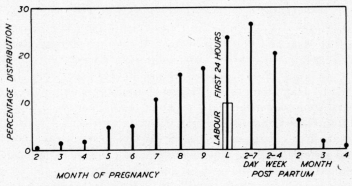

Fig. 21.05—Chart showing when death occurs in fatal cases of heart disease associated with pregnancy.

nearly 24 per cent of the 462 deaths analysed occurring at this time; but the puerperium is also dangerous, 26 per cent of the deaths occurring between the second and seventh day after delivery, and 20 per cent during the next fortnight. Werkö (1954) regards the first 48 hours after delivery as the most dangerous period.

The commonest causes of death are congestive heart failure (36 per cent) and pulmonary œdema (27.5 per cent) (Jensen, 1938). The latter is chiefly responsible for death during pregnancy, the former for death during or after delivery (Morgan Jones, 1951).

General Management

Irrespective of the type of heart disease present the following general rules are widely accepted:

1. Patients with grade 0 to 1 effort intolerance should not ordinarily be dissuaded from having a family and should experience little extra trouble during pregnancy and the puerperium.

2. Patients with grade 2B to 4 effort intolerance, who cannot be radically improved by present methods of treatment, should be advised not to have a family, and pregnancy should be terminated within the first three months if already present. If the nature of the cardiac lesion is beyond foreseeable therapeutic developments sterilisation should also be carried out, but not otherwise. If the pregnancy is already advanced it is usually best to allow it to continue to its natural conclusion.

3. Patients with grade 2A effort intolerance should be considered individually, and social factors may be taken into account.

4. If the cardiac lesion calls for surgical treatment, the operation is best undertaken before pregnancy; if the patient is already pregnant, the operation should be carried out without delay if effort intolerance is grade 2B or more, or deferred for a year or so if effort intolerance is grade 0 to 2A. The pregnancy itself should not be terminated and sterilisation is unjustified.

5. The best means of combating the adverse effect of pregnancy on the cardiovascular system is the low sodium diet, supported if necessary by mercurial diuretics, mictine, diamox or resins. Digitalis is not indicated when pulmonary œdema is due to mitral stenosis, but is helpful in cases of atrial fibrillation and congestive heart failure. Prolonged rest, preferably in bed, should be enforced until the situation is well in control.

RHEUMATIC HEART DISEASE AND PREGNANCY

There are some who maintain that any woman who has rheumatic heart disease should be advised against having any children. They argue that pregnancy affects her adversely and that the strain of bringing up children shortens her life. Others feel that to forfeit so much human happiness on these grounds is both undesirable and unnecessary. Is life so precious to prolong if so much of its meaning is taken away? Moreover, available statistics barely support the first argument. Thus in four combined series collected by Jensen (1938), the average age of death in spinsters or nulliparous women with mitral stenosis was 36.6; in married women with families it was 40.3. Again, Bunim and Rubricius (1948) could find no significant difference in the life histories of 169 rheumatic mothers and 215 rheumatic childless women. Of course, the childless women may have been advised against pregnancy owing to the severity of their condition, so that the two groups may not be strictly comparable: there is insufficient evidence on this point. It is certain, however, that many women with mitral stenosis, unaware that there is anything wrong with them, have large families and lead normal lives, until the lesion is discovered in later life.

Over 90 per cent of all cases of heart disease associated with pregnancy are rheumatic, and at least four-fifths of these have mitral valve disease, usually stenosis. The increased blood volume and raised cardiac output result in further elevation of the left atrial pressure, and since the rapidity of the change leaves little time for the development of physiologically protective mechanisms, hæmoptysis and acute pulmonary œdema are relatively common. Less frequently, and chiefly in those with a high pulmonary vascular resistance, uncontrolled atrial fibrillation, myocardial fibrosis, or active rheumatic carditis, the extra load results in congestive heart failure. Pulmonary embolism increases the mortality during the puerperium.

The majority of patients with uncomplicated mitral stenosis who experience serious trouble during pregnancy *begin* to develop symptoms of increasing pulmonary "congestion" towards the end of the third month; conversely, if all is well at the end of the first trimester without prophylactic treatment, little trouble is likely to arise later. Clinically, when assessing the physiological situation, due allowance must be made for the fact that 60 per cent of normal women experience breathlessness during pregnancy (Hamilton and Thomson, 1942), and that a slight rise of venous pressure is normal.

When considering the question of future pregnancy in cases of rheumatic heart disease it is vitally important to make sure whether surgical treatment is possible or not. In cases of *aortic or mitral incompetence*, for example, pregnancy should be avoided or terminated within the first few months if effort intolerance is grade 2A or more, for these lesions cannot yet be corrected surgically, and any deterioration may well prove disastrous; moreover, both aortic and mitral incompetence must be advanced before grade 2 effort intolerance develops.

Cases of mitral stenosis, on the other hand, are relatively safe: if symptoms are already moderate or severe, valvotomy should be carried out before pregnancy; if effort intolerance is only grade 1 to 2A and the pulmonary vascular resistance normal, valvotomy should be deferred and pregnancy allowed to take its natural course; if serious symptoms then develop valvotomy may be performed during pregnancy, which need not be terminated. Cases of mitral stenosis with a raised pulmonary vascular resistance require valvotomy before pregnancy, irrespective of the grade of effort intolerance, for they are likely to develop congestive heart failure late in pregnancy or during the puerperium, with or without pulmonary embolism. When the patient is already pregnant, valvotomy should be performed as soon as possible and if the operation is technically successful the pregnancy should be allowed to continue.

Although *rheumatic aortic stenosis* may be relieved surgically, the high mortality and relatively indifferent results of the present operation are not reassuring, and patients with this lesion should be managed in respect of pregnancy like patients with aortic incompetence.

Previous statistics showing no difference in the mortality rate from mitral stenosis and the other valve lesions in relation to pregnancy do not apply now that mitral stenosis can be relieved surgically.

Normal pregnancy is safe after technically successful valvotomy in cases with previous mitral stenosis, but toxæmia can be very dangerous when there is mild residual stenosis, pulmonary œdema then occurring very readily. One of the writer's post-operative cases died under just these circumstances and necropsy revealed a partially split valve with an orifice measuring approximately 2.5 × 1 cm.

Retention of sodium and water must be countered strenuously with a rigid low sodium regime.

Cases of active rheumatic carditis are probably best terminated as soon as the state of the heart permits; for there is no knowing what the subsequent course will be, and a relapse later in pregnancy may prove very serious.

When pregnancy is not advised, prevention is best insured by a simple sterilising operation. Termination of pregnancy is by therapeutic abortion in the first three months; by abdominal hysterotomy from the fourth to the sixth month; by induced labour or by Cæsarean section during the seventh and eighth months; by natural means, or by Cæsarean section at term. The choice must rest with the obstetrician.

CONGENITAL HEART DISEASE

Any form of congenital heart disease compatible with adult life may obviously be associated with pregnancy. In practice the more common lesions include atrial septal defect, patent ductus arteriosus, pulmonary stenosis with normal aortic root, coarctation of the aorta, ventricular septal defect and Fallot's tetralogy—in that order of frequency. With the exception of ventricular septal defect all these lesions can now be repaired or relieved surgically, and if severe enough to warrant such treatment the operation should be carried out before pregnancy. If the patient is already pregnant surgical treatment should not be delayed and the pregnancy need not then be terminated. Patients who have had severe congenital heart disease cured, repaired or sufficiently relieved surgically may have one or more babies subsequently without ill effect. Mild congenital lesions are no bar to pregnancy and do not adversely influence obstetrical mortality.

Atrial septal defect of mild or moderate degree is compatible with many normal pregnancies. If severe, however, it should be repaired with the aid of hypothermia, preferably before, but if necessary during the early months of pregnancy.

Patent ductus arteriosus is now treated surgically as a routine, however mild. If a small duct is discovered for the first time during pregnancy it is better to defer operative treatment, but ducts of moderate or large size are better ligated without delay.

Severe pulmonary stenosis has been relieved during pregnancy on several occasions, and patients operated on previously have had normal pregnancies subsequently. The second statement also applies to cases of Fallot's tetralogy who have been successfully relieved by pulmonary valvotomy or infundibular resection.

Coarctation of the aorta may be discovered for the first time during pregnancy on account of the hypertension. Although the majority of cases go through to term safely, a few end disastrously with rupture of the aorta, and to avoid this risk surgical repair is probably best undertaken at once if the condition is diagnosed within the first three months. If not recognised until later, however, it may be better to defer the operation and to allow the pregnancy to proceed, delivering the baby by means of Cæsarian section to avoid the risk of vascular accidents during labour (Benham, 1949).

Since *ventricular septal defect* cannot yet be repaired satisfactorily, severe cases should avoid pregnancy, or should have the pregnancy terminated in the early months. Cases of mild or moderate severity run no special risk. Sterilisation is not justified because successful surgical repair may soon be possible.

BACTERIAL ENDOCARDITIS

Before the introduction of penicillin, the life of the fœtus was the main consideration. The situation is now reversed, however, and every effort should be made to save the mother. As heart failure is now the chief cause of death from bacterial endocarditis, termination of pregnancy may often be desirable.

THYROTOXICOSIS

One of the few known factors that may aggravate or precipitate thyrotoxicosis is pregnancy. It follows that thyrotoxic women should be advised against pregnancy until they are cured. Improvement on rest and iodine or as a result of thiouracil treatment, is not enough; such cases tend to relapse during pregnancy. At least a year should pass after partial thyroidectomy or thiouracil cure before conception should be considered.

If a woman is thyrotoxic and already pregnant, therapeutic abortion should be considered during the first three months; if not seen until gestation is more advanced, it may be wiser to take the patient to term with the aid of thiouracil. Subtotal thyroidectomy is better deferred owing to the risk of relapse. The dose of thiouracil must be the minimum that is effective, for there is some danger of its causing goitre in the fœtus; the simultaneous administration of small doses of iodine or thyroid may prevent this.

HYPERTENSION

High blood pressure discovered during pregnancy may be due to chronic persistent hypertension (usually essential) or to toxæmia of pregnancy. Essential hypertension may be aggravated by pregnancy, but with rest, diet and sedatives mild cases can be taken to term. Nevertheless, women with high basal blood pressures (above 160/100 mm. Hg) should be advised against pregnancy in view of the increased risk of toxæmia, the high infant mortality (66 per cent according to Browne, 1947), and the chances of serious aggravation. For similar reasons pregnancy should be terminated in women with relatively high pressures in the first three months. Hypertension associated with toxæmia of pregnancy is a separate problem and will not be considered here.

ARTERIO-VENOUS FISTULA

Arterio-venous fistula may be congenital (circoid aneurysm) or acquired (usually as a result of a perforating wound), and may occur in any situation, particularly in the brain, limbs or lung.

Physiology

Experimentally, an artificial arterio-venous fistula, between the femoral artery and vein for example, results in an immediate fall of blood pressure, slight elevation of the venous pressure, acceleration of the pulse, and rise of cardiac output, whilst locally the distal part of the leg becomes œdematous, the skin cold, and the toes occasionally gangrenous (Holman, 1937). Physiologically, the fistula acts as a zone of low resistance in the arterial circulation. The drop in blood pressure is due to the fall in total peripheral resistance; the greatly increased blood flow through the fistula tends to raise the venous pressure; the tachycardia is due to the fall in blood pressure acting on carotid and aortic baroreceptors, the rise in venous pressure usually being too slight to stimulate the Bainbridge reflex; the increased cardiac output is due to a combination of the fall in total peripheral resistance which encourages the heart to empty itself more completely, the slight rise of venous filling pressure and the tachycardia. Locally, œdema of the leg has been attributed to great elevation of the femoral venous pressure; coldness, pallor and gangrene to a diminished blood flow distal to the lesion, for it is much easier for blood to pass through the fistula than through the normal channels (Holman, 1937).

After a variable time several important changes take place. The blood volume increases and raises the venous pressure more conspicuously; the cardiac output is thus augmented and the blood pressure gradually restored. The shunt through the fistula is increased by these changes, but sooner or later a state of balance is reached. Locally, the vessels carrying the shunt become dilated, even aneurysmal; the artery below the fistula is affected as well as that above, because blood entering the distal part of the terminal artery from collateral channels is forced backwards by the peripheral resistance to the fistulous zone of lower resistance. The dilated arteries that accommodate the increased flow become thin walled and the veins receiving the flow at a higher pressure than that to which they are accustomed become arterialised; in other words, both become anatomically adjusted to the new pressure. With the increased blood volume and total cardiac output the blood flow to the distal part of the leg is not only restored, but often becomes greater than normal. The leg becomes hot and the veins distended, and when initial œdema has subsided the leg usually remains larger than its fellow (Holman, 1937).

The physiology of congenital and acquired arteriovenous fistula is the same as that found experimentally, both in the initial and later stages of development. Local effects were well described by Reid (1925) amongst others, and Cohen et al. (1948) confirmed that the blood flow in the affected limb distal to the fistula was diminished in early cases and increased in cases of long duration. The increased blood volume was demonstrated by Rowntree and Brown (1929), and the raised cardiac output by Warren et al. (1947), and Cohen et al. (1948). In congenital cases the increased vascularity of ununited epiphyses in the affected limb may lead to considerable hypertrophy of one arm or leg (Horton, 1932).

CONGENITAL CIRCOID ANEURYSM

Circoid aneurysm consists of a twisted mass of dilated vessels in which artery and vein are in direct communication. One or more superficial hæmangiomas may be seen elsewhere, or there may be a family history of such nævi.

The cerebral type may give rise to epilepsy, subarachnoid hæmorrhage, or ophthalmoplegic migraine. Examination may reveal a systolic murmur heard best through the eye-ball on the affected side, or sometimes over the skull. The diagnosis may be proved by finding an unduly high oxygen saturation in samples of blood obtained from the ipsilateral jugular vein. The lesion may be localised by means of angiography, 10 to 20 ml. of 70 per cent diodone or other radio-opaque substance being injected rapidly into the carotid artery and skiagrams of the cerebral vessels being obtained at the appropriate moment. The condition should be distinguished from berry aneurysm, and from Sturge's disease, in which facial and pial nævi without arterio-venous communications are associated with calcification of brain substance, epilepsy, mental retardation, and glaucoma (Nussey and

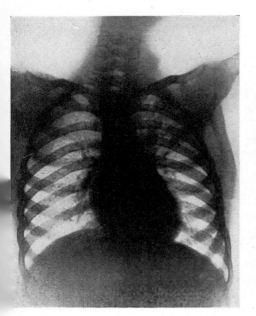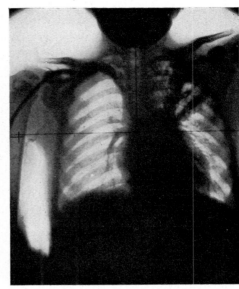

* Fig. 21.06 (a)—Skiagram showing a congenital arterio-venous aneurysm of the lung. The appearances bear some resemblance to those of pulmonary tuberculosis.
(b) Angiocardiogram showing diodone filling the aneurysm.

* *Acknowledgments to Dr. Charles Baker.*

Miller, 1939). Treatment consists of ligation of the common carotid artery on the side of the lesion, if after trial compression hemiplegia or other serious ischæmic symptoms do not occur. The risk of such an untoward event increases progressively with the age of the patient.

Circoid aneurysm in a limb presents similar features to those of its traumatic cousin. It may be situated anywhere from the shoulder or pelvic girdle to the hand or foot. There is usually an increase in blood flow to the limb, which may be longer and larger than its fellow. Occasionally, however, there is ischæmic atrophy in one or more digits distal to an aneurysm in the hand or foot. The veins stand out, are sometimes varicose and may exhibit arterial pulsation, and the skin temperature is raised. It may be possible to locate the aneurysm with precision by observing the effect on the local and general circulation of compressing the various arteries of the limb at appropriate points. An impressive machinery murmur and thrill may be appreciated over the fistula itself. Venous blood from the affected limb may be more saturated with oxygen than venous blood from the unaffected limb. The exact location and construction of the aneurysm may be demonstrated by means of angiography. Treatment is more difficult than in traumatic cases. Excision is usually impossible owing to the diffuse nature of the lesion; moreover, affected vessels are physiologically abnormal and fail to constrict when injured, so that severe and prolonged hæmorrhage may follow surgical interference. Ligation of the main vessels leading to the aneurysm (above and below) may be possible, but deep X-ray therapy is usually best.

Congenital arterio-venous aneurysm in the lung, which is associated with telangiectasis elsewhere in 50 per cent of cases (Baer *et al.*, 1950), causes venous blood from the pulmonary artery to be shunted directly into the pulmonary veins and thence into the arterial circulation; at the same time the blood flow through the rest of the lung may be reduced, the steep pressure gradient through the aneurysm offering the easier pathway. The result is a lowered arterial oxygen saturation in the region of 70 to 75 per cent (Burchell and Clagett, 1947), central cyanosis, polycythæmia and clubbing. Most of the cases reported have been in children or young adults. Hæmoptysis has occurred in 50 per cent. The heart itself is normal, but there may be a continuous machinery murmur over the affected part of the lung. A skiagram may show a rounded or irregular opacity (fig. 21.06a), which on fluoroscopy may be seen to pulsate, tomograms may reveal a dilated artery and vein in close relationship to the abnormal shadow, and angiocardiograms may show the abnormal vessels filled with diodone (fig. 21.06b) (Baker and Trounce, 1949). Lesions may be single or multiple, unilateral or bilateral. Calcification may occur in the wall of an aneurysm (fig. 21.07). One case (a girl aged 9) seen by the author died with cerebral abscess. The condition should be distinguished from patent ductus arteriosus helping to correct pulmonary or tricuspid atresia. Treatment by lobectomy or pneumonectomy is curative unless there are several widely distributed aneurysms (Barnes *et al.*, 1948).

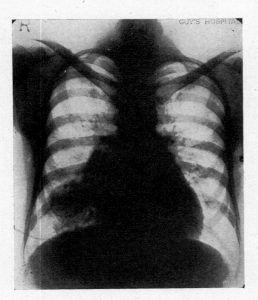

* Fig. 21.07—Calcification in the wall of an arterio-venous aneurysm.

Acknowledgments to Dr. Charles Baker.

Congenital coronary arteriovenous fistula is very rare, but is mentioned in view of its peculiar interest to cardiologists. Details of a few cases that have been reported, including a new one of my own, are given in the accompanying table. It will be noticed that four were symptom free and were detected only because of the continuous thrill and murmur. When this was maximum in the third left space the fistula was between the left circumflex coronary artery and the coronary sinus; when it was maximum low down

AUTHOR	AGE	SEX	SYMPTOMS	SITE OF A-V MURMUR OR THRILL	E.C.G.	X-RAY	CORONARY ARTERY INVOLVED	DIAGNOSIS
Halpert (1930) . .	54	M	Nil	—	—	—	Right	P.M.
Paul *et al* (1949) . .	9	M	Nil	Right sternal edge; 4th and 5th spaces	Normal	Normal	Right	Clinical and operative
Gross (quoted by Paul *et al*) .	16	M	Nil	3rd and 4th left spaces	—	—	? left circumflex	Operation
Davison *et al* (1955) .	58	F	Congestive heart failure	2nd, 3rd, 4th left spaces	A. fib.; QRS balanced	General enlargement "congested" lungs	Left circumflex	P.M.
Wood . .	60	M	Nil	4th and 5th spaces; right sternal edge	Normal	Calcified A-V aneurysm	Right	Clinical X-ray

the right sternal edge the fistula was between the right coronary artery and the coronary sinus. Cardiac catheterisation was carried out in only one instance, and a left to right shunt at atrial level was demonstrated; the pulmonary blood flow was 6.9 litres per minute, the systemic 3.1 (Davison *et al.*, 1955). The diagnosis could have been made had samples from the coronary sinus been obtained. In my own case the diagnosis was obvious clinically and radiologically (fig. 21.08), and catheterisation was not justified. Of these five cases this was the only one with calcification.

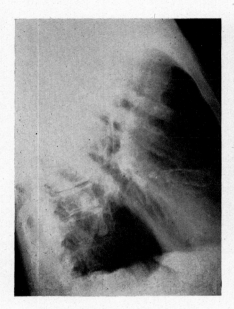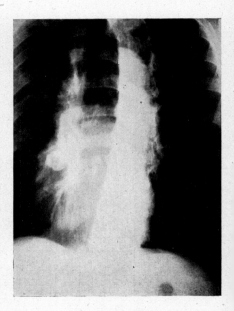

(a) Right anterior oblique view.   (b) Left anterior oblique view.

Fig. 21.08—Calcified arterio-venous fistula between the right coronary artery and coronary sinus.

ACQUIRED ARTERIO-VENOUS ANEURYSM

The great majority of acquired arterio-venous aneurysms are due to perforating gunshot wounds in war, and are seen most often in connexion with the femoral, brachial or carotid arteries. Occasionally they may be syphilitic, mycotic, or artificial. Arterio-venous shunting may also occur in highly vascular structures, such as the thyroid gland in severe thyrotoxicosis or as a result of overdosage with thiouracil (page 879), the uterus in pregnancy (page 903), and the bones in active Paget's disease (page 917).

The local signs and the effect on the general circulation are similar to those in experimental arteriovenous fistula. At first the affected limb swells, the skin becomes cold and there is danger of peripheral gangrene. When a state of balance is reached and compensatory adjustments have been made, the œdema subsides and the limb becomes warmer than its fellow. The veins distend and may pulsate. A coarse machinery murmur and thrill are invariable over the lesion itself.

The general circulation is hyperkinetic, and if the shunt is large enough, paroxysmal cardiac dyspnœa or signs of congestive heart failure may develop, as observed by Reid (1920). If the shunt is temporarily obliterated by digital compression of the femoral artery just above the lesion, the pulse rate falls 10 to 30 beats per minute (Branham's sign), the blood pressure rises 10 to 15 mm. Hg, the venous pressure falls slightly, and the cardiac output falls (Stead and Warren, 1945), but capillary pulsation is accentuated (Lewis and Drury, 1923). Slowing of the pulse is due to the rise in blood pressure, and is abolished by atropine (Kramer and Kahn, 1946).

Cardiac enlargement is almost certainly due to the raised cardiac output and increased stroke volume. The hyperkinetic circulation is maintained by tachycardia and raised venous filling pressure, whilst the peripheral resistance is further reduced by vasodilatation in skin and muscle.

Treatment. Any arterio-venous aneurysm large enough to influence the general circulation should be repaired. Smaller lesions may be left alone if causing no local symptoms, and some of them become obliterated spontaneously. Every effort should be made to repair the artery by lateral suture or graft, so that the normal circulation is preserved (Junghanns, 1943). Ligation of artery and vein above and below the aneurysm is less satisfactory, the resulting circulation through the brain or limb being sometimes inadequate. Simple ligation of the artery above the fistula was condemned as long ago as 1886 by Bramman, for this frequently results in peripheral gangrene.

THE HEART AND CIRCULATION IN BERI-BERI

In modern civilised communities pure beri-beri is rare, the clinical picture being commonly influenced by deficiencies in vitamins other than aneurin (B_1) and by associated conditions, especially chronic alcoholism. Aneurin (thiamine), in association with other components of the vitamin B complex, is found chiefly in unpolished rice, marmite, liver, yeast, wheat, and other grains. It is used by the body in carbohydrate metabolism, its chief known function being concerned with the oxidation of pyruvic acid which is formed from lactate. When there is insufficient aneurin, carbohydrate metabolism is held up at this point, and an excess of pyruvic acid accumulates in the blood (Peters, 1939). It follows that any condition in which carbohydrate metabolism is excessive predisposes to beri-beri, in that aneurin requirements are heavier. When, in addition, the vitamin B intake is reduced at the same time, as in chronic alcoholism, vomiting of pregnancy, and thyrotoxic crises, beri-beri may well develop.

The normal requirement of aneurin is about 1 mg. daily for an adult, and is supplied adequately by the ordinary Europian diet. Special ulcer diets, however, unless supplemented, may be deficient, and psychoneurotic patients with severe anorexia and vomiting may not receive a sufficient supply of the vitamin. Beri-beri was common in German concentration camps and Japanese prison camps during the second world war, although usually complicated by other vitamin deficiencies, and has always been relatively common in the Far East when the basic food has been polished rice.

Aneurin deficiency is rarely gross in civilised communities, and so the presence of some additional factor is commonly needed before the effects of slight deficiencies are brought to light. Under these conditions beri-beri is atypical, for such patients are apt to be middle aged or elderly, and the classical signs may be masked by hypertension, coronary sclerosis, or emphysema; in these mixed cases no clear picture of beri-beri develops (Konstam and Sinclair, 1940).

Behaviour of the heart and circulation. The pure disease was studied in Java by Wenckebach (1928, 1934). The essential features included a hyperkinetic circulation, vasodilatation, enlargement of the heart, and dilatation of the pulmonary artery. Few accurate cardiac output studies have been carried out, but the clinical description and the swift circulation time (Weiss and Wilkins, 1936–37) leave little doubt that it is high. Heart failure may develop suddenly, and fulminating cases occur in which death results within 24 to 48 hours of alleged onset of symptoms (Hashimoto, 1937). Even in Great Britain, cases have been described in which heart failure has occurred remarkably suddenly and unexpectedly, leading to a rapidly fatal issue (Wood, 1939).

The cause of the hyperkinetic circulation is vasodilatation. The drop in peripheral resistance encourages the heart to empty itself more completely, whilst the fall in blood pressure causes reflex tachycardia. As in all hyperkinetic circulatory states associated with a lowered peripheral vascular resistance (except chronic anæmia), retention of sodium and water by the kidneys increases the blood volume, raises the venous pressure, and so further increases the cardiac output. The remarkable quietening of the circulation that follows the injection of 1 ml. of pitressin, and the stormy reaction to 1 mg. of subcutaneous adrenaline (Wenckebach, 1928) confirm the important rôle of vasodilatation. The sudden rise in pulse rate and cardiac output that follow the subcutaneous injection of 10 mg. of mecholin or the inhalation of amyl nitrite, demonstrate clearly the effect of vasodilatation on the circulatory hæmodynamics in normal subjects.

The heart itself shows little specific at necropsy, the disturbance being biochemical, not structural.

Diagnosis. The clinical diagnosis of cardiovascular beri-beri rests on an appropriate dietetic history, the demonstration of a hyperkinetic circulation, radiological appearances showing conspicuous dilatation of the pulmonary artery associated with overaction and general enlargement of the heart, the response to pitressin and adrenaline, associated polyneuritis, and on the finding of a raised blood pyruvic acid or reduced amounts of aneurin in blood (Jansen, 1938; Sinclair, 1938) or urine (Harris *et al.*, 1938; McAlpine and Hills, 1941).

Peripheral neuritis usually begins with pain in the calves on walking, similar in character to intermittent claudication. Associated weakness of the legs, marked tenderness of the calves, numbness and tingling of the fingers and toes, loss of deep tendon jerks, and glove and stocking anæsthesia are usually found.

Evidence of deficiencies in other vitamins, especially of the vitamin B group, is helpful in proving inadequacy of the diet.

Treatment. It must be stressed that the symptoms of beri-beri may begin abruptly, and that the course of the disease may be fulminating, death occurring within a few days of the onset. Once the diagnosis has been made, there may be no time to lose. Again, the possibility of vitamin B_1 deficiency should always be borne in mind in any case of heart failure of obscure origin. Here is one of the fatal forms of heart disease which is curable.

The patient should be put to bed immediately and aneurine hydrochloride should be given at once intravenously in an initial dose of 50 to 100 mg. The effect is dramatic if not given too late. Subsequent doses should be of the order of 10 to 20 mg. per day for a fortnight, orally or parenterally, and followed by an adequate diet. An abundance of the other components of the vitamin B group is also advised.

Fulminating cases should benefit by repeated injections of pitressin (1 ml. 4-hourly) until the vitamin has had time to work; but care must be taken to avoid hydræmia by keeping the salt and water intake as low as possible.

Chronic alcoholics, cases of severe thyrotoxicosis, Simmond's disease or anorexic nervosa, and women vomiting in pregnancy, should be given 2 to 5 mg. of aneurin daily as a precautionary measure.

PAGET'S DISEASE OF BONE

The hyperkinetic circulation associated with extensive active Paget's disease was first clearly demonstrated by Edholm, Howarth and McMichael in 1945. The general cardiovascular findings closely simulate those associated with arterio-venous aneurysm. In the case described by Edholm *et al.*, the blood flow through actively diseased bones was estimated to be 3 to 4 litres per minute, and the total cardiac output was 13 litres per minute. The venous pressure was elevated and there was dependent œdema. Further observations on other cases of active Paget's disease have shown that the heart is not usually overloaded, for it is capable of increasing its output by means of tachycardia or a greater rise of venous filling pressure; on the other hand, paroxysmal cardiac dyspnœa may then occur (McMichael, 1947).

Paget's disease also encourages metastatic calcification, especially Mönckeberg's sclerosis and calcification of the valve rings of the heart.

Extension to the interventricular septum may involve the bundle of His or its branches, with the production of complete heart block or bundle branch block respectively (Harrison and Lennox, 1948).

Cor pulmonale, secondary to thoracic deformity from Paget's disease, has also been described (Wilks, 1869).

Diagnosis. If aortic incompetence and valve calcification are both present, the clinical diagnosis of Paget's disease may be overlooked in favour of atherosclerotic aortic valve disease. As long as the condition is borne in mind, however, diagnosis is easy, for skiagrams of the bones show characteristic changes and the blood alkaline phosphatase is very high.

HEPATIC FAILURE

It has become increasingly evident that advanced disease of the liver may lead to a hyperkinetic circulatory state in addition to the well-known palmar flush and cutaneous spider nævi. The usual cause is secondary carcinoma, but common cirrhosis and even serious infective hepatitis may be responsible. It appears that the liver normally detoxicates some vasodepressor substance, and that this substance accumulates when the organ is failing (Shorr *et al.*, 1945): vasodilatation results in the same chain of physiological adjustments that have been described in arteriovenous fistula and beri-beri. The remarkable effect of hepatic failure on the circulation may be seen sometimes in advanced cases of heart failure when vasodilatation replaces peripheral vasoconstriction.

REFERENCES

THE HEART IN ANÆMIA

Block, C. (1937): "Heart involvement and electrocardiographic findings in anæmia", *Acta. med. Scand.*, 93, 543.

Bouchut, L., and Froment, R. (1934): "Les gros cœurs peu anoxémie a propos des anémics pernicieuses compliquées d'hypertrophie et d'insuffisance cardiaques", *Arch. Mal. du Cœur*, 27, 325.

Cabot, R. C., and Richardson, O. (1919): "Cardiac hypertrophy in pernicious anæmia", *J. Amer. med. Ass.*, 72, 991.

Coombs, C. F. (1926): "The cardiac symptoms of pernicious anæmia, with particular reference to cardiac pain", *Brit. med. J.*, ii, 185.

Forman, M. B., and Daniels, A. L. (1930–1): "Effect of nutritional anæmia on size of the heart", *Proc. Soc. exper. Biol. and Med.*, 28, 479.

Goldstein, B., and Boas, E. P. (1927): "Functional diastolic murmurs and cardiac enlargement in severe anæmias", *Arch. intern. Med.*, 39, 226.

Grunberg, F. W. (1930): "Uber einige Veranderungen von seiten des Herzgefasssystems bei Schweren anamien", *Deutsch. Arch. f. klin. Med.*, 169, 354.

Harrison, T. R. (1935): "Failure of the circulation", Baltimore.

Kraus, F. (1905): "Die klinische Bedentung der fettigen Degeneration des Herzmuskels Schwer anamischer Individuen", *Berl. klin. Wchnschr.*, 42, 5.

Liljestrand, G., and Stenstrom, N. (1925–6): "Work of heart during rest: influence of variations in hæmoglobin content of blood-flow", *Acta. med. Scand.*, 63, 130.

McMichael, J. (1947): "Circulatory failure studies by means of venous catheterization", "Advances in Internal Medicine", 2, 64.

———, Sharpey-Schafer, E. P., Mollison, P. L., and Vaughan, J. M. (1943): "Blood volume in chronic anæmia", Lancet, i, 637.

Nielson, H. E. (1934): "The circulation in anæmic conditions", Acta. med. Scand., 81, 571.

Pickering, G. W., and Wayne, E. J. (1934): "Observations on angina pectoris and intermittent claudication in anæmia", Heart, 1, 3.

Sahli, H. (1895): "Ueber diastolische accidentelle Herzgeransche", Blatt. f. Schweizer Aerzte, 25, 33.

Sharpey-Schafer, E. P. (1944): "Cardiac output in severe anæmia", Clin. Sc., 5, 125.

Smith, K. S. (1933): "Nutrition of heart in relation to electrocardiogram and anginal pain", Lancet, i, 632.

von Noorden, C. (1891): "Untersuchungen uber Schwere Anamien", Charite-Annelen, 16, 217.

THE HEART IN PREGNANCY

Benham, G. H. H. (1949): "Pregnancy and coarctation of the aorta", J. Obs. Gyn. Brit. Emp., 56, 606.

Browne, F. J. (1947): "Chronic hypertension in pregnancy", Brit. med. J., ii, 283.

Bunim, J. J., and Rubricius, J. (1948): "The determination of the prognosis of pregnancy in rheumatic heart disease", Amer. Heart J., 35, 282.

Burwell, C. S. (1937): "Comparison of pressures in arm veins and femoral veins with special reference to changes during pregnancy", Trans. Amer. Ass. Phys., 52, 289.

——— (1938): "Placenta as modified arteriovenous fistula, considered in relation to circulatory adjustments to pregnancy", Amer. J. med. Sc., 195, 1.

———, Strayhorn, W. D., Flickinger, Corlette, M. B., Bowerman, E. P., and Kennedy, J. A. (1938): "Circulation during pregnancy", Arch. intern. Med., 62, 979.

Chesley, L. C. (1943): "Study of extracellular water changes in pregnancy", Surg. Gyn. Obst., 76, 589.

Cohen, M. B., and Thomson, K. J. (1936): "Studies on circulation in pregnancy; velocity of blood flow and related aspects of circulation in normal pregnant women", J. Clin. invest., 15, 607.

Haig, D. C., and Gilchrist, A. R. (1949): "Heart disease complicated by pregnancy", Edin. med. J., 56, 55.

Hamilton, B. E. (1947): "Report from the cardiac clinic of the Boston lying-in hospital for the first twenty-five years", Amer. Heart J., 33, 663.

———, and Thomson, K. J. (1942): "The heart in pregnancy and the childbearing age", Baltimore.

Hamilton, H. F. H. (1949): "The cardiac output in normal pregnancy as determined by the Cournand right heart catheterization technique", J. Obst. Gyn. Brit. Emp., 56, 548.

Jensen, J. (1938): "The heart in pregnancy", London.

Jones, A. M. (1951): "Heart disease in pregnancy", Harvey and Blythe, London.

Palmer, A. J., and Walker, A. H. C. (1949): "The maternal circulation in normal pregnancy", J. Obst. and Gyn. Brit. Emp., 56, 537.

Pardee, H. E. B. (1934): "Cardiac conditions indicating therapeutic abortion", J. Amer. med. Ass., 103, 1899.

Thomson, K. J., Hirsheimer, A., Gibson, J. G., and Evans, W. A. (1938): "Studies on circulation in pregnancy; blood volume changes in normal pregnant women", Amer. J. Obst. Gyn., 36, 48.

Werkö, L. (1954): "Pregnancy and heart disease", Acta Obst. et Gyn. Scandinav., 33, 162.

ARTERIO-VENOUS ANEURYSM

Baer, S., Behrend, A., and Goldburgh, H. L. (1950): "Arteriovenous fistulas of the lungs", *Circulation*, **1**, 602.

Baker, C., and Trounce, J. R. (1949): "Arteriovenous aneurysm of the lung", *Brit. Heart J.*, **11**, 109.

Barnes, C. G., Fatti, L., and Pryce, D. M. (1948): "Arteriovenous aneurysm of the lung", *Thorax*, **3**, 148.

Bramann, F. (1886): "Das arteriellvenose Aneurysma", *Arch. klin. Chir.*, **33**, 1.

Burchell, H. B., and Clagett, O. T. (1947): "The clinical syndrome associated with pulmonary arteriovenous fistulas, including a case report of a surgical cure", *Amer. Heart J.*, **34**, 151.

Cohen, S. M., Edholm, O. G., Howarth, S., McMichael, J., and Sharpey-Schafer, E. P. (1948): "Cardiac output and peripheral blood flow in arteriovenous aneurysm", *Clin. Sc.*, **7**, 35.

Davison, P. H., McCracken, B. H., and McIlveen, D. J. S. (1955): "Congenital coronary arteriovenous aneurysm", *Brit. Heart J.*, **17**, 569.

Halpert, B. (1930): "Arteriovenous communication between the right coronary artery and the coronary sinus", *Heart*, **15**, 129.

Holman, E. (1937): "Arteriovenous aneurysm", The MacMillan Co., New York.

Horton, B. T. (1932): "Hemihypertrophy of extremities associated with congenital arteriovenous fistula", *J. Amer. med. Ass.*, **98**, 373.

Junghanns, H. (1943): "Lateral suture in carotid aneurysm after gunshot wound", *Arch. f. klin. chirurg.*, **205**, 149.

Kramer, M. L., and Kahn, J. W. (1946): "Effect of atropine on the Branham sign in arteriovenous fistula", *Arch. intern. Med.*, **87**, 28.

Lewis, T., and Drury, A. N. (1923): "Observations on arterio-venous aneurysm", *Heart*, **10**, 307.

Nussey, A. M., and Miller, H. H. (1939): "Sturge's disease", *Brit. med. J.*, **i**, 822.

Paul, O., Sweet, R. H., and White, P. D. (1949): "Coronary arteriovenous fistula. Case report", *Amer. Heart J.*, **37**, 441.

Reid, M. R. (1920): "The effect of arteriovenous fistula upon the heart and blood vessels", *Johns Hopk. Hosp. Bull.*, **31**, 43.

—— (1925): "Studies on abnormal arteriovenous communications, acquired and congenital", *Arch. Surg. Chicago*, **10**, 601, 996; **11**, 25, 237.

Rowntree, L. G., and Brown, G. E. (1929): "Diseases of the vascular system. The volume of the blood and plasma", W. B. Saunders Co., Philadelphia.

Stead, E. A., and Warren, J. V. (1945): "Circulation before and after operation for arteriovenous fistula", *Med. Research Bull., New York*, **64**, 711.

Warren, J. V., Brannon, E. S., and Cooper, F. W., Jr. (1947): "The hæmodynamics of rapid changes in cardiac output in man", *J. clin. invest.*, **26**, 1199.

THE HEART AND CIRCULATION IN BERI-BERI

Harris, L. J., Leong, P. C., and Ungley, C. C. (1938): "Measurement of vitamin B_1 in human urine as an index of the nutritional level", *Lancet*, **i**, 539.

Hashimoto, H. (1937): "Acute pernicious form of beri-beri and its treatment by intravenous administration of vitamin B_1, with special reference to electrocardiographic changes", *Amer. Heart J.*, **13**, 580.

Jansen, B. C. P. (1938): "Chemical determination of aneurin (vitamin B_1) in blood", *Acta brev. Neerland.*, **8**, 119.

Konstam, G., and Sinclair, H. M. (1940): "Cardiovascular disturbances caused by deficiency of vitamin B_1", *Brit. Heart J.*, **2**, 231.

McAlpine, D., and Hills, G. M. (1941): "The clinical value of the thiochrome test for aneurin (vitamin B_1) in the urine", *Quart. J. Med.*, 10, 31.

Peters, R. A. (1939): "Discussion on the clinical aspects of the vitamin B complex", *Proc. Roy. Soc. Med.*, 32, 807.

Sinclair, H. M. (1938): "Value of estimation of vitamin B_1 in blood", *Quart. J. Med.*, 7, 591.

Weiss, S., and Wilkins, R. W. (1936): "The nature of the cardiovascular disturbances in vitamin deficiency states", *Trans. Ass. Amer. Phys.*, 2, 341.

——, —— (1937): "Disturbance of the cardiovascular system in nutritional deficiency", *J. Amer. med. Ass.*, 109, 786.

——, —— (1937): "The nature of the cardiovascular disturbances in nutritional deficiency states (beri-beri)", *Ann. intern. Med.*, 2, 104.

Wenckebach, K. F. (1928): "St. Cyres lecture on heart and circulation in tropical avitaminosis (beri-beri)", *Lancet*, ii, 265.

—— (1934): "Das Beriberi Herz", Berlin.

Wood, P. H. (1939): "The effect of vitamin B_1 deficiency upon the cardiovascular system", *Proc. Roy. Soc. Med.*, 32, 817.

PAGET'S DISEASE OF BONE

Edholm, O. G., Howarth, S., and McMichael, J. (1945): "Heart failure and bone blood flow in osteitis deformans", *Clin. Sc.*, 5, 249.

Harrison, C. V., and Lennox, B. (1948): "Heart block in osteitis deformans", *Brit. Heart J.*, 10, 167.

McMichael, J. (1947): "Circulatory failure studies by means of venous catheterisation", "Advances in Internal Medicine", 2, 64.

Wilks, S. (1869): "Case of osteoporosis or spongy hypertrophy of the bones (calvaria, clavicle, os femoris and rib exhibited at the society)", *Trans. path. Soc. of London*, 20, 273.

HEPATIC FAILURE

Shorr, E., Zweifach, B. W., Furchgott, R. F. (1945): "On the occurrence, sites and modes of origin and destruction, of principles affecting the compensatory vascular mechanisms in experimental shock", *Science*, 102, 489.

CHAPTER XXII

TRAUMATIC LESIONS OF THE HEART AND GREAT VESSELS

SPONTANEOUS LESIONS

SPONTANEOUS traumatic lesions of the heart or great vessels include dissecting aneurysm of the aorta, rupture of a hypoplasic aorta or syphilitic aortic aneurysm, ruptured valve cusps in bacterial endocarditis, rupture of a congenital, syphilitic, or mycotic aneurysm of a sinus of Valsalva into the right side of the heart, rupture of chordæ tendineæ in rheumatic or bacterial endocarditis, and rupture or perforation of the heart or ventricular septum secondary to cardiac infarction or ventricular aneurysm. The majority of such lesions have been described elsewhere as complications of the diseases mentioned. Only dissecting aneurysm and rupture of an aneurysm of a sinus of Valsalva into the right side of the heart remain to be considered here.

DISSECTING ANEURYSM

Definition

Dissecting aneurysm was so called by Læennec (1826) and means dissection of the media of the aorta by extravasated blood that has penetrated between its coats from the vasa vasorum or from the lumen of the vessel.

Incidence

About 1 per cent of all sudden deaths are due to dissecting aneurysm (Mote and Carr, 1942). Hospital records, which include relatively few such deaths, give an approximate incidence of one dissecting aneurysm in every 450 necropsies. The Registrar-General's figures for 1953 show it to be responsible for about 0.5 per cent of all cardiac deaths in England and Wales. Men are more susceptible than women in the ratio of 2.5 : 1 (Levinson *et al.*, 1950). Patients are commonly between 50 and 60 years old; but 24 per cent are under 40 (Schnikter and Bayer, 1944), and cases have been recorded in children (e.g. Galbraith, Gardner and Hardwick, 1939). About 50 per cent of dissecting aneurysms in women have occurred during pregnancy (Schnikter and Bayer, 1944).

Etiology and pathology

Virchow's original conception that dissection follows an intimal tear at the site of an atheromatous ulcer is no longer tenable, for a tear at such a site is now known to be rare (Shennan, 1934). Although hypertension and atheroma are usually associated, they are not essential; the intima may be normal, and not even ruptured (Tyson, 1931).

Dissection is always within the media, commonly begins in the ascending aorta, and appears to be closely related to cystic medial necrosis (Erdheim, 1929). The cause of such necrosis is unknown; Tyson's thesis that it was due to obliterative endarteritis of the vasa vasorum has not been confirmed. Cystic necrosis without dissection may be found sometimes in routine necropsies (Moritz, 1932; Rottino, 1939). Whether hæmorrhage into the diseased media commonly follows an intimal tear, or whether it comes from the vasa vasorum (the intimal tear then being due to secondary rupture), remains uncertain. When the intima is intact, hæmorrhage obviously cannot come from the lumen of the aorta. On the other hand, intimal tears may undoubtedly be primary, for they may occur in healthy ascending aortas without subsequent dissection (Peery, 1942). Occasionally, hæmorrhage occurs into an area of cystic necrosis of the media without dissection, the hæmatoma then becoming organised and causing no trouble (Shennan, 1934).

It has recently been suggested that cystic medial necrosis and dissecting aneurysm may be due to defective formation or excessive destruction of chondroitin sulphate, the chief mucopolysaccharide of the ground substance of the aorta (Ponseti and Baird, 1952). These authors noted the high frequency of dissecting aneurysm and kyphoscoliosis in growing rats fed on 50 per cent sweet pea meal, the toxic agent being β-aminoproprionitrile. The fault in the ground substance that results from this agent is believed to be responsible for both skeletal and aortic flaws. Bean and Ponseti (1955) found that seven out of 27 clinical cases of dissecting aneurysm had gross kyphoscoliosis.

Dissection not infrequently complicates congenital hypoplasia of the aorta, usually part of Marfan's syndrome, an inherited mesodermal dyscrasia which may well incorporate faulty ground substance. A similar flaw may explain the frequency of aortic rupture or dissection in cases of coarctation of the aorta.

Dissection may spread proximally and involve the root of the aorta, causing aortic incompetence; occasionally the coronary arteries are dissected and occluded. Dissection usually spreads distally, however, may travel the whole length of the aorta, and may proceed along any of its branches. Ischæmic effects from occluded visceral or parietal vessels are common. The majority of cases die from external rupture, usually into the pericardium (Strassmann, 1947), sometimes into the left pleural cavity or elsewhere. Occasionally, dissection associated with an intimal tear in the ascending aorta ruptures back into the lumen of the vessel at some distal point, forming an alternative or double aortic channel (double-barrelled aorta). This is found in the majority of cases that recover (Shennan, 1934).

Clinical features

Dissection of the aorta may be precipitated by effort (Gager, 1928), but is more often spontaneous. A typical attack begins suddenly with severe pain in the centre of the chest or in the præcordial area. The pain may be gripping, tearing, shooting, or vice-like, and usually lasts for hours; it may radiate to the head and neck, to the back—less often to the arms. Later in the attack it may spread to the lumbar regions or abdomen, and occasion- ally to the legs, depending on the extent of the dissection. In perhaps half the cases, however, pain is slight or absent (Baer and Goldburgh, 1948).

Breathlessness is nearly as common as pain (Hamburger and Ferris, 1938), and syncope occurs in about 10 per cent of cases (Levinson et al., 1950). Attacks may therefore closely resemble coronary thrombosis; but in cases that survive the blood pressure usually remains high and the electrocardiogram normal; moreover, dilatation of the aorta may often be

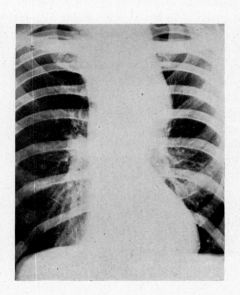

Fig. 22.01—Dissecting aneurysm of the aorta.

seen in skiagrams (fig. 22.01) (Wood, Pendergrass and Ostrum, 1932). Fever and leucocytosis are the rule, not the exception (Baer and Goldburgh, 1948).

Other findings depend upon the site and extent of the dissection, upon which branches of the aorta are occluded, and upon the site of external rupture. Aortic incom- petence may develop when the root of the aorta is dissected (Weiss, 1935), and is being noted with increasing frequency (David et al., 1947); myocardial infarction may occur if the left or right coronary artery is occluded, giving rise to the appropriate electrocardiogra- phic pattern (Wainwright, 1944). Pericardial friction is heard occasionally, and hæmopericar-

dium may be recognised before death.

Dissection of major arteries leads either to occlusion of the vessel, or to increased amplitude of pulsation due to spontaneous periarterial sym- pathectomy (Weisman and Adams, 1944). Occlusion of one or other or both carotid arteries may cause hemiplegia, mental confusion or coma; of the anterior spinal artery, paraplegia; of arteries to the limbs, loss of the peripheral pulse and perhaps ischæmic pain; of the renal artery, hæmaturia —and so on. Occasionally, a pulse that has been absent may re-appear as a result of rupture re-entry (Lawrence, 1935). A systolic murmur and thrill may develop over partly occluded vessels, including the aorta (McGeachy and Paullin, 1937). Left hæmothorax is found in about 12 per cent of cases (Baer and Goldburgh, 1948). Hæmorrhage into the mediastinum may be responsible for cough and dysphagia. An abdominal mass may become palpable. Hæmoptysis, hæmatemesis and hæmaturia occur occasionally.

Cases that survive the original dissection may present themselves later with congestive heart failure associated with aortic incompetence. When there has been no history of pain, such cases have usually been diagnosed erroneously as syphilitic aortic incompetence, despite negative Wassermann reactions (Gouley and Anderson, 1940; Flaxman, 1942).

Angiocardiography may help to prove the diagnosis (Golden and Weens, 1949), but is not advised in the acute or subacute stage.

Prognosis

According to Shennan (1934), about 10 per cent of all cases of dissecting aneurysm recover from the attack, usually owing to rupture re-entry. The majority succumb later to heart failure, either as a result of aortic incompetence or from associated hypertensive heart disease.

Treatment

No treatment is likely to influence the course of dissection. Morphine should be given freely to combat pain. If the patient survives the initial attack, he should be kept in bed for at least a month.

RUPTURE OF AN ANEURYSM OF AN AORTIC SINUS (SINUS OF VALSALVA) INTO THE RIGHT ATRIUM, RIGHT VENTRICLE OR PULMONARY ARTERY

Aneurysm of one of the aortic sinuses may be congenital, syphilitic or mycotic. Rupture of such an aneurysm into the pericardium or left pleural cavity is immediately fatal, but perforation into the right atrium, ventricle or pulmonary artery leads to a well defined clinical syndrome which may be compatible with many years of active life.

Incidence

The condition is rare; indeed, the author has only encountered and investigated four living instances. Congenital cases may occur in young adults, syphilitic cases in later life, and mycotic at any age. About 80 per cent of reported cases have been in men aged 20 to 67 (Oram and East, 1955).

Physiology

Rupture into the right atrium causes a large arteriovenous shunt into that chamber, overloading of the right heart, and the rapid development of congestive failure. Cardiac catheterisation reveals a left to right shunt at atrial level. Perforation into the right ventricle may similarly overload the right heart; blood samples and intracardiac pressures are similar to those in ventricular septal defect (R.A.P. 0, R.V.P. 12, P.A.P. 15 mm. Hg; S.V.C. and R.A. samples 44 to 45, R.V. and P.A. samples 28 ml. oxygen unsat. per litre in a case seen by the author).

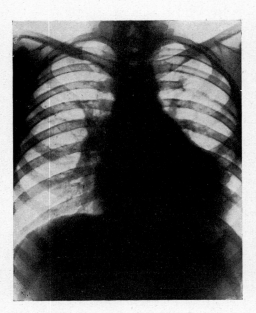 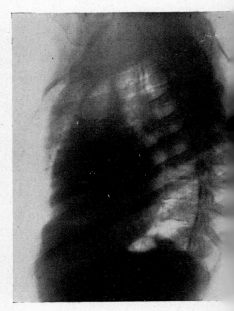

(a) Anterior view, showing engorged pulmonary circulation, enlargement of the left ventricle, and resection of the 5th rib on the left side (the case having been operated on for patent ductus.)

(b) Second oblique view showing enlargement of the left ventricle and dilatation of pulmonary artery.

Fig. 20.02—Case of ruptured mycotic aneurysm of aortic sinus into the pulmonary artery.

Perforation into the pulmonary artery sets up similar features to patent ductus arteriosus (fig. 20.02). In one such case investigated by the author, due to a perforated mycotic aneurysm from bacterial endocarditis (cured by penicillin), samples from the right atrium and ventricle showed 67 to 70 ml. oxygen unsaturation per litre, whereas pulmonary artery samples were only 33 to 36 ml. unsaturated. The mean right ventricular pressure was 31 mm. of Hg above the sternal angle, and the pulmonary artery pressure 63 mm. Hg.

Clinical features

Pain may occur from involvement of the orifice of one or other coronary arteries, but is otherwise absent. The onset is usually signalled by the rapid development of congestive heart failure, but not necessarily. The two cases mentioned above were by no means incapacitated, and one is still alive 15 years after the onset.

The chief signs are a loud machinery murmur, accompanied by a thrill over the base of the heart, but at a lower level than that associated with patent ductus arteriosus; accompanied by signs of aortic incompetence and by features resembling those of ventricular septal defect or patent ductus according to the site of the perforation.

Prognosis

Rapid deterioration to a fatal outcome is said to be the rule (Abbott, 1919), but this may be because the diagnosis is usually only made at autopsy. Three of the author's four cases are not only alive but relatively well; the fourth died of heart failure.

EFFECTS OF DIRECT INJURY

Direct injury to the heart may be caused by stab or gunshot wounds, and very rarely by diagnostic procedures such as needling the pericardium. The literature on the subject has been well surveyed by King (1941) and by Barber (1944).

GUNSHOT WOUNDS

A bullet or piece of shrapnel may perforate the heart through and through, may lodge in the myocardium or pericardium with or without perforation of one or more chambers, or may graze the surface of the heart without causing death. In an analysis of 25 instances of war wounds involving the heart, made in conjunction with Nicholson in 1945, the relative incidence of such lesions was as follows:

Near misses . . .	4
Grazes or tangential wounds .	4
Through and through perforation	3
Foreign body in pericardium .	7
Foreign body in myocardium .	7

Of 1,640 consecutive penetrating chest wounds the heart was directly or indirectly injured in 1.7 per cent. The immediate result is hæmopericardium and the rapid development of cardiac tamponade. If a foreign body passes close to the heart or lodges within half an inch of its surface, a transient pericardial serous effusion may develop. If the patient does not die from cardiac tamponade or hæmorrhage into the pleural cavity, complete recovery may follow, whether or not a metallic foreign body remains in the heart.

The chief complication during convalescence is recurrent acute pericarditis: this is nearly always associated with the presence of a foreign body either in the pericardium or closely connected with it (Wood, 1945); it rarely arises when a bullet is embedded deeply in the myocardium. The attacks tend to be severe, with pain, fever, tachycardia, gross electrocardiographic changes, and the rapid development of a sterile serous effusion which may cause cardiac tamponade. They usually last about a week. The first attack may occur at any time during convalescence up to about three months after the injury, and may recur several times at intervals of about a month. Of five such cases studied by the author in the second world war, all finally recovered, three without interference and two after removal of the foreign body by Nicholson (1945).

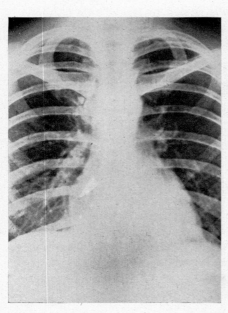

Fig. 22.03—Machine-gun bullet imbedded in the right atrium.

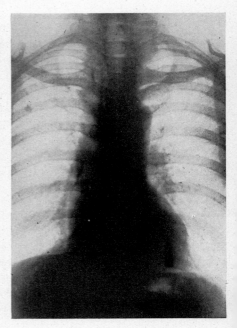

Fig. 22.04—Skiagram taken in 1937 showing machine-gun bullet embedded in the heart since 1917.

A second complication is coronary thrombosis during convalescence, when a pericardial foreign body is in contact with a major coronary vessel; but this was observed only once.

Diagnosis. The possibility of cardiac injury should be considered in all cases of gunshot wounds of the trunk or neck, especially if the missile is judged to have been directed towards the heart, or if its direction is not known for certain. Early diagnosis depends upon recognising the signs of cardiac tamponade or hæmopericardium (page 661). An electrocardiogram may be most helpful by showing the presence or absence of the pericardial T_2 pattern.

Intracardiac or pericardial foreign body may be readily detected by means of fluoroscopy, its movement with the heart beat aiding recognition, but it may be easily overlooked in skiagrams.

Treatment. It is impossible to say how many lives might be saved by early surgical repair of cardiac wounds. In the second world war the majority of cases that survived long enough to be evacuated to general hospitals recovered.

Relief of cardiac tamponade by paracentesis may be life-saving, both in the early stages or during a later attack of acute pericarditis. Metallic foreign bodies lodged in the pericardium are best removed in view of the danger of recurrent pericarditis. Although none of the attacks witnessed proved fatal, the episodes were most alarming. Intracardiac foreign bodies should probably be removed if superficial, and left alone if deep.

Prognosis. Only one of the twenty-five patients mentioned previously died, but as already stated these were favourable cases in that they had survived until evacuated to a general hospital.

Follow-up studies are incomplete, but the worst case, with three attacks of recurrent pericarditis and a machine gun bullet embedded in the wall of the right atrium was alive and well two years after being wounded (fig. 22.03).

In 1937, the author had the opportunity of investigating a healthy man with a machine gun bullet embedded in his heart since 1917. An unsuccessful attempt to remove the bullet was made at the time. An electrocardiogram taken by Sir James MacKenzie showed the usual pericardial T_2 pattern. Twenty years later effort tolerance was excellent, there were no abnormal physical signs, and the electrocardiogram was normal. X-rays showed the bullet still embedded in the heart, in close relationship to the apex of the interventricular septum (fig. 22.04). This case was reported in detail by Grey Turner (1941). On the whole, it seems likely that the ultimate fate of these patients is favourable.

STAB WOUNDS OF THE HEART

Direct injury to the heart in civil life is usually due to single or multiple stab wounds, the majority of which penetrate the right ventricle. The clinical, physiological, radiological, and electrocardiographic features of cases that have survived long enough to receive medical aid have been chiefly those of hæmopericardium (Wood, 1937). Death from hæmorrhage into the pleural cavity or from cardiac tamponade may be prevented by timely surgical repair.

Even when patients appear to be holding their own, it is probably wise to evacuate the blood clot and to repair and sterilise the wound as soon as possible, for hæmorrhage may continue or recur, and serious cardiac tamponade develops in most cases. Moreover, if tamponade is unrelieved too long, acute coronary insufficiency may seriously impair the function of the myocardium, and when it is finally relieved, death may result from acute heart failure. The development of a bulge on the left border of the heart, simulating the appearances of ventricular aneurysm, should not deter the surgeon, for this is likely to prove no more than a localised pericardial hæmatoma (fig. 22.05).

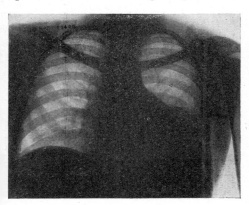

Fig. 20.05—Localised pericardial hæmatoma superficially resembling a cardiac aneurysm.

EFFECTS OF INDIRECT INJURY

Indirect injury to the heart may be caused by crushes, blows, falls or blast. The effects include sudden death from ventricular fibrillation or standstill, rupture of the aorta, rupture of one or more chambers of the heart, rupture of the aortic or mitral valve, hæmopericardium, myocardial bruising, auricular fibrillation and heart block. Coronary occlusion and subsequent angina pectoris or cardiac infarction may also occur, but their relationship to trauma is less well understood.

SUDDEN DEATH

A heavy blow to the region covering the heart may cause sudden death from ventricular fibrillation or cardiac rupture, both naturally and experimentally in dogs (Bright and Beck, 1935).

There have been numerous instances of sudden death resulting from relatively minor trauma of a kind quite incapable of damaging the heart. The catastrophe is then ascribed to ventricular fibrillation or cardiac standstill induced by neurogenic shock. Sudden immersion in icy water, extreme fright, or a blow over the heart insufficient to cause material damage, may each act in this way. This type of death is similar to that which may be caused by a small pulmonary embolism in experiments in dogs, the size of the embolism being quite insufficient to embarrass the circulation, and death being preventable by atropine. The mechanism is probably a vagal reflex.

Rupture of the aorta is more likely to occur from a fall, especially if there is congenital hypoplasia as in many cases of coarctation. Hæmorrhage is usually into the pleural cavity or pericardium.

RUPTURE OF THE HEART

Rupture of one or more chambers of the heart following trauma is not always immediate, nor does it always cause sudden death. A myocardial bruise may result in cardiac aneurysm or delayed rupture, usually during the second week, as described by Bright and Beck. These authors collected over 150 cases of traumatic rupture of the heart from the literature, and found the incidence of the various chambers involved to be as follows:

Left ventricle . . .	37
Right ventricle . . .	31
Left auricle	30
Right auricle	36
More than one chamber . .	13
Interventricular septum . .	11
Interauricular septum . .	1

It will be appreciated that this distribution is very different from that seen with spontaneous rupture secondary to cardiac infarction, when the left ventricle is nearly always responsible.

The latent interval was studied by Warburg (1938). It occurred in 15 out of 51 cases proved at necropsy. A small tear may behave similarly to a direct penetrating wound that causes delayed death from hæmoperi-cardium, usually within a few days. A bruise may rupture at any time within six weeks (Barber, 1938), or occasionally after a longer interval. Cardiac aneurysm resulting from a bruise may rupture years afterwards (Joachim and Mays, 1927).

During the quiescent phase the patient may seem relatively well, any discomfort being attributed to the bruise on the chest, and he may continue his normal activities, including sport (Priest, 1939). In other cases symp-toms may result from hæmopericardium or from any of the other effects to be described presently.

Diagnosis

If the patient is seen alive after cardiac rupture, the signs and symptoms are those of hæmorrhage into the pericardium or pleural cavity. The com-bination of collapse, rapid thready pulse, and a high jugular venous pressure from cardiac tamponade, is very suggestive if discovered within a month of injury. There may be no evidence of external damage to the chest wall, and the history of the accident may not be mentioned, for it may not appear to be connected with the illness. If the possibility of previous trauma is considered, the diagnosis is usually obvious.

Treatment

Immediate surgical repair is the only hope of saving life.

HÆMOPERICARDIUM

Symptoms and signs of pericarditis with or without hæmopericardium are relatively common after indirect cardiac trauma, particularly perhaps after blast injury. They provide useful evidence of cardiac damage, but do not necessarily indicate its nature. Surgical interference is only warranted if there is tamponade, which usually signifies cardiac rupture or serious coronary hæmorrhage. Many cases have recovered spontaneously (Smith and McKeown, 1939).

MYOCARDIAL BRUISING

Crushing of the chest, direct blows over the heart, and blast may all cause myocardial contusion, the clinical picture resembling that of myo-cardial infarction, including the characteristic electrocardiographic changes, or heart failure without pain (Barber, 1940; Barber and Osborn, 1941).

Following a direct blow in the præcordial region, electrocardiographic changes may occur which are indistinguishable from those of posterior myocardial infarction (Anderson, 1940). In these cases it may be assumed that the right coronary artery has been injured anteriorly.

The chief danger of myocardial contusion is delayed rupture, as pre-viously described.

Treatment consists of rest in bed for six weeks, semi-starvation, a low sodium intake, mersalyl if necessary, sedatives, and avoidance of digitalis.

RUPTURED AORTIC CUSP

Indirect trauma sometimes ruptures an aortic cusp. There may or may not be underlying aortic valve disease, congenital or acquired. The lesion results in the abrupt development of aortic incompetence, which throws a heavy burden upon an unprepared left ventricle, so that failure of that chamber is likely to ensue.

The diagnosis is suggested by the sudden onset of orthopnœa, paroxysmal cardiac dyspnœa, or pulmonary œdema, following a serious fall or other violent accident; and is confirmed by the discovery of a loud, harsh, sometimes musical, aortic diastolic murmur, often accompanied by a thrill, especially if the valve was known to have been normal previously.

The prognosis may be good if the patient survives the immediate insult, but death from heart failure within six weeks is a grave risk (Barber, 1938, 1944). Treatment consists of six weeks' rest in bed in order to allow time for adequate compensation, and may have to be directed towards combating left ventricular failure. It must be understood that a degree of aortic incompetence which would be well tolerated and consistent with years of active life if it had developed slowly, may cause death from acute heart failure when it occurs abruptly; just as acute hypertension may cause left ventricular failure and pulmonary œdema, whereas much higher pressures may be tolerated when developing slowly in benign hypertension.

TRAUMATIC MITRAL INCOMPETENCE

A severe fall, or sudden blow over the heart, or other violent accident may occasionally rupture chordæ tendineæ or tear one of the mitral cusps, particularly if already diseased. The lesion is rare, but there are many well authenticated instances (Barber and Osborn, 1937). A clinical diagnosis may be made from the history, if it is known that no murmur was present before the accident, if a loud harsh mitral systolic murmur is heard when the heart is first examined after the accident, if there is no evidence of previous rheumatic valve disease, and if confirmatory signs of organic mitral incompetence develop (page 506).

A number of cases have died from congestive heart failure within a few hours or weeks of the accident, and others have developed mitral stenosis later (Barber, 1938). On the other hand, the accidental discovery of symptomless mitral incompetence attributable to trauma need cause little alarm, such cases behaving like rheumatic mitral incompetence with a healthy myocardium.

HEART BLOCK

There have been a number of instances of asphyxia in which hæmorrhage has taken place around the bundle of His with resulting heart block. Several cases have been seen at necropsy by the author, and a good example was observed during the 1940–1 London air raids.

A woman of about 35, known to have been in previous good health, was rescued in a partly asphyxiated condition from beneath a lot of debris. Examination shortly afterwards revealed not only complete heart block, but also gross signs of hemi-Parkinsonism, presumably due to hæmorrhage into the bundle of His and into the substantia nigra. She declared that she had received no severe blow on her chest, nor significant crush, but had been partly asphyxiated by dust for about one hour.

Heart block may also result from a blow over the heart or from a fall on the chest (Coffen, 1930; Warburg, 1938), and has been so produced experimentally in dogs (Kissane, 1937). Hæmorrhage into the conducting system is presumably responsible. The lesion may be transient or permanent, the prognosis depending on the presence or absence of Stokes-Adams fits, and upon the rate of the idioventricular pace-maker; but on the whole it is fairly good, provided there is no more serious injury, and provided the heart muscle is sound.

AURICULAR FIBRILLATION (OR FLUTTER)

Several cases of auricular fibrillation caused or precipitated by blows have been reported (Kahn and Kahn, 1928), particularly in the elderly (Barber, 1938). Bramwell (1934) records a case in which auricular fibrillation was probably initiated by a head injury, and Hay and Jones (1927) describe one due to electric shock.

The mechanism whereby head injury may cause auricular fibrillation is particularly interesting, though still obscure. There is reason to believe that parasympathetic activity may be culpable. Thus, digitalis, which stimulates the vagus, may cause auricular fibrillation, and there is a form of sinus bradycardia due to vagal influence which is associated with paroxysms of flutter or fibrillation. In experiments on certain animals, fibrillation may be induced by vagal stimulation. Not only head injury, but also meningitis, Ménière's syndrome, and probably other intracranial disturbances may excite this rhythm change.

CARDIAC INFARCTION AND ANGINA PECTORIS

As already described, myocardial contusion may give rise to clinical and electrocardiographic features similar to those of myocardial infarction, and may also result in cardiac rupture or aneurysm. There appears to be a closer relationship, however, between trauma and ischæmic effects. For example, an anterior injury to the chest may cause a posterior left ventricular lesion clinically indistinguishable from a cardiac infarct, and classical angina pectoris may develop for the first time immediately after trauma (Campbell, 1939). Moreover, the subsequent course of these cases may be that of ordinary ischæmic heart disease. It is possible that blows, crush injuries, and blast may injure the anterior coronary vessels, either by causing subintimal hæmorrhage in an atherosclerotic artery, or more directly, and thus cause acute coronary occlusion or secondary thrombosis. After such an event subsequent angina pectoris would be readily understood. Great care must be taken in diagnosing traumatic angina however, for many persistent chest pains following injury represent compensation neurosis.

Treatment consists of three to six weeks' rest in bed, followed by one to three months' convalescence, to allow time for the development of adequate collateral vascularisation. The prognosis depends upon the degree of underlying coronary disease, as well as upon the amount of damage inflicted. On the whole it is not dissimilar to that in ischæmic heart disease in general.

MEDICO-LEGAL ASPECTS

Employees are entitled to compensation if it can be shown that trauma has initiated or aggravated a cardiovascular disability. Even a case of syphilitic aneurysm that ruptures during the course of work receives compensation. Patients with established heart disease may deteriorate after an accident, and this aggravation is equally compensated. The benefit of doubt is always given to the patient, and in a court of Law or a tribunal it is difficult to convince a judge or president that trauma has not adversely affected the cardiovascular system. Yet a firm stand must be taken over the development of cardiac neurosis. Left inframammary pain is especially liable to become persistent and intractable if linked to the idea of compensation, and the physician must be prepared to make a categorical statement to the effect that this is not organic and is not due to the accident: that its origin lies in the mind and in the emotions, and its growth runs parallel with the conscious or subconscious desire for gain.

REFERENCES

SPONTANEOUS LESIONS

Abbott, M. E. (1919): "Clinical and developmental study of a case of ruptured aneurysm of the right anterior aortic sinus of valsalva". Contributions to medical and biological research, New York.

Baer, S., and Goldburgh, H. L. (1948): "The varied clinical syndromes produced by dissecting aneurysm", *Amer. Heart J.*, 35, 198.

Bean, W. B., and Ponseti, I. V. (1955): "Dissecting aneurysm produced by diet", *Circulation*, 12, 185.

David, P., McPeak, E. M., Vivas-Salas, E., and White, P. D. (1947): "Dissecting aneurysm of the aorta; review of 17 autopsied cases of acute dissecting aneurysm of the aorta encountered at the Massachusetts Gen. Hosp. from 1937–46, inc., eight of which were correctly diagnosed ante mortem", *Ann. intern. Med.*, 27, 405.

Erdheim, J. (1929): "Medionecrosis aortæ idiopathica", *Virch. Arch. f. path Anat.*, 273, 454.

Flaxman, N. (1942): "Dissecting aneurysm of aorta", *Amer. Heart J.*, 24, 654

Gager, L. (1928): "Dissecting aneurysm of aorta complicating hypertension", *Ibid.*, 3, 489.

Galbraith, A. J., Gardner, E., and Hardwick, S. (1939): "Huge dissecting aneurysm", *Lancet, ii,* 1019.

Golden, A., and Weens, H. S. (1949): "The diagnosis of dissecting aneurysm of the aorta by angiocardiography. Report of a case", *Amer. Heart J.,* 37, 114.

Gouley, B. A., and Anderson, E. (1940): "Chronic dissecting aneurysm, simulating syphilitic cardiovascular disease: notes on associated aortic murmurs", *Ann. intern. Med.,* 14, 978.

Hamburger, M., and Ferris, E. B. (1938): "Dissecting aneurysm", *Amer. Heart J.,* 16, 1.

Lænnec, R. T. H. (1826): "Traité de l'ausculation médiate", 2nd Edit. Vol. II, 696; 3rd Edit. Vol. III, 295.

Lawrence, J. H. (1935): "Clinical symptoms and signs of dissecting aneurysm of aorta, with report of case diagnosed during life", *Internat. Clin.,* 2, 122.

Levinson, D. C., Edmeades, D. T., and Griffith, G. C. (1950): "Dissecting aneurysm of the aorta: its clinical, electrocardiographic and laboratory features. A report of fifty-eight autopsied cases", *Circulation,* 1, 360.

McGeachy, T. E., and Paullin, J. E. (1937): "Dissecting aneurysm of aorta", *J. Amer. med. Ass.,* 108, 1690.

Moritz, A. R. (1932): "Medionecrosis aortae idiopathica cystica", *Amer. J. Path.,* 8, 717.

Mote, C. D., and Carr, J. L. (1942): "Dissecting aneurysm of the aorta", *Amer. Heart J.,* 24, 65.

Oram, S., and East, T. (1955): "Rupture of aneurysm of aortic sinus (of Valsalva) into the right side of the heart", *Brit. Heart J.,* 17, 541.

Peacock, T. B. (1863): "Report on cases of dissecting aneurysms", *Trans. path. Soc., London,* 14, 87.

Peery, T. M. (1942): "Incomplete rupture of the aorta", *Arch. intern. Med.,* 70, 689.

Ponseti, I. V., and Baird, W. A. (1952): "Scoliosis and dissecting aneurysm of the aorta in rats fed with lathyrus odoratus seeds", *Amer. J. Path.,* 28, 1059.

Rottino, A. (1939): "Medial degeneration of aorta as seen in 12 cases of dissecting aneurysm", *Arch. Path.,* 28, 1.

Schnikter, M. A., and Bayer, C. A. (1944): "Dissecting aneurysm of the aorta in young individuals", *Ann. intern. Med.,* 20, 486.

Shennan, T. (1934): "Dissecting aneurysms", M.R.C. report, London.

Strassmann, G. (1947): "Traumatic rupture of the aorta", *Amer. Jeart J.,* 33, 508.

Taussig, H. (1947): "Congenital malformation of the heart", Commonwealth Fund, New York.

Tyson, M. D. (1931): "Dissecting aneurysms", *Amer. J. Path.,* 7, 581.

Wainwright, C. W. (1944): "Dissecting aneurysm producing coronary occlusion by dissection of coronary artery", *Bull. Johns Hopk. Hosp.,* 75, 81.

Weisman, A. D., and Adams, R. D. (1944): "Neurological complications of dissecting aneurysm", *Brain,* 67, 69.

Weiss, S. (1935): "Clinical course of spontaneous dissecting aneurysm of aorta", *M. Clin. N. Amer.,* 18, 1117.

Wood, F. C., Pendergrass, E. P., and Ostrum, H. W. (1932): "Dissecting aneurysm of aorta with special reference to its roentgenographic features", *Amer. J. Roentgenol.,* 28, 437.

EFFECTS OF DIRECT OR INDIRECT INJURY

Anderson, R. G. (1940): "Non-penetrating injuries of the heart", *Brit. med. J.,* ii, 307.

Barber, H. (1938): "Trauma of the heart", *Ibid.*, i, 433.
—— (1940): "Contusion of the myocardium", *Ibid.*, ii, 520.
—— (1944): "The effects of trauma, direct or indirect, on the heart", *Quart. J. Med.*, **13**, 137.
——, Osborn, G. R. (1937): "Case of mitral stenosis; result of trauma", *Guy's Hosp. Rep.*, **87**, 510.
——, —— (1941): "A fatal case of myocardial contusion", *Brit. Heart J.*, **3**, 127.
Bramwell, C. (1934): "Can a head injury cause auricular fibrillation?", *Lancet*, i, 8.
Bright, E. F., and Beck, C. S. (1935): "Non-penetrating wounds of the heart; a clinical and experimental study", *Amer. Heart J.*, **10**, 293.

Campbell, M. (1939): "Angina pectoris following a crushing accident", *Brit. Heart J.*, **1**, 177.
Coffen, T. H. (1930): "Complete heart block of 7 years' duration in child, resulting from injury", *Amer. Heart J.*, **5**, 667.

Hay, J., and Jones, H. W. (1927): "Trauma as a cause of auricular fibrillation", *Brit. med. J.*, i, 559.

Joachim, H., and Mays, A. T. (1927): "A case of cardiac aneurysm probably of traumatic origin", *Amer. Heart J.*, **2**, 682.

Kahn, M. H., and Kahn, S. (1929): "Cardiovascular lesions following injury to the chest", *Ann. intern. Med.*, **2**, 1013.
King, E. S. J. (1941): "Surgery of the heart", London.
Kissane, R. W. (1937): "Contusion of the heart", Columbus.

Nicholson, W. F. (1945): "War wounds of the heart", Conf. Army Phys., Rome.

Priest, R. (1939): "Notes on three interesting cases. I. Trauma of the heart", *J. Roy. Army Med. C.*, **73**, 125.

Smith, L. B., and McKeown, J. H. (1939): "Contusion of the heart", *Amer. Heart J.*, **17**, 561.

Turner, G. G. (1941): "A bullet in the heart for twenty-three years", *Surg.*, **9**, 832

Warburg, E. (1938): "Traumatic heart lesions", London.
Wood, P. H. (1937): "Electrocardiographic changes of a T_2 pattern in pericardial lesions and in stab wounds of the heart", *Lancet*, ii, 796.
—— (1945): "War wounds of the heart", Conf. Army Phys., Rome.

CHAPTER XXIII

CARDIOVASCULAR DISTURBANCES ASSOCIATED WITH PSYCHIATRIC STATES

THE cardiovascular system may be profoundly influenced by psychological or psychiatric states through the medium of the autonomic nervous system. The stimulus is emotional, and appears to act on the central vegetative nuclei in the region of the hypothalamus. We are all familiar with the uncomfortable thudding of our hearts during moments of fear, and most of us have witnessed a fainting attack provoked by the sight of something that is at once queer and frightening. The physiological basis for such phenomena is relatively simple; sympathetic or adrenergic activity may cause palpitations by accelerating the pulse, elevating the blood pressure, and strengthening the heart beat; parasympathetic or cholinergic activity may induce syncope by retarding the pulse, lowering the blood pressure, and weakening the heart beat.

Cardiovascular upsets of this kind, sufficient to bring the patient to seek medical advice, almost invariably indicate psychiatric disorder; for the effects of emotion within the limits of common physiological experience are too transient and too familiar to disturb a normal individual. Moreover, in psychiatric states such symptoms may be persistent or may be provoked too readily. The syndrome so produced has been called "soldier's heart", irritable heart, disordered action of the heart (D.A.H.), cardiac neurosis, effort syndrome, autonomic imbalance, neurocirculatory asthenia, etc. Such terms should be discarded in favour of the correct psychiatric diagnosis; but the words "effort intolerance" may be added with advantage, preferably in brackets, when clinically important. Historically one may speak of Da Costa's syndrome to cover all previous nomenclature (Wood, 1941).

The syndrome is characterised by a group of symptoms which unduly limit the subject's capacity for effort, or which upset his peace of mind at rest; by a number of signs which depend upon disturbance of the autonomic nervous system; and by an underlying psychiatric disorder. The cardinal symptoms are breathlessness (93 per cent), palpitations (89 per cent), fatigue (88 per cent), left inframammary pain (78 per cent), and dizziness (78 per cent) or syncope (35 per cent). The cardinal signs are those of functional disturbance of the respiratory, vasomotor, sudomotor, and muscular systems. The psychiatric disorder is commonly an anxiety state, but may be almost anything with high emotional content, including the psychoses.

It should be understood that there is no essential difference between "effort syndrome" and "cardiac neurosis", they are merely clothed differ-

937

ently, the former in battle dress, the latter in nylon. In civil life the condition accounts for 10 to 15 per cent of all cases referred to cardio-vascular clinics; it is common in children, and occurs more often in women than in men, the ratio being 3 : 2. It has a preference for the emotional races, especially the Jews and the Italians. In the first world war there were some 60,000 "effort syndrome" casualties in the British forces; in the second a more enlightened view was taken, the majority of these cases receiving appropriate psychiatric labels and management.

CLINICAL FEATURES

The cardinal symptoms and signs have already been mentioned; they will now be discussed in more detail.

Breathlessness. These patients experience a true sensation of breathless-ness in circumstances that would not affect a normal person. It is not only a question of breathlessness on effort, but patients will say they are unable to obtain a satisfying breath, or that they feel a sense of suffocation; and this is confirmed objectively by frequent deep sighs. Sometimes they complain of attacks of nocturnal dyspnœa which may be confused with bronchial asthma or with paroxysmal cardiac dyspnœa; careful question-ing, however, should reveal their psychosomatic nature, especially by probing the precipitating anxiety dream, and by unmasking the associated panic state. Further evidence of functional respiratory disorder may be obtained by noting hurried, irregular, and shallow breathing. A simple and illuminating test is forced hyperventilation. The patient is asked to breathe deeply and rapidly for one minute. A normal individual experiences dizzi-ness, and sometimes slight tingling of the fingers and toes. When told to stop he passes into a state of apnœa lasting about 20 seconds. The psy-choneurotic, especially the hysteric, dramatises his subjective sensations, and when told to desist usually continues forced breathing, explaining later that he felt breathless. Since dizziness is due to cerebral vasoconstriction induced by carbon dioxide washout, it is clear that such psychoneurotics experience breathlessness when the carbon dioxide content of the arterial blood is so low as to cause apnœa in controls. The respiratory stimulus must therefore come from higher centres. The maximum breath-holding time is another useful test. Normal subjects have no difficulty in holding the breath for at least 30 seconds; but patients with Da Costa's syndrome usually give up very quickly, 30 per cent of them in less than 10 seconds; moreover, in contrast to controls, they show little distress when they reach the breaking-point.

Palpitations. Cardiac overaction resulting from emotional stimulation plays an important rôle in the induction of cardiac neurosis. It is a common psychiatric event for some intangible fear to become linked to something more easily understood and remote from the real difficulty. For example, a psychoneurotic with a morbid fear of heights may develop palpitations when ordered to climb a ladder. If the idea that palpitations may denote some disorder of the heart occurs to him, he at once embraces the possibility, and proceeds to advance the theory in all seriousness, for it disguises his true fear which might be thought shameful, and protects him from the danger. Although a successful defence mechanism in these two respects, the manœuvre is baneful because it provokes a new fear: that of heart disease and sudden death; this new fear aggravates the palpitations, and so closes a vicious circle.

The palpitations of anxiety states are associated with sinus tachycardia, elevation of the blood pressure, increase in cardiac output, and probably with strengthening of the heart beat. These features are due essentially to emotional stimulation of a normal adrenergic system.

Fatigue. Patients often complain that they do not feel refreshed when they wake in the morning; that their sleep has been of no benefit to them. They also feel tired and listless during the day, and are unduly fatigued by effort. The symptom is usually attributed to anxiety dreams and to emotional conflicts.

Left inframammary pain. Psychosomatic pain is usually situated in the left inframammary region, but may be higher, lower, more central or more lateral; it may radiate down the left arm. It is commonly described as aching or as sharp and stabbing in quality; but occasionally it is constricting or cramp-like. Although pain may occur during effort, it is more frequent afterwards; it is also common at night and may prevent the patient sleeping on the left side; sometimes it is capricious and bears no relationship to any known factor. Sharp twinges are momentary, and acute stitch-like pain may last several minutes; but the classical ache usually continues for hours. It thus usually differs from angina pectoris in its eccentric site, its quality, relationship to effort, and duration; i.e. in every important respect. Occasionally, however, as may be inferred from the description given above, psychosomatic pain may be situated near the left border of the sternum, referred to the left arm, constricting in quality, and measured in minutes. In such cases it may well be misinterpreted. There is usually some odd remark, however, or something in the patient's manner, which should warn the physician and encourage him to launch a critical cross-examination. The precise history of angina pectoris will not be shaken by this, but that of an anxiety state alters and becomes more complicated and confused when elaborated.

Left inframammary pain is important because it seems to convince the patient that his heart is diseased, and it is not unnatural that he should think thus of a pain arising so close to it. In the psychoneurotic this creates a morbid fear of death and catastrophe, and so closes another vicious circle.

The exact mechanism of the pain is obscure. It is immediately abolished by the intramuscular injection of 2 ml. of novocaine at the site of maximum intensity or tenderness. Cutaneous or subcutaneous anæsthesia has no effect. This indicates that it is not referred, but arises locally in muscle or fascia, and suggests that it is related to "fibrositis" and low back pain. It may be initiated by fatigue or strain of respiratory muscles in cases with respiratory neurosis, by strain of certain muscular attachments involved in such actions as cranking an engine or lifting a heavy weight, by incessant minimum trauma from the light hammer-blows of an overacting heart, or by faulty posture. It is exaggerated and perpetuated by the belief that it arises in the heart.

Dizziness. Dizziness means momentary faintness, transient unsteadiness, "light-headedness", or a "far away feeling". It does not refer to spinning as in vertigo. It may occur on sudden movement of the head, on standing up abruptly, or during effort. It is readily reproduced by hyperventilation, when it is attributed to cerebral vasoconstriction. Orthostatic dizziness is related to orthostatic hypotension, and is due to inadequate circulatory adjustments on assuming the erect posture. It is probable that other forms of dizziness are also due to diminished cerebral blood flow induced by autonomic disturbance. Transient loss of consciousness due to temporary failure of the cerebral circulation occurs at one time or another in 20 to 30 per cent of these cases.

Sweating. Sweating is a helpful diagnostic feature, because in the majority of instances it is confined to the axillæ, the palms of the hands, and the soles of the feet. These are emotional sweat areas. Thermal sweating, and that induced by cholinergic drugs, have a different distribution, being much more widespread. Sweating associated with effort may begin emotionally, but is soon thermal. Thyrotoxic sweating is also thermal. The hands are the best single guide: if sweating is confined to the palms, the stimulus is emotional; if the backs of the hands are also involved other causes should be considered. Undue sweating is mentioned or admitted by 80 per cent of these cases, and is seen objectively in about two-thirds.

Headache. Headache is a common complaint (72 per cent), and is either vague or throbbing. In assessing the reality of the physical basis of the throbbing type it is helpful to ask the patient to count the throb aloud, or better, to tap out the rhythm digitally while the observer checks this against the pulse rate: in true vascular headache they must coincide; in hysteria they do not. Unilateral carotid compression is also useful, for it abolishes vascular headache on the same side, but it either aggravates or has no effect upon hysterical pain. Throbbing vascular headache may be induced by the intravenous injection of 1 mg. of histamine, or by trinitrin or amyl nitrite in some cases. It is closely associated with exaggerated pulsation of the cerebral arteries (Pickering, 1939). It is seen clinically not only in the anxiety states, but also in fevers, and in acute alcoholism. It occurs spontaneously in migraine. Improvement depends upon better autonomic regulation, which in turn depends upon successful treatment of the underlying anxiety state.

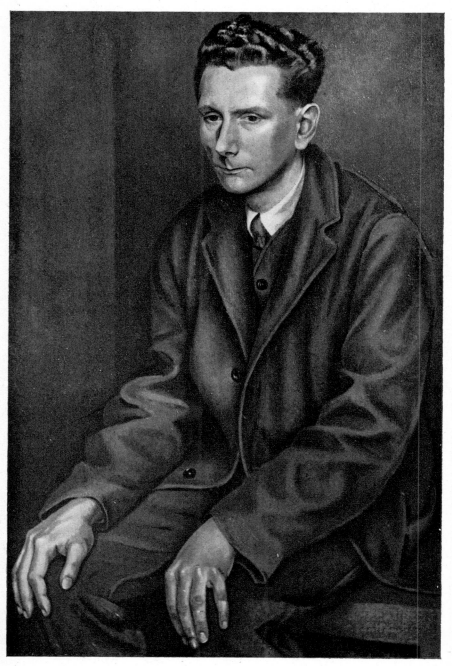

Fig. 23.01—Classical facies, build and posture of a case of Da Costa's syndrome. Painted by Ian Tillard (life-size portrait in the museum of the Post-Graduate Medical School of London).

PHYSICAL SIGNS

Signs of autonomic disturbance serve to check the validity of psychosomatic symptoms. Most have already been mentioned, but they will be recapitulated and grouped here for convenience.

General
    Tense, dejected, or diffident manner
    Dull, weak, or listless, facies
    Soft, quiet, timid voice

Cardiovascular
    Tachycardia (30 per cent)
    Overaction of the heart (44 per cent)
    Blood pressure in the region of 150/90 mm. Hg (27 per cent above)
    Deceleration time over 2 minutes in effort tolerance test (33 per cent)
    Acrocyanosis (44 per cent)
    Flushes (36 per cent)

Respiratory
    Frequent deep sighs (32 per cent)
    Rapid, irregular, or shallow breathing; occasionally hyperventilation (21 per cent)
    Inability to hold the breath for 30 seconds (76 per cent)
    Dyspnœa instead of apnœa after forced breathing

Sudomotor
    Visible sweat on the palms of the hands (67 per cent)
    Sweat trickling from the axillæ (35 per cent)

Skeletal and Muscular
    Tremor of fingers usually coarse, irregular, and inconstant (26 per cent)
    Shakiness of voice and limbs
    Asthenic posture or poor physical development (41 per cent)
    Tenderness in area of left inframammary pain

A life-sized portrait of one of these patients (fig. 23.01) hangs in the library of the Postgraduate Medical School of London and surpasses any description. The effort-tolerance test consists of stepping on and off a chair ten times, and counting the pulse rate before, immediately after, and subsequently at minute intervals until the resting speed is regained. The deceleration time is abnormal (over 2 minutes) in 33 per cent of these patients.

Physical signs of autonomic disturbance are helpful in distinguishing the malingerer, and in assessing the severity of the case. About 90 per cent of normal young adults do not show more than one of these signs, and 50 per cent show none.

PSYCHIATRIC ASPECTS

Although the syndrome described may occur in any psychiatric state with high emotional tone, it is usually associated with an anxiety state. In many there are hysterical features, and a large number show reactive depression.

The family history is tainted with psychoneurosis in 50 to 60 per cent, compared with 5 to 10 per cent in controls with or without organic heart disease. About 66 per cent describe neurotic traits in childhood: morbid fears, especially of the dark, of heights, of water, or of animals, are frequent; bed-wetting, stammering, tics, nightmares, sleep walking, and undue delicacy of health are common. They are timid children, far too dependent upon maternal protection. At school, kindly doctors and soft mothers protect them from the hazards of football, swimming, and the gymnasium.

It is probable that predisposition to psychoneurosis is mainly hereditary, but early environmental factors, such as domestic strife, insecurity, suppression, and maternal coddling, play their part.

There are many factors which may operate to bring about the adult syndrome, and in any particular case one should never be satisfied with the discovery of only one or two. It is fruitful to search for evidence of predisposition, for a state of mind recently prepared for the development of psychoneurosis by external or by endogenous factors, for precipitating agents, for the growth of vicious circles, and for motives for gain that aggravate and perpetuate the syndrome. Proper assessment, management, and prognosis, are impossible if any vital link is overlooked.

Hereditary and environmental predisposition have already been discussed. The mind is especially prepared for the development of psychoneurosis when in a state of confusion and unreality. Head injuries may bring this about; certain acute fevers are often responsible, especially rheumatic fever, influenza, meningitis, and diphtheria; long hours of work in unpleasant and unhappy surroundings may be to blame.

Precipitating factors are often multiple. It is as if one or two could be coped with, but when several occur one on top of the other, mental equilibrium disintegrates. They are usually closely linked with fear in some form or another. The most obvious example is active service, hence the high incidence of the disorder in war. Fear of football, and fear of swimming are common in childhood, and may precipitate anxiety at school. The fear of being unsuccessful, of not being able to shoulder responsibility, is a common cause of breakdown in civil life. Insecurity or fear of the future is also common. The adoption of a line of action contrary to established social custom may cause an anxiety state due to fear of discovery and public criticism. Difficult personal relationships, especially between husband and wife, are often responsible. Sex difficulties are important, but should not be over-emphasised. Financial worry, unemployment, and fear of disease play their part. To a timid sensitive character, the fear of being found out, of being thought a coward, of being proved inadequate, of seeming a fool—and so of losing cast, is a very real and powerful emotional stimulus.

The development of vicious circular patterns is interesting. In this particular syndrome most vicious circles have a common basis, and revolve round the fear of heart disease and sudden death. The combination of breathlessness, dizziness or syncope, fatigue, and especially palpitations and left inframammary pain, provides convincing evidence of heart disease to the lay mind. All these symptoms, which are psychosomatic in mechanism, may be produced by simple anxiety, and may disappear rapidly as soon as the anxiety is resolved. But if the patient takes the fatal step and believes that they are due to heart disease, a vicious circle is at once established, for a new and greater fear develops: that of sudden death at any moment. This constant anxiety, operating consciously or subconsciously every second of the day and night, increases the severity of the psychosomatic symptoms. Under these circumstances the syndrome is maintained long after resolution of the original anxiety. Superimposed upon this pattern or independent of it, there develop various and often complicated conditioned reflexes, until finally distressing autonomic reactions are so ingrained and so divorced from conscious thought as to be practically ineradicable. Correct medical interpretation of early psychosomatic symptoms is of the utmost importance in the prevention of these pernicious grooves. The doctor who misinterprets a boy's fear of water and accepts the pallor and palpitations as signs of heart disease, who mistakes left inframammary pain for angina pectoris, who finding an innocent systolic murmur diagnoses valvular heart disease, who regards syncope or dizziness as a sign of cardiac weakness, is guilty not only of stupidity and ignorance, but is also responsible for turning his patient into a chronic and incurable psychoneurotic. Even so, it may be comforting to know that medical blunders of this kind will influence only 10 per cent of apparently normal individuals, the great majority adversely affected showing evidence of predisposition.

Finally, there is the motive for gain. This is seen in compensation neurosis, and in war it is obvious at every medical board. The inadequate personality of so many of these patients capitalises the symptoms. What timid man, indifferent to higher ideals, will face the dangers of battle, when the very symptoms of his fear offer him protection?

DIFFERENTIAL DIAGNOSIS

The characteristic symptoms and signs associated with psychiatric disorder usually make the diagnosis easy. The physical features have been stressed because the psychiatric state may not be obvious until the mind has been deeply probed. This is well shown by comparing the conclusions drawn at the special investigation centres for "effort syndrome" during the

first two world wars: at Hampstead in world war I, where little attention
was paid to psychiatry, not more than 10 per cent were considered psychoneurotic; at Mill Hill in world war II, a psychiatric basis was proved in
94 per cent. The diagnosis should be positive, not dependent upon a
process of exclusion; it may stand even when organic disease is also found,
especially mild rheumatic heart disease, benign hypertension, and chronic
bronchitis.

Thyrotoxicosis may present difficulty to the inexperienced. The common mistake is to diagnose an anxiety state as thyrotoxicosis, rarely the
reverse. The difference is fully considered on page 874 and 878. Particular attention should be paid to the attitude and behaviour of the patient, to
the expression of the eyes, to the colour and temperature of the hands, to
the distribution of sweating, to the diastolic blood pressure, and to the
appetite.

In children, active rheumatic carditis may cause confusion, vague muscle
pains being mistaken for joint pains, and tics for chorea.

Attacks of violent palpitations in anxiety states are sometimes confused
with paroxysmal tachycardia. Accurate history taking and observation of an
induced attack should prevent error. The special points of difference are
given on page 237.

The distinction between left inframammary pain and angina pectoris
has already been considered, but real difficulty may arise. In both, the
diagnosis depends largely upon the history, and cannot be proved or disproved by the demonstration of psychoneurosis on the one hand, or of
organic heart disease on the other. The matter is further complicated by
the adverse effect of anxiety upon ischæmic heart disease, for it may be so
important a factor that its satisfactory resolution may temporarily relieve
angina pectoris. Occasionally the diagnosis remains doubtful until determined by the future course.

The physician should be on his guard against pulmonary tuberculosis,
chronic undulant fever, juvenile spondylitis, spontaneous hypoglycæmia,
and certain endocrine disorders—especially the menopause. Anæmia should
be more obvious. When the symptoms first arise during convalescence,
simple reassurance should be given and the final diagnosis deferred until
it is clear that rapid recovery has or has not taken place.

TREATMENT

Treatment is never easy, and is the more difficult the longer it is delayed.
Failure is certain if any essential factor in the development of the syndrome
is overlooked, so that a great deal of time must be spent on these patients.
Simple reassurance and some superficial explanation are quite inadequate.

First, the patient must feel that at last he has met a doctor who thoroughly
understands his case; secondly, a complete physical examination, supported
by fluoroscopy and an electrocardiogram, is necessary, so that he will

respect unconditional reassurance. Adequate explanation must follow, and will vary according to the chief symptoms. The object is to convince the patient that the symptoms are emotionally produced. One may point out how sudden fear causes palpitations, sweating, alteration of breathing, and sometimes a fainting attack. He will agree with this, but may object that he feels no such fear. One should then explain that great fear acting for a few seconds may be more than equalled by a tiny remote fear acting over weeks, months, or years; a state called anxiety. This step is difficult, but the point must be carried. Correct interpretation of anxiety dreams is of value in demonstrating the power of subconscious emotion. Enlightenment and conviction may come suddenly if psychosomatic disturbance on some particular occasion or under certain specific circumstances can be explained in the light of emotional experience.

For example, a patient at Mill Hill gave a history of a morbid fear of fireworks in his boyhood, conditioned by London air raids in his infancy. Otherwise he was fit and strong. He was called up in September 1939, was sent to France, and remained well until told one day to unload an ammunition lorry. On handling the shells he became curiously panic stricken, developed gross psychosomatic symptoms, and mis-interpreted them, thinking they meant heart disease. A vicious circle was initiated, he reported sick, and finally arrived at a base hospital with an established "effort syndrome". When the link between his fear of handling fireworks and his handling shells for the first time was pointed out, he was suddenly convinced of the truth of the explanation given for his symptoms, and made a rapid and complete recovery. But his fear of fireworks, shells, and all other explosives was unabated. Treatment had only been directed towards the removal of effort intolerance, by abolishing the misinterpretation and vicious circle that initiated and maintained it.

As a rule, however, it is not enough to reassure and give an adequate explanation, for by the time the patient consults a physician the syndrome is usually highly complex, and conditioned reflexes are well ingrained. To cut across such reflexes and vicious circles, one may encourage the patient to come to better terms with his symptoms. He fears them because he thinks they are injurious, and may result in sudden death. He must be told they are harmless, that they can never be more than a nuisance, that he is already familiar with the worst they can do. Once he appreciates the fact that if he no longer fears his symptoms he will cease to aggravate them, the point is scored.

If there is an hysterical motive for gain it must be mentioned, and then ruthlessly underlined. It is remarkable what little insight these patients have, and disconcerting how little shame.

The methods so far outlined do not touch the underlying psychoneurosis, and the real treatment has yet to begin. The patient may be referred to a psychiatrist, or if the causative factors seem clear the physician may prefer to deal with them himself. There are always three things to consider: the difficulties in which the patient is floundering, his reaction, which is based on his character and intelligence, and his attitude towards his reaction. The difficulties should be taken first, sorted out, and resolved as far as possible. The help of social welfare workers may be enlisted in this respect. The patient's reaction should be analysed, and some psychiatric skill and knowledge are required to do this. It is often possible to show that his reaction is based on false values, ideas, or beliefs. Or one may simply explain just why he so reacts, in order to give him insight. It is impossible to outline precisely just what is required, for every case is different, and needs individual treatment. If the problem has no satisfactory solution, and if the patient's reaction cannot be altered favourably, then at least he may learn to get on better terms with both. Difficulties must be faced, and not hidden away in the dark recesses of the mind; highly personal matters should be fully discussed in a matter of fact way, until they cease to seem so dreadful; if a man is standing on a false pedestal, he must learn humility and honesty, and tread upon the good earth.

Finally, the background must be assessed. With strong hereditary taints and bad early environment, the outlook is poor, and the aim should be to fit the patient into circumstances which will cause the least embarrassment. This is a confession of failure. At the other extreme, if the stock is good, and if there is no evidence of predisposition, and if this is confirmed by the severity of the stress of anxiety causing the breakdown, every effort should be made to cure the patient. In other words, one should deal with the environment when the prognosis is bad, and with the patient when it is good.

REFERENCES

Pickering, G. W. (1939): "Experimental observations on headache", *Brit. med. J.*, i, 907.

Wood, P. H. (1941): "Differential diagnosis of Da Costa's syndrome", *Proc. Roy. Soc. Med.*, **34**, 543.
—— (1941): "El sindrome de Da Costa", *Archiv. Latino Americanos Cardiol. Hematol.*, **11**, 241.
—— (1941): "Da Costa's syndrome", *Brit. med. J.*, i, 767, 805, 845.
(A full bibliography is contained in these three articles.)

Goulstonian lecture to the Royal College of Physicians London 1941

INDEX